Meeting *the* Physical Therapy Needs of Children **Second Edition**

Meeting *the* Physical Therapy Needs of Children

Second Edition

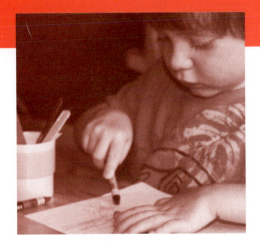

Susan K. Effgen, PT, PhD, FAPTA

Professor
Department of Rehabilitation Sciences
College of Health Sciences
University of Kentucky
Lexington, Kentucky

F.A. Davis Company • Philadelphia

F. A. Davis Company
1915 Arch Street
Philadelphia, PA 19103
www.fadavis.com

Printed in the United States of America

Last digit indicates print number: 10 9 8 7 6 5 4 3

Acquisitions Editor: Melissa Duffield
Developmental Editor: Donna Conaway Morrissey
Manager of Content Development: George Lang
Art and Design Manager: Carolyn O'Brien

As new scientific information becomes available through basic and clinical research, recommended treatments and drug therapies undergo changes. The author(s) and publisher have done everything possible to make this book accurate, up to date, and in accord with accepted standards at the time of publication. The author(s), editors, and publisher are not responsible for errors or omissions or for consequences from application of the book, and make no warranty, expressed or implied, in regard to the contents of the book. Any practice described in this book should be applied by the reader in accordance with professional standards of care used in regard to the unique circumstances that may apply in each situation. The reader is advised always to check product information (package inserts) for changes and new information regarding dose and contraindications before administering any drug. Caution is especially urged when using new or infrequently ordered drugs.

Library of Congress Cataloging-in-Publication Data

Meeting the physical therapy needs of children / [edited by] Susan K. Effgen. — 2nd ed.
   p. ; cm.
 Includes bibliographical references and index.
 ISBN 978-0-8036-1942-5
 I. Effgen, Susan K., 1949–
 [DNLM: 1. Physical Therapy Modalities. 2. Adolescent. 3. Child. 4. Health Facility Environment. 5. Infant. 6. Needs Assessment. 7. Patient Participation. WB 460]

 615.8'2083—dc23

                                             2012017680

Dedication

To those wonderful men in my life:

Arthur, Michael, Brenton, Patrick, and Jonathan

Preface

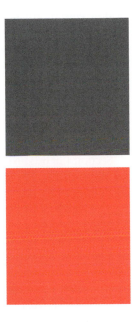

The authors are so pleased to provide present and future physical therapists with a new, totally updated edition of *Meeting the Physical Therapy Needs of Children*. Our diligence and risk in using the International Classification of Functioning, Disability, and Health (ICF; WHO, 2001) in the first edition has been rewarded with nationwide acceptance of this conceptual model that has formed the foundation of both editions of this text. The ICF has been embraced by the American Physical Therapy Association and will be the framework for the 3rd edition of the *Guide to Physical Therapist Practice* (*Guide*; APTA, 2001), the second framework directing this text.

The new *Child and Youth Version* of the ICF (WHO, 2007) has been used in this new edition. Not only has the ICF now been accepted by physical therapists, but they have continued to embrace evidenced-based practice. The authors have been conscientious in reviewing and providing evidence appropriate to the content of each chapter. However, while there have been many new publications related to pediatric physical therapy, there is still a tremendous need for more research as so many questions remain unanswered. There is even conflict over interventions we think we have evidence to support. For example, we have systematic reviews to support the use of strengthening for children with cerebral palsy (Darrah, Fan, Chen, Nunweiler, & Watkins, 1997; Dodd, Taylor, & Damiano, 2002; Mockford & Caulton, 2008), but then a reanalysis of the literature suggested that "strengthening interventions are neither effective nor worthwhile" (Scianni, Butler, Ada, & Teixeira-Salmela, 2009). That was followed by another systematic review suggesting insufficient evidence to support or refute the efficacy of increasing strength in children with cerebral palsy (Verschuren et al., 2011). Those kinds of discord in the literature can leave a clinician questioning the evidence and which interventions to use. That is why in the model of evidenced-based practice there is a place for good clinical judgment.

While our colleagues work to answer the research questions and clinicians review the literature that is available and use their clinical expertise, I want to remind you of an intervention with tremendous face validity and a growing body of evidence: practice, practice, practice, as discussed by Drs. Valvano and LaForme Fiss in Chapter 8. Learning a motor skill requires practice. You did not learn to successfully play a musical instrument, ski, or play computer games without extensive practice. Olympic and professional athletes constantly practice their motor skills, as should a child having trouble with motor skill acquisition. Adolph and Berger (2006) note that early walkers walk the equivalent of 29 football fields a day! Does the average child with a disability learning to walk have the opportunity to walk 29 football fields even in a week? The acceptance of a family-centered model of service delivery in the natural environment will hopefully increase the opportunity for practice and motor skill acquisition in the children we serve.

Section 1 of this text continues to provide a foundation for physical therapy service delivery for children with disabilities and special health-care needs. Chapter 1, Serving the Needs of Children and Their Families, provides a background on pediatric physical therapy, the IFC, the *Guide*'s management plan, models of team interaction, and factors influencing pediatric practice. This is followed by an entirely new chapter on child development, which was added to meet the requests of faculty who wish to have a review of typical development before they address developmental variations seen in the children we serve. Numerous books have been written on child development, so this chapter is but a brief review of development with a focus on motor skill acquisition. Of course, reading about development does not compare to observing development, and readers are encouraged to go out to playgrounds, preschools, and schools to observe the motor skills and interactions of children at a variety of ages. The best environment would be where there are children with disabilities included with children who are typically developing. That allows for comparisons of development and will expose the observer to the benefits of full participation of those with disabilities in the community. These experiences will bring to life the written discussion of the development. There is also a completely new Chapter 3, Child Appraisal: Examination and Evaluation. This includes a review of factors and philosophies influencing examination, tests and measures used in pediatric physical therapy, psychometrics, and documentation. The section ends with a chapter on family-centered care.

This is a critical area of practice and is intentionally placed early in the text to provide an understanding of family-centered care as it is discussed throughout the text.

The second and largest section of the text includes major chapters on the musculoskeletal, neuromuscular, cardiovascular and pulmonary, and integumentary systems consistent with the framework of the *Guide*. For each system, the theoretical foundation and a framework are presented in a review of *structures, functions, examination, evaluation, prognosis, diagnosis,* and *plan of care,* which includes a detailed presentation of evidenced-based *interventions*. Unfortunately, as noted by Dr. Valvano in the first edition and still evident today, "most research on the effectiveness of intervention techniques is limited, sometimes equivocal and sometimes based on studies with small numbers of children . . . [E]ach therapist is encouraged to problem solve for each child, monitor motor function to determine effectiveness . . . and keep current with research findings." A text can summarize only the research evidence to date; it is the professional obligation of therapists to keep abreast of the most recent literature.

Service delivery settings are presented in Section 3. Practice today is very much influenced by the setting. Federal and state laws govern service delivery in early intervention and school-based settings, insurance companies and reimbursement issues govern outpatient services, and the financial limitations of prospective payment impact hospital and rehabilitation services. The infants, toddlers, children, and adolescents seen in each of these environments also differ. Therapists must understand the unique elements of working in each of these settings and how they can provide quality services. These are brief chapters meant to expose the reader to the setting rather than provide extensive information. Originally, there was to be just one chapter on all of the service delivery settings, but that was too limiting, so having relatively concise chapters on each setting was the compromise. Foundational information on assistive technology and the supports available to aid all individuals with disabilities is included in Chapters 17 and 18. Therapists must be knowledgeable in the selection, utilization, and modification of these ever-changing technologies.

The final section of this text is a series of comprehensive case studies. These case studies highlight the multisystem involvement of many common pediatric diagnoses and changes over time. The case studies follow the model of the *Guide* and provide an overall perspective of the role of the therapist in examination, evaluation, diagnosis, prognosis, and intervention throughout the life of the child with a specific medical diagnosis in a variety of service delivery settings. The interventions and life events of each of the children presented in the cases has been updated in this edition to reflect their present status. Since several of these cases cover more than 20 years, the examinations and interventions done at the time the child was seen are outlined. In addition, we have included sections on current practice, which highlights what would be done based on best practice today for examination and intervention. Two new case studies have been added, one involving developmental coordination disorder and one on myelodysplasia.

Ancillary materials are available for both the readers and physical therapy instructors. There are videotapes of children with disabilities being evaluated and receiving intervention. The instructors' materials include additional case studies and a bank of test questions. Also provided is a test construction system that many faculty find very useful in developing and formatting their tests.

As noted in the first edition, *Meeting the Physical Therapy Needs of Children* in the 21st century will involve a continuous process of change and refinement. Therapists must discard deficit models of evaluation and focus on the goals and objectives of the child and family in a culturally sensitive manner. Intervention must be based on evidence supporting its effectiveness or, at the very least, based on sound clinical judgment and experience. Interventions must be discarded if there is no evidence to support continued use. The *Guide*'s emphasis on *coordination, communication, and documentation* as part of the intervention process must be embraced. Services must be coordinated and communicated, and there must be carryover and practice throughout the child's daily routines. These processes assist in making certain that the child receives "appropriate, comprehensive, efficient, and effective quality of care" (APTA, 2001, p. 47/S39) from initial examination to graduation from services.

Susan K. Effgen

References

Adolph, K.E., & Berger, S.E. (2006). Motor development. In W. Damon, R.M. Lerner, D. Kuhn, & R.S. Siegler (Eds.). *Handbook of child psychology, vol. 2: Cognition, perception, and language* (6th ed., pp. 161–213). Hoboken, NJ: John Wiley & Sons.

American Physical Therapy Association (APTA). (2001). Guide to physical therapist practice (2nd ed.). *Physical Therapy, 81*, 9–744.

Darrah, J., Fan, J.S.W., Chen, L.C., Nunweiler, J., & Watkins, B. (1997). Review of the effects of progressive resisted muscle strengthening in children with cerebral palsy: A clinical consensus exercise. *Pediatric Physical Therapy, 9*, 12.

Dodd K.J., Taylor, N.F., & Damiano, D.L. (2002). A systematic review of the effectiveness of strength-training programs for people with cerebral palsy. *Archives of Physical Medicine and Rehabilitation, 83*, 1157–1164.

Mockford, M., & Caulton, J.M. (2008). Systematic review of progressive strength training in children and adolescents with cerebral palsy who are ambulatory. *Pediatric Physical Therapy, 20*(4), 318–333.

Scianni, A., Butler, J.M., Ada, L., & Teixeira-Salmela, L.F. (2009). Muscle strengthening is not effective in children and adolescents with cerebral palsy: A systemic review. *Australian Journal of Physiotherapy, 55*(2), 81–87.

Verschuren, O., Ada, L., Maltais, D.B., Gorter, J.W., Scianni, A., & Ketelaar, M. (2011). Muscle strengthening in children and adolescents with spastic cerebral palsy: Considerations for future resistance training protocols. *Physical Therapy, 91*(7), 1130–1139.

World Health Organization. (2001). *International classification of functioning, disability and health*. Geneva: Author.

World Health Organization. (2007). *International classification of functioning, disability and health. Child and youth version*. Geneva: Author.

Acknowledgments

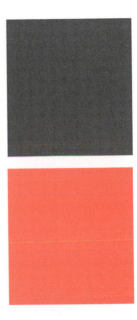

The production of *Meeting the Physical Therapy Needs of Children* is truly a collaborative team effort. Collaborative teamwork is a hallmark of pediatric physical therapy, and it certainly was evident in the writing of this new edition. The new authors who joined the team include Janice Howman, Lindsay Alfano, Jennifer Furze, Alyssa LaForme Fiss, Stacey DiBiaso Caviston, Rachel Unanue Rose, Heather Atkinson, Trina Puddefoot, Marcia Kaminker, Deborah Anderson, and Mary Jo Paris. They have added not only geographic diversity, but their expertise crosses a wide range of pediatric physical therapy practice. A special thanks to Alyssa LaForme Fiss for accepting and editing all of the intervention videotapes. Numerous graduate students have provided valuable assistance to many of the authors over the years. There are just too many to name, but their assistance was invaluable, and we hope they learned from the experience.

They now know that their faculty does not do this work for remuneration—a dollar an hour is not motivation! The service to the profession and the children we serve is what drives these outstanding authors.

The authors have done an amazing job integrating all of the new literature into a manageable publication. Each of the systems chapters could be a text by themselves, so the authors are to be commended for keeping this publication from getting unwieldy. Being concise is very difficult.

The individuals at F. A. Davis Company have been there throughout the publication process. Margaret Biblis and Melissa Duffield have been incredibly supportive, as have the numerous developmental editors, including Donna Conaway-Morrissey, who finally got the text into production. There are certainly more people to thank, and I send apologies to those inadvertently left out.

Contributors

Lindsay Alfano, PT, DPT, PCS
Center for Gene Therapy/Clinical Therapies
Nationwide Children's Hospital
Columbus, Ohio

Deborah Anderson, PT, MS, PCS
Physical Therapy Program
Midwestern University
Downers Grove, Illinois

Heather Atkinson, PT, DPT, NCS
Clinical Specialist
The Children's Hospital *of* Philadelphia
Philadelphia, Pennsylvania

Donna Bernhardt Bainbridge, PT, EdD, ATC
*Special Olympics Senior Global Advisor for FUNfitness
    and Fitness Programming*
Adjunct Faculty
University of Indianapolis

Stacey DiBiaso Caviston, PT, DPT, PCS
Acute Care Team Leader
Physical Therapy Department
The Children's Hospital *of* Philadelphia
Philadelphia, Pennsylvania

Donna J. Cech, PT, DHS, PCS
Program Director and Associate Professor
Physical Therapy Program
Midwestern University
Downers Grove, Illinois

Lisa Ann Chiarello, PT, PhD, PCS
Associate Professor
Department of Physical Therapy and Rehabilitation
    Sciences
Drexel University
Philadelphia, Pennsylvania

Susan K. Effgen, PT, PhD, FAPTA
Professor
Department of Rehabilitation Sciences
College of Health Sciences
University of Kentucky
Lexington, Kentucky

Alyssa LaForme Fiss, PT, PhD, PCS
Assistant Professor
Department of Physical Therapy
Mercer University
Atlanta, Georgia

Jennifer Furze, PT, DPT, PCS
Assistant Professor
Department of Physical Therapy
Creighton University
Omaha, Nebraska

Caroline Goulet, PT, PhD
Professor
Director of Physical Therapy
University of the Incarnate Word
San Antonio, Texas

Janice Howman, PT, DPT, ACCE
Assistant Professor and Academic Coordinator of
    Clinical Education
School of Rehabilitation and Communication Sciences
Division of Physical Therapy
Ohio University
Athens, Ohio

Maria A. Jones, PT, PhD
Clinical Assistant Professor
Department of Rehabilitation Sciences
College of Allied Health
University of Oklahoma Health Sciences Center
Oklahoma City, Oklahoma

Marcia K. Kaminker, PT, DPT, MS, PCS
Physical Therapist
South Brunswick School District
South Brunswick, New Jersey

Jane O'Regan Kleinert, PhD, CCC-SLP
Associate Professor
Department of Rehabilitation Sciences
College of Health Sciences
University of Kentucky
Lexington, Kentucky

Linda Pax Lowes, PT, PhD
Nationwide Children's Hospital
Center for Gene Therapy/Clinical Therapies
Columbus, Ohio

Victoria Gocha Marchese, PT, PhD
Assistant Professor of Physical Therapy
Lebanon Valley College
Annville, Pennsylvania

Suzanne F. Migliore, PT, DPT, PCS
Clinical Practice Coordinator
Center Coordinator for Clinical Education
Coordinator, Residency Program
The Children's Hospital *of* Philadelphia
Philadelphia, Pennsylvania

Margo N. Orlin, PT, PhD
Associate Professor and Interim Chair
Department of Physical Therapy and Rehabilitation
    Sciences
Drexel University
Philadelphia, Pennsylvania

Shree Devi Pandya, PT, DPT
Assistant Professor
Neurology and Physical Medicine and Rehabilitation
University of Rochester
Rochester, New York

Mary Jo Paris, PT, DPT
Physical Therapist
DeKalb County School System
Stone Mountain, Georgia

Trina Puddefoot, PT, MS, PCS, ATP
Program Director
Early Steps Program at Health Planning Council of
    Southwest Florida, Inc.
Fort Myers, Florida

Rachel Unanue Rose, PT, PhD, PCS
Assistant Professor of Physical Therapy
School of Health Professions
Maryville University
St. Louis, Missouri

Carole A. Tucker, PT, PhD, PCS, RCEP
Associate Professor
Department of Physical Therapy
Temple College of Health Professions and
    Social Work
Philadelphia, Pennsylvania

Joanne Valvano, PT, PhD
Assistant Professor
Physical Therapy Program
University of Colorado
Research Coordinator, Center for Gait and
    Movement Analysis
Children's Hospital Colorado
Denver, Colorado

Reviewers

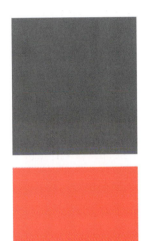

Wendy Bircher, PT, EdD
Director
Physical Therapist Assistant Program
San Juan College
Farmington, NM

Claudia B. Fenderson, PT, EdD, PCS
Professor
Doctor of Physical Therapy Program
Mercy College
Dobbs Ferry, NY

Caroline Goulet, PT, PhD
Professor
Director of Physical Therapy
University of the Incarnate Word
San Antonio, TX

Patricia S. Hodson, PT, DPT, PCS
*Clinical Associate Professor, Director of Clinical
   Education*
Physical Therapy
East Carolina University
Greenville, NC

Kristin J. Krosschell, PT, MA, PCS
Assistant Professor
Department of Physcial Therapy & Human
   Movement Sciences
Northwestern University Feinberg School of
   Medicine
Chicago, IL

Jennifer Lander, EdD, PT
Associate Professor
Physical Therapy Department
Armstrong Atlantic State University
Savannah, GA

Sandra M. Marden-Lokken, MA, PT
Assistant Professor
Physical Therapy
The College of St. Scholastica
Duluth, MN

Marie A. Reilly, PT, PhD
Clinical Associate Professor
Department of Allied Health Science
Division of Physcial Therapy
University of North Carolina
Chapel Hill, NC

Judith C. Vestal, PhD, LOTR
Associate Professor
School of Allied Health Professions
Louisiana State University
Shreveport, LA

Contents

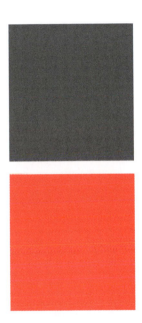

Foundations of Service Delivery

—Susan K. Effgen, PT, PhD, Section Editor

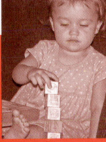
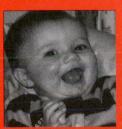
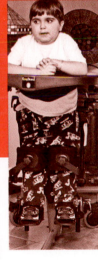
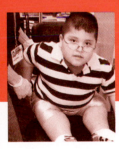
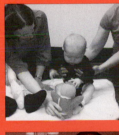
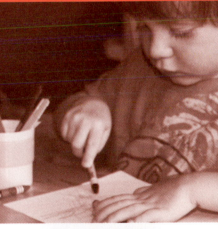
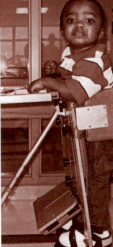

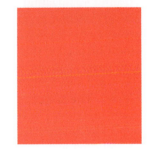

CHAPTER 1

Serving the Needs of Children and Their Families

—Susan K. Effgen, PT, PhD, FAPTA

—Janice Howman, PT, DPT, MEd

The loving mother teaches her child to walk alone. She is far enough from him so that she cannot actually support him, but she holds out her arms to him. She imitates his movements, and if he totters, she swiftly bends as if to seize him, so that the child might believe that he is not walking alone. . . . And yet, she does more. Her face beckons like a reward, an encouragement. Thus, the child walks alone with his eyes fixed on his mother's face, not on the difficulties in his way. He supports himself by the arms that do not hold him and constantly strives towards the refuge in his mother's embrace, little suspecting that in the very same moment that he is emphasizing his need of her, he is proving that he can do without her, because he is walking alone.

—Kierkegaard, 1846

Little did Kierkegaard realize over a century and a half ago that he was describing not only the responsibilities of a mother to nurture her child and then allow the child to go alone but also the role of the physical therapist in serving children. The therapist's responsibility is to provide support, guidance, and specific interventions and also to prepare the child and family for the time when our services are no longer needed. Competent therapists work themselves out of a job. This is not to say that all children achieve their desired goals and objectives, but rather that therapists help them to achieve their greatest potential and then recognize when they can no longer contribute to the advancement of the child's goals and objectives. It is often difficult for therapists to discharge a child from services, especially when the child has not achieved the desired goals, just as it is sometimes difficult for a mother to let her new walker walk alone, or her teenager drive the family car. The therapist's direct role is episodic, although periodic services may be provided over many years.

Throughout this text the role of the physical therapist in meeting the physical therapy needs of children and their families in a culturally appropriate context will be described. Each body system will be discussed in terms of examination, evaluation, diagnosis, prognosis, and intervention for children with a wide range of diagnoses, impairments in body structure and function, limitations in activities, and restrictions in participation in the community. In some areas there is evidence to support the frequency, intensity, and specifics of interventions; however, more commonly there is a dearth of empirical support, and therapists rely on experience and consensus decision making. Throughout the 21st century, physical therapists must strive to obtain the scientific data that will support physical therapy interventions because those who pay for these services are appropriately requiring evidence of the effectiveness of the interventions. Therapists must not only provide intervention but also collect data that will support their continued efforts.

This chapter covers a number of diverse topics that set the stage for meeting the physical therapy needs of children and their families. A brief history of pediatric physical therapy is provided so that the reader can understand the evolution of the profession. The World Health Organization (WHO) *International Classification of Functioning, Disability and Health* (ICF) (2001) serves as the framework for the terminology and classification used in this text, as does the American Physical Therapy Association (APTA) *Guide to Physical Therapist Practice* (2001) (hereafter referred to as the *Guide*). The *Guide's* framework for patient management to achieve optimal outcomes is reviewed as it applies to children. Health care and educational services for children with disabilities require the collaboration of a number of professionals. The models of team interaction are presented, along with models of service delivery. Service delivery has changed over the past several decades in all areas of physical therapy practice, but especially in pediatric physical therapy, in which federal laws play a significant role (see Appendix 1.A). Issues that influence practice conclude the chapter.

Background of Pediatric Physical Therapy

The history of physical therapy is usually traced to the "reconstruction aides" of World War I. However, the significance of poliomyelitis (polio), an inflammation of the gray matter of the spinal cord, in the history of physical therapy cannot be understated. Children and young adults were most likely to contract polio. This disease became a major health-care issue in the United States in 1917, when 27,363 cases were reported and 7,179 deaths occurred (Murphy, 1995, p. 35). It was then that physical therapists began to work with people recovering from polio in addition to those with war injuries.

There were many treatments for polio, and one of the more successful approaches was implemented by Robert W. Lovett, a Boston orthopedist. Assisting Lovett was Wilhelmine Wright, who ran a "gymnasium" clinic at the Boston Children's Hospital. She developed and published a testing procedure called manual muscle testing. The procedures of Lovett and Wright remained among the primary treatments of polio until the 1940s, when an Australian nurse named Sister Elizabeth Kenny arrived in the United States. The standard polio treatment at that time was bed rest and immobilization. Kenny, however, believed in a more aggressive, active treatment that included exercise (Murphy, 1995, p. 123).

Numerous schools, institutions, and clinics for children with polio and other physical disabilities were established by charitable organizations early in the 20th century. Many children lived at these special schools or hospitals for extended periods of time because of the limitations of the transportation and health-care systems and the belief that experts could better meet the children's needs than their families.

The successful development of the polio vaccine in the 1950s ended the need for physical therapists and others to serve children with polio. At the same time, however, the potential for physical therapists to contribute to the treatment of children with cerebral palsy (CP) was beginning to be recognized. CP is a nonprogressive neurological disorder occurring early in life. Children with milder degrees of CP could receive services at special clinics and schools. Those with more serious disabilities that prevented ambulation or included mental retardation were often sent to institutions where they were "taken care of," but they did not receive the services necessary to reach their potential. The growth of these institutions during the early part of the 20th century was tremendous. This growth was stimulated by the misguided beliefs that families could not "handle" children with these conditions and that the child and the family would be better off if the child were "put away." Physical therapists worked in some of these institutions; however, treatment options were very limited. Services did not expand until the deinstitutionalization movement of the 1960s and 1970s.

Some early physical therapists were guided by Bronson Crothers, a pediatric neurologist at the Boston Children's Hospital, who worked with Mary Trainor, a physical therapist. Trainor is the apparent source of the once-famous songs to accompany exercises for children with CP. She would sing "a little descriptive song to the child . . . [so] the child is taught by imitation to go through certain actions" (Mary McMillan, Massage and Therapeutic Exercise, as cited in Murphy, 1995, p. 164). Crothers also trained Dr. Winthrop Phelps, who in 1932 published a now classic paper on CP that emphasized that children with CP were not necessarily mentally retarded, which was a prevailing thought at the time (American Academy for Cerebral Palsy and Developmental Medicine, 1996, p. 9). Crothers and Phelps and others founded the American Academy of Cerebral Palsy in 1946. In 1957, this medical association established an associate category that allowed non-physicians with doctoral degrees, including physical therapists, to join. Today this multidisciplinary organization, called the American Academy of Cerebral Palsy and Developmental Medicine (AACPDM), allows all members full voting privileges. Many therapists are active members who support education and research efforts to find effective interventions for CP and other developmental disabilities.

In the 1940s a group of parents got together to see if there was anything more they could do at home to help meet the needs of their children with CP. In 1947, the national United Cerebral Palsy Association (UCPA) was founded to help people become more aware of the needs of children with CP. Many schools that had once served children with polio, and thus already had physical therapists on staff, now extended their services to children with CP and other disabilities.

Throughout the 1940s, 1950s, and 1960s, therapists sought a neurophysiological foundation to support their clinical interventions. However, the words of Sedwich Mead, in his 1967 presidential address to the American Academy of Cerebral Palsy, were prophetic: "Neurophysiologic doctrine is a most perishable commodity and it is a mistake to pin one's hopes on a current interpretation" (Mead, 1968). Therapists did, however, place their hopes for a scientific rationale for treatment in the rapidly evolving science of neurophysiology. Many of the theoretical foundations of those treatments have not withstood the test of time in light of recent findings in neuroscience. Some techniques have gained a scientific foundation and are presented in this text. Others continue to be accepted because of assumed clinical effectiveness, good salesmanship, and the search by parents to find a cure for their child with a disability.

APTA has always supported the work of pediatric physical therapists, as evidenced by numerous journal articles and conference proceedings. Bud DeHaven, a leader in the advancement of the pediatric physical therapy profession, was instrumental in establishing the APTA Section on Pediatrics in 1973. This component of APTA was one of the first to address the needs of therapists serving a specific clinical population. The APTA Section on Pediatrics continues to support the work of physical therapists in meeting the needs of children and their families, and it is responsible for the publication of the journal *Pediatric Physical Therapy*.

World Health Organization International Classification of Functioning, Disability, and Health

Systems that classify an individual's findings into patterns provide a foundation for examination, evaluation, intervention, and analysis of outcomes of intervention. A number of models have been proposed to study the consequences of diseases. Such models in physical therapy include the Nagi model, which served as the organizational framework for the *Guide* (APTA, 2001), the five-dimension National Center for Medical Rehabilitation Research (NCMRR) model (National Institutes of Health, 1993), and the widely adopted World Health Organization (WHO) **International Classification of Functioning, Disability, and Health (ICF)** model.

The WHO has developed the most widely known models of disablement. In 1980, they published the International Classification of Impairments, Disabilities, and Handicaps (ICIDH), which was later revised and referred to as ICIDH-2. In 2001, after extensive international review, the WHO approved the ICF, which provides a unified and standard language and framework to describe and measure health and health-related states. The WHO ICF Child and Youth Version (ICF-CY), developed in 2007, builds on the ICF conceptual framework to address infancy, childhood, and adolescence as well as the relevant environmental factors associated with these age groups. The ICF-CY attempts to capture the growth and development of a disability, even when the diagnosis does not change. It also helps to identify the wide variability of abilities and levels of functioning seen in children with the same diagnosis and provides a continuity of documentation for transition from child to adult services.

Traditional classification systems focus on mortality; ICF focuses on life. Determining how people can live with their health conditions and be helped to achieve a productive, fulfilling life is more important than noting their inabilities. ICF strives to place all disease and health conditions on an equal footing. An adolescent might miss school because of a cold or a broken leg but also because of depression. ICF takes a neutral approach and places mental disorders on a par with physical illness.

The ICF has two parts, and each part has two components. Part 1, Functioning and Disability, includes (a) Body Functions and Structures and (b) Activities and Participation. Part 2, Contextual Factors, includes (a) Environmental Factors and (b) Personal Factors (Table 1.1). "Each component consists of various domains and, within each domain, categories, which are the units of classification. Health and health-related states of an individual may be recorded by selecting the appropriate category code, or codes, and then adding qualifiers" (WHO, 2001, p. 10–11). The qualifiers are part of a numeric coding system that indicates the degree of the problem ranging from "No problem" to "Complete problem." The ICF codes and qualifiers provide a condensed version of the information found in clinical records. To make the application of the ICF more practical for the clinical environment, Core Sets, which are shortened lists of the ICF categories of functioning related to specific health conditions, are being developed for specific conditions (Escorpizo et al., 2010). Comprehensive Core Sets are useful in interdisciplinary assessment, while brief Core Sets are available for use by a single discipline. The WHO (2008) has also developed an ICF-based assessment instrument for adults, the WHO Disability Assessment Schedule II (WHO DAS II), which provides a summary measure of functioning and disability. Core Sets and assessment schedules are currently being developed for children.

The WHO (2001, p. 10) defines the ICF components as follows:

- **Body functions** are the physiological functions of body systems (including psychological functions).
- **Body structures** are anatomical parts of the body, such as organs, limbs, and their components.
- **Impairments** are problems in body function or structure, such as a significant deviation or loss.
- **Activity** is the execution of a task or an action by an individual.
- **Participation** is involvement in a life situation.
- **Activity limitations** are difficulties an individual may have in executing activities.
- **Participation restrictions** are problems an individual may experience in involvement in life situations.
- **Environmental factors** make up the physical, social, and attitudinal environment in which people live and conduct their lives.

The terminology used in ICF is relatively straightforward; however, the different meanings of similar words among ICF, the NCMRR model, and the *Guide*

Table 1.1 An Overview of the International Classification of Functioning, Disability, and Health

	Part 1: Functioning and Disability		**Part 2: Contextual Factors**	
Components	Body Functions and Structures	Activities and Participation	Environmental Factors	Personal Factors
Domains	Body functions Body structures	Life areas (tasks, actions)	External influences on functioning and disability	Internal influences on functioning and disability
Constructs	Change in body functions (physiological) Change in body structures (anatomical)	Capacity: Executing tasks in a standard environment Performance: Executing tasks in the current environment	Facilitating or hindering impact of features of the physical, social, and attitudinal world	Impact of attributes of the person
Positive aspect	Functional and structural integrity Functioning	Activities: Participation	Facilitators	Not applicable
Negative aspect	Impairment Disability	Activity limitation Participation Restriction	Barriers/hindrances	Not applicable

Source: World Health Organization (2001). *International Classification of Functioning, Disability and Health* (p. 11). Geneva: Author. Copyright by the World Health Organization. Reprinted with permission of the author.

(APTA, 2001) can lead to some confusion. APTA (2008a) has endorsed the ICF, so future editions of the *Guide* will use ICF terminology. Under ICF, function relates to body organ or system function, *not* functional activities. In the ICF model, functional activities, as therapists have used the term in the past, are activities and participation. Impairments are of the body, not of the activity. For example, therapists would discuss limitations in the activity of walking, not impairments, because there might be an impairment of the anatomical structure of the limb influencing the activity of walking. The ICF terminology is used throughout this text.

The ICY-CY (WHO, 2007) recognizes development and disability as parallel processes. For children, changes in functions, activities, and participation reflect the critical role of the environment, the child in context, development, behavioral regulation and organization, the mediating role of temperament, and timing and maturation reflecting developmental delay. The ICF-CY includes a number of new codes reflecting children's issues, such as body function codes for manual and lateral dominance and activity/participation codes for learning through actions and playing, following routines, managing one's own behavior, and indicating the need for eating. There are also now different levels of play codes to reflect the child's main occupation of play.

To provide a comprehensive understanding of the individual's life, ICF includes Contextual Factors, which consist of the components of environmental and personal factors. These factors can be expressed in positive or negative terms. Environmental factors include *individual influences,* such as the immediate environment and the people in that environment, and *societal influences,* such as formal and informal social structures. Environmental factors interact with body functions and structures, activities, and participation. Personal factors include the part of the child's background that is not related to a health condition or health status, as well as demographics and past and current life experiences. There is no classification system of personal factors in ICF (WHO, 2001, p. 17–18). The conceptual model of the interactions among the components of the ICF as presented by the WHO is presented in Figure 1.1A, and Figure 1.1B is an example using the model to describe a child with spastic diplegia cerebral palsy.

Management of Children With Disabilities

Physical therapy practice for children with disabilities previously followed the medical model of determining the symptoms, establishing a diagnosis (usually provided by the physician), determining the child's weaknesses, therapist determination of goals and objectives, and treatment based on the therapist's experience. Over the past few decades, practice has changed substantially. The child and family are primary in determining goals and objectives, the child's and family's strengths are vital in developing appropriate interventions, interventions are increasingly evidence-based, and service settings have shifted from hospital- or center-based environments to the community and home.

Management of children with disabilities is based on clinical decision making and evidence-based practice. Unfortunately, it has been noted that a therapist's decision making is usually based only on expert opinion, advice from a colleague, textbooks, continuing education courses, and personal experience, all of which are subject to bias (Thomson-O'Brien & Moreland, 1998). A stronger foundation for decision-making is provided by evidence-based practice. Evidence based practice or the "evidence-based medicine movement is the conscientious, explicit, and judicious use of current evidence in making decisions about the care of individual patients. The practice of evidence-based medicine means integrating individual clinical expertise with the best available external clinical evidence from systematic research" (Sackett, Rosenberg, Gray, Haynes, & Richardson, 1996).

Evidence-based practice emphasizes findings from sound clinical research and de-emphasizes intuition, unsystematic clinical experience, and explanations based on pathophysiology (Evidence-Based Medical Working Group, 1992). However, it includes a fine balance between "clinical expertise" and "external clinical evidence" (Law & MacDermid, 2008, p. 5). Clinical knowledge is not ignored, but it means critically evaluating what we do. Evidence-based practice strongly supports a client-centered approach; clinical experience is critical because knowledgeable therapists must implement the findings based on the evidence, and it makes use of the best methods of intervention currently available (Law & MacDermid, 2008).

Law and MacDermid (2008, pp. 9,10) note four elements of good evidence-based practice in rehabilitation. The first is *awareness.* The therapist must be aware of the evidence that is available. Unless one is aware of it, evidence cannot be used in clinical decision making. The second is *consultation.* The child and family must be consulted as part of the decision-making process. There must be transparency. We must communicate our knowledge so that they can make informed decisions about various options. *Judgment,* the third element, is important in deciding how and when to apply the recommendations of

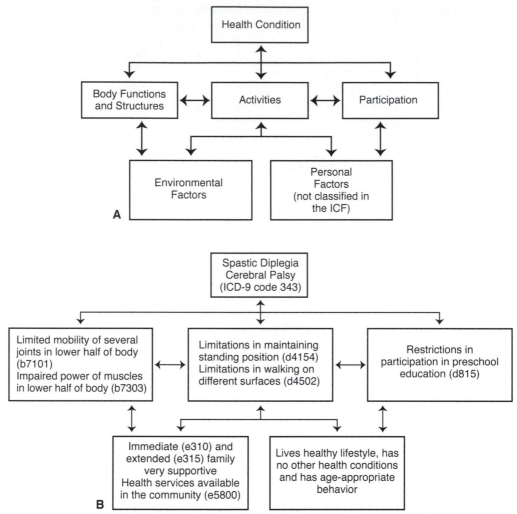

Figure 1.1 (*A*) Interactions between the components of ICF. (*From World Health Organization [2001].* The International Classification of Functioning, Disability, and Health *[p. 18]. Geneva: Author. Copyright 2001 by the World Health Organization. Reprinted with permission.*) (*B*) Interactions between the components of ICF for a preschool-aged child with spastic diplegia cerebral palsy.

evidence-based practice. Information must be analyzed as it applies to a particular child at a particular time. It takes sound professional judgment to avoid blindly embracing evidence. Finally, *creativity* is necessary because even when there is evidence, it must be applied creatively and not in a "cookie-cutter" fashion.

The second edition of the *Guide,* published by APTA in 2001, describes, standardizes, and delineates patient management and preferred practice patterns for physical therapists. The *Guide* divides practice patterns into musculoskeletal, neuromuscular, cardiovascular/pulmonary, and integumentary systems, and is the organizational structure used in this text. The *Guide,* although not geared to the pediatric population, provides

the preferred standards of care and professional terminology to be used by all physical therapists. The *Guide* terminology and practice patterns are used throughout this text, with the exception that ICF language is used to describe health and health-related issues.

According to the *Guide* (APTA, 2001), there are six elements of management of the individual with a disability or illness: examination, evaluation, diagnosis, prognosis, intervention, and outcomes. They are discussed in this section and outlined in Figure 1.2.

Examination

The *Guide* (APTA, 2001) divides the **examination** process into three components: History, Systems Review,

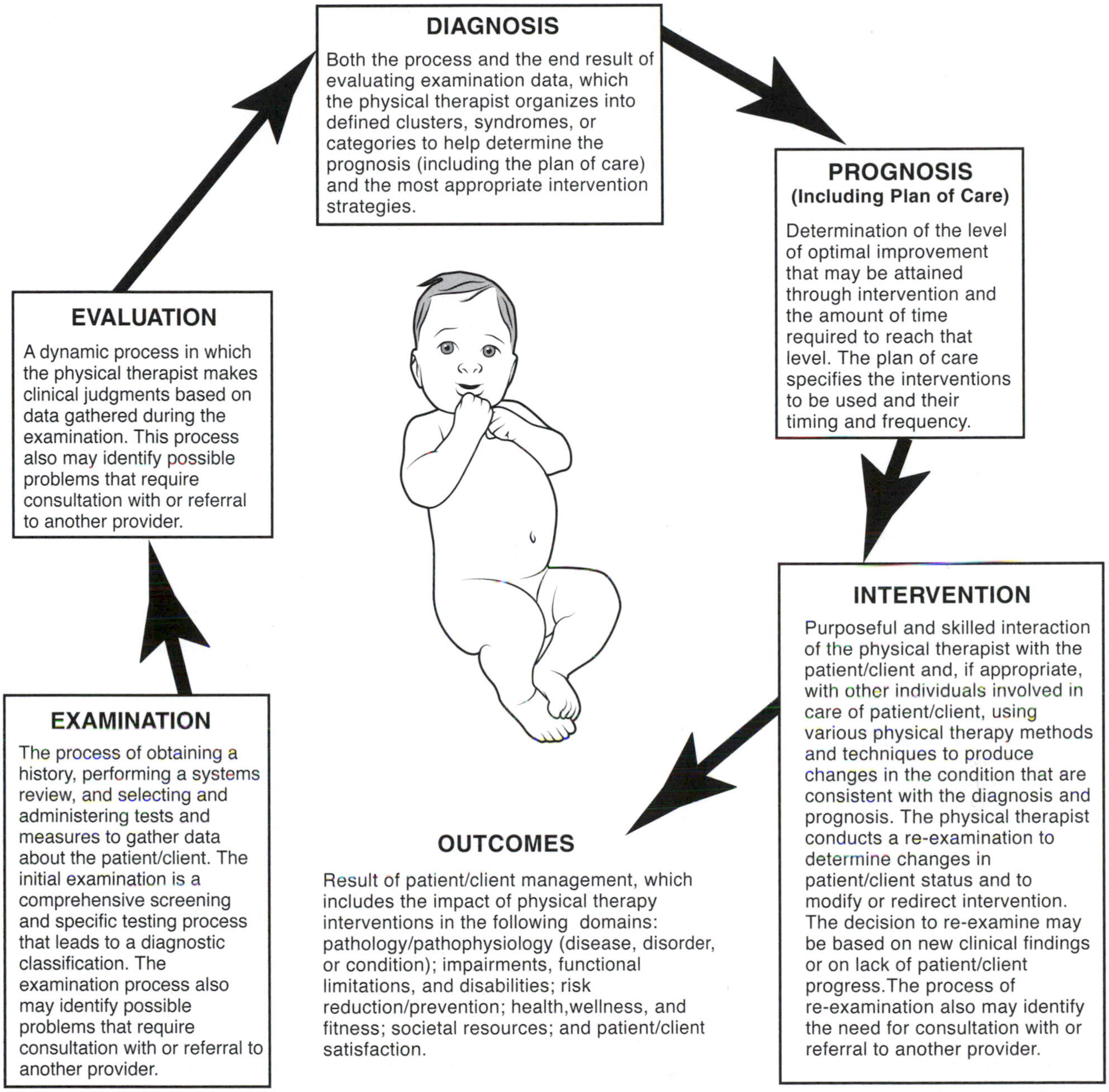

DIAGNOSIS

Both the process and the end result of evaluating examination data, which the physical therapist organizes into defined clusters, syndromes, or categories to help determine the prognosis (including the plan of care) and the most appropriate intervention strategies.

PROGNOSIS
(Including Plan of Care)

Determination of the level of optimal improvement that may be attained through intervention and the amount of time required to reach that level. The plan of care specifies the interventions to be used and their timing and frequency.

EVALUATION

A dynamic process in which the physical therapist makes clinical judgments based on data gathered during the examination. This process also may identify possible problems that require consultation with or referral to another provider.

INTERVENTION

Purposeful and skilled interaction of the physical therapist with the patient/client and, if appropriate, with other individuals involved in care of patient/client, using various physical therapy methods and techniques to produce changes in the condition that are consistent with the diagnosis and prognosis. The physical therapist conducts a re-examination to determine changes in patient/client status and to modify or redirect intervention. The decision to re-examine may be based on new clinical findings or on lack of patient/client progress. The process of re-examination also may identify the need for consultation with or referral to another provider.

EXAMINATION

The process of obtaining a history, performing a systems review, and selecting and administering tests and measures to gather data about the patient/client. The initial examination is a comprehensive screening and specific testing process that leads to a diagnostic classification. The examination process also may identify possible problems that require consultation with or referral to another provider.

OUTCOMES

Result of patient/client management, which includes the impact of physical therapy interventions in the following domains: pathology/pathophysiology (disease, disorder, or condition); impairments, functional limitations, and disabilities; risk reduction/prevention; health, wellness, and fitness; societal resources; and patient/client satisfaction.

Figure 1.2 Elements of child management leading to optimal outcomes. *(From American Physical Therapy Association [2001]. Guide to physical therapist practice [2nd ed.]. Physical Therapy, 81[1], 43. Copyright 2001 by the American Physical Therapy Association. Reprinted with permission of the author.)*

and Tests and Measures. The examination starts with a review of the child's history and a systems review, as outlined in Table 1.2 and Figure 1.3. After analyzing the information gained from the history and systems review, specific tests and measurements are administered by the physical therapist. Tests and measures of development, sensory integration, function, pain, and quality

of life are discussed in Chapter 3 and described in Appendix 3-B. Tests and measures used to examine each body system and activities and participation restrictions related to that body system are presented in the systems section. These tests and measures must be performed and the results evaluated before the plan of care and intervention are developed.

General Demographics
- Age
- Sex
- Race/ethnicity
- Primary language
- Education

Social History
- Cultural beliefs and behaviors
- Family and caregiver resources
- Social interactions, social activities, and support systems

Employment/Work (Job/School/Play)
- Current and prior work(job/school/play), community and leisure actions, tasks, or activities

Growth and Development
- Development history
- Hand dominance

Living Environment
- Devices and equipment (e.g., assistive, adaptive, orthotic, protective, supportive, prosthetic)
- Living environment and community characteristics
- Projected discharge destinations

General Health Status (Self-report, Family Report, Caregiver Report)
- General health perception
- Physical function (e.g., mobility, sleep patterns, restricted bed days)
- Psychological function (e.g., memory, reasoning ability, depression, anxiety)
- Role function (e.g., community, leisure, social, work)
- Social function (e.g., social activity, social interaction, social support)

Social/ Health Habits (Past and Current)
- Behavioral health risks (e.g., smoking, drug abuse)
- Level of physical fitness

Medical/ Surgical History
- Cardiovascular
- Endocrine/metabolic
- Gastrointestinal
- Genitourinary
- Gynecological
- Integumentary
- Musculoskeletal
- Obstetrical
- Prior hospitalizations, surgeries, and preexisting medical and other health-related conditions
- Psychological
- Pulmonary

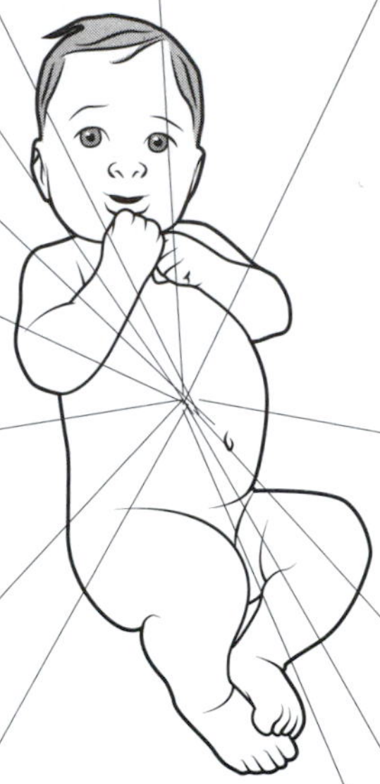

Current Condition(s)/ Chief Complaint(s)
- Concerns that led the patient/ client to seek the services of a physical therapist
- Concerns or needs of patient/ client who requires the services of physical therapist
- Current therapeutic interventions
- Mechanisms of injury or disease, including date of onset and course of events
- Onset and pattern of symptoms
- Patient/client, family, significant other, and caregiver expectations and goals for the therapeutic intervention
- Patient/client, family, significant other, and caregiver perceptions of patient/client's emotional response to the current clinical situation
- Previous occurrences of chief complaint(s)
- Prior therapeutic interventions

Functional Status and Activity Level
- Current and prior functional status in self-care and home management, including activities of daily living (ADL) and instrumental activities of daily living (IADL)
- Current and prior functional status in work (job/school/play), community, and leisure actions, tasks, or activities

Medications
- Medications for current condition
- Medications previously taken for current condition
- Medications for other conditions

Other Clinical Tests
- Laboratory and diagnostic tests
- Review of available records (e.g., medical, education, surgical)
- Review of other clinical findings (e.g., nutrition and hydration)

Family History
- Familial health risks

Figure 1.3 Types of data generated from history. *(From American Physical Therapy Association [2001]. Guide to physical therapist practice [2nd ed.]. Physical Therapy, 81[1], 44. Copyright 2001 by the American Physical Therapy Association. Reprinted with permission of the author.)*

History

Obtaining an acute **history** is a vital part of the examination process. Data are collected from various sources, including medical and educational records, parent and child interviews, and interviews with significant others. The types of data generated are outlined in Figure 1.3. After the history has been obtained and analyzed and the setting and structure of the examination determined, the examination can be started.

Systems Review

According to the *Guide* (APTA, 2001), the **systems review** is a brief or limited examination of the status of the cardiovascular/pulmonary, integumentary, musculoskeletal, and neuromuscular systems, based on pertinent information obtained from the history. In addition, the communication ability, social maturity, cognition, and learning style of the child may be determined.

The *Guide* (APTA, 2001, pp. 42–43) suggests that the systems review include the following:

- For the cardiovascular/pulmonary system, assessment of heart rate, respiratory rate, blood pressure, and edema
- For the integumentary system, assessment of skin integrity, skin color, and presence of scar formation
- For the musculoskeletal system, assessment of gross symmetry, gross range of motion (ROM), gross strength, height, and weight
- For the neuromuscular system, a general assessment of gross coordinated movement (e.g., balance, locomotion, transfers, and transitions)
- For communication ability, affect, cognition, language, and learning style, the assessment of the ability to make needs known, consciousness, orientation (person, place, and time), expected emotional/behavioral responses, and learning preferences (e.g., learning barriers, education needs)

Therapists must also consider a review of the various developmental domains that influence a child's function. "These may include cognition; language and communication; social/emotional development; adaptive function; physical development, including vision and hearing; and play" (APTA, Section on Pediatrics, 2003). The extent of the systems review will depend on the child's age and cognitive ability, the requirements of the setting, and reimbursement issues. The systems review helps determine what specific tests and measures are appropriate to administer and whether consultation with another provider is necessary.

Tests and Measures

The history and systems review help determine what specific tests and measures should be performed to confirm or rule out the causes of impairment in body functions and structures, limitations in activities, and restrictions in participation. They also assist in establishing a diagnosis, prognosis, and plan of care. If a medical diagnosis is available, that will frequently guide the examination. For example, a child with cystic fibrosis will definitely require a comprehensive examination of the cardiopulmonary/vascular system, and the brief systems review might determine that further examination of the integumentary system is not warranted. A child with burns will require a thorough examination of the integumentary system, and the systems review would indicate which other systems require more extensive examination. While using the medical diagnosis to guide the examination process, clinicians must avoid letting it influence their perception of the examination results or their clinical decision making. Clinicians must rely on their own evidence-based knowledge and results of their history, systems review, and examination when developing their conclusions about the child's physical therapy diagnosis, which should be separate from the medical diagnosis.

Tests and measures help confirm or reject a hypothesis regarding what factors are contributing to the child's current level of performance and "support the physical therapist's clinical judgments about appropriate interventions, anticipated goals, and expected outcomes" (APTA, 2001, p. 43). Measurement is the "numeral assigned to an object, event, or person or the class (category) to which an object, event, or person is assigned according to rules" (APTA, 1991). We collect measurements by many methods, including interviewing, observing, and conducting performance-based assessments; taking photographs or videographic recordings; and using scales, indexes, inventories, self-assessments, and logs (APTA, 2001).

Section 2 of this text discusses appropriate tests and measures for each of the body systems. In addition to the examination of specific systems, it is important when working with children to determine their developmental and functional status, sensory processing, presence of pain, and quality of life and health. These tests and measures and other examination issues are the focus of Chapter 3.

Evaluation

After the physical process of performing the examination, the intellectual process of the evaluation is completed. The *Guide* (APTA, 2001, p. 43) states that **evaluation** is a "dynamic process in which the physical therapist makes clinical judgments based on data gathered during the examination." The evaluation involves the synthesis of findings from the history, systems review, and tests and measures of impairments of body structures and functions, limitations in activities, and restrictions in participation. In pediatrics, the terms *evaluation, examination,* and *assessment* are frequently used interchangeably or have different meanings in different settings than indicated in the *Guide* and as discussed in Chapter 3.

There are many approaches to the evaluation of children with disabilities. The theoretical model that serves as the foundation for the process varies based on the setting, diagnoses, resources, payer, and provider. P. H. Campbell (1991) has described both top-down and bottom-up approaches to examination and evaluation. In the **top-down approach** (Fig. 1.4), the desired outcomes (goals or objectives) are determined first, with extensive input from the child and family. Then the strengths and obstacles to achieving the goals are determined through the examination and evaluation process. A plan of care with appropriate interventions is then developed and implemented with ongoing re-examination. This family-centered, top-down approach is commonly used for children with known problems or diagnoses, those with severe limitations in activities, and those in early intervention programs. The **bottom-up approach** is the more traditional approach, in which the child's strengths and weaknesses are identified through the examination process and then the professionals determine the goals and objectives. This approach is more common in medical settings. The evaluation process is influenced by the severity and complexity of the findings, extent of loss of function, family and home situation, school situation, functional level, and activities and participation in the community (APTA, 2001).

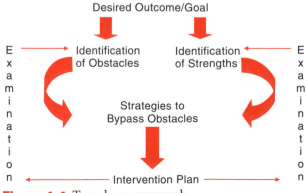

Figure 1.4 Top-down approach.

In a top-down approach, the child and family might identify that being able to climb the stairs at the high-school football stadium is very important to them. It is unlikely that the therapist would have thought about stadium stairs without family input, but with the family's assistance, the therapist can develop a plan of care to help achieve this goal. The therapist would determine what skills and abilities the child has that would assist in performing this task. Strengths might include the ability to walk with crutches on level ground and climb stairs using a railing in an empty stairwell. Possible obstacles might include lacking the balance required for stair climbing without a railing, distractibility in crowded places, and lacking the cardiopulmonary endurance required for the task. The plan of care to achieve this goal would then be developed and provided for the child.

In some settings it is common to include factors affecting function based on the examination results in the evaluation. Internal factors are those within the individual, and include impairments of body structures and functions, limitations in activities, cognitive ability, emotional stability, motivation, and language ability. External factors are personal and environmental factors such as family support, access to health care, financial resources, accessible schools, and so on. Factors that aid and hinder function should be considered and perhaps included in the documentation because they influence intervention. The negative factors affecting function are really a list of problems similar to those used in many physical therapy reporting systems (Kettenbach, 2001).

Diagnosis

Diagnosis is a term used to describe a cluster of signs and symptoms, arranged in syndromes or categories. The diagnosis is based on the results of the examination and evaluation process. Physicians usually use a medical diagnosis to identify a disease, disorder, or condition at the cell, tissue, organ, or system level. A physical therapist, when determining a diagnosis, will use "labels that identify the *impact of a condition on function at the level of the system (especially the movement system) and at the level of the whole person*" (APTA, 2001, p. 45). A physical therapist, after a comprehensive examination and evaluation, will assign a physical therapy diagnostic label based on the specific practice patterns outlined in the *Guide*. Each practice pattern represents a diagnostic classification and "indicates the primary dysfunctions toward which the physical therapist directs intervention" (APTA, 2001, p. 45). The preferred practice patterns can thereby serve as a guide to direct the management and intervention of individuals who are grouped together by clusters of impairments. If this process does not yield an appropriate practice pattern, "the physical therapist may administer interventions for the alleviation of symptoms and remediation of impairments" (APTA, 2001, p. 45) guided by the child's responses.

The concept of determining a physical therapy diagnosis parallels our progression to autonomous practitioners. Historically, physical therapists treated individuals only by referral from a physician and based their treatments on the individual's medical diagnosis. It is not surprising that until recently physical therapy tests and measures "represent[ed] a 'bottom heavy' approach where body structure and function may be over-represented" (Watter et al., 2008, p. 348). It is now recognized that diagnosing and treating only at the impairment level will not automatically translate into the desired functional improvements. This knowledge has spurred the recent development and validation of tests and measures that more functionally assess children's activity and participation. Reviewing the tests and measures and their corresponding ICF-CY classification as discussed in Chapter 3 reveals that there is now a variety of assessment tools available, which should facilitate evaluation of a child's performance at multiple levels.

According to the *Guide* (2001), the primary objective of establishing a physical therapy diagnosis is to identify the gap between a person's desired level of function and the capacity to achieve that level. Categorizing children's functional abilities in this way assists the physical therapist in intervention planning. Through use of the top-down evaluation approach, the desired level of functioning is determined first during the subjective component of the examination, and then the child's current performance capabilities are determined using appropriate tests and measures to assess body structures and functions, activities, and participation. Using the conceptual framework of the ICF, the physical therapist must remember that these dimensions of human function are interrelated and multi-directional, not a simple linear progression with impairments creating activity limitations which in turn lead to participation restrictions (Lollar & Simeonsson, 2005, p. 324).

Systematically applied diagnostic labels provide a common language for communicating information about the child among health-care professionals. Given the interdisciplinary approach to pediatric rehabilitation, having congruent communication across disciplines is essential to coordinating quality care. The WHO advocates using the ICF-CY "as the common language to describe health and disability in the first two decades of life" (Martinuzzi et al., 2010, p. 42). This classification system is being used by pediatric rehabilitation teams and has successfully facilitated team interactions, improved communication of goals, and enhanced effectiveness of interdisciplinary tasks and team conferences (Martinuzzi et al., 2010).

During the diagnostic process, it is important to consider the child's environment to provide holistic interventions and maximize outcomes. Pediatric clinicians have always recognized the importance of environmental influences on children's outcomes. Any practicing therapist can provide examples of children whose functional outcomes were not realized because of environmental barriers or who exceed expectations because of optimal environmental conditions. It is necessary to recognize how environmental influences change over time with the developing child (Simeonsson et al., 2003). Infants and toddlers are more affected by their proximal environment and their immediate family/caregivers, while school-aged children become more influenced by peer, community, and societal factors. The Individuals with Disabilities Education Improvement Act of 2004 (IDEA) for serving infants and children with disabilities in early intervention and schools acknowledges this concept and requires transition planning as the child moves from early intervention services to preschool and from secondary education to postsecondary environments.

Utilization of the ICF-CY framework provides a mechanism for including environmental factors when developing a physical therapy diagnosis. Considering the categories of environmental factors (products and technology, natural environment and human-made changes to environment, supports and relationships, attitudes and services, systems and policies) and labeling the applicable factors as facilitators or barriers during the diagnostic process helps the therapist to focus on the child's participation, which will enhance inclusion in age-appropriate activities, such as toddler reading programs at the local library or community-based sports leagues. Broadening our evaluation and diagnostic process in this fashion not only enhances our physical therapy interventions, it also encourages improvements in children's overall health and wellness, which are necessary as the need for physical fitness and healthy lifestyles for children with disabilities is well established (Fragala-Pinkham, Haley, & Goodgold, 2006; Fowler et al., 2007; Rimmer, 2006).

The diagnostic process is complex and should be systematically addressed, although the notion of "diagnosis has not reached the prominence among therapists working with children that the concept holds for those working in other areas of physical therapy" (VanSant, 2006). This is an area of pediatric practice that requires much more consideration and research.

Prognosis

Once a functional and clinically relevant physical therapy diagnosis has been established, the physical therapist must determine the child's prognosis. **Prognosis** involves determining the "predicted optimal level of improvement in function and the amount of time needed to reach that level, and may also include a prediction of levels of improvement that may be reached at various intervals during the course of therapy" (APTA, 2001, p. 46). This prognostic ability is one of the most difficult tasks for students and new clinicians to develop. Experienced clinicians tend to implicitly integrate examination and evaluation information with past experience to relatively quickly determine the child's diagnosis, prognosis, and plan of care (Bartlett & Palisano, 2000, p. 237).

Plan of Care

The culmination of the examination, evaluation, diagnosis, and prognosis is development of the **plan of care**. The plan is developed in full collaboration with the child, family, and other service providers. Models or frameworks for this clinical decision making that leads to the plan of care have been developed, including the hypothesis-oriented algorithm for clinicians II (HOAC-II) (Rothstein, Echternach, & Riddle, 2003), the Clinical Decision-Making Algorithm for Neonatal Physical Therapy (Sweeney, Heriza, & Blanchard, 2009), the Clinical Decision-Making Algorithm for Pediatric Physical Therapy (as discussed in Chapter 3; Fig. 3.1), and the ICF-CY (WHO, 2007). Incorporating any of these models into clinical practice provides a more transparent approach to the patient management process. Use of the ICF-CY model when developing a plan of care allows the therapist to address multiple domains of health when considering goals, outcomes, and interventions. By evaluating the relationship between these components, the clinician can determine the appropriateness of the plan of care and modify elements as needed. For example, identifying that a child's therapy goals and interventions primarily address decreased ROM, strength, and balance (impairment level deficits) may help the therapist recognize why the family's goal of walking independently at home and preschool (an activity and participation level goal) is not being met, and adjustments to the therapy goals and interventions can be made. We should be cognizant

that "with our clinical interest in improving the functional and participation abilities of children, most of our goals [should be] represented by the ICF component of activity" (Darrah, 2008, p. 148). Making sure that interventions are not all at the impairment level while goals and outcomes are at the activity and participation level will aid the therapist in developing a more contemporary and functional intervention plan.

Table 1.2 provides an outline of a general, comprehensive sample template for documentation of a **Pediatric Physical Therapy Evaluation and Plan of Care** based on the areas suggested in the *Guide* (APTA, 2001), and common pediatric physical therapy practice. While not following the ICF-CY Core Set, the areas of body function and structure, activity, and participation are included. The documentation templates provided in the *Guide* are not generally appropriate to pediatric practice. Table 1.2 provides the basic outline of the major headings, and includes the areas that might be addressed under each heading. The plan of care usually starts with *measurable goals, objectives, and outcomes.*

Goals, Objectives, and Outcomes

The anticipated goals and objectives and predicted outcomes are the intended results of the intervention and guide the interventions. The plan of care indicates in measurable terms the expected changes in impairments of body structures and functions, limitations in activities, and restrictions in participation. The plan might "also address risk reduction, prevention, impact on societal resources and . . . satisfaction" (APTA, 2001, p. 46).

There have been changes in the terminology and definitions used to describe goals, outcomes, and objectives. Goals and objectives might best be considered *expectations* of the intervention, whereas the outcomes are the *results*. This terminology becomes complicated because in the *Guide* (APTA, 2001, p. 46) the word "expected" is placed before outcomes, which would lead one to wonder what the difference is between "anticipated goals" and "expected outcomes." Goals should precede objectives (Alberto & Troutman, 2006). In the past, goals and outcomes were global statements that were usually not measurable (APTA, 1997; Montgomery, 1987). However, in the second edition of the *Guide* (APTA, 2001), it is noted that "anticipated goals and expected outcomes . . . should be measurable and time limited" (p. 48). The term "objective" is not defined in the *Guide*, although it is used in the *Guide* and is standard terminology in physical therapy practice, especially in pediatrics. **Objectives** are measurable

Table 1.2 Documentation of a Pediatric Physical Therapy Evaluation and Plan of Care (most major headings expanded to include potential areas to address under each element; all areas might not be necessary for an individual child)

Child's name:

Physical therapist's name:

Date of examination:

Child's date of birth:

Child's age:

Medical diagnosis:

Parent and Child Issues

What are the family's and child's goals and objectives?

What are the major concerns of the child and family?

What is the child trying to do?

What do the child and parents want the child to be able to do?

What are the child's favorite activities, games, or toys?

Child's History (APTA, 2001, p. 44). See Figure 1.2 for items to include under each heading.

General Demographics
Social History
Employment/Work (Job/School/Play)
Growth and Development (includes birth history and motor milestone)
Living Environment (includes siblings and housing)
General Health Status
Social/Health Habits
Medical/Surgical History
Current Conditions(s)/Chief Complaints(s)
Functional Status and Activity Level
Medications
Other Clinical Tests
Family History

Present Function

Description of present function, preferably in natural environment.

Systems Review

The systems review is a brief or limited examination of each of the systems that will assist in determining what tests and measures to use and in formulating a diagnosis, prognosis, plan of care, and interventions.

Cardiovascular and pulmonary
Integumentary
Musculoskeletal
Neuromuscular
Communication/ cognition/ orientation
Specific to pediatrics
—Language and communication, social/emotional development, adaptive development, physical development including vision and hearing, play behaviors

Tests and Measures:

Activity and Participation

Should address activity and participation in all of the child's environments.

Continued

■
■ **Table 1.2** Documentation of a Pediatric Physical Therapy Evaluation and Plan of Care (most major headings expanded to include potential areas to address under each element; all areas might not be necessary for an individual child)—cont'd

Body Function and Structure

Based on the history and systems review, specific tests and measures are selected to be administered to yield information on limitations in activity and participation and restrictions in body function and structure. The general topic headings of these *Guide* tests and measures, given in alphabetical order, *not* by level of significance, might include the following:

Aerobic Capacity/Endurance
Anthropometric Characteristics
Arousal, Attention, and Cognition
Assistive and Adaptive Devices
Circulation
Cranial and Peripheral Nerve Integrity
Environmental, Home, and Work (Job/School/Play) Barriers
Ergonomics and Body Mechanics
Gait, Location, and Balance
Integumentary Integrity
Joint Integrity and Mobility
Motor Function (Motor Control and Motor Learning)
Muscle Performance (including Strength, Power, and Endurance)
Neuromotor Development and Sensory Integration
Orthotic, Protective, and Supportive Devices
Pain
Posture
Prosthetic Requirements
Range of Motion (including Muscle Length)
Reflex Integrity
Self-Care and Home Management (including Activities of Daily Living [ADL] and Instrumental Activities of Daily Living [IADL])
Sensory Integrity
Ventilation, Respiration, and Circulation
Work (Job/School/Play), Community, and Leisure Integration or Reintegration (including IADL)
Standardized Tests and Measures of neuromotor development, sensory integration, function, and quality of life are commonly used in a pediatric examination and are listed in Appendix 3-B. Tests and Measures of body functions and structures and additional activities are provided in the chapters on body systems.

Evaluation

Clinical judgments are made based on the information gathered during the examination.
In pediatric settings it is common to include a concise "Summary of Findings."

Diagnosis

A label describing a cluster of signs related to impairment of the body systems and the impact of those impairments on activity and participation of the child. A diagnostic label can be assigned using a specific practice pattern (*Guide*, 2001).

Prognosis

The predicted optimal level of improvement in body function and structure, activity, and participation.

Plan of Care
Measurable Goals, Objectives, and Outcomes
Intervention Plan

1. Coordination, Communication, and Documentation
2. Child- and Family-Related Instruction
3. Procedural Interventions

Table 1.2 Documentation of a Pediatric Physical Therapy Evaluation and Plan of Care (most major headings expanded to include potential areas to address under each element; all areas might not be necessary for an individual child)—cont'd

Therapeutic Exercise
Functional Training in Self-Care and Home Management (including ADL and IADL)
Functional Training in Work (Job/School/Play)
Community and Leisure Integration or Reintegration (including IADL, Work Hardening, and Work Conditioning)
Manual Therapy Techniques (including Mobilization/Manipulation)
Prescription, Application, and Fabrication of Devices and Equipment
Airway Clearance Techniques
Integumentary Repair and Protective Techniques
Electrotherapeutic Modalities
Physical Agents and Mechanical Modalities
Re-examination
Criteria for Discharge

statements regarding desired (anticipated/expected) results (goals/outcomes). There appears to be an agreement that **outcomes** are "factors that identify the results of interventions (e.g., functional health status, morbidity, mortality, quality of life, satisfaction, and cost)" (Nicholson, 2002, p. 214). Outcomes at both the impairment of body structure and function level, and at the limitations in activities and participation level may be indicated (Montgomery & Connolly, 2003).

Determining a desired goal, outcome, or objective can be as simple as asking the child what activity he or she wants to perform, or so complex that it requires several interdisciplinary team meetings. The goals, outcomes, and objectives are developed based on the child's and family's desires and the findings of the evaluation.

The ability to measure whether a child has achieved a desired outcome is critical in determining the success of the intervention and the need for continued intervention and program evaluation. Nebulous statements such as "The child will achieve normal motor development" or "The child's tone will normalize" say very little, and it is impossible to know when and if the child attained normal motor development or normal tone. Use of nonmeasurable goal statements hinders the profession's efforts to acquire the data necessary to support the effectiveness of our interventions.

Writing measurable objectives (Table 1.3) is not difficult, but it does require thoughtful consideration of numerous variables. An objective (Effgen, 1991; Mager, 1962) must contain a statement of the behavior that the child is expected to perform, the conditions under which the behavior is performed, and the criteria

expected for ultimate performance. Changes in the behavior may reflect maturation of the behavior itself, progressing from basic skills to more complex skills, or increasing levels of completing the activity. Changes in conditions may be from simple to complex, such as walking at home to walking in a mall filled with people, or transferring with assistance to transferring independently. Progression of criteria may be increased frequency or duration of an activity, or changes in the amount of assistance required. Using criteria, such as three of four trials or 75% of the time, should be considered carefully. For example, successfully transferring into a car 80% of the time could mean that 20% of the time the child ends up on the street! That is not an acceptable outcome or criterion. Selection of the behavior, conditions, and criteria for each objective for each individual child must be based on sound professional judgment. "Cookbooks" of objectives should not replace the judgment of the professional.

Commonly, a long-term objective or goal is determined first and then broken down into several short-term objectives. Short-term objectives are based on a task analysis of the major or long-term objective. In a **task analysis**, the therapist determines the component parts of the task, including activity requirements and prerequisites. For example, a standing transfer from a wheelchair to a car requires the ability to lock the wheelchair, come to a standing position, pivot, and lower oneself to sitting. To perform this activity, the child requires the cognitive ability to understand the activity, the motivation to perform the activity, the motor planning ability to execute the activity, the muscle strength to stand and pivot, the flexion and extension

Table 1.3 Considerations for Objectives

Behavior Examples
- Maintaining sitting position
- Transferring oneself while lying
- Carrying an object from place to place
- Walking on different surfaces

Conditions (might include more than one condition)
- *Equipment:* such as using an assistive device or wearing an orthosis
- *Physical environment:* such as at home or in the school cafeteria
- *Social environment:* such as with the parents or therapist
- *Antecedent stimuli:* such as verbal requests or demonstration

Criteria (might include more than one criterion)
- *Frequency:* number of correct behaviors in a specific number of trials (e.g., 2 of 5 trials) or percentage correct (40% of the time)
- *Duration:* how long a behavior will last (e.g., 3 seconds, 5 minutes, 6 repetitions)
- *Amount of assistance provided:* independent; with supervision; standby assistance; minimal, moderate, or maximum assistance

Examples of Objectives*
- Patrick will ring sit independently on the floor at home for 5 minutes.
- Kathy will transfer from lying on her bed to sitting at the side of her bed with moderate assistance in 3 of 5 trials.
- Julie will carry her books to class from the bus without dropping them 75% of the time.
- Jonathan will walk across his lawn with his walker with standby assistance.

*Examples selected from World Health Organization (2001). *International classification of functioning, disability and health.* Geneva: Author; Mobility Chapter of Activities and Participation.

ROM required to stand and sit, and the balance to sit, stand, and pivot. These are only a few of the components required to perform this complex task. The therapist must select the most important elements for an individual child and systematically develop the objectives.

When possible, each short-term objective should be a desired activity the child wants to perform. There are situations when some short-term objectives relate to impairment of body functions and structures, and when these objectives are attained, they will assist the child in achieving an activity objective. For example,

sitting is an important activity; however, without the prerequisite trunk muscle strength and hip ROM, independent sitting is impossible. In such a case, the therapist might write objectives regarding the ability to sit independently and also write objectives about increasing trunk strength and hip ROM. In educational environments, the activity of sitting and manipulating an object might be an objective placed in the child's Individualized Education Program (IEP), but the impairment level objectives of muscle strengthening and ROM would be part of the plan of care that the therapist writes. Documentation of the achievement of each goal/objective is important, and such achievements should be reported to the child and the family. Many small gains should be recognized and rewarded instead of waiting for the achievement of the major, long-term objective.

Consideration of the level of learning of the activity is also important and is referred to as the hierarchy of response competence (Fig. 1.5) (Alberto & Troutman, 2006). Skill must first be **acquired.** Such skill acquisition might be the initial behavior of propped sitting of an infant, the first few steps with a walker, or a roll from prone to supine. Direct procedural interventions are usually required during the skill acquisition phase (Palisano & Murr, 2009). Acquisition is followed by **fluency** or proficiency, in which the quality and level of learning and performance move beyond merely performance of the task. Fluency occurs when the infant learns to sit without propping, the child can walk around the room with the walker, and the child can roll around from place to place. Fluency may be reflected under conditions or criteria of the objective. Since achieving fluency requires practice and repetition, group therapy and consultation are well suited for fluency (Palisano & Murr, 2009). After fluency there must be **maintenance** of the ability to perform the activities/skills/behaviors over time. The child should be able to perform the activity several days, weeks, or months later. Maintenance is followed by **generalization**, the highest skill level. The child must be able to perform the activity in multiple environments, with different individuals, and with different types of equipment. In the motor learning literature, generalization is referred to as **transfer.** The condition statement may be written to reflect generalization of environments, equipment, and individuals. Acquisition, fluency, maintenance, and generalization of behaviors are terms used by educators and others. Using this terminology is very helpful when we need to convey the rationale for providing services past the initial phase of acquisition of a behavior.

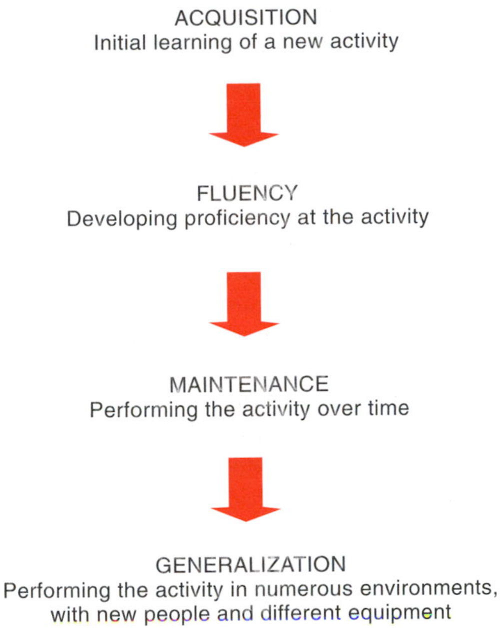

ACQUISITION
Initial learning of a new activity

FLUENCY
Developing proficiency at the activity

MAINTENANCE
Performing the activity over time

GENERALIZATION
Performing the activity in numerous environments,
with new people and different equipment

Figure 1.5 Hierarchy of response competence.

For children, the time stipulated to achieve the long-term objective is setting-specific. In educational settings, the long-term objectives are for 1 year; in early intervention programs, they are generally for 6 months; and in acute-care settings, they might be for 1 week or less. The ability to write realistic objectives that can be achieved in the specified time frame is based, in no

small part, on the skill and experience of the therapist writing the objectives.

A useful method of identifying outcomes relevant to children and families and providing documentation of achievement of increments toward the final goal is Goal Attainment Scaling (GAS) (Brown, Effgen, & Palisano, 1998; King, McDougall, Palisano, Gritzan, & Tucker, 1999; Steenbeek, Ketelaar, Galama, & Gorter, 2007). The therapist writes a specific goal for an individual child and then develops the standard for each level of improvement toward achieving that goal. Specific numeric values are assigned to the expected levels of performance and therefore can be used to evaluate intervention effectiveness and program outcomes (Mailloux et al., 2007; Steenbeek et al., 2007). GAS has demonstrated good content validity, reliability, and responsiveness in studies of children with CP (Law, Dai, & Siu, 2004; Steenbeek, Meester-Delver, Becher, & Lankhorst, 2005). It has been more responsive to changes in motor performance than have standardized measures and is considered more family-centered and child-centered (Palisano, Haley, & Brown, 1992; Rosenbaum, King, Law, King, & Evans, 1998). An example of GAS for the specific objective to ascend and descend four steps is described in Table 1.4.

Different formats for documenting the examination, evaluation findings, and plan of care are used across the nation and service delivery settings. Some of this variation is a result of the purpose of the examination and

Table 1.4 Goal Attainment Scaling Example

Objective (expected outcome): Bill will be able to ascend and descend the 4 steps into his school safely without assistance or holding the railing, 3 out of 3 times by December 1.

Score		Objective Level
–2	Baseline	Bill's current ability is to ascend and descend 2 steps into his school, slowly and safely while holding the railing, 3 out of 3 times.
–1	Less than Expected Outcome	Bill will be able to ascend and descend the *4 steps** into his school, *safely while holding the railing*, 3 out of 3 times by December 1.
0	Expected Outcome	Bill will be able to ascend and descend the 4 steps into his school, *safely without assistance or holding the railing*, 3 out of 3 times by December 1.
+1	Greater than Expected Outcome	Bill will be able to ascend and descend the 4 steps into his school, safely without assistance or holding the railing, *quickly enough to walk to and from his classroom within 5 minutes*, 3 out of 3 times by December 1.
+2	Much Greater than Expected Outcome	Bill will be able to ascend and descend the 4 steps into his school, safely without assistance or holding the railing, *quickly enough to walk to and from his classroom within 2 minutes*, 3 out of 3 times by December 1.

*The italicized portions represent the criteria change of the objective across the different score levels.
N.B.: There can also be additional levels where, for example, a –3 would indicate a regression in current ability level.

the setting. Hospital- and clinic-based therapists must provide daily documentation to reflect the changing status of an ill child, or as required by insurance companies. This documentation is generally concise and typically is in the form of the "SOAP" notes (S = subjective, O = objective, A = assessment, P = plan) (Kettenbach, 2001). Early intervention and school-based therapists must provide documentation that meets the legal requirements of the IDEA and state regulations. While one potential format for the evaluation and plan of care is presented here (see Table 1.2), other formats are discussed in the settings chapters. Documentation is addressed in more detail in Chapter 3. APTA's (2008b) Defensible Documentation for Patient/Client management, Section E: Pediatric Settings also provides useful setting-specific information.

Intervention

Intervention is the term used throughout the *Guide* to describe "the purposeful and skilled interaction of the physical therapist with the patient/client and, if appropriate, with other individuals involved in the care of the patient/client, using various physical therapy methods and techniques to produce changes in the condition that are consistent with the diagnosis and prognosis" (APTA, 2001, p. 43). Judgments regarding intervention are made based on the timely monitoring of the child's responses and progress in achieving the anticipated goals, objectives, and outcomes. The concept of intervention is far more encompassing than just the term "treatment." According to the *Guide,* intervention should be composed of three important components: (1) coordination, communication, and documentation; (2) child- and family-related instruction; and (3) procedural interventions.

Coordination, Communication, and Documentation
Coordination involves the organization and management of services with all parties working together to ensure that the child and family "receive appropriate, comprehensive, efficient, and effective quality of care" (APTA, 2001, p. 47) from the initiation of services to the end of services. The therapist, or a designated case manager, might provide coordination of services. Coordination may involve arranging for durable medical equipment, working with an orthotist or a prosthetist in determining the most appropriate orthotic or prosthesis, arranging transportation, scheduling to avoid medical interventions in the intensive care unit, arranging with teachers about the best time and place to observe a child's classroom performance, and scheduling parent and teacher meetings.

Communication includes written and verbal correspondence to convey information to the child, family, and other approved parties. Therapists must make certain that private health information is released to only those authorized to receive that information as required under the federal Health Insurance Portability and Accountability Act of 1996 (HIPAA). This act limits the nonconsensual use and release of private health information, provides individuals access to their medical records, and restricts disclosure. In school settings, the Family Education Right to Privacy Act (FERPA) also applies. No matter what the setting, professionals must be very careful that information about a child is shared with only those individuals who have a documented need for that information.

Documentation is written information that may include the evaluation report, plan of care, request for approval for services, summary letters to physicians and other service providers, referrals, home and school programs, discharge planning, and information provided to those who pay for the services. Comprehensive documentation is mandatory for reimbursement for services and to meet state practice act standards. HIPAA regulations must be complied with regarding the distribution of these records.

Child- and Family-Related Instruction Along with instruction to other team members, **child- and family-related instruction,** is a critical area of pediatric practice. The family, other professionals, and paraprofessionals are frequently largely responsible for assisting the child in carrying out or practicing many intervention activities. This instruction is to promote and maximize the physical therapy services and expedite achievement of the goals. Physical therapy intervention done once a week (for, perhaps, gait training) will be of little benefit if the family and others are not able to assist the child in practicing this activity daily throughout the week. Positioning devices are of little value if the child is improperly positioned in the device in the classroom or intensive care unit. Instruction given to physical therapist assistants, teachers, aides, and day-care workers is vital if the child is to function on a daily basis by relying on the assistance of others.

Procedural Interventions **Procedural interventions** occur when the physical therapist "selects, applies, or modifies . . . interventions . . . based on examination data, the evaluation, the diagnosis and the prognosis, and the anticipated goals and expected outcomes" (APTA, 2001, p. 47). The type, frequency, and duration of the interventions are based on many factors, including the following:

- Child's age
- Anatomical and physiological changes related to growth and development
- Chronicity or severity of the condition
- Comorbidities
- Degree of limitations and restrictions
- Accessibility and availability of resources
- Concurrent services
- Family desires and degree of participation
- Caregiver ability and expertise
- Community support
- Psychosocial and socioeconomic factors
- Child's level of cognitive ability and cooperation

There are different models and rationales for providing physical therapy procedural interventions. Interventions are determined based not only on the needs of the child but also on the requirements of the settings. For example, physical therapy in an educational environment for school-aged children must be "educationally relevant." If a needed intervention does not relate to an educationally relevant goal, then that intervention, which is needed by the child, should be provided in a different setting such as an outpatient clinic. Some settings will serve a child only with a specific diagnosis, and if the child has an additional diagnosis, services for that secondary diagnosis must be received elsewhere. Some insurance companies limit the number of treatment visits they will pay for, which influences the plan of care.

There has been an increasing trend in health care to use algorithms, clinical practice guidelines, clinical pathways, and clinical prediction rules to increase efficiency and improve quality of care. **Algorithms** are "written guidelines to stepwise evaluation and management strategies that require observations to be made, decisions to be considered, and actions to be taken" (Nicholson, 2002, p. 214). They assist in decision making and make it easier to list essential clinical steps that might later be used to develop clinical practice guidelines. **Clinical practice guidelines** are systematically developed plans to assist in health-care decision making for specific clinical circumstances (Nicholson, 2002). They may be based on focus groups, expert opinion, consensus, or evidence-based practice. They help the service provider determine the most effective and appropriate interventions. The *Guide* (APTA, 2001) is a global clinical practice guideline. More explicit than an algorithm or a clinical practice guideline is the

critical or clinical pathway. **Clinical, critical,** or **care pathways,** as they are frequently named, are predetermined protocols that define the critical steps in examining, evaluating, and providing intervention for a clinical problem to improve quality of care, reduce variability of care, and enhance efficiency (Fleischman et al., 2002). These pathways were initially developed for nurses and physicians; however, there is a trend toward multidisciplinary pathways that will facilitate achievement of expected outcomes in a defined length of time for individuals who require a team approach to intervention.

Clinical practice guidelines have been developed in pediatric physical therapy for congenital muscular torticollis (Burch et al., 2009), spastic diplegia (Chiarello et al., 2005; O'Neil et al., 2006), and osteochondritis dissecans of the knee (Schmitt et al., 2009). Clinical practice guidelines typically provide condition-specific recommendations for examination and evaluation, intervention, goals and outcomes, and frequency and duration as well as discussion of special considerations. These guidelines are not intended to be uniform protocols in which every child is treated exactly the same; rather they provide evidence-based recommendations for managing care. Intervention should still be driven by individualized care plans tailored to meet the needs of each child's impairments, activity limitations, and participation restrictions within the context of his or her unique environmental and personal factors.

Recently **clinical prediction rules (CPR)** have been developed for use in physical therapy, primarily in the musculoskeletal practice patterns. CPRs group clinical findings in a meaningful way to assist the therapist with screening, diagnosing, or prognosticating. These patterns are intended to narrow nonspecific heterogeneous diagnostic groups into smaller, more homogeneous categories that are more likely to respond to a specific intervention approach. With CPRs, the previously described implicit pattern recognition of the experienced clinician becomes "more evidence based and less reliant on unfounded theories and tradition" (Fritz, 2009, p. 159). Development of CPRs entails derivation of the rule through literature review, expert opinion, and/or focus groups and validation through sound statistical study of the relationship between clinical findings (predictor variables) and the likelihood of accurately screening for, diagnosing, or predicting outcomes (Beattie & Nelson, 2006; Stanton, Hancock, Maher, & Koes, 2010). While no formal CPRs have been validated in the area of pediatrics, preliminary work has begun. Research has been conducted to investigate factors that predict ambulation in children with CP (Bartlett & Palisano, 2000; Beckung, Hagberg, Uldall, & Cans, 2008; Montgomery, 1998; Wu, Day, Strauss, & Shavelle, 2004), myelomeningocele (Bartonek & Saraste, 2001), and traumatic brain injury (Dumas, Haley, Ludlow, & Carey, 2004). This evidence can assist therapists in prognosis, establishing realistic goals, and providing guidance for educating families about the potential for achieving important milestones.

Algorithms, CPRs, and clinical practice guidelines/pathways cannot replace sound clinical decision making or professional judgment, but they are useful resources for clinicians. It must also be recognized that development of these tools is still in its infancy, and much more research and development are needed.

The plans of care for children with certain diagnoses might be very similar based on a clinical practice guideline or CPR. However, based on individual variations and circumstances, intervention plans might be very different for children with the same diagnosis. Common impairments in body structure and function are more likely to require similar interventions than a broad diagnostic label. For that reason, this text is organized around the functioning of body systems and not diagnoses, following the IFC model. Children with disabilities frequently present with complex problems involving many systems, all of which must be considered for intervention. A prime example is CP, where the musculoskeletal, neuromuscular, and cardiovascular/pulmonary systems are usually affected, and occasionally the integumentary system as well. Once the impairments in body structures and function in each of the systems are identified, along with restrictions in activities and participation, then an appropriate plan of care for intervention can be determined for an individual child.

Infants and toddlers who present with delay in development and no specific impairment in body structures and functions might have the most straightforward plan of care. They might need to learn the next level of skill or how to move and explore their environment. The therapist and parents would work on encouraging task performance and providing the opportunities to practice the task. Strict adherence to a developmental sequence is not appropriate, but it can be a useful frame of reference with face validity, especially for young children. For older children who have had the time and opportunity to achieve developmental milestones and have not done so, achievement of functional skills in the natural environment is far more important than achieving developmental milestones. Intervention for these older children should focus on achieving specific motor skills and activities that are essential for functioning in the home, school, and community.

Frequency, Intensity, and Duration of Intervention

Determining the appropriate frequency, intensity, and duration of intervention is integral to developing an effective plan of care; however, there is little research evidence to assist in determining what is most appropriate (Palisano & Murr, 2009). The therapist must consider the child's potential to participate and benefit from therapy, the stage of development (i.e., Is the child in a period of potential skill acquisition or regression?), the amount of skill and expertise needed to carry out the plan of care, the environmental opportunities to practice the desired skill/task, and the level of support the child has for achieving the goals.

General guidelines have been developed to assist in determining intervention frequency and intensity for school-based practice by the state education departments in Iowa (2001) and Florida (2010). More recently, the work in schools has been applied to pediatric hospital settings (Bailes, Reder, & Burch, 2008). In hospital settings frequency categories ranged from intensive (3–11 times per week) to periodic or episodic (monthly or less) (outlined in Table 14.1), demonstrating the wide variation in service delivery. Even though research evidence is not available, these guidelines have helped therapists become more aware of the range of service delivery options. A growing trend in service provision is for children to move between different intensity levels as their care transitions across the continuum of care, as they grow and develop, or when they experience plateaus, regressions, illness, exacerbations, or surgeries (Bailes et al., 2008). As children transition from more frequent to perhaps more intermittent service delivery across the life span, it is important to educate families on different service delivery options and our decision-making rationale when initially establishing the child's plan of care. This education enables families to anticipate and understand the rationale for different frequencies of therapy at different times during the course of care and over the child's life time (Bailes et al., 2008). Being deliberate in selecting intervention intensity and continually reassessing the child's progress and current status will assist the therapist in objectively determining the appropriate time to increase or decrease frequency, discontinue, or interrupt therapy services. Practicing clinicians have reported difficulty with reducing intensity or discharging children because of disagreement among team members, fear of complaints from physicians or families (Bailes et al., 2008), and concern about being able to re-enter a child into therapy services (Chiarello et al., 2005). However, experienced, school-based physical therapists report that if the child has met the identified functional goals, then discharging a child from school-based therapy is not difficult (Effgen, 2000). Reassessing progress related to goal attainment and conscientiously educating families will help both therapists and families view decreasing frequencies, discontinuation, or interruption of services as a positive opportunity in which the child can use his or her current functional abilities to participate in life events without the intrusion of ongoing therapy sessions.

Reexamination

The process of reexamination and reevaluation or reappraisal of a child is an ongoing, continual process. Throughout the intervention process, the therapist should constantly be reexamining and reevaluating the child's impairments in body structures and functions, limitations in activities, and restrictions in participation. The child's progress toward achieving the agreed-on goals/outcomes/objectives should be discussed with the parents and other team members. There may also be a need for formal periodic reexaminations. The frequency of reexamination depends on whether the child has an acute or a chronic disability, the requirements of the setting and payor, and the rate of progress. In an acute-care hospital, reexamination might be daily, and in a rehabilitation setting, weekly; in early intervention programs, reexamination occurs at least every 6 months; and in school settings annually for determination of IEP goals. State physical therapy practice acts might also indicate reexamination frequencies.

Outcomes

The final element of the *Guide* (APTA, 2001) is outcomes. Outcomes are the result of the intervention process. Outcomes are usually measured in terms of achievement of the goals and objectives, resulting in reduced limitations in body structures or functions; improved performance in activities and participation; child and family satisfaction; and prevention of secondary problems. Outcomes are measured near the end of the episode of care or during care through reexamination.

According to Guralnick (1997), a leader in early intervention research, outcomes should be measured along three dimensions: child and family characteristics, program/intervention features, and goals and objectives. The interventions done by physical therapists may be successful in terms of achieving the goals and

objectives; however, if the goals and objectives are not meaningful to the child and family, it is unlikely that the child's quality of life will improve, or that the child and family will experience satisfaction. Outcome measures in pediatrics need to expand beyond domains of development and must consider quality of life issues (McLaughlin & Bjornson, 1998). Measurement of quality of life issues is becoming a standard part of practice in many settings. Program evaluation, while important, has not been adequately addressed in the pediatric physical therapy literature.

Criteria for Termination of Physical Therapy

The plan of care must also include plans for discharge or "graduation" from services. The primary criterion for discharge should be achievement of the objectives, not an arbitrary criterion based on number of intervention sessions determined by an insurance company or school administrator. However, physical therapy must not be an ongoing, continuous activity with no discharge plan. Although discharging children from physical therapy services can be difficult, therapists who discuss discharge planning when initiating intervention in school settings do not report problems in "graduating" children from therapy (Effgen, 2000).

Discontinuation of physical therapy occurs when (1) the child or family declines to continue intervention; (2) the child is unable to progress toward the anticipated goals, objectives, and expected outcomes; or (3) the therapist determines that the child and family will no longer benefit from physical therapy (*Guide*, APTA, 2001, p. 49). When termination of services occurs before achievement of the goals, objectives, or outcomes, the rationale for discontinuation must be documented.

Models of Team Interaction

Understanding models of team interaction and the role of the therapist in each model is important for effective and efficient team functioning in health-care and educational settings. The complex needs of the children that therapists serve require the expertise of many disciplines. The terms disciplinary or interprofessional teams suggest that only professionals are involved on the team where in many settings, especially early intervention and schools, the child and the child's family are integral team members. There are different options regarding the best ways for teams to function together. The preferred model of team interaction varies somewhat based on the setting.

The landmark work of Deming (2000) in the manufacturing sector has slowly brought changes in all service delivery, including health-care delivery, over the past several decades. The autocratic, hierarchical model of the "captain of the ship" and the isolated uniprofessional models have evolved into more democratic models. Models of team interaction are presented in Table 1.5. The **unidisciplinary model** is not really a "team" model because it generally involves an individual discipline providing services in isolation from all other disciplines. This is the approach described in the APTA *Guide* (2001) (McEwen, 2000, p. 89). In pediatrics, this might be the only model possible in rural areas where there are no other team members; however, by using current technology, increased team interaction is now possible in most all settings (Wiecha & Pollard, 2004).

The **multidisciplinary model** is the oldest form of teaming and involves the least active interaction among team members. With this model, several professions perform independent evaluations and then meet to discuss their examination and evaluation findings and determine goals, outcomes, and a plan of care. Usually, the interventions are provided individually by each discipline, although communication among providers is maintained. Participants have separate but interrelated roles while they maintain their disciplinary roles (Choi & Pak, 2006).

In the **interdisciplinary model**, the team works together and there is extensive interaction among the team members from the initial examination through the intervention phase. Formal channels of communication are established and all information is shared. There are shared goals and a blurring of disciplinary boundaries (Choi & Pak, 2006). Confusion in terminology occurred when the meaning of multidisciplinary changed because of its use in Public Law (PL) 99-457, Education of the Handicapped Act Amendments of 1986. According to that law, "Multidisciplinary means the involvement of two or more disciplines or professions in the provision of integrated and coordinated services, including evaluation and assessment activities" (Federal Register, June 22, 1989, 303.17, pp. 26, 313). This is consistent with the definition of an interdisciplinary model presented here; therefore, there is sometimes confusion when using these terms. The reauthorization of IDEA PL 108-446 does not provide a definition of multidisciplinary.

Another model of team interaction is the **transdisciplinary model**. In a transdisciplinary model there is work across and beyond several disciplines with permeability of professional boundaries so that communication, interaction, and cooperation are maximized (King et al., 2009). There should be continuous, collaborative sharing of information, terminology, skills, and programming (Zaretsky, 2007). There is usually

Table 1.5 Models of Team Interaction

Unidisciplinary	Professional works independently of others.
Intradisciplinary	Members of the same profession work together without significant communication with members of other professions.
Multidisciplinary	Professionals work independently but recognize and value the contributions of other team members. Draws on knowledge from different disciplines, but there may be little interaction or ongoing communication among professionals.
Interdisciplinary	Individuals from different disciplines work together cooperatively to evaluate and develop programs. Emphasis is on teamwork, and role definitions are relaxed. There is analysis, synthesis, and harmony between disciplines, creating a coordinated and coherent whole (Choi & Pak, 2006).
Transdisciplinary	There is teaching and ongoing work among team members that transcend traditional disciplinary boundaries. Team members work together to develop and carry out interventions. Role release occurs when a team member assumes the responsibilities of other disciplines for service delivery.
Collaborative	All team members work together in equal participation and consensus decision making. The team interaction of the transdisciplinary model is combined with the integrated service delivery model.

joint examination, evaluation, and intervention, coupled with professional role release. Role release involves not merely the sharing of information but also sharing performance competencies and cross-training. Team members teach each other specific interventions to meet the child's needs. This model developed out of the need for consistent services for children with severe disabilities and for infants who would not tolerate being handled by multiple individuals. This is the model most commonly used in early intervention programs. The transdisciplinary model should lead to more effective interventions because the interventions are provided at increased frequencies throughout the day during functional activities. Some professionals are concerned about the liability involved in teaching others to provide interventions, the legal restrictions, the inability of some to properly carry out the interventions, and the watering down of professional involvement in service delivery. However, in 1997, Rainforth examined role release in relation to the legally defined scope of physical therapy practice and found that the roles of evaluation, planning, and supervision may not be delegated, but intervention could be done by others who are trained and supervised by a physical therapist.

As transdisciplinary models of service delivery have evolved and become standard practice, transdisciplinary and translational models of research have become the preferred matrix (Sussman, 2006). Much of the discussion of models of team interaction are now coming out of the research literature (Austin, Park, & Goble, 2008; Choi & Pak, 2006).

As the team process has developed, the use of the terms **collaboration** and **collaborative teamwork** has evolved. A summary of the defining characteristics of collaborative teamwork, first conceptualized by Rainforth and York-Barr (1997), is presented in Table 1.6. Collaborative teamwork involves equal participation in the process by the family and service providers, consensus decision making regarding goals and interventions, skills that are embedded in the intervention program, infusion of knowledge across disciplines, and role release.

Older hierarchical medical or educational models of team interaction dictated the team leaders, but in newer models, the needs of the child determine who is the team leader, if indeed there is a team leader. Dormans and Pellegrino (1998), two leading pediatric orthopedic surgeons, note in *Caring for Children With Cerebral Palsy: A Team Approach* that an effective team requires effective leadership, but that the "specific person and

Table 1.6 Collaborative Teamwork

Collaborative team includes:

- Equal participation on the team by family members and service providers
- Consensus decision making in determining priorities for goals and objectives
- Consensus decision making about the type and amount of intervention
- Motor and communication skills embedded throughout the intervention program
- Design and implementation of the intervention that include infusion of knowledge and skills from different disciplines
- Role release, so team members develop confidence and competence necessary to encourage the child's learning
- A shared framework of trust
- Respectful and empathetic open communication
- Appreciation of diversity
- Solution-focused problem solving

Source: Adapted from Early Intervention Special-Interest Group. (2010). *Team-based service delivery approaches in pediatric practice*. Alexandria, VA: American Physical Therapy Association, Section on Pediatrics. Rainforth, B., & York-Barr, J. (1997). *Collaborative teams for students with severe disabilities* (2nd ed.). Baltimore, MD: Paul H. Brookes.

discipline that provide that leadership are usually determined by the primary mission of the team and by the setting" (p. 59).

Children with severe disabilities (Hunt, Soto, Maier, & Doering, 2003) or complex medical problems generally require the services of an extensive team of professionals. Team members must collaborate to prevent duplication of services and conflicting services and to maximize resources to provide efficient and effective intervention. The different discipline members on teams provide support for each other and enhance each other's problem-solving capabilities. The hopes are that each member of the team will be equally valued and that no member of the team will have inappropriate authority based on personality or self-perceived importance. Unfortunately, Hinojosa and colleagues (2001) in an early intervention study found that team members may not be considered equal and that they did not follow a collaborative process, but the team they studied was nonetheless effective. King and colleagues (2009) note that managerial and team resources are high for a transdisciplinary model; however, the potential benefits for the children, families, and therapists were substantial. They also note that while experienced practitioners might be comfortable with a transdisciplinary approach, novice practitioners may be overwhelmed.

When working in a new setting or joining a new team, you should ask for a clarification and definition of terms regarding models or expectations of team interaction. All individuals involved should have the same understanding to avoid miscommunication and conflict. For example, our colleagues in occupational therapy prefer not to use the term disciplinary and favor interprofessional and transprofessional (Mu & Royeen, 2004).

Models of Service Delivery

The models of physical therapy service delivery are often closely connected with models of team interaction. There is also an array of confusing and conflicting terms used to describe the various models. The framework for these models of service delivery is outlined in Table 1.7 and presented here.

Direct Model

In the **direct model,** the therapist is usually the primary service provider to the child. This is the traditional model used to provide physical therapy. *Direct intervention may be given when specific therapeutic techniques cannot be safely delegated and when there is emphasis on acquisition of new motor skills.* Direct therapy should, when possible, be done in the natural environment. Only when it is in the best interests of the child should the therapy session be in a restrictive environment, such as a treatment room or clinic setting. A restrictive treatment environment might be necessary if specialized equipment is required, if the child is highly distractible, if privacy is needed, or when it is the safest environment for either the therapist or child. Rarely, if ever, should direct intervention be given without instructing and working with the child's parents and other service providers. It is not unusual for a child to receive direct intervention for a specific objective and receive other models of service delivery to achieve other goals. Direct intervention is common in acute-care hospital settings because of the seriousness and complexity of the problems and the usually very short length of stay.

Integrated Model

A number of different definitions of the **integrated model** have been described. These definitions vary by the setting in which they are implemented. The integrated model in educational settings is one in which the therapist's contact is not only with the child but also with the teacher, aide/paraprofessional, and family. The service is generally delivered in the learning environment and the method of intervention is educationally related—activities with an emphasis on practice of newly acquired motor skills during the child's daily routine. *The implementer of the activities may be the teacher, aide/paraprofessional, other professionals, parent, and/or physical therapist or physical therapist assistant* (Iowa Department of Education, 2001).

The integrated model of service delivery can, and frequently does, include direct physical therapy intervention and consultative services. The physical therapist collaborates with all other key individuals serving the child such as the occupational therapist, speech-language pathologist, and teachers. Goals and objectives are jointly developed, and all individuals serving the child are instructed in how to achieve these objectives within their capability. Direct services, when necessary, are provided in the most natural environment; natural environments include the child's home, preschool classroom, regular classroom, and community at large.

Dunn (1991) states that the integrated model also consists of peer integration, functional integration, practice integration, and comprehensive integration. Peer integration occurs when a child with a disability functions in a classroom or at a social event with children without disabilities. The child functions in multiple settings with other peers. Functional integration involves the child's use of a therapeutic strategy or newly acquired skill in the natural environment. Functional integration is one rationale behind providing therapy in natural environments, especially when the objectives involve fluency (refinement of skills) and generalization of skills (ability to perform skills in multiple environments with different individuals and equipment). Practice integration involves the collaboration of professionals to meet a child's individual needs. Comprehensive integration combines all of the areas of integration and is the level to which we must strive.

Consultative Model

In the **consultative model,** the therapist's contact is other health professionals and the teacher, aide/paraprofessional, parent, and child. All personnel, *except the therapist,* implement the activities and interventions. The therapist meets with and demonstrates activities to all appropriate staff so that they can carry out the interventions to help the child achieve the determined goals and objectives. *The responsibility for the outcome lies with the consultee,* the individual receiving the consultation (Dunn, 1991; Iowa Department of Education, 2001). The service is generally provided in the natural environment.

Consultation is usually thought of in terms of a specific child, as outlined in Table 1.7. However, there is also a need for more global, programmatic consultation. Programmatic consultation includes issues related to safety, transportation, architectural barriers, equipment, documentation, continuing education,

and quality improvement (Lindsey, O'Neal, Haas, & Tewey, 1980). These are all very important issues that ultimately relate to successful service provision. In many settings, but especially a school setting, the therapist must consult with the administration regarding overall safety issues, proper positioning during transportation, and the removal of architectural barriers. In programmatic consultation, the therapist makes recommendations but does not necessarily perform the activity, such as removing architectural barriers.

Table 1.7 Physical Therapy Service Delivery Models

	Direct	Integrated	Consultative	Monitoring	Collaborative
Therapist's Primary Contact	Child	Child, team, and family	Family and team	Child	Child, team, and family
Environment for Service Delivery	Hospital, outpatient setting, or home Distraction-free environment Specialized equipment might be needed	Usually early intervention or school-based setting Natural environment Therapy area if necessary for a specific child	Can occur in all intervention settings Natural environment	School-based, early intervention, or outpatient setting Natural environment Therapy area if necessary for a specific child	Can occur in all intervention settings Natural environment
Methods of Intervention	Functional activities and intervention for impairments limiting function Specific therapeutic techniques that cannot safely be delegated Emphasis on acquisition of new motor skills	Functional activities Positioning Emphasis on practice of newly acquired motor skills in the daily routine, activities and participation	Functional activities Positioning Adaptive materials Emphasis on adapting to natural environment and generalization of acquired skills for activities and participation	Emphasis on making certain child maintains functional status for activities and participation	Functional activities Positioning Adaptive materials Emphasis on adapting to natural environment and generalization of acquired skills for activities and participation
Amount of Service Time	Regularly scheduled sessions	Routinely scheduled Flexible amount of time depending on needs of staff or child	Intermittent, depending on needs of staff or child	Intermittent, depending on needs of child, may be as infrequent as once in 6 months	Ongoing intervention Discipline-referenced knowledge shared among team members so relevant activities occur throughout day

Source: Adapted from Effgen, S. K., & Kaminker, M.K. (2012). The educational environment. In S.K. Campbell, R.J. Palisano, & M. Orlin (Eds.), *Physical therapy for children* (4th ed., p. 978). St. Louis: Elsevier Saunders; and Iowa Department of Education (2001). *Iowa guidelines for educationally related physical therapy services.* Des Moines: Author.

Monitoring Model

Another model of indirect service delivery is **monitoring.** Monitoring is an important element of transition from direct or integrated services to no services. In the **monitoring model** the *therapist remains responsible* for the outcome of the intervention. The therapist, although not providing direct intervention, maintains regular contact with the child to check on the child's status and to instruct others. Monitoring is important for the follow-up of children who have impairments that might deteriorate over time or limitations that might require direct, integrated, or consultative intervention at a later date. Monitoring allows the therapist to check on the need for modifications in equipment and to make recommendations quickly. Monitoring provides the family, child, and therapist with a sense that the child is being watched. If the child should then require a change in the model of physical therapy intervention, monitoring generally allows a more rapid transition of services because the child is known to the physical therapist, and justification for services can be expedited to meet the child's immediate needs.

Collaborative Model

The **collaborative model** of service delivery is defined as a combination of transdisciplinary team interaction and an integrated service delivery model. Some would say that it is not a model of service delivery at all and is just the preferred model of professional and family interaction. As noted in Tables 1.6 and 1.7, many team members, as in an integrated model, provide services in a collaborative model but with a greater degree of role release and crossing of disciplinary boundaries than in the integrated model. A key element of this model is that there is collaboration among therapists and others right from the beginning, helping to produce a single integrated plan of care, with individual disciplines contributing based on the needs of the child (Bell, Corfield, Davies, & Richardson, 2009). The team assumes responsibility for consensus decision making on the goals and objectives, and on implementation of the program activities. Any member of the team, including the family, implements the activities in the natural routine of the home, school, and community. The amount of service delivery or therapeutic practice of an activity should be greater than in other models because the entire team is carrying out the activities. In practice, this might not be the case because of the varied levels of skill of the implementers, insufficient "natural" opportunities to practice an activity, competing activities, and the difficulty of some activities (Effgen & Chan,

2009; Ott & Effgen, 2000). Collaborative models in early intervention have led to reductions in waiting times, improved attendance at therapy sessions, and an increased therapist case load (Bell et al., 2009). Teams must strive for collaboration and consensus, even if in some situations there is little actual crossing of discipline boundaries and not all team members are considered equal (Hinojosa et al, 2001).

A variation of the collaborative model of service delivery and transdisciplinary team interaction is **coaching**, practiced in some early childhood programs. A coach guides others to develop competence and should be voluntary, nonjudgmental, and a collaborative partnership between the practitioners and significant others in the young child's life (Hanft, Rush, & Sheldon, 2004, p. 1). By coaching family members and others in how to provide the child with learning and practice opportunities, the child's participation in real-life situations should increase (Hanft et al., 2004, p. 3). This approach seeks to enhance the family's competence in service provision and moves away from hands-on professional intervention (p. 105). While enhancing the family's competence in caring for their child is critical, it should also be noted that new evidenced-based interventions discussed throughout this text require professional involvement and frequently very intensive levels of intervention.

Issues Influencing Practice

Advocacy and Public Policy

In 1961, President John F. Kennedy established a President's Panel on Mental Retardation. On this panel were major proponents for normalization and deinstitutionalization of persons with disabilities. The excellent work of this panel, along with later television documentaries such as the one done on the Willowbrook State Institution by Geraldo Rivera, and Blatt and Kaplan's book, *Christmas in Purgatory: A Photographic Essay on Mental Retardation* (1966), raised national concern for the care and treatment of all people with disabilities, especially those in institutions. This public awareness and concern led to federal legislation that would significantly positively impact those with disabilities (Appendix 1.A). The Developmental Disabilities Act of 1975 (PL 94-103) focused on the need for integration and inclusion of those with developmental disabilities in the community and included a provision that required states to develop and incorporate a "deinstitutionalization and institutional reform" plan. The Rehabilitation Act of 1973 (93-112) guaranteed rights to individuals with disabilities. Included in the Act is

Section 504, which is viewed as the first civil-rights statute for persons with disabilities; this preceded the 1990 American with Disabilities Act (ADA) (PL 101-336). During the 1970s advocacy groups for those with disabilities had gained power, and the location, extent, and type of rehabilitation and educational service delivery, including physical therapy, would see major changes.

As noted, the last quarter of the 20th century has included important federal legislation that has provided rights and services to individuals with disabilities. This legislation includes provisions for early intervention services for infants and toddlers, the right to a free and appropriate public education for all children 3 to 21 years of age, the right to health care for those with disabilities, reduction in discrimination, and access to society. These federal laws are summarized in Appendix 1.A. A review of each of these important pieces of legislation is beyond the scope of this text; however, the listing does serve as a starting point for further study and provides information on the history and sequence of federal legislation. Legislation specific to early intervention and the education of children with disabilities has had a major impact on the provision of physical therapy services and is discussed in Chapters 11 and 12.

Changing Health-Care Delivery System

During the mid-20th century, many Americans had health insurance to cover hospital care and, later, coverage for physicians and other out-of-hospital services. Outpatient physical therapy was one of the benefits of this expanded medical coverage. Before major medical coverage was available, outpatient therapy for children was paid for by the family, provided by charitable organizations, or provided under the federally supported Crippled Children's Services. Under the insurance fee-for-service system, the child's family selected their physicians and therapists and services were paid for in part (usually 80%) or totally by the insurance company. Aside from a large lifetime cap, there was usually no limit on these services, and children with disabilities could receive comprehensive, long-term care. The family could select the physicians and physical therapists of their choice and go to specialists as necessary. Some insurance plans also included durable medical equipment such as wheelchairs.

In the 1950s, a number of small insurance companies began experimenting with what were called health maintenance organizations (HMOs). Groups of physicians and other health professionals provided comprehensive care that included the preventive care not covered under fee-for-service plans. The first such organizations were in Minnesota and California and were nonprofit. They remained relatively small until the 1980s, when there was a vast, nationwide expansion of what are now called managed-care organizations. These organizations are now commonly for profit. Children with disabilities are included; however, the majority of families with children with special needs choose, when possible, to remain in the more costly fee-for-service plans that allow access to medical providers experienced in serving children with disabilities. In managed-care systems, approval to go to a specialist must first be obtained from the primary care provider, usually the pediatrician; then the child goes to a specialist who is part of the plan and who may or may not have experience in the care of children with disabilities.

Although the United States has one of the finest health-care systems in the world, it's also the most expensive. The 1990s saw a dramatic, radical change in the health-care delivery system in the United States. More and more employers found it cost effective to offer their employees only managed-care or other restrictive options, and many states have converted to the less costly care systems for their citizens receiving Medicaid. Congress in 1997 authorized and in 2009 reauthorized the State Children's Health Insurance Plan (SCHIP) to expand and initiate state health insurance coverage for uninsured, low-income children. Children whose parents earned too much to qualify for Medicaid but could not afford private health insurance became eligible for state-run insurance programs. With 11.2% of all American children uninsured and 28.2% of children covered by Medicaid or SCHIP (American Academy of Pediatrics, 2008), therapists must understand that their services are costly, not always supported by outcome studies, and generally not critical to sustaining the life of the child, so reimbursement for services is not guaranteed. Therapists must continue to seek evidence to support their interventions and advocate for the children and families they serve.

Family-Centered Care

One of the major changes in the delivery of physical therapy over the past few decades has been the shift in focus from a child-centered to a family-centered approach. This shift reflects not only changes in health-care service delivery but also an understanding of the importance of the entire family in the habilitative and rehabilitative processes. The input of families was always valued, but now families are considered partners in the habilitation and rehabilitation processes of their child. Therapists need to understand family systems and be sensitive to the unique characteristics and needs of the culturally diverse populations they serve. Issues related to family-centered care and understanding cultural diversity are incorporated throughout this text. All of Chapter 4 is devoted to these topics because of their importance in practice today.

Child Abuse and Neglect

Unfortunately, this text would be remiss if it did not include discussion of the tragic issues of child abuse and neglect. The U.S. Department of Health and Human Services (2010) reported that an estimated 758,289 children were victims of abuse or neglect in 2008. The rate of victimization ranged from 1.5 to 29.1 per 1,000 children. The youngest children had the highest rate of victimization, with 32.6% of all victims younger than 4 years of age. In 2008, 1,740 children died of child abuse in the United States.

Nearly 15% of abused and neglected children have a disability (U.S. Department of Health and Human Services, 2010). Children who have a disability have an increased likelihood of being abused or neglected. They may have difficulty communicating the abuse or neglect to others and may not be able to run away from an abuser. They may also have age-inappropriate dependency, be isolated, need affection and friendship, have a low self-image, and exhibit distressed behavior that could be attributed to their disorder and not to abuse or neglect (Hobbs, Hanks, & Wynn, 1999).

Physical therapists are in a unique position to observe child abuse or neglect first hand (Table 1.8). Therapists typically remove some of a child's clothing to observe muscle activity and movement, and this provides an opportunity to see the results of abuse such as scars and bruises (Gocha, Murphy, Dolakia, Hess, & Effgen, 1999). When handling a child, therapists may also note sensitive areas that have been traumatized. If unexplained bruises, burns, scars, or other signs of trauma are observed, therapists have an obligation to report suspected signs of child abuse to the authorities. The Federal Child Abuse and Prevention and Treatment

---

Table 1.8 Recognizing Child Abuse and Neglect: Signs and Symptoms

The following signs may signal the presence of child abuse or neglect.

The Child:

Shows sudden changes in behavior or school performance

Has not received help for physical or medical problems brought to the parents' attention

Has learning problems (or difficulty concentrating) that cannot be attributed to specific physical or psychological causes

Is always watchful, as though preparing for something bad to happen

Lacks adult supervision

Is overly compliant, passive, or withdrawn

Comes to school or other activities early, stays late, and does not want to go home

The Parent:

Shows little concern for the child

Denies the existence of—or blames the child for—the child's problems in school or at home

Asks teachers or other caregivers to use harsh physical discipline if the child misbehaves

Sees the child as entirely bad, worthless, or burdensome

Demands a level of physical or academic performance the child cannot achieve

Looks primarily to the child for care, attention, and satisfaction of emotional needs

The Parent and Child:

Rarely touch or look at each other

Consider their relationship entirely negative

State that they do not like each other

Types of Abuse

The following are some signs often associated with particular types of child abuse and neglect: physical abuse, neglect, sexual abuse, and emotional abuse. It is important to note, however, that these types of abuse are more typically found in combination than alone.

Table 1.8 Recognizing Child Abuse and Neglect: Signs and Symptoms—cont'd

Signs of Physical Abuse
*Consider the possibility of physical abuse when the **child**:*

Has unexplained burns, bites, bruises, broken bones, or black eyes
Has fading bruises or other marks noticeable after an absence from school
Seems frightened of the parents and protests or cries when it is time to go home
Shrinks at the approach of adults
Reports injury by a parent or another adult caregiver

*Consider the possibility of physical abuse when the **parent or other adult caregiver**:*
Offers conflicting, unconvincing, or no explanation for the child's injury
Describes the child as "evil" or in some other very negative way
Uses harsh physical discipline with the child
Has a history of abuse as a child

Signs of Neglect
*Consider the possibility of neglect when the **child**:*

Is frequently absent from school
Begs or steals food or money
Lacks needed medical or dental care, immunizations, or glasses
Is consistently dirty and has severe body odor
Lacks sufficient clothing for the weather
Abuses alcohol or other drugs
States that there is no one at home to provide care

*Consider the possibility of neglect when the **parent or other adult caregiver**:*

Appears to be indifferent to the child
Seems apathetic or depressed
Behaves irrationally or in a bizarre manner
Is abusing alcohol or other drugs

Signs of Sexual Abuse
*Consider the possibility of sexual abuse when the **child**:*

Has difficulty walking or sitting
Suddenly refuses to change for gym or to participate in physical activities
Reports nightmares or bedwetting
Experiences a sudden change in appetite
Demonstrates bizarre, sophisticated, or unusual sexual knowledge or behavior
Becomes pregnant or contracts a venereal disease, particularly if under age 14
Runs away
Reports sexual abuse by a parent or another adult caregiver

*Consider the possibility of sexual abuse when the **parent or other adult caregiver**:*
Is unduly protective of the child or severely limits the child's contact with other children, especially of the opposite sex
Is secretive and isolated
Is jealous or controlling with family members

Source: Child Welfare Information Gateway. (2007). *Recognizing child abuse and neglect: Signs and symptoms*. Washington, DC: U.S. Department of Health and Human Services. Retrieved from http://www.childwelfare.gov/pubs/factsheets/signs.cfm

Act (PL 93-247), and its amendments, requires every state to have a system for reporting suspected child abuse and neglect. (Child Abuse Reporting telephone numbers are available at http://www.childwelfare.gov/pubs/reslist/rl_dsp.cfm?rs_id=5&rate_chno=11-11172 [last visited Jan. 19, 2012]). The procedures vary from state to state, and therapists should be familiar with the laws in their state. Some states have one central agency and telephone number to contact; other states have individuals report the suspected case to their superiors. Although the professional code of conduct says that the therapist/patient relationship is confidential and that information can be given only with written consent, child abuse mandates a breach of confidentiality that is supported by federal law.

Behavior Management

Somewhat unique to pediatric physical therapy is the need to engage and play with the child to gain participation in the desired therapeutic activities and interventions. Infants, young children, and those with severe cognitive limitations are often unable to follow verbal commands. They must be encouraged to perform activities using therapeutic play, interesting toys and activities, and significant creativity on the part of the therapist and parents. **Play** is the work of children, and it is the milieu in which intervention occurs for most children. Therapeutic play requires extraordinary work on the part of the therapist, and individuals who lack creativity and the ability to "play" will probably have a difficult time working with children.

Some children may choose not to participate in requested tasks, no matter how creative the therapist. These children might require a structured behavior management plan that not only assists with managing their behavior but also facilitates learning. Learning is believed to occur as a result of the consequences of behavior. **Behavioral programming** emphasizes manipulation of the environment through the use of positive reinforcement of desired behaviors and ignoring unwanted behaviors. **Positive reinforcement** might start as a primary reward such as food, then progress to secondary rewards such as toys, favorite activities, or tokens, and then, most important, progress to the nontangible natural rewards of social or natural reinforcers such as verbal praise or a smile. A hug from a parent after taking the first few independent steps encourages many more independent steps. Successfully accessing a computer is reinforcement enough to again perform the task.

Negative reinforcement, which is the removal of an aversive stimulus contingent on the performance of the desired behavior, is generally not an accepted technique in physical therapy. Unfortunately, negative reinforcement is occasionally used, such as when a child is allowed to end a therapy session if he or she performs a specific task. This is not the most appropriate way to reinforce behaviors. It would be far better to provide a positive reinforcement when the child performs a task than to tie performance with ending the session with the therapist.

The goal is to increase the probability that the child will perform the desired behavior. To do this, it may first be necessary to use very frequent primary rewards in what is termed a *continuous schedule of reinforcement.* However, as soon as possible, the frequency of rewards should be decreased or "thinned" to an intermittent schedule of reinforcement and secondary rewards should be used until the behavior is naturally occurring without obvious reinforcement. There is an extensive body of literature on behavioral techniques and reinforcement schedules with which therapists should be familiar if they are going to work with children who are not likely to comply with requests, have behavior disorders (summarized in Alberto & Troutman, 2006) or have autism (summarized in National Autism Center, 2009).

A behavior can be elicited and then improved and elaborated on by using **shaping** or **chaining techniques**. Shaping involves reinforcing behaviors that are increasingly closer to the desired behavior. Chaining links related behaviors to accomplish a more elaborate goal with sequenced elements. Chaining works best with discrete tasks that have a clear beginning and end, such as most activities of daily living, or selected serial tasks that are strung together, such as performing a sliding board transfer. Backward shaping involves teaching and reinforcing behaviors in a step-by-step progression in which the last step is learned first (e.g., performing the task of brushing teeth before learning to put the toothpaste on the brush).

Behavioral techniques should be considered in all areas of physical therapy intervention. Many of the children we serve require considerable time and effort to achieve even the smallest goal. They need to be encouraged and rewarded for their efforts, even if they do not achieve the desired goal. Positive reinforcement will encourage them to keep trying, just as an athlete values the encouragement received from a coach for a good play, even if the team loses the game.

Attaining and Maintaining Clinical Competence

A therapist must have numerous competencies to provide state-of-the-art physical therapy intervention to children. As the body of knowledge regarding the art and science of pediatric physical therapy expands, it becomes more difficult for the generalist clinician to keep up with all areas of practice. Pediatric physical therapy was one of the first areas of physical therapy practice to be recognized by the APTA as a clinical specialty. Pediatric physical therapy is the general area of physical therapy to children, and there is increasing specialization among pediatric physical therapists, for instance, neurological pediatric physical therapy and cardiopulmonary pediatric physical therapy. Some therapists also have special skills and knowledge required to work in specific settings such as the neonatal intensive care unit or sports programs.

To provide the most efficient and effective physical therapy to children, a therapist must work toward achieving clinical competence. Graduating from an entry-level physical therapy program does not fully prepare a therapist to provide quality care for most children. The recent graduate is prepared to serve some children independently and others under supervision; however, therapists should develop a plan to achieve the competence necessary for independent practice with children.

There are published competencies and guidelines for therapists to review in their effort to achieve or maintain clinical competence in various areas of pediatric practice, such as neonatal intensive care nursery (Sweeney et al., 2009), early intervention (Chiarello & Effgen, 2006), and school-based practice (Effgen, Chiarello, & Milbourne, 2007). Material from the American Board of Physical Therapy Specialties (ABPTS) for pediatric clinical specialization also provides an outline of important areas in which a pediatric therapist should achieve competence.

There are a number of ways to attain and maintain clinical competence. The most obvious is on-the-job training. Many clinical sites have excellent in-service training and mentoring programs for new staff. With more children with disabilities now appropriately served in community settings, therapists frequently find themselves working in total isolation or with a few professionals from other disciplines who are equally isolated. Therapists need to join or start journal clubs or special interest groups. Meeting and talking with colleagues is one way to gain and share information

and recognize one's own limitations. One of the problems with working in isolation is that one can acquire a false sense of confidence because there is no one with expertise available to question the therapist's competence.

Therapists should participate in educational programs such as continuing education courses and professional conferences. For more in-depth learning, therapists should consider postprofessional graduate education or residencies. Many universities are attempting to meet the needs of the working clinician by offering courses in the evening, on weekends, or through distance learning. Even with an entry-level doctoral degree, therapists still need to advance their professional competence in pediatrics. Employers have begun to recognize that generalist licensure may not be sufficient to ensure competence to serve children with disabilities. Postprofessional degrees in specialty areas, fellowships, and pediatric clinical certification are ways of documenting advanced clinical competence as a "qualified" physical therapist.

Summary

Pediatric physical therapy has a rich history since the beginnings of the profession. Pediatric physical therapy was one of the first areas of specialization recognized by APTA, and the APTA Section on Pediatrics now has more than 4,000 members. Serving children with disabilities and illnesses and their families is a challenging area of practice that requires diverse skills and knowledge as well as great flexibility and creativity. Therapists must not only be able to examine, evaluate, diagnose, make a prognosis, and provide complex intervention; they must also understand behavior management, developmental theory, family functioning, social trends, reimbursement issues, and the unique requirements of working in environments as diverse as a bone marrow transplant unit and the home of an impoverished inner-city infant born to drug-addicted parents.

Therapists must consider the whole child, the family, and the team of professionals when providing intervention. New developments in neuroscience, motor learning, and motor control are providing the scientific foundation for many of our new and old interventions. Although this text is divided on the basis of the major body systems, therapists must remember that rarely is only one system involved in children with disabilities. Therefore, a thorough understanding of all systems and their interactions is imperative.

DISCUSSION QUESTIONS

1. What are the four elements of good evidence-based practice?

2. Discuss the benefits of naturalistic observation.

3. Discuss the advantages of a transdisciplinary model in meeting the needs of a child with complex problems.

4. Why is collaboration so critical in meeting the needs of children?

5. How has legislation expanded the opportunities for children with disabilities?

6. What signs of child maltreatment should a physical therapist look for?

7. What is your plan for maintaining clinical competence in pediatrics even if it is not your primary area of practice?

References

Alberto, P.A., & Troutman, A.C. (2006). *Applied behavior analysis for teachers* (7th ed.). Upper Saddle River, NJ: Pearson.

American Academy for Cerebral Palsy and Developmental Medicine (1996). *The history of the American Academy for Cerebral Palsy and Developmental Medicine.* Rosemont, IL: Author.

American Academy of Pediatrics. (2008, September 25). *Fact sheet: Children's health insurance.* Retrieved from http://www.aap.org/research/factsheet.pdf

American Physical Therapy Association (APTA) (1991). Standards for tests and measurements in physical therapy practice. *Physical Therapy, 71,* 589–622.

American Physical Therapy Association (APTA) (1997). Guide to physical therapist practice. *Physical Therapy, 77,* 1163–1650.

American Physical Therapy Association (APTA) (2001). Guide to physical therapist practice (2nd ed.). *Physical Therapy, 81,* 6–746.

American Physical Therapy Association (APTA) (2008a). *APTA endorses World Health Organization ICF model.* Alexandria, VA: Author.

American Physical Therapy Association (APTA) (2008b). *APTA's defensible documentation for patient/client management, setting-specific considerations, E. Pediatric settings.* Alexandria, VA: Author.

American Physical Therapy Association (APTA), Section on Pediatrics (2003). *Using APTA's Guide to Physical Therapist Practice in pediatric settings.* Alexandria, VA: Author.

Austin, W., Park, C., & Goble, E. (2008). From interdisciplinary to transdisciplinary research: A case study. *Qualitative Health Research, 18,* 557-564.

Bailes, A.F., Reder, R., & Burch, C. (2008). Development of guidelines for determining frequency of therapy services in a pediatric medical setting. *Pediatric Physical Therapy, 20*(2), 194–198.

Bartlett, D.J., & Palisano, R.J. (2000). A multivariate model of determinants of motor change for children with cerebral palsy. *Physical Therapy, 80*(6), 598–614.

Bartonek, A., & Saraste, H. (2001). Factors influencing ambulation in myelomeningocele: A cross-sectional study. *Developmental Medicine and Child Neurology, 43*(4), 253–260.

Beattie, P., & Nelson, R. (2006). Clinical prediction rules: What are they and what do they tell us? *Australian Journal of Physiotherapy, 52*(3), 157–163.

Beckung, E., Hagberg, G., Uldall, P., & Cans, C. (2008). Probability of walking in children with cerebral palsy in Europe. *Pediatrics, 121*(1), 187–192.

Bell, A., Corfield, M., Davies, J., & Richardson, N. (2009). Collaborative transdisciplinary intervention in early years: Putting theory into practice. *Child: Care, Health & Development, 36*(1), 142–148.

Blatt, B., & Kaplan, F. (1966). *Christmas in purgatory: A photographic essay on mental retardation.* Boston: Allyn & Bacon.

Brown, D.A., Effgen, S., & Palisano, R. (1998). Performance following ability-focused physical therapy intervention in individuals with severely limited physical and cognitive abilities. *Physical Therapy, 78*(9), 934.

Burch, C., Hudson, P., Reder, R., Ritchey, M., Strenk, M., & Woosley, M. (2009). Cincinnati Children's Hospital Medical Center: *Evidence-based clinical care guideline for therapy management of congenital muscular torticollis.* Guideline 33, pages 1–13, Retrieved from http://www.cincinnatichildrens.org/svc/alpha/h/health-policy/ev-based/otpt.htm

Campbell, P.H. (1991). Evaluation and assessment in early intervention for infants and toddlers. *Journal of Early Intervention, 15,* 36–45.

Chiarello, L., & Effgen, S.K. (2006). Updated competencies for physical therapists working in early intervention. *Pediatric Physical Therapy, 18*(2), 148–158.

Chiarello, L.A., O'Neil, M., Dichter, C.G., Westcott, S.L., Orlin, M., Marchese, V.G., Tieman, B., & Rose, R.U. (2005). Exploring physical therapy clinical decision making for children with spastic diplegia: Survey of pediatric practice. *Pediatric Physical Therapy, 17*(1), 46–54.

Child Welfare Information Gateway. (2007). *Recognizing child abuse and neglect: Signs and symptoms.* Washington, DC: Retrieved from http://www.childwelfare.gov/pubs/factsheets/signs.cfm

Choi, B.C.K., & Pak, A.W.P. (2006). Multidisciplinarity, interdisciplinarity and transdisciplinarity in health research, services, education and policy: 1. Definitions, objectives, and evidence of effectiveness. *Clinical & Investigative Medicine, 29*(6), 351–364.

Darrah, J. (2008). Using the ICF as a framework for clinical decision making in pediatric physical therapy. *Advances in Physiotherapy, 10*(3), 146–151.

Deming, W.E. (2000). *The new economics: For industry, government, education* (2nd ed.). Cambridge, MA: MIT Press.

Dormans, J.P., & Pellegrino, L. (Eds.). (1998). *Caring for children with cerebral palsy: A team approach.* Baltimore: Paul H. Brookes.

Dumas, H.M., Haley, S.M., Ludlow, L.H., & Carey, T.M. (2004). Recovery of ambulation during inpatient rehabilitation: Physical therapist prognosis for children and adolescents with traumatic brain injury. *Physical Therapy, 84*(3), 232–242.

Dunn, W. (1991). Integrated related services. In L.H. Meyer, C.A. Peck, & L. Brown (Eds.), *Critical issues in the lives of persons with severe disabilities* (pp. 353–377). Baltimore: Paul H. Brookes.

Early Intervention Special-Interest Group. (2010). *Team-based service delivery approaches in pediatric practice.* Alexandria, VA: American Physical Therapy Association, Section on Pediatrics.

Effgen, S.K. (1991). Systematic delivery and recording of intervention assistance. *Pediatric Physical Therapy, 3,* 63–68.

Effgen, S.K. (2000). Factors affecting the termination of physical therapy services for children in school settings. *Pediatric Physical Therapy, 12,* 121–126.

Effgen, S.K., & Chan, L. (2010). Occurrence of gross motor behaviors and attainment of motor objectives in children with cerebral palsy participating in conductive education. *Physiotherapy Theory & Practice, 26*(1), 22–39.

Effgen, S.K., Chiarello, L., & Milbourne, S. (2007). Updated competencies for physical therapists working in schools. *Pediatric Physical Therapy, 9*(4), 266–274.

Effgen, S.K., & Kaminker, M.K. (2012). The educational environment. In S.K. Campbell, R.J. Palisano, & M. Orlin (Eds.), *Physical therapy for children* (4th ed., p. 978). St. Louis: Elsevier Saunders.

Escorpizo, R., Stucki, G., Cieza, A., Davis, K., Stumbo, T., & Riddle, D.L. (2010). Creating an interface between the international classification of functioning, disability and health and physical therapist practice. *Physical Therapy, 90*(7), 1053–1063.

Evidence-Based Medical Working Group (1992). Evidence-based medicine: A new approach to teaching the practice of medicine. *Journal of the American Medical Association, 268*(17), 2420–2425.

Federal Register, Part III, Department of Education, 32 CFR Part 303. *Early Intervention Program for Infants and Toddlers with Handicaps; Final Regulations,* June 22, 1989 (303.17, p. 26313).

Fleischman, K.E., Goldman, L., Johnson, P.A., Krasuski, R.A., Bohan, J.S., Hartley, L.H., & Lee, T. (2002). Critical pathways for patients with acute chest pain at low risk. *Journal of Thrombosis and Thrombolysis, 13*(2), 89–96.

Florida Department of Education, Exceptional Education & Student Services (2010). *Considerations for Educationally Relevant Therapy (CERT).* Retrieved from http://www.fldoe.org/ESE/cert.asp

Fowler, E.G., Kolobe, T.H., Damiano, D.L., Thorpe, D.E., Morgan, D.W., Brunstrom, J.E., & Section on Pediatrics Research Committee Task Force. (2007). Promotion of physical fitness and prevention of secondary conditions for children with cerebral palsy: Section on Pediatrics research summit proceedings. *Physical Therapy, 87*(11), 1495–1510.

Fragala-Pinkham, M.A., Haley, S.M., & Goodgold, S. (2006). Evaluation of a community-based group fitness program for children with disabilities. *Pediatric Physical Therapy, 18*(2), 159–167.

Fritz, J. (2009). Clinical Prediction Rules in Physical Therapy: Coming of Age? *Journal of Orthopaedic Sports Physical Therapy, 39,* 159–161.

Gocha, V., Murphy, D., Dolakia, K., Hess, A., & Effgen, S. (1999). Child maltreatment: Our responsibility as health care professionals. *Pediatric Physical Therapy, 11,* 133–139.

Guralnick, M.J. (1997). *The effectiveness of early intervention.* Baltimore: Paul H. Brookes.

Hanft, B.E. (1991). Impact of federal policy on pediatric health and education programs. In W. Dunn (Ed.), *Pediatric occupational therapy* (pp. 273–284). Thorofare, NJ: Slack.

Hanft, B.E., Rush, D.D., & Sheldon, M.L. (2004). *Coaching families and colleagues in early childhood.* Baltimore: Paul H. Brookes.

Hinojosa, J., Bedell, G., Buchholz, E.S., Charles, J., Shigaki, I.S., & Bicchieri, S.M. (2001). Team collaboration: A case study of an early intervention team. *Qualitative Health Research, 11,* 206–220.

Hobbs, C.J., Hanks, H.G., & Wynn, J.M. (1999). *Child abuse and neglect: A clinician's handbook.* London: Churchill Livingstone.

Hunt, P., Soto, G., Maier, J., & Doering, K. (2003). Collaborative teaming to support students at risk and students with severe disabilities in general education classrooms. *Exceptional Children, 69*(3), 315–352.

Iowa Department of Education (2001). *Iowa guidelines for educationally related physical therapy services.* Des Moines: Author.

Kettenbach, G. (2001). *Writing SOAP notes* (3rd ed.). Philadelphia: F.A. Davis.

King, G., McDougall, J., Palisano, R. J., Gritzan, J., & Tucker, M.A. (1999). Goal attainment scaling: Its use in evaluating pediatric therapy programs. *Physical and Occupational Therapy in Pediatrics, 19*(2), 31–52.

King, G., Strachan, D., Tucker, M., Duwyn, B., Desserud, S., & Shillington, M. (2009). The application of a transdisciplinary model for early intervention services. *Infants and Young Children, 22*(3), 211–223.

Law, L.S.H., Dai, M.O., & Siu, A. (2004). Applicability of goal attainment scaling in the evaluation of gross motor changes in children with cerebral palsy. *Hong Kong Physiotherapy Journal, 22,* 22–28.

Law, M., & MacDermid, J. (Eds.) (2008). *Evidence-based rehabilitation: A guide to practice* (2nd ed.). Thorofare, NJ: Slack.

Lindsey, D., O'Neal, J., Haas, K., & Tewey, S.M. (1980). Physical therapy services in North Carolina's schools. *Clinical Management in Physical Therapy, 4,* 40–43.

Lollar, D.J., & Simeonsson, R.J. (2005). Diagnosis to function: Classification for children and youths. *Journal of Developmental and Behavioral Pediatrics, 26*(4), 323–330.

Mager, R.F. (1962). *Preparing instructional objectives.* Palo Alto, CA: Fearon Publishers.

Mailloux, Z., May-Benson, T.A., Summers, C.A., Miller, L.J., Brett-Green, B., Burke, J.P., Cohn, E.S., Koomar, J.A., Parham, L.D., Roley, S.S., Schaaf, R.C., & Schoen, S.A. (2007). Goal attainment scaling as a measure of meaningful outcomes for children with sensory integration disorders. *American Journal of Occupational Therapy, 61*(2), 254–259.

Martinuzzi, A., Salghetti, A., Betto, S., Russo, E., Leonardi, M., Raggi, A., et al. (2010). The International Classification of Functioning Disability and Health, version for children and youth as a roadmap for projecting and programming rehabilitation in a neuropaediatric hospital unit. *Journal of Rehabilitation Medicine, 42*(1), 49–55.

McEwen, I. (Ed.). (2000). *Providing physical therapy services under Parts B & C of the Individuals with Disabilities Education Act (IDEA).* Alexandria, VA: Section on Pediatrics, American Physical Therapy Association.

McLaughlin, J., & Bjornson, K.F. (1998). Quality of life and developmental disabilities. *Developmental Medicine and Child Neurology, 40,* 435.

Mead, S. (1968). Presidential address. The treatment of cerebral palsy. *Developmental Medicine and Child Neurology, 10,* 423–436.

Montgomery, P.C. (1987). Treatment planning: Establishing behavior objectives. In B.H. Connolly & P.C. Montgomery (Eds.), *Therapeutic exercise in developmental disabilities* (pp. 21–26). Chattanooga, TN: Chattanooga Corporation.

Montgomery, P.C. (1998). Predicting potential for ambulation in children with cerebral palsy. *Pediatric Physical Therapy, 10*(4), 148–155.

Montgomery, P.C., & Connolly, B.H. (Eds.). (2003). *Clinical applications for motor control* (pp. 1–23). Thorofare, NJ: Slack.

Mu, K., & Royeen, C.B. (2004). Interprofessional vs. interdisciplinary services in school-based occupational therapy practice. *Occupational Therapy International, 11*(4), 244–247.

Murphy, W. (1995). *Healing the generations: A history of physical therapy and the American Physical Therapy Association.* Lyme, CT: Greenwich Publishing Group.

National Autism Center. (2009). *Evidence-based practice and autism in the schools.* Randoph, MA: author.

National Institutes of Health (1993). *Research plan for the National Center for Medical Rehabilitation Research.* NIH Publication No. 93–3509. Bethesda, MD: Author.

Nicholson, D. (2002). Practice guidelines, algorithms, and clinical pathways. In M. Law (Ed.), *Evidence-based rehabilitation: A guide to practice* (pp. 195–219). Thorofare, NJ: Slack.

O'Neil, M.E., Fragala-Pinkham, M.A., Westcott, S.L., Martin, K., Chiarello, L.A., Valvano, J., & Rose, R.U. (2006). Physical therapy clinical management recommendations for children with cerebral palsy—spastic diplegia: Achieving functional mobility outcomes. *Pediatric Physical Therapy, 18*(1), 49–72.

Ott, D., & Effgen, S. (2000). Occurrence of gross motor behaviors in integrated and segregated preschool classrooms. *Pediatric Physical Therapy, 12,* 164–172.

Palisano, R.J., Haley, S.M., & Brown, D.A. (1992). Goal attainment scaling as a measure of change in infants with motor delays. *Physical Therapy, 72*(6), 432–437.

Palisano, R. J., & Murr, S. (2009). Intensity of therapy services: What are the considerations? *Physical & Occupational Therapy in Pediatrics, 29*(2), 107–112.

Rainforth, B. (1997). Analysis of physical therapy practice acts: Implication for role release in educational environments. *Pediatric Physical Therapy, 9,* 54–61.

Rainforth, B., & York-Barr, J. (1997). *Collaborative teams for students with severe disabilities: Integrating therapy and educational services* (2nd ed.). Baltimore: Paul H. Brookes.

Rimmer, J.H. (2006). Use of the ICF in identifying factors that impact participation in physical activity/rehabilitation among people with disabilities. *Disability and Rehabilitation, 28*(17), 1087–1095.

Rosenbaum, P., King, S., Law, M., King, G., & Evans, J. (1998). Family-centered service: A conceptual framework and research review. *Physical and Occupational Therapy in Pediatrics, 18*(1), 1–20.

Rothstein, J.M., Echternach, J.L., & Riddle, D.L. (2003). The hypothesis-oriented algorithm for clinicians II (HOAC II): A guide for patient management. *Physical Therapy, 83*(5), 455–470.

Sackett, D., Rosenberg, W., Gray, J.A.M., Haynes, R.B., & Richardson, W.S. (1996). Evidence-based medicine: What it is and what it isn't. *British Medical Journal, 312,* 71–72.

Schmitt, L., Byrnes, R., Cherny, C., Filipa, A., Harrison, A., Paterno, M., & Smith, T. (2009). Cincinnati Children's Hospital Medical Center: Evidence-based clinical care guideline for management of osteochondritis dissecans of the knee. Guideline 037, pages 1–16. Retrieved from http://www.cincinnatichildrens.org/svc/alpha/h/health-policy/otpt.htm

Simeonsson, R.J., Leonardi, M., Lollar, D., Bjorck-Akesson, E., Hollenweger, J., & Martinuzzi, A. (2003). Applying the International Classification of Functioning, Disability and Health (ICF) to measure childhood disability. *Disability and Rehabilitation, 25*(11–12), 602–610.

Stanton, T.R., Hancock, M.J., Maher, C.G., & Koes, B.W. (2010). Critical appraisal of clinical prediction rules that aim to optimize treatment selection for musculoskeletal conditions. *Physical Therapy, 90*(6), 843–854.

Steenbeek, D., Ketelaar, M., Galama, K., & Gorter, J.W. (2007). Goal attainment scaling in paediatric rehabilitation: a critical review of the literature. *Developmental Medicine and Child Neurology, 49*(7), 550–556.

Steenbeek, D., Meester-Delver, A., Becher, J.G., & Lankhorst, G.J. (2005). The effect of botulinum toxin type A treatment of the lower extremity on the level of functional abilities in children with cerebral palsy: evaluation with goal attainment scaling. *Clinical Rehabilitation, 19*(3), 274–282.

Sussman, S. (2006). The transdisciplinary-translation revolution: Final thoughts. *Evaluation & the Health Professions, 29*(3), 348–352.

Sweeney, J.K., Heriza, C.B., & Blanchard, Y. (2009). Neonatal physical therapy. Part I: Clinical competencies and neonatal intensive care unit clinical training models. *Pediatric Physical Therapy, 21*(4), 296–307.

Thomson-O'Brien, M.A., & Moreland, J. (1998). Evidence-based practice information circle. *Physiotherapy Canada, 50*(3), 184–189.

U.S. Department of Health and Human Services, Administration for Children and Families, Administration on Children, Youth and Families, Children's Bureau. (2010). Child Maltreatment 2008. Retrieved from http://www.acf.hhs.gov/programs/cb/stats_research/index.htm#can

VanSant, A.F. (2006). Physical therapy diagnoses. *Pediatric Physical Therapy, 18*(3), 181.

Watter, P., Rodger, S., Marinac, J., Woodyatt, G., Ziviani, J., & Ozanne, A. (2008). Multidisciplinary assessment of children with developmental coordination disorder: using the ICF framework to inform assessment. *Physical and Occupational Therapy in Pediatrics, 28*(4), 331–352.

Wiecha, J., & Pollard, T. (2004). The interdisciplinary eHealth team: Chronic care for the future. *Journal of Medical Internet Research, 6*(3), e22–e22.

World Health Organization (WHO) (1980). *International classification of impairments, disabilities and handicaps.* Geneva: Author.

World Health Organization (WHO) (2001). *International classi-fication of functioning, disability and health.* Geneva: Author.

World Health Organization (WHO) (2007). *International clas-sification of functioning, disability and health: Children & youth version.* Geneva: Author.

World Health Organization (WHO) (2008). *WHO disability assessment schedule II (WHO DAS 2).* Geneva: Author. Retrieved from http://www.who.int/classifications/icf/whodasii/en/index.html

Wu, Y.W., Day, S.M., Strauss, D.J., & Shavelle, R.M. (2004). Prognosis for ambulation in cerebral palsy: A population-based study. *Pediatrics, 114*(5), 1264–1271.

Zaretsky, L. (2007). A transdisciplinary team approach to achieving moral agency across regular and special educa-tion in K-12 schools. *Journal of Educational Administra-tion, 45*(4), 496.

■ Appendix 1.A Federal Legislation Affecting Children With Disabilities

Year Enacted	Public Law (PL) Number	Name of Legislation	Impact on Children With Disabilities
1963	PL 88-164	Mental Retardation Facilities and Community Mental Health Centers Construction Act	Provided financial aid for building community-based facilities for people with developmental disabilities and mental illness, and authorized research centers and university-affiliated facilities (UAFs).
1963	PL 88-156	Maternal and Child Health and Mental Retardation Planning Act	Expanded the Maternal and Child Health Program to improve prenatal care to high-risk women from low-income families to prevent mental retardation.
1963	PL 88-210	Vocation Education Act of 1963	Recognized that individuals with special needs require assistance to achieve success in regular vocational programs.
1964	PL 88-452	Economic Opportunity Act of 1963	Established Project Head Start, offering health, education, nutritional, and social services to economically deprived preschool children. In 1972, PL 92-424 set aside a minimum of 10% of Head Start enrollment for children with disabilities. Now includes an Early Head Start Program for infants.
1965	PL 89-97	Social Security Amendments	Authorized Medicare/Medicaid to provide public funding for the poor, aged, and disabled. This was one of the reforms recommended by President Kennedy's Panel on Mental Retardation.
1967	PL 90-248	Early and Periodic Screening, Diagnosis, and Treatment (EPSDT) Program, part of the Social Security Act of 1967	Provided early and periodic screening, diagnosis, and treatment for all Medicaid-eligible children. Became mandatory as part of Medicaid in 1972.
1970	PL 91-230	ESEA Amendments of 1970 creates the Education of the Handicapped Act (EHA)	Several special education statutes consolidated into Title VI, referred to as the "Education of the Handicapped Act."

Continued

Appendix 1.A Federal Legislation Affecting Children With Disabilities—cont'd

Year Enacted	Public Law (PL) Number	Name of Legislation	Impact on Children With Disabilities
1970	PL 91-517	Developmental Disabilities Services and Facilities Construction Amendments	Expanded PL 88-164 into a comprehensive statute that required states to establish a governor's council on developmental disabilities. Term "developmental disabilities" replaced "mental retardation." Children with cerebral palsy and epilepsy were now eligible for services under this definition.
1972	PL 92-223	Social Security Amendments	Intermediate care facilities (ICFs) to be reimbursed if states ensured that residents received "active treatment."
1972	PL 92-603	Social Security Amendments	Supplemental Security Income (SSI) provided to people in need, including those with developmental disabilities.
1973	PL 93-112	Rehabilitation Act, Section 504	Extended basic civil rights protections to individuals with disabilities. The rules applied to all institutions, agencies, schools, and organizations that received federal assistance.
1974	PL 93-247	Child Abuse and Prevention and Treatment Act and its later amendments (1992, 1996, & 1997)	Provided protection and treatment for children who were abused or neglected. Included a reporting system.
1975	PL 94-142	Education of All Handicapped Children Act and its later amendments; retitled Individuals with Disabilities Education Improvement Act (IDEA) (1986, 1991, 1997, & 2004)	Provided the right to a free and appropriate public education and related services for all children ages 5/6 to 21 years, regardless of their degree of disability.
1978	PL 95-602	Rehabilitation Comprehensive Services and Developmental Disability Act	"Developmental disabilities" defined in functional terms.
1981	PL 97-35 Section 2176	Omnibus Reconciliation Act, "Home-Based Waiver"	Allowed states to finance a variety of community-based services for those with developmental disabilities instead of institutional settings.
1982	PL 97-248	Social Security Amendments ("Katie Beckett" Amendments)	Permitted states to use Medicaid for certain children with disabilities to stay home rather than be institutionalized.
1984	PL 98-248	Carl Perkins Vocational Technical Education Act	Authorized development of vocational education programs with 10% of the funds used to train individuals with disabilities.
1984	PL 98-527	Developmental Disabilities Act Amendments and later amendments of 1987, PL 100-146	Amended the purpose of the Developmental Disabilities Act to ensure that individuals receive necessary services and to establish a coordination and monitoring system. Later added family support.

Appendix 1.A Federal Legislation Affecting Children With Disabilities—cont'd

Year Enacted	Public Law (PL) Number	Name of Legislation	Impact on Children With Disabilities
1986	PL 99-372	Handicapped Children's Protection Act	Allowed for reasonable attorney's fees incurred by parents who prevailed in hearings related to the child's right to an education under IDEA.
1986	PL 99-401	Temporary Child Care for Handicapped Children and Crisis Nurseries Act and Amendment PL 101-127	Provided funding for temporary respite care for children with disabilities or chronic illness who are at risk of abuse or neglect.
1986	PL 99-457	Education of the Handicapped Act amendments later reauthorized as PL 102-119 Individuals with Disabilities Education Act amendments of 1991	Expanded PL 94-142 to provide special education and related services to preschool children with disabilities, age 3–5 years. Also established early intervention state grant program for infants and toddlers with disabilities age 0 to 36 months and their families.
1986	PL 101-336	Americans with Disabilities Act (ADA)	Ensured full civil rights to individuals with disabilities. Guaranteed equal opportunity in employment, public and private accommodations, transportation, government services, and telecommunications.
1988	PL 100-407	Technology-Related Assistance for Individuals	Provided state funding to develop technology-related assistance programs and to offer assistive technology to individuals with disabilities.
1988	PL 100-360	Medicare Catastrophic Coverage Act	Clarified that Medicaid funds can pay for the cost of "related services" in a school-age child's Individualized Education Program (IEP) or Individualized Family Service Plan (IFSP), if the services would have been paid for if PL 94-142 was not in effect.
1997	PL 105-17	Individuals with Disabilities Education Act Amendments (IDEA)	Refined comprehensive right to education law. Expanded purpose to prepare students for life after school.
1997	PL 105-33	Title XXI of the Social Security Act; State Child Health Insurance Program (SCHIP)	Provided funding for states to initiate and expand health insurance coverage for uninsured, low-income children.
2000	PL 106-402	Developmental Disabilities Assistance and Bill of Rights Act (DD Act)	This reauthorization focuses on the needs of those with developmental disabilities. Ensures full integration and inclusion in their communities. Funds State Developmental Disabilities Councils.
2002	PL 107-110	No Child Left Behind (NCLB) Act of 2001	Education reform for all children, designed to close achievement gap through accountability, increased flexibility, parent options, and evidence-based instruction.

Continued

Appendix 1.A Federal Legislation Affecting Children With Disabilities—cont'd

Year Enacted	Public Law (PL) Number	Name of Legislation	Impact on Children With Disabilities
2004	PL 108-446	Amendments to IDEA	Reauthorization of IDEA. Provided more flexibility for IEP content and meetings. Removed requirements for short-term objectives and benchmarks.
2009	PL 111-3	SCHIP reauthorization	Reauthorization of continued funding for state health insurance for low-income children.

Source: Adapted in part from Hanft, B. E. (1991). Impact of federal policy on pediatric health and education programs. In W. Dunn (Ed.), *Pediatric occupational therapy*. Thorofare, NJ: Slack.

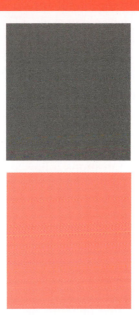

CHAPTER 2

Child Development

—Susan K. Effgen, PT, PhD, FAPTA

The development of a child is a fascinating and complex process involving the interaction between inborn genetic influences and vast environmental influences and experiences. Philosophers and others have spent centuries debating the influence of nature versus nurture on the development of children. Theories of child development abound and numerous books have been written on the topic. The reader is urged to seek more in-depth information beyond what is summarized in this chapter. This chapter briefly reviews theories of child development that have had the greatest impact on pediatric physical therapy. This review is followed by an overview of the development of functional movement from birth through adolescence.

Theories of Child Development

There are numerous theories regarding all aspects of child development. Theories, by definition, are hypotheses or conjectures to explain phenomena.

Therefore, they change and evolve as new information becomes available. However, some general principles of child development are now widely accepted. Development is believed to involve the interaction of three main factors, discussed in this chapter. The first factor is genetic predisposition. Children inherit propensities for certain talents or abilities and genetically transmitted diseases. The second factor is the individual's own role in development, which may include previous experiences, the willingness to persist in a difficult activity, or the tendency to participate or not participate in activities. Finally, environmental factors, such as the family, community, and sociocultural influences, as well as opportunities and experiences, play a role in development. Environmental factors are thought to play a critical role in coordinating the timing and pattern of gene expression (Fox, Levitt, & Nelson, 2010). Therefore, genetic predisposition, the individual's role, and environmental factors all influence development; however, the degree of their importance varies among the developmental theorists.

There is also agreement that all of development is interdependent. The nature of such interaction is not well understood but is an area of expanding research. Shirley (1933) first noted that children mastering motor skills such as reaching for objects, sitting alone, and walking will vocalize much less during active motor periods. Others note "the old adage that children inhibit speech development while working on new motor skills" (Tipps, Mira, & Cairns, 1981). More recently, it has been found that when an infant is learning to walk independently, there is a regression or, as some would say, a reorganization, of reaching skills (Corbetta & Bojczyk, 2002).

For many systems and domains, development generally progresses toward greater complexity through a gradual, continuous process. For some aspects of development, children will experience stages of rapid transitions followed by periods of minimal change. Locomotor development goes through a very rapid transition during the first year of life and is then relatively stable. Physical development also goes through a rapid period of development during the first year of life and again during puberty.

Some areas of development are also thought to have sensitive or critical periods. Certain experiences at one point in development will have a profoundly different effect on future development than the very same experience at another point in time (Bruer, 2001; Ito, 2004). A common example is the ease of learning foreign languages early in life, as opposed to during high school or in adulthood.

The following developmental theories are those of most importance to physical therapists. These are reviewed briefly, and references are suggested for a more in-depth review (Table 2.1). The theories presented are not mutually exclusive; they share different degrees of empirical support, and some are very compatible and complementary.

Neuromaturational View

The **neuromaturational view** uses the framework of central nervous system (CNS) maturation as the foundation for development across all domains. Prerequisite skills are believed to occur in specific, invariant sequences before higher-level skills reflecting a hierarchical development. Shirley (1931), Gesell (1928, 1945, 1952), and McGraw (1932, 1935, 1945) carefully observed child behavior and recorded specific sequences

and periods of motor skill development. They attempted to link the development of motor behaviors with development of the CNS. Believing in a strict hierarchical system of control, they correlated the integration of reflexes and reactions with the time of myelinization of areas of the CNS. Pediatric physical therapy has been heavily influenced by the neuromaturational viewpoint, and many of our assessment tools and some interventions are still based on a neuromaturational view.

From the 1920s to 1950s, Arnold Gesell worked at the Yale Clinic of Child Development. As a physician, he understood neurological, anatomical, and physiological development. This understanding guided his observations and assumptions about the "role of maturation in the pattern of behavior" (Gesell & Thompson, 1934, p. 292). His description of behavior trends and many of his basic tenets have served as the foundation for pediatric physical therapy for the past 60 years. The original tenets purport that development occurs in a cephalocaudal direction; development also occurs in a proximal-to-distal direction; development of one motor skill leads to the development of another, more complex motor skill; motor milestones are invariant in their sequence; motor skills develop from gross to fine; and motor control progresses from reflexive to voluntary movement (Gesell, 1945). However, in Gesell's later work, these tenets are no longer outlined, and he suggests that development occurs in successive epochs with variations that provide a spiral character to the progressions of development (1952, p. 66). The concept of spiral patterns has been further elaborated, and now it is recognized that the developmental sequence is *not* invariant and that his original tenets of development are *not* universal.

During this same period, McGraw (1935) engaged in an intensive, longitudinal study of the development of twins at Columbia University. She, like Gesell, used a new technology, cinematography, to record the development of movement, allowing greater analysis than in the past. She was not as concerned as Gesell with the timing of the achievement of specific skills, but rather with the sequence and patterns from which they developed. Her classic text, *The Neuromuscular Maturation of the Human Infant* (1945), is still a relevant source of information on the common, sequential development of motor behaviors. The works of Gesell and McGraw were the foundation for many of the early neurophysiological or developmental physical therapy intervention approaches, such as those developed by the Bobaths (1980, 1984) and Margaret Rood (Stockmeyer, 1967).

Table 2.1 Selected Child Development Theories

Theory	Basic Concepts	Major Proponents (Physical Therapist Advocates in Italic)
Neuromaturational	• Development follows a set, invariant sequence. • Development is tightly tied to central nervous system development. • Motor development is cephalocaudal and proximal to distal. • Recent modifications acknowledge variations in the sequence and input from all systems.	Gesell, McGraw, Bayley, *Bobath, Bly*
Cognitive	• Thinking develops in stages of increasing complexity. • Children organize mental schemes through the use of mental operations.	Piaget, Vygotsky, Montessori
Behavioral	• Behavior is shaped by the environment. • The stimulus, response, and environmental consequence constitute a contingency of behavior. • Consequences of behavior influence future occurrences of the behavior.	Skinner, Bandura
Psychoanalytic/ psychosocial	• There are biologically determined drives and unconscious conflicts. • The core of these conflicts is sexual. • Initial drives are for survival; when basic needs are met, we seek self-actualization.	Freud, Erikson, Maslow
Ecological, contextual	• The environment has a very strong influence on child development.	Bronfenbrenner, Gibson, Harris, Sameroff
Dynamic systems	• Movement emerges based on the internal milieu, the external environment, and task. • Movement is not directed by one system, but by many dynamic, interacting systems.	Bernstein, Kelso, Thelen, *Heriza, Shumway-Cook, Horak, Valvano*
Neuronal Group Selection	• Infant motor development includes periods of increased and decreased variability due to changes in the central nervous system. • Cortical and subcortical systems dynamically organize into variable neural networks.	Sporns, Edelman, Hadders-Algra, *Helders*

The neuromaturational view supported a sequential pattern of development. This view lent itself to the production of a number of developmental scales to assess infant development. Nancy Bayley (1936), who performed longitudinal studies of infant mental and motor behaviors, published the *Bayley Scales of Infant Development*. The *Bayley Scales of Infant and Toddler Development* (2005) is now in its third edition and is widely used in neonatal intensive care follow-up clinics and early intervention programs. Gesell, in 1949, also published infant scales of motor, adaptive, language, and personal-social development. These comprehensive scales serve as the foundation for many of today's developmental tests.

Neuromaturational concepts were expanded by an occupational therapist, Mary Fiorentino, who studied the stages of normal and abnormal development in relationship to reflex/responses and movement (Fiorentino, 1963, 1972, 1981). She believed that "our total postural behavior is the result of interaction of reflexes and the relative strength of each one of them" (Fiorentino, 1981, p. ix). Her reflex testing methods were standard procedures in pediatric physical and occupational therapy until the 1980s, when the functional and clinical significance of reflexes were seriously questioned, and a greater understanding of CNS development displaced the hierarchical neuromaturational view of the nervous system.

Lois Bly (1994) has provided a comprehensive view of motor skill acquisition and the kinesiological aspects of motor development during the first year of life. She presented a sequential maturational perspective while acknowledging that a "global perspective in which maturation, environment, behavior, biomechanics, kinesiology, perception, learning, and goal direction are considered to be important" (1994, p. xii) in the developmental process. The research of Thelen and colleagues (1985, 1987, 1994), and her protégé Karen Adolph and colleagues (Adolph, Vereijken, & Denny, 1998; Adolph & Berger, 2006; Spencer et al., 2006; Vereijken, 2010), now clearly indicates that motor development is characterized by variation and the development of adaptive variability. Limitations in variation and variability are common in atypical development (Hadders-Algra, 2010). The sequence of infant motor skill acquisition is indeed quite variable, with many infants skipping stages previously thought to be mandatory for achievement of independent walking. As discussed later, the neuromaturational view has been widely replaced by the dynamic systems theory and neuronal group selection theory as the theoretical frameworks for much of pediatric physical therapy.

Cognitive View

The cognitive view refers to the development of "age-appropriate mental functions, especially in perceiving, understanding, and knowing, that is, becoming capable of doing intellectual tasks" (Bowe, 1995, p. 552). As the neuromaturational theories were developing in America, a number of Europeans were studying child development from a cognitive perspective. Jean Piaget (1952), a Swiss psychologist, was interested in the genesis and theory of knowledge (genetic epistemology). He highlighted the importance of the child's active involvement in the environment—not merely neurological maturation—as critical to the infant's development. Piaget's ideas have changed our understanding of human thinking and problem-solving. He believed that thinking developed in stages of increasing complexity. To adapt, children must go through the processes of assimilation, accommodation, and equilibration. Patterns of thoughts, actions, and problem-solving are referred to as schemas that assist a child in dealing with a challenge or situation. His observations of what he called

the sensorimotor period of infant development were important in providing the rationale for some pediatric interventions. Piagetian principles and later variations that are compatible with learning theories are used throughout early childhood education (Case, 1992).

In Russia in the mid-1920s, Vygotsky (1978) was investigating child development and the role of culture and interpersonal communication through social interaction. He also studied the play of children, cultural mediation, and internalization. He defined the concept of the "zone of proximal development" as "the distance between actual developmental level as determined by independent problem solving and the level of potential development as determined through problem solving under adult guidance or in collaboration with more capable peers" (p. 86). This is the zone of what a child can learn with the assistance of another. The zone of proximal development led to the therapeutic principle of **scaffolding.** Scaffolding is the process in which parents and others provide environmental challenges that encourage the child to perform a higher-level skill. The support or guidance helps a child improve his or her ability to perform the task (Case-Smith, Law, Missiuna, Pollock, & Stewart, 2010, p. 29). Just the right amount of challenge allows the child to complete the task and be ready for the next step in skill development.

The cognitive perspective has been used in the development of early childhood learning programs. In the early 1900s, Maria Montessori, an Italian physician, used cognitive and developmental theory to develop a revolutionary teaching strategy, first for children with intellectual disability and later for all young children. In the Montessori approach (Montessori, 1964), a child is given freedom to interact independently with the environment and to choose activities from carefully developed materials. "Sensorial education" was encouraged, involving tasks that required intelligence and movement. This encouragement of both mental and motor development was important for children with physical disabilities who have limited motoric options. Teachers act as facilitators of learning and not directors. This approach to early childhood education is still popular, although some believe it neglects the child's social development (Chattin-McNichols, 1992).

A newer approach to early childhood learning is the Reggio Emilia approach. This approach, led by Loris Malaguzzi, was developed over the past 45 years in the northern Italian region of Reggio Emilia. The child is viewed as competent, capable, curious, creative, and full of potential. The child is encouraged to learn by investigating and exploring things of interest in a carefully prepared, stimulating environment. Development of problem-solving skills is critical as the child learns to predict and reflect. Parent participation is embraced, and the approach provides a supportive environment in which to learn. There is full inclusion of "children with special rights," and therapists work with the child within the school environment. Few, if any, sessions are one-to-one, and therapists instruct teachers on how to integrate therapy into daily classroom activities (Palsha, 2002). This approach has gained in popularity in the United States as preschool educators and others learn more about this child-centered approach (Edwards, Gandini, & Forman, 1993; Lewin-Benham, 2008).

Behavioral/Learning View

Almost simultaneous to the development of the previous theories, another group of individuals were studying human behavior from a very different perspective. In the early 1900s, Ivan Pavlov, a Russian physiologist, recognized the relationship between stimulus and responses in dogs and developed an understanding of what is called classical conditioning. B. F. Skinner (1953), an American psychologist, advanced the concept of operant conditioning. He studied the effects of the stimulus, response, and consequences in animals and humans and showed that environmental manipulation and reinforcement can condition some behaviors. This research provided a greater understanding of the importance of consequences of behaviors and the impact of consequences on recurrence of behavior.

The **behavioral view** assumes that behavior results from an interaction of genetic and environmental events and that most behaviors are learned responses. A behaviorist asserts that positively reinforced behaviors will occur with greater frequency than if the consequence of a behavior is punishment because there is decreased probability that the behavior will reoccur. The primary concepts of the behavioral view, now commonly referred to as **applied behavior analysis**, include positive reinforcement, extinction (planned ignoring), negative reinforcement (the avoidance of an unpleasant event that increases the likelihood of the behavior), and punishment. Positive and negative reinforcement are frequently used in therapy. Children are rewarded with praise, hugs, and perhaps stickers, toys, or food to reinforce positive behaviors. Negative reinforcement is also unintentionally used when a therapy session is allowed to end when a child is crying or uncooperative. By "giving in" to the child's behavior, this negative behavior is reinforced, and it is likely to occur again when the child wants to avoid an unpleasant situation.

Therapists also use Skinner's concept of **shaping.** In shaping, successive approximations of the desired behavior are reinforced until the individual can perform the desired behavior. This is a very useful methodology when working with young children (Bailey & Wolery, 1992; Bowe, 1995, p. 3) and children with severe disabilities (Facon, Sahiri, & Riviere, 2008) who are learning new behaviors. Shaping is also used in many current motor learning approaches such as constraint-induced movement therapy, where it is used to advance the function of the impaired extremity in adults and children with hemiplegia (Charles & Gordon, 2005; Taub, Uswatte, & Pidikiti, 1999).

More recently, Albert Bandura went beyond strict behaviorism to note that behaviors also cause changes in the environment. Reciprocal determinism reflects the premise that environment, behavior, and psychological processes interact to form personality. All learning need not be through reinforcement, but also by observation and modeling. This interest in processes also places Bandura with the cognitivists, and his theory is called the social cognitive theory (Bandura, 2002).

The behavioral view that serves as the foundation of applied behavior analysis is used in education and rehabilitation. Target behaviors that need to be increased or decreased are carefully identified and described in measurable terms. Using the environmental manipulation of providing rewards or, in very selected, carefully controlled situations, punishment, has been successful with young children (Bailey & Wolery, 1992) and with individuals who have severe brain damage, serious behavior disorders, or other disabilities (Alberto & Troutman, 2006). Behavioral interventions have recently been documented as one of eleven established treatments that have been thoroughly researched for children with autism in schools (National Autism Center, 2009, p. 38)

Psychoanalytical/Psychosocial View

Sigmund Freud developed psychoanalytic theories regarding sexual development and the natural state of relationships between individuals of the opposite sex. He believed in biologically determined drives and unconscious conflicts, the core of which was sexual. Erik Erikson expanded Freud's psychoanalytic theory, with its emphasis on psychosexual stages, into a theory based on psychosocial stages of emerging personality and development throughout the life span. Erikson believed that changes are influenced by interrelated forces more than by unconscious drives, including (1) the individual's biological and physical strengths and limitations,

(2) the individual's life circumstances and history, and (3) the social, cultural, and historical forces during one's lifetime (Seifert & Hoffnung, 1997, p. 34). As with neuromaturational and cognitive theories, psychoanalytic/psychosocial views share the concept of successive stages of development. If individuals have problems in the early stages of life, they can have difficulty if a crisis arises in adulthood. Many children with disabilities are delayed or prevented from going through the various stages of development, especially during adolescence where one must establish identity and self-concept. This can have lasting effects into adulthood.

Abraham Maslow developed what is considered a humanistic hierarchical, not stage-dependent, theory of development. He believed that initial drives were for physiological survival and safety, followed by the need for love, affection, and esteem, which culminated in self-actualization. He believed that individuals are motivated not only by "deficiency drives" but also by the drive toward self-actualization. Self-actualization occurs through successful coping with problems in everyday life (Fidler & Fidler, 1978). Understanding a child's position in Maslow's scheme can help a therapist understand how to relate to a child. Highlighting an adolescent's dependence will not help develop self-esteem, and a child seeking safety, love, and affection might not appreciate opportunities for independence.

Ecological Systems Theory, Contextual Views

The environment has a strong influence on all living things. Developmental psychologists have studied how a child's social and cultural environments influence development. Eleanor Gibson and James Gibson considered the interdependence of the child with the environment to be an explanation of perceptual development. Eleanor Gibson studied the perceptions of infants and indicated that perception is an adaptive process and that perceptual learning refers to improvement in performing perceptual tasks as a function of experience. She believed that manipulative play was important for an infant's cognitive development (1988). James Gibson (1950) coined the term "affordance," which refers to the opportunities for action provided by a particular object or the environment. Action and perception are tightly linked. As the infant or child's first actions generate new information about the environment, those actions become the foundation for perceptual development. Eleanor Gibson notes that as "new action systems mature, new affordances open up and new experiments on the world can be undertaken" (1988, p. 7).

The ecological systems theory, proposed by Urie Bronfenbrenner (1995), emphasizes a strong environmental view of the impact of larger social systems on child development and the function of the family unit. He proposes that the child is influenced by five interactive and overlapping ecological systems. As depicted in Figure 2.1, the *microsystem* is the setting in which the child lives. It is the physical and social situations with the family and peer group that directly affect the child. The *mesosystem* involves connections among the child's microsystems that influence the child because of the relationships, such as the relations of family experiences to school experiences and of family experiences to peer experiences. The *exosystem* involves the external settings or situations that influence the child but in which the child does not necessarily have an active role. This might include the government's influence on the school system and, therefore, on the child's education. The values, briefs, and policies of society and culture form the *macrosystem*. The *chronosystem* involves the dimension of time of environmental events and transitions during life and sociohistorical conditions (Santrock, 1998, p. 50). Bronfenbrenner (1995) has added biological influences to his theory, although the ecological and environmental contexts still dominate.

Harris (1998) elucidated the strong influence of the peer group over the parents and biology. This theory has caused some controversy, although it is not a new concept. "The most potent single influence during the adolescent years is the power of group approval. The youth becomes a slave to the conventions of his age group" (Havighurst, 1972, p. 45). The importance, and hopefully positive influence, of a peer group is one of the reasons for encouraging inclusive education of children with disabilities.

The bidirectional nature of the relationship of the child and environment has been addressed by Arnold Sameroff (2009) in his transactional model of development, where he outlines the interplay of nature and nurture in explaining child development. The child's learning and performance also influence the environmental contexts in which the child is learning. Bronfenbrenner's ecological systems theory and Sameroff's transactional model of development have gained wide acceptance in both family therapy and special education, providing support for an ecological approach to family-centered intervention.

Dynamic Systems Theory

The **dynamic systems theory** is a theory of motor development across the life span and has replaced the neuromaturational view as the theoretical framework

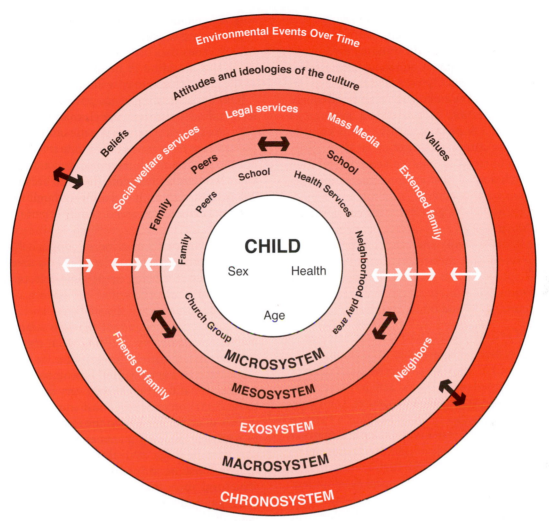

Figure 2.1 Bronfenbrenner's ecological system. *(Adapted from Bronfenbrenner, U. [1979]. The ecology of human development. Cambridge, MA: Harvard University Press.)*

for much of pediatric physical therapy. The theory has its roots in the work of Nicolai Bernstein, a Russian physiologist (1967). It is not one cohesive theory developed by an individual but rather reflects the work of many individuals including Thelen, Smith, Kelso, Fogel, Kugler, and Turvey (Kelso, Holt, Kugler, & Turvey, 1980; Kelso & Tuller, 1984; Thelen, 1985; Thelen, Kelso, & Fogel, 1987; Thelen & Smith, 1994). The work of Thelen and others has been followed by the work of their protégés and other colleagues including several physical therapists (Adolph et al., 1998; Adolph & Berger, 2006; Buchanan & Horak, 2001; Heriza, 1991; Horak, 1991; Shumway-Cook & Woollacott, 2007; Spencer et al., 2006; Thelen & Smith, 1994). Various terms have been used to describe this theory, including systems, dynamic, dynamic action, dynamic action

systems (Shumway-Cook & Woollacott, 2007, p. 16), task-oriented theory, systems approach, and developmental biodynamics (Santrock, 1998, p. 153).

The dynamic systems theory assumes that the individual functions as a complex, dynamic system with many subsystems and that there is an innate organization that occurs between complex particles that is directed by no one system. Development is seen as a complex process that involves multi-leveled and multi-relational changes between the components of the organism and its environment (Corbetta & Bojczyk, 2002; Thelen et al., 1993). Movement emerges based on the child's internal milieu, the external environment, and the motor task to be completed. The concepts about changes in motor behaviors associated with development are derived from principles of nonlinear change that describe many biological and physical systems (Harbourne & Stergiou, 2009; Scholz, 1990; Thelen & Ulrich, 1991). Universal milestones, such as crawling and walking, are learned through a process of adaptation, and movement patterns are modulated as the child explores new movement options to fit a new task. The emergence of new skills might change the organization of established patterns of responses (Corbetta & Bojczyk, 2002). At any point in development, "the critical, rate-limiting factor that triggers the system to reorganize into a new configuration might be a psychological function governed by the CNS (e.g. motivation, balance control), or it might be a more peripheral factor such as gravity or leg fat" (Adolph & Berger, 2006, p. 172).

Dynamic systems theory and other current theories of motor development and motor learning are discussed in Chapters 7 and 8 because they play a major role in determining our intervention strategies for children with neurological and other disabilities.

Neuronal Group Selection Theory

The dynamic systems theory places little emphasis on the role of the CNS. However, Sporns and Edelman (1993) have suggested that repeated activity causes neurons involved in the activity to fire together. Their neuronal group selection theory (NGST) offers a balance between a pure dynamic systems approach and one that recognizes the important role of the CNS in movement at the level of the neuron. NGST highlights variation and variability as key elements of typical development (Hadders-Algra, 2010).

This theory proposes that infant motor development includes two periods of increasing variability due to cell division, migration, and death, and two periods of decreasing variability due to the selection of the most effective response patterns for a particular situation (Helders, 2010). The concepts of variation and variability have application in the diagnosis of infants with, or at risk for, developmental movement disorders and in the study of intervention effectiveness.

Influences on Child Development

Genetic Influences

At conception, the union of the mother's ovum and father's sperm starts an amazing and complex process of development. The ovum and sperm each contain 23 chromosomes consisting of DNA. DNA is a combination of the nucleotide bases cytosine, thymine, adenine, and guanine that form a double-helix structure. These bases of DNA are organized into hundreds to thousands of units called genes. Genes are encoded with the genetic code that determines our physical appearance and biochemical makeup. There are around 30,000 genes that code the proteins of our body. An error or a mutation in the production or translation of the genetic code may result in a genetic disorder.

Our understanding of our genetic code has increased tremendously through the Human Genome Project. This rapid development of genetic information requires therapists to have access to accurate information. Therapists must work closely with genetic professionals when working with families (Sanger, Dave, & Stuberg, 2001). Information is available through the National Human Genome Research Institute (National Institutes of Health, 2011).

Approximately one-third of congenital malformations are attributable to identifiable causes, with approximately 55% being single-gene defects, 25% being chromosomal disorders, and 20% having a genetic etiology but an unknown mechanism (Baird, Anderson, Newcombe, & Lowry, 1988). There is a range of possible genetic disorders resulting from the addition or deletion of an entire chromosome or even the microdeletion of a gene within a chromosome. The clinical manifestations range from very severe limitations in function and activities, most commonly seen in the defects of an addition or a deletion of a chromosome, to relatively minor impairment in body structure, as seen in some single-gene disorders.

Chromosome disorders include **numerical** and **structural abnormalities**. In numerical abnormalities there is an additional chromosome (trisomy), where the individual has 47 chromosomes, or a deletion (monosomy), where there are 45 chromosomes. This addition or deletion of chromosomes is usually due to an error occurring during early cell division, specifically a meiotic error during gametogenesis, and is not hereditary (Sanger et al., 2001).

Between 10% and 15% of all conceptions have a chromosomal abnormality. More than 50% are trisomies, 20% are monosomies, and 15% are triploids (69 chromosomes). The percentage of infants born with chromosomal abnormalities is not that large because 95% of these fetuses do not survive to term (Batshaw, 2007, p. 8).

The most common form of a trisomy is Down syndrome, which is a trisomy of the 21st chromosome. This trisomy, which causes intellectual disability and other impairments, is discussed in Chapters 7 and 21. Other trisomies include Klinefelter syndrome (47XXY), a syndrome in which the male produces inadequate testosterone and has impairments in developing secondary male sexual characteristics, and trisomies 13 and 18, which are rare but involve significant limitation in activities and participation secondary to profound intellectual disability and impaired body function and structure. Monosomy, or deletion of a chromosome, is usually not consistent with life, except for Turner syndrome (45X). This syndrome affects girls, who will have a short stature and webbed neck; 20% have obstruction of the left side of the heart. They usually have normal intellectual functioning but may have visual-perceptual impairments (Batshaw, 2007, p. 7).

Structural abnormalities involve the deletion, translocation, inversion, or other rearrangement of chromosomes. In **deletions**, a portion of a chromosome is missing. For example, in cri-du-chat syndrome, a portion of the short arm of chromosome 5 is missing. The child will have microcephaly (small head size), an unusual facial appearance, and a high-pitched characteristic cry.

Translocations involve a transfer of a portion of one chromosome to another. A form of Down syndrome that involves a partial trisomy of the 21st chromosome is caused by a translocation. Rare rearrangements of chromosomes include inversions, when a chromosome breaks in two places and then reattaches in the reverse order, or a ring chromosome, when deletions occur at both tips of a chromosome and the ends stick together, forming a ring.

These numerical and structural abnormalities can have major consequences for a child's development. Approximately 0.7% of all infants are born with multiple malformations, commonly due to genetic disorders (Jones, 2006, p. 1). Table 2.2 presents a concise overview of genetic disorders commonly encountered by physical therapists. Several of these disorders are presented in more detail throughout the text.

The critical importance of genetic influences on our development is manifested in disorders that are inherited. In **autosomal dominant inheritance**, one parent provides the mutant gene and there is a 50% risk of the offspring inheriting the disorder. The abnormal gene overcomes the normal gene inherited by the other parent.

Table 2.2 Common Genetic Disorders

Disorder	Etiology	Body Function and Structure Impairments	Potential Limitations in Activities and Participation Restrictions
Chromosomal Abnormalities			
Angelman syndrome	Partial deletion of chromosome 15q11q13 (maternal source)	Severe cognitive impairment, microbrachycephaly, seizures, ataxic gait, characteristic arms held with flexed wrists and elbows, and frequent laughter not associated with happiness	Severe limitations in speech, most ADLs, and mobility; requires assistance throughout life
Cri-du-chat syndrome	Partial deletion of short arm of 5th chromosome	Severe cognitive impairment, microcephaly, and abnormal laryngeal development leading to characteristic high-pitched cry	Severe limitations in speech and most ADLs; requires assistance throughout life
Klinefelter syndrome (47XXY)	Sex chromosome abnormality in males	Hypogonadism, infertility, long limbs, and slim stature; possible behavioral or psychiatric problems	Poorly organized motor function, but ambulatory; slight delay in language, possibly affecting some activities, unless other limitations due to behavior
Prader-Willi syndrome	Partial deletion of chromosome 15q11q13 (paternal source)	Mild cognitive impairment, hypotonia in infancy, short stature, and obesity	Limitations with some activities, depending on the degree of cognitive impairment and obesity

Continued

Table 2.2 Common Genetic Disorders—cont'd

Disorder	Etiology	Body Function and Structure Impairments	Potential Limitations in Activities and Participation Restrictions
Chromosomal Abnormalities			
Trisomy 13	Autosomal trisomy of 13th chromosome	Severe CNS abnormalities and defects of eyes, nose, lips, forearms, hands and feet	Severe limitations in speech, most ADLs, and mobility; requires assistance throughout life; only 10% survive the first year of life
Trisomy 18 (Edward's syndrome)	Autosomal trisomy of 18th chromosome	Severe cognitive impairment; significant cardiovascular, skeletal, urogenital, and gastrointestinal anomalies	Severe limitations requiring extensive assistance; frequently die during first year of life
Trisomy 21 (Down syndrome)	Autosomal trisomy of 21st chromosome (95%), others due to translocation or mosaicism	Hypotonia, hyperflexibility, flat facial features, upslanted palpebral fissures, pelvic hypoplasia with shallow acetabular angle, single midpalmar crease (Simian crease), cognitive impairment, and frequent cardiac anomalies	Delay in achieving most gross and fine motor skills and language; will learn most ADLs, attend school with special education and related services; as young adult may work and live outside of home with supports
Turner syndrome (45XO)	Sex chromosome abnormality (females)	Small stature, weblike appearance of the lateral neck, transient congenital lymphedema, gonadal underdevelopment, hearing impairment, bone trabecular abnormalities, possible visuoperceptual limitations, and possible cognitive impairment	Short stature might restrict some activities, otherwise generally few limitations
Single-Gene Abnormalities			
Achondroplasia	Autosomal dominant	Disturbance of endochondral ossification at epiphyseal plate, resulting in short stature, bilateral shortness of humerus and femur, and macrocephaly; may have spinal complications	Possible reduced efficiency in activities due to gait deviation; short stature might require accommodations for some activities
Cystic fibrosis (CF)	Autosomal recessive	Disorder of exocrine glands leading to pancreatic insufficiency, hyperplasia of mucus-producing cells in the lungs, and excessive electrolyte secretion of sweat glands	Endurance may be limited due to pulmonary involvement, but may participate in sports; frequent need for secretion removal from airways may limit time available for some activities; with advances in intervention, many live into adulthood

Table 2.2 Common Genetic Disorders—cont'd

Disorder Single-Gene Abnormalities	Etiology	Body Function and Structure Impairments	Potential Limitations in Activities and Participation Restrictions
Duchenne muscular dystrophy (DMD)	X-linked (mutation of Xp21) (males)	Intrinsic muscle disease, creatine kinase elevated and dystrophin absent; leads to progressive intrinsic muscle weakness (commonly observed by 3 years of age), weakness from proximal to distal muscles	Might have delay in early motor milestones; progressive loss of motor abilities during childhood, leading to wheelchair use and further limitations in activities; death in early adulthood
Fragile X syndrome	X-linked, fragile site at Xq27 (males)	Hypotonia, moderate to borderline cognitive impairment, delayed motor milestones, and emotional lability	Depends on degree of cognitive impairment, but generally few restrictions in activities and participation related to motor skills
Hemophilia	X-linked (males)	Factor VIII (hemophilia A) or factor IX (hemophilia B) deficiency resulting in impaired blood clotting capability; can lead to reduced range of motion and muscle strength in joints into which bleeding occurs, especially the knee, ankle, and elbow	Ambulatory and can perform ADLs; may experience limitations of joint motion and pain; contact sports restricted; intracranial hemorrhage can lead to death
Mucopolysaccharidosis (MPS) (7 forms)	MPS I (previously called Hurler syndrome): autosomal recessive; MPS II (previously called Hunter syndrome): X-linked recessive	Inborn error of metabolism resulting in abnormal storage of mucopolysaccharides in tissues; wide variability. Usually coarse facial features, thick skin, excessive hair, skeletal dysplasia, and cognitive impairment	Depends on form, progressive loss of motor abilities during childhood, leading to wheelchair use and further limitations in activities; deterioration leading to death before adulthood
Lesch-Nyhan syndrome	X-linked recessive	Excessive production of uric acid with serious damage to the brain and liver leading to choreoathetosis, spasticity, growth deficiency, autistic behaviors, and cognitive impairment; tendency to self-mutilate	Serious limitations in all activities and participation including ambulation and ADLs
Neurofibromatosis	Autosomal dominant, gene located in chromosome 17	Wide variance in expression, tumors may cause multiple system involvement, frequently in CNS and skeletal system	Course generally benign; however, as tumors grow and affect more systems, increased limitations in activities and participation

Continued

Table 2.2 Common Genetic Disorders—cont'd

Disorder Single-Gene Abnormalities	Etiology	Body Function and Structure Impairments	Potential Limitations in Activities and Participation Restrictions
Osteogenesis imperfecta (OI) (7 forms)	Generally autosomal dominant	Wide variability in expression. Problem with collagen development; short stature and multiple fractures commonly of long bones, kyphosis, and scoliosis; occasionally adolescent-onset hearing loss	Depends on extent of fractures and secondary complications; most are ambulatory; restrictions in sports, especially contact sports; accommodations for some activities may be needed due to short stature
Phenylketonuria (PKU)	Autosomal recessive	Absence of phenylalanine hydroxylase prevents conversion of phenylalanine to tyrosine, causing abnormal accumulation of phenylalanine; if untreated, leads to cognitive impairment, seizures, and autistic behaviors	Can successfully be treated if detected at birth with no limitations; if untreated, serious limitations in most activities, although should be ambulatory
Rett syndrome	X-linked dominant (Xq28) (females) (lethal in males)	Hypotonia and ataxia; characteristic trunk rocking and stereotyped, repetitive hand wringing, tapping, or mouthing; serious cognitive impairment	Serious limitations in all activities and participation, although some girls may ambulate
Spinal muscular atrophy (SMA)	Autosomal recessive, mutation of SMN gene on 5th chromosome; SMA Type III: X-linked	Anterior horn cell degeneration and flaccid paralysis: SMA Type I (Werdnig-Hoffmann disease) seen at birth; proximal, symmetrical weakness, respiratory and feeding problems SMA Type II (chronic Werdnig-Hoffmann disease), similar pattern as Type I but slower progression, feeding not a problem SMA Type III (Kugelberg-Welander disease) mild, progressive weakness of proximal muscles	SMA Type I: Severely limited motor development affecting all activities; unable to sit without support; power mobility helps in participation; rarely survive beyond 3 years SMA Type II: Not as severe as Type I; may learn to walk with assistance and do many ADLs; computer keyboard use better than pencil use SMA Type III: Mild limitations in activities; can walk unaided but may lose this ability later in life
Tuberous sclerosis	Autosomal dominant; gene located on chromosome 9q34 or 16p13	Brain lesions consist of tubers; depigmented white birthmarks; café-au-lait spots on skin; usually develop seizures and may have cognitive impairment; wide variability in expression	Depends on control of seizures and degree of cognitive impairment

Source: Gordon (2007); Jones (2006).

There are thousands of autosomal dominant disorders; a common example is achondroplasia (short stature).

In **autosomal recessive inheritance**, both parents carry the abnormal gene and the child must inherit the abnormal gene from both the mother and father to manifest the disorder. The parents will not have the disorder and usually there is no family history of the disorder, but there is a 25% chance that their child will inherit the autosomal recessive trait, as shown in Figure 2.2. Cystic fibrosis, a disorder of the exocrine glands (see Chapters 9 and 20), is a common autosomal recessive disorder. The X-linked, or sex-linked, recessive disorders involve mutant genes located in the X (female) chromosome, generally affecting male offspring. Because males have only one X chromosome, the single dose of the abnormal recessive gene will cause the disease, such as hemophilia, Duchenne muscular dystrophy, and fragile X syndrome (see Table 2.2). In females, who have two X chromosomes, the single recessive gene should not cause the disease, although they may manifest the disease through a phenomenon termed *lyonization*, or unequal inactivation of the X chromosomes.

Multifactorial inheritance is a result of the interaction of heredity and the environment. Environmental factors influence the expression of genes. Multifactorial inheritance is thought to be responsible for some forms of diabetes, myelomeningocele (a neural tube defect), and cleft lip and palate.

A limited number of genetic disorders are due to alterations of small mitochondrial DNA fragments. Only the female's ova contain cytoplasm; therefore, all mitochondria are inherited from the mother. As a result, mitochondrial disorders are passed from unaffected mothers to all her children.

Mendelian genetics suggested that the appearance of a child would be the same whether a gene was inherited from the father or mother; however, genomic imprinting indicates that conditions will present differently depending on whether the trait is inherited from the mother or father (Batshaw, 2007, p. 18). An example is a deletion of the long arm of chromosome 15. If it is inherited from the father, the child will have Prader-Willi syndrome (see Table 2.2). If it is inherited from the mother, the child will have Angelman syndrome, a much more serious disability affecting behavior and intelligence.

The exponential increase in genetic knowledge can be overwhelming and is a major area of study and concern for the 21st century. A pressing issue now is how to handle the ethical, legal, and social issues of genetic information. The issues facing any health professional include, but are not limited to, genetic susceptibility, potential for genetic discrimination, access to information, and confidentiality. Although the future holds great promise through genetic diagnosis and biopharmaceuticals, there is the potential for the use and abuse of information (Schaefer, 2001).

Environmental Factors

As important as the genetic factors are in development, the influences of the environment cannot be underestimated, from preconception through adulthood. The physiological well-being of mothers has an impact on fetal development, and the environment that both parents provide to their children has a significant impact on their development. Optimal development requires an appropriate level of external experience and the ability of the sensory mechanism to selectively attune to environmental stimulation (Reznick, 2000). "Rich early experience must be followed by rich and more sophisticated experience later in life, when high-level circuits are maturing, in order for full potential to be achieved" (Fox et al., 2010, p. 35). New empirical evidence regarding the impact of the environment on development continues to evolve.

Prenatal Environmental Factors

Even before conception, a mother's behavior has an influence on the future development of her child. Women should have good nutrition before, during, and after pregnancy to maximize maternal health and reduce the risk of pregnancy complications, birth defects, and chronic disease in their children in adulthood (Kaiser & Allen, 2008). The Centers for Disease Control and Prevention (CDC) (2010) have recommendations for improving preconception health that include the following:

- Daily use of vitamin supplements containing folic acid
- Management of diabetes
- Cessation of alcohol, smoking, and recreational drug use
- Altering the dosage of certain medications
- Receiving vaccinations against or for treatment of infections
- Improving weight status

These preconception recommendations should be followed throughout pregnancy.

Pregnant women must receive early and consistent prenatal care and avoid known threats to the fetus. Diseases, infections, medication, and radiation of the

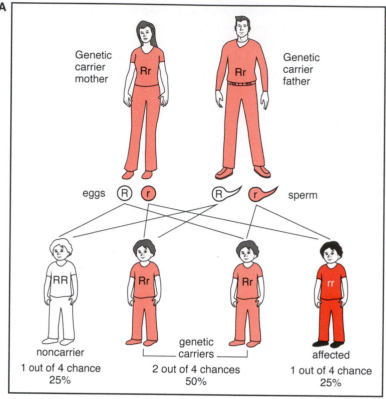

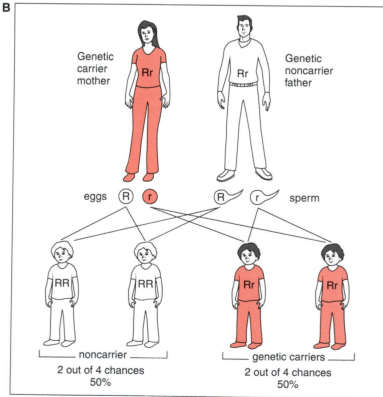

Figure 2.2 Inheritance of autosomal recessive disorders. Two copies of the abnormal gene (aa) are necessary for produce the disease. (*A*) If two carriers mate, usually 25% of the children will be affected, 50% will be carriers, and 25% will not be affected. (*B*) If a carrier and noncarrier mate, 50% of the children will be noncarriers, 50% will be carriers, and no children will have the disease.

mother can all affect the outcome of the pregnancy. The period of greatest risk for a lifetime of severe developmental disabilities is between conception/implantation and birth (Decouflé, Boyle, Paulozzi, & Larry, 2001). Weight gain during pregnancy must be adequate and will influence the infant's birth weight and health. Pregnant women should consume a variety of foods based on sound dietary guidelines and be physically active. They should use appropriate and timely vitamins and mineral supplementations, especially folic acid, iron, calcium, and vitamin D. As already noted, they should cease all use of tobacco, alcohol, caffeine, and illicit drugs. Use of herbal, botanical, and alternative remedies should be restricted because there are limited data regarding their safety and efficacy during pregnancy (Kaiser & Allen, 2008).

Environmental agents that affect fetal development are called **teratogens**. Teratogens include heavy metals, radiation, medications, illicit drugs, infectious agents, and chronic maternal illness. The vulnerability of the fetus to various teratogens depends on a number of factors, such as the timing, magnitude, and duration of the exposure and the ability of the teratogen to cross the placenta (Haffner, 2007, p. 23).

Socioeconomic Status Pregnant woman with low socioeconomic status (SES)—as measured by educational levels—have almost twice as great a risk of having a preterm birth than woman with higher educational levels (Jansen et al., 2009). The educational inequalities that result from low SES result in an unfavorable mixture of pregnancy characteristics, psychosocial factors, and lifestyle practices that lead to preterm births. Lifelong residence in low-income neighborhoods is also a risk factor for low birth weight (LBW) among non-Latino white and African-American women independent of age, education, parity, and prenatal care (Collins, Wambach, David, & Rankin, 2009). Preterm birth is associated with high perinatal mortality, and the infants are vulnerable to complications and morbidity in the neonatal period and throughout life.

Substance Use and Abuse Among pregnant women (ages 12 to 44 years) in the United States, approximately 60.7% used alcohol, with 12% abusing alcohol; 10% smoked cigarettes daily, and 16.6% had smoked in the past week; 10.8% used marijuana; and 1.4% used cocaine in the past 12 months (U.S. Department of Health and Human Services, 2008). All of these behaviors can affect the outcome of the pregnancy. Unfortunately, this trend in substance abuse during pregnancy has remained relatively stable over the past decade.

Use of alcohol during pregnancy has been associated with a group of physical malformations and neurological complications resulting in a spectrum of disorders known as **fetal alcohol spectrum disorders (FASD)**. Children with FASD have a wide range of negative, lifelong problems that include structural malformations and CNS dysfunction resulting from structural brain damage. The CNS dysfunction can range from subtle to very serious. Children with FASD may present with a combination of deficits in memory and information processing as well as learning disabilities that affect academic functioning, including intellectual disability; social skill, attention, motor skill, and executive functioning problems; and significant behavioral and mental health problems (Barr & Streuissguth, 2001; Bertrand, 2009). These children also score significantly more poorly than typically developing children on sensory processing, sensory-motor, and adaptive measures (Jirikowic, Olson, & Kartin, 2008). FASD is reported to have a prevalence of approximately 1 in 100 live births (Burbacher & Grant, 2006). The full spectrum of FASD ranges from the most serious diagnosis of **fetal alcohol syndrome (FAS)**, to partial FAS (pFAS), to alcohol-related neurodevelopmental disorder (ARND) and, finally, alcohol-related birth defects (ARBD).

The criteria for diagnosis of FAS include prenatal and postnatal growth retardation, CNS abnormalities, and distinctive craniofacial abnormalities of microphthalmia (small eyes) and/or short palpebral fissure, thin upper lip, poorly developed groove in the midline of the lips (philtrum), and flat maxillae (Fig. 2.3). Numerous abnormalities coupled with varying degrees of intellectual disability provide a lifetime of challenges for children with FAS. Children with milder intellectual problems and few, if any, of the craniofacial malformations may have pFAS, ARND, or ARBD. They will, however, commonly have the same degree of behavioral abnormalities as those having the more severe FAS (Steinhausen, Metzke, & Spohr, 2003).

The degree of FASD manifestation is influenced by the amount of alcohol consumed by the mother during pregnancy and the timing of consumption. High alcohol intake during the first trimester of pregnancy might lead to FAS; high intake later in the pregnancy or low or moderate intake during the entire pregnancy might lead to other manifestations along the spectrum. Hence, no amount of alcohol intake is considered safe during pregnancy (Jacobson & Jacobson, 1994; Kaiser & Allen, 2008).

Cocaine use during pregnancy has been associated with an increased risk of prematurity, LBW, placental

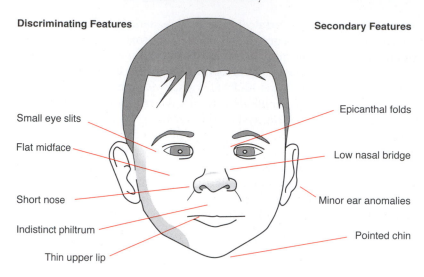

Discriminating Features

Small eye slits
Flat midface
Short nose
Indistinct philtrum
Thin upper lip

Secondary Features

Epicanthal folds
Low nasal bridge
Minor ear anomalies
Pointed chin

Figure 2.3 Characteristics of young child with fetal alcohol syndrome.

abruptions, and neurobehavioral abnormalities. Cocaine is a highly addictive illicit drug and is commonly used concurrently with other drugs and alcohol, so it is difficult to determine the effects of cocaine alone.

Neonatal withdrawal can occur in newborn infants exposed to cocaine. Symptoms might include irritability, restlessness, poor feeding, tremors, increased muscle tone, and lethargy. Withdrawal can last 2 to 3 days, followed by problems related to sleep, feeding, and attention. These infants tend to be irritable, cry frequently, sleep poorly, and have disorganized motor behaviors, making caring for them stressful (Wunsch, Conlon, & Scheidt, 2002).

Tobacco smoking during pregnancy increases the risk of LBW and preterm delivery, both of which can lead to developmental problems. There is also an increased risk of a stillborn infant, the infant dying in the first year of life, cleft lip, cleft palate, clubfoot, and heart defects (CDC, 2011a). The effect of smoking on the fetus is directly related to the amount of smoking, coupled with the use of alcohol or other drugs. Infants prenatally exposed to tobacco average 200 grams lighter than infants born to nonsmokers (Lee, 1998). Cigarette exposure has also been associated with smaller frontal lobe and cerebellar volumes in infants (Ekblad et al., 2010), an increased incidence of infant maltreatment (Wu et al., 2004), and lower global intelligence scores at ages 9 to 12 years (Fried, Watkinson, & Gray, 1998). Women exposed to residential environmental tobacco smoke (second-hand smoke) also have an increased risk of having infants born with LBW (Pogodina, Brunner Huber, Racine, & Platonova, 2009). An association has been shown between maternal smoking during pregnancy and an increased incidence of Legg-Calvé-Perthes disease (avascular necrosis of the ossific nucleus of the femoral head) (Bahmanyar, Montgomery, Weiss, & Ekbom, 2008). Fortunately, cessation of smoking before and during pregnancy can prevent the reduction in birth weight (Li, Windsor, Perkins, Goldenberg, & Lowe, 1993).

Smoking marijuana has not been shown to have the same initial adverse effects as tobacco smoking on the infant (Fried, Watkinson, & Gray, 1999; Lee, 1998). However, by age 10 years, prenatal marijuana exposure was significantly related to increased hyperactivity, impulsivity, and inattentiveness (Goldschmidt, Day, & Richardson, 2000) but not to impaired intellectual functioning (Fried et al., 1998).

Heroin and phencyclidine (PCP), as well as certain prescription drugs, have been linked to perinatal abnormalities. Heroin-exposed neonates have severe withdrawal and frequently require pharmacological intervention to inhibit behavioral manifestations of drug exposure. These infants may have problems with sleep, be resistant to cuddling, have decreased orientation to auditory and visual stimulation, and have growth retardation (Wunsch et al., 2002).

Chemical exposure can also cause abnormalities in the fetus and infant. For example, high-dosage exposure to wood alcohol (methanol), an industrial solvent and potential alternative fuel source for automobiles, can result in severe movement disorder or death. Fetal exposure has only recently been studied but warrants consideration as alternative fuels are developed (Davidson & Myers, 2007, p. 66). The long-term effects of all drug and chemical exposure, which are highly influenced by the environment in which the child is raised, continue to be studied.

Prescription Drugs Pregnant women with medical problems must be under close medical supervision during pregnancy, especially those having diabetes and hypertensive disease (Kaiser & Allen, 2008). Drugs that successfully treat a disease in the mother can have devastating teratogenic effects on the fetus. Therefore, the effect of all pharmacological agents on the fetus must be monitored carefully. The most notorious example of this environmental factor is the morning sickness pill, thalidomide, which caused major fetal limb deficiencies in Europe in the late 1950s. Fortunately, thalidomide was not approved for use in the United States when its devastating effects were unknown. The very controlled use of thalidomide has recently been approved in the United States for the treatment of cancer.

Infections Maternal infections can be passed to the fetus during pregnancy (transplacental infections) or during birth as the fetus passes through the vagina (ascending infections). These infections occur at a time when the fetus is least able to resist them. The most common maternal infections are known as the **STORCH** infections. The letters stand for **s**yphilis, **t**oxoplasmosis, **o**ther (including HIV), **r**ubella, **c**ytomegalovirus (CMV), and **h**erpes simplex (see Table 2.3).

Congenital syphilis can be transmitted during pregnancy or during delivery, whereas toxoplasmosis, rubella, and CMV are transplacental infections, and herpes is an ascending infection. Toxoplasmosis can be transmitted any time in the pregnancy through maternal ingestion of contaminated raw or improperly cooked meat or contact with the feces of infected cats. Stillbirth and death are common, and if the infant survives, there will be serious restrictions in all activities.

Table 2.3 STORCH (Intrauterine) Infections

Diagnosis	Etiology	Impairments of Body Functions and Structures	Potential Activity Limitations and Participation Restrictions
Syphilis	Parabacterial infection (easily treated if diagnosed)	Enlarged liver and spleen, jaundice, anemia, rash, oral lesions, inflammation of the eye, hearing loss	If the infant survives, limitations will depend on the extent of impairments in body function and structure.
Toxoplasmosis	Parasitic infection	Deafness, blindness, intellectual disability, seizures, pneumonia, large liver and spleen	Limitations in activities and participation are serious.
Other infections such as coxsackievirus, varicella-zoster virus, HIV, parvovirus B19	Virus	Varies	Limitations will depend on the extent of impairments in body function and structure.
Rubella	Virus (rubella vaccine has decreased incidence)	Meningitis, hearing loss, cataracts, cardiac problems, intellectual disability, retinal defects	Serious limitations in activities and participation are due to sensory impairments and limitations in cognitive functioning.
Cytomegalovirus	Virus	Hearing loss; in severe form, problems are similar to rubella	Serious limitations in activities and participation are due to deafness and limitations in cognitive functioning.
Herpes simplex	Virus	*Disseminated form*: clotting disorder, liver dysfunction, pneumonia, and shock *Encephalitic form*: attacks CNS, causing intellectual disability, seizures, and other problems *Localized form*: eye or skin lesions	Limitations in activities and participation are serious with the disseminating and encephalitic forms. The localized form is usually successfully treated without limitations in activities.

Source: Hill & Haffner, 2002.

There has been a significant reduction in rubella with the introduction of vaccination programs in the 1970s. Women can be tested for immunity to rubella before becoming pregnant. CMV is the most common cause of congenital viral infections, with an incidence of 0.2 to 2.2% of all live births in the United States (Hill & Haffner, 2002).

A serious threat to the health and development of an infant is the presence of human immunodeficiency virus (HIV) infection or acquired immunodeficiency syndrome (AIDS). Transmission from the mother to the newborn can occur in utero, during the birth process, or through breastfeeding. The majority of infants born to infected mothers are not infected. The intensive use of antiretroviral therapy for the infected mother during pregnancy and delivery of the infant by cesarean section has continued to decrease the incidence (Fiscus et al., 2002) from 25% to 2% (National Institute of Child Health and Human Development, 2004). An estimated 430,000 children worldwide became infected with HIV in 2008, mostly through birth or breastfeeding from an HIV-infected mother (National Institute of Child Health and Human Development, 2010).

Infants who do acquire the HIV infection are grouped into three categories based on the severity of the symptomatology, ranging from no symptoms to severely symptomatic. Regardless of the category, all infants should be treated aggressively with antiretroviral therapy. Infants infected with AIDS have a wide range of symptoms along with slowed growth, delayed overall development, and frequent infections. Family-focused intervention is critical in their care.

Research suggests that conditions present during the fetal period may program the individual's susceptibility to disease that occurs later in life. For example, LBW infants who have very rapid catch-up growth might be at risk for metabolic syndrome as adults (Fagerberg, Bondjers, & Nilsson, 2004). Women who were born weighing less than 2500 grams were reported to have a 23% higher risk of cardiovascular disease than women born weighing more (Rich-Edwards et al., 1997). The small size at birth was reportedly not the problem. The factors in utero that created the suboptimal conditions that caused the infant to be born small for gestational age are thought to be the critical variables in these women who subsequently developed cardiovascular disease. Conversely, women who weighed more than 4000 grams at birth had a greater likelihood of developing early breast cancer than those who weighed 2500 grams at birth (Michels et al., 1996).

Nathanielsz (1999), author of *Life in the Womb*, suggested that there is "compelling proof that the health we enjoy throughout our lives is determined to a large extent by the conditions in which we developed." This is an exciting frontier of scientific research and provides even more support for the need for healthy habits and excellent prenatal care of the mother.

Perinatal Environmental Factors

LBW infants are those with a birth weight less than 2,500 grams (5½ lbs). If they are less than 1,500 grams (3½ lbs) they are considered very low birth weight (VLBW). **Small for gestational age (SGA)** infants can be either full term or preterm. They have a birth weight that is below the 10th percentile for their gestational age. These infants typically appear small and malnourished. Approximately one-half of infants born SGA can be attributed to maternal illness, smoking, or malnutrition (Rais-Bahrami & Short, 2007, p. 108).

In addition to the numerous prenatal environmental factors, such as those discussed already, other factors might cause the infant to be born preterm, LBW, or SGA. These factors include use of assisted reproduction methods, multiple-gestation births, adolescent mothers, a history of previous premature pregnancies, placental bleeding, preeclampsia (maternal hypertension with proteinuria), or congenital anomalies (Rais-Barami & Short, 2007, p.111).

The preterm infant has numerous disadvantages at birth. The transition from the intrauterine to extrauterine environment is complex and the infant faces many potential problems. Most of their organs are immature, especially the lungs. There is decreased production of surfactant, which might cause the serious problem of respiratory distress syndrome (RDS). Administering glucocorticoids to mothers before delivery can improve pulmonary function and the production of surfactant.

The CNS of the preterm infant is also immature, and the infant is at greater risk for intraventricular hemorrhage (IVH), periventricular leukomalacia (PVL), and hydrocephalus (discussed in Chapters 7 and 15). These conditions might lead to developmental disabilities, including cerebral palsy.

The premature infant's kidney function might be inadequate and the infant might have problems with absorption of nutrients. Problems with nutrient absorption and inadequate blood supply to the gastrointestinal track might lead to a very serious condition called necrotizing enterocolitis (NEC), which involves a severe injury to the bowel wall. The mortality rate of LBW infants with NEC is between 16% and 42%, with lower mortality associated with increasing birth weight (Fitzgibbons et al., 2009).

Additionally, the preterm infant's eyes are susceptible to retinopathy of prematurity because of the oxygen used to treat respiratory distress (Rais-Bahrami & Short, 2007). This condition can lead to visual loss.

Preterm, LBW, and SGA status can affect later developmental outcomes, but fortunately the majority of infants do very well. However, severe neonatal brain injury is the strongest predictor of poor intelligence, and children who were born preterm display more behavior problems than controls not born preterm (Luu et al., 2009). O'Keeffe and colleagues (2003) found that adolescents who were born before the 37th week of gestation and were extremely SGA, were more likely to have learning difficulties and lower IQ scores than matching controls.

Very preterm infants and late preterm infants had the same risk of requiring interventional therapies, including physical therapy (Kalia, Visintainer, Brumberg, Pici, & Kase, 2009). Apparently, the morbidities (hypoglycemia, respiratory compromise, apnea, hyperbilirubinemia, and feeding difficulties) of very early or late prematurity have a major influence on developmental outcomes. Children who were born very preterm have also been found to have reduced exercise capacity (Smith, van Asperen, McKay, Selvadurai, & Fitzgerald, 2008). Better cognitive function was associated with antenatal steroid use, higher maternal education, and a two-parent family, whereas minority status was a disadvantage to the outcomes of preterm births (Luu et al., 2009).

Postnatal Environmental Factors

As noted by the developmental theorists, the environment plays a major role in the development of the child. Skinner (1953) emphasized the role of the environment in shaping behavior, and Piaget (1952) emphasized the role of the environment in the development of knowledge. They and others note that the critical element is not just the environment but also the child's interaction with the environment.

David and Weinstein (1987) recommend that the child's environment should fulfill five basic functions:

1. The environment should foster personal identity and help children define their relationship to the world.
2. The environment should foster the development of competence by allowing children opportunities to develop mastery and control over their physical surroundings.
3. The environment should be rich and stimulating.
4. The environment should foster a sense of security and trust.
5. The environment should provide opportunities for social contact and privacy.

For physical development, the child needs the opportunity to practice universal skills, such as sitting, crawling, and walking; and advanced, culturally dependent skills, such as riding a bicycle or horse, playing tennis, or snow boarding. The amount of practice necessary to master a specific skill is dictated by innate ability and environmental variables. Adolph and colleagues (Adolph & Berger, 2006; Adolph et al., 1998) note that infants without disabilities practice gross motor skills with great variety and intensity. They found that early walkers walk the equivalent distance of more than 29 football fields per day! They also note that infants walk over almost a dozen different surfaces—indoors and outdoors—with varying surface friction, rigidity, and texture. Rarely do children with disabilities have the opportunity for such extensive and varied practice of motor skills, which probably contributes to their motor impairments and limitations in activities.

For a child with disabilities, the physical environment can have a significant influence on performance. Not only should the environment be accessible, but it must also be responsive to the needs of the child. Historically, society and especially parents have been overprotective toward children with disabilities. This attitude can result in adults doing almost everything for the child and thereby imparting that the child has little control over the environment (Bailey & Wolery, 1992, p. 200). Children easily perceive that they lack control over their lives and are unintentionally taught "learned helplessness" (DeVellis, 1977; Seligman, 1975). A physically responsive environment may help to increase perceptions of control (Bailey & Wolery, 1992, p. 200) that may carry over to other situations.

Physical therapists must understand the impact of the environment in which they treat children. Some children respond and learn very well in very stimulating environments, and others are overwhelmed and withdraw from the stimulation and do not interact. A clinical setting might be exciting for one child and totally overwhelming to another. The focus on home-based services for young children is based on the recognition that children generally respond best in their natural environment. However, not all natural or home environments are appropriately stimulating and supportive to children, and interventionists must recognize that, on occasion, other environments are more appropriate for the child's learning.

Socioeconomic Status The child's physical environment is significantly influenced by the family's SES. Children raised in poverty are far less likely to have appropriate toys, reading material, and personal space than those raised by families with greater means, not to mention the basic necessities of food, clothing, and shelter. In the United States, one in six or 18% of all children live in poverty (1 in 3 African American, 1 in 4 Latino American, and 1 in 10 European American children). More than 25% of children younger than age 18 years in Louisiana, Mississippi, Arkansas, and New Mexico live in poverty (Children's Defense Fund, 2008). This percentage is almost twice as high as in other developed nations. The environments of children raised in poverty are frequently more chaotic and more stressful, and the children lack the social and psychological supports needed to develop successfully. Children raised in poverty are more likely than children raised in more affluent families to:

- Have a disability
- Have no health insurance
- Have poor-quality child care
- Have inadequate housing
- Live in areas with high crime rates
- Change schools frequently
- Watch more television
- Not read
- Live in single-parent families (Morales & Sheafor, 2001)
- Be maltreated (Scarborough & McCrae, 2010)

Children raised in poverty are more likely to have a number of negative health-related behaviors such as aggressive/delinquent behavior, with increased levels of smoking and alcohol consumption (Najman et al., 2010). Poverty and educational level of the parents are closely connected. Children's success in school has a direct relationship to the educational attainment of their parents (Case, Griffin, & Kelly, 2001) and especially the maternal literacy level in low-income families (Green et al., 2009).

Nutrition Nutrition plays an important part in normal growth and development. Culture, poverty, and lifestyle influence nutrition. During the first few years of life, children are completely dependent on their caregivers for their nutrition, as are some children with disabilities throughout their lives. For infants, the advantages of breast milk "include health, nutritional, immunological, developmental, psychologic, social, economic, and environmental benefits" (American Academy of Pediatrics (AAP) (2005, p. 496). Recent research indicates improved cognitive development in infants who are breastfed, especially children born preterm (Quigley et al., 2012). Breastfeeding during the first months of life is strongly recommended by the AAP (2005) and the American Dietetic Association (Kaiser & Allen, 2008). Breastfeeding also may protect against maternally perpetrated child abuse and neglect (Strathearn, Mamun, Najman, & O'Callaghan, 2009) and reduce the incidence of sudden infant death syndrome (SIDS) (Vennemann et al., 2009). Preterm infants and those with oral motor problems, who are unable to nurse adequately, can still be fed breast milk that has been expressed by the mother.

Undernutrition involves the underconsumption of nutrients and may lead to malnutrition. Malnutrition leads to severe failure to thrive and failure to meet expected growth standards. Inadequate intake of nutrition may lead to neurodevelopmental problems and lack of energy to explore and learn from the environment. The other extreme is the excessive intake of food relative to the metabolic needs of the child that leads to obesity. In developed countries of the world, increasing numbers of children are becoming obese (Steinberger & Daniels, 2003). This trend is caused by the increased consumption of fatty foods, increased time sitting watching television or playing video games, and decreased physical activity in general. Overweight infants and young toddlers have high rates of respiratory problems, snoring, and delayed gross motor skills (Shibli, Rubin, Akons, & Shaoul, 2008).

Children with disabilities have a higher likelihood of becoming obese than the general population. Children with Down syndrome have lower metabolic rates, which increases the likelihood of weight gain. Children with Prader-Willi syndrome have a compulsive eating problem. Those with muscular dystrophy or high-level myelomeningocele, disorders that can lead to restricted mobility and inactivity, also have problems with obesity. Obesity can lead to secondary medical problems associated with musculoskeletal pain, cardiopulmonary insufficiency, diabetes, and sleep apnea.

Physical therapists should be supportive of proper nutrition and work closely with nutritionists, nurses, and physicians to make certain children have an appropriate balance of proper caloric input and exercise. Directing fitness programs for children with and without disabilities is becoming an expanded area of practice for physical therapists and is discussed in Chapters 9 and 13.

Culture and Ethnicity Child development is significantly influenced by the environmental factors of **culture** and ethnicity. "Culture is the behavior, patterns, beliefs and all other products of a particular group of people that are passed on from generation to generation" (Santrock, 1998, p. 579) and forms an "integrated system of learned patterns of behavior" (Low, 1984, p. 14). The characteristics of culture are complex and evolving. Adolescents and young adults might reject their cultural upbringing, only to embrace their culture when raising their own children. Cultural values influence child-rearing behaviors for children with and without disabilities.

Understanding cultural variations in child rearing will assist the therapist in providing culturally sensitive, competent intervention, as discussed in Chapter 4. One need only read Anne Fadiman's (1997) award-winning book, *The Spirit Catches You and You Fall Down*, to see what can go wrong when American health-care professionals fail to understand the collision of cultures. In this anthropology text, a young Hmong child with a serious seizure disorder eventually falls into a persistent vegetative state after years of misunderstanding and misinterpretation of the family and the family's culture by American health-care professionals.

Ethnicity is based not only on cultural heritage but also on nationality characteristics, race, religion, and language. There is wide diversity among individuals within those of a specific ethnic group. Failure to recognize this heterogeneity can result in inappropriate stereotyping. This stereotyping has, unfortunately, been common in research on ethnic minority children where the influences of SES have not been properly accounted for in drawing conclusions about ethnic issues. Researchers are now beginning to document the strong influence of poverty on what were previously considered factors related to ethnicity (Low, 1984; Morales & Sheafor, 2001).

Sensitive Periods Sensitive or critical periods in development have been discussed throughout the 20th century, and there is now renewed interest in this concept of "windows of opportunity" due to the revolution in neuroscience and greater understanding of neuroplasticity. Some scientists use "critical periods" to define a time during which a system requires specific experiences if development is to proceed normally. The presence or absence of an experience results in irreversible change (Fox et al., 2010). A "sensitive period" is a time when normal development is most sensitive to abnormal environmental conditions (Bruer, 2001) and is the time in development during which the brain is particularly responsive to experience (Elman et al., 1997). Experiences at one point in development will have a profoundly

different effect on future development than the very same experience at another point in time (Bruer, 2001). There is reduced responsivity before and after the sensitive period (Farran, 2001, p. 240). Common examples include the ease of learning a second language in the first decade of life compared with during adolescence or adult life and the classic work on the effect of visual deprivation early in the life of kittens. Depriving kittens of visual input to one eye for the first 6 weeks of life led to blindness in that eye (Hubel & Wiesel, 1970). Multiple sensitive periods for visual development in children are now noted (Lewis & Maurer, 2005), as are sensitive periods of language development. Children who are deaf and receive cochlear implants before the age of 3 years have better speech perception outcomes than children implanted later. Children implanted during the first year of life have better vocabulary outcomes than those implanted in the second year of life (Houston & Miyamoto, 2010).

Initially, scientists believed that critical or sensitive periods were short, well-defined periods of development. Now it is realized they are rarely brief and seldom sharply defined; rather the impact of experience peaks and then gradually declines (Bruer, 2001). Each sensory and cognitive system has its own unique sensitive period and the same environmental conditions, depending on the age of the child, will result in very different cognitive and emotional experiences (Fox et al., 2010).

Edward Taub, a rehabilitation researcher, has noted that the exciting aspect of his work is not merely that the immature brain has plasticity but that the mature brain also has plasticity (Bruer, 2001, p. 21). Taub and colleagues (Taub & Morris, 2001; Taub & Wolf, 1997) have successfully demonstrated the neuroplasticity of mature nervous systems in adults post-stroke using constraint-induced movement therapy (CIT). CIT is now a promising intervention for improving hand function (Charles & Gordon, 2005, 2007) and gait function (Coker, Karakostas, Dodds, & Hsiang, 2010) in children with hemiplegia. There is even a case study showing neuroplasticity with cortical reorganization after modified CIT in a child with hemiplegic cerebral palsy (Sutcliffe, Gaetz, Logan, Cheyne, & Fehlings, 2007).

An excellent review of this evolving topic, of vital importance to pediatric physical therapy, can be found in *Critical Thinking About Critical Periods* (Bailey, Bruer, Symons, & Lichtman, 2001). In the conclusion of the book, Bailey and Symons write that "when a window of opportunity opens, we should take advantage of it, even if we don't have evidence that doing so now is necessarily better than later" (2001, p. 290). They note the need for further research but provide the following considerations for practice:

First, different windows open at different times. . . . Second, each child follows a unique developmental course. . . . Third, there is no point in trying to teach something if the window is not yet open. . . . Finally, it is clear that inequity exists in our society in the extent to which children have opportunities for access to various experiences after a certain window opens.

Developmental Domains

Volumes upon volumes have been written regarding all aspects of child development, and the reader is encouraged to learn as much as possible about the development of children to successfully work with children with disabilities. This section of the chapter provides a brief overview of each of the developmental domains, with an emphasis on the development of functional movement. Movement is the domain of physical therapists and it's necessary to have a thorough understanding of the normal acquisition, fluency, maintenance, and generalization of motor skills to better understand their influence on activities and participation.

Any movement can be functional, depending on the context. A child with severely limited muscular activation produces functional movement with his eyes when he activates an environmental control unit that assists in operating his television. On the other hand, a child with autism who runs consistently in circles is not participating in true functional movement. **Functional movement** has been defined as a complex activity directed toward performing a behavioral task. Behaviors that are efficient in achieving the task are considered optimal. Movement involves the complex interaction of the environment, individual, and task. The child generates a movement based on innate capabilities in response to the demands of the task within the limitations set by the environment. Movement is proactive and reactive based on the needs of the task, the environment, and previous experience with that movement.

Historically, the development of postural control and mobility was considered gross motor development and the development of reach, grasp, and manipulation was considered fine motor development. However, movements of the entire body can be very fine and accurate, such as those seen in an Olympic skier or ice skater. Movements of the arm and hand can be rather gross and crude, such as a physical therapy student drawing the Mona Lisa. Leg movements are not necessarily "gross"

and hand movements need not be "fine." This division into fine and gross motor development is not accurate and is being used somewhat less in the literature, although tests and measures of development and many professionals still use this division following common convention.

The study and discussion of the development of children are usually divided into specific age periods, reflecting not only major periods of growth and development but also times of major transitions in the life of the child. Following this convention, the discussion of child development is divided into the following stages: prenatal, neonatal/infant, toddler, preschooler, primary school age, and adolescence. These stages are not mutually exclusive; there is tremendous overlap. Outlines of the usual or customary development of functional movement, reflexes, and cognitive, language, and play development appear in Tables 2.4 to 2.10. The common age of attainment is provided; however, these are average ages and ranges of attainment. Remember that there is a wide range of normal variability influenced by genetics, the environment, child-rearing practices, and cultural expectations. Toilet training in China, for example, is commonly completed by about 6 months of age while in America some 3-year-olds still use diapers.

Prenatal Stage

Movement occurs during the earliest stages of embryonic development. Mothers first become aware of these movements of the fetus at about 16 to 18 weeks' gestation. Three- and four-dimensional ultrasound technology has, however, documented extensive, refined movement much earlier in fetal life. Fetal movement reflects the development of the CNS. As summarized by Kurjak and colleagues (2008), first trimester movements emerge between 7 and 15 weeks' gestation. The head first moves toward the body, followed by the startle (rapid contractions of all limb muscles) by 8 to 9 weeks' gestation. After the ninth week of gestation, the type and amount of movement greatly expands. Isolated limb movements are seen with the simultaneous onset of arm and leg movements. This is an unexpected finding "because of the long-held principle of a cephalocaudal development in spinal motor functions" (Kurjak et al., 2008).

Hand-to-face contact and various head movements are seen after 10 weeks. By 11 weeks, opening of the jaw is seen, along with bending of the head and stretching movements. By 12 weeks, the fetus makes breathing movements and two-thirds of the fetus's arm movements are directed toward objects in the uterus (e.g., the face and body, the uterus and umbilical cord) (Sparling, van Tol, & Chescheir, 1999). There is an increased frequency of movement with increased gestational age during this first trimester.

During the second trimester development continues, but no new movements appear. The incidence of hiccups, startles, and stretches decrease (Kurjak et al., 2008). The most active movement is arm movement, then leg movement. The least active movement is mouth movement, followed by trunk movement, which, as noted by Kuno and colleagues (2001), is contrary to a medial to lateral developmental sequence.

In the third trimester generalized movement decreases as the fetus's body occupies more space in the uterus. Facial movements increase (opening/closing the jaw, swallowing, chewing, eyelid movement, and mouthing) and the complexity of movements increase in the absence of more generalized movements (Kurjak et al., 2008). Distal to proximal development of the extremities is observed, with an unexpected linear decrease in the hand-to-face or head movement (Sparling et al, 1999). Sleep and sleep cycles appear around 26 to 28 weeks' gestation and are considered essential for the development of the neurosensory and motor systems of the fetus and neonate (Graven & Browne, 2008). Usually between 37 and 40 weeks' gestation the fetus begins the birth process. For some fetuses, this process starts earlier, which can have serious consequences.

Neonatal/Infant Stage

The neonate does not look like the pictures in baby books; those adorable infants are generally 3 to 4 months old. The neonate's face is usually puffy and bluish, the ears and head may be pressed into odd shapes, the nose flattened, and the skin covered in a fine hair called lanugo. At birth the neonate fluctuates between bursts of energy and deep sleep.

The neonate is dependent on others for continued existence. Caregivers must provide nutrition and make certain that the neonate is kept clean and warm. Sucking, which began prenatally, is now used for feeding. There is an established relationship of breathing, swallowing, and sucking movements. Problems in this relationship are seen commonly in preterm infants with feeding problems. In addition to nutritive sucking, infants display nonnutritive sucking while sleeping or sucking a finger or pacifier.

Infant feeding is monitored by physical growth, because extremely large and extremely small infants might indicate problems requiring medical attention.

The CDC and the WHO have child growth standards. The CDC (Grummer-Strawn, Reinold, & Krebs, 2010) recommends the WHO (2011) standards for children ages 0 to 2 years and the CDC charts for older children (2011b). Standards and charts are provided by sex for length/height for age, weight for age, weight for height, body mass index for age, and head circumference for age (CDC, 2011b; WHO, 2011). The infant's measurements should be plotted on these growth charts and compared with the standards. Usually growth is consistent along a specific percentile. In Figure 2.4, the growth curves of an infant boy are charted during the first months of his life. Note that he is generally in the 50th percentile for height, weight, and head circumference, except at birth his weight was above the 95th percentile. His weight soon adjusted to around the 50th percentile, consistent with the other parameters. If his weight had remained above the 95th percentile, that would have been reason for concern. When the infant is in the outer limits of the curves/percentiles, or when there are radical fluctuations, the infant must be carefully monitored by the pediatrician. Consistent measures below the 10th percentile might indicate malnutrition, failure to thrive, or other problems. It can be difficult to evaluate the growth of children with known disabilities using the standard norms, so some specialized charts have been developed for children with disabilities such as Down syndrome (Cronk et al., 1988; Toledo, Alembik, Aguirre Jaime, & Stoll, 1999) and cerebral palsy (Krick, Murphy-Miller, Zeger, & Wright, 1996; Stevenson et al., 2006).

The critical importance of development during infancy has been highlighted by legislation in at least 120 countries, allowing for paid maternity leave from work so the mother can stay home from work with her infant. Many nations also allow paternal leave. Australia was the last developed nation to provide parental leave, starting in 2011 (Australian Government, 2011). The only developed nation of the world that does not provide paid maternity leave is the United States (Brown, 2009; Human Rights and Equal Opportunity Commission, 2003). In the United States, the Family Medical Leave Act of 1993 does allow for 12 weeks of unpaid leave for mothers or fathers, and California, New Jersey, and Washington have paid-leave programs (Brown, 2009).

Development of Postural Control and Locomotion

During the first year of life the infant progresses through a rapid transformation in postural control and locomotion, advancing from seemingly random

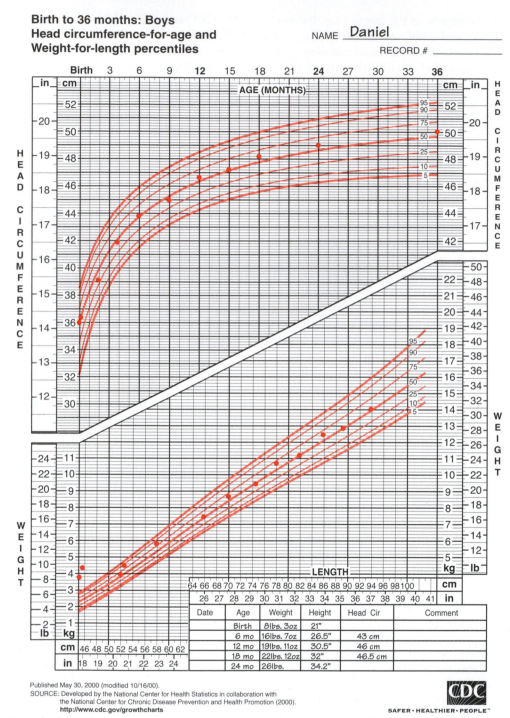

Birth to 36 months: Boys
Head circumference-for-age and
Weight-for-length percentiles

NAME __Daniel__

RECORD # _____

Date	Age	Weight	Height	Head Cir	Comment
	Birth	8lbs. 3oz	21"		
	6 mo	16lbs. 7oz	26.5"	43 cm	
	12 mo	19lbs. 11oz	30.5"	46 cm	
	18 mo	22lbs. 12oz	32"	46.5 cm	
	24 mo	26lbs.	34.2"		

Published May 30, 2000 (modified 10/16/00).
SOURCE: Developed by the National Center for Health Statistics in collaboration with
the National Center for Chronic Disease Prevention and Health Promotion (2000).
http://www.cdc.gov/growthcharts

CDC
SAFER • HEALTHIER • PEOPLE™

Figure 2.4 Growth charts for length/stature for age and weight for a 12-month-old boy. *(Growth charts for girls and boys age birth to 20 years are available from the Centers for Disease Control and Prevention [2011b]. National Center for Health Statistics, National Health and Nutrition Examination Survey, 2000 CDC Growth Charts for the United States at http://www.cdc.gov/growthcharts)*

limb movements to independent ambulation without any appreciable differences between boys and girls (WHO, 2006). The sequence of the development of postural control and motor skill acquisition can be viewed linearly and nonlinearly. From the linear perspective, postural responses are considered innate, genetically determined behaviors that are perhaps driven by a central pattern generator for the activation of muscle groups (Hadders-Algra, Brogren, & Forssberg, 1996). Another perspective, in keeping with Bernstein's dynamic systems theory, views postural control and motor skill acquisition as a nonlinear process of coordinating the many and redundant degrees of freedom of the body, with skill emerging as the result of interactions with the environment. If one views postural control as an emergent dynamic skill of nonlinear progression, then as the skill progresses to a more mature form, the degrees of freedom would increase for more adaptable and flexible coordination of the body (Harbourne & Stergiou, 2003).

Reflexes

The motor characteristics of neonates are limited and relatively predictable, as outlined in Tables 2.4 to 2.7. Their reflexes (see Fig. 2.5; Table 2.6) are thought to be protective, allowing them to withdraw from noxious stimuli. In addition to responding reflexively to environmental stimuli, the neonate displays important independent responses to stimuli. Neonates will suck in a specific pattern once they learn that certain sucking patterns are reinforcing. They will kick in a particular way if a ribbon tied to their leg causes a mobile to juggle (Rovee-Collier, Sullivan, Enright, Lucus, & Fagen, 1980). They will respond in a similar vocal pattern to the rhythmic voice of their parents. They will babble differently to each parent; using a lower pitch when babbling to their father (Reich, 1986, p. 29). Hand-to-mouth behavior, observed during fetal development, is used for self-calming in the postnatal period.

After the first few weeks of life, infants start to have longer periods of wakefulness and begin to amuse and comfort themselves. Finger or hand sucking is common and the infant shows joy at the sight of a familiar face. Cycles of wakefulness and sleep are more established and the family settles into a routine that is very important for the infant.

During infancy, the primitive reflexes (Table 2.6) that dominated the first few weeks of life begin to lessen in prominence. The rooting reflex is replaced by an active visual search for the mother's breast or bottle. The asymmetrical tonic neck reflex (ATNR), which should never be dominant, is easily overcome. The Moro reflex is no longer present; however, an infant might display a similar movement pattern to the Moro when startled by an irritating noise. Postural reactions that assist in the progression of movement begin to appear.

Rolling Over

The infant joyously begins to discover and experience the environment and movement during the first few

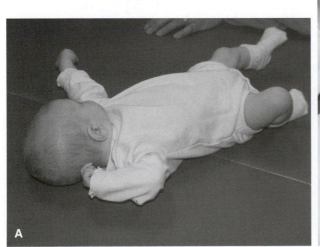
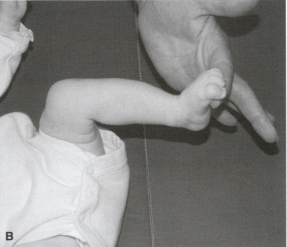

Figure 2.5 Reflexes commonly seen in infants. (*A*) Asymmetrical tonic neck reflex (ATNR). (*B*) Plantar grasp tested in supine position.

Table 2.4 Development of Functional Movement by Age and Position*

Rolling	
3–4 months	Rolls from supine to side lying, rolls from prone to side accidentally
5–7 months	Rolls from prone to supine with right and left leg performing independent movements
6–14 months	Rolls segmentally prone to supine and back with roll initiated by the head, shoulder, or hips
Crawling/Creeping	
7 months	Crawls forward on belly; assumes quadruped position on hands and knees
7–10 months [8.5 months (SD 1.7) (WHO, 2006)]**	Reciprocal creep on all fours (opposite/contralateral upper and lower extremities move simultaneously)
10–11 months	Creeps on hands and feet (plantigrade)
10–12 months	Creeps well, over, around, and on objects
Sitting	
0–3 months (held in sitting position)	Initially head bobs in sitting, back rounded, hips are apart, turned out, and bent; then head is steady; chin tucks; able to gaze at floor; sits with less support; hips are bent and shoulders are in front of hips
5–6 months (supports self in sitting position)	Sits alone momentarily with increased back extension, wide base, bent legs, and periodic use of "high guard" position with arms; sits by propping forward on arms; protective responses with arms present when falling to the front
5–10 months (sits alone) [6.0 months (SD 1.1) (WHO, 2006)]	Sits alone steadily, can flex head and keep cervical extension, initially wide base of support; able to play with toys in sitting position
6–11 months	Goes from sitting to quadruped or prone; gets to sitting position from prone
7–8 months	Equilibrium reactions are present; able to rotate upper body while lower body remains stationary; protective responses using arms are present when falling to the side; plays with toy in sitting
8–10 months	Sits well without support; legs are closer; full upright position, knees straight; increased variety of sitting positions, including "w" sit and side sit; difficult fine motor tasks may prompt return to wide base of support
9–18 months	Rises from supine position by rolling over to stomach then pushing up into four-point position, then to sitting
10–12 months	Protective extension backwards, first with bent elbows then straight elbows; able to move freely in and out of sitting position into other positions
11–12 months	Trunk control and equilibrium responses are fully developed in sitting, further increase in variety of positions
11–24+ months	Rises from supine by first rolling to side then pushing up into sitting position
Standing	
0–3 months	When held in standing position, takes some weight on legs
2–3 months	When held in standing position, legs may give way
3–4 months	Bears some weight on legs, but must be held proximally; head is up in midline, no chin tuck; pelvis and hips are behind shoulders; legs are apart and turned outward
5–10 months [stands with assistance 7.6 months (SD 1.4) (WHO, 2006)]	Increased capability to bear weight; decreased support needed; may be held by arms or hands; legs spread apart and turned outward; bounces in standing position; stands while holding on to furniture
6–12 months	Pulls to standing position at furniture
8–9 months	Rotates the trunk over the leg; legs are more active when pulled to a standing position; pulls to standing by kneeling, then half-kneeling

Standing

9–13 months *[stands alone 11.0 months (SD 1.9) (WHO, 2006)]*	Pulls to standing with legs only, no longer needs to use arms; stands alone momentarily
12 months	Equilibrium reactions are present in standing
31–32 months	Stands on one foot for 1–2 seconds
43–52 months	Stands on tiptoes
53–60 months	Stands on one foot for 10 seconds without swaying more than 20 degrees

Walking

8 months	Cruises sideways at furniture using arms for support
8–18 months	Walks with two hands held
9–10 months	Cruises around furniture, turning slightly in intended direction
9–17 months *[walks alone 12.1 months (SD 1.8) (WHO, 2006)]*	Takes independent steps, falls easily; initial independent walking characterized by excessive hip flexion, external rotation, abduction with wide base of support, knee flexion through stance, no heel strike, hyperextension of swing leg, short stride length and swing phase and scapular adduction and high hand guard (Fig. 2.6L)
10–14 months	Walking: stoops and recovers in play
11 months	Walks with one hand held; reaches for furniture out of reach when cruising; cruises in either direction, no hesitation
18–20 months	Seldom falls; runs stiffly with eyes on ground
25–26 months	Walks backward 10 feet
27–28 months	Walks three steps on a taped line
29–30 months	Runs 30 feet in 6 seconds
41–42 months	Runs with arms moving back and forth, balls of feet used to push forward, high knee and heel lift and trunk leans forward

Stair Climbing

8–14 months	Climbs up stairs on hands, knees, and feet
15–16 months	Walks up stairs while holding on
17–18 months	Walks down stairs while holding on
12–20 months	Crawls/creeps backwards down stairs
24–30 months	Walks up and down stairs without support, marking time
30–36 months	Walks up stairs, alternating feet
36–42 months	Walks down stairs, alternating feet

Jumping and Hopping

2 years	Jumps down from step
2½+ years	Hops on one foot, few steps
3 years	Jumps off floor with both feet
3–5 years	Jumps over objects, hops on one foot
3–4 years	Gallops, leading with one foot and transferring weight smoothly and evenly
5 years	Hops in straight line
5–6 years	Skips on alternating feet, maintaining balance

*Generally, age ranges start with the youngest reported average age and end with the oldest reported average age of typically developing children. All ages and sequences are approximations, as there is wide individual variation.

**Italic ages are averages from the WHO Motor Development Study (2006). SD = standard deviation

Source: References include Bayley (2005); Berger, Theuring, & Adolph (2007); Bly (1994); Case-Smith (2010); Folio & Fewell (2000); and Knobloch & Pasamanick (1974).

Table 2.5 Development of Manipulation by Age and Activity*

Reaching	
Reaching	
0–2 months	Visual regard of objects
1–3 months	Swipes at objects
1–4½ months	Alternating glance from hand to object
2–6 months	Inspects own hands; reaches for, but may not contact, object
3½–4½ months	Visually directed reaching
3½–6 months	Hands are oriented to object, rapid reach for object without contact
4 months	Shoulders come down to natural level; hands are together in space; in sitting bilateral backhand approach with wrist turned so thumb is down
5 months	In prone bilateral approach, hands slide forward; two-handed corralling of object
5–6 months	Elbow is in front of shoulder joint; developing isolated voluntary control of forearm rotation
6 months	In prone, reaches with one hand while weight bearing on the other forearm; elbow is extended, wrist is straight, midway between supination and pronation
7 months	Prone: reaches with one hand while weight bearing on the other extended arm
8–9 months	Unilateral direct approach, reach and grasp single continuous movement
9 months	Controls supination with upper arm in any position, if trunk is stable
10 months	Wrist extended, appropriate finger extension
11–12 months	Voluntary supination, upper arm in any position
Grasp	
0–3 months	Hands are predominantly closed
2–7 months	Object is clutched between little and ring fingers and palm
3–3½ months	Hands clasped together often
4 months	Able to grasp rattle within 3 inches of hand
3–7 months	Able to hold a small object in each hand
4 months	Hands are partly open
4–6 months	Hands are predominantly open
4–8 months	Partial thumb opposition on a cube; attempts to secure tiny objects; picks up cube with ease
5–9 months	Rakes or scoops tiny objects using ulnar grasp
6–7 months	Objects held in palm by finger and opposed thumb (radial palmar grasp)
6–10 months	Picks up tiny objects with several fingers and thumb
7–12 months	Precisely picks up tiny objects
8 months	Tiny objects are held between the side of index finger and thumb (lateral scissors)
8–9 months	Objects are held with opposed thumb and fingertips; space is visible between palm and object
9–10 months	Small objects are held between the thumb and index finger, first near middle of index (inferior pincer) finger; later between pads of thumb and index finger with thumb opposed (pincer)
10 months	Pokes with index finger
12 months	Small objects are held between the thumb and index finger, near tips, thumbs opposed (fine pincer)
12–18 months	Crayon is held in the fist with thumb up
2 years	Crayon is held with fingers, hands on top of tool, forearm turned so thumb is directed downward (digital pronate)

Table 2.5 Development of Manipulation by Age and Activity—cont'd

Release	
0–1 month	No release, grasp reflex is strong
1–4 months	Involuntary release
4 months	Mutual fingering in midline
4–8 months	Transfers object from hand to hand
5–6 months	Taking hand grasps before releasing hand lets go
6–7 months	Taking hand and releasing hand perform actions simultaneously
7–9 months	Volitional release
7–10 months	Presses down on surface to release
8 months	Releases above a surface with wrist flexion
9–10 months	Releases into a container with wrist straight
10–14 months	Clumsy release into small container; hand rests on edge of container
12–15 months	Precise, controlled release into small container with wrist extended
Feeding	Very dependent on environmental affordances
Birth–1 month	Rooting, sucking, and swallowing reflexes
3–4 months	Sucking-swallowing in sequence; mouth poises for nipple
4–6 months	Brings head to mouth; pats bottle or nibble; brings both hands to bottle
6–7½ months	Grasps and draws bottle to mouth; grasps spoon and pulls food off spoon with lips; sucks liquid from cup; keeps lips closed while chewing; explores things with mouth
9–10 months	Feeds self cracker; holds feeding bottle
10–12 months	Tries to feed self using spoon; holds and drinks from cup with spilling; lateral motion of tongue; pincer grasp of finger foods; choosy about food

*Generally, age ranges start with the youngest reported average age and end with the oldest reported average age of typically developing children. All ages and sequences are approximations, as there is wide individual variation.

Source: References: Bayley (2005); Case-Smith (2010); Erhardt (1994); Folio & Fewell (2000); Gesell & Amatruda (1947); Halverson (1931); Knobloch & Pasamanick (1974).

Table 2.6 Selected Primitive Reflexes

Reflex	Weeks of Gestation at Which Reflex Appears	Integrates After Birth*	Stimulus	Response
Asymmetrical tonic neck (ATNR)	20	4–5 months	Turning of head	Facial arm extends and abducts, occipital arm flexes and abducts
Rooting	28	3 months	Touch to perioral area of hungry infant	Turns head and lips toward stimulus
Suck-swallow	28–34	5 months	Touch to lips and inside mouth for suckling and liquid for swallowing	Rhythmic excursions of jaw; tongue rides up and down with jaw; then swallow
Palmar grasp	28	4–7 months	Pressure on palm of hand	Flexion of fingers

Continued

Table 2.6 Selected Primitive Reflexes—cont'd

Reflex	Weeks of Gestation at Which Reflex Appears	Integrates After Birth*	Stimulus	Response
Plantar grasp	28	9 months	Supported standing on feet or pressure to sole of the foot just distal to metatarsal heads	Flexion of toes
Flexor withdrawal	28	1–2 months	Noxious stimulus to sole of foot	Flexion withdrawal of leg
Crossed extension	28	1–2 months, inconsistent	Noxious stimulus to sole of foot	Flexion of stimulated leg and then extension of opposite leg with adduction
Galant (trunk incurvation)	28	3 months, inconsistent	In prone, stroke paravertebral skin	Lateral curvature of trunk on stimulated side
Moro	28	3–5 months	Head drop backward (stimulus for the startle reflex is loud noise with same response)	Abduction and extension of arms, splaying of fingers, may be followed by arm flexion and adduction
Positive support	35	1–2 months, inconsistent	Balls of feet in contact with firm surface	Legs extend to support weight
Automatic walking/reflex stepping	37	3–4 months	Hold upright with feet on support	High stepping movements with regular rhythm
Symmetrical tonic neck (STNR)	4–6 months after full-term delivery	8–12 months	Flexion or extension of head	With head flexion, arms flex and hips extend, with head extension arms extend and hips flex

*A weaker response to the stimulus might generally occur for a few more months.
Source: Peiper (1963); Touwen (1976).

months of life (Fig. 2.6, Table 2.7), first by a mere head turn, then by causing actions such as hitting an object with arms or legs. Tying a bell to an infant's hand or foot can produce endless enjoyment. Slowly the infant learns to turn his body and finally achieves the ability to roll over. This is a monumental event. The infant can now roll off the bed or changing table, much to the parents' concern! McGraw (1945) noted that for initial rolling the infant turns the face laterally and then extends the neck. This raises the shoulder on the side the occiput is turned, and leads to spinal extension. The rolling movement is generally initiated by the movement of the shoulder girdle. Later the initial movement might occur at the pelvic area and the shoulder lags behind (McGraw, 1945). Eventually, there is trunk rotation instead of spinal extension and the infant flexes his legs and raises his abdomen to come to a creeping or

sitting position. Rolling becomes deliberate and is a very important activity because the infant can now roll to reach a desired object or person.

The sequence or direction of infant rolling appears to be culturally dependent. In western cultures, infants have been reported consistently to first roll prone to supine at about 3.6 months (Capute, Shapiro, Palmer, Ross, & Watchel, 1985; Davis, Moon, Sachs, & Ottolini, 1998; Piper & Darrah, 1994). Chinese infants, however, first roll supine to prone (Nelson, Yu, Wong, Wong, & Yim, 2004). Japanese and Chinese mothers do not use the prone position for sleep or play and Asian infants usually learn to roll in any direction later than those reported in the United States (Nelson et al., 2004). Now, with the success of the back-to-sleep campaign to prevent SIDS, there are reports of the reverse order of learning to roll for infants in the United States, with

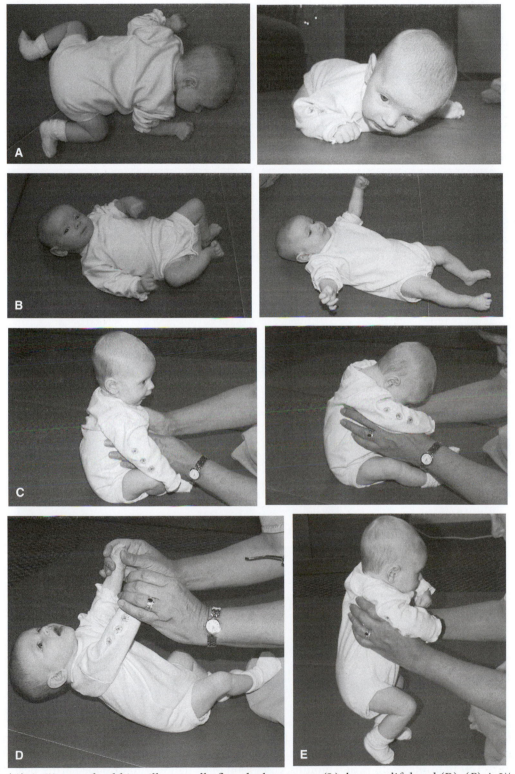

Figure 2.6 (*A*) A 2½-month-old is still generally flexed when prone (L), but can lift head (R). (*B*) A 2½-month-old can alternate between flexion (L) and extension (R) in supine position. (*C*) In supported sitting at 2½ months, the back is still somewhat flexed, but the head is erect or flexed. (*D*) Head lag is still present at 2½ months when infant is pulled to sitting. (*E*) At 2½ months in standing position, the infant might choose to not bear weight. This is called *astasia*.

Continued

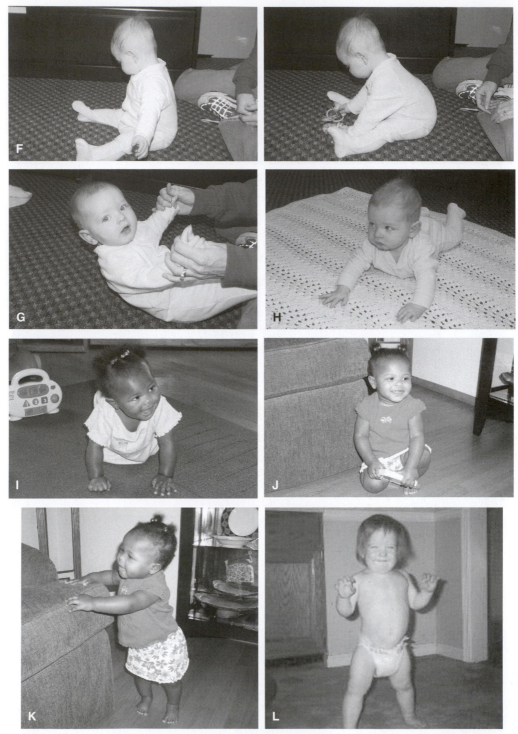

Figure 2.6 cont'd (*F*) At 6 months child can sit independently with erect trunk (L). Can also sit and reach for a toy within basis support (R). (*G*) At 6 months, when child is pulled to sitting, there is antigravity flexion of head, arms, and trunk. (*H*) In prone position at 6 months, child is on open hands with extended arms, head erect, and trunk extended. (*I*) Between 7 to 10 months of age, the infant starts to use creeping on all fours to explore the environment. (*J*) By 11 months, a variety of erect sitting positions are possible, allowing easy and rapid transitions. (*K*) Standing and beginning to cruise at a support surface are common for many, although not all, 11-month-old children. (*L*) When the child is standing independently at 12 months, the arms and legs are abducted and externally rotated.

Table 2.7 Customary Infant Development by Age

	Prone	Supine	Sitting	Upper Extremity	Mobility	Social	Language
1 month	Slightly elevates and rotates head	Reciprocal and symmetrical kicking	Forward flexion of trunk; head in line with trunk	Opens and closes hands; reaching depends on body position and visual gaze on object	Turns head	Visual preferences for humans;	Moves in response to a voice; vocalizes to caregiver's smile and voice
2–3 months	Elbows in line with shoulders for forearm support; lateral weight-shifting; arcs back in pivot prone (Fig. 2.6A)	Symmetrical posture predominates; kicking movements (Fig. 2.6B)	Midline head alignment; minimal head lag during pull-to-sitting; propped sitting with support (Fig. 2.6C)	Reaches and grasps with eye-hand coordination; finger play in mouth	May roll supine to prone	Listens to voices; smiles purposely in response to caregiver's face or voice	Coos; cries to get attention; crying decreases with adult eye contact; vocalizes to express displeasure
4–5 months	Weight-shifting to free arm and reach with one hand	Brings feet to mouth; attempts roll to side with leg or arm leading	No head lag when pulled to sit; static ring sitting emerging; attempts lateral weight-shift to support body with one arm and grasp toy with the other	Arms extend up in supine to reach in midline; palmar grasp on cube; holds toy with two hands	Pivot-prone rotation; may attempt rocking in quadruped and pushing backward; in standing bears weight	Laughs, excited by food; smiles at self in mirror	Turns head toward a voice; vocalizes; laughs and babbles
6–7 months	Elevates trunk with elbow extension; may rock on hands and knees; transitions to sitting; pushes backward (Fig. 2.6H)	Brings feet to chin or mouth; rolls to prone; attempts to raise self to sit	Sits without support while manipulating a toy; weight-shifting with lateral and anterior arm support (Fig. 2.6F)	Brings objects to midline; holds bottle with two hands; rakes for small objects; objects held in palm by fingers and opposed thumb (radial palmar grasp)	Moves forward with arms with or without abdomen elevated; rolls; stands with assistance	Enjoys mirror; lively response to familiar people	Babbles; vocalizes four different syllables; has two syllable combinations; responds to name

Continued

Table 2.7 Customary Infant Development by Age—cont'd

	Prone	Supine	Sitting	Upper Extremity	Mobility	Social	Language
8–9 months	Transitions in and out of sitting to quadruped or prone; pulls to stand with support	Raises self to sit	Manipulates toy in sitting position; anterior, lateral protective reactions present and backward emerging	Controlled release; transfers objects; radial digital grasp	Crawls; creeps; pulls to stand at support (Fig. 2.6I); walks with assistance	Shows initial separation concern; desires to be with people; waves bye	Shouts or vocalizes to gain attention; vocalizes syllables; responds to "no" most of time
10–11 months	Pulls to stand through half-kneeling	Transitions to sitting and quadruped; rarely supine	Rotates or pivots while sitting to reach	Small objects held between thumb and middle of index finger (inferior pincer) later between pads of thumb and index finger (pincer)	Sidesteps or cruises with external support; stands alone; walks with one hand held (Fig. 2.6K)	Plays peek-a-boo and patty-cake; waves bye-bye; has fear of strangers; performs for attention	Says repetitive consonant sounds like mama, dada; gives objects upon verbal request
12 months	Stands up through quadruped	Moves rapidly into sitting or quadruped to standing	Wide variety of sitting positions	Small objects held between tips of thumb and index finger (fine or superior pincer); rolls a ball; scoops with spoon; finger feeds	Independent walking with high hand guard and wide base of support; lowers self with control from standing; may move in and out of full squat position	Actively engages in play, understands and follows simple commands; performs for social attention;	Points to 3 body parts; imitates name of familiar objects; vocalizes with intent; uses a word to call a person; understands simple commands; identifies two body parts

Source: Bly (1994); Case-Smith (2010); Folio & Fewell (2000); Long & Toscano (2002); Rossetti (2005); and WHO (2006).

rolling supine to prone likely to occur first (Liao, Zawacki, & Campbell, 2005). Unfortunately, many infants who spend much of their time in supine might not like prone (Dudek-Shriber & Zelazny, 2007) and therefore are reluctant to roll to prone. This trend might account for the reported delays in achieving the important motor skills of tripod sitting, crawling, creeping, and pulling to stand in a timely manner (Davis et al., 1998; Dewey, Fleming, Golding, & the ALSPAC Study Team, 1998). Four-month-old infants who spend more time in prone while awake are reported to achieve many motor milestones in prone, supine, and sitting before infants who spend less time awake in prone (Dudek-Shriber & Zelazny, 2007).

Sitting

While infants are learning to roll, their parents are placing them in supported sitting in which their heads are flexed and their spines are rounded in a "c" curve. As sitting skills progress, many systems will be involved as body proportions and dimensions change, perceptual abilities develop, and the ability to generate forces to maintain an erect head and trunk advances. Environmental factors also influence sitting. Harbourne and Stergiou (2003) note that infants "dynamically assemble the sitting posture by increasing the stability and regularity of their strategy, and controlling the degrees of freedom first to approximate the skill, then to explore adaptations to function in the environment" (p. 376).

In supported upright vertical positions, the infant's head begins to right itself using a combination of visual, proprioceptive, and labyrinthine inputs, traditionally referred to as reflexes (Fiorentino, 1972). The infant uses those inputs to maintain head-upright positions in supported sitting. Initially, the care provider must support the sitting infant's trunk to prevent the infant from falling over. Slowly the infant learns to use the trunk musculature and controls the degrees of freedom to maintain the upright position with less and less outside support. As the infant advances in sitting ability, there is an increase in the degrees of freedom of the body (Harbourne & Stergiou, 2003). By 5 months of age, just prior to achieving independent sitting, the infant begins to display directionally appropriate muscle responses during movement of the support surface (Hadders-Algra et al., 1996).

At approximately 6 months of age, infants learn to sit independently (WHO, 2006). Initially they will use their arms for support. Soon their heads and trunks become more erect and they can turn their heads, showing dynamic stabilization of the linked segments of the body. With practice, infants are able to slowly lift up one, then two hands, and then play with a toy in their lap while sitting. Their balance ability is controlled mainly by their hips, within their cone of stability. They have stable postural control. Eventually, they will rotate in sitting to reach toys on either side and then behind themselves. This ability to shift positions in sitting shows increased complexity of movement and increasing dynamic control of the sitting posture (Harbourne & Stergiou, 2003). Infants at this age will also learn to protect themselves from falling by extending their arms using a **protective reaction** (parachute). By 9 months, they can protect themselves in all directions, including backward, the last protective reaction to emerge in sitting (Haley, 1986; Milani-Comparetti & Gidoni, 1967).

Crawling, Creeping, and Prone Positions

As the infant's skill in sitting further develops, infants in Western cultures usually learn to move around on their stomachs. They use a wide variety of interlimb patterns. They might use a combat/amphibian crawl by flexing and extending all extremities or a homolateral crawling pattern where both the arm and leg on the same side of the body flex or extend in synchrony.* This skill is usually followed by the more advanced pattern of reciprocal arm and leg movements, also called contralateral crawling, where the opposite arm and leg flex and extend together.

Some infants never crawl on their bellies (Adolph et al., 1998) but will learn to get up on hands and knees and rock, perhaps falling backward instead of forward. Soon they learn to creep on all fours. Creeping is far more efficient than rolling or crawling. Initially they might move one limb at a time to maintain a stable posture, followed perhaps by a homolateral creep in which the arm and leg on the same side of the body flex or extend at the same time and then the **reciprocal creeping pattern** (also called diagonal or contralateral pattern) in which the opposite arm and leg flex and extend together.

McGraw noted in 1945 that no other neuromuscular function of the infant had greater individual variation than the prone progression of crawling and creeping. Research by Adolph and colleagues (1998) found no strict, stage-like progression, although most infants did display most milestones. Some infants skipped expected

---

*Historically, when reading international literature, the term creeping is used for movement on the belly and *crawling* is used for on all fours, which is the reverse of the usual United States professional terminology. In recent years, there is much greater inconsistency in United States professional terminology, and it is now best to add descriptive terms when discussing crawling and creeping, such as crawling on the belly or creeping on the hands and knees.

stages such as crawling on their belly altogether, and there was a wide range of onset of belly crawling and creeping on hands and knees. Experience in belly crawling did not affect the age of onset of creeping on hands and knees. Smaller, slimmer, and more maturely proportioned infants did begin to creep on hands and knees earlier than bigger, fatter, top-heavy infants. They also found that infants used different crawling/creeping patterns from week to week and even test cycle to test cycle. Although infants who crawled on their bellies did not start to creep on hands and knees any earlier than those who never crawled, the former belly crawlers were more proficient on hands and knees compared with the nonbelly crawlers. Superiority in velocity and cycle times lasted for 7 to 20 weeks after onset of creeping (Adolph, 2003). Thus, motoric experience did play a role in quality of the execution of the motor task but not in initial achievement of the task. A study by the WHO (2006) done in five diverse nations noted that 4.3% of the infants never exhibited hands and knees creeping and there was a wide range for achieving this milestone, between 5.2 and 13.5 months. Adolph (2003) also reported that infants who crawl or creep spend about 5 hours per day on the floor, and move 27 to 43 meters per hour, 60 to 188 meters per day, a total of about the length of two football fields! Compare that statistic with the total dearth of active movement activities, less than 10 minutes per morning, seen in children with disabilities in preschool classrooms (Effgen & Chan, 2010; Ott & Effgen, 2000).

As infants crawl and creep exploring the environment they will, by around 11 months, ascend stairs and several weeks later descend stairs (13 months). Children who have stairs in the home ascend stairs at a slightly younger age and use a backing strategy to descend, but there is no difference in the overall age of ascent and descent (Berger, Theuring, & Adolph, 2007). When descending, 76% of the infants studied turned around and crawled or slid down backward, feet first, while others scooted in a sitting position and a few crawled or slid down face first in prone (Berger et al., 2007).

In 1992, a correlation was made between SIDS and sleeping in prone. The American Academy of Pediatrics (1992) recommended that all healthy infants be positioned on their backs for sleeping. As a result of this national effort to have all children sleep supine, the incidence of SIDS has decreased 50%. However, an unexpected consequence of encouraging supine sleeping is that many infants spend little, if any, time awake in prone position. This trend has led to secondary

problems of plagiocephaly (head deformity), acquired torticollis, and delayed development of the prone progression of rolling, crawling, and creeping (Davis et al., 1998; Dewey et al., 1998; Jantz, Blosser, & Fruechting, 1997; Mildred, Beard, Dallwitz, & Unwin, 1995). Prone positioning for play while awake is not a risk factor for SIDS, and parents need to be encouraged to play with their infants in prone during supervised "tummy time" (American Academy of Pediatrics, 2000). The American Physical Therapy Association, Section on Pediatrics and many children's hospitals now have fact sheets for parents explaining the back to sleep program and the need for tummy time. Unfortunately, national magazines geared toward woman of childbearing age rarely portray appropriate sleep environments (Joyner, Gill-Bailey, & Moon, 2009), so one must overcome the media to provide appropriate information for the best sleeping and awake positions.

Pulling Up, Cruising, Standing, and Walking

Once infants learn to creep, they will attempt to pull to standing. The success of this effort will depend on the integration of many systems and the person or object used to pull to standing. Trying to pull to standing at a flat wall is usually unsuccessful, but the sides of a crib, low table, or sofa are commonly the first places infants pull to standing. The problem is then how to get down! This is when infants call for help, either when they recognize they cannot get down, or after they have an uncontrolled fall from standing. These can be trying times for parents because infants insist on using their new skill of pulling to standing but might still require assistance to come safely down again.

Infants usually stand with assistance at 7.6 months (WHO, 2006). While in standing they will begin to shift weight and might even lift a leg. This weight shift is not only the start of upright balancing but also the start of upright mobility, because infants will soon learn to cruise along a supporting surface. **Cruising** along an object such as a sofa or low table is an important developmental skill because of the unilateral weight bearing, weight shifting, balance, and synergistic hip abduction/adduction required for movement. Cruising apparently is controlled by the arms, and infants do not initially take their legs and the floor into account to balance and respond adaptively (Adolph, 2003).

As infants freely creep and cruise, there are also initial attempts at standing independently, walking with support, and taking independent steps. There is great variability in achievement of these upright movements. Independent standing occurs around 10 to 11 months

(Folio & Fewell, 2000; Piper & Darrah, 1994; WHO, 2006), although as many as 10% of infants may not stand alone at 13 months (Piper & Darrah, 1994; WHO, 2006). Independent walking occurs at about 12 months ±3 months (Folio & Fewell, 2000; Sutherland, Olshen, Biden, & Wyatt, 1988; WHO, 2006) but African American children tend to walk at 10.9 months (Capute et al., 1985). Piper and Darrah (1994) found that 90% of children walk by 14 months. Some American children do not walk until 15.5 months (Bayley, 2005), and the WHO (2006) international study found 17.6 months as the upper limit of normal variation in walking alone. Gait development is a complex interaction of neurological, musculoskeletal, and biomechanical factors, which is presented from a developmental perspective here and from a biomechanical perspective in Chapter 5.

The infant's first steps are an exciting time for the infant and family, and this is an important milestone in most cultures. Sutherland, Statham, and their colleagues (Statham & Murray, 1971; Sutherland, Olshen, Cooper & Woo, 1980; Sutherland et al., 1988) note that **early walking** (Table 2.8) is characterized by a wide base of support, and arms are held in "high hand guard"

(abduction, external rotation, and flexion with scapular adduction), unless they are outstretched, such as when reaching forward for a parent. The hips are abducted, flexed, and slightly externally rotated; knee flexion occurs at foot contact and remains flexed through midstance and then knee extension occurs. At the ankle, there is no heel strike, and floor contact is usually with a flat foot followed by ankle dorsiflexion until midstance, where it decreases. There is no plantar flexion for push-off. Sufficient extensor strength is considered critical for independent ambulation (Thelen, Ulrich, & Jensen, 1989).

It is interesting to note that when just learning to walk independently, infants return to an earlier two-handed reaching behavior (Corbetta & Bojczyk, 2002). When they achieve better balance in walking, the two-handed reaching declined. It is possible that "the postural reorganization and development of new coordination skills associated with the transition to upright locomotion temporarily affect infants' ability to reach adaptively" (p. 84).

Three requirements for locomotion are noted by Shumway-Cook and Woollacott (2007, p. 336): (1) a

Table 2.8 Development of Walking

Initial Walking *First 3-6 months after learning to walk*	Immature Walking *Approximately 2 years of age*	Mature Walking *7 years of age; approximates adult gait*
Unpredictable loss of balance	Occasionally loses balance	Rarely loses balance without perturbation
Rigid, halting stepping	Gradual smoothing of pattern	Relaxed, elongated gait
Short step length (22 cm)	Increased step length (28 cm at 2 years and 33 cm at 3 years)	Increased step length (48 cm)
High hand guard/outstretched arms	Reciprocal arm swing*	Reciprocal arm swing
Flat-foot contact	Heel strike*	Heel strike
Wide base of support	Base of support within lateral dimensions of the trunk	Narrow base of support
Toes turned out/external rotation	Minimal out toeing/external rotation	
	Vertical lift	Minimal vertical lift
Brief single limb stance (32% of gait cycle)	Longer single limb stance (34% of gait cycle)	38% of gait cycle single limb stance
Knee flexion in stance	Greater knee flexion after foot strike and then extends before toe-off*	

Source: Adapted from Shumway-Cook & Woollacott, 2007; Sutherland et al., 1980; Sutherland et al., 1988).
*All should be present by 18 months and their absence at age 2 years may indicate a pathological gait (Sutherland et al., 1980, p. 351; Sutherland et al., 1988, p. 151).

rhythmic stepping pattern, (2) the ability to balance, and (3) the ability to modify and adapt gait to needs of the environment. Rhythmic stepping develops first and is seen in the neonate. Then the stability required to balance develops as the child learns to walk during the end of the first year and beginning of the second year of life. In addition, the child must want to walk. There needs to be a reason or desire to use upright movement. Some children with disabilities do not initially display a desire to walk and must be motivated. Last, the adaptability required for generalization of ambulation across environments is refined during the second year of life.

As the child gains experience in walking and learns to control balance, the step length increases rapidly over the first few months of independent walking, the lateral distance between the feet decreases, there is increased single limb support time, velocity increases and the child can move slower and start and stop (Sutherland et al., 1988). Infants also occasionally begin to take steps that exceed their leg length, which reflects more balance and strength than originally expected in early infant walkers (Badaly & Adolph, 2008).

Shortly after learning to walk unsupported, the infant will use walking as the primary means of locomotion; creeping will greatly decrease. This initial phase of learning to walk occurs for 3 to 6 months after the onset of walking. Contemporary researchers plot walking skills by time post–walking onset and not by age as was done by the early infant researchers (Adolph & Berger, 2006).

The ability of infants to adapt their movements to changes in the environment has been studied by Adolph and colleagues. They changed the degree of slope on the walking path of infants (Gill, Adolph, & Vereijken, 2009) and changed the infants' body dimensions by adding weights to their chests (Adolph & Avolio, 2000). The infants generally overestimated their ability but were able to adjust their gait based on the degree of slope. The success rate decreased as the degree of slant increased; however, the more experienced walkers could handle the steeper slopes. In fact, experience in walking, not age, could predict their walking boundaries on the slopes. An interesting finding was that initially when wearing the weights, many babies weaved and staggered, but by the end of the first session they became "stiffer" and their gait appeared more normal. They adapted to the task by perhaps limiting their degrees of freedom and using more muscle contraction. Adolph and Avolio suggest that adaptation occurred on many levels, including behavioral, kinematic, and muscular, demonstrating the complex interacting processes of a dynamic system.

Development of Upper Extremity Function

Development of upper extremity function involving reach, grasp, and release are critical for environmental exploration, learning, and self-feeding as outlined in Table 2.5 and shown in Figure 2.7. For the first 2 months of life, whenever an infant extends the arm, the hand opens at the same time. This movement makes it difficult to grasp an object, unless an appropriate sized object is pressed into the palm of the hand eliciting a palmar grasp reflex. By age 2 months, the arm can extend and the fingers can flex, allowing for voluntary grasping of an object.

One way to view reaching is to look at its functional components. The first component is the transportation phase, which serves to bring the hand to the target. This component and early reaching in general are controlled largely by the proximal shoulder muscles (Halverson, 1933; Spencer & Thelen, 2000), suggesting a proximodistal nature of development for this activity (Berthier, Clifton, McCall, & Robin, 1999); however, infants reach first with their feet (Galloway & Thelen, 2004). The second component of reaching is the grasp phase, where the hand anticipates the object. This component involves primarily the distal joints and muscles. The complexity of the movement is controlled by limiting the degrees of freedom at the elbow. In early reaching there is little change in elbow angle (Berthier et al., 1999). Because joint stiffness decreases the abilities of the arm and increases energetic cost of the movement, joint stiffening is seen only in the initial phases of the learning process (Berthier & Keen, 2006). By 6 months of age the infant no longer locks the elbow and freely uses it in reaching.

Successful, goal-directed reaching typically starts at about 16 weeks of age. Berthier and Keen (2006) indicate several factors that influence early reaching including: speed/jerk, number of speed peaks/duration, time of peak speed, distance of the reach, and straightness of the reach. The variables are highly intercorrelated. The infant reaches are significantly curved and become straighter and less jerky with age. With development, the time of maximum hand speed during reach movement moves closer to the beginning of the reach; however, there are some inconsistencies in studies regarding the speed of reaching and peaks or number of movement units. Halverson (1933) originally noted that the speed of reaching increases with the age of the infant; however, studies using modern technology have shown a significant

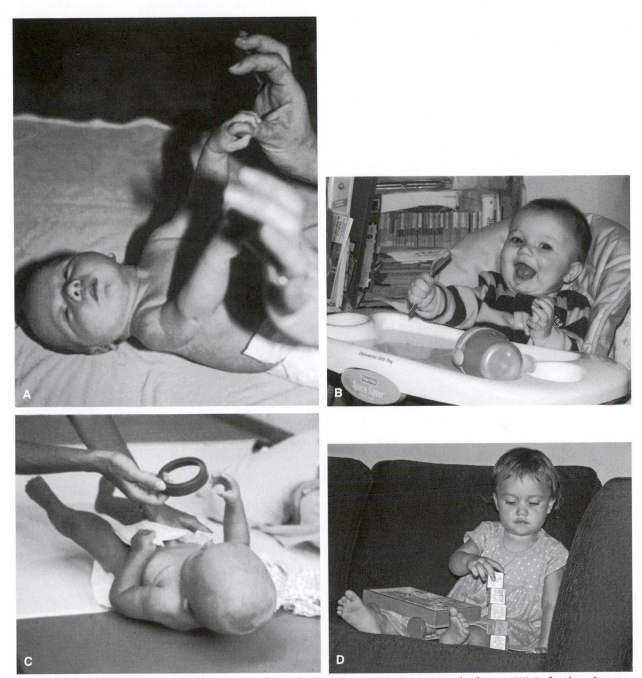

Figure 2.7 Development of Manipulation. (*A*) Newborn infant's palmar grasp of a finger. (*B*) Infant's voluntary palmar grasp of a spoon. (*C*) Infant reaching for an object with hand open. (*D*) Radial digital grasp of block with opposed thumb and fingertips.

Continued

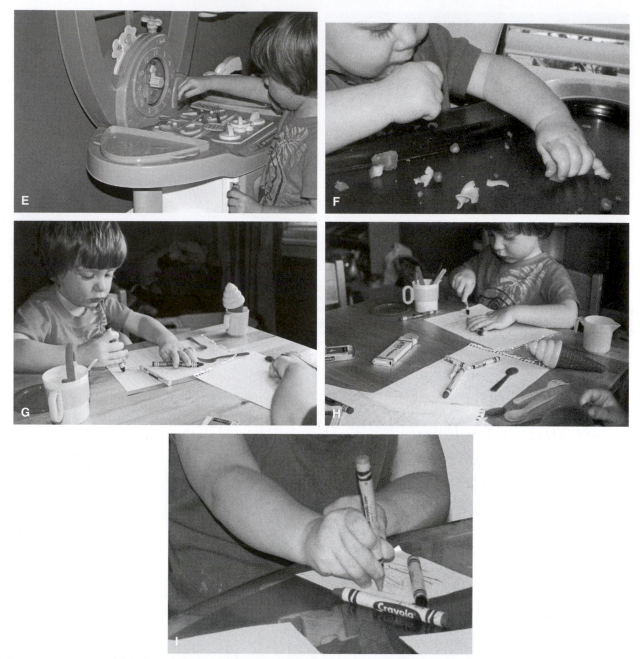

Figure 2.7 cont'd (*E*) Inferior pincer grasp using thumb and side of index finger. (*F*) An attempt at a superior pincer grasp using tip of index finger and almost tip of thumb. (*G*) Palmar-supinate grasp of crayon. (*H*) Digital-pronate grasp of crayon with extended index finger. Same child at same age as in Figure 2.7G, but having switched to a more mature grasp of the crayon. (*I*) Static tripod grasp of crayon.

decrease in speed (Berthier & Keen, 2006; Fetters & Todd, 1987: Thelen, Corbetta, & Spencer, 1996), or no change (Konczak & Dichgans, 1997). Berthier and Keen (2006) note that the decrease in speed is probably a reflection of the increase in smoothness of reaching and that reaching depends on the ability, motivation, and goals of the infant. This is in line with Thelen and colleagues, who noted that reaching is probably not a preexisting motor program, but depends on the opportunities and intention of hand use (Thelen et al., 1993).

Postural stability is an important component in reaching. As infants start to reach, there is increased postural activity. Postural muscle activation accompanies goal-directed reaching in infants 3 to 6 months of age before the onset of successful reaching at 4 to 6 months of age (van der Fits, Klip, van Eykern, & Hadders-Algra, 1999). The young infant will tend to use both hands in a symmetric and synergistic manner with the hands meeting at midline to reach the object; only later is there a one-handed reach (Rochat, 1992). Rochat also noted that when infants first achieved the ability to sit without support, they used a one-handed reach and used the other hand to maintain balance. In nonindependent sitters, the quality of reaching was improved when a firm postural support for sitting was provided (Hopkins & Rönnqvist, 2002). The postural control is anticipatory and by 10 months of age, when infants are sitting independently and have relatively mature reaching movements, they will activate the muscles of their trunk before making arm movements (von Hofsten & Woollacott, 1989).

Grasp and Release   Neonates, who initially can grasp a parent's finger using a palmar grasp reflex, soon can bring their hands to midline and keep them open. By 4 months, infants have learned to voluntarily hold and then involuntarily release an appropriately sized object. They hold the object in the palm of their hands initially without using the thumb. By 4 to 5 months the fingers flex and the thumb adducts. The infant can transfer objects from hand to hand, hold a bottle with two hands, and use a "raking and scooping" **ulnar palmar grasp** of smaller objects by 6 months of age. The infant then progresses from an ulnar palmar grasp to a more refined palmar grasp and then a **radial palmar grasp** (Fig. 2.7F) where objects are grasped from the radial side of the hand. Eventually the infant will need to use only the fingers to grasp small objects. Unfortunately, release of objects is not well developed until around 9 months, so although 6-month-old infants can grasp and enjoy rattles, they can also get very frustrated because they may not yet be able to voluntarily release the rattle.

Between 7 and 12 months grasp continues to change rapidly. By 10 months, a **"three-jaw chuck"** grasp is used involving the distal pads of the thumb and the index and middle fingers. The infant should also have a crude voluntary release of objects into a large container. Infants will have problems properly orienting objects such as a spoon in their hands. The 12-month-old infant usually has a **superior pincer grasp** (also called fine pincer grasp) and can pick up small items such as pieces of cereal or raisins using the tips of the index finger and thumb. The 12-month-old infant will use various grasping patterns depending on the object. Between 12 and 15 months the infant also has a precise, controlled release of objects into a small container with the wrist extended. The infant can now finger-feed foods, hold a bottle independently, and hold and drink from a cup with some spilling. The ability to drink from a cup without a lid will depend on the opportunity the infant has to learn this skill. The frequent use of covered cups and continued bottle drinking can delay acquisition of independent cup-drinking skills.

Parents must now be very cautious about what is available in the environment for children to pick up and put in their mouths or other body openings. Noses and ears are all too common receptacles! Choking on small objects becomes a serious risk.

During this period of infant development, there is great variability among infants as evidenced in the wide age ranges of normal achievement of motor skills seen in standardized assessments. Some infants will display accelerated hand manipulation while seemingly lagging behind in mobility skills. Others display wonderful social skills while preferring to sit still in one place for extended periods. Great care must be taken when determining if there is a true deviation in development, delay in development, or merely typical variation. A number of standardized tests and measures are available to help examine many aspects of development and are discussed in the next chapter.

Development of Language, Social, and Play Skills

From smiling to laughing to responding to familiar people, infants continue to advance in their interaction with others. The infant learns to communicate very early in life by crying to get attention and convey needs. The 4- to 5-month-old will vocalize, laugh, and babble. Babbling continues, and by about 10 months infants will make repetitive consonant sounds such as the all important "mama" and "dada." They start to imitate words and sounds and use real words. Fear of strangers may present itself late in the first year of life. By 12 months, the infant can point to three body parts, imitate names of familiar objects, vocalize with intent, use a word to call a person, and follow a simple command. They also use pointing in prelinguistic communication to influence adult interactions involving multiple layers of intentionality (Tomasello, Carpenter, & Liszkowski, 2007). Language will be based on experiences and interaction with people and the environment.

Twelve-month-olds will engage in sensorimotor play as they discover their bodies and use their bodies in action. They can play alone in solitary play and eventually their play evolves into functional play. Infants who reach developmental milestones sooner in their first year of life, such as learning to stand alone, and have three or more words at 1 year of age are reported to fare better and have higher educational levels in adolescence and adulthood than slower developers (Taanila, Murray, Isohanni, & Rantakallio, 2005).

Toddlers

Toddlers, 1 to 3 years of age, are wonderful bundles of energy, trying even the most patient of parents. They want and need to explore everything! They learn by doing. Their ability to adapt to the demands of the environment continues to advance. Toddlers learn to run everywhere, climb up and over everything, and climb stairs. They must be watched very carefully. Some, however, are content to sit and perform manipulative tasks or look through picture books for extended periods. Extremely active or sedentary behavior may just be a variation of typical development, may reflect the temperament common to their ethnic group, or may be an indication of possible abnormality. Children who prefer manipulative activities tend to excel in them and might need encouragement to participate in mobility activities. Research suggests a relationship between high stimulation-seeking behaviors at age 3 years and higher IQs at 11 years of age (Raine, Reynolds, Venables, & Mednick, 2002). Perhaps toddlers who seek stimulation create an enriched environment that stimulates their cognitive development (Fig. 2.8; Tables 2.4 and 2.9).

Between birth and 2 years of age the infant's body dimensions become more evenly proportioned; height nearly doubles and weight more than quadruples (CDC, 2011b). The leg length increases by 130%, but head circumference increases by only 50%. These changes in body dimensions and proportions are important because of the impact on physical constraints and balance ability. As the center of mass lowers, the body becomes more stable and less muscle force is required to stand; however there are inconsistent findings on the effect of body dimension on walking skills (Adolph & Avolio, 2000).

Development of Postural Control and Locomotion

Toddlers continue to advance their skills in walking. In gait, the length of time in double-limb support decreases, as does step width, pelvic tilt, abduction, and external rotation (Table 2.8) (Sutherland et al., 1988).

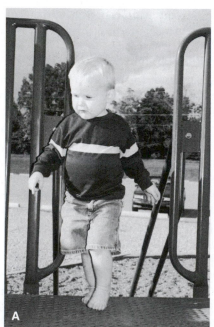 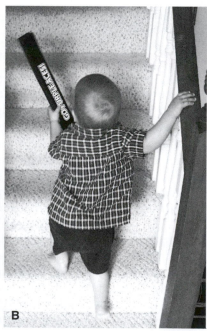 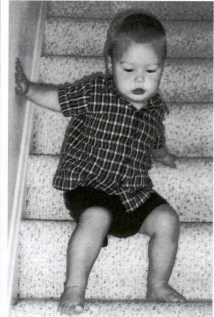

Figure 2.8 Toddler development. (*A*) Walking is mastered, with hands down at sides swinging, and a narrow base of support. (*B*) Going upstairs holding on and standing is easy, but going down is frequently more easily done in the sitting position.

Continued

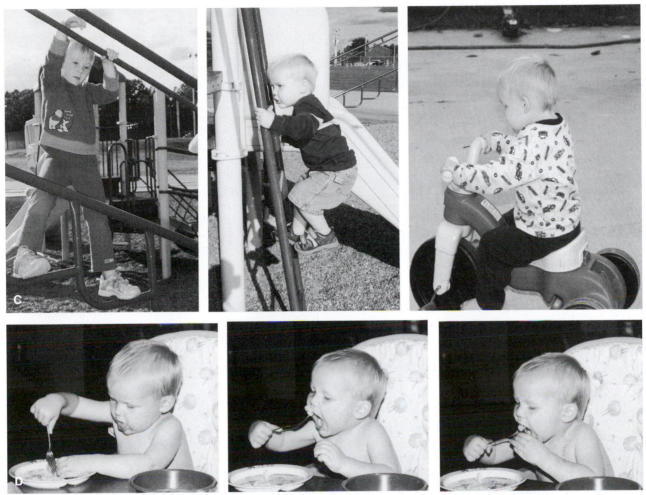

Figure 2.8 cont'd (*C*) Climbing and playing at the playground is fun and excellent for gross motor development. (*D*) Independent feeding is an important and enjoyable activity. Note the open mouth and protruding tongue as the child tries to get food on the fork. Then a bit of a miss before successfully getting the food in his mouth!

Ankle dorsiflexion appears during the swing phase of the gait cycle, and by age 2 years, toddlers begin to have push-off in stance. Adaptation to environmental influences occurs at the behavioral, kinematic, and muscular levels. Toddlers can adjust their judgments to sudden, adverse changes in body dimension such as the introduction of a weighted vest when walking (Adolph & Avolio, 2000). By 15 to 17 months, they show consistent anticipatory postural control in standing; after 3 months of walking experience 80% of trials included anticipatory activation of the leg muscles (Witherington et al., 2002).

Toddlers now start to run (Fig. 2.9), but it is really a fast walk. Initially, they run with a short, limited leg swing; stiff, uneven stride; no flight phase; incomplete extension of the support leg; short arm swing; and wide base of support (Gallahue & Ozmum, 2006). A flight phase, which characterizes running, will not be seen until around the second birthday. At that point in time there is an increase in stride length, arm swing, and speed, along with more complete extension of the support leg. Two-year-olds will also jump up and down from a step. According to Gallahue and Ozmum (2006), when engaged in horizontal jumping, toddlers initially have limited arm swing, the trunk moves vertically, they have difficulty using both feet, and they have limited extension of the ankles, knees, and hips at takeoff (Fig. 2.10). As toddlers mature, their horizontal jump progresses, so the arms initiate the jumping action and remain toward the front of the body during the preparatory crouch. The arms move out to the side to maintain balance during flight, and the preparatory

Table 2.9 Customary Child Development by Age Across Domains

	Mobility	Manipulation	Cognitive	Language	Social-Emotional
13–18 months	Walks freely; creeps up stairs; stoops to pick up objects and regains standing	Imitative scribble; palmar-supinate grasp of pencil; precise release of pellet into small container	Understands and follows simple commands; includes others as recipients of play behaviors; points to three body parts	Uses expressive jargon; talks rather than gestures; recessive language greater than expressive; shakes head "no"; says 15 meaningful words	Experiences peak of separation distress; imitates other children
18–24 months	Begins to run; creeps backwards down stairs or climbs stairs using railing (Fig. 2.7B)	Spontaneous scribble	Demonstrates invention of new means through mental combinations; finds hidden objects through invisible displacement; shows deferred imitation; activates toy or doll in pretend play	Understands multiword utterances; uses multiword utterance to express complex thoughts, e.g., "Mommy go," "Baby up"; 50-200+ word vocabulary; identifies pictures when named	Demonstrates less separation distress; begins to show empathic responses to another's distress; uses words to protest
24–36 months	Jumps off low step; begins to ride a tricycle; kicks small ball; throws over hand (Fig. 2.7C)	Digital-pronate grasp of pencil; imitates vertical then horizontal stroke	Shows ability to substitute objects in pretend play; matches objects; responds to 2 or 3 commands; sings songs	Rapid increase in language; uses verb strategies to start a conversation; uses two-part sentences ("me go home"); demands response from others, 250+ word vocabulary	Begins to respond verbally to another's distress; includes others in pretend plan; pretends to perform caregiver's routines
3 years	Demonstrates true run, with both feet leaving ground; walks upstairs alternating feet; walks downstairs using marking time; jumps off step and over 2-inch object	Copies circle	Tells simple story; knows conventional counting words up to 5; tells action in pictures; puts together puzzle; follows a 3-step unrelated command	Is versatile in language use; speaks in more complete sentences; distinguishes graphics as writing versus picture graphics; begins to overgeneralize rules creating verb tenses and plurals; uses adult syntax and grammar	Uses physical aggression more than verbal aggression; shows an interest in why and how things work

Table 2.9 Customary Child Development by Age Across Domains—cont'd

	Mobility	Manipulation	Cognitive	Language	Social-Emotional
3½ years	Can hop a few steps on preferred foot; kicks ball; mounts, pedals and dismounts 3-wheel riding vehicle	Traces diamond with angles rounded	Can't easily distinguish reality from fantasy; can count 5 objects	Might use syllable hypothesis to create written words; rereads favorite storybooks using picture-governed strategies; often uses scribble-writing	Has difficulty generating alternatives in a conflict situation; will learn aggressive behavior rapidly if initially successful
4 years	Walks downstairs alternating feet; gallops; stands on tip toes; rotation of body follows throw of ball	Cuts straight line with scissors; copies cross; uses static tripod grasp of pencil	Makes row of objects equal to another row by matching; gives age; makes opposite analogies; matches and names 4 colors	Creates questions and negative sentences using correct word arrangement; imitation of parents' intonation pattern; voice well modulated and firm	Watches, on average, 2–4 hours of TV per day
4½ years	Catches ball if prepared; jumps 2–3 inches; leans forward when jumping from a height	May begin to hold writing tool in finger grip; can button small buttons; copies square	Knows conventional counting up to 15; better able to distinguish reality from fantasy	Often reverses letter when writing; understands beside, between, and back; does not notice or grasp print conventions	
5 years	Can stop and change directions quickly when running; can hop 8–10 steps on 1 foot; throws ball and hits target at 10 ft; roller skates; rides bike	Uses dynamic tripod grasp of pencil; copies triangle	Appreciates past, present and future; creates classes of objects based on a single defining attribute; counts to 20	Understands passive sentences; may begin to use invented spellings	Is still poor at self-control; success depends on removal of temptation or diversion by others

Continued

■ **Table 2.9** Customary Child Development by Age Across Domains—cont'd

	Mobility	Manipulation	Cognitive	Language	Social-Emotional
6 years	Can skip	Can connect a zipper on a coat; may tie shoes; moves a writing tool with fingers while side of hand rests on table; copies diamond	Begins to demonstrate concrete operational thinking	Appreciates jokes and riddles based on phonological ambiguity	Feels one way only about a situation; has some difficulty detecting intentions accurately in situations where damage occurs
7 years		Makes small, controlled marks with pencils due to more refined finger dexterity	Begins to use some rehearsal strategies to aid memory; better able to play strategy games; may demonstrate conservation of mass and length	Appreciates jokes and riddles based on lexical ambiguity; might have begun to read	May express two emotions about one situation, but these will be same valence; understands gender constancy
8 years	Jumps rope skillfully; throws and bats a ball more skillfully	Plays games requiring considerable fine motor skill and good reaction time	Difficulty judging if a passage is relevant to a specific theme; may demonstrate conservation of area	Begins to sort out more complex syntactic difficulties such as "ask" and "tell"; might integrate cueing systems for smooth reading; becomes more conventional speller	May express 2 same-valence emotions about different targets simultaneously; understands people may interpret situation differently but thinks this is due to different information
9 years		Enjoys hobbies requiring high levels of fine-motor skill (sewing, model building)	May demonstrate conservation of weight	Interprets "ask" and "tell" correctly	Can think about own thinking or another person's thinking but not both at the same time.
10 years	Jumping distance continues to increase		Makes better judgments about relevance of a text; begins to delete unimportant information when summarizing	Becomes more sophisticated conventional speller	Can take own view and view of another as if a disinterested third party

■ **Table 2.9** Customary Child Development by Age Across Domains—cont'd

	Mobility	Manipulation	Cognitive	Language	Social-Emotional
11 years	Running speed stabilizes for girls		May demonstrate conservation of volume	Begins to appreciate jokes and riddles based on syntactic ambiguity	Still has trouble detecting deception; spends more time with friends
12 years	Plays ball more skillfully due to improved reaction time		Shows skill in summarizing and outlining		
13 years	Males continue to increase running speed and jumping distance		May demonstrate formal operational thinking	Speaks in longer sentences, uses principles of subordination; understands metaphors, multiple levels of meaning; increases vocabulary	Still has weak sense of individual identity, is easily influenced by peer group; spends more time with friends, usually of same sex; may begin sexual relationships, especially if male
14 years	Standing long jump distance continues to increase for males, but stabilizes for females		Continues to gain metacognitive abilities and improve study skills	Improves reading comprehension abilities; writes longer, more complex sentences	Seeks increasing emotional autonomy from parents
15 years	May reach fastest reaction time		Can think in terms of abstract principles; may demonstrate dogmatism-skepticism		Seeks intimate friendships and relationships
16 years	May reach peak performance level in sports		Can argue either side in a debate; shows growing interest in social and philosophical problems		Is actively involved in search for personal identity; is likely to be sexually active; may use alcohol and cigarettes

Source: Child Development Institute (2010); Erhardt (1994); Gallahue & Ozmum (2006); Long & Toscano (2002); Owens (2001); Rossetti (2005); Schickendanz, Schickendanz, Hansen, & Forsyth (1993).

Initial

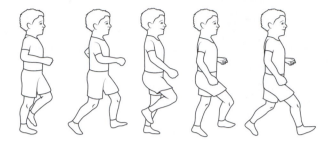

Elementary

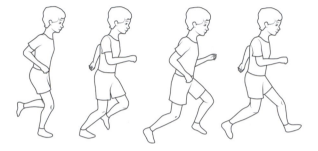

Mature

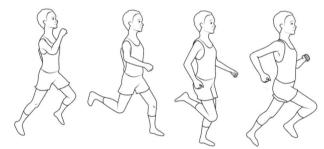

Figure 2.9 Stages of running pattern.*(Gallahue & Ozmum, 2006, p. 211)*

crouch is deeper and more consistent. Knee and hip extension are almost complete at takeoff and the hips are flexed during flight.

Toddlers will creep up and down stairs; however, if they do not have stairs in their homes, they will most likely already be walking when they go up their first flight of stairs (Berger et al., 2007). By 18 months they will first learn to walk up stairs using a railing and then downstairs using a railing.

Development of Upper Extremity Function

In the second year of life, toddlers refine all grasping patterns. The manipulation of objects is more dynamic because the toddler has distal finger control and understands which end of an object to grasp to use it easily,

such as grasping a spoon at the proper end and orienting the other end toward the month. Toddlers will imitate a scribble using a **palmar-supinate grasp** (object held with fisted hand and flexed, slightly supinated wrist) (Fig. 2.7I). Many grasping patterns will be used depending on the object's size and intended use. By 15 to 18 months, toddlers will release a raisin into a small bottle and stack two cubes, both standard items on many developmental tests. They progress to a **digital-palmar grasp** (object held with all fingers, and a straight, pronated wrist) of a crayon or pencil as they begin to learn to imitate vertical then horizontal strokes. By 2 to 3 years of life, the toddler shows dramatic increases in upper extremity function as outlined in Table 2.9 and Figure 2.7. There is increased straightness and smoothness of reaching with decreases in reaching speed and jerk (Berthier & Keen, 2006). The toddler should be independent in self-feeding but cannot yet cut food.

Development of Language, Social, and Play Skills

When toddlers have mastered the locomotor and upper extremity skills required to walk and manipulate objects, language and social skills appear to advance exponentially. Once children walk independently, they will spend more time interacting with toys and their mothers (Clearfield, 2011). They start to use nonverbal and verbal output together and use a variety of vocabulary based on referents and a variety of intents. By 18 to 24 months toddlers are using two-word combinations and indicating an understanding of basic semantic relations. The two-word combinations usually involve persons, places, things, actions, and position/locations (e.g. "mommy sock," "daddy up"). They should have at least a vocabulary of between 50 words (Rossetti, 2005) to 300 words (Child Development Institute, 2010; Owens, 2001) by 24 months. If they do not have at least a 50-word vocabulary, they are considered "late talkers" (D'Odorico & Jacob, 2006). They will comprehend (receptive language) a greater number of words than the words they can produce (expressive language) (Reich, 1986, 42). By 24 months of age, toddlers should be using multiword utterances to express complex needs. Speech becomes more accurate, but toddlers may still leave off ending sounds and strangers might not understand everything they say.

As language develops, multiword combinations will depend on concept development, information/language processing (including memory), sequencing, direction following, and discrimination. Delay in language development is seen in approximately 15% of

Initial

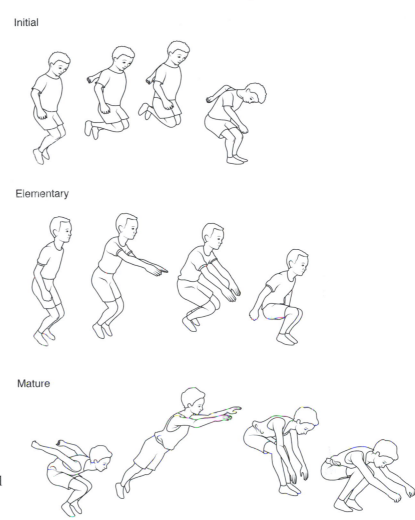

Elementary

Mature

Figure 2.10 Stages of the horizontal jumping pattern. *(Gallahue & Ozmum, 2006, p. 217)*

toddlers between the age of 24 to 29 months (Horwitz et al., 2003). Of toddlers with language delays, 22% also tend to have associated neurodevelopmental problems (Buschmann et al., 2008) and show social withdrawal compared to typically developing peers (Rescorda, Ross, & McClue, 2007),

Play, which is the work of children, advances greatly during the second year of life (Table 2.10). Toddlers use **exploratory play,** which is sensory rich and involves much repetition that is necessary for mastery. Toddlers have increased body awareness and they use play to explore all aspects of the environment. Toddlers engage in **parallel play,** where children play adjacent to each other but not necessarily together and do not try to influence each other's behavior. It is highly social and contains some cooperative interaction. **Social play** starts out as parallel play with others next to the child,

whom the child watches and then imitates, but this is not yet associative with true interactions.

Preschoolers

The preschool period is generally considered to be from 3 to 5 years of age whether the child is at home or participates in community programs. Preschoolers are ready to experience the world beyond their home. In preschool, the focus of the curriculum is development in all domains, but especially social development. In some Asian cultures, 3-year-olds might begin to learn to read and write. In other cultures, the focus might be discovery and exploration.

Development of Advanced Motor Skills

Active movement throughout the environment characterizes the preschooler. Muscle amplitudes and durations

Table 2.10 Development of Play

Age	Type of Play	Associated Actions
Infants		
0–6 months	Exploratory	• Sensorimotor play predominates
	Social	• Focused on attachment and bonding
6–12 months	Exploratory	• Sensorimotor play evolves into functional play
	Functional	• Begins to use toys based on their functional purpose
	Social	• Attachment to parents or caregivers
12–18 months	Relational and functional	• Simple pretend play directed toward self (will pretend to eat, dress) • Links two to three schemes in simple combinations • Exhibits imitative play from an immediate model
	Gross motor	• Explores all aspects of a room • Rolls and crawls in play
	Social	• Beginning of peer interactions during play • Parallel play next to a peer
Toddlers		
19–24 months	Functional	• Performs multiple related actions together
	Gross motor	• Might enjoy the sensory input
	Pretend or symbolic	• Makes inanimate objects real (will feed and dress dolls or action figures) • Pretends objects are real or symbolize another object
	Social	• Parallel play • Imitates others in play • Participates with several children • Watches other children • Beginning to take turns
Preschoolers		
2–3 years	Symbolic	• Links multiple scheme combinations into meaningful sequence of pretend play • Uses objects for multiple pretend ideas • Uses toys to represent animals or people • Plays out drama with stuffed animals or imaginary friends • Plays house
	Constructive	• Participates in drawing and puzzles • Imitates adults using toys
	Gross motor	• Likes jumping, tumbling
	Social	• Associative, parallel play predominates
3–4 years	Complex Imaginary	• Creates scripts for play where pretend objects have actions reflecting roles in real or imaginary life
	Constructive	• Creates art product with supervision • Completes puzzles and blocks
	Rough and tumble	• Enjoys physical play, swinging, jumping, running
	Social	• Participates in circle time, games, drawing, and art time at preschool • Singing and dancing in groups • Associative play with other children, sharing, and talking

■ **Table 2.10** Development of Play—cont'd

Age Preschoolers	Type of Play	Associated Actions
4–5 years	Games with rules	• Begins group games with single rules • Organized play with prescribed roles • Participates in an organized gross motor games
	Constructive	• Interested in the goal of the art activity • Constructs complex structures • Takes pride in products
	Social/dramatic	• Role plays with other children • Participates in dress up • Tells stories • Continues with pretend play that involves scripts with imaginary characters
Kindergartners		
5–6 years	Games with rules	• Computer, card, and board games with rules
	Dramatic	• Elaborate imaginary play • Reconstructs real world play
	Sports	• Cooperative play in groups/ teams of children
	Social play	• Participates in organized play in groups

Source: Case-Smith, J. (2010, pp. 65–75); Linder (2008); Park (2007).

increase, and children will refine their gait pattern until age 5 to 7 years, when their patterns become fully mature. By age 3 years their running pattern has matured with a true, consistent flight phase requiring more strength and balance than walking. Preschoolers by age 30 months climb up stairs alternating feet, but might still go down step by step (Bayley, 2005).

By 4 years of age, preschoolers can hop, which requires a great deal of coordination and balance ability. Initially in hopping, the unsupported leg is flexed to 90 degrees or less and is parallel to the ground with the body upright. The arms are flexed at the elbows and held slightly at the side, there is little height or distance generated in a hop, and balance is lost easily (Gallahue & Ozmum, 2006) (Fig. 2.11). The preschooler will also learn to gallop (a step and a hop with the same foot leading), walk alternating down stairs, and stand on tiptoes. Motor skills continue to be refined and are important in social interactions. However, many children are already spending too much time in sedentary activities, and they must not be allowed to become "couch potatoes" at this early age (Patrick, Spear, Holt, & Sofka, 2001). Exercise is important for fitness, and with obesity on the rise with children, therapists should be mindful of the very early signs of a sedentary lifestyle.

Manipulation skills are advancing with more sophistication in fine motor play, including pasting, coloring, and drawing. There is isolation of the thumb and fingers and rotation of the wrist. Between $3\frac{1}{2}$ years and 4 years of age the preschooler will hold a crayon or pencil with a **static tripod** (crude approximation of the thumb, index, and middle fingers and the hand moves as a unit) (Fig. 2.7I). The preschooler will then progress to the **dynamic tripod** in the use of writing instruments. In a dynamic tripod the crayon is held with precise opposition of the distal phalanges of the thumb, index, and middle fingers; the ring and middle fingers flex to form a stable arch; the wrist is slightly extended; and, in an important distinction from a static tripod, the metacarpal phalangeal joints stabilize and there are localized movement of the proximal interphalangeal joints (Erhardt, 1994). The shoulder, elbow, forearm, and wrist function as stabilizers along with the core trunk muscles, providing a foundation for the precise movement of the hand and fingers.

Development of Language, Social, and Play Skills

The preschooler is a very social individual who is now making friends and exploring the world. Language skills, which are very closely tied to social ability, are developing exponentially. Children can understand

Initial

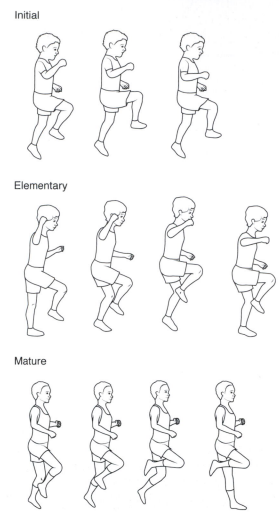

Elementary

Mature

Figure 2.11 Stages of the hopping pattern. *(Gallahue & Ozmum, 2006, p. 219)*

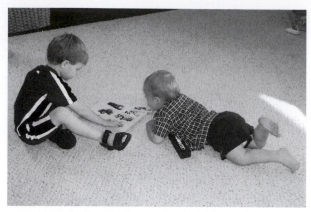

Figure 2.12 Play is the work of children. Note the different postures assumed for this activity.

past and future events, and they begin to emerge as conversational partners. A 3-year-old will speak in more complete sentences, and begins to overgeneralize rules, creating verb tenses and plurals. Adult syntax and grammar is present. By age 4 years, the preschooler readily converses and asks an endless stream of questions; however, approximately 6% to 8% of preschoolers may have speech and language difficulties (Boyle, Gillham, & Smith, 1996; Tomblin, Smith, & Zhang, 1997).

Play is a major activity of the preschooler whether at home or in the community (Table 2.10 and Fig. 2.12). **Play** as defined by Blanche (1999) as spontaneous, exciting, energy-producing or -expending, physically and mentally activating, relaxing, or perhaps even stressful. Play might include creativity, imagination, and a sense

of freedom but may not have a clear purpose and is performed for oneself. Three types of play have been identified in early childhood: (1) **pretend** or **symbolic play** (the child pretends that dolls or figurines are real; toys are used to represent people or animals), (2) **constructive play** (involves building and constructing things, drawing, and puzzles), and (3) **physical** or **rough-tumble play** (active movement that frequently involves other children; might include jumping, running, swinging, and sliding) (Case-Smith, 2010, p. 73). As children develop, their play becomes more elaborate and they concentrate for longer periods of time. Some children prefer play as a social activity, whereas others prefer solitary play. Understanding a child's preferences for play and the latest songs, toys, games, and action figures can assist the therapist in more easily establishing rapport with a child and gaining cooperation.

The preschool period is an excellent time for children with disabilities and typically developing children to learn about each other and interact in a playful environment. Children with disabilities learn to model typical behavior and develop friendships and typically developing children learn about children with special needs. Inclusive preschools have been shown to be beneficial for the development of social skills and other behaviors in children with disabilities (Buysse & Bailey, 1993; Guralnick, 1999, 2001). Additionally, typically developing children develop a sensitivity to the needs of others with disabilities (Diamond & Carpenter, 2000). A **naturalistic curriculum model** is advocated, which enhances the "young child's environmental control, participation, and interaction in natural experiences consistent with the cultural values and expectations of the family" (Noonan, 2006, p. 82).

Elementary School-Age Child

School is the principal environment of children 5 to 18 years of age (or sometimes 21 years of age if the child has a disability). Elementary school is usually from kindergarten through eighth grade, although many school systems add the distinction of middle school or junior high school. Children also engage in multiple community environments; they belong to religious organizations, sports groups, scouts, and endless activities based on their resources and community. Development continues in all domains with experiences and opportunities influencing outcomes.

Development of Advanced Motor Skills

When children enter school, all of the basic motor skills required to function throughout life are present and will be refined and advanced based on the needs of their cultures and environment (Table 2.9). Children will learn the advanced motor skills required of the activities and sports in which they want to engage. Eye-hand coordination will advance if the child wants to play baseball and video games; running speeds might increase if the child plays soccer; strength will increase if the child does gymnastics; and coordination improves if the child plays musical instruments. Children will learn to swim, water or snow ski, snowboard, skate, or horseback ride depending on their interests and resources. Their degree of proficiency will depend on a genetic predisposition, opportunity, instruction, and desire.

By 9 years of age children have achieved adult-like timing and accuracy in their reaching behaviors (Favilla, 2006). They will refine their writing and drawing throughout their school years, achieving varying degrees of competence. Practice is the critical factor in the level of skill development, although some children have a natural propensity for athletics, art, or musical ability and might rapidly exceed the norm. A tendency for sedentary activities and inactivity must be examined with the rise in obesity and poor physical fitness of our youth. Obesity impacts multiple areas of a child's development and functioning. Increased fitness, especially aerobic capacity, is associated with academic success (Wittberg, Northrup, & Cottrel, 2009).

Some children will continue to have immature movement patterns, especially noticeable during physical education class or sports. Characteristics of **immature movement patterns** include the following:

- Inconsistency of performance
- Perseveration-response repetition, the inability to stop when appropriate
- Extraneous movements
- Mirroring or the inability to transpose right-left visual cues
- Asymmetry and difficulty in bilateral coordination
- Loss of dynamic balance and falling after finishing a motor task
- Inability to maintain rhythm or movement pattern
- Inability to control force, whether unable to generate enough force or using too much force
- Inappropriate motor planning (Sherrill, 1993)

Children with these problems may have a developmental coordination disorder, as discussed in Chapters 7 and 24, or other developmental disabilities.

Development of Language, Social, and Play Skills

Cognitive and written and oral language skills continue to advance throughout childhood and as different languages are learned. Play continues to be an important activity for school-age children. In the early school years (ages 7 to 12 years), the child's play is frequently focused on games with rules such as computer games and card games that require problem solving and abstract thinking. Crafts and hobbies might also be important activities. Participation in organized sports is very common during these years when advanced skill is not yet required and the focus is on cooperation. Soon, however, winning and skill become very important, and children who do not live up to the team's or their own expectations will drop out of the sport. When this happens, it is critical for children to find other sports or activities that will help maintain their physical fitness and help prevent obesity. Activities such as biking, hiking, and swimming along with computer activities that involve physical participation, such as Nintendo Wii and Wii Fit games, should be encouraged to increase energy expenditure (Graves, Stratton, Ridgers, & Cable, 2007).

During middle childhood Havighurst (1972) notes the growth of the following developmental tasks: (1) building wholesome attitudes toward oneself, (2) learning an appropriate masculine or feminine social role, (3) developing fundamental skills and concepts for everyday living, (4) developing conscience, morality, and a scale of values, and (5) developing attitudes toward social groups. How the child learns these tasks is a reflection of their physical, social, and cultural environment.

School-age children having disabilities or special health-care needs should be attending their local school according to federal law and best practices. As discussed in Chapter 12, all children are to be educated in the least restrictive environment in their local school.

Children are adaptable and accepting, and if the adults in the environment model behavior appropriately, inclusive education has proved to be very successful for both children with disabilities and typically developing children (Giangreco, Dennis, Cloninger, Edelman, & Schattman, 1993; Hunt, Doering, Hirose-Hatae, Maier, & Goetz, 2001; Hunt, Soto, Maier, & Doering, 2003; Peck, Donaldson, & Pezzoli, 1990; Soto, Muller, Hunt, & Goetz, 2001).

Adolescent

Adolescence, usually ages 11 to 18 years, is a time of rapid physical growth, onset of sexual maturation, activation of new drives and motivations, and social challenges (Forbes & Dahl, 2010). School is the predominant part of the adolescent's life and academic and social development continues. There is further brain development and gradual increases in capacities for cognitive control and executive function (Luna, Padmanabhan, & O'Hearn, 2010). The adolescent is seeking mature relationships with age-mates of both sexes, learning a masculine or feminine role, going through puberty, achieving an adult physique, seeking emotional independence from parents, and preparing for adult life (Havighurst, 1972). This time of transition can be a trying time for the adolescent and the parents because the desire and need for independence and separation from the family occurs at a time when they are also more likely to engage in high-risk behaviors. Parents may find themselves trying to balance providing their teens with the independence they seek with the need to be even more aware of their child's activities.

Adolescents continue to develop in all domains depending on their needs, desires, and opportunities. During adolescence there are numerous body changes, comparable only to those of the first year of life. Changes in sleep patterns appear, which predate the bodily changes associated with puberty (Sadeh, Dahl, Shahar, & Rosenblat-Stein, 2009). The onset and progression of puberty is quite variable and can be influenced by environmental factors such as endocrine-disrupting chemicals, nutrition, and body size (Sadeh et al., 2009). Physically, the mean peak height velocity in females is at $11\frac{1}{2}$ years and menarche occurs around $12\frac{1}{2}$ years. Males begin their puberty growth spurt 2 years after the females, and their mean peak height velocity is at $13\frac{1}{2}$ years (Patrick et al., 2001). Mexican American and African American youth, especially girls, go through puberty earlier than European American youth (Himes, 2006).

Adolescents often find great enjoyment in sports participation or observation and community activities (Fig. 2.13). Their motor skills continue to develop based on need and practice. Without proper training and fitness, there can be a tendency toward injury. Adolescents with injuries can be easy to motivate if they wish to return to their sport. However, they can be very difficult to motivate if the goal is improved physical fitness for obese teenagers or meeting the complex needs of teenagers with disabilities. Adolescents who participate in sports or who require fitness programs have unique physical therapy needs. In Chapter 13, the specific roles and responsibilities of therapists who work in this area are discussed.

Adolescence is one of the healthiest periods of the life span; however, 18% of adolescents aged 12 to 19 are obese (Ogden, Carroll, Curtin, Lamb, & Flegal, 2010), and morbidity and mortality rates increase 200% (CDC, 2009). During this period, the incidence of motor vehicle accidents, suicide, homicide, alcohol and substance abuse, HIV, hepatitis C, unplanned pregnancies, and eating disorders increases (Forbes & Dahl, 2010). These health consequences suggest problems with control of emotion and behavior. They also reflect the sensation-seeking behaviors seen in adolescence. The positive thrill of sensation-seeking or risk-taking behaviors appears to have a greater influence on behavioral choice than a cognitive understanding of the negative consequences of the behavior (Forbes & Dahl, 2010). Sensation-seeking behaviors apparently increase between 13 to 16 years and then decrease in a curvilinear pattern linked to pubertal maturation. On the other hand, impulsivity, which has been connected to sensation-seeking behaviors, is unrelated to puberty, and follows a linear pattern declining steadily after age 10 years (Steinberg et al., 2008).

Adolescence is a time for acquiring social and personal values as the teenager starts the transition into adulthood. Plans are now being made for future vocations and post–secondary school pursuits. For adolescents with disabilities, this is an especially complicated period. They may now have to consider possible limitations in career options and ability to move away from the family. The stresses of school and determining future options can be a heavy burden on any adolescent.

As their bodies grow, adolescents with disabilities may face new limitations and restrictions due to increased body mass and shortening of muscles as bones grow. It is not uncommon for an adolescent with a disability, who was ambulatory at home and school, to decide that the effort and energy requirements of ambulation are too great, and a decision is made to use a wheelchair for the majority of the day (Dudgeon,

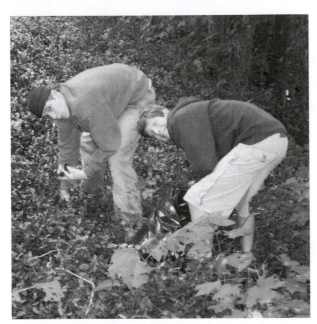

Figure 2.13 High school students participating in community service learning project.

Jaffe, & Shurtleff, 1991). Others are able to enjoy the opportunity to further explore their environment and achieve independence by driving a car using a variety of assistive devices as necessary.

Adolescents are also developing sexually. They and their parents must address issues of birth control and prevention of sexually transmitted diseases. This is particularly important for females with disabilities, because they are especially vulnerable to sexual abuse. Adolescents with disabilities also indulge in risky sexual behaviors and should receive health promotion and sex education (Maart & Jelsma, 2010). Participation in the community might become more restricted as the adolescent with a disability, who was once well accepted in the community, is no longer the "cute" little child, and inappropriate behaviors are no longer socially acceptable. For others, it is a time to separate from parents as they achieve independence, which might be difficult for parents to accept.

Atypical Motor Behaviors

The majority of infants and children develop in the progressions noted in Tables 2.4 to 2.10. Their rates of development in various domains may differ, and areas of early aptitude may continue throughout life. Some infants and children do not follow a customary developmental progression. This may be common in their culture or family and not a matter of concern. On the

other hand, atypical or delayed development may indicate a disability or detrimental environmental influences. Common indicators of atypical development seen frequently in children later diagnosed with cerebral palsy and other developmental disabilities are presented in Table 2.11. Therapists should carefully determine the presence of atypical or delayed motor development as discussed throughout this text, and it should be monitored by the therapist with intervention provided as appropriate. If it is observed during a developmental screening, then the child should receive a more comprehensive examination and, as appropriate, be referred to an early intervention program and pediatrician. If a problem is observed in a school-age child, the child should be referred to the school system's advisory and examination committee, and reported to the child's pediatrician. In the following chapter we will discuss the methods of examination and evaluation to determine variations in motor development.

Because the development of play has been discussed in this chapter, it is important to mention play and participation in leisure activities by children with atypical or delayed motor development or disabilities. In general, these children tend to engage in less varied play, engage in more quiet recreation than active recreation, have fewer social activities, participate and move at a slower tempo, play indoors more than outside, have less interaction with peers than children without disabilities, and play with adults more than with other children (Brown & Gordon, 1987; Howard, 1996; Tamm & Skär, 2000). During social play, children with restricted mobility seldom initiated play and were given "lower status" play roles by their peers (Tamm & Skär, 2000). Children aged 9 to 13 years with cerebral palsy reported that their major play activity was watching television and listening to music (Malkawi, 2009). Shikako-Thomas and colleagues (2008) did a systematic review of the literature to determine participation in leisure activities in children and youth with cerebral palsy. Child factors that influenced play included age, gender, degree of limitation in motor function, and interests and preferences. Environmental factors included the physical environment (lack of equipment and structural barriers), social environment (policies, segregation, lack of information and peer support), and attitudinal issues (bullying, staring, and dependence on adults). Family factors included SES, parents' educational level (lower family income and lower parental education level associated with lower participation), and family functioning. Engagement in play is a major life area under the ICF-CY. Physical therapists must

![] **Table 2.11** Possible Indications of Atypical Development

Age	Possible Indications of Atypical Development
Month 1	• Serious impairment of body functions and structures, such as intraventricular hemorrhage of grades III or IV, perinatal asphyxia, myelomeningocele, genetic abnormalities. • Impaired age-appropriate activities, such as feeding problems, lack of leg movement; being "stuck" in head, neck, and trunk hyperextension (opisthotonus); extremely floppy.
Month 4	• Serious impairment of body functions and structures will continue to affect motor development depending on the impairment. • Impaired age-appropriate activities, such as maintaining rigid postures; inability to alternate between flexion and extension; consistent asymmetrical postures; inability to achieve midline orientation of head and extremities; lack of reaching behaviors or only unilateral movement. • Quiet, unresponsive baby.
Month 6	• Serious impairment of body functions and structures will continue to affect motor development, such as strong hip extensor, adductor, internal rotation, and ankle plantar flexor activity, especially in combination when held in standing or the opposite combination of extreme external rotation, abduction, and dorsiflexion with eversion, especially in supine. • Impaired age-appropriate activities, such as lack of a wide variety of movements; inability to laterally flex in prone or side lying or bring feet to mouth in supine; inability to roll; rolling using extension; poor upper extremity weight bearing in prone; inability to maintain propped sitting; or problems reaching and grasping toy.
Month 9	• Serious impairment of body functions and structures will continue to affect motor development. • Impaired age-appropriate activities such as those mentioned above and inability to move forward in prone; get in or out of sitting or stand with support; use of a "bunny hopping" pattern in creeping; or lack of a controlled release of a cube. • Little or no babbling
Month 12	• Serious impairment of body functions and structures will continue to affect motor development. There should be balance of muscle activation and neither restricted nor excessive range of motion or strong asymmetrical postures. • Impaired age-appropriate activities such as those mentioned above including not walking with support with good weight shift; not climbing; lack of inferior pincer grasp; or stereotyped hand movements restricting function. • No words by age 12 to 15 months
Month 15	• Serious impairment of body functions and structures will continue to affect motor development. • Impaired age-appropriate activities such as those mentioned above including not attempting to walk independently; or walking on toes with adducted legs; lack of a fine pincer grasp; or lack of controlled release of a pellet into a container. • Comprehension problems, limited social interaction or social avoidance, ritualistic behaviors, unintelligible speech

Source: Bly (1994); Erhardt (1994).

recognize the importance of play in a child's life, in the child's development, and in successful therapeutic intervention.

Summary

Neuromaturational theory has provided us with important information regarding common, although not invariant, sequences of development in all domains.

An individual's genetic base provides a foundation for their development, and the environment provides the stimulus and setting in which to learn and develop. Behavioral theory provides an understanding of human behavior and cognitive theory provides information on the process of development and learning. Dynamic systems theory is helping to reshape intervention strategies for children with disabilities by emphasizing the interdependence and importance of all body systems and the environment and task. NGST has expanded our understanding of variation and variability in human development.

The theories of development help physical therapists shape their thinking regarding expectations in child development and to understand deviations in development that influence their interventions. The importance of the environment from preconception to adulthood on all aspects of development needs to be recognized. Environmental factors are especially important for children with disabilities because they are frequently dependent on others for many environmental experiences. Therapists must understand and appreciate the importance of the environment and use the opportunities afforded through enriched environments to maximize the child's learning and functioning.

The study of child development is a dynamic, ongoing process. Courses and excellent texts are available to help you fully appreciate the complexity of child development. Physical therapists must not only be experts in motor development but also understand the overall development of child and family dynamics to be able to perform a thorough examination and evaluation and to provide appropriate and effective intervention.

DISCUSSION QUESTIONS

1. What are the theories presently guiding physical therapy interventions? Why are they important to intervention?

2. Describe the most common features of the gait pattern of early walkers.

3. Why is knowledge of the customary sequence of early motor development important if there is so much variation in the sequence?

4. At a neighborhood get-together, several mothers ask you if their children are developing normally. What skills would you expect to see in infants at 4, 6, 9, 12, or 18 months of age?

5. Besides delays in motor skill acquisition, what are some of the limitations in body structures and functions and restrictions in activities that might indicate atypical motor development throughout the first year of life?

Recommended Readings

Adolph, K.E., & Berger, S.E. (2006). Motor development. In W. Damon, R.M. Lerner, D. Kuhn, & R.S. Siegler (Eds.), *Handbook of child psychology, vol. 2, Cognition, perception, and language* (6th ed. pp. 161–213). Hoboken, NJ: John Wiley & Sons.

Batshaw, M.L., Pellegrino, L., & Roizen, N.J. (Eds.). (2007). *Children with disabilities* (6th ed.). Baltimore: Paul H. Brookes.

Bly, L. (1994). *Motor skills acquisition in the first year: An illustrated guide to normal movement*. San Antonio, TX: Therapy Skill Builders.

Brazelton, T.B., & Sparrow, J.D. (2006). *Touchpoints: Birth to three, your child's emotional and behavioral development* (2nd ed.). Cambridge, MA: Da Capo Press.

Cech, D.J., & Martin, S.T. (2012). *Functional movement development across the life span* (3rd ed.). St. Louis: Elsevier Saunders.

Hadders-Algra, M. (2010). Variation and variability: Key words in human motor development. *Physical Therapy, 90*(12), 1823–1837.

Henderson, A., & Pehoski, C. (2006). *Hand function in the child: Foundations for remediation*. St. Louis: Mosby Elsevier.

Vereijken, B. (2010). The complexity of childhood development: Variability in perspective. *Physical Therapy, 90*(12), 1850–1859.

Web-Based Resources

American Academy of Pediatrics
www.aap.org/
Parent information, practice guidelines, and articles on health, childhood diseases and treatments.

Centers for Disease Control and Prevention (CDC), National Center on Birth Defects and Developmental Disabilities (NCBDDD)
www.cdc.gov/ncbddd/actearly/index.html
Information on preventing birth defects, developmental disabilities, developmental screening, developmental milestones, and an interactive developmental checklist.

American Physical Therapy Association, Section on Pediatrics
www.pediatricapta.org/consumer-patient-information/resources.cfm
Information for families, physical therapists, and other service providers.

Developmental Milestones for Babies (0–2 yrs.) from the March of Dimes
www.marchofdimes.com/pnhec/298_10203.asp

Growth Milestones from KidsGrowth.com

> www.kidsgrowth.com/stages/guide/index.cfm

Speech and Language Developmental Milestones from the National Institute on Deafness and Other Communication Disorders

> http://www.nidcd.nih.gov/Pages/default.aspx

Is My Baby Developing on Schedule? from Pathways Awareness Foundation

> www.pathwaysawareness.org/?q=monthlymile-stones/developing

References

Adolph, K. (2003). Advances in research on infant motor development. Paper presented at APTA Combined Sections Meeting 2003, Tampa, FL (Cassette Recording No. CSM03-122). Englewood, CO: Sound Images. Handouts retrieved from http://apta.org

Adolph, K., & Avolio, A. (2000). Walking infants adapt locomotion to changing body dimensions. *Journal of Experimental Psychology: Human Perception and Performance, 26*(3), 1148–1166.

Adolph, K.E., & Berger, S.E. (2006). Motor development. In W. Damon, R.M. Lerner, D. Kuhn, & R.S. Siegler (Eds.), *Handbook of child psychology, vol. 2, Cognition, perception, and language* (6th ed., pp. 161–213). Hoboken, NJ: John Wiley & Sons.

Adolph, K., Vereijken, B., & Denny, M.A. (1998). Learning to crawl. *Child Development, 69*(5), 1299–1312.

Alberto, P.A., & Troutman, A.C. (2006). *Applied behavior analysis for teachers* (7th ed.). Upper Saddle River, NJ: Pearson Education Inc.

American Academy of Pediatrics (AAP), (2005). Breastfeeding and the use of human milk. *Pediatrics, 115*(2), 496–506. doi:10.1542/peds.2004-2491

American Academy of Pediatrics (AAP), Task Force on Infant Positioning and SIDS (1992). Positioning and SIDS. *Pediatrics, 89*(6 Pt 1), 1120–1126.

American Academy of Pediatrics (AAP), Task Force on Infant Sleep Position and SIDS (2000). Changing concepts of sudden infant death syndrome: Implications for infant sleeping environment and sleep position. *Pediatrics, 105,* 650–656.

Australian Government. (2011). How the paid parental leave comparison estimator works. Retrieved from http://www.centrelink.gov.au/internet/internet.nsf/individuals/ppl_working_parents_estimator.htm

Badaly, D., & Adolph, K.E. (2008). Beyond the average: Walking infants take steps longer than their leg length. *Infant Behavior & Development, 31*(3), 554–558.

Bahmanyar, S., Montgomery, S M., Weiss, R.J., & Ekbom, A. (2008). Maternal smoking during pregnancy, other prenatal and perinatal factors, and the risk of Legg-Calvé-Perthes disease. *Pediatrics, 122*(2), e459–464.

Bailey, D.B., Bruer, J.T., Symons, F.J., & Lichtman, J.W. (Eds.). (2001). *Critical thinking about critical periods.* Baltimore: Paul H. Brookes.

Bailey, D.B., & Symons, F.J. (2001). Critical periods. In D.B. Bailey, J.T. Bruer, F.J. Symons, & J.W. Lichtman (Eds.),

Critical thinking about critical periods (pp. 289–292). Baltimore: Paul H. Brookes.

Bailey, D.B., & Wolery, M. (1992). *Teaching infants and preschoolers with disabilities* (2nd ed.). New York: Merrill.

Baird, P.A., Anderson, T.W., Newcombe, H.B., & Lowry, R.B. (1988). Genetic disorders in children and young adults: A population study. *American Journal of Human Genetics, 42*(5), 677–693.

Bandura, A. (2002). Social cognitive theory in cultural context. *Applied Psychology: An International Review, 51*(2), 269–290.

Barr, H.M., & Streuissguth, A.P. (2001). Identifying maternal self-reported alcohol use associated with fetal alcohol spectrum disorders. *Alcoholism: Clinical and Experimental Research, 25*(2), 283–287.

Batshaw, M.L. (2007). Genetics and developmental disabilities. In M.L. Batshaw, L. Pellegrino, & N.J. Roizen, (Eds.), *Children with disabilities* (6th ed., p. 7). Baltimore: Paul H. Brookes.

Bayley, N. (1936). *The California infant scale of motor development.* Berkeley: University of California.

Bayley, N. (2005). *Bayley scales of infant and toddler development* (3rd ed.). San Antonio, TX: Pearson.

Berger, S.E., Theuring, C., & Adolph, K.E. (2007). How and when infants learn to climb stairs. *Infant Behavior & Development, 30*(1), 36–49. doi: 10.1016/j.infbeh.2006.11.002

Bernstein, N. (1967). *The coordination and regulation of movement.* London: Pergamon Press.

Berthier, N.E., Clifton, R.K., McCall, D.D., & Robin, D.J. (1999). Proximodistal structure of early reaching in human infants. *Experimental Brain Research, 127*(3), 259–269.

Berthier, N.E., & Keen, R. (2006). Development of reaching in infancy. *Experimental Brain Research, 169*(4), 507–518.

Bertrand, J. (2009). Interventions for children with fetal alcohol spectrum disorders (FASDs): Overview of findings for five innovative research projects. *Research in Developmental Disabilities, 30*(5), 986–1006.

Blanche, E. (1999). *Play and process: The experience of play in the life of the adult.* Ann Arbor, MI: University of Michigan.

Bly, L. (1994). *Motor skills acquisition in the first year: An illustrated guide to normal development.* San Antonio, TX: Therapy Skill Builders.

Bobath. K. (1980). The neurophysiological basis for the treatment of cerebral palsy. *Clinics in Developmental Medicine, 75.* Philadelphia: J.B. Lippincott.

Bobath, K., & Bobath, B. (1984). The neuro-developmental treatment. In D. Scrutton (Ed.), *Management of the motor disorders of children with cerebral palsy* (pp. 6–18). Philadelphia: J.B. Lippincott.

Bowe, F.G. (1995). *Birth to five: Early childhood special education.* New York: Delmar Publishers.

Boyle, J., Gillham, B., & Smith, N. (1996). Screening for early language delay in the 18–36 month age-range: The predictive validity of tests of production and implications for practice. *Child Language Teaching and Therapy, 12,* 113–127.

Bronfenbrenner, U. (1979). *The ecology of human development: Experiments by nature and design.* Cambridge, MA: Harvard University Press.

Bronfenbrenner, U. (1995). The bioecological model from a life course perspective. In P. Moen, G.H. Elder, & K. Lusher

(Eds.), *Examining lives in context*. Washington, DC: American Psychological Association.

Brown, H. (2009). U.S. maternity leave benefits are still dismal. *Forbes.com, 05.04.09*. Retrieved from http://www.forbes.com/2009/05/04/maternity-leave-laws-forbes-woman-wellbeing-pregnancy.html

Brown, M., & Gordon, W. (1987). Impact of impairments on activity patterns of children. *Archives of Physical Medicine and Rehabilitation, 68*, 828–832.

Bruer, J.T. (2001). A critical and sensitive period primer. In D.B. Bailey, J.T. Bruer, F.J. Symons, & J.W. Lichtman (Eds.), *Critical thinking about critical periods* (pp. 1–26). Baltimore: Paul H. Brookes.

Buchanan, J.J., & Horak, F.B. (2001). Transition in a postural task: Do the recruitment and suppression of degrees of freedom stabilize posture? *Experimental Brain Research, 139*, 482–494.

Burbacher, T.M., & Grant, K.S. (2006). Neurodevelopmental effects of alcohol. In P.W. Davidson, G.J. Myers, & B. Weiss (Eds.), *International review of mental retardation research: Vol. 30. Neurotoxicology and developmental disabilities* (pp. 1–46). San Diego: Elsevier Academic Press.

Buschmann, A., Jooss, B., Rupp, A., Dockter, S., Blaschtikowitz, H., Heggen, I., & Pietz, J. (2008). Children with developmental language delay at 24 months of age: Results of a diagnostic work-up. *Developmental Medicine and Child Neurology, 50*(3), 223–229.

Buysse, V., & Bailey, D.B. (1993). Behavioral and developmental outcomes in young children with disabilities in integrated and segregated settings: A review of comparative studies. *Journal of Special Education, 26*, 434–461.

Capute, A.J., Shapiro, B.K., Palmer, F.B., Ross, A., & Wachtel, R.C. (1985). Normal gross motor development: The influences of race, sex and socio-economic status. *Developmental Medicine and Child Neurology, 27*, 635–643.

Case, R. (1992). Potential contributions of neo-Piagetian theory to the art and science of instruction. In M. Carretero, M. Pope, R.J. Simons, & J.I. Pozo, *Learning and instruction: European research in an international context* (pp. 1–25). Elmsford, NY: Pergamon Press.

Case, R., Griffin, S., & Kelly, W.M. (2001). Socioeconomic differences in children's early cognitive development and their readiness for schooling (pp. 37–63). In S. Golbeck (Ed.), *Psychological perspectives on early childhood education: Reframing dilemmas in research and practice*. Mahwah, NJ: Lawrence Erlbaum Associates.

Case-Smith, J. (2010). Development of childhood occupations. In J. Case-Smith & J. Clifford O'Brien (Eds.), *Occupational therapy for children* (6th ed., pp. 56–83). Maryland Heights, MS: Mosby Elsevier.

Case-Smith, J., Law, M., Missiuna, C., Pollock, N., & Stewart, D. (2010). Foundations of occupational therapy practice in children. In J. Case-Smith & J. Clifford O'Brien (Eds.), *Occupational therapy for children* (6th ed., pp. 22–55). Maryland Heights, MS: Mosby Elsevier.

Centers for Disease Control and Prevention (CDC). (2009). Surveillance for violent deaths: National violent death reporting system, 16 States, 2006. *Morbidity and Mortality Weekly Report: Surveillance Summaries, 58*(SS-1). Retrieved from http://www.cdc.gov/mmwr/PDF/ss/ss5801.pdf

Centers for Disease Control and Prevention (CDC) (2010). *Preconception care*. Retrieved from http://www.cdc.gov/ncbddd/preconception/QandA_providers.htm#1

Centers for Disease Control and Prevention (CDC) (2011a). Pregnant? Don't smoke! Retrieved from http://www.cdc.gov/Features/PregnantDontSmok

Centers for Disease Control and Prevention (CDC) (2011b). *National Center for Health Statistics, Clinical Growth Charts*. Retrieved from http://www.cdc.gov/growthcharts/clinical_charts.htm

Charles, J., & Gordon, A.M. (2005). A critical review of constraint-induced movement therapy and forced use in children with hemiplegia. *Neural Plasticity, 12*, 245–261.

Charles, J.R., & Gordon, A.M. (2007). A repeated course of constraint-induced movement therapy results in further improvement. *Developmental Medicine and Child Neurology, 49*(10), 770–773.

Chattin-McNichols, J. (1992). *The Montessori controversy*. Albany, NY: Delmar.

Child Development Institute (2010). *Language development in children*. Retrieved from http://www.childdevelopmentinfo.com/development/language_development.shtml

Children's Defense Fund (2008). *Children in poverty*. Retrieved from http://www.childrensdefense.org

Clearfield, M.W. (2011). Learning to walk changes infants' social interactions. *Infant Behavior and Development, 34*(1), 15–25.

Coker, P., Karakostas, T., Dodds, C., & Hsiang, S. (2010). Gait characteristics of children with hemiplegic cerebral palsy before and after modified constraint-induced movement therapy. *Disability and Rehabilitation, 32*(5), 402–408.

Collins, J.W., Jr., Wambach, J., David, R.J., & Rankin, K.M. (2009). Women's lifelong exposure to neighborhood poverty and low birth weight: A population-based study. *Maternal and Child Health Journal, 13*(3), 326–333.

Corbetta, D., & Bojczyk, K.E. (2002). Infants return to two-handed reaching when they are learning to walk. *Journal of Motor Behavior, 34*(1), 83.

Cronk, C., Crocker, A.C., Pueschel, S.M., Shea, A.M., Zackai, E., & Reed, R.B. (1988). Growth charts for children with Down syndrome: 1 month to 18 years of age. *Pediatrics, 81*, 102–110.

David, T.B., & Weinstein, C.S. (1987). The built environment and children's development. In C.S. Weinstein & T.C. David (Eds.), *Spaces for children: The built environment and child development* (pp. 3–18). New York: Plenum Press.

Davidson, P.W., & Myers, G.J., (2007). Environmental toxins. In M.L. Batshaw, L. Pellegrino, & N.J. Roizen (Eds.), *Children with disabilities* (6th ed., pp. 1–70). Baltimore: Paul H. Brookes.

Davis, B.E., Moon, R.Y., Sachs, H.C., & Ottolini, M.C. (1998). Effects of sleep position on infant motor development. *Pediatrics, 102*(5), 1135–1140.

Decouflé, P., Boyle, C.A., Paulozzi, L.J., & Larry, J.M. (2001). Increased risk for developmental disabilities in children who have major birth defects: A population-based study. *Pediatrics, 108*, 728–734.

DeVellis, R.F. (1977). Learned helplessness in institutions. *Mental Retardation, 15*(5), 10–13.

Dewey, C., Fleming, P., Golding, J., & the ALSPAC Study Team. (1998). Does the supine sleeping position have any adverse effects on the child? II. Development in the first 18 months. *Pediatrics, 101*(1), 1–5.

Diamond, K.E., & Carpenter, E.S. (2000). Participation in inclusive preschool programs and sensitivity to the needs of others. *Journal of Early Intervention, 23*(2), 81–91.

D'Odorico, L., & Jacob, V. (2006). Prosodic and lexical aspects of maternal linguistic input to late-talking toddlers. *International Journal of Language and Communication Disorders, 41*(3), 293–311.

Dudek-Shriber, L., & Zelazny, S. (2007). The effects of prone positioning on the quality and acquisition of developmental milestones in four-month-old infants. *Pediatric Physical Therapy, 19*(1), 48–55.

Dudgeon, B.J., Jaffe, K.M., & Shurtleff, D.B. (1991). Variations in midlumbar myelomeningocele: Implications for ambulation. *Pediatric Physical Therapy, 3*, 57–62.

Edwards, C., Gandini, L., & Forman, G. (Eds.). (1993). *The hundred languages of children: The Reggio Emilia approach to early childhood education.* Norwood, NJ: Ablex Publishing.

Effgen, S.K., & Chan, L. (2010). Relationship between occurrence of gross motor behaviors and attainment of objectives in children with cerebral palsy participating in conductive education. *Physiotherapy Theory and Practice, 26*(1), 1–18.

Ekblad, M., Korkeila, J., Parkkola, R., Lapinleimu, H., Haataja, L., & Lehtonen, L. (2010). Maternal smoking during pregnancy and regional brain volumes in preterm infants. *The Journal of Pediatrics, 156*(2), 185–190.

Elman, J., Bates, E., Johnson, M., Karmiloff-Smith, A., Parisi, D., & Plunkett, K. (1997). *Rethinking innateness.* Cambridge, MA: The MIT Press.

Erhardt, R.P. (1994). *Developmental hand dysfunction: Theory, assessment, treatment* (2nd ed.). Austin: Pro-Ed, Inc.

Facon, B., Sahiri, S., & Riviere, V. (2008). A controlled single-case treatment of severe long-term selective mutism in a child with mental retardation. *Behavior Therapy, 39*(4), 313–321.

Fadiman, A. (1997). *The spirit catches you and you fall down.* New York: Noonday Press.

Fagerberg, B., Bondjers, L., & Nilsson, P. (2004). Low birth weight in combination with catch-up growth predicts the occurrence of the metabolic syndrome in men at late middle age: The atherosclerosis and insulin resistance study. *Journal of Internal Medicine, 256*(3), 254–259.

Farran, D.C. (2001). Critical periods and early intervention. In D.B. Bailey, J.T. Bruer, F.J. Symons, & J.W. Lichtman (Eds.), *Critical thinking about critical periods* (pp. 233–266). Baltimore: Paul H. Brookes.

Favilla, M. (2006). Reaching movements in children: Accuracy and reaction time development. *Experimental Brain Research, 169*, 122–125.

Fetters, L., & Todd, J. (1987). Quantitative assessment of infant reaching movements. *Journal of Motor Behavior, 19*(2), 147–166.

Fidler, G.S., & Fidler, J.W. (1978). Doing and becoming: Purposeful action and self-actualization. *American Journal of Occupational Therapy, 32*, 305–310.

Fiorentino, M.R. (1963). *Reflex testing methods for evaluating C.N.S. development.* Springfield, IL: Charles C. Thomas.

Fiorentino, M.R. (1972). *Normal and abnormal development.* Springfield, IL: Charles C. Thomas.

Fiorentino, M.R. (1981). *A basis for sensorimotor development: Normal and abnormal.* Springfield, IL: Charles C. Thomas.

Fiscus, S.A., Adimora, A.A., Funk, M.L., Schoenbach, V.J., Tristram, D., Lim, W., & Wilfert, C. (2002). Trends in interventions to reduce perinatal human immunodeficiency virus type 1 transmission in North Carolina. *The Journal of Pediatric Infectious Disease, 21*(7), 664–668.

Fitzgibbons, S.C., Ching, Y., Yu, D., Carpenter, J., Kenny, M., Weldon, C., & Jaksic, T. (2009). Mortality of necrotizing enterocolitis expressed by birth weight categories. *Journal of Pediatric Surgery, 44*(6), 1072–1076. doi: DOI: 10.1016/j.jpedsurg.2009.02.013

Folio, M.R., & Fewell, R.R. (2000). *Peabody Developmental Motor Scales* (PDMS-2). Austin, TX: Pro-Ed, Inc.

Forbes, E.E., & Dahl, R.E. (2010). Pubertal development and behavior: Hormonal activation of social and motivational tendencies. *Brain and Cognition, 72*(1), 66–72.

Fox, S.E., Levitt, P., & Nelson, C.A., III. (2010). How the timing and quality of early experiences influence the development of brain architecture. *Child Development, 81*(1), 28–40. doi: 10.1111/j.1467-8624.2009.01380.x

Fried, P.A., Watkinson, B., & Gray, R. (1998). Differential effects on cognitive functioning in 9–12-year-olds prenatally exposed to cigarettes and marihuana. *Neurotoxicology and Teratology, 20*, 293–306.

Fried, P.A., Watkinson, B., & Gray, R. (1999). Growth from birth to early adolescence in offspring prenatally exposed to cigarettes and marijuana. *Neurotoxicology and Teratology, 21*, 513–525.

Gallahue, D.L., & Ozmum, J.C. (2006). *Understanding motor development: Infants, children, adolescents, adults* (6th ed.). Boston: McGraw Hill.

Galloway, J.C., & Thelen, E. (2004). Feet first: object exploration in young infants. *Infant Behavior & Development, 27*, 107–112.

Gesell, A. (1928). *Infancy and human growth.* New York: Macmillan.

Gesell, A. (1945). *The embryology of behavior* (p. 169). New York: Harper.

Gesell, A. (1949). *Gesell developmental scales.* New York: Psychological Corp.

Gesell, A. (1952). *Infant development.* Westport, CT: Greenwood Press.

Gesell, A., & Amatruda, C.S. (1947). *Developmental diagnosis: Normal and abnormal child development, clinical methods and pediatric applications.* New York: Harper & Row.

Gesell, A., & Thompson, H. (1934). *Infant behavior: Its genesis and growth.* New York: McGraw-Hill.

Giangreco, M.E., Dennis, R., Cloninger, C.J., Edelman, S., & Schattman, R. (1993). "I've counted Jon": Transformational experiences of teachers educating students with disabilities. *Exceptional Children, 59*, 359–372.

Gibson, E. (1988). Exploratory behavior in the development of perceiving, acting, and acquiring knowledge. *Annual Review of Psychology, 39*, 1–41.

Gibson, J.J. (1950). *The perception of the visual world.* Boston: Houghton Mifflin.

Gill, S.V., Adolph, K.E., & Vereijken, B. (2009). Change in action: How infants learn to walk down slopes. *Developmental Science, 12*(6), 888–902.

Goldschmidt, L., Day, N.L., & Richardson, G.A. (2000). Effects of prenatal marijuana exposure on child behavior problems at age 10. *Neurotoxicology and Tetralogy, 22,* 325–336.

Gordon, E.S. (2007). Syndromes and inborn errors of metabolism. In M.L. Batshaw, L. Pellegrino, & N.J. Roizen (Eds.), *Children with disabilities* (6th ed., pp. 663–697). Baltimore: Paul H. Brookes.

Graven, S.N., & Browne, J.V. (2008). Sleep and brain development: The critical role of sleep in fetal and early neonatal brain development. *Newborn & Infant Nursing Reviews, 8*(4), 173–179.

Graves, L., Stratton, G., Ridgers, N.D., & Cable, N.T. (2007). Comparison of energy expenditure in adolescents when playing new generation and sedentary computer games: cross sectional study. *British Medical Journal, 335,* 1282–1284. doi:10.1136/bmj.3 9415.632951.80

Green, C.M., Berkule, S.B., Dreyer, B.P., Fierman, A.H., Huberman, H.S., Klass, P.E., Tomopulos, S., & Mendelsohn, A.L. (2009). Maternal literacy and associations between education and the cognitive home environment in low-income families. *Archives of Pediatrics & Adolescent Medicine, 163*(9), 832–837.

Grummer-Strawn, L.M., Reinold, C., & Krebs, N.F. (2010). Use of World Health Organization and CDC Growth Charts for Children aged 0–59 months in the United States. *Morbidity and Mortality Weekly Report, 59*(rr09), 1–15. Retrieved from http://www.cdc.gov/mmwr/preview/mmwrhtml/rr5909a1.htm

Guralnick, M.J. (1999). The nature and meaning of social integration for young children with mild developmental delays in inclusive settings. *Journal of Early Intervention, 22,* 70–86.

Guralnick, M.J. (2001). *Early childhood inclusion: Focus on change.* Baltimore: Paul H. Brookes.

Hadders-Algra, M. (2010). Variation and variability: Key words in human motor development. *Physical Therapy, 90*(12), 1823–1837.

Hadders-Algra, M., Brogren, E., & Forssberg, H. (1996). Ontogeny of postural adjustments during sitting in infancy: Variation, selection and modulation. *Journal of Physiology, 493,* 273–288.

Haffner, W.H.J. (2007). Development before birth. In M.L. Batshaw, L. Pellegrino, & N.J. Roizen (Eds.), *Children with disabilities* (6th ed., p. 23). Baltimore: Paul H. Brookes.

Haley, S.M. (1986). Sequential analysis of postural reactions in non-handicapped infants. *Physical Therapy, 66,* 531–536.

Halverson, H.M. (1931). An experimental study of prehension in infants by means of systematic cinema records. *Genetic Psychology Monographs, 10,* 107–286.

Halverson, H.M. (1933). The acquisition of skill in infancy. *Journal of Genetic Psychology, 43,* 3–48.

Harbourne, R.T., & Stergiou, N. (2003). Nonlinear analysis of the development of sitting postural control. *Developmental Psychobiology, 3*(42), 368–377.

Harbourne, R.T., & Stergiou, N. (2009). Movement variability and the use of nonlinear tools: Principles to guide physical therapist practice. *Physical Therapy, 89*(3), 267–280.

Harris, J.R. (1998). *The nurture assumption: Why children turn out the way they do.* New York: Free Press.

Havighurst, R.J. (1972). *Developmental tasks and education* (3rd ed.). New York: David McKay Company, Inc.

Helders, P.J.M. (2010). Variability in childhood development. *Physical Therapy, 90*(12), 1708–1709.

Heriza, C. (1991). Motor development: Traditional and contemporary theories. In M. Lister (Ed.), *Contemporary management of motor control problems. Proceedings of the II Step Conference* (pp. 99–126). Alexandria, VA: Foundation for Physical Therapy.

Hill, J.B., & Haffner, W.H.J. (2002). Growth before birth. In M.L. Batshaw (Ed.), *Children with disabilities* (5th ed., pp. 43–53). Baltimore: Paul H. Brookes.

Himes, J.H. (2006). Examining the evidence for recent secular changes in the timing of puberty in US children in light of increases in the prevalence of obesity. *Molecular and Cellular Endocrinology, 254–255,* 13–21.

Hopkins, B., & Rönnqvist, L. (2002). Facilitating postural control: Effect of reaching behavior of 6-month-old infants. *Developmental Psychobiology, 40,* 168–182.

Horak, F.B. (1991). Assumptions underlying motor control for neurologic rehabilitation. In M. Lister (Ed.), *Contemporary management of motor control problems. Proceedings of the II Step Conference* (pp. 11–27). Alexandria, VA: Foundation for Physical Therapy.

Horwitz, S.M., Irwin, J.R., Briggs-Gowan, M., Heenan, J., Mendoza, J., & Carter, A. (2003). Language delay in a community cohort of young children. *American Academy of Child and Adolescent Psychiatry, 42,* 932–940.

Houston, D.M., & Miyamoto, R.T. (2010). Effects of early auditory experience on word learning and speech perception in deaf children with cochlear implants: implications for sensitive periods of language development. *Otology and Neurotology, 31*(8), 1248–1253.

Howard, L. (1996). A comparison of leisure time activities between able bodied children and children with physical disabilities. *British Journal of Occupational Therapy, 59*(12), 570–574.

Hubel, D.H., & Wiesel, T.N. (1970). The period of susceptibility to the physiological effects of unilateral eye closure in kittens. *Journal of Physiology, 206,* 419–436.

Human Rights and Equal Opportunity Commission (2003). Goward applauds introduction of 12 weeks paid paternal leave in New Zealand.

Hunt, P., Doering, K., Hirose-Hatae, A., Maier J., & Goetz, L. (2001). Across-program collaboration to support students with and without disabilities in a general education classroom. *Journal for the Association for Persons with Severe Handicaps, 26,* 240–256.

Hunt, P., Soto, G., Maier, J., & Doering, K. (2003). Collaborative teaming to support students at risk and students with severe disabilities in general education classrooms. *Exceptional Children, 69*(3), 315–332.

Ito, M. (2004). 'Nurturing the brain' as an emerging research field involving child neurology. *Brain & Development, 26*(7), 429-433. doi: 10.1016/j.braindev.2003.02.001

Jacobson, J.L., & Jacobson, S.W. (1994). Prenatal alcohol exposure and neurobehavioral development: Where is the threshold? *Alcohol Health and Research World, 18,* 30–36.

Jansen, P.W., Tiemeier, H., Jaddoe, V.W., Hofman, A., Steegers, E.A., Verhulst, F.C., & Raat, H. (2009). Explaining educational inequalities in preterm birth: The generation R study. *Archives of Disease in Childhood. Fetal and Neonatal Edition, 94*(1), F28–34.

Jantz, J.W., Blosser, C.D., & Fruechting, L.A. (1997). A motor milestone change noted with a change in sleep position. *Archives of Pediatrics and Adolescent Medicine, 151,* 565–568.

Jirikowic, T., Olson, H.C., & Kartin, D. (2008). Sensory processing, school performance, and adaptive behavior of young school-aged children with fetal alcohol spectrum disorders. *Physical & Occupational Therapy in Pediatrics, 28*(2), 117–136.

Jones, K.L. (2006). *Smith's recognizable patterns of human malformation* (6th ed.). Philadelphia: Elsevier Saunders.

Joyner, B.L., Gill-Bailey, C., & Moon, R.Y. (2009). Infant sleep environments depicted in magazines targeted to women of childbearing age. *Pediatrics, 124*(3), e416–422.

Kaiser, L., & Allen, L.H. (2008). Position of the American Dietetic Association: Nutrition and lifestyle for a healthy pregnancy outcome. *Journal of the American Dietetic Association, 108*(3), 553–561.

Kalia, J.L., Visintainer, P., Brumberg, H.L., Pici, M., & Kase, J. (2009). Comparison of enrollment in interventional therapies between late-preterm and very preterm infants at 12 months' corrected age. *Pediatrics, 123*(3), 804–809.

Kelso, J.A.S., Holt, K.G., Kugler, P.N., & Turvey, M.T. (1980). On the concept of coordinative structures as dissipative structures: II. Empirical lines of convergence. In G.E. Stelmach & J. Requin (Eds.), *Tutorials in motor behavior* (pp. 49–70). New York: North Holland.

Kelso, J.A.S., & Tuller, B. (1984). A dynamical basis for action systems. In M. Gassaniga (Ed.), *Handbook of cognitive neuroscience.* New York: Plenum Press.

Knobloch, H., & Pasamanick, B. (Eds.). (1974). *Gesell and Amatruda's manual of developmental diagnosis* (3rd ed.). New York: Harper & Row Publishing.

Konczak, J., & Dichgans, J. (1997). The development toward stereotypic arm kinematics during reaching in the first 3 years of life. *Experimental Brain Research, 117*(2), 346–354.

Krick, J., Murphy-Miller, P., Zeger, S., & Wright, E. (1996). Patterns of growth in children with cerebral palsy. *Journal of the American Dietetic Association, 96,* 680–685.

Kuno, A., Akiyama, M., Yamashiro, C., Tanaka, H., Yanagihara, T., & Hata, T. (2001). Three-dimensional sonographic assessment of fetal behavior in the early second trimester of pregnancy. *Journal of Ultrasound in Medicine, 20*(12), 1271–1275.

Kurjak, A., Tikvica, A., Stanojevic, M., Miskovic, B., Ahmed, B., Azumendi, G., Di Renzo, G.C. (2008). The assessment of fetal neurobehavior by three-dimensional and four-dimensional ultrasound. *The Journal of Maternal-Fetal & Neonatal Medicine, 21*(10), 675–684.

Lee, M. (1998). Substance abuse in pregnancy. *Obstetrics and Gynecology Clinics, 25,* 65–83.

Lewin-Benham, A. (2008). *Powerful children: Understanding how to teach and learn using the Reggio Approach.* New York: Teachers College Press.

Lewis, T.L., & Maurer, D. (2005). Multiple sensitive periods in human visual development: Evidence from visually deprived children. *Developmental Psychobiology, 46*(3), 163–183. doi: 10.1002/dev.20055

Li, C.Q., Windsor, R.A. Perkins, I., Goldenberg, R.L., & Lowe, J.B. (1993). The impact on infant birth weight and gestational age of cotinine-validated smoking reduction during pregnancy. *Journal of the American Medical Association, 269,* 1519–1524.

Liao, P.J.M., Zawacki, L., & Campbell, S.K. (2005). Annotated bibliography: Effects of sleep position and play position on motor development in early infancy. *Physical & Occupational Therapy in Pediatrics, 25*(1–2), 149–160.

Linder, T. (2008). *Transdisciplinary play-based assessment* (2nd ed.). Baltimore: Brookes.

Long, T.M., & Toscano, K. (2002). *Handbook of pediatric physical therapy* (2nd ed.). Philadelphia: Lippincott Williams & Wilkins.

Low, S.M. (1984). The cultural basis of health, illness and disease. *Social Work in Health Care, 9*(3), 13–23.

Luna, B., Padmanabhan, A., & O'Hearn, K. (2010). What has fMRI told us about the development of cognitive control through adolescence? *Brain and Cognition, 72*(1), 101–113.

Luu, T.M., Ment, L.R., Schneider, K.C., Katz, K.H., Allan, W.C., & Vohr, B.R. (2009). Lasting effects of preterm birth and neonatal brain hemorrhage at 12 years of age. *Pediatrics, 123*(3), 1037–1044.

Maart, S., & Jelsma, J. (2010). The sexual behaviour of physically disabled adolescents. *Disability and Rehabilitation, 32*(6), 438–443.

Malkawi, S.H. (2009). *Participation in play activities of children with cerebral palsy.* Unpublished doctoral dissertation. University of Kentucky, Lexington, KY.

McGraw, M.B. (1932). From reflex to muscular control in the assumption of erect posture and ambulation in the human infant. *Child Development, 3,* 291–297.

McGraw, M.B. (1935). *Growth: A study of Johnny and Jimmy.* New York: Appleton-Century.

McGraw, M.B. (1945). *The neuromuscular maturation of the human infant.* New York: Columbia University Press.

Michels, K.B., Trichopoulos, D., Robins, J.M., Rosner, B.A., Manson, J.E., Hunter, D.J., & Willett, W.C. (1996). Birthweight as a risk factor for breast cancer. *Lancet, 348*(9041), 1542–1546.

Milani-Comparetti, A., & Gidoni, E.A. (1967). Routine developmental examination in normal and retarded children. *Developmental Medicine and Child Neurology, 9,* 631–638.

Mildred, J., Beard, K., Dallwitz, A., & Unwin, J. (1995). Play position is influenced by knowledge of SIDS sleep position recommendations. *Journal of Paediatric Child Health, 31,* 499–502.

Montessori, M. (1964). *The Montessori method.* New York: Schocken Books.

Morales, A.T., & Sheafor, B.W. (2001). *Social work* (9th ed.). Needham Heights, MA: Pearson Education.

Najman, J.M., Clavarino, A., McGee, T.R., Bor, W., Williams, G.M., & Hayatbakhsh, M.R. (2010). Timing and chronicity of family poverty and development of unhealthy behaviors in children: A longitudinal study. *Journal of Adolescent Health, 46*(6), 538–544. doi: 10.1016/j.jadohealth.2009.12.001

Nathanielsz, P. (1999). *Life in the womb: The origins of health and disease.* Ithaca, NY: Promethean Press.

National Autism Center (2009). *Evidence-based practice and autism in the schools: A guide to providing appropriate interventions to students with autism spectrum disorders.* (p. 38). Randolph, MA: Author.

National Institute of Child Health and Human Development (2004). *Thai study shows that inexpensive treatment reduces risk of mother to child HIV transmission.* Retrieved from http://www.nichd.nih.gov/news/releases/maternal_AIDS.cfm

National Institute of Child Health and Human Development (2010). *The "PROMISE" of research.* Retrieved from http://www.nichd.nih.gov/news/resources/spotlight/012210-promise.cfm

National Institutes of Health (2011). *National Human Genome Research Institute.* Retrieved from http://www.genome.gov/

Nelson, E.A.S., Yu, L.M., Wong, D., Wong, H.Y.E., & Yim, L. (2004). Rolling over in infants: Age, ethnicity, and cultural differences. *Developmental Medicine and Child Neurology, 46*(10), 706–709.

Noonan, M.J. (2006). Naturalistic curriculum model. In M.J. Noonan and L. McCormick, *Young children with disabilities in natural environments* (pp. 77–98). Baltimore: Paul H. Brookes.

Ogden, C.L., Carroll, M.D., Curtin, L.R., Lamb, M.M., & Flegal, K.M. (2010). Prevalence of high body mass index in US children and adolescents, 2007–2008. *Journal of the American Medical Association, 303*(3), 242–249.

O'Keeffe, M.J., O'Callaghan, M., Williams, G.M., Najman, J.M., & Bor, W. (2003). Learning, cognitive, and attentional problems in adolescents born small for gestational age. *Pediatrics, 112*(2), 301–307.

Ott, D.A.D., & Effgen, S.K. (2000). Occurrence of gross motor behaviors in integrated and segregated preschool classrooms. *Pediatric Physical Therapy, 12,* 164–172.

Owens, R. E. (2001) *Language development: An introduction* (5th ed., p. 92). Boston: Allyn & Bacon.

Palsha, S. (2002). An outstanding education for ALL children: Learning from Reggio Emilia's approach to inclusion. In V.R. Fu, A.J. Stemmel, & L.T. Hill (Eds.), *Teaching and learning: Collaborative exploration of the Reggio Emilia approach* (pp. 109–130). Upper Saddle River, NJ: Merrill Prentice Hall.

Park, S. (2007). *HELP Strands.* Palo Alto, CA: VORT Corporation.

Patrick, K., Spear, B., Holt, K., & Sofka, D. (Eds.). (2001). *Bright futures in practice: Physical activity.* Arlington, VA: National Center for Education in Maternal and Child Health.

Peck, C.A., Donaldson, J., & Pezzoli, M. (1990). Some benefits nonhandicapped adolescents perceive for themselves from their social relationships with peers who have severe handicaps. *Journal of the Association for Persons with Severe Handicaps, 15,* 241–249.

Peiper, A. (1963). *Cerebral function in infancy and childhood.* New York: Consultants' Bureau.

Piaget, J. (1952). *The origins of intelligence in children.* New York: International University Press.

Piper, M.C., & Darrah, J. (1994). *Motor assessment of the developing infant.* Philadelphia: W.B. Saunders.

Pogodina, C., Brunner Huber, L.R., Racine, E.F., & Platonova, E. (2009). Smoke-free homes for smoke-free babies: the role of residential environmental tobacco smoke on low birth weight. *Journal of Community Health, 34*(5), 376–382.

Quigley, M.A., Hockley, C., Carson, C., Kelly, Y., Renfrew, M.J., & Sacker, A. (2012). Breastfeeding is associated with improved child cognitive development: A population-based cohort study. *Journal of Pediatrics, 160*(1), 25–32.

Raine, A., Reynolds, C., Venables, P.H., & Mednick, S. (2002). Stimulation seeking and intelligence: A prospective longitudinal study. *Journal of Personality and Social Psychology, 82*(4), 663–674.

Rais-Bahrami, K., & Short, B.L. (2007). Premature and small-for-dates infants. In M.L. Batshaw, L. Pellegrino, & N.J. Roizen (Eds.), *Children with disabilities* (6th ed., pp. 107–122). Baltimore: Paul H. Brookes.

Reich, P.A. (1986). *Language development.* Englewood Cliffs, NJ: Prentice-Hall.

Rescorda, L., Ross, G.S., & McClue, S. (2007). Language delay and behavioral/emotional problems in toddlers: Findings from two developmental clinics. *Journal of Speech, Language, and Hearing Research, 50,* 1063–1078.

Reznick, J.S. (2000). Biology versus experience: Balancing the equation. *Developmental Science, 3,* 133–134.

Rich-Edwards, J.W., Stampfer, M.J., Manson, J.E., Rosner, B., Hankinson, S.E., Colditz, G.A., & Hennekens, C.H. (1997). Birthweight and risk of cardiovascular disease in a cohort of women followed up since 1976. *British Medical Journal, 315*(7105), 396–400.

Rochat, P. (1992). Self-sitting and reaching in 5- to 8-month-old infants: The impact of posture and its development on eye-hand coordination. *Journal of Motor Behavior, 24,* 210–220.

Rossetti, L. (2005). *The Rossetti Infant-Toddler Language Scale.* East Moline, IL: Lingui Systems, Inc.

Rovee-Collier, C.K., Sullivan, M., Enright, M.K., Lucus, D., & Fagen, J.W. (1980). Reactivation of infant memory. *Science, 208,* 1159–1161.

Sadeh, A., Dahl, R.E., Shahar, G., & Rosenblat-Stein, S. (2009). Sleep and the transition to adolescence: a longitudinal study. *Sleep, 1*(32), 1602–1609.

Sameroff, A. (2009). *The transactional model of development: How children and contexts shape each other.* Washington, DC: American Psychological Association.

Sanger, W.G., Dave, B., & Stuberg, W. (2001). Overview of genetics and role of the pediatric physical therapist in diagnostic process. *Pediatric Physical Therapy, 13,* 164–168.

Santrock, J.W. (1998). *Child development* (8th ed., pp. 35–71). Boston: McGraw-Hill.

Scarborough, A.A., & McCrae, J.S. (2010). School-age special education outcomes of infants and toddlers investigated for maltreatment. *Children and Youth Services Review, 32*(1), 80–88.

Schaefer, G.B. (2001). Clinical genetics in pediatric physical therapy practice? The future. *Pediatric Physical Therapy, 13,* 182–184.

Schickendanz, J., Schickendanz, D., Hansen, K., & Forsyth, P.D. (1993). *Understanding children.* Mountain View, CA: Mayfield Publishing.

Scholz, J.P. (1990). Dynamic pattern theory: Some implications for therapeutics. *Physical Therapy, 70*(12), 827–843.

Seifert, K.L., & Hoffnung, R.J. (1997). *Child and adolescent development* (4th ed., pp. 29–55). New York: Houghton Mifflin Co.

Seligman, M.E.P. (1975). *Helplessness: On depression, development, and death.* San Francisco: W.H. Freeman.

Sherrill, C. (1993). *Adapted physical activity, recreation and sport: Cross disciplinary and life span* (Chapters 5, 10, 11, and 12). Dubuque, IA: W.C. Brown.

Shibli, R., Rubin, L., Akons, H., & Shaoul, R. (2008). Morbidity of overweight (>=85th percentile) in the first 2 years of life. *Pediatrics, 122*(2), 267–272.

Shikako-Thomas, K., Majnemer, A., Law, M., & Lach, L. (2008). Determinants of participation in leisure activities in children and youth with cerebral palsy: Systematic review. *Physical and Occupational Therapy in Pediatrics, 28*(2), 155–163.

Shirley, M.M. (1931). *The first two years: A study of twenty-five babies,* Vol. I. Minneapolis: University of Minnesota Press.

Shirley, M.M. (1933*).* The first two years, a study of twenty-five babies. In *Intellectual Development* (Vol. 2). Minneapolis: University of Minnesota Press.

Shumway-Cook, A., & Woollacott, M. (2007). *Motor control theory and practical applications* (3rd ed.). Philadelphia: Lippincott Williams & Wilkins.

Skinner, B.F. (1953). *Science and human behavior.* New York: Macmillan.

Smith, L.J., van Asperen, P.P., McKay, K.O., Selvadurai, H., & Fitzgerald, D.A. (2008). Reduced exercise capacity in children born very preterm. *Pediatrics, 122*(2), e287–293.

Soto, G., Muller, E., Hunt, P., & Goetz, L. (2001). Critical issues in the inclusion of students who use AAC: An educational team perspective. *Augmentative and Alternative Communication, 17*(3), 62–72.

Sparling, J.W., van Tol, J., & Chescheir, N.C. (1999). Fetal and neonatal hand movement. *Physical Therapy, 79*(10), 195–200.

Spencer, J. P., Clearfield, M., Corbetta, D., Ulrich, B., Buchanan, P., & Schoner, G. (2006). Moving toward a grand theory of development: In memory of Esther Thelen. *Child Development, 77*(6), 1521–1538.

Spencer, J.P., & Thelen, E. (2000). Spatially specific changes in infants' muscle co-activity as they learn to reach. *Infancy, 1,* 275–302.

Sporns, O., & Edelman, G.M. (1993). Solving Bernstein's problem: Proposal for the development of coordinated movement by selection. *Child Development, 64,* 960–981.

Statham, L., & Murray, M. (1971). Early walking patterns of normal children. *Clinical Orthopaedics and Related Research, 79,* 8–24.

Steinberg, L., Albert, D., Cauffman, E., Banich, M., Graham, S., & Woolard, J. (2008). Age differences in sensation seeking and impulsivity as indexed by behavior and self-report: Evidence for a dual systems model, *Developmental Psychology, 44*(6), 1764–1778.

Steinberger, J., & Daniels, S.R. (2003). Obesity, insulin resistance, diabetes, and cardiovascular risk in children: An American Heart Association scientific statement from the Atherosclerosis, Hypertension, and Obesity in the Young Committee (Council on Cardiovascular Disease in the Young), and the Diabetes Committee (Council on Nutrition, Physical Activity, and Metabolism). *Circulation, 107*(10), 1448–1453.

Steinhausen, H., Metzke, C.W., & Spohr, H. (2003). Behavioral phenotype in foetal alcohol syndrome and foetal alcohol effects. *Developmental Medicine and Child Neurology, 45,* 179–182.

Stevenson, R.D., Conaway, M., Chumlea, W.C., Rosenbaum, P., Fung, E.B., Henderson, R.C., & North American Growth in Cerebral Palsy Study. (2006). Growth and health in children with moderate-to-severe cerebral palsy. *Pediatrics, 118*(3), 1010–1018.

Stockmeyer, S.A. (1967). An interpretation of the approach of Rood to the treatment of neuromuscular dysfunction. *American Journal of Physical Medicine, 46*(1), 900–961.

Strathearn, L., Mamun, A.A., Najman, J.M., & O'Callaghan, M.J. (2009). Does breastfeeding protect against substantiated child abuse and neglect? A 15-year cohort study. *Pediatrics, 123*(2), 483–493.

Sutcliffe, T.L., Gaetz, W.C., Logan, W.J., Cheyne, D.O., & Fehlings, D.L. (2007). Cortical reorganization after modified constraint-induced movement therapy in pediatric hemiplegic cerebral palsy. *Journal of Child Neurology, 22*(11), 1281–1287.

Sutherland, D., Olshen, R., Biden, E., & Wyatt, M. (1988). The development of mature gait. *Clinics in Developmental Medicine,* No. 104/105. Philadelphia: J.B. Lippincott.

Sutherland, D., Olshen, R., Cooper, L., & Woo, S. (1980). The development of mature gait. *The Journal of Bone and Joint Surgery, 62-A*(3), 336–353.

Taanila, A., Murray, G.K., Isohanni, M., & Rantakallio, P. (2005). Infant developmental milestones: A 31-year follow-up. *Developmental Medicine and Child Neurology, 47,* 581–586.

Tamm, M., & Skär, L. (2000). How I play: Roles and relations in the play situations of children with restricted mobility. *Scandinavian Journal of Occupational Therapy, 7*(4), 174–182.

Taub, E., & Morris, D.M. (2001). Constraint-induced movement therapy to enhance recovery after stroke. *Current Atherosclerosis Reports, 3,* 279–286.

Taub, E., Uswatte, G., & Pidikiti, R. (1999). Constraint-induced movement therapy: A new family of techniques with broad application to physical rehabilitation—A clinical review. *Journal of Rehabilitation Research and Development, 36*(3), 237–251.

Taub, E., & Wolf, S.L. (1997). Constraint-induced (CI) movement techniques to facilitate upper extremity use in stroke patients. *Topics in Stroke Rehabilitation, 3,* 38–61.

Thelen, E. (1985). Developmental origins of motor coordination: Leg movements in human infants. *Developmental Psychobiology, 18,* 1–22.

Thelen, E., Corbetta, D., Kamm, K., Spencer, J.P., Schneider, K., & Zernicke, R.F. (1993). The transition to reaching: Mapping intention and intrinsic dynamics. *Child Development, 64*(4), 1058–1098.

Thelen, E., Corbetta, D., & Spencer, J.P. (1996). Development of reaching during the first year: Role of movement speed. *Journal of Experimental Psychology. Human Perception and Performance, 22*(5), 1059–1076.

Thelen, E., Kelso, J.A., & Fogel, A. (1987). Self-organizing systems and infant motor development. *Developmental Review, 7,* 39–65.

Thelen, E., & Smith, L.B. (1994). *A dynamic systems approach to the development of cognition and action.* Cambridge, MA: The MIT Press.

Thelen, E., & Ulrich, B.D. (1991). Hidden skills: A dynamic systems analysis of treadmill stepping during the first year. *Monographs of the Society for Research in Child Development, 56*(1, Serial No. 223).

Thelen, E., Ulrich, B.D., & Jensen, J.L. (1989). The developmental origins of locomotion. In M.H. Woollacott & A. Shumway-Cook (Eds.), *Development of posture and gait across the life span* (pp. 25–47). Columbia, SC: University of South Carolina Press.

Tipps, S.T., Mira, M.P., & Cairns, G.F. (1981). Concurrent tracking of infant motor and speech development. *Genetic Psychology Monographs, 104*, 303–324.

Toledo, C., Alembik, Y., Aguirre Jaime, A., & Stoll, C. (1999). Growth curves of children with Down syndrome. *Annales De Génétique, 42*(2), 81–90.

Tomasello, M., Carpenter, M., & Liszkowski, U. (2007). A new look at infant pointing. *Child Development, 78*(3), 705–722.

Tomblin, J.B., Smith, E., & Zhang, X. (1997). Epidemiology of specific language impairment: Prenatal and perinatal risk factors. *Journal of Communication Disorders, 30*, 325–344.

Touwen, B. (1976). Neurological development in infancy. *Clinics in Developmental Medicine*, No. 58. Philadelphia: J.B. Lippincott.

U.S. Department of Health and Human Services, Substance Abuse and Mental Health Services Administration, Office of Applied Studies. (2008). *National survey on drug use and health*. ICPSR26701-v1. Research Triangle Park, NC: Research Triangle Institute [producer], 2009. Ann Arbor, MI: Inter-university Consortium for Political and Social Research [distributor], 2009-11-16. Retrieved from http://www.icpsr.umich.edu/quicktables/quickconfig.do?26701-0001_du

van der Fits, I.B.M., Klip, A.W.J., van Eykern, L.A., & Hadders-Algra, M. (1999). Postural adjustments during spontaneous and goal-directed arm movements in the first half year of life. *Behavioral Brain Research, 106*, 75–90.

Vennemann, M.M., Bajanowski, T., Brinkmann, B., Jorch, G., Yücesan, K., Sauerland, C., & GeSID Study Group (2009). Does breastfeeding reduce the risk of sudden infant death syndrome? *Pediatrics, 123*(3), e406–410.

Vereijken, B. (2010). The complexity of childhood development: Variability in perspective. *Physical Therapy, 90*(12), 1850–1859.

von Hofsten, C., & Woollacott, H.M. (1989). Anticipatory postural adjustments during infant reaching. *Neuroscience Abstracts, 15*, 1199.

Vygotsky, L.S. (1978). *Mind in society: The development of higher psychological processes*. Cambridge, MA: Cambridge University Press.

Witherington, D.C., von Hofsten, C., Rosander, K., Robinette, A., Woollacott, M.H., & Bertenthal, B.I. (2002). The development of anticipatory postural adjustments in infancy. *Infancy, 3*(4), 495–517.

Wittberg, R.A., Northrup, K.L., & Cottrel, L. (2009). Children's physical fitness and academic performance. *American Journal of Health Education, 40*(1), 30–36.

World Health Organization (WHO) (2006). Motor development study: Windows of achievement for six gross motor development milestones. *Acta Paediatrica, Supplement, 450*, 86–95.

World Health Organization (WHO) (2011). WHO Child Growth Standards: Methods and development: Length/height-for-age, weight-for-age, weight-for-length, weight-for-height and body mass index-for-age. Retrieved from http://www.who.int/childgrowth/publications/technical_report_pub/en/index.html

Wu, S. S., Ma, C.-X., Carter, R.L., Ariet, M., Feaver, E.A., Resnick, M.B., Roth, J. (2004). Risk factors for infant maltreatment: a population-based study. *Child Abuse & Neglect, 28*(12), 1253–1264.

Wunsch, M.J., Conlon, C.J., & Scheidt, P.C. (2002). Substance abuse. In M.L. Batshaw (Ed.), *Children with disabilities* (5th ed., pp. 107–122). Baltimore: Paul H. Brookes.

CHAPTER 3

Child Appraisal: Examination and Evaluation

—Susan K. Effgen, PT, PhD, FAPTA

—Janice Howman, PT, DPT, MEd

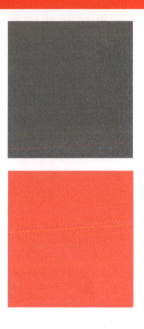

Physical therapists should understand the pathology, etiology, impairments in body structures and functions, and restrictions in activities and participation for all the individuals they serve. Those working with children must also understand all domains of child development and behavior and family functioning to provide appropriate examination, evaluation, diagnosis, prognosis, and intervention. The examination and evaluation processes are complex with children because almost everything is influenced by the child's developmental, functional, and behavioral level, which are in turn significantly influenced by environmental and personal contextual factors. Additionally, when obtaining information regarding the child's status, the therapist must usually disguise the examination as "play." The child generally must be cooperative and actively engaged to display the highest level of performance. Therapists must be experts

at eliciting best performance and making it all fun, thus making the examination process more complex and difficult than in other areas of physical therapy practice.

There are a variety of terms used to describe what the American Physical Therapy Association (APTA) *Guide to Physical Therapist Practice* (hereafter referred to as the *Guide*) (2001) labels "examination" and "evaluation." As discussed in Chapter 1, many professionals, especially in pediatrics, continue to use the terms *examination*, *evaluation*, and *assessment* interchangeably. Others consider *evaluation* the process used to diagnose and identify atypical development or movement, whereas *assessment* is used to describe the process of collecting and organizing relevant information (Brenneman, 1999, p. 28), and some make no distinction at all. The Individuals with Disabilities Education Improvement Act (IDEA) (PL 108-446, 2004), the U.S.

right-to-education law, uses the term *evaluation* to refer to the processes of examination and evaluation for eligibility for services, and *assessment* for program planning purposes.

This text uses the *Guide*'s (APTA, 2001) terminology of *examination* for the physical process and *evaluation* for the dynamic, intellectual process of clinical decision making to determine the level of functioning of body functions and structures, activities, and participation. Under most situations, both processes occur simultaneously, so the terms are usually used together, except when there is a real distinction between the physical activity of the examination and the clinical judgment process of evaluation. In all settings, it is important to clarify the terminology used to avoid misunderstandings.

Factors Influencing Examination and Evaluation

Regardless of why a child comes to physical therapy for examination and evaluation, multiple factors must be considered to maximize the effectiveness of the process. Often these factors intertwine, resulting in overlapping and sometimes conflicting influences. The therapist must thoughtfully consider all applicable factors, then rely on his or her knowledge and clinical judgment to provide a skilled examination that is in the best interest of the child. Understanding the following factors will assist the therapist in determining location, time, style, and focus of examination, choosing which team members will be involved, selecting tests and measures to perform, and sequencing the components of examination. These skills are foundational for determining an accurate diagnosis and developing a relevant plan of care through sound clinical reasoning and decision making, which is the desired outcome of the examination and evaluation process.

Serving children with disabilities or special healthcare needs usually requires a team approach. Collaboration by team members is critical for a comprehensive examination and evaluation and for the provision of coordinated, integrated services. To facilitate this collaboration, team members commonly perform the examination together. Any member of the team might collect the history data and perform portions of the examination. For example, blood pressure, pulse, and respiration should be collected only once, unless there is a need to collect this information under different conditions, such as after stair climbing. Many professionals from different disciplines are trained to collect these data; duplication of examination procedures is avoided by a coordinated plan.

Purpose of the Examination and Evaluation

The purpose of the evaluation is critical in determining the examination procedures and what tests and measures to use. The tests and measures used will be different for a screening examination, a diagnostic examination, or a prescriptive examination. A screening examination is done to determine whether a problem exists that requires further detailed assessment. A screening test should generally be brief and cost effective, with minimal false-negative results.

Children who screen positive then receive a more comprehensive test as part of the examination. Screenings are commonly done for infants and young children who might require early intervention services or to determine the presence of a specific disability or characteristic. After the screening, a determination is made if more detailed examination is required and in what specific domains. If problems in the physical/motor domain are suggested, a physical therapist would then be asked to do a comprehensive examination to help determine eligibility for services, provide a referral to a medical agency, or develop a physical therapy plan of care.

A diagnostic examination is used to determine whether a child has a specific disability or is at risk for developing one. Completing a diagnostic examination for the purpose of developing a differential diagnosis is less common in pediatric practice than in other areas of physical therapy, but it is necessary for some children. For example, examination of an infant with torticollis requires distinguishing between congenital muscular torticollis and ocular, bony, or neurologic abnormalities to ensure proper intervention (Gray & Tasso, 2009)

A common purpose of examination in pediatrics, especially in early intervention, is to determine eligibility for services. Once the child is determined eligible for services, the prescriptive examination can be completed. A prescriptive examination is used to assist in determining the plan of care and most appropriate intervention. It is usually quite comprehensive. The purpose of the examination might also be to evaluate the magnitude of longitudinal change within subjects over time or to evaluate the effectiveness of interventions. Selecting the correct tests and measures for the examination is critical for determining services, documenting outcomes, and receiving reimbursement for services.

The diagnostic and prescriptive examinations, and sometimes a screening examination, usually start with a review of the child's history and a systems review. Table 1.2 and Figure 1.3 outline the content of the *Guide*'s (APTA, 2001) history and systems review. The important items that should be part of the history for a child are outlined in Table 3.1. While obtaining the child's history, it is also an excellent time to observe the child during natural play and the interactions of the child and parent. After collecting relevant history data, a systems review is completed. The systems review is a "brief or limited examination of (1) the anatomical and physiological status of the cardiovascular/pulmonary, integumentary, musculoskeletal, and neuromuscular systems; and (2) the communication ability, affect, cognition, language, and learning style of the patient" (APTA, 2001, p. 42). This coincides generally with the ICF-CY domains of body function and body structures. Basic system areas to be screened in children are presented in Table 3.2.

The systems review will assist the therapist in determining whether referral to another provider is necessary (APTA, 2001, p. 42) and what tests and measures should then be performed. Tests and measures should be limited to those necessary to determine the factors that contribute to making the child's current level of function less than optimal and those required to support the clinical judgments of the therapist regarding appropriate intervention, anticipated goals, and expected outcomes (p. 43). The tests and measures selected will depend on the complexity of the condition, the directives of the agency, and funding/insurance issues.

While professional judgment based on the condition and apparent needs of the child should drive the examination, some agencies might require the use of specific tests and measures, which might not be otherwise indicated or reliable and valid. State early intervention programs frequently mandate what tests a physical therapist must use for determination of eligibility. Usually, the therapist can administer additional tests and measures as long as the mandated tests are also used.

The classic work of Bailey and Wolery (1992) suggests that the evaluation process should achieve specific goals. While these goals were developed for preschoolers with disabilities, the process can be applied across the pediatric life span. They suggest (1992, pp. 97–99) that the evaluation process should achieve the following goals:

- Determine eligibility for services and the best place to receive those services
- "Identify developmentally appropriate and functional intervention goals" that are useful within the context of specific environments
- "Identify the unique styles, strengths, and coping strategies of each child"
- "Identify the parents' goals for their children and their needs for themselves," as in the top-down approach

Table 3.1 Data to be Obtained from Child's History

Past Medical History

- Mother's history related to pregnancy, labor, delivery
- Child's history related to pregnancy, labor, delivery
- Significant medical history of biological parents and relatives including siblings
- General health status
- Immunizations
- History of major childhood/adolescent illnesses
- History of any surgical or medical procedures
- Diagnostic or medical tests related to past history

Current Medical History

- Current signs and symptoms
- Onset, duration, and severity of presenting problem
- Current health-care practitioners involved with child's care (physicians, therapists, psychologists, orthotists, etc.)
- Current medications: purpose, dosage, history of adverse reactions
- Date and results of recent medical and diagnostic testing
- Current and planned medical and surgical interventions
- Current functional and activity levels
- Known allergies to food, medications, substances, etc.
- Use of adaptive equipment or devices

Developmental History

- Growth and nutrition (including rate of growth in height, weight, head circumference; timing of tooth eruption)
- Feeding: daily routine, preferences, difficulties
- Achievement of major milestones (including motor, social-emotional, cognitive, language, self-care)
- Bowel and bladder control/toilet training
- Infant/child temperament

Social and Education History

- Child-caregiver interactions
- Parents/caregivers' employment status
- Home layout and environment (including safety issues/childproofing)
- Sleep routine, child's sleeping position
- Early intervention/child care/school history
- Reports from early intervention team, child care providers, or teachers
- Use of car seat
- Signs of abuse or neglect

Source: Adapted from Dole, R.L., & Chafetz, R. (2010). *Peds Rehab Notes* (pp. 8, 9). Philadelphia: F.A. Davis. Copyright 2010 by F.A. Davis. Reprinted with permission of the authors.

Table 3.2 Systems Review/Basic Screening*

Cardiovascular-Pulmonary System

- *Vital signs*: heart rate, respiratory rate, blood pressure, temperature, pain
- *Observation*: difficulty breathing or crying, excessive crying, cyanosis, retractions, nasal flaring, cough, response to change in position or activity, fatigue, weight loss or gain
- *Palpation*: peripheral pulses, tactile fremitus
- *Auscultation*: heart and lung sounds
- *Percussion*: any areas of dullness over lung fields

Neuromuscular System

- *Newborns*: APGAR, gestational age, birth weight; suck and swallow, irritability/consolability, state regulation
- *Observation:* general resistance to passive movement; is it velocity-dependent?
- *Observation:* ability to make eye contact and track objects

Musculoskeletal System

- *Anthropometrics*: height, weight, head circumference
- *Observation*: size and shape of head, face, skull; any abnormalities of eyes, ears, nose, mouth, palate, teeth; skeletal asymmetry; swelling; bruising
- *Complaints:* pain; refusal to bear weight, walk, move; fever; night pain

Integumentary System

- *Observation/palpitation*: texture, temperature, color and pigmentation, scarring, presence of hair, turgor/hydration, swelling
- *Observation*: presence of skin lesions, rash, skin infection, change in a mole (color, size, shape, pain, itching, bleeding)

Endocrine System

- *Complaints:* increased thirst, frequent urination (especially at night), decreased activity, persistent constipation or diarrhea, increased sweating, hunger or decreased appetite, headache, dizziness or light-headedness, emotional lability, alterations to menstrual cycle
- *Observation*: short stature, precocious puberty, swollen gums, delayed healing time with typical sores/abrasions, weight loss or gain

Gastrointestinal System

- *Complaints*: nausea, vomiting, fever, reflux, colic, abdominal pain, chronic hunger or refusal to eat, abnormal stools or diarrhea, change in urine/output
- *Observation:* excessive mucus in mouth and nose, posturing neck extension or movement of head during feeding, signs of dehydration, weight loss or gain

Lymphatic/Immune System

- *Complaints:* fever, sore throat, rash, general malaise, night sweats, joint swelling or pain, weight loss
- *Palpation:* lymph nodes (neck, clavicular area, axilla, groin) spleen (1–2 cm below left costal margin), liver (≤2 cm below right costal margin)—check for enlargements

Genitourinary System

- *Complaints:* problems or changes in bowel/bladder function; frequent urinary tract infection; fever; vomiting; chills; abdominal pain; pain with urination; referred pain patterns to low back, flank, inner thigh, leg, ipsilateral shoulder; alterations to menstrual cycle
- *Observation:* fluid retention, dehydration, weight loss or gain, edema, irritability, unusual odor, discharge, signs of abuse
- *Vital signs:* blood pressure, fever

*See system chapters for more detailed information.

Source: From Dole, R.L., & Chafetz, R. (2010). *Peds Rehab Notes* (pp. 9, 10). Philadelphia: F.A. Davis. Copyright 2010 by F.A. Davis. Reprinted with permission of the authors.

- "Build and reinforce parents' sense of competence and worth"
- "Develop a shared and integrated perspective (across professionals and between professionals and family members) on the child and family needs and resources"
- "Create a shared commitment to the intervention goals" among the professionals and parents
- Evaluate the effectiveness and outcomes of the services and interventions

The focus on families noted by Bailey and Wolery (1992) has evolved since the enactment of Public Law 94-142, the Education for All Handicapped Children's Act, in 1975. This family-centered approach is now a clearly established perspective to serving children with disabilities and their families, as noted throughout the text and elaborated in Chapter 4.

Frameworks and Philosophies

Physical therapists use the APTA *Guide to Physical Therapist Practice* (2001), the APTA *Code of Ethics for the Physical Therapist* (2010a), individual state practice acts, the Hypothesis-Oriented Algorithm for Clinicians II (HOAC II) (Rothstein, Echternach, & Riddle, 2003), and the International Classification of Functioning, Disability and Health—Children and Youth Version (ICF-CY) (World Health Organization [WHO], 2007) to help guide their independent and objective professional judgment of their appraisal of a child's needs based on their scope of practice and level of expertise (APTA, 2010b). While the *Guide* is in the process of being updated to include the ICF, the ICF has already been incorporated in many areas of pediatric physical therapy practice.

When performing an examination, it is common to follow the sequence outlined in the *Guide* (APTA, 2001), starting with the history, then a systems review, and then performance of appropriate tests and measures. This is followed by an evaluation based on the information obtained during the examination. There are two common ways of focusing the examination. In HOAC II, a problem list is usually generated first, and then an examination strategy is developed, followed by the examination.

HOAC II indicates that there are two types of patient problems that are important to consider. The first are those problems that exist when the child is initially seen, labeled patient-identified problems. The second includes those problems that may occur in the future based on the diagnosis or developmental influences and might require prevention, or those problems that the child and family might not recognize as problems, labeled non-patient-identified problems (Rothstein et al., 2003). For child and family-identified problems, the therapist must generate hypotheses as to what caused the problems and then establish criteria that can be used to determine whether the interventions that will be used are successful. A non-patient-identified problem might be prevented by anticipating the problem and providing correct management. Determining measurable outcomes and prognosis are a critical aspect of the plan of care. Therapists must have considerable expertise with similar problems to achieve a high level of accuracy in prognosis and outcomes.

This approach of initially establishing a problem list is common in adult care and in pediatric acute care settings. However, in community-based pediatric practice, the outcome-driven, **top-down approach** (see Fig. 1.4) to examination and evaluation, first elaborated by Philippa Campbell (1991), has become the usual standard of practice (McEwen, Meiser, & Hansen, 2012, p. 549). This approach to examination and evaluation is especially evident in early intervention programs and schools. The desired outcomes and goals of intervention are determined first, preferably with the parents, the child if appropriate, and other team members, and then the examination is done to identify strengths that will assist in achieving the goals and the obstacles that must be overcome. The child and family are vital team members in this usually interdisciplinary or transdisciplinary team process. An example of a Clinical Decision-Making Algorithm for Pediatric Physical Therapy is presented in Fig. 3.1. This example includes the top-down approach but also incorporates the existing and anticipated problem lists of HOAC II. Rarely is the unidisciplinary, deficit-driven model, using a bottom-up approach in which the examination is used to determine the needs and deficits, the approach of choice in pediatrics, but it still might be used in other areas of physical therapy practice.

Therapists must understand these differences in the approach to examination and evaluation and how they reflect the different focus and priorities of different service delivery settings. Both approaches have merit based on the clinical situation and can even be combined. In a pediatric intensive care unit, the parents' general priority is the child's life. While the parents' input is valued, the medical team generally determines the specific priorities and goals, whereas in early intervention, the parents' specific goals take priority. For example, if the parent wants to focus on the child's

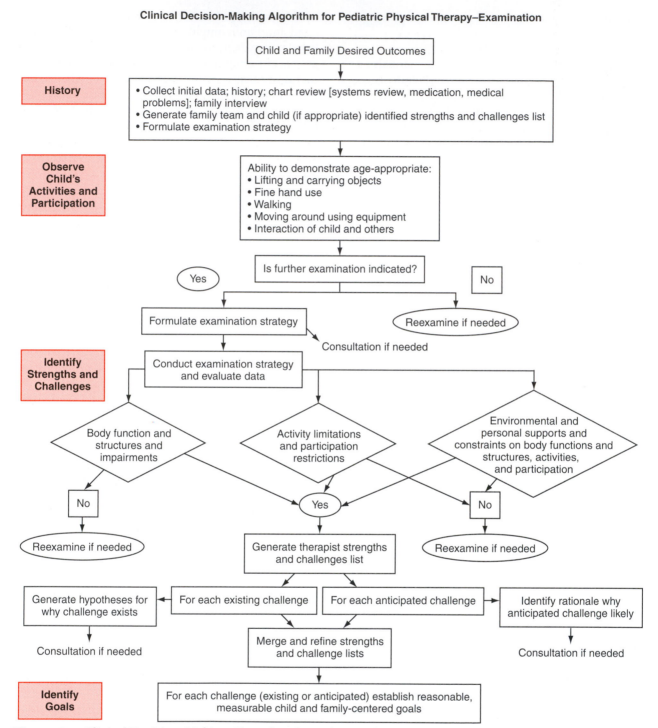

Figure 3.1 Clinical Decision-Making Algorithm for Pediatric Physical Therapy—Examination.

sitting skills over creeping, even though the therapist thinks focusing on creeping might be more important at the present time, the therapist will work on the parents' sitting goal with the child. However, as noted in *Code of Ethics for the Physical Therapist* (APTA, 2010a), the physical therapist must be accountable for making sound professional judgments, which include being independent and objective. Therefore, the therapist has an obligation to inform the family about what he or she considers in the child's best interest. The therapist in this example might try to persuade the parents of the importance of the creeping goal in overall development and environmental exploration, while also working on the parents' goal of sitting.

Environmental Considerations

A comprehensive examination and evaluation is a complicated process that is highly influenced by the requirements of the specific service delivery setting. The sequence and focus of an examination and evaluation can be very different in an acute care children's hospital versus the home setting of an early intervention program. Children are served in a wide variety of settings as discussed in Section 3. Therapists must understand the unique needs and demands of each setting and recognize the rationale for the differences in priorities and service delivery.

Careful consideration must be given to the setting and conditions under which the examination will be performed. One of the first issues to consider is the time of day of the examination. This timing is especially important for an infant or a young child. Testing near naptime or just before feeding will not encourage optimal results. Taking school-age children out of their favorite class is also not a good way to establish rapport. One must also consider the effects of long commutes to the examination and multiple examinations by several professionals. When possible, both parents should be present, so therapists should consider nontraditional work hours. Although evenings may be best for parents, it is generally not best for children. Saturdays may be the best day to get all of the participants together.

The setting of the examination is important because it influences the child's performance. If the child is fearful in a strange clinical environment, he or she may not participate at all; even when comfortable, the child may not be able to generalize skills to a new environment. As a result, the findings might be inaccurate. When possible, the best place to conduct an examination is in the child's **natural environment** (Bagnato, 2007). Natural environments are settings where children live,

learn, and play. The setting will vary depending on the age, medical status, and disability of the child. If the child is not a hospital inpatient, the home, day-care center, or educational setting is frequently the natural environment of choice. In early intervention for children from birth to 3 years of age, the most common natural environment is the home (Campbell, Sawyer, & Muhlenhaupt, 2009). Familiarity with the physical environment and people in that environment helps the child and family to be more comfortable and allows the therapist to observe the child's best performance.

The examination should first include **naturalistic observation.** During naturalistic observation, the therapist observes the child functioning in the regular environment—be it home, day-care center, or school—doing whatever is normally done in that environment. Naturalistic observation has a number of advantages. How and when the child typically moves under normal circumstances is observed. Information is learned regarding the child's behavior, interaction with adults and children (if available), mobility, preferred positions and movement patterns, use of verbal and nonverbal language, indications of cognitive ability based on play behaviors and communication, manipulation of objects, and indications of endurance. The more comfortable and enriched the environment, the more likely it is that typical behaviors will be observed. Very "clinical" settings do not promote observation of optimal, typical behaviors. Observation of the child in the waiting room might provide a more realistic view of the child's behavior than other clinic rooms. During the observation, the therapist must not handle the child, a very difficult restriction for some experienced therapists! As the child becomes comfortable with the setting, the therapist slowly starts to interact with the child, providing objects to play with to encourage natural movement. With an older, cooperative child, the therapist can ask the child to perform tasks while the therapist observes.

Therapists have a number of systematic techniques available for observation and recording of movement (Bailey & Wolery, 1992, pp. 104–110; Effgen, 1991; Effgen & Chan, 2010). Observation of the child's best performance in the natural environment allows accurate determination of environmental obstacles, needed supports, and the child's strengths, which encourages realistic remediation. For example, suggesting that a child practice stair climbing in a home without stairs is not realistic, nor is cruising along a sofa if there is no sofa. In a clinical setting, parents are frequently reluctant to admit that they do not have certain items. Knowing the resources in the home allows the therapist to best determine what realistic and practical activities can be done in the home. If specialized examination equipment is necessary, a portion of the examination can be done in a setting that has the equipment; however, one should first consider selecting portable equipment and alternative means of measurement. For example, instead of using a computerized isokinetic system, a handheld dynamometer is a reliable tool to measure muscle force production (Effgen & Brown, 1992; Katz-Leurer, Rottem, & Meyer, 2008) and is easily carried into homes and schools.

During the observation, the therapist determines areas of development and functioning that warrant further examination. In addition, the observation provides rich information that may be included in the tests-and-measures portion of the examination. When working with children, especially young children, their schedule and desires must be followed, not the predetermined examination plans of the therapist. The examination data are frequently obtained in a random order based on the child's activity and cooperation, unless a specific sequence must be followed for a standardized test. With infants, toddlers, and children with severe disabilities, it is generally best to perform an examination in one position at a time and to not request frequent position changes. Therapists will, for example, observe all activities in prone before observing and testing in sitting position. An example of a developmental observation by position is provided in Table 3.3. Many therapists also take the individual items of the tests they need to administer and list each item by position, thus minimizing position changes and increasing efficiency.

Play-based assessment is a form of naturalistic observation of young children popular in early childhood education (Linder, 2008). Professionals watch as the child interacts with selected play materials and with other children. Materials are carefully arranged to encourage the child's participation in activities that will provide the observers with information needed to evaluate the child's strengths and weaknesses based on their profession's frame of reference. An occupational therapist might evaluate the play behaviors, including sensorimotor, imaginary, constructional, and gross and fine motor game play (Olson, 1999). An educator might focus on creativity, social skills, and spontaneous language; the speech-language pathologist would note articulation and word usage. Play-based assessment has resulted in higher language performance scores than more formal, standardized measures (Calhoon, 1997).

The physical therapist focuses on spontaneity and ease of movement during functional skills, movement

Table 3.3 Partial List of Body Movement Functions and Activities That Can Be Observed in Different Positions

Supine

Head position

Head turning to follow object or sounds

Position and movement of arms, legs, and trunk

Prone

Head position

Head lifting and turning

Propping on elbows or hands

Reaching for toys

Forward progression (rolling, crawling, creeping)

Sitting

Head posture

Head turning

Trunk posture and weight bearing

Arm position (used to prop, used to play)

Maintains sitting position (with support, propping, independently)

Type of sitting position (ring, tailor, long, bench)

All Fours

Maintains position on hands and knees

Rocks on hands and knees

Moves forward on hands and knees (homolateral, reciprocal)

Kneeling

Maintains tall kneeling

Tall kneeling to half kneeling

Comes to standing

Standing

Stands with hands held or at support surface

Stands independently

Transitional Movements

Rolling in all directions

Horizontal to sitting

Sitting to all fours

Assumes tall kneeling to half kneeling

Assumes standing

Walking

Position of head, trunk, arms, and legs in each phase of gait cycle

activities, and transitions between play activities and positions. The strength of play-based assessment is that it is very functional and activity based; however, it provides limited information about impairment of body structures or functions, such as range of motion (ROM) and muscle strength, which can be important in understanding the cause of activity limitations.

Arena assessments are commonly used in examination of infants in early intervention and for children with severe disabilities. This assessment involves team members, including the parents, observing the child at the same time. One team member usually does the majority of the handling, and others provide direction, take notes, and talk with the parents. Play-based arena assessments may also be done via televideo. A facilitator performs the assessment in the child's home while communicating with other team members who are viewing the assessment on a televideo monitor at another site (Smith, 1997).

When an examination is done in the child's home, generally the full team will not participate, and a decision must be made regarding which professionals will participate in the examination. If all team members are necessary, the examination might initially be done in the home with a few professionals present, with a follow-up by members of other disciplines at the home or in a center. Center-based assessment is generally considered artificial and not as likely to provide an accurate picture of the child's abilities (Rainforth & York-Barr, 1997); however, it is appropriate in some practice settings.

Part of the examination and evaluation process involves the administration of objective tests and measures. What tests and measures to use will depend on the outcome of the systems review, the practice setting requirements, and professional judgment, as discussed in the following section.

Tests and Measures

The examination and evaluation of children includes an appraisal of their body structures and functions (systems), as well as activity and participation restrictions, which might include determination of the child's developmental level. Knowledge of the child's level of development and functioning can be critical in determining eligibility for services and developing the plan of care. The tests and measurements used in the examination of a specific body system to determine impairments in body functions and structures are presented in chapters on each system in this text. Based on the child's needs, tests and measures for several systems might be performed. Tests and measures used to determine activities such as general task demands, mobility, and self-care are addressed both in this chapter and in the system chapters.

It is also important to determine whether there are problems with the child's sensory processing, whether the child is experiencing any pain, and what the child's feelings are about his or her quality of life, all of which will influence services and development of the plan of care. Tests and measures of neuromotor development, sensory integration, function, pain, and quality of life are not system dependent and are reviewed in this chapter and in the systems chapters as appropriate.

Physical therapists working in pediatrics have a long tradition of using tests and measures to assess the development and overall functioning of the children they serve. Therapists working at special centers serving children with disabilities have developed many "home-grown" tests; however, those tests do not have the psychometric properties now considered the standard for approved tests and measures. Test construction is a very difficult, complex, time-consuming, and expensive process, and the rigor in the development of different tests and measures varies greatly. As a result, the psychometric quality of tests and measures varies. Not all of the tests discussed in this text would necessarily withstand rigorous review; however, because they are commonly used and may be in the process of rigorous revision, they are introduced.

Selecting the right test for the right purpose is critical. The therapist must consider what the test measures, the age group of children for which the test was developed, the psychometric properties of the test, how well the test correlates with other "gold standard" tests, the time and cost involved in administering the test, and why the test is being given. Therapists must become knowledgeable regarding the strengths, weaknesses, and psychometric qualities of the tests they administer. A test should be used for the purpose for which it was developed. An **evaluative measure** can be used to determine a child's performance against previous performance on the same measure, whereas a **discriminative measure** is used to determine if a child displays deviations from the normal standard. **Predictive measures** are used to forecast future outcomes, behaviors or prognosis.

APTA now offers an online guide (2010b) that provides current information on a wide range of tests and measures commonly used by physical therapists. This is an important resource that should be consulted by therapists considering using an unfamiliar test or measure or defending test selection.

Hanna and colleagues (2007) found that 59% of therapists working in children's rehabilitation programs in Ontario, Canada, reported using standardized measures in their practice daily to weekly; only 10.7% use standardized measures only a few times a year. They found that the most commonly used measure was the

Gross Motor Function Measure, followed by the Alberta Infant Motor Scale, goniometry, and the Peabody Developmental Motor Scales. They also found that the only predictor related to self-reported frequency of measurement use was a positive attitude toward measurement. Developing a positive attitude toward tests and measures is therefore critical, since there is increasing pressure on clinicians to use standardized tests and measures to provide an accurate and reliable foundation for documenting a child's current status, evaluating services, and measuring intervention outcomes (APTA, 2001; PL 108-446).

Psychometrics

The tests and measurements that therapists use should be **reliable** (produce consistent, repeatable results) and **valid** (measure what they are supposed to measure). Reliability and validity are not necessarily linked. A test might be reliable but not valid for the construct it is supposed to be measuring, and vice versa. For example a goniometric measure of knee range of motion might be very reliable, but it is not a valid measure of knee function or strength.

A diagnostic test or measure indicates the presence or absence of a disease or injury. A test or measurement should have the **sensitivity** to detect dysfunction or a disorder in individuals who actually have the disorder. Tests with high sensitivity are good for ruling out a disorder with few false-negative results. **Specificity**, on the other hand, indicates normality, or the absence of a disorder. If a test has high specificity, there should be few false-positives. Once a test suggests that an individual has a particular diagnosis, the sensitivity and specificity of the test can be used to form a measure called the likelihood ratio. The **likelihood ratio** indicates the probability of the existence of a diagnosis. A positive likelihood ratio suggests the existence of the disorder and a negative likelihood ratio suggests the absence of the disorder. Likelihood ratios greater than 5.0 and lower than 0.2 indicate relatively important effects. Likelihood ratios between 0.2 and 0.5 and between 2.0 and 5.0 might be important, while values near 1.0 suggest unimportant effects (Portney & Watkins, 2009, p. 627). Likelihood ratios are now being reported more frequently in the literature. If a study does not report a test's likelihood ratio, it can be calculated from the test's reported sensitivity and specificity.

Tests and measures must be administered as directed in test manuals or standardized protocols if they are to be reliable. Results of standardized tests and measures are reported in several ways, depending on how the test was developed. The **raw score** indicates the total number of items passed on a test. When providing raw scores, usually the basal and ceiling levels are indicated. The **basal level** is the item preceding the earliest failed item, and the **ceiling level** is the item representing the most difficult success. For an age-equivalent score, the performance of a child is compared with the mean age when 50% of children would have mastered those skills. For example, an infant of 12 months chronological age (CA) may be described as having an age-equivalent score of 6 months because the infant has just learned to sit and has other skills common to most 6-month-olds as noted on a developmental test. The **age equivalent score** is not a truly accurate appraisal of the child's ability, but most families easily understand it.

The **developmental quotient** is the ratio between the child's actual score based on the developmental age achieved on a test and the child's CA. The developmental quotient in the previous example would be 6 months/ 12 months = 0.5, or 50%. This would indicate a significant delay in development. If the child had scored at the 12-month level and was 12 months old, the developmental quotient would be 12 months/12 months = 1, or 100%, indicating no delay at all.

Descriptive statistics are used to compare an individual to other individuals based on a normal distribution called the normal, or bell-shaped, curve (Fig. 3.2). **Standard scores** are used to express deviation or variations from the mean score of a group and include Z-scores, T-scores, IQ scores, developmental index scores, percentile scores, and age-equivalent scores (Richardson, 2001). **Percentile scores** are used to indicate the number of children of the same age expected to score lower than the subject child. A child scoring in the 75th percentile on a norm-referenced test would be scoring *above* 75% of the children in the normative sample of the test. The Z-score and T-score are computed using standard deviation scores. The Z-score is determined by subtracting the mean for a test from the child's score and then dividing it by the published standard deviation for the test. The equation would be as follows:

$$Z = \frac{\text{child's score} - \text{test mean score}}{\text{test standard deviation}}$$

The T-score is derived from the Z-score; however, the mean is always 50 and the standard deviation is always 10. The equation would be as follows:

$$T = 10(Z) + 50$$

The T-score is always a positive value, and any result below 50 indicates a score below the mean.

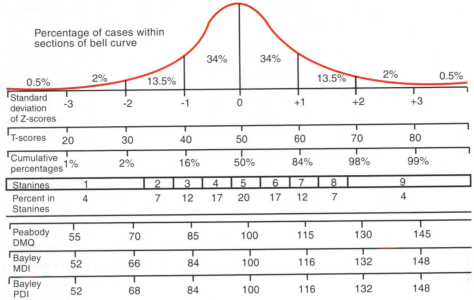

Standard deviation of Z-scores	-3		-2		-1		0		+1		+2		+3
T-scores	20		30		40		50		60		70		80
Cumulative percentages	1%		2%		16%		50%		84%		98%		99%
Stanines	1		2	3	4		5	6	7	8		9	
Percent in Stanines	4		7	12	17		20	17	12	7		4	
Peabody DMQ	55		70		85		100		115		130		145
Bayley MDI	52		66		84		100		116		132		148
Bayley PDI	52		68		84		100		116		132		148

Figure 3.2 Normal curve and associated standard scores. *(From Richardson, P.K. (2001). Use of standardized tests in pediatric practice. In J. Case-Smith (Ed.): Occupational therapy for children, 4th ed. , p. 336. St. Louis: Mosby. Reprinted with permission of the author.)*

Another important issue to consider regarding tests and measures is the standard error of measurement and confidence intervals. The **standard error of measurement** reflects the reliability of the response if a test were administered a number of times simultaneously with no practice or fatigue effects. It is the expected range of error for the test score. The more reliable the measurement, the smaller the errors will be. The standard error of measurement is calculated for a test using the standard deviation and reliability coefficient for the test. Once one knows the standard error of measurement for a test, that value is added and subtracted from the child's score. This gives the range of expected scores for that child, referred to as a **confidence interval.** A confidence interval is the range of scores with specific boundaries or limits based on the sample mean and its standard deviation. The degree of confidence is noted as a probability percentage, usually reported as a 95% confidence interval, which means that the therapist can be 95% sure that the test score obtained lies within the range indicated by the confidence interval. While there is no identified limit to the range of an acceptable confidence interval, it is important to recognize that a narrower interval indicates a more precise score (Jewell, 2008).

The standard error of measurement and confidence intervals are important reminders that measurement error is inherent in all test scores. This is an especially important issue when scores are used to evaluate changes over time. If the confidence intervals of two test scores overlap, it might be wrong to conclude that any change has occurred. An example reported by Hanna and colleagues (2007) notes that if a clinician gives a child the Grasping Subtest of the Peabody Developmental Motor Scale before and after intervention and reports a score of 40 before intervention and a score of 43 after intervention, one might think that this reflects positive improvement. However, these scores are estimates, influenced by many factors unrelated to the intervention effects, including the reliability of the measure. The standard error of measurement reflects the test's reliability and measures how much a child's observed score is expected to vary. It is used to produce a confidence interval on the difference between the two scores. In the Grasping Subtest, the standard error of measurement is 1 point. This means that the confidence interval around each score is plus or minus 2 points. The high end of the confidence interval in this example for the pre-test would be 40 +2, which means that it overlaps with the low end of the confidence interval for the post-test score of 43 − 2. This would suggest that the apparent change in scores could easily be due to a chance variation that was not related to the intervention.

Frequently in clinical practice, a test is used that is within the performance level of the child, but the test's norms were determined on a younger population of children. In this situation, the standard norms are invalid because the child's age is outside the test's age norms, even though the child scores within the test's range. The test score is not valid, but the results can provide a standardized indication of performance and an indication of developmental level. For example, the normative standard scores of the Pediatric Evaluation of Disability Inventory (PEDI) go up to only age 7.5 years; however, the PEDI can still be used if the child is older than 7.5 years but is functioning at a lower level. In this situation, the scaled scores, not the normative standard scores, can be used to indicate functional ability (Haley, Coster, Ludlow, Haltiwanger, & Andrellos, 1998, p. 6).

Most tests are either **criterion referenced** or **norm referenced**. Criterion-referenced tests are standardized tests that consist of a series of skills or behaviors measured against a set criteria for performance. The items are selected for the test because of their importance in the everyday life of the child. Criterion-referenced tests are common in physical therapy practice and especially in early intervention. The items of these tests are frequently used as the goal of intervention because of their functional significance. Cut-off scores are used to compare individual performance against a defined standard (description of desired performance) and not against group performance. Criterion-referenced tests, such as the Functional Independence Measure for Children (WEEFIM) or PEDI, are used in ongoing examination and for program planning because they are sensitive to the effects of intervention. Obtaining repeated measures over time allows the therapist to evaluate a child's performance against previous scores to document progress and effectiveness of interventions; therefore, most criterion-referenced tests are considered evaluative measures. Norm-referenced tests compare individual performance against a known group performance, and deviations from the normal distribution are determined. IQ tests and SATs are common norm-referenced tests. Other norm-referenced tests, such as the Bayley Scales of Infant Development and Peabody Developmental Motor Scales, are frequently used to determine the program eligibility of young children. Norm-referenced tests are considered discriminative measures since they can identify children with delays. They are not sensitive to the effects of intervention but have all too frequently been used inappropriately to evaluate intervention outcomes.

A therapist must be skilled in observation of behavior and movement. Although the formal, standardized tests and measures are most highly valued in practice, skilled observation also offers important information

(Stewart, 2010, p. 207). Dunn (2000, as noted in Stewart, 2010, p. 208), a noted pediatric occupational therapist, has reported that the key elements of skilled observation should include the following: (1) do not interfere with the natural course of events, (2) pay attention to the physical and social features of the environment that support or limit a child's performance, and (3) record the child's behavior. The antecedent and consequences of the behavior should also be noted. For example, when a child climbs to the top of the stairs, does the parent panic and "rescue" the child or clap and praise the child? Future outcomes of the stair climbing behavior will be influenced by the parent's response. Another common example is when a child is just learning to walk, does the parent immediately run and pick up the child when he or she safely falls, or does the parent encourage the child to stand up and try again? This information will not be provided in a standardized test but offers valuable information for the intervention program.

Computer Adaptive Testing

Measure development has progressed to now allow the introduction of technologies such as item response theory and a **computer adaptive testing (CAT)** algorithm. This is a promising area in the development of tests and measures. In an effort to reduce the amount of time it takes to administer a standardized assessment and to increase the likelihood that an assessment will be used, CAT has been investigated by Haley and colleagues for assessing physical functioning in children and adolescents with disabilities (Coster, Haley, Ni, Dumas, & Fragala-Pinkham, 2008; Dumas et al., 2010; Haley et al., 2009; Haley, Ni, Fragala-Pinkham, Skrinar, & Corzo, 2005; Haley, Ni, Hambleton, Slavin, & Jette, 2006).

Presently, most items on a test must be scored to properly administer a test; this can be a very time consuming, costly, and sometimes unpleasant process. CAT is a method of test administration that uses the child's ability level, based on previous responses to select questions, to maximize test precision. Items are skipped that are either too easy or too difficult. CAT requires fewer test items but has accurate scores comparable to the full-length test (Coster et al., 2008; Dumas et al., 2010; Haley et al., 2005, 2009). The brief administration time of CAT allows a more focused examination of a child's functional status and reduces the time required for the examination. This is an area of increasing research, and therapists should stay abreast of developments using CAT technology for tests and measures and patient reported outcomes (Tucker, 2011).

Domains of Tests and Measures

ICF-CY Movement Functions and Mobility

To examine and study movement functions and mobility systematically, a framework and classification system are needed help to unify terminology and establish objective criteria. Under the International Classification of Functioning, Disability and Health— Children and Youth Version (ICF-CY), introduced in Chapter 1, the WHO (2007) has developed a broad-based definition of body functions that includes the physiological and psychological functions of body systems. Body functions are divided into eight categories related to the systems of the body. The body function category *neuromusculoskeletal and movement-related functions* is the most critical to physical therapy intervention. This body function category is further divided into three sections: *functions of the joints and bones, muscle functions,* and *movement functions.* The functions of joints, bones, and muscles and their examination are discussed in Chapter 5; however, an understanding of *movement functions* (Table 3.4) is

necessary to understand the development of all functional movement and mobility.

The first movement functions are *motor reflex functions.* These are best displayed in the neonate and infant. Many reflexes observed in infants, such as the Moro reflex, asymmetrical tonic neck reflex, and palmar and plantar grasp reflexes, slowly fade or integrate until they are no longer observed in toddlers. Other motor reflexes, such as the withdrawal reflex, and biceps and patellar reflexes, remain throughout life when the appropriate stimuli are presented. While assessment of motor reflexes is no longer central to examination and evaluation of infants and children, it is still prudent to make note of atypical reflex activity. Some developmental and sensory integration tests and measures include items or an entire section to assess reflex functions.

The *involuntary movement reaction functions* are induced by body position, balance needs, and threatening stimuli. They include the postural reactions that develop during the first years of life. Facilitating the development and refinement of these reactions in a functional context is an important aspect of physical therapy intervention. For a child to explore the environment,

---

■ **Table 3.4** ICF-CY Body Function Categories for Movement Functions

Motor reflex functions (b750)	"Functions of involuntary contraction of muscles automatically induced by specific stimuli"
Involuntary movement reaction functions (b755)	"Functions of involuntary contractions of large muscles or the whole body induced by body position, balance, and threatening stimuli"
Control of voluntary movement functions (b760)	"Functions associated with the control over and coordination of voluntary movement"
Involuntary movement functions (b765)	"Functions of unintentional, non- or semi-purposive involuntary contractions of a muscle or group of muscles"
Gait pattern functions (b770)	"Functions of movement patterns associated with walking, running or other whole body movement"
Sensations related to muscles and movement functions (b780)	"Sensations associated with the muscles or muscle groups of the body and their movement. Includes: sensations of muscle stiffness and tightness of muscles, muscle spasm or constriction and heaviness of muscles"
Movement functions, other specified and unspecified (b789)	
Neuromusculoskeletal and movement-related function, other specified (b798)	
Neuromusculoskeletal and movement-related function, unspecified (b799)	

Source: World Health Organization (2007). *International classification of functioning, disability and health—children and youth version* (pp. 99–103). Geneva: Author.

whether by rolling, crawling, or walking, a series of continual movements and postural adjustments are necessary. Adjustments allow a child to move freely and respond rapidly to the demands of the environment. As a child matures, a number of distinct movements and reactions develop, which orient the head and body in space, protect the child from falls, and assist in maintaining balance. The development of involuntary movement results from the complex interaction and evolution of the numerous subsystems and interactions with the environment. Postural reactions develop in infants in a relatively set sequence. Impaired development of these involuntary movement reactions may indicate neuromotor delay or disability and aid in the diagnosis of central nervous system disorders. Testing for their presence is commonly part of a comprehensive examination.

Control of voluntary movement functions includes the control of simple and complex voluntary movement, and coordination of movements of the arms, legs, and eyes. Development of this control is an ongoing process throughout life; however, the peak developmental period is during the first several years of life. Many of these voluntary movement functions are examined as part of the developmental and functional examination process.

Involuntary movement functions include nonpurposive movements such as tremors, tics, stereotypies, chorea, athetosis, dystonic movements, and dyskinesia. These involuntary movements can significantly interfere with functional movement. Under what conditions involuntary movement functions appear, or worsen, should be carefully considered. Some involuntary movements become worse during periods of stress or when performing difficult movement activities. They can also be common symptoms of disabilities, such as the hand wringing seen in Rett syndrome, or the side effect of some medications.

Acquiring the *gait pattern functions* is of primary importance to many parents and is the focus of much intervention. These abilities are important for the next level of functioning—activities and participation in the category of *mobility*. As discussed in Chapter 1, "activity is the execution of a task or action by an individual" and "activity limitations are difficulties an individual may have in executing activities." "Participation is involvement in a life situation" and "participation restrictions are problems an individual may have in executing activities" (WHO, 2007, p. 9). The nine major areas of activities and participation are listed in Table 3.5. These areas should be assessed based on the needs of the individual child. The health and health-related status of a child may be documented by selecting the appropriate category code, or codes, and then adding qualifiers (WHO, 2007, p. 10).

Table 3.5 ICF-CY Activities and Participation for Mobility

Changing and Maintaining Body Position (d410–d429)*

Changing basic body position (d410)
Lying down (d4100)
Squatting (d4101)
Kneeling (d4102)
Sitting (d4103)
Standing (d4104)
Bending (d4105)
Shifting the body's center of gravity (d4106)
Rolling over (d4107)
Changing basic body position, other specified (d4108)
Changing basic body position, unspecified (d4109)

Maintaining a body position (d415)
Maintaining a lying position (d4150)
Maintaining a squatting position (d4151)
Maintaining a kneeling position (d4125)
Maintaining a sitting position (d4153)
Maintaining a standing position (d4154)
Maintaining a head position (d4155)
Maintaining a body position, other specified (d4158)
Maintaining a body position, unspecified (d4159)

Transferring oneself (d420)
Transferring oneself while sitting (d4200)
Transferring oneself while lying (d4201)
Transferring oneself, other specified (d4208)
Transferring oneself, unspecified (d4209)

Changing and maintaining body position, other specified and unspecified (d429)

Carrying, Moving, and Handling Objects (d430–d449)*

Lifting and carrying objects (d430)
Lifting (d4300)
Carrying in the hands (d4301)
Carrying in the arms (d4302)
Carrying on shoulders, hip, and back (d4303)
Carrying on the head (d4304)
Putting down objects (d4305)
Lifting and carrying, other specified (d4308)
Lifting and carrying, unspecified (d4309)

Moving objects with lower extremities (d435)
Pushing with lower extremities (d4350)
Kicking (d4351)
Moving objects with lower extremities, other specified (d4358)
Moving objects with lower extremities, unspecified (d4359)

*Numbers in parentheses refer to ICF-CY classification.

Table 3.5 ICF-CY Activities and Participation for Mobility—cont'd

Fine hand use (d440)
Picking up (d4400)
Grasping (d4401)
Manipulating (d4402)
Releasing (d4403)
Fine hand use, other specified (d4408)
Fine hand use, unspecified (d4409)

Hand and arm use (d445)
Pulling (d4450)
Pushing (d4451)
Reaching (d4452)
Turning or twisting the hands or arms (d4453)
Throwing (d4454)
Catching (d4455)
Hand and arm use, other specified (d4458)
Hand and arm use, unspecified (d4459)

Carrying, moving, and handling objects, other specified and unspecified (d449)

Walking and Moving (d450–d469)*

Walking (d450)
Walking short distances (d4500)
Walking long distances (d4501)
Walking on different surfaces (d4502)
Walking around obstacles (d4503)
Walking, other specified (d4508)
Walking, unspecified (d4509)

Moving around (d455)
Crawling (d4550)
Climbing (d4551)
Running (d4552)
Jumping (d4553)
Swimming (d4554)
Scooting and rolling (d4555)
Shuffling (d4556)
Moving around, other specified (d4558)
Moving around, unspecified (d4559)

Moving around in different locations (d460)
Moving around within the home (d4600)
Moving around within buildings other than home (d4601)
Moving around outside the home and other buildings (d4602)
Moving around in different locations, other specified (d4608)
Moving around in different locations, unspecified (d4609)

Moving around using equipment (d465)
Walking and moving, other specified and unspecified (d469)
Moving Around Using Transportation (d470–489)*

Using transportation (d470)
Using human-powered vehicles (d4700)
Using private motorized transportation (d4701)
Using public transportation (d4702)
Using humans for transportation (d4703)
Using transportation, other specified (d4708)
Using transportation, unspecified (d4709)

Driving (d475)
Driving human-powered transportation (d4750)
Driving motorized vehicles (d4751)
Driving animal-powered vehicles (d4752)
Driving, other specified (d4758)
Driving, unspecified (d4759)

Riding animals for transportation (d480)
Moving around using transportation, other specified and unspecified (d489)
Mobility, other specified (d498)
Mobility, unspecified (d499)

*Numbers in parentheses refer to ICF-CY classification.
Source: World Health Organization (2007). *International classification of functioning, disability and health—children and youth version* (pp. 150–160). Geneva: Author.

The qualifiers are a numeric coding system that indicates the degree of the problem ranging from *No problem* to *Complete problem* (Table 3.6). The ICF codes and qualifiers provide a "condensed version" of the information found in clinical records. Two qualifiers, *performance* and *capacity*, qualify the ICF-CY domains for activity and participation. The *performance* qualifier describes what a child does in the current environment and includes societal context. The *capacity* qualifier describes the child's ability to execute a task or action in a standardized or neutral environment. The highest probable level of functioning at the moment is indicated (WHO, 2007, p. 13). The difference between *capacity* and *performance* reflects the gap between what the child can do and what the child does in the current environment. This provides a guide to improving performance.

The WHO (2010) has also developed an ICF-based assessment instrument, the WHO Disability Assessment Schedule 2.0 (WHODAS), which provides a generic summary measure of functioning and disability. This measure covers the domains of cognition, mobility, self-care, getting along, life activities, and participation. The WHO is also developing and testing

■ **Table 3.6** ICF Scoring System

If an impairment in body functions or body structure, limitation in activity, or restriction in participation is present, the following generic performance qualifiers may be used to indicate degree of difficulty in accomplishing an activity.

Code (comes after the ICF code)	Impairment, Limitation, or Restriction Level	Description	Magnitude of Impairment
.0	No problem	Functioning is within expected norms (none, absent, negligible)	0–4%
.1	Mild problem	Slight deviation from expected norm and functioning (slight, low)	5–24%
.2	Moderate problem	Significant impairment of functioning, person likely to need assistance (medium, fair)	25–49%
.3	Severe problem	Seriously compromised functioning, person may be unable to perform functions, even with assistance (high, extreme)	50–95%
.4	Complete problem	Total loss of function (total)	96–100%
.8	Not specified	Insufficient data	
.9	Not applicable	Qualifier not applicable in this instance	

This performance qualifier can be used in conjunction with another qualifier that implies the level of difficulty, such as using an assistive device or personal help. Additional qualifiers can be used to describe the individual's ability to perform the task. All three components of the ICF (Body Functions and Structures, Activities and Participation, and Environmental Factors) are qualified using the same scale.

Source: Adapted from World Health Organization (2001). *International Classification of Functioning, Disability and Health* (p. 222). Geneva: Author. Copyright by the World Health Organization. Reprinted with permission of the author. Adapted from American Psychological Association (APA) and World Health Organization (2003). *International classification of functioning, disability and health procedural manual and guide for a standardized application of the ICF: A manual for health professionals.* Washington, DC: Author.

ICF Comprehensive Core Sets for specific health conditions to guide multidisciplinary assessments of all individuals with that condition. Brief ICF Core Sets are also being developed to include as few categories as possible but as many as necessary to sufficiently describe the typical spectrum of the specific problem. The development of core sets for conditions common in children and youth is just beginning.

Numerous other published tests and measures can be used to assess many of these *movement-related functions* and *mobility* as addressed in Appendix 3.A and throughout this text. The Preferred Practice Patterns in the *Guide* (APTA, 2001) also provide recommendations to assist in examination of movement functions.

Developmental and Functional Tests and Measures

In addition to determining the performance of each body system (body functions and structures), it is important to determine the level of neuromotor development and functional performance of the child covered under the ICF activities and participation headings of general task demands, mobility, and self care specific to the child's culture (see Table 3.7).

Using standardized tests and measures provides an excellent foundation for learning about child development for a therapist new to pediatrics. Numerous tests and measures have been developed to assist in this process. Most developmental and functional tests assess a child's activity and participation, although some also have items to evaluate body structures and functions as well. Common tests and measures are listed by category and ICF-CY classification of the test in Table 3.8, and more detailed information is provided in Appendix 3.A. Several of these tests also cross categories but are listed in only the main category.

Some developmental or functional tests have very specific applications. The School Function Assessment (SFA) (Coster, Deeney, Haltiwanger, & Haley, 1998) provides an exemplary model of test development and

Table 3.7 ICF Short Checklist of Activities and Participation Domains

Learning and Applying Knowledge
Watching
Listening
Learning to read
Learning to write
Learning to calculate
Solving problems

General Tasks and Demands
Undertaking a single task
Undertaking multiple tasks

Communication
Communicating with—receiving—spoken messages
Communicating with—receiving—nonverbal messages
Speaking
Producing nonverbal messages
Conversation

Mobility
Lifting and carrying objects
Fine hand use (picking up, grasping)
Walking
Moving around using equipment (wheelchairs, skates, etc.)
Using transportation (car, bus, train, plane, etc.)
Driving (riding bicycle or motorbike, driving car, etc.)

Self Care
Washing oneself (bathing, drying, washing hands, etc.)
Caring for body parts (brushing teeth, shaving, grooming, etc.)
Toileting
Dressing
Eating
Drinking
Looking after one's health

Domestic Life
Acquisition of goods and services (shopping, etc.)
Preparation of meals (cooking, etc.)
Doing housework (cleaning house, washing dishes, doing laundry, ironing, etc.)
Assisting others

Interpersonal Interactions and Relationships
Basic interpersonal interactions
Complex interpersonal interactions
Relating with strangers
Formal relationships
Informal social relationships
Family relationships
Intimate relationships

Major Life Areas
Informal education
School education
Higher education
Remunerative employment
Basic economic transactions
Economic self-sufficiency

Community, Social, and Civil Life
Community life
Recreation and leisure
Religion and spirituality
Human rights
Political life and citizenship

Any Other Activity and Participation

Source: From World Health Organization (2003). *ICF checklist, version 2.1a: Clinician form*. Geneva: Author. Available from http://www.who.int/classifications/icf/training/icfchecklist.pdf

application using a top-down, problem-solving approach based on the ICF model. The child's current level of activity and participation in the school setting is determined, which provides an excellent guide for developing a plan of care specific to the needs of the child in a school setting. The Gross Motor Function Measure (GMFM) (Russell, Rosenbaum, Avery, & Lane, 2002) is an example of a test developed and validated for a specific population. This test is used to evaluate changes in gross motor function, not quality of movement, in children with cerebral palsy. The GMFM has also been validated for children with Down syndrome (Russell et al., 1998).

Canadian Occupational Performance Measure

The **Canadian Occupational Performance Measure (COPM)** is an individualized outcome measure that uses a structured interview to obtain information on the child and family's goals, performance, and satisfaction in the areas of self care, leisure, and productivity using a top-down model (Law et al., 2005). This well-researched tool helps the therapist identify the focus of intervention based on what is most important to the child and family across developmental and functional areas. The child, with the help of the family as necessary, identifies what is most important for him or her to learn and then rates his or her *performance* and *satisfaction* with the task. This information is used to help the child and family prioritize the intervention goals.

The COPM has good content, structural, and external validity (Law et al., 2005). It should be used with caution in assessing children younger than 6 years and those with intellectual disabilities. The COPM and Goal Attainment Scaling (GAS) were the only two measures that reported adequate responsiveness to detect clinically significant change in a study of participation measures (Sakzewski, Boyd, & Ziviani, 2007), and both were sensitive in detecting change in a study of children with cerebral palsy (Cusick, McIntrye, Novak, Lannin, & Lowe, 2006). While developed for use by occupational therapists, this measure is appropriate for use by all members of the pediatric rehabilitation team (Chiarello et al., 2010). Chiarello and colleagues (2010) note that interviewing families and listening to their priorities for their children, which is integral to the COPM, are essential to guiding service delivery plans.

Sensory Functioning and Pain Tests and Measures

In addition to determining the developmental and mobility abilities of children, the subjective history frequently leads a pediatric physical therapist to assess how the child's body structures and functions are performing with regard to sensory functioning and pain. This includes the ICF-CY domains of seeing, hearing and vestibular functions, and pain. Sensory processing/integration might also be assessed, since the ability of our senses to work together is critical for the production of coordinated movement and appropriately modulated behaviors. Several tests that evaluate visual perception and visual motor skills are also included in Table 3.8 and Appendix 3.A.

Determination of pain is another aspect of child appraisal that should be part of any examination and evaluation. **Pain** has been called the fifth vital sign (American Pain Society, 1995), and its assessment is required in hospitals under the Joint Commission, Standard PC.01.02.07 (2010). Pain should be assessed in addition to the vital signs of pulse, blood pressure, core temperature, and respiration. Pain must be assessed for each child. Children with the same tissue damage will experience different levels of pain. The nature of

Table 3.8 Common Tests and Measures of Development, Function, Sensory Integration, Pain, Quality of Life, and Participation

Developmental Tests and Measures	ICF-CY Classification
Ages & Stages Questionnaire, 3rd edition (ASQ-3)	Activity, Participation
Alberta Infant Motor Scale (AIMS) and Motor Assessment of the Developing Infant	Activity
Assessment, Evaluation, and Programming System for Infants and Children (AEPS), 2nd edition	Activity, Participation
Battelle Developmental Inventory, 2nd edition (BDI-2)	Activity, Participation
Bayley Infant Neurodevelopmental Screener (BINS)	Body structures and functions, Activity
Bayley Scales of Infant and Toddler Development, 3rd edition (BSID-III)	Activity, Participation
Brigance Inventory of Early Development II (BIED-II)	Activity, Participation
Bruininks Oseretsky Test of Motor Proficiency, 2nd edition(BOT-2)	Body structures and functions, Activity
Carolina Curriculum for Infants and Toddlers with Special Needs (CCITSM), 3rd edition, and Carolina Curriculum for Preschoolers with Special Needs (CCPSN), 2nd edition	Activity, Participation
Denver Developmental Screening TestII (DDST-II)	Activity, Participation
Developmental Assessment of Young Children (DAYC)	Activity, Participation
Developmental Hand Dysfunction, 2nd edition	Activity
Developmental Observation Checklist System (DOCS)	Activity, Participation
Developmental Programming for Infants and Young Children—Revised (DPIYC)	Activity
FirstSTEp: Screening Test for Evaluating Preschoolers (FirstSTEp)	Activity, Participation
Harris Infant Neuromotor Test	Activity
Hawaii Early Learning Profile (HELP 0-3 and HELP 3-6), 2nd edition	Activity, Participation

Table 3.8 Common Tests and Measures of Development, Function, Sensory Integration, Pain, Quality of Life, and Participation—cont'd

Developmental Tests and Measures	ICF-CY Classification
Infanib	Body structures and functions
Infant Motor Profile (IMP)	Activity
Infant-Toddler Developmental Assessment (IDA)—Provence Profile	Activity, Participation
Meade Movement Checklist (MMCL)	Body structures and functions, Activity, Participation
Merrill-Palmer Revised Scales of Development (M-P-R)	Activity, Participation
Milani-Comparetti Motor Development Screening Test, 3rd edition	Body structures and functions, Activity
Miller Assessment of Preschoolers (MAP)	Body structures and functions, Activity
Motor Skills Acquisition in the First Year and Checklist	Activity
Movement Assessment Battery for Children, 2nd edition (MOVEMENT ABC-2)	Body structures and functions, Activity, Participation
Movement Assessment of Infants (MAI)	Body structures and functions
Mullen Scales of Early Learning	Activity
Neonatal Behavioral Assessment Scale, 3rd edition (NBAS-3)	Body structures and functions, Participation
Neonatal Individualized Developmental Care and Assessment Program (NIDCAP)	Body structures and functions, Activity
Neurobehavioral Assessment of the Preterm Infant (NAPI)	Body structures and functions, Activity
Neurological Assessment of the Preterm and Full-term Born Infant, 2nd edition (NAPFI-2)	Body structures and functions
Neurological Exam of the Full Term Infant (NEFTI), 2nd edition	Body structures and functions
Peabody Development Motor Scales, 2nd edition (PDMS-2)	Activity
Posture and Fine Motor Assessment of Infants	Activity
Scales of Independent Behavior—Revised (SIB-R)	Activity, Participation
Test of Gross Motor Development, 2nd edition (TGMD2)	Activity
Test of Infant Motor Performance (TIMP)	Activity
Toddler and Infant Motor Evaluation (TIME)	Activity, Participation
Transdisciplinary Play-Based Assessment, 2nd edition (TPBA2)	Activity, Participation
Vulpe Assessment Battery—Revised (VAB-R)	Body structures and functions, Activity, Participation
Functional Tests and Measures	**ICF-CY Classification**
ABILITIES Index	Body structures and functions, Activity, Participation
Canadian Occupational Performance Measure (COPM), 4th edition	Activity, Participation
Childhood Health Assessment Questionnaire (C-HAQ)	Activity, Participation
Gross Motor Function Measure (GMFM)	Activity
Gross Motor Performance Measure (GMPM)	Body structures and functions, Activity
Pediatric Balance Scale	Body structures and functions, Activity
Pediatric Evaluation of Disability Inventory (PEDI)	Activity, Participation
Pediatric Reach Test	Body structures and functions, Activity
Physical and Neurological Exam for Subtle Signs (PANESS)	Activity
School Function Assessment (SFA)	Activity, Participation

Continued

Table 3.8 Common Tests and Measures of Development, Function, Sensory Integration, Pain, Quality of Life, and Participation—cont'd

Functional Tests and Measures	ICF-CY Classification
Timed Up and Down Stairs (TUDS)	Body structures and functions, Activity
Timed Up and Go (TUG)	Body structures and functions, Activity
Vineland Adaptive Behavior Scales, 2nd edition (Vineland-II)	Activity, Participation
WEEFIM: Functional Independence Measure for Children	Activity, Participation
Sensory Integration Tests and Measures	**ICF-CY Classification**
Clinical Observations of Motor and Postural Skills (COMPS), 2nd edition	Body structures and functions
DeGangi-Berk Test of Sensory Integration (TSI)	Body structures and functions
Developmental Test of Visual-Motor Integration (VMI), 6th edition	Body structures and functions
Developmental Test of Visual Perception, 2nd edition (DTVP-2)	Body structures and functions
Early Coping Inventory (ECI) and Coping Inventories	Activity, Participation
Infant/Toddler Symptom Checklist	Activity, Participation
Pediatric Clinical Test for Sensory Interaction in Balance (P-CTSIB)	Body structures and function
Sensory Integration and Praxis Tests (SIPT)	Body structures and functions
Sensory Profile and Infant/Toddler Sensory Profile	Body structures and functions
Test of Sensory Function in Infants (TSFI)	Body structures and functions
Test of Visual-Motor Skills-3 (TVMS-3)	Body structures and functions
Pain Scales	**ICF-CY Classification**
Children's Hospital of Eastern Ontario Pain Scale (CHEOPS)	Body structures and functions
Children's and Infants' Postoperative Pain Scale (CHIPPS)	Body structures and functions
Cry, Requires O_2, Increased vital signs, Expression, and Sleeplessness (CRIES)	Body structures and functions
Face, Legs, Activity, Cry, and Consolability (FLACC) behavioral pain scale	Body structures and functions
Faces Pain Scale – Revised (FPS-R)	Body structures and functions
Neonatal Infant Pain Scale (NIPS)	Body structures and functions
Oucher Scales	Body structures and functions
Riley Infant Pain Scale	Body structures and functions
Visual Analog Scale	Body structures and functions
Wong-Baker Faces Scale	Body structures and functions
Quality of Life, Health-Related Quality of Life, and Participation	**ICF-CY Classification**
Activities Scale for Kids (ASK)	Activity
Assessment of Life Habits (LIFE-H)	Participation
Child Health and Illness Profile—Child and Parent Edition (CHIP-CE) and Adolescent Edition (CHIP-AE)	Activity, Participation
Child Health Questionnaire (CHQ)	Activity, Participation
Children's Assessment of Participation and Enjoyment (CAPE) and Preferences for Activities of Children (PAC)	Participation
Home Observation for Measurement of the Environment (HOME)	Participation
KIDSCREEN	Activity, Participation
Pediatric Quality of Life Inventory (PedsQL)	Activity, Participation
POSNA Pediatric Musculoskeletal Functional Health Questionnaire	Activity, Participation
Quality of Well-Being Scale (QWB)	Activity, Participation
Youth Quality of Life Instrument—Research Version (YQOL-R)	Participation

the child's pain includes cognitive, behavioral, and emotional factors (McGrath, 1995). Cognitive factors include the child's understanding of the source of the pain, ability to control what happened, and expectations regarding the pain. Behavioral factors include the child's overt actions such as crying, the response of parents and others, use of restraint, and the implications of the pain/injury in the child's life. The emotional factors include the ability to understand and cope with what has happened. All of these factors have an impact on the child's perception of pain.

The assessment of a child's pain depends on the age and cognitive ability of the child. Commonly used pain assessments are discussed below and are listed in Table 3.8 and Appendix 3.A. Because pain can significantly influence the child's quality of life and physical therapy intervention, its management must be carefully monitored

Neonatal Pain Scales

Neonatal neuroanatomy and chemistry studies indicate that neonates respond to painful stimuli; therefore, neonatal pain should be evaluated and treated. Use of an objective tool to measure pain is necessary for caregivers to administer in a reliable manner. The most valid, reliable, specific, and practical pain scales for use in the clinical setting for this population include the Cry, Requires O_2, Increased vital signs, Expression, and Sleeplessness (CRIES), the Children's and Infants' Postoperative Pain Scale (CHIPPS), and the Neonatal Infant Pain Scale (NIPS) (Suraseranivongse et al., 2006). These three pain scales have excellent inter-rater reliability, demonstrate concurrent and construct validity, exhibit good predictive validity, and are appropriate for evaluating neonatal pain (Suraseranivongse et al., 2006). The NIPS is the most practical scale due to the ease of scoring.

Behavioral Pain Scales

For a child who is preverbal or nonverbal and cannot participate in a self-reporting scale, a behavioral pain scale is needed. Two such scales are the Face, Legs, Activity, Cry, and Consolability (FLACC) behavioral pain scale and the Children's Hospital of Eastern Ontario Pain Scale (CHEOPS). The CHEOPS, which assesses six areas, was developed by McGrath and colleagues (1985) and was validated for children 1–7 years of age. The CHEOPS is considered by some to be too complex to use in a busy setting. The FLACC has five categories (see above) and has good inter-rater reliability and validity for evaluating pain after surgery, trauma, and other diseases for children up to age 7 years (Merkel, Voepel-Lewis, Shayevitz, & Malviya, 1997). Nilsson and colleagues (2008) found the FLACC to be a valid and reliable tool for assessing procedural pain in children aged 5–16 years.

Self-Reporting Scales

For children who are cognitively intact and able to participate in reporting their pain, there are several scales to choose from. The Wong-Baker Faces scale was developed for children between 3 and 7 years of age. The child is asked to pick from 5 different faces according to the pain level. The scores range from 0 to 10 (Wong & Baker, 1988). Other scales include a numeric reporting scale from 0 to 10, the visual analog scale (use of a 100-mm line with a mark made on the line indicating pain score), and a color analog scale (using a mechanical slide rule with gradations of pain in color from white to red to black). Bailey and colleagues (2007) compared these four pain scales on children with acute abdominal pain in a pediatric emergency department. While the age ranges for each scale varied, the color analog scale and the visual analog scale were in agreement. They found that the numeric scale overestimated pain values in one-third of the children.

Quality of Life, Health-Related Quality of Life, and Participation Measures

Another area of assessment and outcome that has come into predominance is the child's perceived quality of life (QOL), health-related quality of life (HRQOL), and the IFC-CY domain of participation. **QOL** is the "individual's perceptions of their position in life in the context of the culture and value system in which they live, and in relation to their goals, expectations and concerns" (WHO, 1993) or, in other words, "an overall assessment of well-being across various domains" (Bjornson& McLaughlin, 2001). It is an individual's self-reported, subjective perception of his or her place in the world and society (Colver, 2009). The dimensions of QOL include these perceptions:

- Emotional well-being
- Social well-being
- Material well-being
- Physical well-being
- Self-esteem
- Self-determination (Colver, 2009)

QOL cannot be measured directly and is usually captured by calculating from a group of questions the value of the underlying dimension. There is no normal range or standard mean. Two types of instruments are used for assessment of QOL, a generic and a condition-specific QOL measure. Generic instruments address a broad array of domains of well-being, whereas condition-specific instruments address characteristics related to a condition. A potential limitation of generic QOL measures might be the lack of sensitivity to detect subtle facets of specific disorders; however, they allow comparison across demographic and clinical populations (Waters et al., 2009). Condition-specific QOL instruments include domains important for children having that condition. For example, the QOL instrument for children with cerebral palsy would include elements found in generic instruments, such as social well-being, emotional well-being, self-esteem, and self-determination, and domains specific to the child with cerebral palsy, such as pain and the impact of disability and functioning. HRQOL is a subdomain of the more global construct of QOL and includes the domains of physical, mental, and social well-being.

QOL instruments should focus on the child's perception of well-being or feelings about life, not on functioning, impairment, and health status (Waters et al., 2009). Functioning has an influence on QOL but is a separate concept and should not be mixed with well-being, as in many measures currently used (Waters et al., 2009). QOL measures should provide the opportunity for self-report, especially for children over age 8 years. If self-reports cannot be collected for a child or adolescent due to age, disability, or intellectual impairment, then a parent-proxy can be used. The level of agreement between child self-report and parent-proxy depends on the domain being assessed. Usually there is good agreement for the domains of physical activity, physical health, and functioning, with less agreement related to social and emotional domains and school functioning (Eiser & Morse, 2001; Majnemer, Shevell, Law, Poulin, & Rosenbaum, 2008).

The number of QOL and health-related outcome measures for children is not as extensive as those for adults, but the number and quality are increasing. Waters and colleagues (2009) have done a systematic review of generic and condition-specific QOL instruments for children and adolescents with neurodisabilities. They note that some instruments have sound psychometric properties; however, many were developed with minimal involvement from families and focus on functioning rather than well-being. Additionally, many have items that might produce an emotional upset due to negative wording. Several QOL instruments are listed in Table 3.8 and Appendix 3.A; however,

as with all tests and measures, their psychometric properties and appropriateness for specific populations and purposes must be considered before using them.

The ICF-CY (WHO, 2007, p. 9) definition of participation is "involvement in a life situation." It is combined with the activity as a domain of the ICF; however, new tests and measures are being developed to assess just participation. "Participation is the context in which children develop skills and competences, experience socialization, and foster initiative and self-efficacy. . . . Meaningful and intrinsically motivated leisure activities foster mental and physical health benefits, provide opportunities for social relationships, and may improve quality of life." (Orlin et al., 2010, p. 160). Therefore, to achieve optimal outcomes for interventions with children, successful participation in daily activities is critical and should be evaluated.

There are differences in participation between children with and without physical disabilities. Children with physical disabilities, such as cerebral palsy, participate in less diverse leisure activities, spend more time at home and on quiet activities, have fewer social and physical activities, and experience social isolation and loneliness (Imms, Reilly, Carlin, & Dodd, 2008; Orlin et al., 2010). There is a positive relationship between gross motor function and participation in daily activities (King et al., 2007, Orlin et al., 2010). This is important, since low participation in physical activities has implications for fitness and health, especially for children and adolescences with more serious impairments of motor functioning.

One measure of participation used frequently in the recent literature (Orlin et al., 2010; Palisano et al., 2009, 2011) is the Children's Assessment of Participation and Enjoyment (CAPE), which is used to explore the day-to-day participation in children ages 6 to 21 years (King et al., 2004). The CAPE is a direct measure of participation and can help in program planning and measuring outcomes. It is used to examine the influence of skill, support, and opportunity-based interventions on children's participation as well as the influence of impairments and environmental factors. Also included with the CAPE for a similar age range is the Preferences for Activities for Children (PAC). The CAPE and PAC explore the following dimensions of participation: diversity, intensity, with whom, where, enjoyment, and preference. They were designed to be child friendly, using pictures and minimal verbiage.

Diagnosis and Prognosis or Outcomes of the Examination and Evaluation Process

Given the multitude of impairments and limitations presented by the children therapists serve, therapists must have a thorough understanding of all available tests and measures in order to select and correctly utilize multiple assessment tools during the examination and evaluation process. Recognizing that the results from one test or measure usually cannot adequately describe a child's impairments and performance capabilities across all domains, the therapist must continually adapt the examination based on the subjective information being provided and the results of each objective test and measure performed. It is from the synthesis and analysis of all the examination and evaluation findings that the therapist is able to consider a child's impairments of body structures and functions, activity limitations, and participation restrictions and arrive at a functional physical therapy diagnosis. The physical therapist will assign a physical therapy diagnostic label, usually based on the practice patterns in the *Guide* (APTA, 2001). Based on this clinically relevant physical therapy diagnosis, a prognosis should be determined and a plan of care developed. This is a difficult task for students and new clinicians, and they especially should rely on the literature to support their statements.

To illustrate integration of examination and evaluation results to determine a diagnosis and prognosis, consider the following scenario. Examination of a 9-month-old infant born prematurely, whose parents report is not sitting independently like age-matched peers at the daycare center, reveals hypotonia on initial observation. While this observation alone could serve as a diagnostic label, it does not provide enough information to guide clinical decision making. Developing a more functional diagnosis requires information obtained from a detailed history as outlined in Chapter 1 and a comprehensive examination. Systems review should provide information about the infant's vital signs, muscle tone, antigravity movements, reflex function, and postural reactions. Objective data regarding this infant's developmental and functional abilities can be gathered using a combination of tools such as the Alberta Infant Motor Scale (AIMS) and the PEDI. Incorporating a quality of life or health-related outcomes measure such as the Pediatric Quality of Life Inventory (PedsQL) Infant Scales will provide additional information about the infant's functioning within the context of the family and community. Synthesizing the results from this comprehensive examination assists the therapist in distinguishing between central versus peripheral nervous system involvement; congenital, hereditary, infectious, environmental, or traumatic causes; and the progressive versus non-progressive nature of the disorder, leading the therapist to a more clinically relevant diagnosis, which in this example might be Impaired Motor Function Associated with Nonprogressive Disorders of the Central Nervous System—Congenital Origin (APTA, 2001, Practice Pattern 5C).

In this example, the parent's desired goal may be for the child to sit independently. Using the environment as a facilitator, the therapist can obtain or fabricate adaptive seating to accomplish this functional goal. Coupling this with parent education will allow the equipment to be used within the home and daycare center for participation in age-appropriate activities with family and peers. Intervening at the activity and participation levels and providing opportunities for practice may lead to improved trunk strength and an improvement at the impairment level, as well as enhancing performance of the sitting task itself.

The culmination of the examination, evaluation, diagnosis, and prognosis is development of the plan of care. The plan is developed in full collaboration with the child, family, and other service providers. The development of appropriate and meaningful, measurable goals and objectives are addressed throughout this text, as are evidence-based interventions. The results of the examination, evaluation, diagnosis, prognosis, and plan of care must be written down with appropriate documentation, as must all components of patient management.

Mini-Case Study 3.1: Examination, Evaluation, Diagnosis, and Prognosis of a Child Who Walks on His Toes

Name: Zachary X—
Date of Birth:
Age: 44 months
Parents' Concerns: Why is Zachary walking on his toes all the time?
History: Zachary, aged 44 months, was referred to an outpatient physical therapy clinic by a local pediatrician because of concerns about persistent toe walking. As is common in outpatient clinics, only the child's name, age, contact information, and primary reason for seeking evaluation were known prior to the therapist's examination; therefore, a thorough subjective history was obtained from the child's biological parents, who attended the examination with

Continued

him. Zachary's mom described her pregnancy as healthy and uncomplicated. Zachary was born by vaginal delivery at full-term and weighed 8 pounds, 2 ounces. No complications were reported post delivery. The family history is negative for congenital neuromuscular disease, but his dad and uncle were reported to have walked on their toes when they were little, and his dad had to wear "braces" when he was a toddler. Zachary has never had any surgeries, significant illnesses, accidents, or previous intervention for his toe walking. The only medication that he takes regularly is Zyrtec for his allergies to dust, cats, and pollen. Zachary sat up independently by the time he was 6 months old, crawled by 10 months, and started walking at 15 months of age. His parents report that he has walked on his toes "on and off" ever since he started walking, but it has become a more consistent pattern in the last year. When questioned about balance, his parents did not report excessive "clumsiness," falls or injuries. Zachary lives with his parents and older sister, and he just started attending preschool two days per week. Zachary reportedly eats and sleeps well. He is described as being "picky" about what he eats and pretty routine in his daily activities. He enjoys bath time, looking at picture books, and playing with his toy cars and trains, but he does not like to play outside in the sandbox or to get "messy."

Systems Review, Present Function, and Tests and Measures:

Based on the information from the history, a review of the integumentary, musculoskeletal, and neuromuscular systems and a screening of communication skills and behavior were completed. No calluses, blisters, or skin breakdown were noted on Zachary's ankles or feet. Screening of joint mobility revealed stiffness in bilateral ankles with subsequent dorsiflexion goniometric measures as follows: –10 degrees, knee extended, and –2 degrees, knee flexed, on the right; –5 degrees, knee extended, and 0 degrees, knee flexed, on the left. Strength screening revealed active dorsiflexion through approximately 75% of his available range bilaterally, observed in short sitting on his dad's lap while kicking a balloon, indicating 3-/5 strength. When asked about pain, Zachary pointed to the "1" on the Oucher Scale. Muscle tone was screened by assessing velocity-dependent resistance to passive stretch. No clonus was elicited and Zachary scored a "0" on the Modified Ashworth Scale (see Chapter 7), indicating normal muscle tone. Lower extremity deep tendon reflexes demonstrated a normal 2+ response. To screen communication and behavior, the therapist had Zachary's parents complete the Ages and Stages Questionnaire: Social-Emotional (ASQ:SE) while he was being evaluated. The therapist noted that Zachary demonstrated good eye contact while interacting with her, easily followed multiple step directions, and answered and asked questions spontaneously and without hesitation. Scoring of the ASQ:SE was completed at the end of the evaluation session and revealed that his communication and behavior were age-appropriate. Had this parent-reported screening tool or Zachary's behaviors during the evaluation revealed any concerns, the therapist would have completed further testing, utilizing tools such as the DeGangi-Berk Test of Sensory Integration, the Sensory Integration and Praxis Test, or the Sensory Profile at the next session or referred Zachary to speech or occupational therapy for further testing.

To fully assess Zachary's gross motor skills, the therapist completed the gross motor sections of the Peabody Developmental Motor Scales. Zachary scored at the 50th percentile for the Stationary and Locomotion sections and at the 95th percentile for Object Manipulation, which placed Zachary in the 77th percentile overall for his gross motor development. While this demonstrates typical performance, the therapist did make note of Zachary's difficulty with the single leg stance, jumping, and hopping items. Other developmental tests that the therapist could have chosen to use with Zachary include the Brigance Inventory of Early Development II, Bruininks Oseretsky Test of Motor Proficiency, Revised Merrill-Palmer Scale, Movement Assessment Battery for Children, and Test of Gross Motor Development.

In addition to evaluating the level of Zachary's gross motor development, the therapist observed the quality of his gait. Observational analysis revealed lack of heel contact throughout all phases of gait bilaterally, mild out-toeing, pronation and knee hyperextension bilaterally, minimal forward trunk lean with hip flexion and increased lumbar lordosis, equal stride lengths, and smooth reciprocal arm swing. Based on the gait deviations observed, the therapist determined further evaluation of lower extremity alignment was indicated. Zachary was found to have a negative Thomas test and his thigh-foot angle, sacral angle, standing knee extension, hindfoot and forefoot alignment and leg length discrepancy measures (see Chapter 5) were all within age-appropriate norms.

Evaluation, Diagnosis, and Prognosis:

Because toe walking can be a symptom of multiple conditions, the therapist must systematically consider the various causes and associated conditions when determining a diagnosis for Zachary. Upon hearing about Zachary's "routine" behavior, "picky" eating habits, and dislike of being "messy," the therapist knew to screen his communication skills and adaptive behaviors since toe walking can be associated with autism-spectrum disorders (Le Cras, Bouck, Brausch & Taylor-Hass, 2011; Newman, Ziegler, Jeannet, Roulet-Perez, & Deonna, 2006; Sala, Shulman, Kennedy, Grant, & Chu, 1999). It was also prudent to assess Zachary's neuromuscular system since toe walking is frequently associated with nervous system disorders, such as cerebral palsy (Le Cras et al., 2011; Lundequam & Willis, 2009; Newman et al., 2006; Sala et al., 1999). Because Zachary passed these screenings, it is feasible to assume that his toe walking is not related to these types of disorders. Because Zachary's development is within age appropriate limits and his gait, although posturally atypical, is symmetrical and coordinated, it is safe to assume that his toe walking is more idiopathic and musculoskeletal in nature (Sala et al., 1999). Given Zachary's family history and the results of his musculoskeletal exam, it is most likely that the increased frequency and severity of his toe walking is related to the plantar flexion contractures. Using the *Guide* (APTA, 2001), the therapist would list Zachary's diagnosis as Impaired Posture (Pattern 4B) and could use the ICD-9-CM codes of 719.5 (stiffness of joint, not elsewhere classified), 781.92 (abnormal posture), or 781.2 (abnormality of gait) for billing purposes.

Plan of Care

With this diagnostic information, the therapist can then establish a plan of care that will be best suited for Zachary's impairments and activity limitations. The plan of care would include specific measurable objectives and interventions. Examples of goals for Zachary include the following: (1) Zachary will achieve 10 degrees of active ankle dorsiflexion with knee extended bilaterally and (2) Zachary will demonstrate heel contact while walking, running, and playing at preschool during 3 of 4 10-minute observation periods. Educational and procedural interventions are indicated to address Zachary's postural issues. His parents would be instructed in stretching activities, such as standing on a wedge and lunges, and strengthening activities, such as tapping his toes and kicking a balloon in short sitting (Le Cras et al., 2011). Procedural interventions would include serial casting or dynamic splinting, manual stretching, and strengthening along with consideration of referral for Botox injections and/or bracing (Le Cras et al., 2011; Lundequam & Willis, 2009; Sala et al., 1999). The therapist might schedule Zachary for weekly sessions with an anticipated duration of 4–6 weeks for this episode of care with further intervention or referral indicated depending on Zachary's response to the initial interventions (Le Cras et al., 2011).

Documentation

Most pediatric clinicians enjoy interacting with the infants and children they treat more than completing the documentation required by employers, state and federal law, accrediting and regulatory bodies, and third-party payers. Despite this, documentation is a skill that must be attended to as diligently as examination and intervention skills. Maintaining accurate records assists the therapist in planning services, monitoring progress toward goals and outcomes, ensuring quality and continuity of services, facilitating communication among healthcare workers, validating the need for skilled services, justifying reimbursement for service provision, and supplying legal evidence when needed (APTA, 2010c). While the requirement to document is universal, the process for completing and maintaining records varies due to differences in rules and regulations across practice settings and state physical therapy practice acts.

In general, some form of documentation is required for every physical therapy visit or encounter and a mechanism for recording cancellations and absences should be available (APTA, 2011a). This may range from a chart for logging attendance to completing a lengthy narrative note for every visit. While charts and flow sheets are convenient to use, it is important to remember that they cannot be used in isolation; they should supplement, not replace, physical therapy records (APTA, 2011b). All components of the patient/client management model should be documented, and most practice settings have established forms for recording initial examinations/evaluations, daily or progress notes, re-examinations, and discharges or discontinuations.

Typically, examination/evaluation documentation includes the following information: (1) the subjective history provided by the child and/or family, (2) the infant or child's current level of functioning and development determined from results of a systems review and appropriate tests and measures, (3) the physical therapy diagnosis and prognosis, which includes the plan of care describing interventions to be provided and mutually developed, measurable goals, and frequency and duration of services, and (4) anticipated discharge plans (APTA, n.d.). Daily notes, which are done for every encounter, or progress notes, which are completed at set intervals such as every week or school term, generally record the actual interventions performed, the infant or child's response to the interventions, progress toward established goals and outcomes, any new subjective information reported by the child or family, and any changes the therapist made to the current plan of care.

Requirements for documentation of a comprehensive re-examination vary considerably in terms of how frequently it should to be done, who is to be involved, and what must be included, depending on the practice setting and how the services are being funded. Re-examinations may range from discipline-specific monthly re-certifications to annual reviews by the full team. In early intervention, for example, re-examination is documented through a team review of the Individualized Family Service Plan (IFSP) every 6 months (APTA, 2011c). Discharge or discontinuation summaries are usually required upon termination of an episode of care and should include objective comparison of the infant or child's initial functional and developmental status with current status, a report on goal and outcome attainment, and discharge disposition details such as transition planning or recommendations for referral to other services (APTA, n.d.).

Documentation may be completed and stored in a variety of ways, depending on the practice setting and model of service delivery. In some settings, usually those that are more medically based, each discipline completes the documentation independently. An infant or child's record is then stored in a discipline-specific chart, a multidisciplinary medical or rehabilitation chart, or as an electronic record. Use of electronic records is becoming increasingly more prevalent, especially in hospital settings. In other settings, usually those that are more educationally based, documentation is developed through integrated service delivery and consensus decision-making. In early intervention and school settings, documentation is frequently done collaboratively, with all team members contributing to the final document, such as the IFSP or Individualized Education Program (IEP). Even with collaborative documentation, the physical therapist may maintain discipline-specific records to keep track of more detailed and technical information, such as relevant biomechanical measurements of the musculoskeletal system and achievement of specific objectives that relate to the child's interdisciplinary goals, as required by state practice acts (APTA, 2011c).

A challenge in documenting therapy services for children is balancing the inclusion of professional judgment and decision-making rationale to substantiate the need and evidence base for skilled therapy (APTA, 2011d) with family-friendly, lay language, which is necessary to promote comprehension and communication with other team members, including the child and their family (APTA, 2011c). One example for achieving this balance is to report results of valid and reliable standardized developmental testing in lay terms using percentile scores or age equivalents instead of referring to developmental quotients or standard scores, which are more difficult for families to understand. Emphasizing the child's activity and participation (i.e., their functional abilities) rather than their impairments also helps the therapist document in terms that are more relevant and understandable to families. Referring to the "infant" or "child" in documentation instead of using the labels "patient" or "client," as recommended in APTA's Defensible Documentation: Setting Specific Considerations in Documentation (2011c), makes reports more personable and fosters family participation.

The emphasis on family participation, naturally occurring environments, play-based interventions, and less use of technical jargon in pediatric documentation does give a more relaxed feeling to service delivery. With this approach to pediatric physical therapy, the therapist must be even more alert to maintaining confidentiality of an infant or child's records. Physical therapists must know and conform with all state and federal laws related to confidentiality including the Health Insurance Portability and Accountability Act (HIPAA) in medical settings and the Family Educational Rights and Privacy Act (FERPA) in federally funded school settings (APTA, 2011e).

Summary

The examination of children is exciting and challenging. The examination process with a child is not easy and requires creativity and flexibility on the part of the therapist. A careful, comprehensive initial examination is mandatory. Therapists must perform developmental and functional tests and measures of activities along with more traditional tests and measures of body structures and functions. The goals, outcomes, and objectives should be based on the desires of the family and child. The examination and evaluation lead to the diagnostic process, prognosis, plan of care, intervention, and outcomes. The specific examination methods, tests, and measures, along with interventions for each body system, are presented separately in the major chapters of this text; however, children frequently have involvement of more than one system and require coordinated intervention to address impairments of body functions and structures of each system and restrictions in activities and participation. The separation of systems into chapters is necessary for organizational purposes, but the child must be considered as a whole, with an understanding and appreciation that all systems interact at all times and that development is context dependent.

DISCUSSION QUESTIONS

1. Select a test used with children with disabilities that you have been exposed to. What is the sensitivity and specificity of the test? Is the standard error of measurement reported?

2. Why is knowing the standard error of measurement of a test so important in determining the outcome of intervention?

3. Discuss the benefits of naturalistic observation as part of the examination process.

4. Why is including a quality of life measure such an important part of the examination and evaluation process?

Recommended Readings

American Physical Therapy Association (APTA). (2011). *Defensible documentation: Setting specific considerations in documentation.* Retrieved from http://www.apta.org/Documentation/Defensible-Documentation/

American Physical Therapy Association (APTA). (2010). *Online guide to physical therapist practice.* Retrieved from http://guidetoptpractice.apta.org

Chiarello, L.A., Palisano, R.J., Maggs, J.M., Orlin, M.N., Almasri, N., Lin-Ju, K., & Chang, H. (2010). Family priorities for activity and participation of children and youth with cerebral palsy. *Physical Therapy, 90*(9), 1254–1264.

Waters, E., Davis, E., Ronen, G.M., Rosenbaum, P., Livingston, M., & Saigal, S. (2009). Quality of life

instruments for children and adolescents with neurodisabilities: How to choose the appropriate instrument. *Developmental Medicine and Child Neurology, 51*(8), 660–669.

References

American Pain Society (1995). *Pain: The fifth vital sign.* Glenview, IL: Author.

American Physical Therapy Association (APTA) (2001). Guide to physical therapist practice (2nd ed.). *Physical Therapy, 81*(1).

American Physical Therapy Association (APTA) (2010a). *Code of ethics for the physical therapist.* Alexandria, VA: Author. Retrieved from http://www.apta.org/uploadedFiles/APTAorg/About_Us/Policies/HOD/Ethics/CodeofEthics.pdf

American Physical Therapy Association (APTA) (2010b). *Online guide to physical therapist practice.* ISBN: 978-1-887759-87-8. Retrieved from http://guidetoptpractice.apta.org

American Physical Therapy Association (APTA). (2010c). *Introduction to defensible documentation.* Retrieved from http://www.apta.org/Documentation/Defensible Documentation/

American Physical Therapy Association (APTA). (2011a). *Defensible documentation: General guidelines.* Retrieved from http://www.apta.org/Documentation/Defensible Documentation/

American Physical Therapy Association (APTA). (2011b). *Defensible documentation: Definitions and references.* Retrieved from http://www.apta.org/Documentation/DefensibleDocumentation/

American Physical Therapy Association (APTA). (2011c). *Defensible documentation: Setting specific considerations in documentation.* Retrieved from http://www.apta.org/Documentation/DefensibleDocumentation/

American Physical Therapy Association (APTA). (2011d). *Defensible documentation: Current concerns in physical therapy documentation.* Retrieved from http://www.apta.org/Documentation/DefensibleDocumentation/

American Physical Therapy Association (APTA). (2011e). *Defensible documentation: other considerations.* Retrieved from http://www.apta.org/Documentation/Defensible Documentation/

American Physical Therapy Association (APTA). (n.d.) *Defensible documentation: Elements.* Retrieved from http://www.apta.org/Documentation/Defensible Documentation/

American Psychological Association (APA) & World Health Organization (2003). *International classification of functioning, disability, and health procedural manual and guide for a standardized application of the ICF: A manual for health professionals.* Washington, DC: Author.

Bagnato, S.J. (2007). *Authentic assessment for early childhood intervention: Best Practices.* New York: Guilford Press.

Bailey, D.B., & Wolery, M. (1992). *Teaching infants and preschoolers with disabilities* (2nd ed.). New York: Merrill.

Baily, B., Bergeron, S., Gravel, J., & Daoust, R. (2007). Comparison of four pain scales in children with acute abdominal pain in a pediatric emergency department. *Annals of Emergency Medicine, 50*(4), 379–383.

Bjornson, K.F., & McLaughlin, J.F. (2001). The measurement of health-related quality of life (HRQL) in children with cerebral palsy. *European Journal of Neurology, 8,* 183–193.

Brenneman, S.K. (1999). Assessment and testing of infant and child development. In J.S. Tecklin (Ed.), *Pediatric physical therapy* (3rd ed., pp. 28–70). Philadelphia: Lippincott.

Calhoon, J.M. (1997). Comparison of assessment results between a formal standardized measure and a play-based format. *Infant-Toddler Intervention, 7*(3), 201–214.

Campbell, P.H. (1991). Evaluation and assessment in early intervention for infants and toddlers. *Journal of Early Intervention, 15,* 36–45.

Campbell, P.H., Sawyer. B., & Muhlenhaupt, M. (2009). The meaning of natural environments for parents and professionals. *Infants & Young Children: An Interdisciplinary Journal of Special Care Practices, 22*(4), 264–278.

Chiarello, L.A., Palisano, R.J., Maggs, J.M., Orlin, M.N., Almasri, N., Lin-Ju, K., & Chang, H. (2010). Family priorities for activity and participation of children and youth with cerebral palsy. *Physical Therapy, 90*(9), 1254–1264.

Colver, A. (2009). Quality of life and participation. *Developmental Medicine and Child Neurology, 51*(8), 656–659.

Coster, W., Deeney, T., Haltiwanger, J., & Haley, S. (1998). *School function assessment.* San Antonio, TX: The Psychological Corporation.

Coster, W.J., Haley, S.M., Ni, P., Dumas, H.M., & Fragala-Pinkham, M.A. (2008). Assessing self-care and social function using a computer adaptive testing version of the pediatric evaluation of disability inventory. *Archives of Physical Medicine and Rehabilitation, 89*(4), 622–629.

Cusick, A., McIntyre, S., Novak, I., Lannin, N., & Lowe, K. (2006). A comparison of goal attainment scaling and the Canadian occupational performance measure for paediatric rehabilitation research. *Pediatric Rehabilitation, 9*(2), 149–157.

Dole, R.L., & Chafetz, R. (2010). *Peds Rehab Notes.* Philadelphia: F.A. Davis.

Dumas, H.M., Rosen, E.L., Haley, S.M., Fragala-Pinkham, M.A., Ni, P., & O'Brien, J.E. (2010). Measuring physical function in children with airway support: a pilot study using computer adaptive testing. *Developmental Neurorehabilitation, 13*(2), 95–102.

Effgen, S. (1991). Systematic delivery and recording of intervention assistance. *Pediatric Physical Therapy, 3,* 63–68.

Effgen, S., & Brown, D. (1992). Long-term stability of hand-held dynamometric measurements in children who have myelomeningocele. *Physical Therapy, 72*(6), 458–465.

Effgen, S.K., & Chan, L. (2010). Relationship between occurrence of gross motor behaviors and attainment of objectives in children with cerebral palsy participating in conductive education. *Physiotherapy Theory and Practice, 26*(1), 1–18.

Eiser, C., & Morse, R. (2001). Can parents rate their child's health-related quality of life? Results of a systematic review. *Quality of Life Research, 10*(4), 347–357.

Gray, G.M., & Tasso, K.H. (2009). Differential diagnosis of torticollis: A case report. *Pediatric Physical Therapy, 21*(4), 369–374.

Haley, S.M., Coster, W.J., Ludlow, L.H., Haltiwanger, J.T., & Andrellos, P.J. (1998). *Pediatric Evaluation of Disability Inventory (PEDI).* Boston, MA: PEDI Research Group, Boston University.

Haley, S.M., Fragala-Pinkham, M.A., Dumas, H.M., Ni, P., Gorton, G.E., Watson, K., Montpetit, K, Bilodeau, N, Hambleton, R.K., & Tucker, C.A. (2009). Evaluation of an item bank for a computerized adaptive test of activity in children with cerebral palsy. *Physical Therapy, 89*(6), 589–600.

Haley, S.M., Ni, P., Fragala-Pinkham, M.A., Skrinar, A.M., & Corzo, D. (2005). A computer adaptive testing approach for assessing physical functioning in children and adolescents. *Developmental Medicine and Child Neurology, 47*(2), 113–120.

Haley, S.M., Ni, P., Hambleton, R.K., Slavin, M.D., & Jette, A.M. (2006). Computer adaptive testing improved accuracy and precision of scores over random item selection in a physical functioning item bank. *Journal of Clinical Epidemiology, 59*(11), 1174–1182.

Hanna, S.E., Russell, D.J., Bartlett, D.J., Kertoy, M.L., Rosenbaum, P.L., & Wynn, K. (2007). Measurement practices in pediatric rehabilitation: a survey of physical therapists, occupational therapists, and speech-language pathologists in Ontario. *Physical & Occupational Therapy in Pediatrics, 27*(2), 25–42.

Imms, C., Reilly, S., Carlin, J., & Dodd, K. (2008). Diversity of participation in children with cerebral palsy. *Developmental Medicine and Child Neurology, 50*(5), 363–369.

Jewell, D.V. (2008). *Guide to evidence-based physical therapist practice.* Sudbury, MA: Jones & Bartlett.

Joint Commission Resources. (2010). Standards and Elements of Performance. PC.01.02.07: The hospital assesses and manages the patient's pain. Retrieved from https://ecm.jcrinc.com/Login.aspx?msg=TO

Katz-Leurer, M., Rottem, H., & Meyer, S. (2008). Hand-held dynamometry in children with traumatic brain injury: Within-session reliability. *Pediatric Physical Therapy, 20*(3), 259–263.

King, G.A., Law, M., King, S., Hurley, P., Hanna, S., Kertoy, M., & Rosenbaum, P. (2007). Measuring children's participation in recreation and leisure activities: construct validation of the CAPE and PAC. *Child: Care, Health and Development, 33,* 28–39.

King, G., Law, M., King, S., Hurley, P., Rosenbaum, P., Hanna, S., Kertoy, M., & Young, N. (2004). *Children's Assessment of Participation and Enjoyment (CAPE) and Preferences for Activities of Children (PAC).* San Antonio, TX: Pearson.

Law, M., Baptiste, S., Carswell, A., McColl, M., Polatajko, H., & Pollock, P. (2005). *Canadian Occupational Performance Measure (COPM)* (4th ed.). Ottawa, OH: Canadian Association of Occupational Therapy Publications.

Le Cras, S., Bouck, J., Brausch, S., Taylor-Haas, A. Cincinnati Children's Hospital Medical Center. (2011). Evidence-based clinical care guideline for Management of Idiopathic Toe Walking, http://www.cincinnatichildrens.org/service/j/anderson-center/evidence-based-care/occupational-therapy-physical-therapy/, Guideline 040, pages 1–17, February 15, 2011.

Linder, T. (2008). *Transdisciplinary play-based assessment* (2nd ed.). Baltimore: Brookes.

Lundequam, P., & Willis, F.B. (2009). Dynamic splinting home therapy for toe walking: A case report. *Cases Journal, 2,* 188–188.

Majnemer, A., Shevell, M., Law, M., Poulin, C., & Rosenbaum, P. (2008). Reliability in the ratings of quality of life between parents and their children of school age with cerebral palsy. *Quality of Life Research, 17*(9), 1163–1171.

McEwen, I.R., Meiser, M.J., & Hansen, L.H. (2012). Children with motor and intellectual disabilities. In S.K. Campbell, R.J. Palisano, & M.N. Orlin (Eds.), *Physical therapy for children* (4th ed., pp. 539–576). St. Louis: Elsevier Saunders.

McGrath, P. A. (1995). Pain in the pediatric patient: practical aspects of assessment. *Pediatric Annals, 24*(3), 126.

McGrath, P.J., Johnston, G., Goodman, J.T., Schillinger, J., Dunn, J., & Chapman, J. (1985). CHEOPS: A behavioral scale for rating postoperative pain in children. In H.L. Fields, R. Dubner & F. Cereri (Eds.), *Advances in pain research and therapy* (pp. 395–402). New York: Raven Press.

Merkel, S.I., Voepel-Lewis, T., Shayevitz, J.R., & Malviya, S. (1997). The FLACC: A behavioral scale for scoring postoperative pain in young children. *Pediatric Nursing, 23,* 293–297.

Newman, C.J., Ziegler, A.-L., Jeannet, P.-Y., Roulet-Perez, E., & Deonna, T.W. (2006). Transient dystonic toe-walking: differentiation from cerebral palsy and a rare explanation for some unexplained cases of idiopathic toe-walking. *Developmental Medicine and Child Neurology, 48*(2), 96–102.

Nilsson, S., Finnstrom, B., & Kokinsky, E. (2008). The FLACC behavioral scale for procedural pain assessment in children age 5–16 years. *Pediatric Anesthesia, 18,* 767–774.

Olson, L. J. (1999). Psychosocial frame of reference. In P. Kramer & J. Hinojosa (Eds.), *Frames of reference for pediatric occupational therapy* (2nd ed., pp. 323–375). Philadelphia: Lippincott Williams & Wilkins.

Orlin, M.N., Palisano, R.J., Chiarello, L.A., Kang, L.J., Polansky, M., Almasri, N., & Maggs, J. (2010). Participation in home, extracurricular, and community activities among children and young people with cerebral palsy. *Developmental Medicine and Child Neurology, 52*(2), 160–166.

Palisano, R.J., Chiarello, L.A., Orlin, M., Oeffinger, D., Polansky, M., Maggs, J., Bagley, A., Gorton, G., & The Children's Activity and Participation Group. (2011). Determinants of intensity of participation in leisure and recreational activities by children with cerebral palsy. *Developmental Medicine and Child Neurology, 53*(2), 142–147.

Palisano, R.J., Kang, L.J., Chiarello, L.A., Orlin, M., Oeffinger, D., & Maggs, J. (2009). Social and community participation of children and youth with cerebral palsy is associated with age and gross motor function classification. *Physical Therapy, 89*(12), 1304–1314.

PL 108-446, Individuals with Disabilities Education Improvement Act of 2004. Retrieved from http://www.copyright.gov/legislation/pl108-446.pdf

Portney, L.G., & Watkins, M.P. (2009). *Foundation of clinical research: Application to practice* (3rd. ed.). Upper Saddle River, NJ: Pearson Prentice Hall.

Rainforth, B., & York-Barr, J. (1997). *Collaborative teams for students with severe disabilities: Integrating therapy and educational services* (2nd ed.). Baltimore: Paul H. Brookes.

Richardson, P.K. (2001). Use of standardized tests in pediatric practice. In J. Case-Smith (Ed.). *Occupational therapy for children* (4th ed., p. 336). St. Louis: Mosby.

Rothstein, J.M., Echternach, J.L., & Riddle, D.L. (2003). The Hypothesis-Oriented Algorithm for Clinicians II (HOAC II): A guide for patient management. *Physical Therapy, 83*(5), 455–470.

Russell, D., Palisano, R., Walter, S., Rosenbaum, P., Gemus, M., Gowland, C., Galuppi, B., & Lane, M. (1998). Evaluating motor function in children with Down syndrome: Validity of the GMFM. *Developmental Medicine and Child Neurology, 40,* 693–701.

Russell, D., Rosenbaum, P., Avery, L., & Lane, M. (2002). Gross Motor Function Measure (GMFM-66 & GMFM-88) User's Manual. *Clinics in Developmental Medicine, 159,* London: MacKeith Press.

Sakzewski, L., Boyd, R., & Ziviani, J. (2007). Clinimetric properties of participation measures for 5- to 13-year-old children with cerebral palsy: A systematic review. *Developmental Medicine and Child Neurology, 49*(3), 232–240.

Sala, D.A., Shulman, L.H., Kennedy, R.F., Grant, A.D., & Chu, M.L. (1999). Idiopathic toe-walking: A review. *Developmental Medicine and Child Neurology, 41*(12), 846–848.

Smith, D.L. (1997). Technology. Teleassessment: A model for team developmental assessment of high-risk infants using a televideo network. *Infants & Young Children: An Interdisciplinary Journal of Special Care Practices, 9*(4), 58–61.

Stewart, K.B. (2010). Purposes, processes and methods of evaluation. In J. Case-Smith (Ed.). *Occupational therapy for children* (6th ed., pp. 193–215). St. Louis: Mosby Elsevier.

Suraseranivongse, S., Kaosaard, R., Intakong, P., Pornsiriprasert, S., Karnchana, Y., Koapinpruck, J., & Sangjeen, K. (2006) A comparison of postoperative pain scales in neonates. *British Journal of Anesthesia, 97*(4), 540–544.

Tucker, C.A. (2011). Computer adaptive testing for patient-reported outcomes: Resources for clinical research. *Journal of Physical Therapy Education, 25*(1), 54–58.

Waters, E., Davis, E., Ronen, G.M., Rosenbaum, P., Livingston, M., & Saigal, S. (2009). Quality of life instruments for children and adolescents with neurodisabilities: How to choose the appropriate instrument. *Developmental Medicine and Child Neurology, 51*(8), 660–669.

Wong, D., & Baker, C. (1988). Pain in children: Comparison of assessment scales. *Pediatric nursing, 14* (1), 9–17.

World Health Organization (1993). WHOQOL Group. Study protocol for the World Health Organization project to develop a quality of life assessment instrument. *Quality of Life Research, 2,* 153–159.

World Health Organization (2001). *International classification of functioning, disability and health.* Geneva: Author.

World Health Organization (WHO) (2003). *ICF checklist version 2.1a: Clinician form.* Geneva: Author. Retrieved from http://www.who.int/classifications/icf/training/icfchecklist.pdf

World Health Organization (WHO) (2007). *International classification of functioning, disability and health—children and youth version* (pp. 150–160). Geneva: Author. Portions available at http://apps.who.int/classifications/icfbrowser/

World Health Organization (WHO) (2010). *WHO Disability Assessment Schedule 2.0 (WHODAS 2.0).* Geneva: Author. Retrieved from: http://www.who.int/classifications/icf/whodasii/en/index.html

Appendix 3.A Common Tests and Measures of Development, Function, Sensory Integration, Pain, Quality of Life, and Participation*

Test/Measure and Author/ Reference or Publisher	Age Range	Areas Tested and ICF-CY Classification	Primary Use
ABILITIES Index Simeonsson, R.J., Bailey, D., Smith, T., & Buyssee, V. (1995). Young children with disabilities: Functional assessment by teachers. *Journal of Developmental Physical Disabilities, 7,* 267–284.	36–69 months	Index of 9 domains: audition, behavior, intelligence, limbs, intentional communication, tonicity, integrity of health, eyes, and structure. ICF-CY body structures and functions, activity, participation	Documents the nature and extent of the functional characteristics of childhood disability. Has potential to identify discrete profiles of functional characteristics.
Activities Scale for Kids (ASK) Young, N.L., Williams, J.I., Yoshida, K.K., & Wright, J.G. (2000). Measurement properties of the Activities Scale for Kids. *Journal of Clinical Epidemiology, 53*(2), 125–137.	5–15 years, children experiencing limitations in physical activity due to musculoskeletal disorders	Self-reported 30-item measure of physical functioning with capability and performance versions. ICF-CY activity	Performance version measures what the child "did do" and capability version measures what the child "could do." Explores the nature of the child's activity limitations
Ages & Stages Questionnaire (ASQ-3), 3rd edition Squires, J.,& Bricker, D.	1–66 months	Norm-referenced, standardized parent report of communication, gross motor, fine motor, problem-solving and personal-social development. ICF-CY activity, participation	Screening tool to determine if areas require further testing. Encourages family participation, commonly used in Early Head Start programs. Ages & Stages Questionnaires: Social Emotional (ASQ:SE) also available.
Alberta Infant Motor Scale (AIMS) and Motor Assessment of the Developing Infant Piper, M.,& Darrah, J.	Birth–18 months	Standardized observation of spontaneous gross motor skills in four positions: prone, supine, sitting, and standing. ICF-CY activity	Identifies infants and toddlers with gross motor delay and evaluates gross motor skill maturation.
Assessment, Evaluation, and Programming System for Infants and Children (AEPS), 2nd edition Bricker, D.	Birth–3years and 3–6 years	Criterion-referenced assessment done through observation of naturally occurring activities. Areas observed include fine motor, gross motor, cognitive, adaptive, social-communication, and social. ICF-CY activity, participation	Identifies skill attainment and assist in program planning and monitoring of outcomes. No standard scores or age equivalents provided; it is linked to a curriculum. Web-based electronic management system available for scoring and reporting.

Appendix 3.A Common Tests and Measures of Development, Function, Sensory Integration, Pain, Quality of Life, and Participation—cont'd

Test/Measure and Author/ Reference or Publisher	Age Range	Areas Tested and ICF-CY Classification	Primary Use
Assessment of Life Habits (LIFE-H) Noreau, L., Lepage, C., Boissiere, L., Picard, R., Fougeyrollas, P., Mathieu, J., Desmarais, G., & Nadeau, L. (2007). Measuring participation in children with disabilities using the Assessment of Life Habits. *Journal of Developmental Medicine and Child Neurology, 49*(9), 666–671.	Children with disabilities 5–13 years	Level of difficulty and type of assistance are measured for daily activities (nutrition, fitness, personal care, communication, housing, mobility) and social roles (responsibility, interpersonal relations, community life, education, employment, recreation). ICF-CY participation	Description of participation of children with disabilities
Battelle Developmental Inventory (BDI-2), 2nd edition Newborg, J.	Birth–8 years	Norm-referenced, standardized assessment of personal-social, adaptive, motor, communication, and cognition skills completed by interview or observation. A screening tool is also available. ICF-CY activity, participation	Commonly used tool to determine developmental delay or dysfunction in infants and young children for eligibility for early intervention services. Unfortunately, there are few items in each domain at each age level.
Bayley Infant Neurodevelopmental Screener (BINS) Aylward, G.	3–24 months	Norm-referenced screening of basic neurological, visual, auditory, gross motor, fine motor, verbal and cognitive functions. ICF-CY body structures and functions, activity	Determines level of risk by age in 1-month intervals.
Bayley Scales of Infant and Toddler Development (BSID-III), 3rd edition Bayley, N.	1–42 months	Norm-referenced, standardized assessment of adaptive behavior, cognitive, language, motor and social-emotional development. Motor scale includes fine and gross motor function. ICF-CY activity, participation	Commonly used assessment in early intervention and research to determine developmental delay. Requires training in assessment.
Brigance Inventory of Early Development II (BIED-II) Brigance, A.	Birth–7 years	Criterion-referenced test of: psychomotor, self-help, speech and language, general knowledge and comprehension, early academic skills, and social-emotional development. ICF-CY activity, participation	Commonly used assessment in early intervention and preschool programs to determine developmental delay in several domains and for program planning.

Continued

Appendix 3.A Common Tests and Measures of Development, Function, Sensory Integration, Pain, Quality of Life, and Participation—cont'd

Test/Measure and Author/ Reference or Publisher	Age Range	Areas Tested and ICF-CY Classification	Primary Use
Bruininks Oseretsky Test of Motor Proficiency, 2nd edition (BOT-2) Bruininks, R., & Bruininks, B.	4–21 years	Norm-referenced, standardized test of gross and fine motor skills. Subscales for running speed and agility, balance, bilateral coordination, strength, upper limb coordination, response speed, visual-motor control, and upper limb speed and dexterity. ICF-CY body structures and functions, activity	Common assessment tool for higher-level motor skills and to evaluate motor training programs.
Canadian Occupational Performance Measure (COPM), 4th edition Law, M., Baptiste, S., Carswell, A., McColl, M.A., Polatajko, H., & Pollock, N.	8 years–adult	Child identifies areas of concern regarding perception of self-care, productivity, and leisure occupations. ICF-CY activity, participation	Functional, client-centered approach, especially useful with child or adolescent who is able to participate in program planning.
Carolina Curriculum for Infants and Toddlers with Special Needs (CCITSN), 3rd edition, and Carolina Curriculum for Preschoolers with Special Needs (CCPSN), 2nd edition Johnson-Martin, N., Attermeier, S., & Hacker, B.	Birth–36 months (CCITSN) and 2–5 years (CCCPSN)	Criterion-referenced test of cognition, communication, social adaptation, and fine and gross motor skills. ICF-CY activity, participation	Assesses infants, toddlers, and preschoolers with disabilities to determine developmental level and assist in curriculum planning. Not used for eligibility because there is no standardized score.
Child Health and Illness Profile—Child and Parent Edition (CHIP-CE) and Adolescent Edition (CHIP-AE) Starfield, B., Bergner, M., Ensminger, M., Riley, A., Ryan, S., Green, B., McGauhey, P., Skinner, A., & Kim, S. (1993). Adolescent health status measurement: Development of the Child Health and Illness Profile. *Pediatrics, 91*, 430–435.	6–11 years and 11–17 years	Younger version completed by children and parent. Adolescent edition is a self-administered questionnaire of health assessment. Domains covered: comfort, satisfaction with health, risk avoidance, disorder, achievement of social expectations, and resilience. ICF-CY activity, participation	Detects differences in health status among children with chronic illness.

■ **Appendix 3.A** Common Tests and Measures of Development, Function, Sensory Integration, Pain,
■ Quality of Life, and Participation—cont'd

Test/Measure and Author/ Reference or Publisher	Age Range	Areas Tested and ICF-CY Classification	Primary Use
Child Health Questionnaire (CHQ) Landgraf, J., Abetz, L., & Ware, J.	5–18 years, parent-report	Questionnaire covers concepts of physical functioning; bodily pain; limitations in schoolwork and activities due to behavioral difficulties; mental health; general behavior; and self-esteem. ICF-CY activity, participation	Measures general health and emotional impact of the child's health on the parent and family activities.
Childhood Health Assessment Questionnaire (C-HAQ) Singh, G., Athreya, B.A., Fries, J.F., & Goldsmith, D.P. (1994). Measurement of health status in children with juvenile rheumatoid arthritis. *Arthritis and Rheumatism 37,* 1761–1769.	Children with juvenile rheumatoid arthritis	Parent or child reports limitations in domains of eating, dressing and grooming, walking, arising from bed, hygiene, reach, grip and general activities. Also includes a visual analog scale to assess pain. ICF-CY activity, participation	Adapted for children from the *Stanford Health Assessment Questionnaire* (HAQ)
Children's Assessment of Participation and Enjoyment (CAPE) and Preference for Activity of Children (PAC) King, G., Law, M., King, S., Hurley, P., Rosenbaum, P., Hanna, S., Kertoy, M., & Young. N. (2004).	6–21 years	Discriminate measurement tool of five dimensions of participation: diversity, intensity, with whom, where, and enjoyment. Scores reflect participation in formal and informal activities, and reflect participation in 5 types of activities (recreational, active physical, social, skill-based, and self improvement activities). PAC assesses preference for involvement in activities. ICF-CY participation	Explore the individual day-to-day participation in children. The CAPE is a direct measure of participation and can help determine a rehabilitation program. CAPE and PAC are sold together and can be used together or separately.
Children's Hospital of Eastern Ontario Pain Scale (CHEOPS) McGrath, P.J., Johnston, G., Goodman, J.T., Schillinger, J., Dunn, J., & Chapman, J. (1985). CHEOPS: A behavioral scale for rating postoperative pain in children (pp. 395–402). In H.L. Fields (Ed.). *Advances in pain research and therapy.* New York: Raven Press.	1–7 years	Observational scale for measuring postoperative pain in six categories associated with medical procedures. ICF-CY body structures and functions	Used to monitor the effectiveness of interventions to reduce pain.

Continued

■ **Appendix 3.A** Common Tests and Measures of Development, Function, Sensory Integration, Pain, Quality of Life, and Participation—cont'd

Test/Measure and Author/ Reference or Publisher	Age Range	Areas Tested and ICF-CY Classification	Primary Use
Children's and Infants' Postoperative Pain Scale (CHIPPS) Büttner, W., & Finke, W. (2000). Analysis of behavioral and physiological parameters for the assessment of postoperative analgesic demand in newborns, infants and young children. *Paediatric Anaesthesia, 10*, 303–318.	0–4 years	Scale to assess postoperative pain across five items. ICF-CY body structures and functions	Used in hospital settings to measure postoperative pain
Clinical Observations of Motor and Postural Skills (COMPS), 2nd edition Wilson, B., Pollack, N., Kaplan, B., & Law, M.	5–15 years	Tests subtle motor coordination during slow movements, arm rotation, finger-nose touching, prone extension posture, asymmetrical tonic neck reflex, and supine flexion posture. ICF-CY body structures and functions	Screens for subtle motor coordination problems.
Cry, Requires O₂, Increased vital signs, Expression, Sleeplessness (CRIES) Krechel, S.W., & Bildner, J. (1995). CRIES: A new neonatal postoperative pain measurement score. Initial testing of validity and reliability. *Paediatric Anaesthesia, 5*, 53–61.	Neonates	Neonatal post-operative pain measurement of the five domains. ICF-CY body structures and functions	Used in hospital settings to measure postoperative pain
DeGangi-Berk Test of Sensory Integration (TSI) DeGangi, G., & Berk, R.	3–5 years	Criterion-referenced test of postural control, bilateral motor integration, and reflex integration. ICF-CY body structures and functions	Screens for sensory integration dysfunction in preschoolers.
Denver Developmental Screening Test—II (DDST-II) Frankenburg, W., Dodds, J., Archer, P., Bresnick, B., Maschka, P., Edelman, N., & Shapiro, H.	1 week–6½ years	Norm-referenced, standardized test of development in: personal-social, fine motor-adaptive, language, gross motor, and behavior. ICF-CY activity, participation	Commonly used screening test to determine developmental delay, although the specificity is weak and the sample population may be biased.

■ **Appendix 3.A** Common Tests and Measures of Development, Function, Sensory Integration, Pain, ■ Quality of Life, and Participation—cont'd

Test/Measure and Author/ Reference or Publisher	Age Range	Areas Tested and ICF-CY Classification	Primary Use
Developmental Assessment of Young Children (DAYC) Voress, J.,& Maddox, T.	Birth–5 years	Norm-referenced assessment of cognition, communication, social-emotional, physical development and adaptive behavior. Subtests can be used independently or in combination. ICF-CY activity, participation	Used to identify delays in areas assessed. Information collected through observation, caregiver interview and direct assessment in 10-20 minutes.
Developmental Hand Dysfunction, 2nd edition Erhardt, R.	Birth–adult	Criterion-referenced assessment of prehension including positional-reflexive, cognitively directed movement, and prewriting skills. ICF-CY activity	Used to determine delay or dysfunction in prehension skills, but without standardized scores. Useful tool in intervention planning.
Developmental Observation Checklist System (DOCS) Hresko, W.P., Shirley Miguel, S., Sherbenou, R., & Burton, S.	Birth–6 years	Norm-referenced checklist covering language, motor, social, and cognitive development. Also includes adjustment behavior and parent stress and support. ICF-CY activity, participation	Provides general developmental assessment.
Developmental Programming for Infants and Young Children—Revised (DPIYC) Schafer, S., Martha Moersch, M., & D'Eugenio, D.	0–36 months: Early Intervention Developmental Profile (EIDP) 36–60 months: Preschool Developmental Profile (PDP)	Criterion-referenced test of cognition, gross motor, fine motor, language, social-emotional, and self-care. ICF-CY activity	Used to describe the developmental status of a child with a disability across domains. Used for program planning, not to determine eligibility.
Developmental Test of Visual-Motor Integration (VMI), 6th edition Beery, K., Buktenica, N. & Beery, N.	2–8 years (short form) 2–18 years (long form)	Norm-referenced test of visual perception, motor coordination, and integration. ICF-CY body structures and functions	Easy test to determine problems in visual-motor integration important in writing and reading.
Developmental Test of Visual Perception, 2nd edition (DTVP-2) Hammil, D., Person, N., & Voress, J.	4–10 years	Norm-referenced test of form consistency, figure ground, position in space, and spatial relation. ICF-CY body structures and functions	Assists in distinguishing between problems in visual perception versus visual-motor problems.

Continued

■ **Appendix 3.A** Common Tests and Measures of Development, Function, Sensory Integration, Pain,
■ Quality of Life, and Participation—cont'd

Test/Measure and Author/ Reference or Publisher	Age Range	Areas Tested and ICF-CY Classification	Primary Use
Early Coping Inventory (ECI) and Coping Inventories Zeitlin, S.	4–36 months, developmental age (ECI) 3–16 years (Coping Inventories)	ECI is an observational assessment of adaptive behaviors related to Sensorimotor Organization, Reactive Behavior and Self-Initiated Behavior. Coping Inventories assess behavior in 2 categories, Self and Environment. ICF-CY activity, participation	Used to design strategies for intervention based on coping styles.
Face, Legs, Activity, Cry, and Consolability (FLACC) Behavioral Pain Scale Merkel, S., Voepel-Lewis, T., Shayevitz, J.R., & Malviya, S. (1997). The FLACC: A behavioral scale for scoring postoperative pain in young children. *Pediatric Nurse, 23*(3), 293–297.	2–7 years	Measurement of pain in five categories in children who are unable to communicate their pain. ICF-CY body structures and functions	Observational pain assessment.
Faces Pain Scale— Revised (FPS-R) Hicks, C.L., von Baeyer, C.L., Spafford, P., van Korlaar, I., & Goodenough, B. (2001). The *Faces Pain Scale— Revised:* Toward a common metric in pediatric pain measurement. *Pain, 93,* 173–183.	4–16 years	Pain intensity rating scale using pictures of faces in parallel with a numeric scale rating (0 to 10). ICF-CY body structures and functions	Measures self-reporting of pain intensity. Translations available in 47 different languages.
FirstSTEp: Screening Test for Evaluating Preschoolers (FirstSTEp) Miller, L.J.	2.9–6.2 years	Norm-referenced screening test of cognition, communication, motor, social-emotional, and adaptive behavior. ICF-CY activity, participation	Determines delay in all developmental areas.
Gross Motor Function Measure (GMFM) Russell, D., Rosenbaum, P., Avery, L., & Lane, M. (2002).	5 months–16 years for children with cerebral palsy and Down Syndrome (probably best at 1–5 years)	Gross motor function along the dimensions of lying and rolling, sitting, crawling, standing, and walking, running, and jumping. ICF-CY activity	Common assessment to determine quantity of movement in children with cerebral palsy or Down syndrome.

Appendix 3.A Common Tests and Measures of Development, Function, Sensory Integration, Pain, Quality of Life, and Participation—cont'd

Test/Measure and Author/ Reference or Publisher	Age Range	Areas Tested and ICF-CY Classification	Primary Use
Gross Motor Performance Measure (GMPM) Boyce, W., Gowland, C., Rosenbaum, P., Hardy, S., Lane, C., Plews, N., Goldsmith, C., Russell, D., Wright, V., Potter, S., & Harding, D.	5 months–12 years for children with cerebral palsy	Criterion-referenced, observational assessment of the quality of gross motor function based on the attributes of alignment, coordination, dissociated movements, stability and weight shifts. ICF-CY body structures and functions, activity	Intended for use with the Gross Motor Function Measure (GMFM)
Hawaii Early Learning Profile (HELP 0-3 and HELP 3-6), 2nd edition Parks, S.	Birth–36 months and 3–6 years	Criterion-referenced assessment of regulatory/sensory organization, cognition, language, gross motor, fine motor, social-emotional, and self-help. ICF-CY activity, participation	Complements the very popular HELP curriculum and assessment materials by providing guidelines for administration and scoring. Used to determine delay and program planning, but without a standardized score
Harris Infant Neuromotor Test (HINT) Harris, S.R., Megens, A.M., & Daniels, L.E. (2010).	2.5–12.5 months	Tests neuromotor development of infants, and includes parental questions regarding infant's movement and play. ICF-CY activity	Neuromotor screening test for low- and high-risk infants. Used to categorize infant's level of motor delay.
Home Observation for Measurement of the Environment (HOME) Caldwell, B.M., & Bradley, R.H.	Birth–3years (Infant/Toddler), 3–6 years (Early Childhood), 6–10 years (Middle Childhood), 10–15 years (Early Adolescent)	A semi-structured observation and interview to measure quality and quantity of stimulation and support available in the home. ICF-CY participation	Versions also available to assess child in other home settings (Child Care HOME) and to assess environment of children with disabilities (Disability HOME).
Infant-Toddler Developmental Assessment (IDA)—Provence Profile Provence, S., Erikson, J., Vater, S., & Palmeri, S. (1995)	Birth–3 years	A criterion-referenced assessment of gross and fine motor, cognition, communication, self-help, relationships to persons, emotion and feeling states, and coping through naturalistic observation and parent report. ICF-CY activity, participation	Provence Profile is part of a comprehensive and holistic evaluation process that includes a health and family component. Training is required.
The Infant Neurological International Battery (Infanib) Ellison, P.H.	1–18 months, at-risk infants, including those born prematurely	Tests spasticity, vestibular function, head and trunk control, French angles, and legs. ICF-CY body structures and functions	To determine normal and abnormal neuromotor function.

Continued

■ **Appendix 3.A** Common Tests and Measures of Development, Function, Sensory Integration, Pain,
■ Quality of Life, and Participation—cont'd

Test/Measure and Author/ Reference or Publisher	Age Range	Areas Tested and ICF-CY Classification	Primary Use
Infant Motor Profile (IMP) Heineman, K.R., Bos, A.F., & Hadders-Algra, M. (2008). The Infant Motor Profile: A standardized and qualitative method to assess motor behavior in infancy. *Developmental Medicine and Child Neurology, 50*(4), 275–282.	3–18 months or until child has walked several months independently	Video-based assessment focusing on the quality of motor behaviors using five domains: size of movement repertoire, ability to select movement pattern, symmetry, fluency and performance. ICF-CY activity	Demonstrates promising ability for early identification of developmental motor deficits.
Infant/Toddler Symptom Checklist DeGangi, G., Poisson, S., Sickel, R., & Wiener, A.	7–30 months	Criterion-referenced checklist for assessing behavior in 9 domains: self-regulation; attention; sleep; eating or feeding; dressing, bathing and touch; movement; listening and language; looking and sight; attachment/emotional functioning. ICF-CY activity, participation	Quick screening tool to determine if a child may have a predisposition for development of sensory integrative disorders, attention deficits or emotional, behavioral or learning difficulties.
KIDSCREEN The KIDSCREEN Group	8–18 years	Self-reported measure of physical, psychological and social well-being and financial resources with 52-, 27-, or 10-item instruments. ICF-CY activity and participation	To determine quality of life of healthy children and those with chronic illness.
Meade Movement Checklist (MMCL) Meade, V.	4–6 months	Observational assessment of vision, attention, fine and gross motor movements, personal-social and communication. ICF-CY body structures and functions, activity, participation	Screening for early signs of developmental delay. Parents/ caregivers involved with handling of infant during screening.
Merrill-Palmer-Revised Scales of Development (M-P-R) Roid, G., & Sampers, J.	1–78 months	Norm-referenced, standardized measure of cognitive (reasoning, memory, visual, etc.), language and motor (fine and gross), self-help/adaptive, and social-emotional development. Patterns of development are assessed. Includes supplemental parent and examiner ratings. ICF-CY activity, participation	The new addition of the motor measures makes this a comprehensive assessment that can be used from birth to kindergarten to determine delay or dysfunction and evaluate intervention effectiveness.

Appendix 3.A Common Tests and Measures of Development, Function, Sensory Integration, Pain, Quality of Life, and Participation—cont'd

Test/Measure and Author/ Reference or Publisher	Age Range	Areas Tested and ICF-CY Classification	Primary Use
Milani-Comparetti Motor Development Screening Test, 3rd edition Milani-Comparetti, A., & Gidoni, E.A., (Stuberg, W., revised edition)	Birth–2 years	Standardized screening of spontaneous motor behaviors including locomotion, sitting, and standing, and evoked responses, including equilibrium reactions, protective reactions, righting reactions, and primitive reflexes. ICF-CY body structures and functions, activity	Helpful in describing an infant's motor development, but no total score obtained. Relies on the integration of primitive reflexes for the development of postural control.
Miller Assessment of Preschoolers (MAP) Miller, L.J.	2 years 9 months–5 years 8 months	Norm-referenced test of sensory and motor foundations and coordination, verbal and nonverbal cognitive skills, and complex tasks. ICF-CY body structures and functions, activity	Determination of preschoolers, without major problems, who are at risk for preacademic problems.
Motor Skills Acquisition in the First Year and Checklist Bly, L.	Birth–12 months	Detailed explanation with photographs and checklist of gross motor development and indications of possible disturbances in motor development. ICF-CY activity	To monitor motor development and assist in intervention planning for infants with motor delays or dysfunction.
Movement Assessment Battery for Children, 2nd Edition (MOVEMENT ABC-2) Henderson, S., Sugden, D., & Barnett, A.	3–16 years (checklist 5–12 years)	Norm-referenced standardized performance test of manual dexterity, ball skills, and static and dynamic balance. Also included is a checklist of daily routine activities, consideration of the context of performance, and behavioral attributes. ICF-CY body structures and functions, activity, participation	Identifies impairments in motor function of children with milder movement disorders. Includes qualitative and quantitative information.
Movement Assessment of Infants (MAI) Chandler, L., Andrews, M., & Sanson, M.	Birth–12 months	Criterion-referenced assessment of muscle tone, reflexes, automatic reactions, and volitional movement. ICF-CY body structures and functions	A risk score is calculated for identification of infants at risk for motor dysfunction. High-risk profiles are provided for only 4- and 8-month-old infants.
Mullen Scales of Early Learning Mullen, E.	Birth–68 months	Standardized assessment of gross and fine motor, expressive and receptive language and visual reception. ICF-CY activity	Identifies strengths/weaknesses and assesses readiness for school.

Continued

■ **Appendix 3.A** Common Tests and Measures of Development, Function, Sensory Integration, Pain,
■ Quality of Life, and Participation—cont'd

Test/Measure and Author/ Reference or Publisher	Age Range	Areas Tested and ICF-CY Classification	Primary Use
Neonatal Behavioral Assessment Scale, 3rd edition (NBAS-3) Brazelton, T.B., & Nugent, J.K.	Full-term neonates 37–48 weeks post conceptional age	Criterion-referenced test of habituation, motor-oral responses, truncal and vestibular function, and social-interactive behaviors. ICF-CY body structures and functions, participation	Provides information on the infant's interactive patterns that can be used to assist parents and caregivers. Training program recommended to become reliable in test administration.
Neonatal Individualized Developmental Care and Assessment Program (NIDCAP) Als, H.	Neonates–4 weeks postterm	Criterion-referenced assessment of physiological and behavioral responses in the areas of autonomic, motor, and attention. ICF-CY body structures and functions, activity	Used to determine the infant's physiological and behavioral responses to the environment to assist parents and caregivers. Training program recommended to become reliable in test administration.
Neonatal Infant Pain Scale (NIPS) Lawrence, J., Alcock, D., McGrath, P., Kay, J., MacMurray, B., & Dulberg, C. (1993). The development of a tool to assess neonatal pain. *Neonatal Network, 12,* 59–66.	Pre- and full-term neonates	Behavioral assessment tool measuring five parameters: facial expression, cry, breathing patterns, arms, legs and state of arousal. ICF-CY body structures and functions	Observational pain assessment
Neurobehavioral Assessment of the Preterm Infant (NAPI) Korner, A., & Thom, V.	Medically stable preterm infants from 32 weeks post-conceptional age to term	Assesses infant behavior in 7 clusters: motor development and vigor; scarf sign; popliteal angle; alertness and orientation; irritability; quality of crying; and percent sleep ratings. ICF-CY body structures and functions, activity	Used to monitor developmental progress, identify persistent lags in development and assess effectiveness of interventions.
Neurological Assessment of the Preterm and Full-Term Newborn Infant, 2nd edition (NAPFI-2) Dubowitz, L., Dubowitz, V., & Mercuri, E.	Full-term infants and stable preterm infants up to 3rd day of life	Criterion-referenced test of neurological maturation. Tests habituation, movement and tone, reflexes, and neurobehavioral responses. ICF-CY body structures and functions	Classic assessment to determine maturation and deviations in neurological development of infants. Commonly used though limited psychometric data available.
Neurological Exam of the Full-Term Infant (NEFTI), 2nd edition Prechtl, H.	Full-term and preterm infants 38–42 weeks gestation	Norm-referenced, standardized examination of posture, eyes, power and passive movement, spontaneous and voluntary movements, and state. ICF-CY body structures and functions	Classic test to determine neurological dysfunction in young infants.

Appendix 3.A Common Tests and Measures of Development, Function, Sensory Integration, Pain, Quality of Life, and Participation—cont'd

Test/Measure and Author/ Reference or Publisher	Age Range	Areas Tested and ICF-CY Classification	Primary Use
Oucher Scales Beyer, J.E., Villarruel A.M., & Denyes, M.J.	3–12 years	Pain intensity rating scale using actual pictures and a numeric scale. ICF-CY body structures and functions	Measures self-reporting of pain intensity.
Peabody Development Motor Scales, 2nd edition (PDMS-2) Folio, M.R., & Fewell, R.R.	1–72 months	Norm-referenced, standardized assessment of gross motor and fine motor skills divided into 6 subtests: reflexes, stationary, locomotion, object manipulation, grasping, and visual-motor integration. ICF-CY activity	Motor quotients are determined to estimate overall motor abilities. Commonly used in early intervention programs to determine eligibility for services. Has accompanying Motor Activities Program to assist in teaching skills.
Pediatric Balance Scale Franjoine, M.R., Gunther, J.S., & Taylor, M.J. (2003). Pediatric Balance Scale: A modified version of the Berg Balance Scale for the school-age child with mild to moderate motor impairment. *Pediatric Physical Therapy, 15*(2), 114–28.	5–15 years with mild to moderate motor impairments	Assesses balance in functional activities including sit to stand, transfers, sitting and standing unsupported, standing with eyes closed, standing on one foot, turning, retrieving object from floor, placing foot on stool and reaching forward. ICF-CY body structures and functions, activity	Used for screening or evaluation of functional balance skills.
Pediatric Clinical Test of Sensory Interaction for Balance (P-CTSIB) Westcott, S.L., Crowe, T.K., Deitz, J.C., & Richardson, P. (1994). Test-retest reliability of the Pediatric Clinical Test of Sensory Interaction for Balance (P-CTSIB). *Physical & Occupational Therapy in Pediatrics, 14*(1), 1–22.	4–9 years	Measures the influence of sensory information on balance by testing balance under six different sensory conditions. ICF-CY body structures and functions	Requires use of specialized equipment.

Continued

Appendix 3.A Common Tests and Measures of Development, Function, Sensory Integration, Pain, Quality of Life, and Participation—cont'd

Test/Measure and Author/ Reference or Publisher	Age Range	Areas Tested and ICF-CY Classification	Primary Use
Pediatric Evaluation of Disability Inventory (PEDI) Haley, S.M., Coster, W.J., Ludlow, L.H., Haltiwanger, J.T.,& Andrellas, P.J.	6 months–7.5 years and those whose functional abilities are lower than those of a 7-year-old	Norm-referenced, standardized assessment based on parent interview to determine self-care (eating, grooming, dressing, bathing, and toileting); mobility including transfers; social function (communication, social interaction, household and community tasks); and need for modifications and assistance. ICF-CY activity, participation	Identifies the functional and activity capabilities of infants and children with disabilities. Used to monitor change in activities and functional skills and evaluate program outcomes.
Pediatric Quality of Life Inventory (PedsQL) Varni, J.W.	2–18 years	Measures physical, emotional, social, school functioning and global health. ICF-CY activity, participation	Forms available for healthy school and community populations as well as disease-specific questionnaires.
Pediatric Reach Test Bartlett, D., & Birmingham, T. (2003). Validity and Reliability of a Pediatric Reach Test. *Pediatric Physical Therapy, 15*(2), 84–92.	2.5–14 years	Modification of Functional Reach Test. Measures balance and postural control in sitting and standing through forward and side reaching. ICF-CY body structures and functions, activity	Inclusion of sitting position allows for use with more involved children.
Physical and Neurological Exam for Subtle Signs (PANESS) Denckla, M.B., (1985). Revised Neurological Examination for Subtle Signs. *Psychopharmacology Bulletin, 21*(4), 773–800.	School-aged children	Measures components of motor function including lateral preference of hand, foot and eye; stressed gaits such as heel and toe walking; balance; motor persistence; coordination and patterned and repetitive timed movements. ICF-CY activity	Four summary variables' scores quantify subtle neurologic signs and can be used to demonstrate change over time. Minimal equipment and administration time required.
POSNA Pediatric Musculoskeletal Functional Health Questionnaire Daltroy, L.H., Liang, M.H., Fossel, A.H., & Goldberg, M.J. (1998). Pediatric Outcomes Instrument Development Group. Pediatric Orthopaedic Society of North America. *Journal of Pediatric Orthopedics, 18*, 561–571.	2–18 years with musculoskeletal disorders	Scales completed by child and parent to measure upper extremity function, transfers and mobility, physical function and sports, comfort (pain free), happiness and satisfaction, and expectations for treatment. ICF-CY activity, participation	Used to assess functional health outcomes, generally postorthopedic surgery. Can also examine child-parent agreement.

Appendix 3.A Common Tests and Measures of Development, Function, Sensory Integration, Pain, Quality of Life, and Participation—cont'd

Test/Measure and Author/ Reference or Publisher	Age Range	Areas Tested and ICF-CY Classification	Primary Use
Posture and Fine Motor Assessment of Infants Case-Smith, J., & Bigsby, R.	2–12 months	Fine motor scales addressing infant's reaching and grasping patterns, finger and thumb movements, release, and manipulation. ICF-CY activity	Assists in intervention planning and documenting progress over brief periods of time.
Quality of Well-Being Scale (QWB) Kaplan, R.M., Bush, J.W., & Berry, C.C. (1976). Health status: Types of validity and the index of well-being. *Health Services Research, 11,* 478–507.	14+ years Some studies have used scale in children as young as 4–7years	Four scales focus on the physical impact of an illness related to symptoms, functions, and social and mobility levels. ICF-CY activity, participation	Summarizes health-related quality of life across symptoms, problems, and functional states.
Riley Infant Pain Scale Schare, J., Joyce, B., Gerkensmeyer, J., & Keck, J. (1996). Comparison of three preverbal scales for postoperative pain assessment in a diverse pediatric sample. *Journal of Pain and Symptom Management, 12*(6), 348–359.	Infants and preverbal or nonverbal children	Behavioral observation as an indication of pain. ICF-CY body structures and functions	Indication of pain in infants and preverbal or nonverbal children.
Scales of Independent Behavior—Revised (SIB-R) Bruininks, R., Woodcock, R., Weatherman, R., & Hill, B.	3 months–adult	Norm-referenced, standardized test using interviews to determine motor skills, social interaction and communication skills, personal living skills, and problem behaviors. ICF-CY activity, participation	Measure functional independence and adaptive functioning across settings. Is used with the Adaptive Living Skills Assessment Intervention System.
School Function Assessment (SFA) Coster, W., Deeney, T., Haltiwanger, J., & Haley, S.	Children with disabilities in grades K–6	Criterion-referenced, standardized, judgment-based interview to determine the child's participation in all aspects of the school environment; task supports needed to function in school; activity performance of school-related activities; physical tasks such as changing position, manipulation, using materials, eating, and written work; and cognitive and behavioral tasks. ICF-CY activity, participation	Comprehensive assessment of activity and functional capabilities of children with disabilities in school setting. While not tied to a curriculum, information obtained assists in determining eligibility for service and in development of educationally relevant objectives.

Continued

■ Appendix 3.A Common Tests and Measures of Development, Function, Sensory Integration, Pain,
■ Quality of Life, and Participation—cont'd

Test/Measure and Author/ Reference or Publisher	Age Range	Areas Tested and ICF-CY Classification	Primary Use
Sensory Integration and Praxis Tests (SIPT) Ayres, A.J.	4 years–8 years 11 months	Measure sensory integration of form and space perception, somatic and vestibular processing, praxis, and bilateral integration and sequencing. ICF-CY body structures and functions	Determine presence and type of sensory integrative disorder. Require advanced training to properly administer and interpret.
Sensory Profile and Infant/ Toddler Sensory Profile Dunn, W.	3–10 years and birth–36 months (Infant/Toddler)	Questionnaire used to determine basic sensory processing in daily life; sensory processing modulation and behavioral and emotional responses. ICF-CY body structures and functions, participation	Links strengths and barriers in sensory processing with daily life.
Test of Gross Motor Development, 2nd edition (TGMD2) Ulrich, D.	3–10 years	Norm-referenced test of 12 gross motor skills involving locomotion and object control. ICF-CY activity	Used to identify children who are significantly behind their peers in gross motor skill development.
Test of Infant Motor Performance (TIMP) Campbell, S., Kolobe, G., Girolami, G., Osten, E., & Lenke, M.	Prematurely born infants 34 weeks post conceptual age– 4 months post term	Functional movements of head and trunk control in prone, supine and upright positions. 28 items scored dichotomously and 31 scaled items. ICF-CY activity	Discriminates infants with risk of poor motor outcome; sensitive to effects of intervention.
Test of Sensory Function in Infants (TSFI) DeGangi, G., & Greenspan, S.	4–18 months	Criterion-referenced test of reactivity to tactile pressure, adaptive motor function, visual-tactile integration, ocular motor control, and reactivity to vestibular stimulation. ICF-CY body structures and functions	Identifies sensory processing and reactivity dysfunction in infants.
Test of Visual-Motor Skills-3 (TVMS-3) Martin, N.	3–90+ years	Norm-referenced tests of visual perception, motor planning and execution. ICF-CY body structures and functions	Simple test of visual-motor skills.
Toddler and Infant Motor Evaluation (TIME) Miller, L.J., & Roid, G.	Birth–3½ years with suspected motor delay or dysfunction	Comprehensive qualitative assessment of mobility, motor organization, stability-functional performance, and social-emotional abilities. Items indicating motor organization are observed during parent-child interaction. ICF-CY activity, participation	Track development over time to determine extent of motor delay or dysfunction and to link function with quality of movement.

■ Appendix 3.A Common Tests and Measures of Development, Function, Sensory Integration, Pain,
■ Quality of Life, and Participation—cont'd

Test/Measure and Author/ Reference or Publisher	Age Range	Areas Tested and ICF-CY Classification	Primary Use
Timed Up and Down Stairs (TUDS) Zaino, C.A., Marchese, V.G., & Westcott, S.L. (2004). Timed up and down stairs test: Preliminary reliability and validity of a new measure of functional mobility. *Pediatric Physical Therapy, 16*(2), 90–98.	8–14 years	Measure of functional mobility and postural control. ICF-CY body structures and functions, activity	Children may ascend or descend stairs using any method as long as they face forward (e.g.,reciprocal, non-reciprocal, running, skipping steps, etc.).
Timed Up and Go (TUG) Williams, E.N., Carroll, S.G., Reddihough, D.S., Phillips, B.A., & Galea, M.P. (2005). Investigation of the timed "up & go" test in children. *Developmental Medicine and Child Neurology, 47*(8), 518–524.	3 years–adult, excluding those with cognitive impairment or unable to follow directions	Measure of functional ambulatory mobility and dynamic balance. ICF-CY body structures and functions, activity	Modifications for children include use of concrete task (e.g., touch target on wall), seat with back but no arm rests, sitting position with 90° knee flexion, and timing from moment child's bottom leaves seat until returns to seat.
Transdisciplinary Play-Based Assessment, 2nd edition (TPBA2) Linder, T.W.	Birth–6 years	Criterion-referenced assessment based in observations of the child at play. Areas observed include cognitive, social-emotional, communication and language, and sensorimotor development. ICF-CY activity, participation	Used to identify intervention needs and evaluate progress of children with disabilities. Scores do not compare the child to others. An intervention volume is also available.
Vineland Adaptive Behavior Scales, 2nd edition (Vineland-II) Sparrow, S.S., Cicchetti, D.V., & Balla, D.A.	Birth–90 years	Semi-structured interview of parent/caregiver to measure adaptive behavior in 5 domains: communication, daily living skills, socialization, motor skills, and maladaptive behavior index. ICF-CY activity, participation	Assists in identifying intellectual and developmental disabilities, autism spectrum disorders, and developmental delays. Parent/ Caregiver Rating Form, Expanded Interview Form and Teacher Rating Form available. Software to assist with scoring and reporting.
Visual Analog Scale Shields, B., Cohen, D., Harbeck-Weber, C., Powers, J., & Smith, G. (2003). Pediatric pain measurement using a visual analogue scale. *Clinical Pediatrics*, April.	5 years and above, over 11 years	Pain intensity rating scale using numerical scale on a vertical or horizontal continuum. ICF-CY body structures and functions	Measures self-report of pain intensity.

Continued

Appendix 3.A Common Tests and Measures of Development, Function, Sensory Integration, Pain, Quality of Life, and Participation—cont'd

Test/Measure and Author/ Reference or Publisher	Age Range	Areas Tested and ICF-CY Classification	Primary Use
Vulpe Assessment Battery— Revised (VAB-R) Vulpe, S.G.	Birth–6 years for children with disabilities	One of the first criterion-referenced tests with enough items/task analysis to be useful in assessing children with significant delay or dysfunction. Includes assessment of basic senses and function, development behavior, environment and performance analysis system. ICF-CY body structures and functions, activity, participation	Identifies areas of skill performance, strengths, and needs for children with moderate to severe disability. Includes environment's influence on task performance. Psychometric data are incomplete.
WEEFIM: Functional Independence Measure for Children Granger, C., Braun, S., Griswood, K., Heyer, N., McCabe, M., Msau, M., & Hamilton, B.	6 months–8 years, but can be used up to 12 years with children with disabilities	Comprehensive, criterion-referenced assessment based on observation of motor function of 18 items in 6 subscales including self-care, sphincter control, transfers, locomotion, and cognitive function including communication and social cognition. This is the child version of the Functional Independence Measure (FIM). ICF-CY activity, participation	Determines degree of a child's disability, ability to accomplish tasks, and caregiver assistance required. Must use their data collection and outcome reporting system.
Wong-Baker Faces Scale Wong, D., & Baker, C.	3 years and older	Child indicates one of six faces from very happy, no pain, to hurt as much as you can imagine. ICF-CY body structures and functions	Measures self-report of pain intensity.
Youth Quality of Life Instrument-Research Version (YQOL-R) Seattle Quality of Life Group	11–18 years with and without disabilities	Self-report measure in four domains: sense of self, social relationships, environment, and general quality of life. ICF-CY participation	To assess quality of life with an emphasis on aspects of positive health.

*If a test or measure is published in a journal, the full reference is provided. Some tests and measures can be obtained from their publisher, while others are carried by multiple vendors. An online search for a specific instrument will provide the most current information regarding availability.

CHAPTER 4

Family-Centered Care

—Lisa Ann Chiarello, PT, PhD, PCS

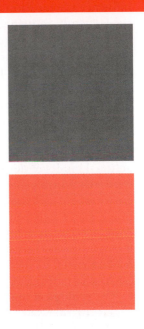

Overview and Theoretical Foundation of Family-Centered Care

Family-centered care is a service delivery philosophy and approach that respects the rights, roles, and abilities of family members. Services are provided through a collaboration with the family and child to support their outcomes and promote their well-being and quality of life.

Physical therapists have identified the need for professional and post-professional training to foster competency in collaborating with families (Cochrane & Farley, 1990; Iversen, Shimmel, Ciacera, & Prabhakar, 2003; Sparling & Sekerak, 1992). While professionals value family-centered care, there can be challenges when implementing this philosophy (Bruce et al., 2002).

The purpose of this chapter is to provide an introduction to issues related to family-centered care to support physical therapists in their interactions and interventions with the children and families they serve.

Family-centered care is not restricted to the pediatric specialty area; it is a life-span approach. The World Health Organization's model on functioning, disability, and health supports a family-centered approach (2001). Cherry (1991) identified that in pediatric physical therapy, "there is a greater need for a holistic approach that encompasses the total child, the family, and the natural settings where children live, learn, and play" (p. 70). This need especially continues during the transition into adulthood (Gall, Kingsnorth, & Healy, 2006; Rubin & Quinn-Curran, 1983).

In addition, family-centered care is not restricted to one practice setting. Family-centered care is a standard of practice for both hospital and community-based services. Family-centered care provides an opportunity for a preventive and supportive approach to wellness across the life span and along the entire continuum of care.

The foundation for family-centered practice is based on the synthesis of many theoretical frameworks. The fundamental premise of family-centered care is that a person does not exist in isolation but functions within a family as well as within larger and more complex social systems. Social systems, including the family unit, influence the function of that person, and that person subsequently influences the function of the systems to which he or she belongs. This proposition is central to systems theory. The **family systems theory** views individual and family functioning as an interactional dynamic process (Becvar & Becvar, 1988). Interventions for the family can indirectly influence the child's development and function.

In pediatric physical therapy, the needs of children can best be met by involving their families. The **transactional model of development** emphasizes the reciprocal relationship between the child and caregiving environment and stresses the importance of an appropriate match between the child and the environment. A supportive environment may minimize the effects of biological risks (Sameroff & Chandler, 1975; Sameroff & MacKenzie, 2003). The child's characteristics and the environment together influence functional outcomes.

The **ecological model of human development** discusses the role that larger social systems have on the function of the family unit (Bronfenbrenner, 1977). Support from social networks and the political and economical culture can influence how a family interacts with and cares for their child. Research in early intervention has emphasized that family patterns (parent-child relationship, family arranged experiences, and health and safety) have the greatest impact on child outcomes (Guralnick, 1998). Family-centered care in pediatrics is based on the philosophy that the family plays the central role in the life of a child.

To develop an understanding of family-centered care, it is essential to understand what is meant by a family. Therapists must broaden their conceptualization of the traditional family configuration, for the contemporary family in America is diverse (Sparling, 1991). Family is defined more by emotional or functional elements than by structural or legal elements. A family is a group of people who love and care for each other. The family is the base for caring and nurturing and is the place where values are taught and learned.

With family-centered care being practiced by multiple disciplines, in various settings, and for diverse populations, several definitions, perspectives, and models have been presented. Edleman defined *family-centered care* "as a collaborative relationship between families and professionals in the continual pursuit of being responsive to the priorities and choices of families" (cited in Leviton, Mueller, & Kauffman, 1992, p. 1). This definition, along with those from major organizations that advocate for family-centered care (CanChild Centre for Childhood Disability Research, cited in Law, Rosenbaum, King, et al., 2003; Institute for Family-Centered Care, 2009; Maternal and Child Health Bureau, 2005; Orelena Hawks Puckett Institute, cited in Dunst, Trivette, & Hamby, 2008), emphasizes **family-professional collaboration** as the key component. In addition, the various models acknowledge core beliefs of respect for children and families and appreciation of the family's impact on the child's well-being.

The primary goals of family-centered care are interrelated. The first goal is the one with which therapists are most familiar—enhance the health, development, and functional independence of the child through a partnership with the family and child. Dunst, Trivette, and Snyder define parent-professional partnership as follows:

Parents and other family members working together with professionals in pursuit of a common goal where the relationship between the family and the professional is based on shared decision-making and responsibility and mutual trust and respect. (2000, p. 32)

This partnership entails a commitment of shared responsibility toward the accomplishment of an outcome. Care is directed toward goals that are important and relevant to the family and child in order to support the child in being a child and to prepare him or her for adulthood.

The second goal is to promote quality of life for the family. This goal is accomplished by supporting the family (Brewer, McPherson, Magrab, & Hutchins, 1989). This includes protecting the integrity of the family and respecting the subunits of the family, and the developmental goals of each of its members. These subunits include the adult-adult relationship, caregiver-child relationship, sibling-sibling relationship, and extended family relationship. Professionals support the family by promoting **family competence** and participation in their community (Dunst, Johanson, Trivette, & Hamby, 1991). This process recognizes the strengths of families and includes proactively providing information and helping families identify and mobilize both informal and formal resources and support.

History of Family-Centered Services

Historically, services for children with disabilities were limited, and families were solely responsible for their children's care, education, and treatment. In the early part of the 20th century, families were encouraged to institutionalize children with disabilities. From the middle of the 20th century, through humanitarian efforts, charitable organizations began providing services to children (Newman, 1983), but most families had a passive role. In the late 1950s and early 1960s, professionals and parents alike began to advocate for a more family-oriented approach for children in hospital care. The Platt Report in 1959 revealed the negative effects on children when separated from their mothers, and the National Association for the Welfare of Children in Hospitals advocated for the role of parents in their children's hospital care (as cited in Palmer, 1993). Around this same time, Head Start programs were instituted to address the needs of select groups and families by organizing major advocacy groups and fighting for educational rights and services for children.

Traditionally, the medical model was a child-centered approach, and parents did not assume an active role. Professionals were viewed as the experts and were responsible for developing and implementing medical treatment or an intervention plan. In hospital settings, parent visitations were limited and parents were not involved in their children's medical care (Palmer, 1993). In education settings, intervention techniques were aimed at enhancing the development of the child, and outcomes were based on achievement of developmental skills (Bricker & Veltman, 1990).

Caregiver-focused intervention programs became popular in the 1970s, and interventions were aimed at training caregivers to promote their child's development. This decade was marked by increased family involvement as well as advocacy. In many cases, families were leading advocates for the rights of and services for children with disabilities. The passage of landmark federal legislation in the United States, the Education of All Handicapped Children Act of 1975 (PL 94-142, 1975), included a mandate for family involvement in children's education. According to the legislation, families were to be involved in the decision-making process, to help plan and coordinate their child's education, to be advocates for their child's rights, and to assume a teaching role at home.

Caregiver training and home programs became an integral component of intervention programs (Bazak, 1989). Families wanted to have opportunities for decision making, be kept informed of their child's test results and progress, and actively participate in their child's intervention (Redman-Bentley, 1982). Parents began to publish articles and books and to participate in support groups in which they shared their personal experiences and provided guidance for other families.

While this legislation acknowledged the competence and importance of families, implementation practices had some negative consequences. The federal mandate set forth the practices that public agencies must perform to involve families; however, the degree and type of family participation vary. The degree of involvement may be overwhelming to some families, and there has been controversy regarding how much responsibility should be put on the caregivers (Turnbull & Turnbull, 1982).

Caregivers assuming the primary roles of teacher and therapist may negatively influence the **caregiver-child relationship**. Another concern was that the practice of family involvement was a formality on paper only and that the actual degree of family/professional partnership was limited.

As models of service delivery evolved into a family-centered approach, a model developed in early intervention that was identified as relationship focused. The goal of the relationship-focused model was to guide caregivers in understanding and responding to their child's behaviors, interests, and needs. The relationship-focused model in early intervention strove to enhance positive caregiver-child interactions and emphasized that these interactions provide the foundation for a satisfying relationship, as well as the development of the child and caregiver (Affleck, McGrade, McQueeney, & Allen, 1982; Bromwich, 1981). Family-centered intervention emerged with a shift of emphasis from only the child or caregiver to the larger context of the family and social environment.

In early intervention, the Education of the Handicapped Act Amendment (PL 99-457, 1986) and its reauthorizations clearly mandate services to meet the needs of the family related to enhancing their child's development. Assessment of the family's concerns, priorities, and resources; family training and counseling; intervention in the child's natural environment; and social work were some of the services identified in the law that particularly relate to this concept of family-centered care. Physical therapists need to be familiar with federal and state laws and their rules and regulations to provide service that reflects legal, ethical, and best-practice standards (see Chapters 1, 11, and 12).

A family-centered philosophy can still be integrated with more traditional client-centered approaches (Deardorff, 1992). "Family-centered practices are how child-centered interventions are implemented" (Dunst et al., 2008, p. 38). Recent trends in child-centered intervention emphasize approaches that are more aligned with a family-centered philosophy. These approaches include child-initiated activities, use of daily routines, and natural contexts (Bricker & Veltman, 1990; Hanft & Pilkington, 2000).

Families acknowledge that they want some portion of the intervention to be child centered. Child-centered intervention does not have to be viewed as though it is at the opposite end of the spectrum from a family-centered approach. Health-care professionals can provide direct intervention to the child and support the family. Family education is a vital component of family-centered care when it is practiced in a respectful manner and there is a reciprocal exchange of information.

Child-centered, caregiver-centered, and family-centered models each have their own values and limitations. In practice, therapists use a variety of models throughout a child's intervention because it is very difficult to provide service to only the child without involving the caregivers or to only the caregivers without involving the child. Family-centered intervention is the most comprehensive model of service delivery. When family-centered care is individualized, it may include aspects of both child- and caregiver-centered service delivery models to meet the needs of the family and promote the child's development and function (Fig. 4.1).

In pediatric physical therapy, families have long been recognized as an important factor in the child's response to intervention. Decades ago clinicians and researchers expressed their subjective insights that physical therapy appears to positively affect family well-being (Ferry, 1986; Wright & Nicholson, 1973). Family information is collected at the initial examination and is used to guide intervention planning, family education, home exercise and activity programs, and discharge and transition planning. Physical therapists are concerned about the structure of the home environment, the family's understanding of the disability, and the family's daily routines. The question therapists must answer is, how is it most appropriate to foster caregiver involvement and provide family-centered care? The most respectful approach involves flexibility and individualization based on the family's concerns, priorities, and resources and on the strengths and needs of the child.

Factors in a Family Unit That Influence Family-Centered Intervention

The concept of family is broad, and family structure, family function, and a family's life cycle are very individual. Awareness of this variability is important when developing a family-centered intervention plan. Based on the 2001 National Survey of 38,366 Children with

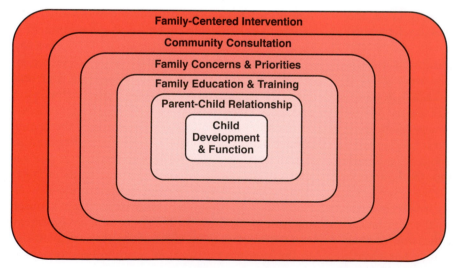

Figure 4.1 Family-centered intervention.

Special Health-Care Needs, Denboba and colleagues (2006) found that various subgroups of families were more at risk for experiencing a lack of partnership with their children's doctors and health-care providers. These subgroups included families with limited financial resources, no health insurance, minority racial/ethnic status, children with functional limitations, and older children. This was of particular significance given that a family's sense of partnership with their health-care providers was related to access to care, their child's well-being, and having their needs met.

Family structure and function may be identified by the family as a strength or a need in terms of influencing the intervention process. If these factors are identified as strengths, family structure and function could be capitalized on to promote opportunities to enhance the child's development and function. If these factors are identified as concerns, professionals and the family can work collaboratively to access avenues of resources and support.

Family Structure

The structure of the family can include family members, caregivers, and extended family and friends. Some families include a large number of people resources, and in others the number may be very small. Demographic statistics reveal the decrease in family size across all ethnic groups in the United States, an increase in the number of children living with only their mothers, and an increase in the number of children with working mothers (Bureau of Labor Statistics, 2008; Simmons & O'Neil, 2001; U.S. House of Representatives, 1989). It is important for professionals to understand and support the role of extended family members in childrearing (Ochieng, 2003).

In addition to the human resources in a family, the structure of the home, the material resources, and the neighboring environment are also changing. Inner-city environments, housing conditions, and poverty are dimensions of family life that influence family function. Material resources may or may not be adequate to provide the necessities for daily function and development. Socioeconomic status and the organization of the home, including the provision of appropriate play materials, have been shown to positively correlate with child development (Poresky & Henderson, 1982; Ramey, Mills, Campbell, & O'Brien, 1975). Shannon (2004) recommends addressing family basic needs as the first strategy to overcoming barriers to family-centered care. Professionals need to be aware of the influence that family members, home environment, and material

resources may have on the intervention process to recommend appropriate intervention strategies that promote family-identified outcomes.

Family Function

In addition to the actual constitution of a family and home, how a family functions needs to be considered when developing a family-centered intervention plan. In discussing the transition from child-centered to family-centered care, Stuberg and Harbourne (1994) stated that therapists need to understand how **family dynamics** influence functional outcomes. Therapists first need an understanding about the roles and responsibilities of family members as defined by each individual family. In addition, an awareness of individual family members' attitudes toward themselves and others in the family will help the therapist guide the intervention process. For example, a parent with low self-esteem regarding his or her parenting skills may benefit from a therapist acknowledging his or her appropriate carrying and holding of the child.

Therapists need to be aware of the roles of the mother, father, siblings, and other caregivers in child care. Numerous studies have documented the positive influence that maternal involvement has on child development (Ainsworth & Bell, 1974; Clarke-Stewart, 1973; Mahoney, Finger, & Powell, 1985; Yarrow, Rubenstein, Pedersen, & Jankowski, 1972). However, it is important to remember that both mothers and fathers influence their child's development (Lamb, 1983). The role that the father plays in the family is diverse and changing, and paternal involvement is increasing in child care tasks (Fig. 4.2).

In addition, professionals need to acknowledge the importance of the sibling bond. Seligman and Darling (1989) emphasized that siblings have a need for accurate and appropriate information, a balance between caregiving responsibility and age-appropriate tasks, and individual parental attention. Professionals need to consider that the appropriate amount of involvement of a sibling will vary from family to family and that the intervention plan may need to include steps to foster sibling adjustment. With family consent, it may be appropriate to include the mother, father, siblings, or other "family members" in the intervention plan (Fig. 4.3).

Family Life Cycle

Family function and personal development of all family members are interdependent with the family's life cycle (Minuchin, 1985). The life-span process is no longer viewed just as the traditional stages that people pass

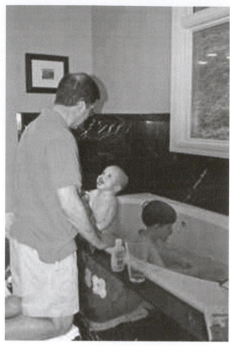

Figure 4.2 Dad giving child a bath: It is important for therapists to partner with fathers to provide support for their caregiving tasks.

through as they marry, establish a career, have children, send their children off into the world, and retire. The pattern of the family life cycle is variable and depends on many life events and life circumstances. Factors such as culture, economics, political contexts, health, lower birth rate, longer life expectancy, the changing role of women, and increasing divorce and remarriage rates shape an individual family's life cycle pattern (Carter & McGoldrick, 1989).

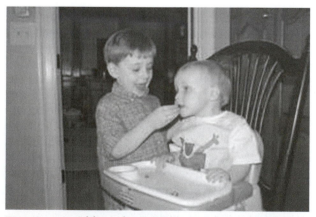

Figure 4.3 Siblings have important roles in being playmates as well as participating in daily care activities.

The family life cycle involves several generations, and the process influences each individual member. Where a family is in the life-span process, as well as the developmental tasks of the individual family members, will influence how they make meaning of their life circumstances and how they respond to the disability and intervention. Knowing and respecting the developmental tasks of the family as a whole, as well as the individual members, and how these two interrelate will allow the therapist to make the intervention process more meaningful to the family.

Family Culture

A family's **culture** provides a foundation for their expectations and actions. Low (1984, p. 14) defined *culture* as "the integrated system of learned patterns of behavior." A person's cultural identify is influenced by many variables, including ethnicity, race, age, gender, family, vocation, religion, and disability. An earnest assessment of a family's culture will provide valuable information that may be a resource for intervention. Culture affects intervention through three processes: (a) communication of information between the family and the provider, (b) lifestyle of the family and the provider, and (c) societal environment in terms of regulations for health care (Hill, Fortenberry, & Stein, 1989). The family's ethnic heritage, lifestyle, child-rearing practices, values, and beliefs make the process and content of intervention very individualized.

The family ecology of ethnic minority groups and the traditional American lifestyle have been generalized, compared, and contrasted (McGoldrick, 1989; Sparling, 1991). While it is helpful to be aware that differences may be present in terms of relationships, extended family, role flexibility, and rules of family life, families deserve respect to allow them to teach therapists about their individual family perspective before any assumptions can be made.

Gerhard (1995) recommended that therapists demonstrate respect for individual family culture by careful observation and by following the lead of the family. An awareness of the family's communication and problem-solving style will help a therapist to optimize sharing of information and learning. A therapist may choose to use an interpreter to help bridge language barriers but may also want to become skillful in appropriate nonverbal communication methods to develop a relationship with the family.

It is particularly important for therapists to explore and acknowledge the family's values regarding childhood, independence, work ethics, health care, decision making, and disability and to be aware of how these values may have an impact on intervention outcomes. Child-rearing practices and parental expectations are of particular importance to physical therapists because these factors have been related to motor development (Cintas, 1995). The family practices of ethnic groups, including African Americans, Hispanic Americans, Asian Americans/Pacific Islanders, and Native Americans/Alaskan natives have more heavily emphasized the role of the extended family as a resource and support compared to traditional European American practices. In addition, the child-rearing philosophies of these groups promote interdependency and cooperation as opposed to independence and competitiveness (Harrison, Wilson, Pine, Chan, & Buriel, 1990). The family's values may guide a therapist's recommendations for resources, such as extended family members, as well as for intervention strategies, such as independent play activities versus interactive play activities.

Hanson (1992) recommended that interventionists need to consider (1) how a family views their child's disability, (2) how receptive a family is to intervention, and (3) the family's preferences for location, method, type, agent, and style of service delivery. In reference to the current model of family-centered care, therapists need to be sensitive to the family's beliefs about family participation. As emphasized by Lynch (1992), a family-professional partnership is not common in many cultures, and families may not be ready to fully participate in a collaborative process. Therapists need to respect the position of the family and at the same time provide informal opportunities for the family to share their opinions and priorities. Mini-Case Study 4.1 provides a clinical scenario regarding the influence that culture has on the intervention process.

Mini-Case Study 4.1
Family Culture and Physical Therapy Intervention

A physical therapist went to conduct an initial home visit for a 1-year-old girl with Down syndrome and her family, who were of Asian descent. The visit was scheduled at mid-day, with the older sibling, a pre-schooler, and the mother present. When the therapist entered the home, she noticed that shoes were lined up in the foyer by the door. The therapist quietly slipped off her shoes when she entered the foyer. After introductions were made, the mother offered the therapist some lunch. The therapist politely declined the offer; however, the mother persisted. The mother, although very quiet, was able to explain to the therapist that it was important to her to be able to share some food with the therapist as a way of

showing her appreciation. The therapist decided that it was more important to build a trusting relationship with the family than to abide by policy, which required that therapists not accept gifts of any nature from clients. The therapist sat down at the table that was prepared and shared a brief meal with the mother.

During the initial meeting, the therapist encouraged family input as well as participation from the mother. However, the mother always placed herself several feet behind the therapist and commented that the therapist should do what she felt was right. The therapist did not push the matter any further and spent the rest of the session playing with the child. The therapist made sure to make an occasional connection with the mother by commenting on the child's abilities. During subsequent visits, the therapist was able to make comments on mother-child interactions, as the therapist observed the mother carry and comfort the child. The therapist was able to convey to the mother that she respected the mother's abilities and would be happy if the mother felt comfortable participating in part of the sessions. The mother's participation started out very slowly, but collaboration was developing. After several weeks, the mother asked if it would be okay if the father came home for lunch so that he could be part of the therapy session. The therapist and family achieved a trusting partnership that was founded on mutual respect.

Therapists must make a commitment to achieve **cultural competence**. Thorpe and Baker (1995) defined *cultural competence* as "the ability to think and behave in ways that enable a member of one culture to work effectively with members of another culture" (p. 143). An awareness of one's own beliefs will help therapists be open to and respectful of cultural variations. Therapists then need to make a concerted effort to gain knowledge of the culture of the families that they serve. Lynch (1992) recommended avenues through which to gain this information: reading, talking, and working with individuals from other cultures, sharing the daily routines of another culture, and learning other languages. This knowledge then needs to be put into action as the therapist learns the skills to most effectively interact with each family as well as using cultural resources as part of the intervention process.

Family Stress, Resources, and Adaptation

Family stress and **coping skills** influence a family's ability to function and develop. While it is necessary to acknowledge a family's daily stress, it is important to be aware that family stress is not necessarily related to raising a child with a disability (Chiarello, 1993; Hanson & Hanline, 1990). The presence of a child with a disability does not necessarily mean that the family will have problems (Petersen & Wikoff, 1987). The family's role in society has changed, and contemporary family life has many challenges that can be a source of stress (Petersen & Wikoff, 1987; Sparling, 1991). The range of these challenges includes dual-career families, teenage pregnancy, single-parent families, violence and substance abuse in the family, absence of extended family, geographic mobility, and financial constraints. Time constraints may limit family members' rest, fitness activities, social interactions, and leisure activities. All of these factors may influence the family's overall satisfaction and happiness.

Even though physical therapists are not the primary professionals dealing with the issues of daily stress and coping, physical therapists do come in contact with these issues because they interact with the family on a routine and frequent basis. Physical therapists can be helpful by providing the family with opportunities to articulate concerns, supporting the family's coping strategies, respecting the family's privacy, and being flexible. However, the field of psychology and family therapy is beyond the scope of the practice of physical therapy. Specialized study is needed in these fields to have the in-depth knowledge necessary to intervene at that level of professional practice, and physical therapists should refer families when appropriate.

The process of **family adaptation** when a child has a special health-care need is beyond the scope of this chapter. The therapist should be cognizant that the process is complex and influenced by many variables, including the nature of the disability, the time of onset, the family's personal belief system, and the family's support network and resources (Roberts, 1984; Yau & Li-Tsang, 1999). It is important to remember that family members will vary in how they perceive and react to stress. In addition, the number and quality of stressors as well as the extent of the **family's resources and support systems** will influence the family's response to any particular stress. As indicated by Sparling, Kolobe, and Ezzelle (1994), "support for family members appears to be an important mediating variable in adaptation, yet generic support is not easily described. The unique constellation of stressors experienced by contemporary families requires a combination of support ranging from financial and intellectual support to social support" (p. 830).

Social support has been defined as "mutually rewarding personal interactions from which an individual derives feelings of being needed, valued, and esteemed"

(Sparling et al., p. 832). Dunst, Trivette, and Cross (1986) found that social support had a positive influence on parent and family well-being, parent-infant play opportunities, and child development for families with young children in early intervention. The interrelationship between stress and support influences how a family adapts and how they are able to participate in an intervention program.

Three common stresses often associated with raising a child with a disability have been acknowledged. These are lack of information, dealing with the health-care system, and extended caregiving (Dura & Kiecolt-Glaser, 1991). Limited knowledge of their child's condition and standards of care creates an uncertainty for parents that can be stressful. Parents may not be aware of federal, state, and local resources. Dealing with the complexity of the health-care system, school environment, and special services requires energy, time, and skills.

The complexities of daily care management can also add to the primary stresses of contemporary life. Prolonged caregiving can dramatically alter the family's way of functioning and may have negative physiological and psychological effects (Dura & Kiecolt-Glaser, 1991). The family must balance the amount of time needed to care for a child with special needs with the amount of time for other family members and work responsibilities. Issues such as loss of privacy and loss of freedom to individuate must be handled. In addition, the parents must cope with their own fears regarding the child's health and future.

The degree to which the caregiving "burden" influences family function and development appears to be related more to a family's subjective perception, as opposed to direct objective issues of caregiving. An understanding of this relationship is helpful for a therapist to avoid a judgment or a direct comparison between families. For example, some families may decide on residential care for their children. Therapists need to be supportive and respectful of each family's personal decision and not view the decision as a failure of the family or the service-delivery system.

Transitional periods in the family life cycle have also been identified as stressful times. How a family adapts to a transition can be influenced by their personal family history; the nature, duration, and timing of the transition itself; and the family's perception of the transition (Elder, 1991). Special birthdays, events, and celebrations may evoke mixed feelings—happiness for the occasion but sadness for the loss of normalcy.

Therapists can acknowledge the normal aspects of the developmental transition and create the opportunity for the family to celebrate the event (Roberts, 1984). Therapists can assist with preparations for attending a dance (see Fig. 4.4) or the first day at a new school. Adapting to a new school, classroom, teacher, classmates, therapists, and administrators can be overwhelming. Parents have to deal with the uncertainty regarding the appropriateness of the educational placement, the philosophy of care, intervention services, and equipment needs. In the educational system, transition plans are now required to be proactive in helping families meet these challenges.

Service Factors

In addition to family factors, service system factors, including the therapist's personality, also influence

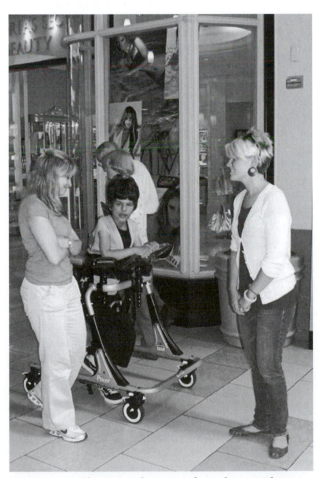

Figure 4.4 Therapist shopping for a dress with an adolescent: Supporting special occasions such as a prom respects the youth and her family and provides a meaningful opportunity to problem-solve and practice mobility strategies while shopping for a dress at the mall.

family-centered care. Funding, administrative policies, and administrative issues such as caseloads impact day-to-day service provision and can be a barrier to implementation of behaviors that are family-centered. Examples include policies on parents staying in the waiting room during outpatient therapy sessions and prohibition of physical and occupation therapy co-visits in early intervention. Advocacy by the therapist and the ability to effectively create change are important skills to promote family-centered care.

Therapists need to be aware that their own personal histories, experiences, beliefs, and personalities may influence their interactions with families and their ability to be family-centered. Parents value providers who are caring individuals with positive interpersonal and communication skills with families and children (MacKean, Thurston, & Scott, 2005). Various self-assessment tools, such as the Family-Professional Partnership Self Assessment (Beach Center on Disability, 2003), the Are We Really Family Centered fact sheet (Law, Rosenbaum, King, et al., 2003), and the Family-Centered Practices Checklist (Wilson & Dunst, 2005) are available to guide therapists in self-reflection on their implementation of family-centered care.

Guidelines for Family-Centered Services

To provide family-centered services, therapists need to individualize their care to respect families' unique abilities, needs, and preferences (Rosenbaum, King, Law, King, & Evans, 1998; Nijhuis et al., 2007; Viscardis, 1998). Family-centered care requires an understanding of who the family is and what is important for them, and planning collaboratively with the family on how best to provide supports and services with the whole family in mind. Therapists need to embrace the idea that supports and services are provided to all members of the family, not only the child (Shields, Pratt, & Hunter, 2006). The therapist's role is to honor the beliefs and goals of family-centered care through his or her behaviors and practices within the service delivery system. Therapists bring part of themselves to any partnership, and the **therapist-family/child relationship** is the avenue through which family-centered practice is provided (MacKean et al., 2005).

Supporting the Family

One of the tenets of family-centered care outlined by Shelton and Stepanek (1995, p. 363) is "appreciating families as families and children as children." Professionals need to respect the caregiver's primary role as a source of nurturing and love, not as teacher or therapist. "All families need time to relax, to play without an objective in mind, and simply to enjoy life together" (Raver, 2005, p. 12) (Fig. 4.5). In hospital settings, efforts are made to enable parents and children to participate together in typical daily activities.

The family is recognized as the key member of the intervention team, the one who is "the constant in the child's life; and . . . the experts on the child's ability and needs" (Law et al., 2003). The family is the consumer of services and retains the ultimate decision-making authority. Historically, there had been an erroneous assumption that experts were better able to decide what was in the best interest of the child and family. In family-centered care, it is the professionals' responsibility to provide information that the caregivers can use to make informed decisions and to give informed consent. This concept has been referred to as "empowering" (Dunst, Trivette, Davis, & Cornwell, 1988).

Professionals provide families with information on federal and state legislation and local policies related to service provision for children with disabilities, thorough explanations regarding evaluation findings, and flexible and individualized service options. The family-professional partnership forms the foundation of service delivery. This partnership includes learning from each other, sharing responsibility, and accepting each other's perspective.

Positive family-provider relationships are related to a range of child, family, and provider outcomes (Forry et al., 2011). Dunst and Dempsey found that higher parent's self-efficacy and sense of control were associated

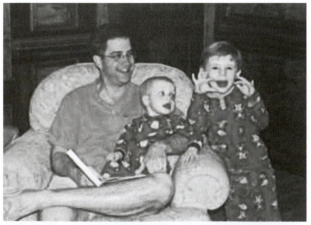

Figure 4.5 Dad reading to sons: It is important for therapists to acknowledge family time to read together, cuddle, and enjoy smiles and pleasures of family life.

with a positive parent-professional partnership (Dunst & Dempsey, 2007). Particular attention to promoting partnership with the family is warranted because professionals have rated this aspect of family-centered care as the lowest in terms of both their beliefs and actual practice (Bruce et al., 2002) and have indicated that they are more comfortable interacting with children than with families (Iversen et al., 2003).

Communication is a crucial key to establishing the family-professional partnership. Therapists have the responsibility of sharing information with families in a thorough, honest and supportive manner. Families have acknowledged that they respect the professionals' knowledge and clinical expertise regarding recommendations for their children.

However, it is important for professionals to value the family's expertise in knowing whether the recommendation is appropriate for their individual circumstances (Leviton et al., 1992). Families know their child in the most intimate way and have valuable information to share. When professionals acknowledge family competence, they help create an environment in which the family can be successful. This concept has been referred to as "enabling" (Dunst et al., 1988).

Through empowering and enabling, therapists acknowledge the family's competence, strengths, and ability to mobilize resources to meet their needs (Dunst et al., 1988). The relationship between the professional and family will change and develop over time. Andrews and Andrews (1995) viewed this evolution "as the family teaching the clinician how to help them even as the clinician is teaching the family how to help their child. The process is a mutual one, each teaching the other, and each learning to be more effective in carrying out his or her responsibility relative to the child with a disability" (p. 66).

More recent discussions on family-centered care have raised the concern that in its implementation, professionals may be expecting too much from families and potentially adding to family stress (Leiter, 2004; MacKean et al., 2005). Providing support for families is a critical component of family-centered care. Therapists can strive to achieve a balance between acknowledging a family's unique realities and acknowledging their right to be a "typical" family. Therapists show respect by accepting families as they balance their many responsibilities at home and work. The role of the professional in this process is to be flexible, because the degree and type of professional involvement will vary depending on the family's needs at any particular time (Leviton et al., 1992; Strickland, 1983). Support may include being an active listener, accompanying care-givers to meetings, providing information, providing guidelines on accessing community services and collaboration strategies, conducting a variety of training programs, providing direct service for their child, and making referrals to appropriate community resources. Pediatric physical therapists must advocate for the needs of children with disabilities and their families (Cherry, 1991), offer families options and opportunities, and ultimately support the level of involvement the family chooses.

Supporting the Child

In a family-centered model, it is important not to lose sight of the therapist's role in providing support for the child (Bazak, 1989). The child is respected as an individual and is involved in intervention planning and decision making. The child's roles as a member of a family, as a sibling, as a friend, and as a student need to be acknowledged and promoted (Bazak, 1989). Therapists may be in a unique role to collaborate with the family in identifying and discussing the child's perspective and goals for their care and future. In family-centered care, it is important for providers to find the balance to support both the child and the family (Franck & Callery, 2004).

Evidence for Family-Centered Care

The guidelines presented are based on the philosophical model of family-centered service delivery. In a meta-analysis of the effectiveness of early intervention, over 20 years ago, Shonkoff and Hauser-Cram (1987) concluded that the programs that focused intervention on the caregiver and child together appeared to be the most effective. And in 1990, Harris promoted efficacy research in pediatric physical therapy on family-focused outcomes. Today, evidence is beginning to accumulate on the process and outcomes of family-centered care.

In early intervention, the philosophies and behaviors of service providers who strive to be family centered have been examined. The components of family-centered services that were identified were (1) family orientation, positiveness, thinking the best of families; (2) sensitivity, putting themselves in the parents' shoes; (3) responsiveness, doing whatever needs to be done; (4) friendliness, treating parents as friends; and (5) child and community skills (McWilliam, Tocci, & Harbin, 1998). A more recent study (MacKean et al., 2005) of

families of children receiving developmental services documented similar findings: Families acknowledge a need for technical competence but value "relational competencies of health-care providers"—providers who are caring, demonstrate compassion and respect, provide personalized care, and have strong skills in communication and interacting with children.

Examining the evidence for family-centered care poses several challenges because the construct of family-centered care is broad, inclusive of a magnitude of provider behaviors and services, and there is also a multitude of child and family outcomes that may be influenced by this approach. Parent satisfaction with services has consistently been related to family-centered practices in a variety of settings across various populations (Dunst et al., 2008; Forry et al., 2011; Law et al., 2003; Stein & Jessop, 1984). A review of the literature on family-centered care for children with neurodevelopmental disabilities in community-based rehabilitation or health-care services summarizes positive results on outcomes related to the improvement in children's developmental skills, maternal knowledge of child development and participation in intervention programs, developmental appropriateness of the home environment, and psychosocial well-being of children and mothers (King, Teplicky, King, & Rosenbaum, 2004; Rosenbaum et al., 1998). While it is difficult to specifically identify key behaviors responsible for these effects, the authors identify the following consistent characteristics: communication, information sharing, collaboration, strength base, and provision of support.

Dunst and colleagues (2008) conducted a research synthesis and meta-analysis of 52 studies that examined the relationship between family-centered practices and family and child functioning. These studies were inclusive of various practice settings, service providers, and recipients of care. The children of the families participating in these studies ranged in age from 1 month through adulthood. Family-centered practices were categorized into a **relational component**, practices that foster the parent-professional relationship, and a **participatory component**, practices that foster family involvement and choice. Outcomes were categorized as either proximal or distal, with proximal outcomes referring to outcomes that were the focus of the intervention.

Family-centered practices had both a direct and indirect effect on family and child behavior and functioning. Participants, mostly mothers, reported higher benefits to themselves and their children when they rated services to be more family-centered. Indirect effects were mediated by participants' self-efficacy beliefs.

Family-centered practices had stronger relationships with outcomes that were categorized as proximal. Practices categorized as participatory generally were more strongly related to outcomes than those that were categorized as relational. In discussing the implications of the findings, the authors highlight the need to advocate for the adoption of family-centered practices along with an appropriate understanding of the outcomes that can be expected.

A recent review, sponsored by the U. S. Department of Health and Human Services (Forry et al., 2011), sought to identify the key components of family engagement and family-sensitive care in early care and education settings. Quality practices in family-provider relationships were categorized as relational practices and goal-oriented practices. Relational practices included behaviors that build on family strengths, support families, respond to family and child needs and preferences, and communicate with families in a reciprocal and frequent exchange. Goal-oriented practices included providing information, advocating for and connecting families with peers and the community, collaborating with families in goal-setting and decision making, providing family-friendly facilities and special events. These practices were associated with children's health and well-being, improved academic and social skills, and decrease in problem behaviors; families' satisfaction, engagement with children's services and education, efficacy, improved mental health, and enhance parent-child relationships; and providers' perceptions and interactions with children, confidence, and relationships with families.

Despite the positive findings of these previous reviews, more research is needed to examine the effects of family-centered care prospectively and systematically. In their review of family-centered care for children in hospital settings, Shields and colleagues (2007) were unable to derive a conclusion on the effectiveness of this approach because no studies met the scientific rigor to be included in the review.

Furthermore, in the past 5 years, several publications have noted the possible negative consequences that may have arisen as professionals have attempted to implement family-centered care. Leiter (2004) cautions that providers need to be aware that the implementation of family-centered care may be fostering inappropriate expectations for the family, especially mothers, to carry out therapeutic strategies with their children. In Leiter's qualitative study, mothers indicated that in relation to the expectation to implement therapeutic recommendations, they did not have adequate knowledge, believed

that the therapist's input was of more value, and did not always feel that they wanted or were able to take on this role.

Similarly, Franck and Callery (2004) challenge providers to "rethink" family-centered care. These authors reviewed discrepancies between parents' and providers' understanding of parent participation and the struggles in integrating parent and professional knowledge. MacKean and colleagues (2005) advocate that recent research and practice related to family-centered care does not highlight the importance of a true collaborative relationship, but rather focuses on educating parents to take more responsibility. Parents in their study described wanting more guidance from health-care providers in making decisions and implementing and coordinating a care plan. Likewise, in a review article on qualitative studies of hospital-based family-centered medical care, Shields and colleagues (2006) note the increase in responsibility expected of families, often without appropriate support and resources.

Family-centered care is complex. Research is needed both to identify the specific behaviors that characterize an effective family-centered approach as well as to understand the comprehensive processes that promote improved outcomes for children and their families.

Family-Centered Physical Therapy

Sokoly and Dokecki (1992) observed that "despite the expressed willingness of professionals to regard families as partners in the care of children with developmental disabilities, partnership thinking has not always prevailed at the level of practice" (p. 23). In discussing future considerations for pediatric physical therapy practice, Stuberg and Harbourne (1994) stated:

It is becoming clearer that pediatric physical therapy can no longer focus primarily on the developmental and neuromotor aspects of patient care. We must now address all levels of the disablement continuum and health-related quality of life issues. Family-centered services with a focus on the consumer and not the provider will be the trend of the future; new theoretical concepts, assessment methods; and perhaps new physical therapy intervention techniques need to address this area of practice. (p. 124)

These are still the challenges for the pediatric physical therapist today—that is, to embrace a scope of practice that includes family-centered care, to advocate for family-centered care within the constraints of service delivery systems, and to apply current philosophy regarding respect for and partnership with families to actual, meaningful practice.

Pediatric Physical Therapy Competencies

Practice guidelines are available for pediatric physical therapists practicing in the neonatal intensive care unit (Sweeney, Heriza, & Blanchard, 2009; Sweeney, Heriza, Blanchard, & Dusing, 2010), in early intervention (Chiarello & Effgen, 2006), and in the school system (Effgen, Chiarello, & Milbourne, 2007). All of the documents include competencies related to family-centered care.

The Competencies for Physical Therapists in Early Intervention identifies family-centered care as the context for therapy. Even though the competencies are focused on early intervention, they can be applied to other areas of pediatric practice, though the exact nature of their implementation may need to be adapted to various practice settings. The competencies can serve as a guide for therapists as they strive to develop the knowledge and skills necessary to provide quality service.

The competencies and behavior indicators specific to family-centered care are listed in Table 4.1. One criticism that has been raised in anecdotal conversations

---

Table 4.1 Family-Centered Intervention Competencies for Physical Therapists in Early Intervention

---

1. **Demonstrate knowledge of family systems theory, recognize the central importance of the family, and be able to provide family-centered services.**
   a. Identify and discuss how the following factors may affect a child's and family's experience with an early intervention program:
      i. cultural
      ii. socioeconomic
      iii. ethical
      iv. historical
      v. personal values
   b. Conduct a family interview using active listening skills to gather information on family's knowledge, strengths, concerns, and priorities regarding their
      i. child
      ii. family lifestyle and beliefs
      iii. services and outcomes desired
   c. Respect the family and acknowledge that the family is the most significant member of the team.
   d. Advocate that children are best understood in the contexts of family, culture, and community.
2. **Recognize the impact of a child with special needs on a family unit throughout the family life cycle.**
   a. Describe a typical daily routine and activities that families may encounter.
   b. Implement basic strategies to support the family unit, including the parents, parent-child relationships, and sibling subsystems.
3. **Support the parents' primary roles as mother and father to the child.**
   a. Assist the family in identifying and developing:
      i. internal and external resources
      ii. a social support network
      iii. advocacy skills
   b. Advocate the right of parents to be decision makers in the early intervention process.
   c. Provide parents with the information and options needed for informed decisions.
   d. Respect parents' choices and goals for their children.
4. **Collaborate and encourage family involvement with the early intervention process.**
   a. Implement a range of family-oriented services based on the family's identified resources, priorities, and concerns.
   b. Provide information on family-oriented conferences and support groups in the community.
   c. Demonstrate people-first and family-friendly communication and interaction skills.
   d. Communicate effectively with parents about curriculum and child's progress.

Source: Chiarello, L., & Effgen, S.K. (2006). Update of competencies for physical therapists working in early intervention. *Pediatric Physical Therapy, 18*(2), 148–158.

as well as in the literature (Franck & Callery, 2004) is the question of whether providers can "do it all." Meeting both child and family needs requires an art and dedication to advocacy and coordinated care.

Clinical Prevention and Population Health

The physical therapy profession's focus on health promotion and disease prevention is consistent with family-centered care. Therapists need to make a commitment to develop or become involved in a variety of community efforts to promote health and well-being. Prevention programs vary in structure, content, and process. Many community hospitals provide families of newborns with a gift bag that includes information on child care, immunization schedules, and developmental milestones, as well as sample baby products such as a toy tester that alerts parents of the choking hazards of small toys.

Typically, physical therapists consult to neonatal intensive care units and high-risk follow-up clinics to provide preventive information and guidance to caregivers on motor and functional development and early warning signs of developmental problems. Their role as a consultant also includes conducting screenings to identify infants who may need to be monitored or referred to early intervention. Physical therapists may also be involved in school- or community-based prevention programs or health fairs to advocate for injury prevention such as campaigns for use of bicycle helmets, to promote fitness, or to identify musculoskeletal problems such as scoliosis.

In addition to community efforts, when therapists are serving a child and his or her family, therapists can provide general education and guidance on health promotion for the family such as information on postpartum depression or environmental hazards related to lead-based paint. While health-care objectives now emphasize the importance of prevention efforts, physical therapists need to make the commitment to put these programs into practice.

Physical Therapy Examination and Evaluation

There are many points to consider when applying the principles of family-centered care to the performance of a physical therapy examination. The first point is that the purpose and process of the child and family assessment need to be discussed and agreed on before the examination and evaluation begin. In today's health-care arena, therapists may not be able to meet all of the requests of families, but families should have the opportunity to provide their recommendations regarding the format, content, time, and place of the examination and evaluation. Therapists also need to ask families how they want to be involved in the actual examination. Do family members want to be the facilitator, assist with activities, observe, or exchange ideas (Leviton et al., 1992)? Families provide accurate and valid information regarding their children, and this information is valuable to the team (Long, 1992; Wilson, Kaplan, Crawford, Campbell, & Dewey, 2000). Therapists need to voice their belief and trust for the family's perspective and knowledge.

If the child's development is being examined in more than one area, the team may consider an arena model for the examination and evaluation (Connor, Williamson, & Siepp, 1978). This model is consistent with many family-centered principles. One team member may lead the examination, thus not overwhelming the child, while other team members observe. The child is typically observed in a variety of contexts, such as interactive play and feeding, allowing the child's abilities to be viewed in natural situations. The family does not have to repeat background information to a variety of professionals, and the arena model fosters team interactions. However, a family may be uncomfortable if many professionals are in the room. Such factors as the child's age and degree of impairment may also influence the decision regarding an appropriate format for the examination and evaluation. Providers need to be flexible in their approach.

A second point to consider when applying the principles of family-centered care to physical therapy examination is respect for the child's rights and sensitivity to the child's age and temperament. Therapists need to think about the child's interests and how these interests can be used to promote motor function. Ideally, some portion of the examination should be in the child's **natural setting** during activities of daily living, play, interactions between the child and the family members, and interactions between the child and his or her peers (Comfort & Farran, 1994).

Practically, simulating natural situations may be more feasible, but therapists need to obtain information regarding the child's home, school, and community environments. Observing family-child interactions during play or snack time will provide valuable information regarding the child's sensorimotor function and the family's strengths and needs. Therapists are concerned about how a child uses his or her skill to function, which is to play and interact with his or her environment, not just the ability to perform the skill. Multiple observations and sources of information will provide a more representative picture of the child and family (Comfort & Farran, 1994). Physical therapy examination reflects the expertise of the physical therapist in physical and adaptive development and is child centered. However, recognition during the examination of the way that the child uses those physical and adaptive skills within his or her environment reflects the family-centered approach to physical therapy.

A third point to consider is the need for a family assessment. Family assessment is a voluntary, interactive process between the professionals and family members to determine the concerns, priorities, and resources of the family related to enhancing the development of the child. The focus of the assessment is determined by the concerns of the family, the relevance of the information to the family's ability to enhance the child's development, and the scope of practice of the professional. A physical therapist will be involved in some aspects of family assessment and will recommend consultation with other professionals or human service agencies when it is appropriate (Chiarello, Effgen, & Levinson, 1992; Effgen & Chiarello, 2000).

Family assessment is generally performed by way of a personal interview and/or self-report survey instruments. Typically, the family assessment and child examination are not two different entities but are often interwoven. As a therapist is observing the child at play, she or he will ask the family about a typical day, the home environment, the child's interests and preferences, the child's strengths, and what they would like the child to accomplish. The interview provides an opportunity to gather essential information about the family's culture, beliefs, and everyday life that can guide intervention activities (Rhoades, 2007).

Bernheimer and Keogh (1995) advocate for an ecological framework for a family assessment that provides a direct link to intervention. Their approach to the family assessment is based on developing an understanding of how families organize their life, who does what, and how family members spend their time. Information is gathered on characteristics of the child, physical and social context of the home and family, goals and beliefs of family members, and family daily routines.

The therapist usually guides the interview, but it is important for the therapist to be an active listener and let the family do the talking. Communication style needs to be tailored to capture both mothers and fathers (Turbiville, Turnbull, & Turnbull, 1995). Table 4.2 provides information on important interviewing skills.

Table 4.2 Recommended Interviewing Skills

- Be aware of eye contact.
- Respect personal space.
- Use inviting facial expressions and gestures.
- Give your full attention to the speaker.
- Respect pauses and provide family time to reflect on the discussion.
- Ask for clarification or examples.
- Acknowledge information, concerns, and suggestions shared by the family.
- Provide requested information.
- Adapt interviewing skills to respect the family's culture.

Caregivers and professionals have identified information as one of the primary needs of families (Summers et al., 1990). Therefore, in a family assessment it is crucial to ascertain what knowledge the family has regarding their child's condition and what additional information they want. It is important to discuss the family's awareness of, use of, and satisfaction with medical, therapeutic, educational, and other community services. In addition, professionals need to inquire about which family members are involved in caregiving and about what strategies the family is using to help their child (Kolobe, Sparling, & Daniels, 2000). Andrews and Andrews (1995) recommended asking families to describe what they have done that appears most helpful for the child. This question acknowledges the family's abilities and provides the therapist with vital information for intervention planning. The family assessment includes having the caregivers identify their formal, informal, and material supports as well as their competing needs (Seligman & Darling, 1989). Knowledge of the family's basic needs in regard to nutrition, health care, clothing, and shelter, as well as the availability of professional and informal support networks, provides a realistic and essential starting point for any intervention plan. Table 4.3 provides examples of specific interview questions that reflect a family-centered approach.

Many family-oriented assessments that measure areas of family routines, support, strengths, resources, and stress are available. Some of these assessments are self-report paper and pencil questionnaires. As therapists review these instruments to determine the appropriateness for their setting, they will also gain an awareness of the variety of issues that may be important to an intervention program. If a standardized assessment is

■ **Table 4.3** Sample Family-Centered Interview
■ Questions

- "Tell me about your child."
- "Tell me about your family and friends who are an important part of your child's life."
- "What is a typical day like for your family and your child?"
- "How would you describe your child's personality?"
- "How does your child like to interact with other people?"
- "How does your child like to play?"
- "What are your child's interests and preferences?"
- "What are your family's interests?"
- "Share with me something your child does that you like."
- "What is the one thing that has helped your child the most?"
- "What would you like your child to learn to do in the immediate future?"
- "What would you like help with in the immediate future?"
- "What supports and resources can you rely on?"

used, clinicians need to become knowledgeable in administration and interpretation of the information. The team collaboratively interprets the information from family assessments in context with other child and family information. Assessments include the Family Routines Inventory (Gallagher, Beckman, & Cross, 1983), Family Needs Survey (Bailey & Simeonsson, 1988), Family Celebrations, Traditions, Routines, and Strengths Questionnaire (McCubbin, Thompson, Pirner, & McCubbin, 1988), Family Resource Scale (Dunst & Leet, 1987), Family Support Scale (Dunst, Jenkins, & Trivette, 1994), Parenting Stress Index—Short Form (Abidin, 1995), Scale for Assessment of Family Enjoyment Within Routines (Scott & McWilliam, 2000), and the Routines-Based Interview (McWilliam, 2003).

Intervention Planning

In family-centered care, intervention planning is a collaborative effort among the child, family, and providers to design an intervention process that is suited to the child's and family's needs and style. Before the plan is delineated, therapists need to provide the family with information obtained from the examination. The family's concerns, priorities, strengths, and resources, as well as the child's strengths and needs, are reviewed with the family. Professionals acknowledge the child's

strengths so families can celebrate their child's abilities. Relaying the information from the examination is crucial because it will help families make informed recommendations and decisions. Verbal feedback should be given to the family immediately after the examination, and more detailed information can be given to the family during the intervention planning process. During this process professionals also need to ask the family how they perceived the examination, what information they gained from the examination, and whether they have any additional information not addressed in the examination. Caregivers' observations of their child's abilities have validity and need to be respected (Leviton et al., 1992). Discussions related to the child's diagnosis and prognosis are conducted with honesty, respect, and hope.

Professionals need to set a positive tone for **collaboration**. All team members, including the family, should be addressed with the same degree of formality or informality (Leviton et al., 1992). Eliciting the perspectives of all those involved may expand the intervention options and provide opportunities for family participation (Andrews & Andrews, 1995; Leviton et al., 1992). Caregivers will vary in their ability to participate, and professionals need to encourage all families to provide their input.

An effective approach is to directly ask the family how they want to be involved, what they see as their role, and how they want the professionals to be involved (Leviton et al., 1992). Families are invited to provide their requests and recommendations. Collaboration should not be viewed as negotiation, but that does not mean that negotiations will not be part of the process. Professionals need to be active listeners. If therapists are uncertain about information the family provides, clarification or examples should be requested instead of making assumptions.

When talking to families, the therapist must avoid using jargon. The therapist may present options for the intervention plan, but when making a recommendation, it is important to phrase it as an "I statement" (Meilahn, 1993). For example, "I believe that Susan would benefit from a preschool program" is more acceptable than "You need to put Susan into preschool." Professionals need to present themselves in a dignified manner, but at the same time they need to establish a relaxed and friendly environment. Courteous conversation and light humor can be used effectively to accomplish this goal.

Discussions for intervention planning should be **solution focused** as opposed to problem focused

(Andrews & Andrews, 1995; Deardorff, 1992). Globally, the plan includes services necessary to enhance the development of the child and the capacity of the family to meet the needs of the child. Leviton and colleagues (1992) recommended the use of exploratory questions to inquire about what resources would be the most helpful for families to reduce stress. In a family-centered framework, the plan may include use of family and community resources, consultative services between professionals and the family (Hanft, 1989), and direct professional service for the child or family.

Community resources that may benefit both the child and family should be identified. "Children with special health care needs should have the opportunity to live at home and to share in the everyday family and community experiences that those without such needs take for granted" (Brewer et al., 1989, p. 1056). These may include recreation activities such as YMCA programs, swimming, horseback riding, dance, fitness programs, music, and sports organizations, in addition to special resources such as therapeutic services, special education, nutrition, family-to-family networking, vocational rehabilitation, transportation, housing, and financial assistance.

The intervention plan should be specific enough to provide the family with the following information: summary of the child's present level of functioning, type and method of service delivery, payment arrangements, location of intervention, frequency, intensity, duration, strategies, and expected outcomes. Efforts must be made to ensure that the method and location of service delivery are family oriented. Intervention in natural community environments, as well as the least restricted environment, are preferred and supported by federal legislation in the Individuals with Disabilities Education Improvement Act (IDEA) (PL 108-446, 2004). Outcomes should be meaningful to the child and family. They should not be goals that address impairments but rather functional goals and objectives. There is an important difference between "the child will be able to hold his arms antigravity" and "the child will be able to reach his arms toward his parents when indicating that he wants to be picked up from the crib."

If during the course of the upcoming year the child is transitioning from one agency to another, a specific plan on the transitioning process must be included. This plan outlines procedures to (1) review service options with the family, (2) communicate information between agencies, (3) orient the child and family to the new agency, and (4) determine what abilities are needed before the transition. The goal of the plan is to avoid disruption of services, ensure appropriate placement, ease the process for the family, and enhance adaptation. This transition plan is especially crucial when a child is transitioning from a pediatric to an adult care agency.

A written intervention plan serves as a communication vehicle among team members, a guide for intervention, and a standard for program evaluation. Caregivers need assurance that the intervention plan will be implemented and that the family will be informed and involved with revisions when circumstances change. Written and electronic communication, telephone calls, and meetings can be used to exchange information on an ongoing basis.

Presently in early intervention, the intervention planning process is outlined and mandated as an **Individualized Family Service Plan (IFSP)** (PL 108-446, 2004). The mandate includes guidelines for the child evaluation and family assessment, an annual meeting with the family, persons involved with the evaluation, persons who will be providing service, and an assigned service coordinator. As part of the collaboration process, the family has the opportunity to decide who they wish to invite to the meeting. This option is especially important for families of cultures where other family or community members are valued in the decision-making process. Even though the intervention planning process is most clearly defined for the early intervention years, family collaboration during this process is crucial for all ages and establishes a family-professional partnership of mutual trust and respect.

While the legislation related to early intervention clearly requires family participation, and current practice endorses family empowerment, the process of family-centered intervention is not meant to imply that the family is to take sole responsibility for the education and therapeutic needs of their child. Families have the option of deciding on their level of involvement and professionals must not be judgmental.

Physical Therapy Intervention
Communication, Coordination, and Documentation

Communication is the skill needed to receive and provide knowledge and information among team members to facilitate coordination and implementation of services. All communications need to be respectful. It is unacceptable to talk in front of children without acknowledging them. This rule is frequently abused when discussing issues with the family, other health-care/educational professionals, or student interns. During the course of a session, communications with the family often include general social conversation as well as opportunities to share information. Mothers have identified communication skills as a necessary factor for promoting positive outcomes for families and children (Washington & Schwartz, 1996). When therapists see children in a school setting, it is very important to send short notes home to the families because in this setting, families can feel isolated from the day-to-day interactions between their children and the therapists.

Therapists also make the commitment to reach out to other providers in their setting as well as professionals in other systems of care serving the child to ensure coordination of care. Care **coordination** among service providers and families is particularly critical to meet the complex needs of children with disabilities and their families. Families of children with disabilities expend considerable time and resources to meet their children's health, education, and development needs.

Services for children with special needs and their families are often complex, dispersed through a variety of agencies, organizations, and facilities, and have varying eligibility and financial requirements. Administrative bureaucracy can undermine an atmosphere of support and respect. "Appropriate, flexible, and reasonable ways must be found to link them together to provide maximum benefit to these children and their families" (Brewer et al., 1989, p. 1056).

Care coordination is based on the assumption that integrated services will result in efficient and effective service delivery toward common goals for the child and family, while reducing duplication of services or conflicting approaches. This component of service delivery reflects the tenets of family-centered care, including facilitating parent/professional relationships and designing health-care delivery systems that are feasible, accessible, and responsive to family needs (Shelton & Stepanek, 1995). Unfortunately, studies have reported the struggles therapists face in providing care coordination both within and across practice settings (Campbell & Halbert, 2002; Mullins et al., 1997; O'Neil, Ideishi, Nixon-Cave, & Kohrt, 2008), such as inadequate knowledge about available services, limited opportunities for teaming, and lack of time and resources. Agencies' policies, procedures, and resources for service delivery should reflect a family-centered philosophy (Leviton et al., 1992; Shelton & Stepanek, 1995) that promotes timely communication, coordination and documentation.

For coordination to be effective, providers and families not only need to share information, but also must synthesize the information to decide on a focus of services, specific intervention strategies, and an action plan to ensure implementation. Therapists identify formal team meetings, home visits, co-intervention sessions with other disciplines, and education on service delivery systems and teaming as strategies to improve care coordination (Campbell & Halbert, 2002; Mullins et al., 1997; O'Neil et al., 2008). In all practice settings, it is essential that families be present for team care meetings to collaborate in the coordination process.

In educational systems, service coordinators and case managers organize services for children and their families; however, throughout all areas of pediatrics, physical therapists can be instrumental in promoting coordinated care and ease of entry into their community's intervention systems. Physical therapists can consult with local agencies to help establish an efficient and effective system for service delivery with appropriate health care, education, and recreational providers. Physical therapists can help form the link between the social worker or case manager in the health-care center with the service coordinator in the educational center. Coordination of services is an important function of family-centered care. Time constraints often leave this job undone, and families and professionals may be frustrated by gaps in the care plan.

Respite care is temporary care for a person with a disability or chronic illness, providing rest for the primary caregiver. This is one service often needed and requested by families, and should be part of family-centered service coordination. Family-centered care supports children living in their home; however, this process must be assisted and must not be just a philosophical agreement. Physical therapists can become involved in a respite program on many levels, including being aware of community programs and making referrals, assisting with the development or administration of a respite program, being on the advisory board of a respite program, educating staff involved with the program, and providing direct service in a respite program (Short-DeGraff & Kologinsky, 1988; Warren & Cohen, 1986).

Physical therapists can be instrumental in increasing professional and community awareness of the needs of families. Political involvement is needed to support legislation that assists families with financing and availability of services. Physical therapists can provide consultation to community-based rehabilitation programs, and they can become involved in developing resource directories and conducting parent workshops. Topics frequently requested by parents include availability of financial resources, legislative mandates affecting service delivery, and how to collaborate within the school system. While successful support groups are led by the participants, physical therapists can be instrumental in helping families develop formal parent, sibling, and peer support groups or connect with other parents for informal support or networking.

Meaningful **documentation** of services communicates vital information to the family, service providers, and agencies to promote coordination. Therapists can be creative to ensure that documentation is family-friendly by perhaps defining difficult medical terminology in parentheses or by appending supplemental technical reports with explanations in lay terms. Families can participate in the documentation process to ensure that it accurately reflects their child's and family's status, accomplishments, and needs.

Patient/Client-Related Instruction

While the terminology for the component of intervention entitled "patient/client-related instruction" as presented in the *Guide to Physical Therapist Practice* (APTA, 2001) does not fully reflect a family-centered approach, the construct of the intervention is a critical aspect of family-centered care. Families have identified meeting information needs as a key outcome of intervention (Bailey et al., 1992; King et al., 1999; McWilliam & Scott, 2001).

Exchanging information is the process by which families and providers share knowledge, skills, and expertise related to meeting child and family needs. Within early intervention, the topic of "parent education" has been controversial, and a redefined focus of "partnership education" (Turnbull, Blue-Banning, Turbiville, & Park, 1999) promotes a family-centered approach.

Information sharing is reciprocal and acknowledges that families know their children best. Families provide therapists with vital information on how their child functions in a variety of contexts and have insights on what strategies are or are not effective for their child. Therapists meet the families' requests for information on general areas such as child development and community resources as well as specific information and guidance related to areas such as their child's condition and how to position and carry their child. This information is provided to enhance family competence in caring and nurturing their child. Families have the opportunity to evaluate this information in order to make informed decisions for their children. It is through this collaborative sharing of knowledge, skill, experience, and resources that appropriate interventions and home

activities are selected and implemented to achieve child and family outcomes (Case-Smith, 1998; Dunst, Bruder, Trivette, Raab, & McLean, 2001; Kaiser & Hancock, 2003; Viscardis, 1998).

Therapists need to ask families how they would like information presented to them. Some families like to keep a journal and others prefer written information such as books or articles. Explanations and demonstrations are two important ways to help make information meaningful to the family. Families have indicated that it is important for them to learn simple tasks they can be successful at in order to promote self-esteem and empowerment (Shannon, 2004).

Home recommendations are essential if an intervention plan is to incorporate practice and to promote generalization of skill into the natural environment. In a family-centered philosophy, therapists do not prescribe home programs (Bazak, 1989); rather, home programs are established in collaboration with the family. Therapists need to be sensitive to the unique situations within each family. An elder caregiver may not be able to participate in a program geared to play time on the floor, or a single parent may have limited time and energy.

Home activities should be functional and incorporated into activities of daily living and the family's daily routine (Rainforth & Salisbury, 1988). Therapists collaborate with the family to identify naturally occurring intervention opportunities (Kaiser & Hancock, 2003). The family and child choose program activities that are realistic and meaningful to them. Therapists use the information gathered during the family interview to pursue appropriate activities with various family members. If a father mentioned that he gives the children their baths at night, then the therapist works with the father on strategies that can be incorporated during bath time.

It is the therapist's responsibility to ensure that the family is comfortable with the techniques and activities. Therapists need to ask the family how they would best learn a therapeutic technique. The many avenues of learning include modeling, participatory demonstrations, photographs, videos, diagrams, and written instruction (Fig. 4.6). It is important to remember to find out if the activity worked. Bazak (1989) urges therapists to stop using the term *noncompliance*. Families and children may not be able to adhere to recommendations for a variety of reasons, not because they are choosing to disregard instructions willfully. If the activity has not been used at home, then the therapist and family need to revisit appropriate and realistic home activities.

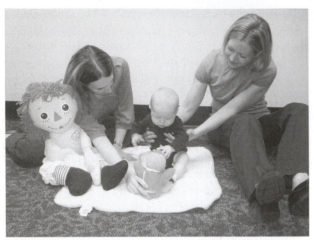

Figure 4.6 Parents are invited and encouraged to engage their children in functional tasks and try intervention strategies during therapy sessions. Therapists can provide guidance and support and families can provide feedback on their insights and comfort level with using a particular strategy.

Procedural Interventions

Family-centered intervention does not preclude **direct service delivery** from a professional (Hanft, 1989). Direct physical therapy service is indicated to address neuromuscular, musculoskeletal, integumentary, cardiovascular, and pulmonary impairments that limit function, and to enhance activity and participation of children. Direct service is especially indicated when specialized intervention procedures are needed and when the child is learning a new skill. Family-centered intervention means that direct service is provided in a manner that respects the child and family and fosters their competence. Family members and the child are active participants during therapy sessions. The availability of appointments, such as the option of some evening and weekend hours, respects the family's lifestyle and may provide the opportunity for a variety of family members and caregivers to participate in the intervention. As health-care providers, therapists need to put consumer-focused services into practice.

The initial focus of intervention should be in an area where success is most likely. Achievement of outcomes acknowledges the child's and family's competence and may give them the confidence to work on more challenging tasks (Andrews & Andrews, 1995). The initial focus should also be on an area that is important to the child and family, and not necessarily the therapist's first priority (Fig. 4.7). Goals and interventions should

address *functional skills* needed for the child to be an active participant in *social relationships*. For example, functional cruising for a 6-year-old may provide the child with the responsibility for a household chore, such as setting the table or the ability to collect lunch money at school.

Interventions are provided within the natural environment of the child as appropriate. Federal legislation supports the provision of early intervention services in the natural environment. With infants and toddlers in early intervention, the context of learning is their home or child care facility. These environments foster spontaneous use of skills by providing natural cues and reinforcement (Grabowski, 1991). Even though home-based services may not be feasible in all instances, home visits should be an integral component to an intervention plan. Families have acknowledged that home visits are one of the most helpful aspects of early intervention (Upshur, 1991). During home visits for children of all ages, therapists can gain valuable information about the child's natural environment that can guide intervention plans and recommendations for *task adaptations, environmental modifications,* and *assistive technology*. In addition to home visits, therapists may need to consult in a variety of settings in the child's community, such as child care, community groups, and recreation. In the clinic, therapists can set up simulations to address functional skills needed in the home, school, and community. As an example, a family member may be asked to

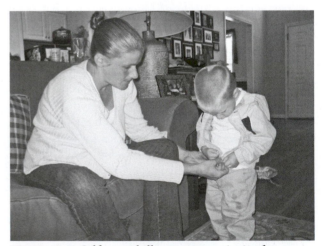

Figure 4.7 Self-care skills are a top priority for parents of children with disabilities, and therapists respect this priority by focusing intervention on tasks such as dressing.

measure the height of furniture at home so that transfer training in the clinic can simulate the chair-to-bed transfer that is needed in the home.

The natural environment goes beyond the actual location of the intervention and requires that the intervention be provided within the context of the child's and family's *daily activities and routines* while promoting learning opportunities for the child (Dunst et al., 2001; Dunst & Bruder, 2002). The settings where children live and play afford many opportunities for therapists to address family interests and priorities (Dunst et al., 2001; McWilliam & Scott, 2001). Therapists assist the family with developing the skills and resources they will need to provide specialized daily care for their children and support the children's participation in *self-care*. When therapists work with young children, therapists can involve the family by setting up opportunities for reciprocal and enjoyable caregiver-child interactions. For preschool and school-aged children, opportunities for developmentally appropriate interactions with siblings and peers and application of their motor behaviors in meaningful contexts become important. Providing guidance for playground and extracurricular activities will enable children to more fully participate in their natural environments (Fig. 4.8).

Therapists can promote motor function, playfulness, and self-esteem by using *play* as a context for therapy (Chiarello & Palisano, 1998; Fewell & Glick, 1993; Schaaf & Mulrooney, 1989). Play includes sensory,

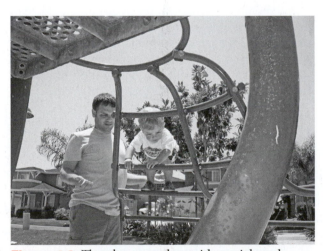

Figure 4.8 The playground provides a rich and meaningful environment for therapists to support children's participation in physical and social recreation.

neuromuscular, and mental processes. Play with motion is an integral part of physical therapy. Play makes therapy more meaningful; it elicits a child's attention, motivation, cooperation, and initiation. A motor skill for a play activity is an understandable goal for the child. Play provides an avenue for motor learning and also affords a relaxed and enjoyable atmosphere. More importantly, through play, physical therapists support children's playfulness, their enjoyment, and their engagement with activities (Bundy, 1997). Physical therapists provide the family with the physical resources, such as positioning equipment and adaptive switches, to make play time happen at home. Therapists encourage active participation of the child and sensitivity to the child's interests, cues, and needs. When choices are available, they should be offered to the child. Even simple choices provide the child with the opportunity to direct an interaction and to be a leader. Physical therapists are concerned not only with teaching a child a motor skill but also with helping the child gain the confidence to use that skill in his or her daily interactions. A range of activities should be used to provide a balance among interactive play, exploration, and independent play.

Two contemporary therapy practice models, family-centered functional therapy (Law et al., 1998) and activity-focused motor interventions (Valvano, 2004; Chapter 8) offer guidelines for provision of intervention in a manner consistent with family-centered care. Both models highlight (1) family and child priorities and involvement, (2) selecting goals for which the child is ready to achieve, (3) task adaptations, (4) environmental modifications, (5) practice of functional activities, and (6) embedding procedural interventions for body structure and function within activities. Law et al. (1998) performed a single group pilot study on the effects of family-centered functional therapy for young children with cerebral palsy and reported that children improved in functional performance after the intervention. Upon analysis of the interventions, the authors found that more interventions focused on promoting changes within the child and recommended further development of specific intervention strategies that focus on the task and environment. This finding suggests that when implementing family-centered therapy, therapists may need to consider a comprehensive approach to supporting children and families.

Mini-Case Studies 4.2 and 4.3 provide clinical scenarios highlighting some of the family-centered principles discussed.

Mini-Case Study 4.2
Family-Centered Intervention for a Young Child

A therapist was providing service for a 5-year-old boy with a diagnosis of global developmental delay. His gross motor age equivalent was 12 months, and the child had limited standing balance and was not ambulating independently. He had limited expressive communication. His parents worked and he had two older siblings. The *first step* in developing an intervention plan was to determine the family's goals and objectives. The family identified four skills for the child to learn that were important to them: (1) the ability to stand up from the potty chair, (2) the ability to climb into the bathtub, (3) the ability to walk safely in the house and outside in the yard, and (4) the ability to shake hands.

The *second step* was to discuss the method of intervention. The family requested home-based services in the early evening or Saturday morning. They expressed their desire to participate during part of the session, but they also believed that their son should work alone with the therapist for part of the time. This balance enabled the family members to participate in some positive play and functional activities and also to have some independent time while their son was working one-on-one with the therapist during a challenging activity. The therapist was able to try new interventions and determine their success before teaching the family.

The *third step* was to discuss the family's typical routine to identify opportunities for integrating intervention techniques. The family acknowledged their busy schedule but identified Saturday morning as a relaxed time when the children sometimes climbed into the parents' bed for some cuddling and play. This time was hallmarked as a fun way to work on climbing. The home setting enabled the therapist to work on functional mobility on the stairs, in the bathroom, and outside in the yard.

Mini-Case Study 4.3
Family-Centered Intervention for an Adolescent

A 15-year-old boy with a diagnosis of juvenile rheumatoid arthritis was referred to outpatient pediatric rehabilitation. During the intake telephone call, a description of the facility and pediatric rehabilitation program was provided to the mother. The therapist requested that this information be shared with her son. Both the mother and son made an informed decision that the son would be comfortable being served in a pediatric facility. The therapist made an effort to redesign a portion of the therapy gym to respect the interests of older children.

During the initial evaluation, the adolescent was asked what he wanted to gain from therapy and what he enjoyed most and least about therapy in the past. The adolescent was able to clearly identify three goals: (1) he wanted to maintain his range of motion to avoid surgery, (2) he wanted to be able to walk short distances in his home, but he was comfortable using his wheelchair for long distances, and (3) he wanted to have enough energy to participate in after-school activities such as throwing some basketball shots.

The adolescent was very open in his communication style and shared that he had been angry during previous episodes of therapy when the therapist did not believe his subjective reports of pain. The therapist and adolescent agreed on a contract in which the therapist would stop any activity if the adolescent used a designated time-out signal. This agreement was upheld throughout the therapy process and was an essential element in building a trustful relationship. Based on the adolescent's goals, an intervention program consisting of range of motion, positioning, ambulation activities, strengthening, and endurance training was developed.

The therapist discussed with the family how other family members wanted to be involved. The adolescent wanted to be treated without his parents present, but it was agreed that at the end of the session the adolescent and therapist would provide the parents with an update on any changes in status or recommended activities for home. The mother and adolescent did discuss involving his younger sister during an occasional session. The mother believed that it was important for her daughter to be involved in a positive experience with her brother. At the end of therapy sessions, his sister was often invited to participate in a sports activity with her brother. A brief, daily range-of-motion program at home was recommended. The rest of the movement activities were integrated into the adolescent's responsibilities and routines, such as clearing the dinner table and eventually walking to the mailbox to get the mail. This approach respected the adolescent's academic demands and social needs.

The adolescent was followed for periodic therapy over the course of the next few years. During his senior year in high school, he was involved in the decision-making process of obtaining powered mobility in preparation for the locomotion demands of a college campus. The therapist, parents, and adolescent talked openly of transitioning his care to the college health center as well as to an adult rheumatologist. The family scheduled several consultation visits before selecting an adult specialist. After the discharge from the pediatric facility, the therapist made a follow-up call to both the young adult and the parents to make sure that there were no gaps in the service-delivery process. The young adult was on his way to being an advocate for himself to receive appropriate, respectful care.

Outcomes

Continuous quality improvement needs to be an essential part of family-centered care. Use of customer satisfaction surveys or focus groups may be effective methods of collecting information on the family's perspective on intervention services they receive. It is important to share the results of the surveys or focus groups with the families and to develop and implement action plans to modify the program to address their recommendations. This process is effective in identifying and improving issues that are important to families, such as greater ease in accessibility and decreased waiting time for appointments (Odle, 1988).

Person-Centered Care

As pediatric physical therapists serving children along a continuum of care and preparing them for the transition to adulthood, we need to be cognizant of models of service delivery in adult care. The Beach Center on Disability (2012) defines person-centered planning as a "process that focuses on realizing the visions of individuals with disabilities and their families through collaborative partnerships among the individual, family members, friends, professionals, and community members." Common names for person-centered care approaches include Individual Service Design, Lifestyle Planning, Personal Futures Planning, Essential Lifestyles Planning, and Making Action Plans (MAPS). These models have also been utilized with school-age children during the Individualized Education Program process and in preparation for transition (Meadan, Shelden, Appel, & DeGrazia,

2010). Person-centered planning approaches are founded on the principle of self-determination, the process of taking responsibility and providing direction for one's life.

Therapists can promote the development of self-determination in young children by supporting their self-awareness, problem-solving, decision making, and goal setting. Consistent with family centered care, in person-centered care the individual and the people important in his or her life are respected and recognized as the authority and decision makers (O'Brien & Lovett, 1992). Principles of person-centered care may be useful when therapists are trying to balance respect for the child and the family. Therapists serving adolescents and youth are encouraged to learn more about this approach.

Summary

Family-centered care honors families and children and supports their priorities for their lives. Evidence suggests that family-centered care has a positive influence on families and children. Future research, especially within physical therapy, is needed to identify the specific strategies that are effective and to explore the scope of child and family outcomes that can realistically be expected. Family-centered care requires the integration of the science of family systems with other behavioral, biological, and clinical sciences (Sparling & Sekerak, 1992).

Therapists can apply the principles of family-centered care to all aspects of pediatric physical therapy practice. These principles can be integrated within a person-centered care approach as therapists serve adolescents and adults. Family-centered care is challenging; it takes time and consideration. In the clinical arena, with the never-ending demands of high caseloads, productivity standards, and funding, it is at times difficult to meet all the responsibilities; however, not using a family-centered approach is a disservice to the children and families.

Therapists need to consider how their belief system matches accepted state-of-the-art practice principles of family-centered care, as well as how to integrate these practices in a clinical arena with many payor constraints. Physical therapists have an important role in advocating for quality standards in practice. "Only through collaborative efforts between parents, professionals, and service providers can the goal of family-centered, community-based, coordinated care for these families and their children become a reality" (Odle, 1988, p. 85). It is well worth the effort.

DISCUSSION QUESTIONS

1. How do your values and behaviors reflect a family-centered perspective?

2. What are some stumbling blocks that could prevent a therapist-family partnership from developing? What are some communication skills you can use to prevent this from happening? What can be done to prevent or minimize additional stressors that a family may be facing? What administrative supports or policies are needed to assist you in implementing family-centered care in your practice?

3. What is the therapist's role when presented with other team members who do not embrace this philosophy?

Recommended Readings

Dunst, C.J., Trivette, C.M., & Hamby, D.W. (2008). *Research synthesis and meta-analysis of studies of family-centered practices.* Asheville, NC: Winterberry Press.

King, S., Teplicky, R., King, G., & Rosenbaum, P. (2004). Family-centered service for children with cerebral palsy and their families: A review of the literature. *Seminars in Pediatric Neurology, 11*(1), 78–86.

Viscardis, L. (1998). The family-centered approach to providing services: A parent perspective. *Physical and Occupational Therapy in Pediatrics, 18*(1), 41–53.

References

Abidin, R. (1995). *Parenting Stress Index: Short Form.* Lutz, FL: Psychological Assessment Resources.

Affleck, G., McGrade, B.J., McQueeney, M., & Allen, D. (1982). Promise of relationship-focused early intervention in developmental disabilities. *Journal of Special Education, 16,* 413–430.

Ainsworth, M.D., & Bell, S.M. (1974). Mother-infant interaction and the development of competence. In K. Connolly & J. Brunner (Eds.). *The growth of competence* (pp. 97–118). New York: Academic Press.

American Physical Therapy Association (APTA). (2001). Guide to physical therapist practice (2nd ed.). *Physical Therapy, 81*(1), 9–744.

Andrews, J.R., & Andrews, M.A. (1995). Solution-focused assumptions that support family-centered early intervention. *Infants and Young Children, 8*(1), 60–67.

Bailey, D.B., Blasco, P.M., & Simeonsson, R.J. (1992). Needs expressed by mothers and fathers of young children with disabilities. *American Journal of Mental Retardation, 97*(1), 1–10.

Bailey, D.B., & Simeonsson, R.J. (1988). Assessing needs of families with handicapped infants. *Journal of Special Education, 22,* 117–127.

Bazak, S. (1989). Changes in attitudes and beliefs regarding parent participation and home programs: An update. *American Journal of Occupational Therapy, 43*(11), 723–728.

Beach Center on Disability. (2003). *Family-professional partnership self-assessment.* Retrieved from http://www.beachcenter.org/common/cms/documents/Partnership%20Self%20Assessment%20form.pdf

Beach Center on Disability. (2012). *Person-centered planning.* Retrieved from http://www.beachcenter.org/families/person-centered_planning.aspx?JScript=1

Becvar, D.S., & Becvar, R.J. (1988). *Family therapy: A systemic integration.* Boston: Allyn & Bacon.

Bernheimer, L., & Keogh, B. (1995). Weaving interventions into the fabric of everyday life: An approach to family assessment. *Topics in Early Childhood Special Education, 15,* 415–433.

Brewer, E.J., McPherson, M., Magrab, P.T., & Hutchins, V.L. (1989). Family-centered, community-based, coordinated care for children with special health care needs. *Pediatrics, 83*(6), 1055–1060.

Bricker, D., & Veltman, M. (1990). Early intervention programs: Child-focused approaches. In S.J. Meisels & J.P. Shonkoff (Eds.), *Handbook of early childhood intervention* (pp. 373–399). New York: Cambridge University Press.

Bromwich, R. (1981). *Working with parents and infants: An interactional approach.* Baltimore: University Park Press.

Bronfenbrenner, U. (1977). Toward an experimental ecology of human development. *American Psychologist, 32,* 513–531.

Bruce, B., Letourneau, N., Ritchie, J., Larocque, S., Dennis, C., & Elliott, M.R. (2002). A multisite study of health professionals' perceptions and practices of family-centered care. *Journal of Family Nursing, 8*(4), 408–429.

Bundy, A. (1997). Play and playfulness: What to look for. In L. Parham & L. Fazio (Eds.), *Play and occupational therapy for children.* (pp. 52–66). Philadelphia: Mosby.

Bureau of Labor Statistics. (2008). *Women in the labor force: A data book.* Washington, DC: U.S. Department of Labor.

Campbell, P., & Halbert, J. (2002). Between research and practice: Provider perspectives on early intervention. *Topics in Early Childhood Special Education, 22*(4), 213–226.

Carter, B., & McGoldrick, M. (1989). Overview: The changing family life cycle: A framework for family therapy. In B. Carter & M. McGoldrick (Eds.), *The changing family life cycle: A framework for family therapy* (2nd ed., pp. 3–28). Boston: Allyn & Bacon.

Case-Smith, J. (1998). *Pediatric occupational therapy and early intervention* (2nd ed.). Boston: Butterworth-Heinemann.

Cherry, D. (1991). Pediatric physical therapy: Philosophy, science, and techniques. *Pediatric Physical Therapy, 3,* 70–76.

Chiarello, L. (1993-). Influence of physical therapy on the motor and interactive behaviors of mothers and their children with motor delay during play (Doctoral dissertation, MCP Hahnemann University). *Dissertation Abstracts International, 54/07-B,* 3572.

Chiarello L., & Effgen, S. (2006). Update of Competencies for Physical Therapists Working in Early Intervention. *Pediatric Physical Therapy, 18*(2), 148–158.

Chiarello, L., Effgen, S., & Levinson, M. (1992). Parent-professional partnership in evaluation and development of individual family service plans. *Pediatric Physical Therapy, 4,* 64–69.

Chiarello, L., & Palisano, R. (1998). Investigation of the effects of a model of physical therapy on mother-child interactions and the motor behaviors of children with motor delay. *Physical Therapy, 78*(2), 180–194.

Cintas, H.L. (1995). Cross-cultural similarities and differences in development: Impact of parental expectations on motor behavior. *Pediatric Physical Therapy, 7*(3), 103–111.

Clarke-Stewart, K.A. (1973). Interactions between mothers and their young children: Characteristics and consequences. *Monographs of the Society for Research in Child Development, 38*(6–7, Serial # 153).

Cochrane, C.C., & Farley, B.G. (1990). Preparation of physical therapists to work with handicapped infants and their families: Current status and training needs. *Physical Therapy, 70,* 372–380.

Comfort, M., & Farran, D.C. (1994). Parent-child interaction assessment in family-centered intervention. *Infants and Young Children, 6*(4), 33–45.

Connor, F.P., Williamson, G.G., & Siepp, J.M. (1978). *Program guide for infants and toddlers with neuromotor and other developmental disabilities.* New York: Teachers College Press.

Deardorff, C.A. (1992). Use of the double ABCX model of family adaptation in the early intervention process. *Infants and Young Children, 4*(3), 75–83.

Denboba, D., McPherson, M.G., Kenney, M.K., Strickland, B., & Newacheck, P.W. (2006). Achieving family and provider partnerships for children with special health care needs. *Pediatrics, 118,* 1607–1615.

Dunst, C.J., & Bruder, M.B. (2002). Valued outcomes of service coordination, early intervention, and natural environments. *Exceptional Children, 68*(3), 361–375.

Dunst, C.J., Bruder, M.B., Trivette, C.M., Hamby, D., Raab, M., & McLean, M. (2001). Characteristics and consequences of everyday natural learning opportunities. *Topics in Early Childhood Special Education, 21*(2), 68–92.

Dunst, C.J., Bruder, M.B., Trivette, C.M., Raab, M., & McLean, M. (2001). Natural learning opportunities for infants, toddlers, and preschoolers. *Young Exceptional Children, 4*(3), 18–25.

Dunst, C.J., & Dempsey, I. (2007). Family/professional partnerships and parenting competence, confidence and enjoyment. *International Journal of Disability, Development and Education, 54,* 305–318.

Dunst, C.J., Jenkins, V., & Trivette, C.M. (1994). Measuring social support in families with young children with disabilities. In C.J. Dunst, C.M. Trivette, & A.G. Deal (Eds.), *Supporting and strengthening families. Volume 1. Methods, strategies, and practices* (pp. 152–160). Cambridge, MA: Brookline Books.

Dunst, C.J., Johanson, C., Trivette, C.M., & Hamby, D. (1991). Family-oriented intervention policies and practices: Family-centered or not? *Exceptional Children, 58*(2), 115–126.

Dunst, C.J., & Leet, H.E. (1987). Measuring the adequacy of resources in households with young children. *Child: Care, Health and Development, 13,* 111–125.

Dunst, C.J., Trivette, C.M., & Cross, A. H. (1986). Mediating influences of social support: Personal, family, and child outcomes. *American Journal of Mental Deficiency, 90,* 403–417.

Dunst, C.J., Trivette, C.M., Davis, M., & Cornwell, J. (1988). Enabling and empowering families of children with health impairments. *Children's Health Care, 17*(2), 71–81.

Dunst, C.J., Trivette, C.M., & Hamby, D.W. (2008). *Research synthesis and meta-analysis of studies of family-centered practices.* Asheville, NC: Winterberry Press.

Dunst, C.J., Trivette, C.M., & Snyder, D.M. (2000). Family-professional partnerships: A behavioral science perspective. In M.J. Fine & R.L. Simpson (Eds.), *Collaboration with parents and families of children and youth with exceptionalities* (2nd ed., pp. 27–48). Austin, TX: PRO-ED.

Dura, J.R., & Kiecolt-Glaser, J.K. (1991). Family transitions, stress, and health. In P.A. Cowan & M. Hetherington (Eds.), *Family transitions* (pp. 59–76). Hillsdale, NJ: Lawrence Erlbaum Associates.

Effgen, S.K., & Chiarello. L.A. (2000). Physical therapist education for service in early intervention. *Infants and Young Children, 12*(4), 63–76.

Effgen, S., Chiarello, L., & Milbourne, S. (2007). Update of competencies for physical therapists working in schools. *Pediatric Physical Therapy, 19*(4), 266–274.

Elder, G.H. (1991). Family transitions, cycles, and social change. In P.A. Cowan & M. Hetherington (Eds.), *Family transitions* (pp. 31–57). Hillsdale, NJ: Lawrence Erlbaum Associates.

Ferry, P.C. (1986). Infant stimulation programs: A neurological shell game? *Archives of Neurology, 43,* 281–282.

Fewell, R., & Glick, M.P. (1993). Observing play: An appropriate process for learning and assessment. *Infants and Young Children, 5,* 35–43.

Forry, N.D., Moodie, S., Simkin, S. & Rothenberg, L. (2011). *Family-provider relationships: A multidisciplinary review of high quality practices and associations with family, child, and provider outcomes,* Issue Brief OPRE 2011-26a. Washington, DC: Office of Planning, Research and Evaluation, Administration for Children and Families, U.S. Department of Health and Human Services.

Franck, L.S., & Callery, P. (2004). Re-thinking family-centred care across the continuum of children's healthcare. *Child: Care, Health & Development, 30*(3), 265–277.

Gall, C., Kingsnorth, S., & Healy, H. (2006). Growing up ready: A shared management approach. *Physical and Occupational Therapy in Pediatrics, 26*(4), 47–62.

Gallagher, J., Beckman, P., & Cross, A. (1983). Families of handicapped children: Sources of stress and its amelioration. *Exceptional Children, 50,* 10–19.

Gerhard, M. (1995). Perspective: Home-based early intervention in a multicultural community. *Pediatric Physical Therapy, 7*(3), 133–134.

Grabowski, K. (1991). *Best practices for therapy in preschool settings.* Morgantown, NC: North Carolina Division for Early Childhood of the Council for Exceptional Children.

Guralnick, M.J. (1998). Effectiveness of early intervention for vulnerable children: A developmental perspective. *American Journal of Mental Retardation, 102*(4), 319–345.

Hanft, B.E. (1989). Early intervention: Issues in specialization. *American Journal of Occupational Therapy, 43*(7), 431–434.

Hanft, B.E., & Pilkington K.O. (2000). Therapy in natural environments: The means or end goal for early intervention? *Infants and Young Children, 12*(4), 1–13.

Hanson, M.J. (1992). Ethnic, cultural, and language diversity in intervention settings. In E. Lynch & M. Hanson (Eds.), *Developing cross-cultural competence* (pp. 3–18). Baltimore: Paul H. Brookes.

Hanson, M.J., & Hanline, M.F. (1990). Parenting a child with a disability: A longitudinal study of parental stress and adaptation. *Journal of Early Intervention, 14,* 234–248.

Harris, S. (1990). Efficacy of physical therapy in promoting family functioning and functional independence for children with cerebral palsy. *Pediatric Physical Therapy, 2*(3), 160–164.

Harrison, A.O., Wilson, M.N., Pine, C.J., Chan, S.Q., & Buriel, R. (1990). Family ecologies of ethnic minority children. *Child Development, 61,* 347–362.

Hill, R.F., Fortenberry, J.D., & Stein, H.F. (1989). Culture in clinical medicine. *Southern Medical Journal, 83*(9), 1071–1080.

Institute for Family-Centered Care. (2009). *Patient and family-centered care.* Retrieved from http://www.familycentered-care.org/pdf/CoreConcepts.pdf

Iversen, M.D., Shimmel, J.P., Ciacera, S.L., & Prabhakar, M. (2003). Creating a family-centered approach to early intervention services: Perceptions of parents and professionals. *Pediatric Physical Therapy, 15,* 23–31.

Kaiser, A.P., & Hancock, T.B. (2003). Teaching parents new skills to support their young children's development. *Infants and Young Children, 16*(1), 9–21.

King, G., King, S., Rosenbaum, P., & Goffin, R. (1999). Family-centered care giving and well being of parents of children with disabilities: Linking process with outcome. *Journal of Pediatric Psychology, 24*(1), 41–53.

King, S., Teplicky, R., King, G., & Rosenbaum, P. (2004). Family-centered service for children with cerebral palsy and their families: A review of the literature. *Seminars in Pediatric Neurology, 11*(1), 78–86.

Kolobe, T.H.A., Sparling, J., & Daniels, L.E. (2000). Family-centered intervention. In S.K. Campbell, D.W. Vander Linden, & R.J. Palisano (Eds.), *Physical therapy for children* (2nd ed.). Philadelphia: W.B. Saunders.

Lamb, M. (1983). Fathers of exceptional children. In M. Seligman (Ed.). *The family with a handicapped child: Understanding and treatment* (pp. 125–146). New York: Grune & Stratton.

Law, M., Darrah, J., Pollock, N., King, G., Rosenbaum, P., Russell, Palisano, R., Harris, S., Armstrong, R., & Watt, J. (1998). Family-centered functional therapy for children with cerebral palsy: An emerging practice model. *Physical and Occupational Therapy in Pediatrics, 18*(1), 82–102.

Law, M., Hanna, S., King, G., Hurley, P., King, S., Kertoy, M., & Rosenbaum, P. (2003). Factors affecting family-centred service delivery for children with disabilities. *Child: Care, Health & Development, 29*(5), 357–366.

Law, M., Rosenbaum, P., King, G., et al. (2003). Family-centered service sheets: 18 educational materials designed from parents, service providers, and organizations. Hamilton, ON, Canada: McMaster University, CanChild Centre for Childhood Disability Research.

Leiter, V. (2004). Dilemmas in sharing care: Maternal provision of professionally driven therapy for children with disabilities. *Social Science & Medicine, 58,* 837–849.

Leviton, A., Mueller, M., & Kauffman, C. (1992). The family-centered consultation model: Practical applications for professionals. *Infants and Young Children, 4*(3), 1–8.

Long, T.M. (1992). The use of parent report measures to assess infant development. *Pediatric Physical Therapy, 4*(2), 74–77.

Low, S.M. (1984). The cultural basis of health, illness and disease. *Social Work Health Care, 9*(3), 13–23.

Lynch, E.W. (1992). From culture shock to culture learning. In E. Lynch & M. Hanson (Eds.), *Developing cross-cultural competence* (pp. 19–34). Baltimore: Paul H. Brookes.

MacKean, G.L., Thurston, W.E., & Scott, C.M. (2005). Bridging the divide between families and health professionals' perspectives on family-centred care. *Health Expectations, 8,* 74–85.

Mahoney, G., Finger, I., & Powell, A. (1985). Relationship of maternal behavioral style to the development of organically impaired mentally retarded infants. *American Journal of Mental Deficiency, 90,* 296–302.

Maternal and Child Health Bureau. (2005). *Definition and principles of family-centered care.* Rockville, MD: Department of Health and Human Services.

McCubbin, H., Thompson, A., Pirner, P., & McCubbin, M. (1988). *Family types and strengths: A life cycle and ecological perspective.* Edina, MN: Bellwether Press.

McGoldrick, M. (1989). Ethnicity and the family life cycle. In B. Carter & M. McGoldrick (Eds.), *The changing family life cycle: A framework for family therapy* (2nd. ed., pp. 69–90). Boston: Allyn & Bacon.

McWilliam, R.A. (2003). *RBI report form.* Nashville, TN: Center for Child Development, Vanderbilt University Medical Center.

McWilliam, R.A., & Scott, S. (2001). A support approach to early intervention: A three-part framework. *Infants and Young Children, 13*(4), 55–66.

McWilliam, R.A., Tocci, L., & Harbin, G.L. (1998). Family-centered services: Service providers' discourse and behavior. *Topics in Early Childhood Special Education, 18*(4), 206–221.

Meadan, H., Shelden, D.L., Appel, K., & DeGrazia, R.L. (2010). Developing a long-term vision. *Teaching Exceptional Children, 43*(2), 8–14.

Meilahn, K. (1993). Promoting partnerships between health care providers and parents of children with special health care needs. *Nutrition Focus, 8*(3), 1–6.

Minuchin, P. (1985). Families and individual development: Provocations from the field of family therapy. *Child Development, 56,* 289–302.

Mullins, L.L., Balderson, B.H.K., Sanders, N., Chaney, J.M., & Whatley, P.R. (1997). Therapists' perceptions of team functioning in rehabilitation contexts. *International Journal of Rehabilitation and Health, 3*(4), 281–288.

Newman, J. (1983). Handicapped persons and their families: Philosophical, historical, and legislative perspectives. In M. Seligman (Ed.), *The family with a handicapped child: Understanding and treatment* (pp. 3–25). New York: Grune & Stratton.

Nijhuis, B.J.G., Reinders-Messelink, H.A., de Blécourt, A.C.E., Hitters, W.M.G.C., Groothoff, J.W., & Postema, K. (2007). Family-centred care in family-specific teams. *Clinical Rehabilitation, 21,* 660–671.

O'Brien, J., & Lovett, H. (1992). *Finding a way toward everyday lives: The contribution of person centered planning.* Harrisburg, PA: Pennsylvania Office of Mental Retardation.

Ochieng, B. (2003). Minority ethnic families and family-centred care. *Journal of Child Health Care, 7*(2), 123–132.

Odle, K. (1988). In my opinion: Partnership for family-centered care: Reality or fantasy? *Children's Health Care, 17*(2), 85–86.

O'Neil, M., Ideishi, R., Nixon-Cave, K., & Kohrt, A. (2008). Care coordination between medical and early intervention services: Family and provider perspectives. *Families, Systems & Health, 26*(2), 119–134.

Palmer, S.J. (1993). Care of sick children by parents: A meaningful role. *Journal of Advanced Nursing, 18*, 185–191.

Petersen, P., & Wikoff, R.L. (1987). Home environment and adjustment in families with handicapped children: A canonical correlation study. *Occupational Therapy Journal of Research, 7*(2), 67–82.

PL 94-142, Education of All Handicapped Children Act (1975). 20 U.S.C. 14.

PL 99-457, Education of the Handicapped Act Amendments of (1986). 20 U.S.C. 1400–1485.

PL 108-446, Individuals with Disabilities Education Improvement Act of 2004 (2004). Retrieved from http://www.copyright.gov/legislation/pl108-446.pdf

Poresky, R.H., & Henderson, M.L. (1982). Infants' mental and motor development: Effects of home environment, maternal attitudes, marital adjustment, and socioeconomic status. *Perceptual and Motor Skills, 54*, 695–702.

Rainforth, B., & Salisbury, C.L. (1988). Functional home programs: A model for therapists. *Topics in Early Childhood Education, 7*(4), 33–45.

Ramey, C.T., Mills, P., Campbell, F.A., & O'Brien, C. (1975). Infants' home environments: A comparison of high-risk families and families from the general population. *American Journal of Mental Deficiency, 80*, 40–42.

Raver, S.A. (2005). Using family-based practices for young children with special needs in preschool programs. *Childhood Education, 82*(1), 9–13.

Redman-Bentley, D. (1982). Parent expectation for professionals providing services to their handicapped children. *Physical and Occupational Therapy in Pediatrics, 2*, 13–27.

Rhoades, E.A. (2007). Setting the stage for culturally responsive intervention. *Volta Voices, 14*(4), 10–13.

Roberts, J. (1984). Families with infants and young children with special needs. In J.C. Hansen & E.I. Coppersmith (Eds.), *Families with handicapped members* (pp. 1–17). Rockville, MD: Aspen.

Rosenbaum, P., King, S., Law, M., King, G., & Evans, J. (1998). Family-centered service: A conceptual framework and research review. *Physical and Occupational Therapy in Pediatrics, 18*(1), 1–20.

Rubin, S., & Quinn-Curran, N. (1983). Lost, then found: Parents' journey through the community service maze. In M. Seligman (Ed.), *The family with a handicapped child: Understanding and treatment* (pp. 63–94). New York: Grune & Stratton.

Sameroff, A.J., & Chandler, M.J. (1975). Reproductive risk and the continuum of care-taking casualty. In F.D. Horowitz, M. Hetherington, S. Scarr-Salapatek, & G. Siegel (Eds.), *Review of child development research* (vol. 4). Chicago: University of Chicago Press.

Sameroff, A.J., & MacKenzie, M.J. (2003). A quarter-century of the transactional model: How have things changed. *Zero to Three, 24*(1), 14–22.

Schaaf, R.C., & Mulrooney, L.L. (1989). Occupational therapy in early intervention: A family-centered approach. *American Journal of Occupational therapy, 43*(11), 745–754.

Scott, S., & McWilliam, R.A. (2000). *Scale for Assessment of Family Enjoyment within Routines (SAFER)*. Chapel Hill, NC: Frank Porter Graham Child Development Center, University of North Carolina at Chapel Hill.

Seligman, M., & Darling, R.B. (1989). *Ordinary families, special children*. New York: Guilford Press.

Shannon, P. (2004). Barriers to family-centered services for infants and toddlers with developmental delays. *Social Work, 49*(2), 301–308.

Shelton, T.L., & Stepanek, J.S. (1995). Excerpts from family centered care for children needing specialized health and developmental services. *Pediatric Nursing, 21*(4), 362–364.

Shields, L., Pratt, J., Davis, L.M., & Hunter, J. (2007). *Family-centred care for children in hospital*. Cochrane Database of Systematic Reviews, 4.

Shields, L., Pratt, J., & Hunter, J. (2006). Family centred care: A review of qualitative studies. *Journal of Clinical Nursing, 15*, 1317–1323.

Shonkoff, J.P., & Hauser-Cram, P. (1987). Early intervention for disabled infants and their families: A quantitative analysis. *Pediatrics, 80*, 650–658.

Short-DeGraff, M.A., & Kologinsky, E. (1988). Respite care: Roles for therapist in support of families with handicapped children. *Physical and Occupational Therapy in Pediatrics, 7*(4), 3–18.

Simmons, T., & O'Neil, G. (2001). *Households and families: 2000*. Census 2000 Brief. U.S. Department of Commerce.

Sokoly, M.M., & Dokecki, P.R. (1992). Ethical perspectives on family-centered early intervention. *Infants and Young Children, 4*(4), 23–32.

Sparling, J.W. (1991). The cultural definition of the family. *Physical and Occupational Therapy in Pediatrics, 11*(4), 17–29.

Sparling, J.W., Kolobe, T., & Ezzelle, L. (1994). Family-centered intervention. In S.K. Campbell (Ed.), *Physical therapy for children* (pp. 823–846). Philadelphia: W.B. Saunders Company.

Sparling, J.W., & Sekerak, D.K. (1992). Embedding the family perspective in a physical therapy curriculum. *Pediatric Physical Therapy, 4*, 116–121.

Stein, R.E.K., & Jessop, D.J. (1984). Does pediatric home care make a difference for children with chronic illness? Findings from the pediatric ambulatory care treatment study. *Pediatrics, 73*, 845–853.

Strickland, B. (1983). Legal issues that affect parents. In M. Seligman (Ed.), *The family with a handicapped child: Understanding and treatment* (pp. 27–59). New York: Grune & Stratton.

Stuberg, W., & Harbourne, R. (1994). Theoretical practice in pediatric physical therapy: Past, present, and future considerations. *Pediatric Physical Therapy, 6*, 119–125.

Summers, J.A., DellOliver, C., Turnbull, A.P., Benson, H.A., Santelli, E., Campbell, M., & Siegel-Causey, E. (1990). Examining the individualized family service plan process: What are family and practitioner preferences? *Topics in Early Childhood Special Education, 10*, 78–99.

Sweeney, J.K., Heriza, C.B., & Blanchard, Y. (2009). Neonatal physical therapy. Part I: Clinical competencies and neonatal intensive care unit clinical training models. *Pediatric Physical Therapy, 21*(4), 296–307.

Sweeney, J.K., Heriza, C.B., Blanchard, Y., & Dusing, S.C. (2010). Neonatal physical therapy. Part II: practice frameworks and evidence-based practice guidelines. *Pediatric Physical Therapy, 22*(1), 2–16.

Thorpe, D.E., & Baker, C.P. (1995). Perspective: Addressing "cultural competence" in health care education. *Pediatric Physical Therapy, 7*(3), 143–145.

Turbiville, V.P., Turnbull, A.P., & Turnbull, H.R. (1995). Fathers and family-centered early intervention. *Infants and Young Children, 7*(4), 12–19.

Turnbull, A.P., Blue-Banning, M., Turbiville, V., & Park, J. (1999). From parent education to partnership education: A call for a transformed focus. *Topics in Early Childhood Special Education, 19*(3), 164–172.

Turnbull, A.P., & Turnbull, H.R. (1982). Parent involvement in the education of handicapped children: A critique. *Mental Retardation, 20*, 115–120.

United States House of Representatives Select Committee on Children, Youth, and Families (1989). *U.S. Children and Their Families: Current Conditions and Recent Trends, 1989.* Washington, DC: U.S. Government Printing Office.

Upshur, C.C. (1991). Mothers' and fathers' ratings of the benefits of early intervention services. *Journal of Early Intervention, 15*, 345–357.

Valvano, J. (2004). Activity-focused motor interventions for children with neurological conditions. *Physical and Occupational Therapy in Pediatrics, 24*(1/2), 79–107.

Viscardis, L. (1998). The family-centered approach to providing services: A parent perspective. *Physical and Occupational Therapy in Pediatrics, 18*(1), 41–53.

Warren, R.D., & Cohen, S. (1986). Respite care services: A role for physical therapist. *Clinical Management, 6*, 20–23.

Washington, K., & Schwartz, I.S. (1996). Maternal perceptions of the effects of physical and occupational therapy services on caregiving competency. *Physical and Occupational Therapy in Pediatrics, 16*(3), 33–54.

Wilson, B.N., Kaplan, B.J., Crawford, S.G., Campbell, A., & Dewey, D. (2000). Reliability and validity of a parent questionnaire on childhood motor skills. *American Journal of Occupational Therapy, 54*(5), 484–493.

Wilson, L.L., & Dunst, C.J. (2005). Checklist for assessing adherence to family-centered practices. *CASEtools, 1*(1), 1-6. Retrieved from www.fippcase.org/casetools/casetools_vol1_no1.pdf

World Health Organization (2001). *International classification of functioning, disability, and health.* Geneva, Switzerland.

Wright, T., & Nicholson, J. (1973). Physiotherapy for the spastic child: An evaluation. *Developmental Medicine and Child Neurology, 15*, 146–163.

Yarrow, L.J., Rubenstein, J.L., Pedersen, F.A., & Jankowski, J.J. (1972). Dimensions of early stimulation and their differential effects on infant development. *Merril-Palmer Quarterly, 18*, 205–218.

Yau, M.K., & Li-Tsang, C.W.P. (1999). Adjustment and adaptation in parents of children with developmental disability in two-parent families: A review of the characteristics and attributes. *British Journal of Developmental Disabilities, 45*(88), 38–51.

Systems

—SUSAN K. EFFGEN, PT, PHD, SECTION EDITOR

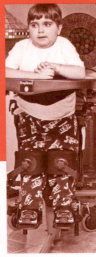
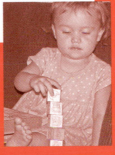
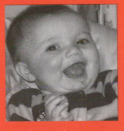
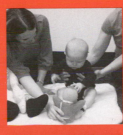
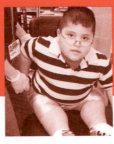
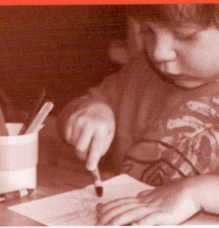

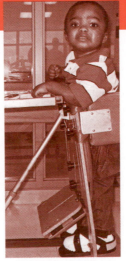
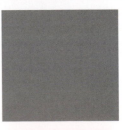

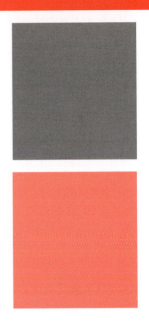

CHAPTER 5

Musculoskeletal System: Structure, Function, and Evaluation

—Margo N. Orlin, PT, PhD

—Linda Pax Lowes, PT, PhD

This chapter is designed to present information on the musculoskeletal system in childhood and adolescence and to relate this information to pediatric disorders commonly seen by the physical therapist. The chapter is divided into three main sections. The first section contains information on developmental biomechanics, including principles of growth and musculoskeletal development during childhood and adolescence. The second section reviews the histology and anatomy of the main musculoskeletal tissue systems—connective tissue, bone, and muscle—relating each to specific pediatric disorders. The third section discusses the comprehensive pediatric musculoskeletal examination process, including specific procedures and their evaluation.

Developmental Biomechanics

Developmental biomechanics is defined as "the effects of forces on the musculoskeletal system during the entire life span" (LeVeau & Bernhardt, 1984, p. 1874). Understanding how the musculoskeletal system changes and reacts to internal and external forces provides a framework to evaluate musculoskeletal examination data and develop a plan of care. This section highlights the major principles of musculoskeletal growth and discusses the changes that occur from birth and throughout childhood.

Principles of Growth and Development

In this section, the basic structure and function of three key tissues in the musculoskeletal system—connective tissue, bone, and muscle—are discussed as they affect child development and function. During development and, to a lesser extent, throughout life, biological tissue is created, shaped, and remodeled through external or internal forces. Tissues respond not only to the different types of forces to which they are exposed in the intrauterine and extrauterine environments, but also to the direction and amount of force. In addition to force, which is only one factor that influences body size, shape, genetics, nutrition, drugs, and hormones also influence body structure. An appreciation of the typical sequence of development and the impact of pathological influences on these tissues will assist the physical therapist in identifying deviations from typical development and may allow prevention or remediation of impairments and limit disability. Principles of growth and development will also be applied to the key musculoskeletal tissue systems.

Musculoskeletal Tissue Systems

Connective Tissue

There are two general types of connective tissue—dense ordinary connective tissue and cartilage. **Dense ordinary connective tissue** can have a regular or irregular arrangement. Tendons and ligaments have regular arrangements of dense ordinary connective tissue, which is best suited to withstand tension only in the direction of the fibers. This arrangement makes them strong to resist the pull of muscles. The connective tissue that surrounds the bones, muscles, heart, and other areas is irregularly aligned and withstands tension in a number of directions.

Tendons are composed of tightly packed bundles of parallel collagen fibers. If the tendon rubs over a bone or other friction-producing surface, **synovia** (synovial fluid) acts as a lubricant. The synovial sheath is made up of an inner sheath that is attached to the tendon and an outer sheath that attaches to the object that is rubbing against the tendon. Synovial fluid fills the space between the two sheaths and allows the surfaces to glide past one another.

Ligaments are composed primarily of tightly packed parallel bundles of collagen, but they also have elastic fibers interwoven within the main fibers. This construction provides the stability for strong support around articulating joints while allowing flexibility to permit appropriate joint motion.

Both tendons and ligaments can heal if torn or surgically cut. Tendon regeneration is mediated by the fibroblasts in the inner tendon sheath or surrounding loose connective tissue. The new fibroblasts become oriented along the tendon axis, and then collagen is produced. A common complication of tendon regeneration is the development of fibrous adhesions between the tendon and surrounding tissues. These adhesions can prevent the return of normal movement. Early, gentle range of motion (ROM) can disrupt production of adhesions in undesired directions and help speed recovery (Mortensen, Skov, & Jensen, 1999).

Cartilage, the second type of connective tissue, is found at the site of articulating joints and provides a smooth surface for movement. Cartilage provides the initial prenatal structure for bone development. Cartilage is a gel-like substance with fine collagen fibrils distributed in the gel to add tensile strength.

Bones

Bone is similar to cartilage except that bone has more collagen, is heavily mineralized, and is covered by a fibrous connective tissue called periosteum. These differences make bone much harder and less supple than cartilage. Bone cells, or osteocytes, are found in lacunae (little caves) throughout the rigid bone. The heavy mineralization of bone precludes long-range diffusion of nutrients; therefore, osteocytes must be in close proximity to blood capillaries. Canaliculi are narrow, fluid-filled channels that interconnect the osteocyte lacunae with nutrients from the capillaries.

Most bones develop from a cartilaginous model formed of mesenchyme early in the embryonic period. Mesenchyme is part of the mesoderm layer of the embryo found between the outer ectoderm and inner endoderm layers. Bone, cartilage, and muscle are all derived from the mesoderm. Bone growth occurs through apposition, or the deposition of additional bone on preexisting surfaces. There are two methods of bone appositional growth. The clavicle, mandible, and facial and cranial flat bones develop directly in vascularized mesenchyme through a process called *intramembranous ossification*. Intramembranous ossification begins near the end of the second month of gestation.

The remaining bones of the body develop through *endochondral ossification,* or the deposition of bone on a cartilaginous model. A limb bud, or mesodermal outgrowth, develops on the embryo where the extremities are going to form. The mesenchymal cells condense and determine the shape of the future bone and then begin the process of bone development by differentiating into chondroblasts that produce a framework of hyaline cartilage. Mesenchymal cells can differentiate into either chondroblasts or osteoblasts. Determination of the type of cells produced is dependent on vascularization. The differentiation of mesenchymal cells into osteoblasts, or bone precursor cells, is dependent on the availability of oxygen. Therefore, bone is produced only in areas that are vascularized, whereas cartilage can be produced in avascular areas.

Around the end of the second month of gestation, periosteal capillaries begin to invade the cartilage near the middle of the model, bringing with it osteogenic cells. This area begins the process of bone matrix deposition over the cartilage and is the primary center of ossification. As the bony matrix is deposited, the central portion of the model undergoes resorption and the medullary cavity is developed. The middle section, or diaphysis, of the bone is therefore formed first while the ends of the bone, or epiphyses, are still cartilaginous.

Calcification of fetal bone increases as the fetus increases in weight. Neonates born prematurely, therefore, have significantly less calcified bones (Walker, 1991). Long bones will eventually develop secondary centers of ossification in the epiphyseal region. The majority of secondary centers of ossification develop postnatally. The secondary centers in the lower end of the femur and the upper end of the tibia are the only centers present at birth. Following the development of the secondary centers of ossification, the epiphysis begins the process of conversion to bone, except that cartilage remains on the articulating surfaces of the bone and a transverse disc of hyaline cartilage remains on the border of the diaphysis. These regions of cartilage, called the **epiphyseal plates**, allow the bone to grow until adult stature is attained.

Postnatal longitudinal bone growth occurs on the diaphyseal sides of both epiphyseal plates. During this process, capillaries are sprouting and invade the spaces vacated by the chondrocytes. The capillaries can be injured as they grow and a small amount of blood can leak into the lacunae. If a child has a bacterial infection in another part of the body, it may be transmitted to the bone and result in juvenile osteomyelitis, which commonly begins at the diaphysis.

The width of the epiphysis is wider than the width of the diaphysis. The tapered area that connects the wide epiphysis to the narrow diaphysis is referred to as the *metaphysis*. The metaphysis retains a tapered shape through the process of resorption. As the shaft is lengthened, bone is resorbed in the area that was previously adjacent to the epiphysis to match the diameter of the diaphysis (Fig. 5.1). Resorption is also involved in the process of growth in the diameter of the bone. Successive layers of osteoblasts are deposited to the outer surface of the diaphysis. This process is accompanied by absorption on the inner surface, which allows widening of the medullary cavity to prevent the bone from becoming too thick and heavy.

Mechanical forces influence the rate of bone deposition or resorption. Early in the prenatal period, the

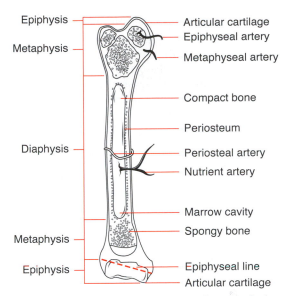

Figure 5.1 Schematic drawing of parts of a bone. *(From Pratt, N. [1991]. Clinical musculoskeletal anatomy [p. 6]. Philadelphia: Lippincott. Copyright 1991 by the J.B. Lippincott Company. Reprinted with permission.)*

role of mechanical forces on the fetus is minimal because the uterus and embryonic fluid suspend the fetus in a "weightless" environment. As the fetus grows, the confines of the uterus can have an impact on development, especially if there is a size discrepancy between a small uterus and large baby or if the fetus is positioned atypically. Abnormal facies and talipes equinovarus (congenital clubfoot) are examples of atypical bone structure caused by uterine crowding (Walker, 1991). Breech positioning also puts atypical stresses on the fetus and has been related to musculoskeletal changes such as torticollis and hip dysplasia (Davids, Wenger, & Mubarak, 1993). Decreased joint movement also affects the developing fetus and may delay the formation of secondary ossification centers (Trueta, 1968). This could result in fragile, misshapen bones.

After initial development, bone shape can be changed through a process called **modeling,** which includes bone formation and resorption. These two factors serve to increase the amount of bone and determine its shape. Remodeling is a process that replaces immature and old bone with no net gain, but possibly a decrease in bone. These processes of bone formation and adaptation are influenced by several factors, including nutrition and heredity. Another factor is expressed by **Wolff's law**, first proposed in the 1870s, which suggests that bones develop a particular internal trabecular structure in response to the mechanical forces that are placed on them (Mullender & Huiskes, 1995). The type of loading and stress (or force per bone area) in different situations affect bones differently.

Loading a bone longitudinally, parallel to the direction of growth, results in either compression or tension. Either type of loading, applied intermittently with appropriate force, such as with weight bearing or muscle pull, stimulates bone growth. Intermittent compression forces appear to stimulate more growth than tension (LeVeau & Bernhardt, 1984; Nigg & Grimston, 1994). Animal studies have also shown that weight bearing has a beneficial effect on fracture healing (O'Sullivan, Bronk, Chao, & Kelly, 1994) and improves the density and trabecular network of osteopenic bone when coupled with active exercise (Bourrin, Palle, Genty, & Alexandre, 1995).

Constant or excessive static loading, however, causes bone material to decrease, and thus can be detrimental to bone integrity and strength (Lanyon & Rubin, 1984). This concept is demonstrated by the **Hueter-Volkmann principle** of bone growth regulation. This principle states that growth plates produce increased growth in response to tension and decreased growth in response to excessive compression (Zaleske, 2001). Growth plates line up to be perpendicular to the direction of the forces across them, and in the case of a malaligned fracture, this is a mechanism for remodeling to take place (Grasco & de Pablos, 1997). Therefore, if the forces are directed unequally or abnormally across an epiphyseal plate because of malalignment, growth may be uneven and increase the malalignment. In the lower extremities, this malalignment could result in **genu valgum** ("knock-knees") or **genu varum** ("bowlegs"). In the spine, this mechanism has been shown to contribute to the uneven growth of the vertebrae in scoliosis, a lateral curvature of the spine (Stokes, 1997) and to the kyphosis seen in Scheuermann Disease (Zaleske, 2001).

Asymmetrical growth can also occur during fracture healing. However, bone is able to straighten some degree of malalignment through a process known as **flexure drift**. This remodeling mechanism outlined by Frost in 1964 describes a process whereby strain on a curved bone wall applied by repeated loading tends to move the bone surface in the direction of the concavity to straighten the bone (Cusick, 1990; Nigg & Grimston, 1994). Bone is resorbed from the convex side and laid down on the concave side. This process is seen in the femur and tibia during development as the child loses the initial genu valgum posture (Fig. 5.2).

In addition to stimulating growth, dynamic mechanical loading promotes bone density and normal developmental remodeling. Children who do not participate in normal physical activities can experience osteopenia, or decreased bone density, which leads to weaker bones (Apkon, 2002; Bourrin et al., 1995; King, Levin, Schmidt, Oestreich, & Heubi, 2003). Commonly, children with neuromuscular disorders, such as cerebral palsy (CP), do not participate in as much physical activity as do peers without disorders (Van Den Berg-Emons, Van Baak, Speth, & Saris, 1998). Inability to walk is one of the risk factors for faulty hip joint alignment in CP (Horstmann & Bleck, 2007). Chronic inflammatory diseases such as rheumatoid arthritis can lead to osteoporosis (Cimaz, 2002). Intervention strategies for maintaining and improving bone mineralization are discussed in Chapter 6.

Development of Musculoskeletal Alignment During Childhood

The principles of reshaping the musculoskeletal system will now be applied to the developing fetus and child. A neonate has a skeletal structure and alignment that is uniquely different from that of an adult. Intrauterine positioning for 40 weeks and the posture of

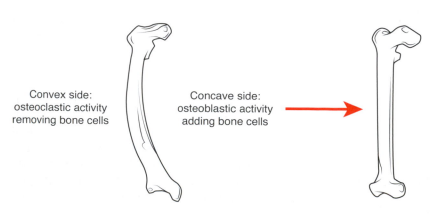

Convex side: osteoclastic activity removing bone cells

Concave side: osteoblastic activity adding bone cells

Figure 5.2 Schematic drawing of the process of flexure drift using an example of a femur in varus alignment.

"physiological flexion" profoundly affect the alignment of the newborn. Physiological flexion refers to the normal hip, knee, and elbow flexion contractures or "physiological limitation of motion" seen in newborns (Walker, 1991, p. 887). The term *contracture*, as used here, is not pathological but refers to the normal flexed posture that develops toward the end of gestation as the fetus grows and becomes cramped in the uterus. Compare the infant in Figure 5.3, who was born prematurely, with the infant in Figure 5.4, who was born at full term. The preterm infant has not had the full 40-week gestation to develop the flexed posture of the full-term infant. Note how the upper and lower extremities of the infant in Figure 5.3 are more extended, with fewer "normal" joint restrictions than the full-term infant.

The physical therapist must always be aware of the wide variability of reported norms for ROM within typical populations. Average values of joint ROM vary within different samples of children and with measurement methodology. Understanding musculoskeletal development is more important than knowing specific joint ROM values. Age-based ROM values are available for the therapist to evaluate examination findings relative to normative samples when making a differential diagnosis or planning intervention. Charts with joint ROM means and ranges can be found in Tables 5.1, 5.2A & 5.2B, and 5.3. The following paragraphs provide a review of both classic and some newer papers that describe the alignment of the newborn lower extremity and how it changes over time throughout childhood. Although much of this research was done in the 1970s and 1980s, it is still valid and in use today.

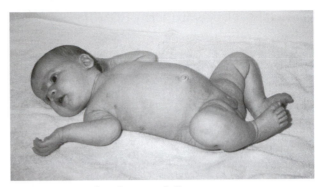

Figure 5.4 Infant born at full term.

Spine

The infant's spine is initially in a kyphotic position, but as the infant begins to hold its head up and prop on its forearms in prone position, cervical and lumbar lordosis begin to develop. The lumbar lordosis is further accentuated as the infant begins to attain the quadruped position with gravity pulling down on the normally weak abdominal area (LeVeau & Bernhardt, 1984). The lumbar lordosis continues to increase from childhood through adolescence (Widhe, 2001; Wright & Bell, 1991).

Pelvis

The infant has a posterior pelvic tilt at birth. The increase in lumbar lordosis over time, as discussed above, coupled with the hip flexion contracture, positions the pelvis in an anterior tilt. This anterior tilt continues to increase over childhood (Mac-Thiong, Berthonnaud, Dimar, Betz, & Labelle, 2004).

At birth, the neonate's hip is unstable. Both the acetabulum and the femur contribute to this instability. The acetabulum is largely cartilaginous and shallow (Walker, 1991), whereas the femoral head is flat, has a high femoral neck-shaft angle, and is anteverted. Despite this instability, the femoral head is normally seated within the acetabulum at birth because of bony structure as well as the surface tension of the synovial fluid (Weinstein, 2001). The modeling process is described in more detail in Chapter 6.

Hip and Femur

Neonates present with a hip flexion contracture of about 30° as a result of intrauterine positioning (Cusick, 1990; Drews, Vraciu, & Pellino, 1984). The range of contracture reported at birth varies between 50° and 120° because of measuring differences and tester variability (Hensinger & Jones, 1982). In a study of 86 typical healthy infants, the hip flexion contracture

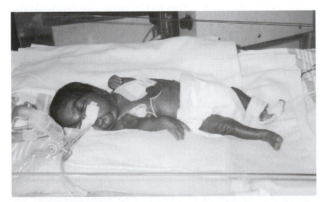

Figure 5.3 Infant born prematurely. Note extended posture.

Table 5.1 Upper Extremity ROM Ranges or Means (in degrees, unless otherwise noted)

		Birth	Birth–2 yrs	3 yrs	5–10 yrs	11–30 yrs	12 yrs
Shoulder	Flexion		172–180[b]				
	Extension		79–89[b]				
	Abduction	70–130[c]	177–187[b]				
	Behind the back reach test				−2.4cm female[a] −0.6cm male[a]	−6.1cm female[a] −4.2cm male[a]	
Elbow	Flexion Contracture	0–30[c]					
	Flexion		148–158[b]				
	Hyperextension			17[d]			10[d]
Wrist	Flexion		88–96[b]				
	Extension		82–89[b]				
	Pronation		90–96[b]				
	Supination		81–93[b]				

Source: Table developed by Gina C. Siconolfi-Morris, PT, MPT.
[a] Phillips, V.A., Chang, D.E., Hartigan, C., Smith, J.F., & Edlich, R.F. (1987). Influence of gender and age on the behind-the-back reach test. *Journal of Burn Care and Rehabilitation, 8*(3), 228–232.
[b] Watanabe, H., Ogata, K., Amano, T., & Okabe, T. (1979). The range of joint motions of the extremities in health Japanese people: The difference according to age. *Nippon Seikeigeka Gakkai Zasshi, 53,* 275–291.
[c] Hoffer, M.M. (1980). Joint motion limitations in newborns. *Clinical Orthopaedics and Related Research, 148,* 94–96.
[d] Cheng, J.C.Y., Chan, P.S., & Hui, P.W. (1991). Joint laxity in children. *Journal of Pediatric Orthopaedics, 11,* 752–756.

diminished from a mean of 10° (SD = 2.6°) at 9 months to 9° (SD = 4.8°) at 12 months, 4° (SD = 3.2°) at 18 months, and 3° (SD = 3.0°) at 24 months (Phelps, Smith, & Hallum, 1985).

It is interesting to note that the standard deviations increase as children age, suggesting that variability may increase with age. Sutherland and colleagues (1988) report that during gait, 1-year-old children lack approximately 8° of hip extension, 1½-year-olds lack approximately 4°, and by age 2, the hip reaches 0° flexion. The change in hip ROM occurs as the young child attempts to attain and maintain positions against gravity. As the iliopsoas muscle stretches out, the anterior hip joint capsule also elongates, allowing anterior glide of the head of the femur and permitting increasing extension (Cusick, 1990). Action of the major hip extensor, the gluteus maximus, during antigravity activities is also essential for decreasing the normal hip flexion contracture of the infant.

In the frontal plane, neonates have large amounts of hip abduction, again because of the influence of intrauterine positioning. The amount of hip abduction differs depending on whether the hip was held in a more extended position (within the limits of available extension) or in a flexed position. In a flexed position, more hip abduction is available. Published hip abduction mean values range between 69° and 76° (Drews et al., 1984; Haas, Epps, & Adams, 1973). Hip abduction range decreases to a mean of 60° at age 2 years (Phelps et al., 1985) and continues to decrease over time to the typical adult value of 45°. This extreme abduction range decreases in conjunction with the development of upright postures, such as quadruped (all fours), kneeling, standing, and walking, and the need for the lower extremities to be in a position that will support weight bearing (Hensinger & Jones, 1982) with a stable pelvis.

In the transverse plane, more lateral rotation than medial rotation is present in the first few months of life. The reported mean for lateral hip rotation in the newborn is between 89° (Haas et al., 1973) and 114° (Drews et al., 1984). Medial rotation means are reported between 62° (Haas et al., 1973) and 80° (Drews et al., 1984). The large amount of lateral hip rotation is quite apparent in supported standing when the young child

Table 5.2A Lower Extremity ROM Ranges or Means (in degrees, unless otherwise noted) from Birth to 3 Years

	Birth	4 wks	6 wks	3 mo	4-8 mo	6 mo	8-12 mo	9 mo	12 mo	15 mo	18 mo	2 yrs	1-3 yrs
Hip													
Flexion Contracture	20[l]–34[s]	12[f]	19[b]	7[b]–19[s]	4[f]	7[b]–8[s]							
Flexion	120[f,l]	138[f]			136[f]	138[f]	138[f]		141[f]			143[f]	
Extension							3[f]		15[f]			21[f]	
Abduction (flexion)	69[g]–79[e]												
Abduction (extension)	39[e]–56[g]							59[q]	54[q]		59[q]	60[q]	
Adduction	6[g]–17[e]												
Internal Rotation (flexion)	40[h]–80[g]			40-80[h]				41[q]	40-80[h]	40-80[h]	45[q]	52[q]	
External Rotation (flexion)	80[l]–114[g]							56[q]	58[q]		52[q]	47[q]	
Internal Rotation (extension)			24[b]	26[b]		21[b]							
External Rotation (extension)			48[b]	45[b]		46[b]							
Knee													
Flexion Contracture	15[l]–21[s]	25[f]		11[s]	4[f]	3[s]	1[f]						
Flexion Female/Male	150[l]–151[s]			146[s]		142[s]							
Extension Female/Male									4[f]			7[f]	6[k]
Hyperextension Female/Male													
Popliteal Angle Female/Male	27[r]–29[i]	25[r]		18[r]		11[r]		2[r]	0[r]				
Ankle													
Plantarflexion	26[i]–50[g]				60[f]		60[f]	45[j]	62[f]			62[f]	
Dorsiflexion	54[f]–80[h]				51[f]		50[f]		45[f]			41[f]	
Inversion	99[g]												
Eversion	82[g]												

Continued

Table 5.2B Lower Extremity ROM Ranges or Means (in degrees, unless otherwise noted) from 3 Years to 19 Years

	3-5 yrs	4 yrs	5 yrs	6 yrs	6-15 yrs	7 yrs	8 yrs	9 yrs	9-13 yrs	10	11	12	13	14	14-16 yrs	16-19 yrs
Hip																
Flexion			147[a]	141[a]		137[a]	137[a]	138[a]		137[a]	135[a]	135[a]	132[a]	129[a]		
Extension			26[a]	25[a]		20[a]	19[a]	21[a]		21[a]	22[a]	20[a]	22[a]	20[a]		
Abduction (flexion)			80[a]	71[a]		62[a]	63[a]	65[a]		65[a]	57[a]	60[a]	62[a]	62[a]		
Abduction (extension)																
Adduction			33[a]	29[a]		26[a]	28[a]	29[a]		29[a]	28[a]	26[a]	27[a]	26[a]		
Internal Rotation (flexion)			56[a]	49[a]		47[a]	47[a]	47[a]		45[a]	43[a]	43[a]	41[a]	38[a]		
External Rotation (flexion)			60[a]	60[a]		54[a]	54[a]	55[a]		53[a]	52[a]	51[a]	50[a]	49[a]		
Internal Rotation (extension)			52[a]	43[a]		43[a]	44[a]	44[a]		42[a]	40[a]	40[a]	39[a]	36[a]		
External Rotation (extension)			55[a]	51[a]		48[a]	48[a]	50[a]		48[a]	46[a]	46[a]	47[a]	47[a]		
Knee																
Flexion																
Female														143[d]		
Male														140[d]		
Extension																
Female														0[d]		
Male														0[d]		
Hyperextension																
Female														6[d]		
Male														5[d]		
Popliteal Angle																
Female	30[p]	17[k]	26[k]	25[m]	45[p]											30[p]
Male	40[p]	27[k]			50[p]											40[p]
Plantarflexion									43[o]						44[o]	
Ankle																
Dorsiflexion									27[o]						28[o]	
Inversion									27[o]						29[o]	
Eversion									11[o]						13[o]	

■ **Table 5.2B** Lower Extremity ROM Ranges or Means (in degrees, unless otherwise noted) from 3 Years to 19 Years—cont'd

Source: Tables developed by Gina C. Siconolfi-Morris, PT, MPT.

[a] Rao, K.N., & Joseph, B. (2001). Value of measurement of hip movements in childhood hip disorders. *Journal of Pediatric Orthopaedics, 21*, 495–501.

[b] Coon, V., Donato, G., Houser, C., & Bleck, E.E. (1975). Normal ranges of hip motion in infants six weeks, three month and six months of age. *Clinical Orthopaedics and Related Research, 110,* 256–260.

[c] Haas, S.S., Epps, C.H., & Adams, J.P. (1973). Normal ranges of hip motion in the newborn. *Clinical Orthopaedics and Related Research, 91*, 114–118.

[d] De Carlo, M.S., & Sell, K.E. (1997). Normative data for range of motion and single-leg hop in high school athletes. *Journal of Sports Rehabilitation, 6*, 246–255.

[e] Forero, N., Okamura, L.A., & Larson, M.A. (1989). Normal ranges of hip motion in neonates. *Journal of Pediatric Orthopedics, 9,* 391–395.

[f] Watanabe, H., Ogata, K., Amano, T., & Okabe, T. (1979). The range of joint motions of the extremities in health Japanese people: The difference according to age. *Nippon Seikeigeka Gakkai Zasshi, 53*, 275–291.

[g] Drews, J.E., Vraciu, J.K., & Pellino, G. (1984). Range of motion of the joints of the lower extremities of newborns. *Physical and Occupational Therapy in Pediatrics, 4*(2), 49–63.

[h] Hoffer, M.M. (1980). Joint motion limitations in newborns. *Clinical Orthopaedics and Related Research, 148*, 94–96.

[i] Waugh, K.G., Minkel, J.L., Parker, R., & Coon, V.A. (1983). Measurement of selected hip, knee, and ankle joint motions in newborns. *Physical Therapy, 63*(10), 1616–1621.

[j] Wong, S., Ada, L., & Butler, J. (1998). Differences in ankle range of motion between pre-walking and walking infants. *Australian Journal of Physiotherapy, 44*(1), 57–60.

[k] Katz, K., Rosenthal, A., & Yosipovitch, Z. (1992). Normal ranges of popliteal angle in children. *Journal of Pediatric Orthopaedics, 12*, 229–231.

[l] Schwarze, D.J., & Denton, J.R. (1993). Normal values of neonatal lower limbs: An evaluation of 1,000 neonates. *Journal of Pediatric Orthopaedics, 13*, 758–760.

[m] Kuo, L., Chung, W., Bates, E., & Stephen, J. (1997). The hamstring index. *Journal of Pediatric Orthopaedics, 17*(1), 78–88.

[n] Cheng, J.C.Y., Chan, P.S., & Hui, P.W. (1991). Joint laxity in children. *Journal of Pediatric Orthopaedics, 11*, 752–756.

[o] Grimston, S.K., Nigg, B.M., Hanley, D.A., & Engsberg, J.R. (1993). Differences in ankle joint complex range of motion as a function of age. *Foot & Ankle, 14*(4), 215–222.

[p] Jozwiak, M., Pietrzak, S., & Tobjasz, F. (1997). The epidemiology and clinical manifestations of hamstring muscle and plantar foot flexor shortening. *Developmental Medicine and Child Neurology, 39*, 481–483.

[q] Phelps, E., Smith, L.J., & Hallum, A. (1985). Normal ranges of hip motion of infants between nine and 24 months of age. *Developmental Medicine and Child Neurology, 27*, 785–792.

[r] Reade, E., Hom, L., Hallum, A., & Lopopolo, R. (1984). Changes in popliteal angle measurement in infants up to one year of age. *Developmental Medicine and Child Neurology, 26*, 774–780.

[s] Broughton, N.S., Wright, J., & Menelaus, M.B. (1993). Range of knee motion in normal neonates. *Journal of Pediatric Orthopaedics, 13*, 263–264.

stands with toes pointed outward. During the first 2 years of life, lateral rotation decreases to a mean value of 47° and medial rotation increases to a mean value of 52° (Drews et al., 1984).

Decreased lateral rotation is related to increased hip extension. As the hip joint stretches out into extension, this lateral rotation pull diminishes (Phelps et al., 1985). The mechanism for the decrease in lateral rotation is similar to that of hip abduction. As the infant assumes standing, decreasing lateral rotation allows the greater trochanter to lie in a more lateral position, so that the hip abductors work more efficiently to stabilize the pelvis in standing (Pitkow, 1975).

At birth, the femur is in a position of **coxa valga**, which is defined as an increased angle of inclination or neck-shaft angle. The **angle of inclination** is the angle formed by the long axis of the femur and an axis drawn

through the head and neck of the femur (Fig. 5.5). The typical neonatal value ranges from 135° to 145° (McCrea, 1985) and decreases to the adult value of 125° to 135° during late adolescence (Staheli, 2008). This angle decreases as a result of the compression and tension forces placed on the proximal end of the femur through normal weight bearing and muscle pull (LeVeau & Bernhardt, 1984).

To understand the position of the femur, the terms *torsion* and *version* require discussion. **Torsion** refers to the normal amount of rotation present in a long bone (Fig. 5.6). Femoral torsion is the angle formed by an axis drawn through the head and neck of the femur and an axis through the femoral condyles. The easiest way to visualize this angle is to actually look down the long axis of a femur. Line up the posterior surfaces of the femoral condyles with a horizontal surface such as a

Table 5.3 Mandibular and Spinal Range of Motion Mean Values (in degrees unless otherwise noted)

		3–5 yrs	5 yrs	6–8 yrs	7 yrs	8–12 yrs	9 yrs	10–13 yrs	11 yrs	14–17 yrs
Mandibular	Maximum Opening							50mm[d]		51mm[d]
	Laterotrusion right							10mm[d]		10mm[d]
	Laterotrusion left							10mm[d]		11mm[d]
	Protrusion							9mm[d]		8mm[d]
Cervical	Flexion	56[b]		60[b]		63[b]-66[a]				
	Extension	75[b]		77[b]		75[b]- 85[a]				
	Right horizontal rotation	68[b]		74[b]		77[b]				
	Left horizontal rotation	69[b]		74[b]		76[b]				
	Right lateral bending	51[b]		51[b]		48[b]				
	Left lateral bending	48[b]		50[b]		47[b]				
Lumbar	Flexion									
	Female		24[c]		25[c]		22[c]		20[c]	
	Male		22[c]		24[c]		24[c]		21[c]	
	Extension									
	Female		17[c]		16[c]		13[c]		15[c]	
	Male		17[c]		14[c]		15[c]		16[c]	
	Right Side-Bending									
	Female		25[c]		20[c]		18[c]		16[c]	
	Male		24[c]		20[c]		16[c]		20[c]	
	Left Side-Bending									
	Female		26[c]		20[c]		17[c]		15[c]	
	Male		23[c]		20[c]		18[c]		21[c]	
	Right Rotation									
	Female		24[c]		20[c]		16[c]		13[c]	
	Male		19[c]		20[c]		19[c]		14[c]	
	Left Rotation									
	Female		24[c]		17[c]		17[c]		14[c]	
	Male		18[c]		22[c]		20[c]		14[c]	

Source: Table developed by Gina C. Siconolfi-Morris, PT, MPT.

[a] Lynch-Caris, T., Majeske, K.D., et al. (2008). Establishing reference values for cervical spinal range of motion in pre-pubescent children. *Journal of Biomechanics, 41,* 2714–2719.

[b] Arbogast, K.B., Gholve, P.A., et al. (2007). Normal cervical spinal range of motion in children 3–12 years old. *Spine, 32*(10), E309–E315.

[c] Kondratek, M., Krauss, J., & Stiller, C. (2007). Normative values for active lumbar range of motion in children. *Pediatric Physical Therapy, 19,* 236–244.

[d] Hirsch, C., John, M.T., Lautenschlager, C., & List, T. (2006). Mandibular jaw movement capacity in 10–17-yr-old children and adolescents: Normative values and the influence of gender, age and temporomandibular disorders. *European Journal of Oral Sciences, 114,* 465–470.

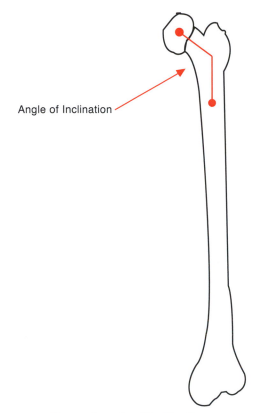

Angle of Inclination

Figure 5.5 Femoral angle of inclination.

table. Then look down the bone toward the head of the femur and note that the head and neck of the femur are angled upward from the table approximately 15°. This is the angle of torsion.

Antetorsion occurs when the head and neck of the femur are rotated forward in the sagittal plane relative to the axis through the femoral condyles. If the head and neck of the femur are backwardly rotated, the femur is said to be in **retrotorsion**. The femur has maximum antetorsion, approximately 30° to 40°, at birth (McCrea, 1985; Phelps et al., 1985; Rang, 1993c). This angle decreases from birth through adolescence. The derotation progresses rapidly between birth and the first year, more slowly between 1 and 8 years, and then rapidly again through adolescence to reach an adult mean of 10° to 15° by approximately age 14 to 16 years (Staheli, 2008). Femoral antetorsion decreases over this time due to hip external rotation and an increase in hip extension (Horstmann & Bleck, 2007) as well as growth (Staheli, 2004).

Femoral antetorsion can cause a lower extremity posture of **in-toeing**. In-toeing is not seen in an infant when the infant is placed in supported stance because the excessive lateral hip rotation and femoral anteversion overcompensate for the inward rotation of the shaft of the femur and result in an appearance of out-toeing. If the normal antetorsion does not reduce with development, the child may have an in-toeing gait pattern when the normal reduction in the lateral rotation occurs with age. The majority of children with in-toeing caused by a normal amount of "persistent fetal antetorsion," in the absence of other disease processes, will improve as the hips spontaneously realign (Rang, 1993c; Staheli, 2004). In less than 1% of these children, antetorsion fails to resolve and the children warrant treatment (Staheli, 2004). In children with CP, however, persistent fetal antetorsion is a causative factor in the development of hip instability. This is discussed later in this chapter.

Unlike persistent fetal antetorsion, in which the child starts out with a normal amount of antetorsion that does not reduce over time, some infants have excessive fetal femoral antetorsion. In a large follow-up study, these children retained a higher amount of femoral torsion through skeletal maturity. However, the in-toeing that accompanies excessive femoral antetorsion disappeared over time in 50% of the children. This is attributed to the development of compensatory external tibial torsion (lateral rotation through the shaft of the tibia) rather than to a decrease in femoral torsion (Fabry, MacEwen, & Shands, 1973). This compensatory tibial rotation tends to lead the foot to an out-toed posture even though the femur continues to have excessive antetorsion.

Femoral **version** refers to the position of the head of the femur in the acetabulum relative to the posterior pelvis (frontal plane). Anteversion positions the head of the femur anteriorly in the acetabulum and results in a position of thigh external rotation. Conversely, retroversion positions the head of the femur posteriorly in the acetabulum and results in thigh internal rotation. At birth, a neonate has 60° of anteversion. By adulthood, femoral version has reduced to 12°. At birth, anteversion (60°) is greater than antetorsion (30°), with a net result of an external rotated femur. This is why a newborn has an externally rotated lower extremity posture at rest.

Knee and Tibia

In the sagittal plane, the newborn demonstrates a knee flexion contracture of approximately 20° to 30° (Drews et al., 1984; Hensinger & Jones, 1982), as demonstrated in Figure 5.7. Again, this is caused by physiological flexion as a result of intrauterine positioning. This will gradually stretch out with elongation of the hamstrings

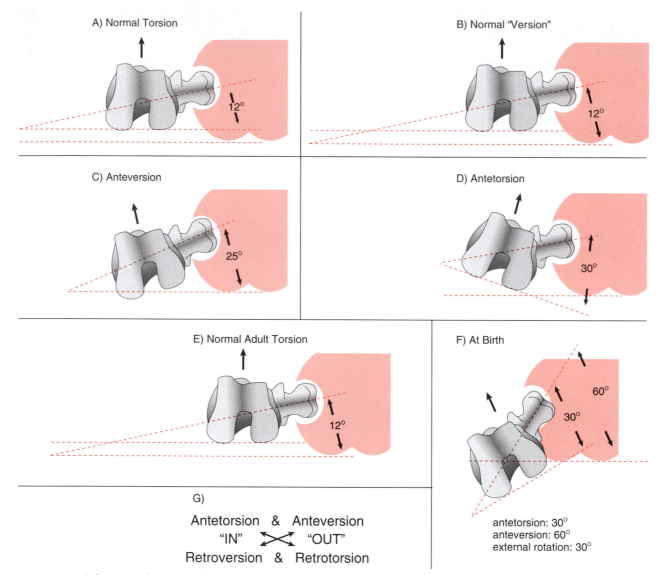

A) Normal Torsion
12°

B) Normal "Version"
12°

C) Anteversion
25°

D) Antetorsion
30°

E) Normal Adult Torsion
12°

F) At Birth
60°
30°

antetorsion: 30°
anteversion: 60°
external rotation: 30°

G)
Antetorsion & Anteversion
"IN" ⋈ "OUT"
Retroversion & Retrotorsion

Figure 5.6 Schematic drawing of femoral version.

through activities such as the infant bringing hands to feet and feet to mouth in supine position and positions such as weight bearing on extended arms, one foot, or one knee, and bear walking (weight bearing on both extended arms and both feet).

Katz, Rosenthal, and Yosipovitch (1992) documented the popliteal angles of 482 typical children from 1 to 10 years of age and found from 1 to 3 years a mean angle of approximately 6° (range of 0–15°). At age 4, the angle increased to a mean of 24°, which was consistent until age 10. They suggested that the increase at age 4 is related to the increase in pelvic tilt discussed previously.

In the frontal plane, the tibia appears outwardly bowed in a position called **apparent physiological bowing.** The entire tibia is rotated slightly forward, which places the larger lateral head of the gastrocnemius muscle in a more forward position. This gives the appearance of a bowed tibia even though the bone itself is only mildly bowed. This "apparent bowing," caused by the forwardly rotated position of the tibia, results from the contracture of the medial knee structures due to intrauterine positioning (Wilkins, 1986).

The tibiofemoral angle of the infant is in a varus position, also called genu varum. The tibiofemoral

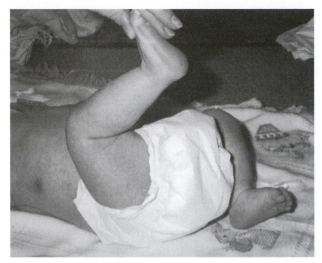

Figure 5.7 Maximum knee extension in a newborn infant.

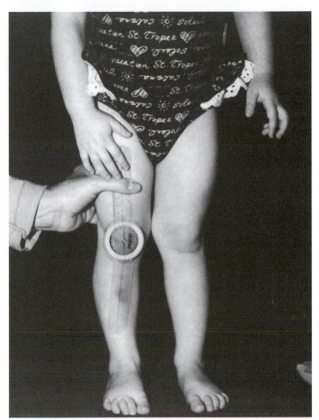

Figure 5.8 Tibiofemoral angle measurement.

angle is formed by the longitudinal axes of the femur and the tibia (Engel & Staheli, 1974) (Fig. 5.8). The apex of the angle is the knee, with the femur and tibia forming the distal segments. The angle may be in genu varum (the distal segments are more medial than the apex), genu valgum (the distal segments are more lateral than the apex), or neutral. Figure 5.9A shows a 4-year-old child in a position of genu valgum. As can be seen, the distal portion of the tibia is more lateral than the apex of the angle. In Figure 5.9B the genu valgum that was evident in the younger child is resolving in the child who is 2 years older.

A natural progression of this angle has been documented. At birth, genu varum may be as high as 15° but decreases approximately 5° during the first year of life (Salenius & Vankka, 1975). Bowing of the knee joint during the first 1 to 2 years of life is likely because of a number of factors, including medial knee joint capsule tightness caused by intrauterine positioning, coxa valga angle of the femur, and lateral hip rotation contracture (Beeson, 1999; Cusick, 1990; Hensinger & Jones, 1982). As weight bearing during standing increases on the lower extremities between 12 and 24 months of age, both the coxa valga angle of the femur (distal end of the femur is more lateral/bowleg) and the femoral anteversion resolve. Additionally, between 3 and 4 years of age, the genu varum shifts into about 10° to 15° of genu valgum (Beeson, 1999; Hensinger & Jones, 1982). After this peak of valgus, the knee angle decreases until it stabilizes at approximately 6 to 7 years of age, at about 5° valgus (Bleck, 1982; Salenius & Vankka, 1975). In

prepubescent children, there is no gender difference in angulation; however, during puberty, males typically tend to have more coxa valga (bowlegged) posture than females (Beeson, 1999).

There are various opinions about when or if genu varum or valgum in young children warrants treatment. Both Bleck (1982) and McDade (1977) state that if the varus position of the knees is not decreasing by age 18 months to 2 years, either bilaterally or unilaterally, further investigation is warranted, particularly if the value is at or beyond 25° (Bleck, 1982). Likewise, if the genu valgum position does not reduce to the typical value of 5° to 7° but remains excessive bilaterally or presents unilaterally, further evaluation may be necessary.

The neonatal tibia is in a position of slight external torsion (approximately 5°). The distal end is externally rotated with respect to the proximal end. The external torsion increases to 18° by age 14 years (Engel & Staheli, 1974) and 23° to 25° of external rotation by skeletal maturity (LeVeau & Bernhardt, 1984). Therefore, since the tibia begins in a position of slight external torsion that

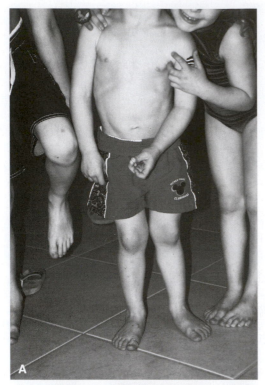

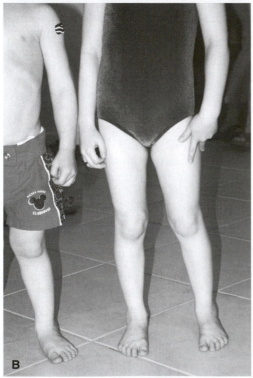

Figure 5.9 (*A*) Genu valgum typical of a 4-year-old child. (*B*) Resolving genu valgum typical of a 6-year-old child.

continues to increase, internal tibial torsion is not a common finding during typical development. If internal tibial torsion is found during childhood, adolescence, or adulthood, it may have resulted from a lack of progression of typical tibial external rotation during early childhood or may be a compensation for rotational malalignment in the femur, hip, or foot.

Ankle and Foot

In general, the newborn foot is very flexible. The newborn talocrural (talus articulation with ankle mortice) joint rests in dorsiflexion and may have a plantar flexion limitation (Cusick, 1990). This dorsiflexed position is, again, the result of intrauterine posture, particularly during the last 2 to 3 months of gestation (LeVeau & Bernhardt, 1984). As gravity begins to have an effect on ankle motion, and as the child begins to move the ankle joint, the amount of plantar flexion increases quickly during the first year of life (Cusick, 1990).

The calcaneus and talus in the newborn foot are inclined medially as a result of intrauterine positioning and shortening of the medial structures (Cusick, 1990). The foot follows this medial slant so that the forefoot is also slightly inverted in the non-weight-bearing position (Bernhardt, 1988; McCrea, 1985). Therefore, both the rear foot and the forefoot are in varus positions in non–weight bearing. Despite this inverted posture, the infant's foot will appear everted when in supported stance. This appearance is caused by the medial forces placed on the foot in standing caused by the posture of hip abduction and lateral rotation, tibiofemoral varus, and the normal fat pad in the midfoot area.

The foot should have a straight lateral border regardless of its weight-bearing status. A foot that has a lateral border that is curved like a "C" has a metatarsus adductus, with an atypical adduction of the metatarsals. This is called a "packaging" problem attributed to intrauterine positioning and is differentiated from a "manufacturing" problem with a structural malformation or genetic cause (Williams, 1982).

Newborns have **flat feet** because of a thick fat pad covering the longitudinal arch of the midfoot and laxity of the joints of the midfoot (Staheli, Chew, & Corbett, 1987). The arch develops through early childhood and is generally observable in stance by approximately 4 years of age (Engel & Staheli, 1974). Flat feet in children up to 4 to 5 years of age are normal and do not require intervention; however, there is some controversy about whether to intervene in older children. The child with a pathological flat foot with pain or one that occurs along with a neuromuscular or musculoskeletal disorder such as Down syndrome or cerebral palsy may require intervention. This flat foot should be differentiated from the flexible flat foot of a young child or that of an older child with no other disability. Most authors agree that these flat feet do not require intervention. A recent study of children aged 11 to 15 years with flexible flat feet found that they did not differ from children without flat feet on athletic performance and motor skills (Tudor, Ruzic, Sestan, Sirola, & Prpic, 2009). Figure 5.10 is a picture of a child aged 4 years who is just beginning to show a longitudinal arch but still has a slight flat foot typical of this age.

Development of Gait

The development of independent walking is one of the most well studied motor activities in young children. Gait, like alignment, changes sequentially over time in a predictable fashion through growth, development, and practice. The postures seen in early gait are directly related to the alignment and postures described in the previous section as well as to growth and neurological maturation.

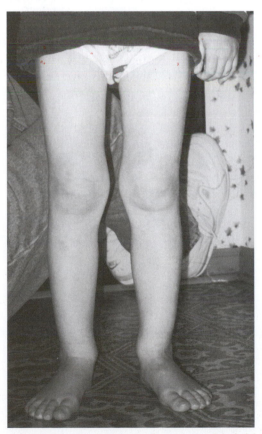

Figure 5.10 Flat feet typical of a 4-year-old child.

As with all developmental processes, there is variability in gait, some that are within typical limits and some that are not. When observing and examining gait in young children, it is important to know whether the variability in the joint or extremity under examination during gait is within the expected variability for appropriate clinical decisions. The intent of this section is to provide a brief description of the expected joint and extremity alignment changes during gait that evolve during childhood to assist the therapist in gait examination and decision making. Variability in joint angle, or kinematic patterns, is the highest in the youngest independent walkers and decreases rapidly with gait maturation (Ivanenko, Dominici, & Lacquaniti, 2007). Some of the variability is surprising. For example, although new walkers tend to have very short step lengths, it has been shown recently that infants occasionally take large steps, where step length is actually longer than leg length (Badaly & Adolph, 2008), suggesting that some infants have more balance and strength ability than traditionally thought.

For physical therapists, knowledge of the typical processes and variability of gait development is critical since walking is so often one of the main objectives of therapy. The purpose of this section is to provide a general foundation of how and when gait develops in young children. Gait development is a complex interaction of neurological, musculoskeletal, and biomechanical factors. Experience and opportunities for practice have also been shown to be important (Badaly & Adolph, 2008; Adolph, Vereijken, & Shrout, 2003) but there is also an innate maturational pattern.

The average age of walking is 12 months ± 3 months (Sutherland, Olshen, Biden, & Wyatt, 1988). Sutherland (1997) has reported that temporal-spatial gait parameters such as stride and step lengths and cadence are modified over time by both maturation and growth until approximately 4 years. After that point, changes in these temporal spatial characteristics are due mainly to changes in leg length. The kinematics, or joint angles, of children also mature and change over time. These changes have been well described by several authors, but most completely in children ages 1–7 years by Sutherland and colleagues in the 1988 monograph *The Development of Mature Walking*. The reader is directed to this volume for a detailed description of gait maturation.

According to Sutherland and colleagues (1980), there are five major indicators of mature gait:

1. *Single-leg stance.* Long one-leg stance time is an indication of increasing stability and balance. This variable increases the most rapidly between 1½ and

3½ to 4 years, when it reaches the adult value (Sutherland et al., 1997).

2. *Velocity, measured as distance/time.* As gait matures, velocity increases. The increase is linear between 1 and 7 years of age, but the rate of increase is greater from 1 to 3 years than from 4 to 7 years.

3. *Cadence, measured in number of steps per minute.* Cadence is very high in 1-year-old walkers and decreases with age the most rapidly between 1 and 2 years. It continues to decrease over time into adulthood. (Sutherland et al., 1988)

4. *Step length measured in distance.* Like velocity, step length increases linearly throughout childhood but most rapidly between 1 and 4 years compared to between 4 and 7 years (Dusing & Thorpe, 2007; Sutherland et al., 1997). This is because lower limb growth slows down after age 4 years (Kelly & Dimeglio, 2008; Sutherland et al., 1988). The youngest walkers take very short steps because of their leg lengths (Fig. 5.11A), but this increases with growth (Fig. 5.11B).

5. *Pelvic span to ankle spread ratio.* This is a gait laboratory measurement that defines the base of support by comparing the width of the pelvis to the width from ankle to ankle. This ratio increases over time, indicating that the base of support is narrowing with increases in time in single-limb stance and improving balance. Clinically, early walkers have a wide base of support during gait, which gradually changes as hip abduction and hip external rotation biases decrease and as stability in stance increases (Fig. 5.12). Joint angle parameters or kinematics during gait mature to adult levels by age 3½ to 4 years of age. (Sutherland, 1997)

In the following section, the joint positions and major changes that occur in the pelvis, hip, knee, and ankle during walking are described. The descriptions start at 1 year and are based on several classic works including

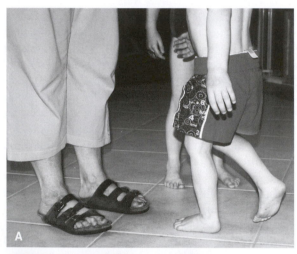

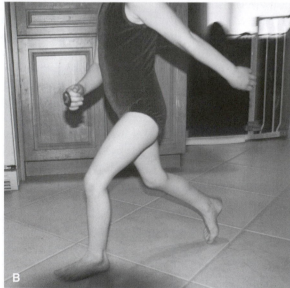

Figure 5.11 (*A*) Typical early walker with characteristically short step lengths. (*B*) Typical older walker with longer step lengths.

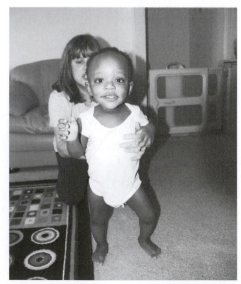

Figure 5.12 Externally rotated and abducted hips in a typical early walker.

Sutherland (1997; 1988). As you will see, these segmental and joint positions and motions are clearly reflective of the age-related developmental alignment detailed in the previous section.

Pelvis

The pelvis in the 1-year-old is anteriorly tilted and rotated during walking. Both of these decrease gradually to age 3 years. The anterior tilt in standing and during early walking is likely in part related to the presence of the typical hip flexion "contracture" as already described. Pelvic obliquity is quite different than that of the more mature child and adult. In the 1-year-old walker, the pelvis reaches its highest point during swing, not during stance as it does with a more mature gait. One of the reasons for this may be that the younger child has more hip abduction, effectively limiting the amount of pelvic elevation that can occur during stance. By age 3 years, this pattern reverses and becomes mature.

Hip

The hip stays flexed throughout the gait cycle in the 1-year-old and reaches approximately 0° of flexion by age 2 years. This occurs at approximately 50% of the gait cycle, when the other foot contacts the floor. Hip external rotation and abduction are also increased throughout the gait cycle (Fig 5.12). External rotation is greatest between ages 1 and 2 years. It continues to decrease after that but very little. Similarly, hip abduction is the greatest between ages 1 and 2½ years, with small changes thereafter. Both of these joint position biases change as the available joint ranges change through growth and maturity. As the hip external rotation and abduction positioning decreases, the child is better able to shift weight onto each leg, contributing to the increased time spent in single-leg stance and the building of stability and balance.

Knee

In the sagittal plane, the major change at the knee joint is the development of the flexion wave that occurs during loading response (LR), an important motion necessary for shock absorption in early stance. In the 1-year-old, the flexion wave is present, but the amount of flexion is small compared to the mature pattern, and the knee stays somewhat flexed after LR has ended. Gradually, the knee joint flexes a few more degrees at the beginning of LR and is followed by more extension. This creates a more developed and mature flexion wave. The pattern is similar to that of

an adult by age 4 years. As described above, the tibiofemoral angle in the 1-year-old is in slight varus but begins to take on a valgus attitude by age 2 years (Salenius & Vankka, 1975). This increases to approximately age 3–5 years, when it begins to resolve (Fig 5.9A & B).

Ankle

Several changes occur in the ankle from the early walker to the mature pattern. Heel contact is absent in the 1-year-old, who strikes the ground with a flat foot. A heel contact pattern is evident by approximately 2 years of age, which produces the more mature plantarflexion motion that lowers the foot to the floor directly after contact. The second change relates to dorsiflexion during swing. In the 1-year-old the amount of dorsiflexion is decreased, resulting, effectively, in a foot drop posture. However as already described, also during this time the pelvis is at its highest point, which assists the foot in clearing the floor. By age 1½ years the ankle begins to develop dorsiflexion in swing, while at the same time the high pelvic position is beginning to decrease.

One more interesting difference in the young walker compared to the more mature walker is the absence of a reciprocal arm swing in the young walker. The 1-year-old walker does not display an arm swing, but instead holds both arms in a fixed position called "**high guard.**" There is some variation in this pattern, but in general, the arms are held in some shoulder and elbow flexion, external rotation, and horizontal abduction (Fig. 5.13). Sutherland (1988) indicated that by age 1½ years the arms begin to come down and reciprocal arm swing begins to emerge. By age 3½ to 4 years, it was seen in all children. It has been suggested that the high guard pattern assists the child with balance and stability during upright forward locomotion. Additionally, the emergence of a reciprocal arm swing though walking experience is correlated with the decrease in the base of support, indicating improvement in balance (Ledebt, 2000).

Muscle

There are three general types of muscle tissue: skeletal, cardiac, and smooth. **Skeletal muscle**, also known as striated or voluntary muscle, is the focus of this section. Skeletal muscle fibers are developed from embryonic myoblast cells. The majority of human muscle fibers are present before birth, with the remainder being formed during the first year of life. After the first 4 years of life, the muscles need to continue to grow to match

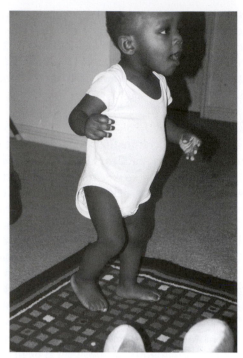

Figure 5.13 "High guard" position of the arms in a typical early walker.

increasing skeletal size; however, this is done entirely through hypertrophy of the existing muscle fibers, rather than addition of more fibers. Each muscle fiber is made up of smaller myofibrils. Additional myofibrils can be added to individual muscle fibers, and this process accounts for the majority of the circumferential growth of a muscle. New myofibrils are added to the periphery, expand, and then split to create more myofibrils. In addition to genetic predetermination, the demands put on the muscle through exercise will ultimately determine the muscle size. Longitudinal growth of muscle fibers is accomplished by adding additional sarcomeres to the muscle fiber at the ends of the muscle. A sarcomere is the contractile unit of a muscle and is composed of actin (thin) and myosin (thick) filaments.

There are two basic types of muscle fibers, which are classified by the speed of contraction and method for generating energy to perform the contraction:

● Type 1 slow-twitch oxidative fibers have a slow contraction time and a low level of anaerobic energy production. Type 1 fibers primarily use oxidative activity, which is best suited for low-level sustained activity.

● Type 2 muscle fibers have faster contraction speeds. The type 2 fibers are subdivided into two groups.
  • Type 2A fibers are considered intermediate fibers because they use both aerobic and anaerobic energy production and have a greater resistance to fatigue than the type 2B fibers.
  • Type 2B fibers are the most rapidly contracting fiber type and use primarily anaerobic energy production.

The percentage of each fiber type in any given muscle is dependent on the function of the muscle. The soleus muscle, for example, is primarily a postural muscle, which requires it to perform slow, prolonged contraction rather than bursts of high-intensity activity. The soleus muscle therefore has a higher concentration of type 1 fibers (Haggmark & Eriksson, 1979). The distribution of fiber types differs between individuals. Elite athletes have a higher proportion of the fiber type best suited for their sport. For example, sprinters have a higher proportion of type 2 fibers, whereas distance runners have more type 1 fibers (Pitman & Peterson, 1989). Genetic predisposition of fiber type distribution may be partially responsible for the natural selection of elite athletes (Pitman & Peterson, 1989).

Although there can be a mixture of fiber types in each muscle, a single nerve branch innervates only one fiber type. The impulse a muscle receives from a nerve appears to influence the type of muscle fiber. Sending external electrical impulses through a nerve (Munsat, McNeal, & Waters, 1976) or surgically transecting the nerve from one muscle to another (Dubowitz, 1967) has been shown to change fiber type orientation. This would suggest that fiber type distribution might be changed therapeutically to optimize motor performance.

Musculoskeletal Examination

There are many examination procedures for the child with musculoskeletal concerns. This portion of the chapter will discuss procedures used across many different impairments and the most important procedures for particular disorders. It is not possible to detail all available procedures, however, so the reader is encouraged to review the recommended readings at the end of the chapter.

Several principles should be followed regardless of the procedure. The examination should follow a consistent, logical sequence that is dictated by a careful, detailed history, observation of the child, discussion of present and historical symptoms, and determination of the child's and caregiver's goals. Children may not always be forthcoming with information, so the therapist must pay attention to the child's expressions and behavior during the examination to detect pain or discomfort with any procedures and ask questions if the child is able to answer.

The examination should be comprehensive but focused, so all salient procedures can be performed. This requires knowledge of the natural history of pediatric conditions so the therapist can focus the examination on critical areas. The age and developmental expectations of the child should form a framework for the examination to ensure there is appropriate evaluation of examination data. For example, when examining a neonate, the therapist must take into account the normal ROM limitations seen in newborns to avoid erroneous conclusions. In addition, the therapist needs to develop unusual and entertaining ways to keep the child engaged during the examination process. This involves establishing a rapport with the child, family, and other caregivers before beginning the examination. Preferably the examination can be done in the child's home or other familiar environment or, if a natural environment is not possible, a clinic area with age-appropriate decorations and toys to help put the child at ease. Getting onto the floor and playing with a young child, or talking to an older child about school or hobbies before the examination also helps develop rapport. Family members and caregivers can be valuable assistants during the examination in a number of ways, such as holding young children on their laps when possible, and helping older children feel comfortable sharing information with the therapist.

Once the examination has begun, the therapist must develop a systematic way of accurately recording and evaluating the data. Time is often limited by the child's endurance or clinic scheduling, so information must be gathered efficiently. The therapist must accurately document the examination results while trying to keep the child engaged. Having equipment readily available and a flexible strategy outlined will help the therapist proceed quickly from one activity to the next while keeping the child's attention and cooperation.

The therapist working with children must recognize that the examination and intervention will both need to be performed in ways that make the child feel as comfortable as possible. When a child is uncooperative, it is difficult to determine whether the child cannot or simply will not perform the activity. The use of games, toys, stickers, songs, and other age-appropriate activities will significantly improve cooperation and provide a more representative picture of the child's abilities. The caregiver can give you an idea of a young child's personality and favorite toys or activities so that you can best tailor the examination to the child. Finally, it is important when giving directions to talk directly to the child at a level appropriate for his or her age and understanding. In the following discussion of specific examination procedures, some ideas for implementation with children will be presented to assist in making the examination process a success.

Child and Family Goals

Family-centered care will allow the therapist to complete a succinct evaluation by first determining the child's and family's goals for the therapy. The therapist should always ask families why they are seeking physical therapy and what they hope to gain by intervention. Leading questions will enable the entire family to articulate their concerns, rather than just repeating something they were told by another professional. For example, asking the child or parent about what a typical day is like may start a discussion about a variety of important issues that impact daily life and that may be able to be addressed with therapy. For example, a child or parent is rarely worried about decreased ROM but could be bothered by having difficulty in putting on a shirt that makes getting ready for school problematic. Making the evaluation and intervention meaningful to the child should improve cooperation and adherence. Through the initial discussion, the therapist should determine the activities that are important to the child and family. Physical therapy goals and intervention should consider how impairments in body function and structure impact the child's participation in activities that are valued.

The therapist must also be culturally sensitive and family focused. Except in cases of abuse or neglect, the family is entitled to make decisions for the child that best meet the needs of the family, regardless of whether these decisions are in line with the therapist's values. For example, the therapist may want a child to begin to use powered mobility on a regular basis. If the parents are not ready to move forward with that plan, the therapist needs to respect their decision and continue to be available with support and information for a later time when they may be more ready to take that step. The family is in the best position to take into account all factors surrounding the current situation and to make the best overall decision. The therapist's job is to provide information about the medical condition, treatment potential, and complications. The therapist may try to guide the family toward a decision by providing information but must respect the family's decision unless the child is being put in danger.

History

A detailed history includes information gathered from many sources. In a pediatric examination, the therapist must listen carefully to the parents or other caregivers and, if the child is able to answer questions, ask questions of the child at the developmentally appropriate level. The therapist should allow enough time for the interview so that it can be done in a sympathetic, caring, and sensitive manner. Many families go through a grieving period when a child is diagnosed with a disorder and may display a range of emotions, such as sadness or anger. Sensitive interview techniques will allow the therapist to gain information without unnecessarily distressing the family.

Here is a short list of do's and don'ts for therapists to remember when interviewing parents and children:
   DO:

- Make eye contact.
- Use body language that shows that you are interested and actively listening.
- Use probing questions when necessary.
- Use lay language.
- Ask appropriate questions of the child in child-friendly language.
- Try to engage everyone who is part of the interview.
- Take notes if necessary.
- Always use people-first language.

DON'T:

- Repeat questions.
- Use technical jargon–laden language.
- Use judgmental language.
- Continue to probe an issue if the family has indicated that they are not willing to share any more information.

Birth history and developmental history are particularly important if the child has a multisystem disorder such as CP, Down syndrome, or myelomeningocele. However, even in a child with a specific segment disorder, such as limping, in- or out-toeing, torticollis, or knee pain, the birth and developmental histories may assist in differential diagnosis of the problem. History of illness and injury can assist in differential diagnosis of conditions that require referral for further orthopedic

evaluation. Determining developmental and functional status, as addressed in Chapters 2 and 3, is an important part of a comprehensive examination. The therapist documents pertinent historical information such as illnesses, medications, operations, school history, and previous therapies. Family history is also important since there are pediatric conditions that may be familial, such as scoliosis, back pain, and flat feet (Staheli, 2008). If the child presents with musculoskeletal pain, the therapist must carefully document the pain location, severity, and history. For each body segment, there are specific diagnoses that may present with pain. In the hip, for example, slipped capital femoral epiphysis (see Chapter 6) often presents with pain in the groin and anteromedial thigh and knee, along with an antalgic limp. The pain history is critical for the appropriate differential diagnosis and intervention or referral. Children who present with back pain should be taken seriously. There are many potential causes of back pain, but the following features are cause for concern and physician referral: night pain, interference with normal functional activities, persistence over 4 weeks, onset prior to age 4 years, neurological symptoms, recent onset of scoliosis, pain that is increasing, and systemic symptoms (Staheli, 2008). Make sure the parent has the opportunity to provide this information if the child cannot.

Observation

Before beginning any musculoskeletal examination, the child should be observed while playing and moving around spontaneously, unless the movements are limited by pain. This will help the therapist determine how the child's musculoskeletal status may be affecting functional activities and will allow the child time to acclimate to the examination setting. The therapist should interact with the child while playing to establish a nonthreatening rapport. During any spontaneous motion such as walking, observe the child's alignment, look for signs of pain, compensations, and gait deviations such as any type of limping, equinus or toe walking, or crouched gait. An astute, knowledgeable observer is able to assess quickly the child's movements and determine the most important tests and measures to perform. For example, a child who stands with one shoulder higher than the other should have a spine examination since this can be an indication of scoliosis. A child who stands with one leg in external rotation and abduction may have a leg length discrepancy. Another example is a child who presents with a limping gait, a common orthopedic complaint that is readily observed. The type of limping should be noted (i.e., antalgic versus Trendelenburg) since there are different causes of limping based on the type of limp and the age of the child. Existing algorithms can and should be utilized to categorize and organize the examination (Flynn & Widman, 2001). This can be done for different clinical conditions such as limping (Fig. 5.14) so that the therapist can utilize the appropriate tests and measures and plan for the correct intervention or referral. As an example, limping may be caused by trauma, hip dysplasia, or foot pain, all which have different physical findings and different gait patterns (Staheli, 2008).

Specific Musculoskeletal Tests and Measures

Leg Length

Leg length is an important measurement when the child presents with a limp, a pelvic obliquity, back pain, or an asymmetrical gait pattern. Leg length asymmetries are frequently seen in children with neuromuscular involvement.

Physical therapists traditionally have used either a tape measure or the block method for assessing leg length discrepancy. The most accurate method for documenting limb length is to use a tape measure

(Fig. 5.15). Beattie and colleagues (1990) compared tape measurements with measurements obtained through radiographs and found that the tape measurement technique yielded valid results. The child lies supine with hips and knees extended, and the measurement is taken between the most prominent point on the anterior superior iliac spine and the medial malleolus. It is important that the child lie quietly for tests of leg length, so before beginning, give the child a quiet toy to manipulate or a video to watch during the test. It may be helpful to talk to the child, tell a story, or sing a song to make sure that the supine position is maintained throughout the measurements. Parents and siblings can also assist during tests like this to keep the child interested and lying quietly. To improve accuracy, use a washable marker to identify bone landmarks, and use the average of two measurements (Beattie, Isaacson, Riddle, & Rothstein, 1990).

The block method is not advocated because of its poor reliability. In the block method, the child stands with his or her back to the therapist. The therapist palpates the iliac crests and determines visually if they are level. In a study by Mann, Glasheen-Wray, and Nyberg (1984), therapists were unable to consistently identify which side was higher. After the tape measure method is used to identify a leg length discrepancy, blocks might provide supplemental information about the

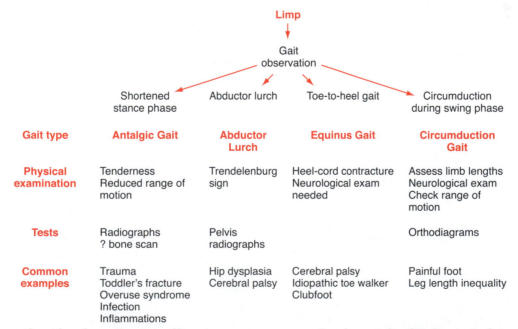

Gait type	Antalgic Gait	Abductor Lurch	Equinus Gait	Circumduction Gait
Physical examination	Tenderness Reduced range of motion	Trendelenburg sign	Heel-cord contracture Neurological exam needed	Assess limb lengths Neurological exam Check range of motion
Tests	Radiographs ? bone scan	Pelvis radiographs		Orthodiagrams
Common examples	Trauma Toddler's fracture Overuse syndrome Infection Inflammations	Hip dysplasia Cerebral palsy	Cerebral palsy Idiopathic toe walker Clubfoot	Painful foot Leg length inequality

Figure 5.14 Algorithm for evaluation of limping. *(Staheli, L. [2008].* Fundamentals of Pediatric Orthopedics *[p. 136]. Philadelphia: Lippincott Williams and Wilkins. Copyright 2008 by Staheli, Inc. Reprinted with permission.)*

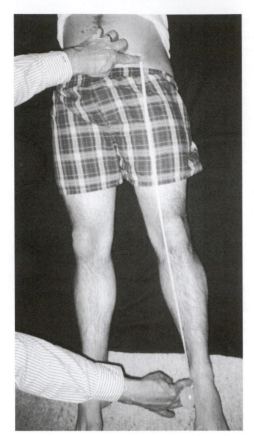

Figure 5.15 Measurement of leg length with a tape measure.

combined effects of other factors contributing to a functional leg length discrepancy, such as posture or lower extremity joint contractures.

The **Galeazzi sign,** or Allis test, is a quick screening method to assist in the determination of leg length equality. The Galeazzi sign is performed with the child supine, the hips and knees flexed, and the feet flat on the table (Fig. 5.16). The anterior-superior iliac spines are held level so a pelvic obliquity does not appear to cause a difference in the knee heights. Look to see if one knee is higher than the other; if so, this may be evidence that the legs need to be measured to quantify the difference. The therapist can also use a gravity-assisted angle finder placed across the knees to determine whether the knees are level. The Galeazzi sign is also used as one indication of hip joint integrity. If a child has a dislocated hip, the femur will slide posteriorly when the child is in the testing position, and therefore that femur will appear shorter than the other one. Tape measurements can be used to differentiate between a leg length discrepancy and a dislocated hip.

Range of Motion (ROM)

Joint ROM is an important component of any musculoskeletal examination. The therapist is attempting to find joints that have motion limitations, contractures, or excessive motion (see Tables 5.1, 5.2, and 5.3). A ROM examination can be difficult to achieve in children who are very young, apprehensive, and active or who generally have difficulty with the demands of the examination process. There are some ways in which the therapist can help the child tolerate the testing situation. One, as mentioned earlier, is to distract the child with songs, to provide small toys, and to enlist the help of caregivers to provide distraction. Another is to structure the ROM examination to cover all tests in one position before moving the child to another position. For example, perform all supine ROM tests and additional tests such as leg length measurements before moving to prone. In addition, if the examination is performed in a consistent order, it is less likely that tests will be missed or forgotten even when working with distractible youngsters. This is particularly important for the novice clinician.

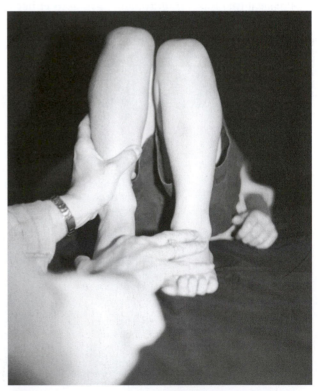

Figure 5.16 The Galeazzi sign, or Allis test. The lower knee of this child may indicate a leg length discrepancy and should be measured using the tape measure method.

Children with hypertonicity frequently have ROM deficits. Hypertonicity presents unique measurement difficulties. Illness, temperament, medication, and speed of movement can all affect the ROM of a child with hypertonicity (Gajdosik & Bohannon, 1987; Harris, Harthun-Smith, & Krukowski, 1985; Stuberg, Fuchs, & Miedaner, 1988). Both interrater and test-retest reliability in children with CP is difficult to achieve. Harris and colleagues (1985) examined goniometric reliability on a child with spastic quadriplegia. Measurements were within 10° of each other 57% to 100% of the time. Often clinical decisions are made based on a change of ROM of 10° or less. This study suggests that decisions based on ROM should be considered carefully, as the data may not be accurate. This study also suggests that therapists must evaluate their goniometric reliability.

Frequently, the therapist is measuring an angle to indicate the severity of the limitation and how it compares with a normative sample. Because there are age-related changes, measurements must be compared with an appropriate-age sample. Understanding that there is a wide range of normal values is critical. ROM tests relevant to children with common musculoskeletal disabilities will be discussed by segment, beginning proximally with the spine.

Spine

The spine should always be screened for scoliosis, a lateral spinal curvature, and excessive kyphosis, a forward curvature of the spine. The spine should be examined in standing and using the **Adams forward bend test** (Fig. 5.17).

To perform the forward bend test, the child bends forward with the arms hanging in front and the knees straight. The therapist stands behind and then in front of the child and assesses back symmetry. Asymmetry may be indicated by a prominence on one side of the back or the spine appearing curved when viewed from the top to the bottom. The forward bend is a screening procedure, not a definitive diagnostic test, so children with asymmetries should be referred for an examination including a scoliometer, which will help to quantify the curve and determine the need for further examination by a physician (Newton & Wenger, 2001). Additional findings on observation may be uneven iliac crest heights or shoulder heights. The child should also be viewed from the side to determine whether excessive kyphosis is seen. Some forward curvature is normally present, as is seen in the young man in Figure 5.17. However, excessive kyphosis is seen when the curve is

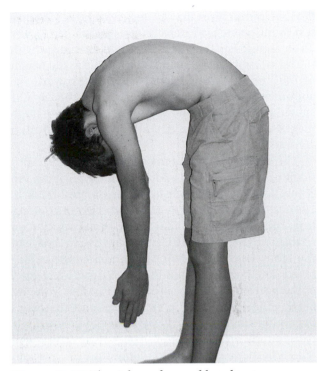

Figure 5.17 The Adams forward bend test.

more severe and angular. Other symptoms such as pain, lumbar muscle spasms, and hamstring tightness as well as pain during straight-leg raising are indications for a referral for further testing. These may be indicative of nerve root pathology (Newton & Wenger, 2001).

Idiopathic scoliosis refers to scoliosis of an unknown cause, and it may occur at any age in children without specific disabilities. Idiopathic scoliosis accounts for a majority of scoliosis cases; however, scoliosis may be indicative of an underlying cause such as a spinal tumor or congenital malformation (Newton & Wenger, 2001). Scoliosis also frequently develops in children with neuromuscular disorders, such as CP, Down syndrome, or myelomeningocele, so it is important that children with these disorders always be screened for scoliosis. Many school districts regularly screen school children for scoliosis, and a physical therapist employed by a school district may be involved in administering scoliosis screening.

Hip

In the sagittal plane, lack of hip extension is often a problem in children with CP caused by the tightness of the iliopsoas muscle group. Hip flexion contractures may also occur in children with juvenile rheumatoid arthritis and myelomeningocele. The presence of hip flexion contractures may be tested with the **Thomas test** or the prone hip extension test (Staheli, 1977). The Thomas test is done with the child in supine with the leg being tested hanging off the table at the height of the knee. The opposite hip is flexed toward the abdomen and held there to flatten out the lumbar spine, and the resulting angle that the other thigh makes with the surface is the amount of hip flexion contracture (Fig. 5.18).

The Thomas test is commonly used but may be difficult to do reliably in children with CP (Horstmann & Bleck, 2007). The **prone hip extension test** (Staheli, 1977) can also be used to assess hip flexion contracture. In this test, the child is in the prone position on a table with the opposite leg hanging over the edge of the table. In this position, the lumbar spine is flattened. The examiner holds the pelvis down at the level of the posterior superior iliac spines and pulls the leg being examined into hip extension until the pelvis begins to move anteriorly. At that point, the angle between the femur and the surface is measured and reflects the degree of hip flexion contracture (Horstmann & Bleck, 2007; Gross, 1995). It can be difficult to perform this test with large children because the therapist needs to hold the leg while simultaneously holding the goniometer and measuring the angle. However, this test has been shown to have better reliability than the Thomas test in children with spastic diplegic CP (Bartlett, Wolf, Shurtless, & Staheli, 1985) (Fig. 5.19).

Hip adduction and abduction ROM are both frontal plane motions. Hip adduction contractures (limitations in hip adduction), seen in certain types of CP, can result

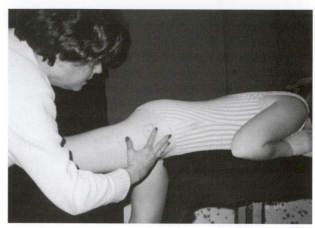

Figure 5.19 The Staheli test for hip flexion contracture.

from spasticity in the hip adductor muscles, often adductor longus and gracilis. These limitations can interfere with sitting balance, hygiene, and activities of daily living (Horstmann & Bleck, 2007). Hip abduction limitation is an important factor in the development of spastic hip disease and subluxed or dislocated hips in the child with CP (Miller, Dias, Dabney, Lipton, & Trianna, 1997; Reimers, 1980). The mechanics of hip problems in children with CP are discussed in more detail in Chapter 6. Adequate hip abduction allows the head of the femur to move into the acetabulum and is frequently limited in children with slipped capital femoral epiphysis and Legg-Calvé-Perthes disease.

Hip adduction limitations are frequently seen in juvenile rheumatoid arthritis (Scull, 2001). One method of assessing the amount of hip adduction is the **Ober test,** which indirectly measures contracture of the iliotibial band. The iliotibial band is the large flat band of thick fascia on the lateral border of the thigh that extends from the gluteal fascia from the iliac crest and the inferior border of the tensor fasciae latae muscle caudally to the fascia surrounding the popliteal area. This fascia may become tight and restricted with excessive hip external rotation or hip abduction, as seen in the gait of children with juvenile rheumatoid arthritis.

To perform the Ober test, the child is in sidelying position with the bottom hip flexed toward the chest. The top hip being measured is slightly flexed and abducted. The knee is either in extension or flexed to 90°. The hip is then pulled into extension and allowed to fall into adduction. If contracture is present, the hip is unable to adduct. As with many orthopedic tests,

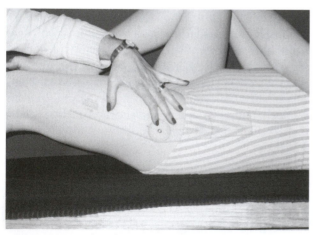

Figure 5.18 The Thomas test for hip flexion contracture.

achieving adequate reliability depends on using a consistent protocol. In adults, if the knee is flexed to 90°, it limits adduction more than if the knee is extended (Gajdosik, Sandler, & Marr, 2003; Melchione & Sullivan, 1993). Allowing the hip to move into flexion also distorts results. Therapists need to develop a consistent protocol for testing and document this with their results.

Measurement of the Ober test using a goniometer is shown in Figure 5.20. Instead of a goniometer, this may also be done with a gravity-referenced angle finder, as is shown in Figure 5.21. This gravity reference is very helpful in referencing either the horizontal or vertical axis or abduction.

Hip internal and external rotations are transverse plane motions that may be measured with the child in the sitting, supine, or prone position. The prone position, with the hip extended and the knees flexed to 90° with the tibia vertical, is the preferred position (Schoenecker & Rich, 2001). In prone, the pelvis can be held down, avoiding inaccurate rotation measures caused by upward and downward rolling of the pelvis during leg movement. The examiner holds one hand across the pelvis while the leg is rotated and the ranges are measured. A gravity-assisted angle finder may be used (Fig. 5.22).

Ryder's test, also called **Craig's test** and the **Trochanteric Prominence Angle Test**, is an estimation of the amount of femoral torsion. The objective of this test is to rotate the hip until the head and the neck of

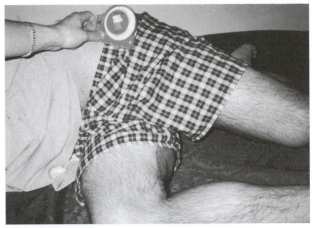

Figure 5.21 The Ober test measurement using a gravity-assisted angle finder.

the femur are on the frontal plane and then to measure the resulting hip rotation. To perform this test, the child may be prone, supine, or sitting. Figure 5.23 shows this test being performed in the sitting position. The hip may be flexed or extended, but the knee is flexed to 90°. The examiner holds the leg proximal to the ankle and rotates the hip medially and laterally while palpating the greater trochanter. When the trochanter reaches its most prominent lateral position, it is assumed that the head and the neck of the femur are on the frontal plane. The amount of hip rotation is measured at this point. Comparisons between this technique and computed tomography scans have shown that there is actually 20° more medial femoral torsion than the value obtained from this test (Cusick & Stuberg, 1992; Stuberg, Koehler, Witicha, Temme, & Kaplan, 1989), so 20° of internal rotation is added to the goniometric reading to

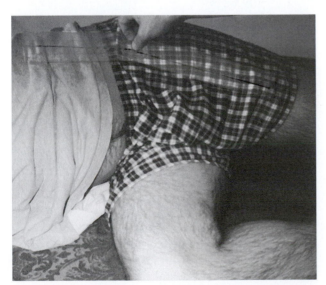

Figure 5.20 The Ober test measurement using a goniometer.

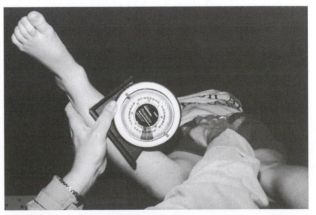

Figure 5.22 Measurement of hip internal rotation using a gravity-assisted angle finder.

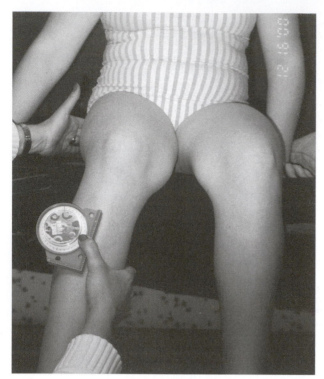

Figure 5.23 Ryder's test done sitting at the edge of a table.

determine a more accurate measure of femoral torsion. Therefore, if the obtained reading was 10° of internal rotation, the estimated measurement would be 30° femoral antetorsion. Similarly, if the examiner measures 25° of external hip rotation when the lateral trochanter is at its most prominent point, then when 20° is added, it would result in a negative number. This would be interpreted as –5° of femoral antetorsion or 5° of retrotorsion.

Knee

In the sagittal plane at the knee joint, it is important to measure knee extension, because hamstring flexibility may be a problem. A knee flexion contracture can be due to several factors including short hamstrings, anterior pelvic tilt, reduced ankle dorsiflexion ROM, and capsular limitation (Gage, Schwartz, Koop & Novacheck, 2009). To measure the length of the hamstring muscle group and estimate the amount of knee flexion contracture, the straight leg test, popliteal angle test, or hamstring length test may be performed. The popliteal angle test is typically done with neonates and is a measure of physiological flexion. The test is

performed in supine with the hip and knee of the leg being measured flexed to 90° (Fig. 5.24). The contralateral leg is stabilized down against the surface while the testing leg is extended up into the air. The goniometer is placed with the axis at the knee joint and the arms along the long axes of the leg and thigh. The angle that is measured is that between the leg and the thigh.

The procedure for the **hamstring length test** is the same as the popliteal angle test with the exception that the angle recorded is the amount of ROM that is *missing* or lacking from full knee extension. The angle measured by the goniometer is subtracted from 180° to yield the hamstring length test. This test measures the length of the hamstring muscles because they are stretched over both the hip and knee joints in this test. The amount of the measured popliteal angle that is due to anterior pelvic tilt can be assessed with the **bilateral**

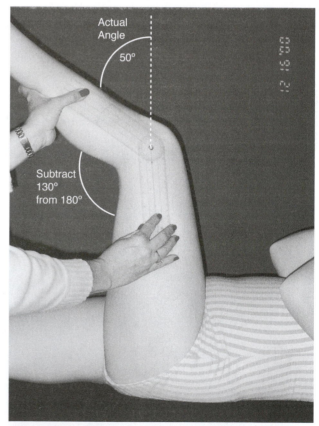

Figure 5.24 Measurement of hamstring length test. The measured angle is subtracted from the full vertical of 180° to yield the actual angle. In this case, the angle would be 50°.

popliteal angle test (Gage et al., 2009, p. 193). This test is performed in supine by flexing the test leg to 90° of hip and knee flexion as described above, but instead of stabilizing the contralateral leg against the table, it is placed so that the pelvis is in neutral, flat against the table. If the position of the pelvis is a significant contributor to the hamstring length, there will be more hamstring length as the pelvis moves posteriorly. This "hamstring shift" suggests that the true or anatomical amount of hamstring length is best measured with the pelvis flat against the table; however, the functional measure of hamstring length is best evaluated with the pelvis in the relaxed, lordotic position (Gage et al., 2009). This is a useful test for children with cerebral palsy who often have an excessive posterior pelvic tilt that can produce functionally shortened hamstrings in the upright position.

When there is a limitation in knee flexion ROM, the hamstring test evaluates the contribution of the hamstring length to the problem. To evaluate the contribution of other structures in the knee to the limitation, the **straight-leg test** can be used. In neutral hip extension, the hamstrings are in a slackened state and the knee flexion contracture is attributed to other causes (Fig. 5.25). The child is placed in a relaxed supine position with the hips in neutral rotation. The knee should rest against the table except in the young infant, who will have a normal, temporary flexion contracture as discussed previously.

In the frontal plane at the knee joint, varus and valgus should be measured. This test should begin with an observation of the knees in the supine position to delete the effects of rotation, weakness, and knee flexion (Rang, 1993a). There are two methods for measuring varus and valgus. In the standing position, if valgus is present, the distance between the medial malleoli is measured with a tape measure with the patella directly forward and the knees touching; if varus is present, the distance between the femoral condyles is measured with the malleoli touching (Fig. 5.26).

Another method in standing or supine position is to line up the patellae facing forward, with the axis of the goniometer over the knee joint. One arm of the goniometer is placed over the long axis of the thigh pointing toward the anterior superior iliac spine (ASIS) and the other arm along the long axis of the tibia pointing toward the middle of the ankle (Cahuzac, Vardon, & Sales de Gauzy, 1995; Heath & Staheli, 1993) (Fig. 5.27).

In the transverse plane, tibial torsion should be measured. Tibial torsion is the normal rotation between the proximal and distal ends of the tibia and, again, values greater than two standard deviations from the mean for an age group are considered atypical. This is measured in two ways. The **thigh-foot angle test** is an estimate of tibial torsion because it measures the angular difference between the thigh and foot axes (Schoenecker & Rich, 2001; Staheli, 1992). The child is in the

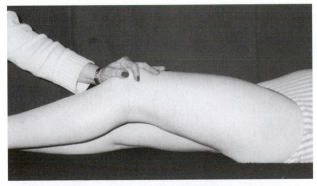

Figure 5.25 Example of knee flexion contracture seen with hip extension to slacken hamstrings.

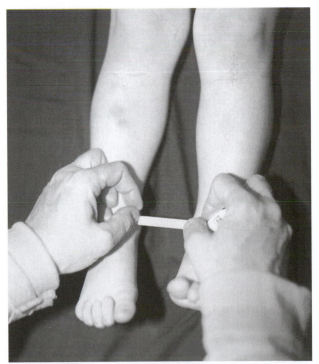

Figure 5.26 The distance between malleoli is measured with the knees touching in supine or standing, yielding a measure of knee valgus.

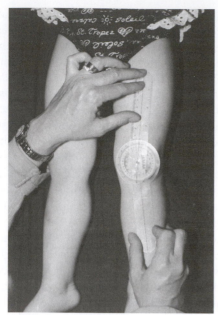

Figure 5.27 Measurement of knee valgus using a goniometer in supine position.

prone position with the thighs parallel, in neutral rotation, the hips extended, and the knee flexed to 90°, and the ankle is allowed to fall into a neutral position of 90° (Staheli, 1992). The axis of the goniometer is placed over the center of the calcaneus, the stationary arm is placed along a visual bisection of the thigh, and the moveable arm is placed on the long axis of the foot along the second metatarsal (Fig. 5.28). The resulting angle is measured. The convention is to assign a negative value to a measurement that points in toward the midline (internal tibial version or torsion) and a

positive value to a measurement that points away from the midline (external tibial version or torsion).

The thigh-foot angle test, although it is a quick and relatively accurate screen, may present validity problems if there is a foot deformity (such as a metatarsus adductus) (Lee, Chung, Park, Choi, & Cho, 2009; Tolo, 1996). In this case, the **transmalleolar angle test** should be performed. The transmalleolar angle test uses the same position but different landmarks. A line is drawn that connects the medial and lateral malleoli (the transmalleolar axis). A second line perpendicular to the first that bisects the calcaneus is drawn and a line through the long axis of the femur is visualized. Figure 5.29 shows the landmarks drawn onto a schematic of the foot and thigh and the resulting angle that is measured. This angle would be measured with a goniometer. The angle measured is between the long axis of the femur and the bisection of the calcaneus. This eliminates the forefoot from the measurement so that forefoot problems will not cause an invalid measurement. The negative and positive conventions are the same as for the thigh-foot angle test; that is, a measurement that points toward the midline is a negative value and a measurement that points away from the midline is a positive value. The interrater reliability and concurrent validity of these two methods were compared recently against a CT scan. The reliability of the transmalleolar test was greater than that of the thigh-foot angle test, and both had acceptable validity with the transmalleolar axis test having a somewhat higher value than the thigh-foot angle test (Lee et al., 2009).

Knee joint stability can also be assessed with tests commonly used on adults. Examples are the Lachman test to examine for tears of the anterior cruciate ligament and tests for collateral ligaments and varus/valgus. These tests are also useful when assessing

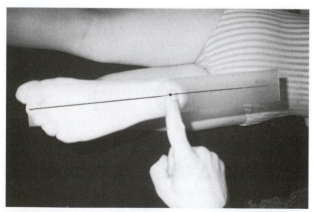

Figure 5.28 Measurement of the thigh-foot angle.

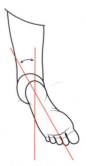

Figure 5.29 Landmarks for the measurement of the transmalleolar angle, indicated by the black arrow.

the knee joint in athletes as well as in children with disorders such as Down syndrome or Ehlers-Danlos syndrome. In children with known or suspected hypermobility syndromes, the therapist must perform these tests carefully since less force is required and tissues are more fragile (Simmonds & Keer, 2007). When there is anterior knee pain or a history of ligamentous laxity, patellar stability can also be examined using the patellar apprehension test. This test is performed with the child in sitting with the knee flexed to 30°. The patella is moved gently laterally while watching the child for signs of discomfort. If this is uncomfortable, the finding is positive for patellar instability. Patellar instability and dislocation are common in children with Down syndrome but are usually asymptomatic and do not require intervention (Dugdale & Renshaw, 1986). If they are symptomatic, nonsurgical intervention is generally the first course of intervention, followed by surgery if conservative measures are not successful (Caird, Wills, & Dormans, 2006).

Foot and Ankle

Measurements of a child's foot and ankle can be difficult to make. Ankle dorsiflexion is measured as in adults; however, extra care should be taken to hold the foot in slight inversion and not allow the midfoot to move independently of the rear foot. If there is a limitation in the length of the gastrocnemius-soleus complex, the foot may bend at the midfoot (talocalcaneonavicular and calcaneocuboid joints) and incorrectly appear as dorsiflexion. Holding the ankle in slight inversion locks the midtarsal joint so that midfoot bending will not occur (Horstmann & Bleck, 2007; Mosca, 2001). If there is a limitation of motion with the knee extended, then the test should also be performed with the knee flexed. This will assist in differentiating whether the limitation is in the soleus, the gastrocnemius, or the talocrural joint. If the ROM is more limited with the knee in extension, the gastrocnemius muscle is responsible for the limitation (Gage et al., 2009; Horstmann & Bleck, 2007). This is called the Silverskiöld test.

There are many ways to examine the foot. In general, the foot posture should be observed in both weight bearing and non–weight bearing. The lateral border of the foot should be straight, not curved. A curvature may indicate a metatarsus adductus that occurs when the metatarsals are adducted toward the midline. The amount of metatarsus adductus can be classified by drawing a straight line that bisects the heel and continues through the long axis of the foot (Horstmann &

Bleck, 2007). In a normally aligned foot, this line should pass between the second and third toes. In metatarsus adductus, the toes are medial to the line. If the distal projection of the line passes between the third and fourth toes, it is considered moderate, and if the line passes through the fourth and fifth toes, it is considered severe metatarsus adductus. In mild cases, there is often a spontaneous resolution; however, in moderate or severe cases, intervention with stretching, corrective shoes, or casting may be required (Staheli, 2008; Wenger, 1993a). These are used to reverse the excessive compressive forces on the tarsal and metatarsal bones because, according to the Hueter-Volkmann principle discussed earlier, these abnormal compressive forces will alter growth (Wenger, 1993a).

The position during weight bearing should be observed for arch development and position of the rear foot. As discussed in developmental biomechanics, children younger than 3 to 4 years will not have a longitudinal arch, so flat feet are typical in this age group. To estimate the arch height, the arch index, developed for adults (Cavanagh & Rogers, 1987) has been used with children (Gilmour & Burns, 2001; Kanatli et al., 2006; Mickle, Steele, & Munro, 2006). For a static measure of arch height, the bottom of the foot is inked and the child stands with even weight distribution on both feet. The footprint is then divided into thirds, excluding the toes. To calculate the arch index, the area of the middle third is divided by the total foot print area. This can also be done during gait for a dynamic measure. For the full instructions, refer to Cavanagh and Rogers (1987). It should be noted that recent literature suggests that this measure may be confounded by increased body adiposity in adults. Therefore, the results should be interpreted carefully in children who are overweight or obese (Wearing et al., 2004). It is also important to remember that young children will have a more medial weight-bearing pattern until the arch forms, as discussed earlier. Another arch index measure using a footprint is calculated by dividing the width of the arch by the width of the heel (Staheli et al., 1987).

Flat feet in older children may be flexible or rigid. **Flexible flat feet** have little or no arch when standing, caused by calcaneal valgus. Extension of the great toe or standing on tiptoes will cause the arch to reappear (Gage et al., 2009), and the heel will realign into slight varus (Wenger, 1993b). If an arch cannot be elicited and there is limited subtalar ROM, it is a **rigid flat foot**. A rigid flat foot signals a problem such as a vertical talus or a tarsal coalition and should be examined in more detail by an orthopedic surgeon. When examining children, the use of a treatment algorithm can assist the physical therapist in determining which flat foot should be referred for further medical evaluation and management (Staheli, 2008). A *congenital vertical talus,* a rare condition in children (Scoles, 1988), is more prevalent in children with CP or myelomeningocele and is defined as a superior dislocation of the talonavicular joint (Rang, 1993b). The head of the talus lies below the navicular bone, producing what is termed a "rocker-bottom foot deformity." In a **rocker-bottom foot deformity,** there is no arch and the foot curves downward where the arch would typically be present. This deformity should be evaluated by an orthopedic surgeon and is generally treated by surgery. A **tarsal coalition** is a congenital fusion of tarsal bones and may involve several different tarsal bones. The two most common tarsal coalitions are calcaneonavicular and talocalcaneal (Nalaboff & Schweitzer, 2008). The fusion can be fibrous, cartilaginous, or osseous. The incidence of tarsal coalitions has been noted to be approximately 1% (Stormont & Peterson, 1983), but more current literature indicates that those numbers are for those of osseous origin only. When those of fibrous and cartilaginous origin are added, the incidence increases to approximately 12% (Nalaboff & Schweitzer, 2008), making these more common than previously thought. These can cause foot pain and are the most common causes of rigid flat feet in children (Cass & Camasta, 2010). These may be asymptomatic but need to be treated if they cause pain (Staheli, 2008).

The decision to treat a flexible flat foot is somewhat controversial; however, there is little scientific evidence that intervention for asymptomatic flat feet is warranted (Pfeiffer, Kotz, Ledl, Hauser, & Sluga, 2006; Staheli et al., 1987; Wenger, Mauldin, Speck, Morgan, & Lieber, 1989). Children who are overweight or obese have been shown to have lower arches than their counterparts who are not overweight, suggesting that there may be changes in foot structure in these children (Dowling, Steele, & Baur, 2004; Gilmour & Burns, 2001; Mickle, Steele, & Munro, 2006). The physical therapist should consider a foot structure examination in children who are obese if they present with foot pain. If persistent pain is present or gross motor skills are affected, further examination is necessary to rule out a deformity such as a tarsal coalition or a vertical talus, as discussed previously. It is important to measure the ROM of the gastrocnemius-soleus complex in children with flat feet, because limitation is shown to be a causative factor in the development of flat feet with calcaneal valgus (Harris & Beath, 1948). If limitations are noted, the parents and child should be instructed in passive and self-stretching techniques.

Strength

Strength is an extremely important component of function and the ability of the child to perform age-appropriate gross motor activities. In children with typical development, many skills have a component of strength that is needed for competency in that task. For example, the ability of a young child to ride a tricycle is partly attributed to having the strength to push the pedals. The abilities to jump, hop, and climb stairs all need muscular strength for achievement in addition to all of the other components needed, such as adequate ROM, balance, and sensory processing. Improvement in strength has been shown to improve ambulation ability in children with CP (Damiano, Kelly, & Vaughn, 1995; Kramer & MacPhail, 1994). In addition, children with CP were able to show improvements in gross motor abilities (Dodd, Taylor, & Damiano, 2002; Kramer & MacPhail, 1994) after strength training, indicating the importance of strength to daily activities.

The examination of strength capabilities gives the therapist more information for a physical therapy diagnosis. There are many ways to test strength. In very young babies, movement against gravity, such as kicking in the air, the pull-to-sit maneuver, and the ability to lift the head in the prone position, are all indications of strength. In the toddler and preschool child, strength-assessing maneuvers include getting up from the floor using a half-kneeling, jumping, standing on one foot, ascending and descending stairs, and standing on tiptoes. It is useful to look at these functional measures of strength because they give the examiner an idea of how the child uses his or her strength. Games such as "Simon Says" help ensure that the child understands the task, cooperates, and gives the most representative effort. A demonstration is also helpful.

Manual muscle testing can be done with children who are old enough to understand the directions and remain in test positions, generally by age 3 to 4 years. When testing young children, the grades of 0 (no activity), 1 (contraction is palpated but no movement), 2 (full ROM with gravity eliminated), and 3 (full ROM) are used as with adults. There is more subjectivity in grades 4 (full ROM with some resistance) and 5 (full ROM with full resistance), because force must be adjusted based on the child's age. If more objective measurement is needed, handheld dynamometry is preferred (Connolly, 1995).

Children aged 3 to 4 years may be tested reliably with a standard handheld dynamometer as long as they understand the directions and are given verbal praise to help them put forth their best effort (Gajdosik, Nelson, & Gleason, 1994). It has also been shown to be reliable in children with CP (Pax Lowes, Westcott, Palisano, Effgen, & Orlin, 2004), spina bifida (Effgen & Brown, 1992), juvenile rheumatoid arthritis (Wessel et al., 1999), spinal muscular atrophy (Merlini, Mazzone, Solari, & Morandi, 2002), and muscular dystrophy (Stuberg & Metcalf, 1988), and in adolescents with intellectual disabilities (Horvat, Croce, & Roswal, 1994). It is important that the child be given clear instructions and the opportunity to practice the desired movement. Handheld dynamometry eliminates the need to estimate resistance based on the child's age and is therefore more objective than manual muscle testing when resistance is possible. Several studies have published standardized positions and methods for lower extremity dynamometry for children (Berry, Giuliani, & Damiano, 2004; Crompton, Galea, & Phillips, 2007; Wiley & Damiano, 1998).

Average values for handheld dynamometry for a small sample of children aged 4 to 16 years without motor impairment are presented in Table 5.4. The study had only a small sample at each age (n = 9 to 13). The size of the standard deviation should also be noted. A large standard deviation suggests that there is variability in the normal sample. In general, a child would have to fall two standard deviations below the mean to be considered "abnormal." In a small sample size, the standard deviations may be unusually large. So the numbers and standard deviations are only general guidelines until a more normative database is generated. In general, force abilities in this study were similar between girls and boys until about age 14 years, with the exception that 10-year-old girls showed a growth spurt and were stronger than the boys (Beenakker, van der Hoeven, Fock, & Maurits, 2001). The authors found a strong correlation between force and the child's weight (Beenakker et al., 2001). This should be considered when testing children with disabilities, because they can be significantly lighter than typically developing peers.

Summary

The musculoskeletal system is an integral part of the overall health and well-being of children both with and without neurological complications. A systematic assessment of the musculoskeletal system, guided by patient complaints, will allow the therapist to formulate orthopedic-based intervention strategies that will complement neurological techniques.

Working with children requires the ability to play while being organized to maximize the child's attention span and assess as many items as possible. The therapist must remain flexible and change the routine if the child is hesitant to cooperate. By establishing rapport with the child and performing assessments in the natural environment or at least in a child-friendly environment, the therapist should be able to examine and evaluate the child's typical performance.

DISCUSSION QUESTIONS

1. How would you organize an initial assessment of a 2-year-old child?

2. Describe how decreased lower extremity weight bearing would affect hip joint development.

3. How would you assess a 4-year-old with flat feet? What factors would influence your recommendations to the family?

4. What are the most important factors related to the development of a "typical" walking pattern in a young child?

5. What motor experiences do you think are critical to provide to a child who is just learning to walk?

Recommended Readings

Horstmann, H.M., & Bleck, E.E. (2007). *Orthopedic management in cerebral palsy* (2nd ed.). London: Mac Keith Press.

Magee, D. (2008), *Orthopedic physical assessment atlas and video: Selected special tests and movements.* St. Louis: Elsevier.

Staheli, L.T. (2008). *Fundamentals of pediatric orthopedics* (4th ed., p. 177). Philadelphia: Wolters Kluwer, Lippincott Williams & Wilkins.

Stout, J. (2012). Chapter E1: Gait, development and analysis. In S.K. Campbell, R.J. Palisano, & M.N. Orlin (Eds.), *Physical therapy for children* (4th ed.). St. Louis: Elsevier.

Sutherland, D.H., Olshen, R.A., Biden, E.N., & Wyatt, M.P. (1988). *The development of mature walking.* Oxford: Mac Keith Press

Table 5.4 Force Output in Newtons (kg • m • s^2) for Boys and Girls Aged 4 to 16 Years

Muscle Group		4	5	6	7	8	9	10	11	12	13	14	15	16
Neck flexors	Boys			48 (9)*	64 (11)	56 (8)	66 (9)	74 (20)	67 (13)	70 (16)	98 (40)	129 (42)	143 (36)	141 (33)
	Girls			55 (8)	60 (7)	56 (10)	55 (12)	55 (25)	67 (15)	76 (15)	92 (17)	96 (15)	108 (27)	87 (14)
Shoulder abductors	Boys	62 (20)	55 (10)	97 (27)	92 (29)	98 (19)	110 (31)	136 (26)	110 (39)	118 (29)	159 (46)	205 (44)	219 (36)	253 (54)
	Girls	68 (26)	47 (9)	75 (17)	91 (18)	94 (25)	91 (27)	81 (17)	129 (25)	123 (27)	154 (26)	178 (18)	173 (29)	173 (38)
Elbow extensors	Boys			73 (8)	85 (16)	90 (18)	89 (22)	120 (18)	103 (31)	104 (31)	128 (42)	158 (42)	175 (46)	182 (64)
	Girls			73 (8)	85 (14)	82 (10)	91 (24)	84 (20)	108 (25)	117 (24)	118 (26)	129 (23)	141 (37)	107 (36)
Elbow flexors	Boys	78 (24)	70 (12)	103 (21)	121 (32)	124 (23)	134 (24)	173 (19)	153 (30)	160 (25)	195 (26)	253 (50)	287 (55)	276 (68)
	Girls	69 (21)	66 (12)	105 (9)	103 (20)	115 (16)	125 (28)	134 (21)	172 (25)	168 (28)	201 (23)	193 (32)	198 (48)	215 (30)
Wrist extensors	Boys			77 (11)	89 (26)	87 (15)	97 (15)	121 (21)	100 (19)	108 (21)	153 (42)	195 (41)	218 (49)	237 (58)
	Girls			66 (6)	74 (13)	75 (11)	80 (21)	80 (17)	112 (16)	127 (23)	152 (14)	155 (6)	166 (26)	147 (28)
Hip flexors	Boys			182 (39)	182 (57)	225 (40)	232 (53)	261 (74)	245 (65)	198 (38)	289 (60)	337 (66)	301 (69)	395 (102)
	Girls			162 (31)	184 (50)	175 (36)	195 (48)	177 (25)	264 (55)	232 (61)	308 (51)	281 (72)	288 (70)	301 (42)
Hip abductors	Boys			128 (40)	124 (32)	131 (30)	153 (33)	174 (47)	151 (63)	158 (41)	225 (58)	306 (83)	356 (87)	312 (106)
	Girls			109 (26)	122 (24)	117 (18)	124 (35)	104 (25)	140 (22)	171 (44)	227 (52)	244 (30)	257 (68)	244 (59)
Knee extensors	Boys			156 (33)	157 (38)	185 (41)	194 (30)	267 (47)	239 (65)	225 (43)	296 (70)	370 (61)	362 (76)	396 (90)
	Girls			148 (24)	177 (47)	166 (30)	173 (57)	198 (57)	265 (36)	250 (71)	346 (49)	280 (69)	325 (79)	373 (81)
Knee flexors	Boys	111 (15)	105 (20)	158 (38)	180 (45)	185 (20)	195 (40)	268 (48)	218 (64)	201 (34)	273 (59)	307 (64)	327 (76)	382 (80)
	Girls	92 (25)	99 (15)	154 (33)	171 (35)	160 (23)	180 (54)	175 (29)	246 (52)	221 (54)	301 (38)	271 (76)	282 (61)	336 (57)
Ankle dorsiflexors	Boys	71 (22)	76 (23)	104 (11)	130 (26)	137 (24)	141 (31)	154 (18)	149 (26)	170 (28)	218 (55)	257 (60)	267 (50)	291 (60)
	Girls	75 (20)	76 (15)	95 (17)	114 (18)	121 (17)	137 (32)	130 (21)	178 (25)	177 (34)	214 (29)	207 (31)	220 (40)	232 (30)

*Values given as mean (SD) in Newtons (kg • m • s^2) (n = 7 to 13 per age group).

Source: Beenakker, E.A., van der Hoeven, J.H., Fock, J.M., & Maurits, N.M. (2001). Reference values of maximum isometric muscle force obtained in 270 children aged 4–16 years by hand-held dynamometry. *Neuromuscular Disorders, 11*(5), 441–446. Copyright 2001 by Elsevier. Reprinted with permission.

References

Adolph, K.E., Vereijken, B., & Shrout, P.E. (2003). What changes in infant walking and why. *Child Development, 74*(2), 475–479.

Apkon, S.D. (2002). Osteoporosis in children who have disabilities. *Physical Medicine and Rehabilitation Clinics of North America, 13*(4), 839–855.

Badaly, E., & Adolph, K.E. (2008). Beyond the average: Walking infants take steps longer than their leg length. *Infant Behavior & Development, 31*, 554–558.

Bartlett, M.D., Wolf, L.S., Shurtless, D.B., & Staheli, L.T. (1985). Hip flexion contractures: A comparison of measurement methods. *Archives of Physical Medicine and Rehabilitation, 66*, 620–625.

Beattie, P., Isaacson, K., Riddle, D.L., & Rothstein, J. (1990). Validity of derived measurements of leg-length differences obtained by use of a tape measure. *Physical Therapy, 70*(3), 150–157.

Beenakker, E.A., van der Hoeven, J.H., Fock, J.M., & Maurits, N.M. (2001). Reference values of maximum isometric muscle force obtained in 270 children aged 4–16 years by hand-held dynamometry. *Neuromuscular Disorders, 11*(5), 441–446.

Beeson, P. (1999). Frontal plane configuration of the knee in children. *The Foot, 9*, 18–26.

Bernhardt, D. (1988). Prenatal and postnatal growth and development of the foot and ankle. *Physical Therapy, 68*(12), 1831–1839.

Berry, E.T., Giuliani, C.A., & Damiano, D.L. (2004). Intrasession and intersession reliability of handheld dynamometery in children with cerebral palsy. *Pediatric Physical Therapy, 16*(4), 191–198.

Bleck, E.E. (1982). The shoeing of children: Sham or science. *Developmental Medicine and Child Neurology, 13*, 188–195.

Bourrin, S., Palle, S., Genty, C., & Alexandre, C. (1995). Physical exercise during remobilization restores a normal bone trabecular network after tail suspension-induced osteopenia in young rats. *Journal of Bone and Mineral Research, 10*(5), 820–828.

Cahuzac, J.P., Vardon, D., & Sales de Gauzy, J. (1995). Development of the clinical tibiofemoral angle in normal adolescents: A study of 427 normal subjects from 10 to 16 years of age. *Journal of Bone and Joint Surgery (British), 77*(5), 729–732.

Caird, M.S., Wills, B.P.D., & Dormans, J.P. (2006). Down syndrome in children: The role of the orthopedic surgeon. *Journal of the American Academy of Orthopedic Surgeons, 14*, 610–619.

Cass, A.D., & Camasta, C.A. (2010). A review of tarsal coalition and pes planovalgus: Clinical examination, diagnostic imaging and surgical planning. *The Journal of Foot & Ankle Surgery, 49*, 274–293.

Cavanagh, P.R., & Rodgers, M.M. (1987). The arch index: A useful measure from footprints. *Journal of Biomechanics, 20*, 547-51

Cimaz, R. (2002). Osteoporosis in childhood rheumatic diseases: Prevention and therapy. *Best Practice & Research in Clinical Rheumatology, 16*(3), 397–409.

Connolly, B. (1995). Testing in infants and children. In H.J. Hislop & J. Montgomery (Eds.), *Daniels and Worthingham's muscle testing* (6th ed., pp. 235–260). Philadelphia: W.B. Saunders.

Crompton, J., Galea, M.P., Phillips, B. (2007). Hand-held dynamometry for muscle strength measurement in children with cerebral palsy. *Developmental Medicine & Child Neurology, 49*, 106–111.

Cusick, B. (1990). *Progressive casting and splinting for lower extremity deformities in children with neuromotor dysfunction.* Tucson, AZ: Therapy Skill Builders.

Cusick, B.D., & Stuberg, W.A. (1992). Assessment of lower-extremity alignment in the transverse plane: Implications for management of children with neuromotor dysfunction. *Physical Therapy, 72*, 3–15.

Damiano, D.L., Kelly, L.E., & Vaughn, C.L. (1995). Effects of quadriceps femoris muscle strengthening on crouch gait in children with spastic diplegia. *Physical Therapy, 75*, 658–667.

Davids, J.R., Wenger, D.R., & Mubarak, S.J. (1993). Congenital muscular torticollis: Sequela of intrauterine or perinatal compartment syndrome. *Journal of Pediatric Orthopedics, 13*, 1–7.

Dodd, K.J., Taylor, N.F., & Damiano, D.L. (2002). A systematic review of the effectiveness of strength-training programs for people with cerebral palsy. *Archives of Physical Medicine and Rehabilitation, 83*, 1157–1164.

Dowling, A.M., Steele, J.R., & Baur, L.A. (2004). What are the effects of obesity in children on plantar pressure distributions? *International Journal of Obesity and Related Metabolic Disorders, 28*(11), 1514–1519.

Drews, J.E., Vraciu, J.K., & Pellino, G. (1984). Range of motion of the joints of the lower extremities of newborns. *Physical and Occupational Therapy in Pediatrics, 4*(2), 49–62.

Dubowitz, V. (1967). Pathology of experimentally re-innervated skeletal muscle. *Journal of Neurology, Neurosurgery and Psychiatry, 30*(2), 99–110.

Dugdale, T.W., & Renshaw, T.S. (1986). Instability of the patellofemoral joint in Down syndrome. *Journal of Bone & Joint Surgery, American, 68*, 405–413.

Dusing, S.C., & Thorpe, D.E. (2007). A normative sample of temporal and spatial gait parameters in children using the GAITRite® electronic walkway. *Gait & Posture, 25*, 135–139.

Effgen, S.K., & Brown, D.A. (1992). Long-term stability of hand-held dynamometric measurements in children who have myelomeningocele. *Physical Therapy, 72*, 458–465.

Engel, G.M., & Staheli, L.T. (1974). The natural history of torsion and other factors influencing gait in childhood. *Clinical Orthopedics and Related Research, 99*, 12–17.

Fabry, G., MacEwen, G.D., & Shands, A.R., Jr. (1973). Torsion of the femur. A follow-up study in normal and abnormal conditions. *Journal of Bone and Joint Surgery, 55-A*(8), 1726–1738.

Flynn, J.M., & Widman, R.F. (2001). The limping child: Evaluation and diagnosis. *Journal of the American Academy of Orthopedic Surgery, 9*(2), 89–98.

Frost, H.M. (1964). *The laws of bone structure.* Springfield, IL: Charles C. Thomas Publishers.

Gage, J.R., Schwartz, M.H., Koop, S.E., & Novacheck, T.F. (2009). *The identification and treatment of gait problems in cerebral palsy.* London: Mac Keith Press.

Gajdosik, R.L., & Bohannon, R.W. (1987). Clinical measurement of range of motion: Review of goniometry emphasizing reliability and validity. *Physical Therapy, 67*, 1867–1872.

Gajdosik, C.G., Nelson, S.A., & Gleason, D.K. (1994). Reliability of isometric measurements of girls ages 3–5 years: A preliminary study. *Pediatric Physical Therapy, 6,* 206.

Gajdosik, R.L., Sandler, M.M., & Marr, H.L. (2003). Influence of knee positions and gender on the Ober test for length of the iliotibial band. *Clinical Biomechanics, 18*(1), 77–79.

Gilmour, J.C., & Burns, Y. (2001). The measurement of the medial longitudinal arch in children. *Foot and Ankle International, 22,* 493–498.

Grasco, J., & de Pablos, J. (1997). Bone remodeling in malunited fractures in children. *Journal of Pediatric Orthopedics, Part B, 6,* 126–132.

Gross, M.T. (1995). Lower quarter screening for skeletal malalignments: Suggestions for orthotics and shoewear. *Journal of Orthopedics and Sports Physical Therapy, 21,* 389–405.

Haas, S.S., Epps, C.H., & Adams, J.P. (1973). Normal ranges of hip motion in the newborn. *Clinical Orthopedics, 91,* 114–118.

Haggmark, T., & Eriksson, E. (1979). Hypotrophy of the soleus muscle in man after Achilles tendon rupture. Discussion of findings obtained by computed tomography and morphologic studies. *American Journal of Sports Medicine, 7*(2), 121–126.

Harris, R.I., & Beath, T. (1948). Hypermobile flat-foot with short tendon Achilles. *Journal of Bone and Joint Surgery, 30-A,* 116–150.

Harris, S.R., Harthun-Smith, L., & Krukowski, L. (1985). Goniometric reliability for a child with spastic quadriplegia. *Journal of Pediatric Orthopedics, 5,* 348–351.

Heath, C.H., & Staheli, L.T. (1993). Normal limits of knee angle in white children—genu varum and genu valgum. *Journal of Pediatric Orthopedics, 13*(2), 259–266.

Hensinger, R.N., & Jones, E.T. (1982). Developmental orthopedics. I: The lower limb. *Developmental Medicine and Child Neurology, 24,* 95–116.

Horstmann, H.M., & Bleck, E.E. (2007). *Orthopedic management in cerebral palsy* (2nd ed.). London: Mac Keith Press.

Horvat, M., Croce, R., & Roswal, G. (1994). Intratester reliability of the Nicholas Manual Muscle Tester on individuals with intellectual disabilities by a tester having minimal experience. *Archives of Physical Medicine and Rehabilitation, 76,* 808–811.

Ivanenko, Y.P., Dominici, N., & Lacquaniti, F. (2007). Development of independent walking in toddlers. *Exercise and Sport Sciences Reviews, 35*(2), 67–73.

Kanatli, U., Gözil, R, Besli, K., Yetkin, H., & Bölökasi, S. (2006). The relationship between the hindfoot angle and the medial longitudinal arch of the foot. *Foot & Ankle International, 27*(8), 623–627.

Katz, K., Rosenthal, A., & Yosipovitch, Z. (1992). Normal ranges of popliteal angle in children. *Journal of Pediatric Orthopaedics, 12,* 229–231.

Kelly, P.M., & Dimeglio, A. (2008). Lower limb growth: How predictable are predictions? *Journal of Childhood Orthopedics, 2,* 407–415.

King, W., Levin, R., Schmidt, R., Oestreich, A., & Heubi, J.E. (2003). Prevalence of reduced bone mass in children and adults with spastic quadriplegia. *Developmental Medicine and Child Neurology, 45*(1), 12–16.

Kramer, J.F., & MacPhail, A. (1994). Relationships among measures of walking efficiency, gross motor ability, and isokinetic strength in adolescents with cerebral palsy. *Pediatric Physical Therapy, 6,* 3–8.

Lanyon, L.E., & Rubin, C.T. (1984). Static vs dynamic loads as an influence on bone remodelling. *Journal of Biomechanics, 17,* 897–905.

Ledebt, A. (2000). Changes in arm posture during the early acquisition of walking. *Infant Behavior & Development, 23,* 79–89.

Lee, S.H., Chung, C.Y., Park, M.S., Choi, I.H., & Cho, T.J. (2009). Tibial torsion in cerebral palsy: Validity and reliability of measurement. *Clinical Orthopedics & Related Research* (published online, January 22, 2009).

LeVeau, B.F., & Bernhardt, D.B. (1984). Developmental biomechanics. *Physical Therapy, 64*(12), 1874–1881.

Mac-Thiong, J.M., Berthonnaud, E., Dimar, J.R., Betz, R.R., & Labelle, H. (2004). Sagittal alignment of the spine and pelvis during growth. *Spine, 29*(15), 1642–1647.

Mann, M., Glasheen-Wray, M., & Nyberg, R. (1984). Therapist agreement for palpation and observation of iliac crest heights. *Physical Therapy, 64*(3), 334–338.

McCrea, J.D. (1985). *Pediatric orthopedics of the lower extremity. An instructional handbook.* Mount Kisco, NY: Futura Publishing Co.

McDade, W. (1977). Bow legs and knock knees. *Pediatric Clinics of North America, 24*(4), 825–839.

Melchione, W.E., & Sullivan, M.S. (1993). Reliability of measurements obtained by use of an instrument designed to indirectly measure iliotibial band length. *Journal of Orthopaedic and Sports Physical Therapy, 18*(3), 511–515.

Merlini, L., Mazzone, E.S., Solari, A., & Morandi, L. (2002). Reliability of hand-held dynamometry in spinal muscular atrophy. *Muscle and Nerve, 26,* 64–67.

Mickle, K.J., Steele, J.R., & Munro, B.J. (2006). The feet of overweight and obese young children: Are they flat or fat? *Obesity, 14*(11), 1949–1953.

Miller, F., Dias, R.C., Dabney, K.W., Lipton, G., & Trianna, M. (1997). Soft-tissue release for spastic hip subluxation in cerebral palsy. *Journal of Pediatric Orthopaedics, 17*(5), 571–584.

Mortensen, H.M., Skov, O., & Jensen, P.E. (1999). Early motion of the ankle after operative treatment of a rupture of the Achilles tendon. A prospective, randomized clinical and radiographic study. *Journal of Bone and Joint Surgery (American), 81*(7), 983–990.

Mosca, V.S. (2001). The foot. In R.T. Morrissey & S.L. Weinstein (Eds.), *Lovell and Winter's pediatric orthopedics* (pp. 1051–1215). Philadelphia: Lippincott Williams & Wilkins.

Mullender, M.G., & Huiskes, R. (1995). Proposal for the regulatory mechanism of Wolff's law. *Journal of Orthopedic Research, 13*(4), 503–512.

Munsat, T.L., McNeal, D., & Waters, R. (1976). Effects of nerve stimulation on human muscle. *Archives of Neurology, 33*(9), 608–617.

Nalaboff, K.M., & Schweitzer, M.E. (2008). MRI of tarsal coalition. *Bulletin of the NYU Hospital for Joint Diseases, 66*(1), 14–21.

Newton, P.O., & Wenger, D.O. (2001). Idiopathic and congenital scoliosis. In R.T. Morrissey & S.L. Weinstein (Eds.). *Lovell and Winter's pediatric orthopedics* (pp. 677–740). Philadelphia: Lippincott Williams & Wilkins.

Nigg, B.M., & Grimston, S.K. (1994). Bone. In B.M. Nigg & W. Herzog (Eds.), *Biomechanics of the musculoskeletal system.* Chichester, England: Wiley & Sons.

O'Sullivan, M.E., Bronk, J.T., Chao, E.Y.S., & Kelly, P.J. (1994). Experimental study of the effect of weight bearing on fracture healing in the canine tibia. *Clinical Orthopedics and Related Research, 302,* 273–283.

Pax Lowes, L., Westcott, S.L., Palisano, R.J., Effgen, S.K., & Orlin, M.N. (2004). Muscle force and range of motion as predictors of standing balance in children with cerebral palsy. *Physical and Occupational Therapy in Pediatrics,* 24(1/2), 57–77.

Pfeiffer, M., Kotz, R., Ledl, T., Hauser, G., & Sluga, M. (2006). Prevalence of flat foot in preschool-aged children. *Pediatrics,* 118(2), 634–639.

Phelps, E., Smith, L.J., & Hallum, A. (1985). Normal ranges of hip motion of infants between nine and 24 months of age. *Developmental Medicine and Child Neurology, 27,* 785–792.

Pitkow, R.B. (1975). External rotation contracture of the extended hip. *Clinical Orthopedics and Related Research, 110,* 139–145.

Pitman, M.I., & Peterson, L. (1989). Biomechanics of skeletal muscle. In M. Nordkin & V.H. Frankel (Eds.), *Basic biomechanics of the musculoskeletal system* (pp. 89–107). Philadelphia: Lippincott.

Pratt, N. (1991). *Clinical musculoskeletal anatomy.* Philadelphia: Lippincott.

Rang, M. (1993a). Bow-legs and knock knees. In D.R. Wenger & M. Rang (Eds.), *The art and practice of children's orthopedics* (pp. 201–219). New York: Raven Press.

Rang, M. (1993b). Other feet. In D.R. Wenger & M. Rang (Eds.), *The art and practice of children's orthopedics* (pp. 168–200). New York: Raven Press.

Rang, M. (1993c). Toeing in and toeing out: Gait disorders. In D.R. Wenger & M. Rang (Eds.), *The art and practice of children's orthopedics* (pp. 50–76). New York: Raven Press.

Reimers, J. (1980). The stability of the hip joint in children. A radiological study of the results of muscle surgery in cerebral palsy. *Acta Orthopaedica Scandinavica Supplementum, 184,* 1–100.

Salenius, P., & Vankka, E. (1975). Development of the tibiofemoral angle in children. *Journal of Bone and Joint Surgery, 57-A,* 259–261.

Schoenecker, P.L., & Rich, M.M. (2001). The lower extremity. In R.T. Morrissey & S.L. Weinstein (Eds.), *Lovell and Winter's pediatric orthopedics* (pp. 1059–1104). Philadelphia: Lippincott Williams &Wilkins.

Scoles, P.V. (1988*). Pediatric orthopedics in clinical practice* (2nd ed.). Chicago: Year Book Medical Publishers, Inc.

Scull, S. (2001). Juvenile rheumatoid arthritis. In S.K. Campbell, R.J. Palisano, & D.W. Vander Linden (Eds.), *Physical therapy for children* (2nd ed., pp. 227–246). Philadelphia: W.B. Saunders.

Simmonds, J.V., & Keer, R.J. (2007). Hypermobility and the hypermobility syndrome. *Manual Therapy, 12,* 298–309.

Staheli, L.T. (1977). The prone hip extension test. *Clinical Orthopedics and Related Research, 12,* 12–15.

Staheli, L.T. (2008). *Fundamentals of pediatric orthopedics.* (4th ed., pp. 177). Philadelphia: Wolters Kluwer, Lippincott Williams & Wilkins.

Staheli, L. T. (1992). *Fundamentals of pediatric orthopedics.* New York: Raven Press.

Staheli, L.T., Chew, D.E., & Corbett, M. (1987). The longitudinal arch. *Journal of Bone and Joint Surgery, 69-A*(3), 426–428.

Stokes, I.A. (1997). Analysis of symmetry of vertebral body loading consequent to lateral spinal curvature. *Spine,* 22(21), 2495–2503.

Stormont, D.M., & Peterson, H.A. (1983). The relative incidence of tarsal coalition. *Clinical Orthopedics and Related Research, 181,* 28–35.

Stuberg, W.A., Fuchs, R.H., & Miedaner, J.A. (1988). Reliability of goniometric measurements of children with cerebral palsy. *Developmental Medicine and Child Neurology, 30,* 657–666.

Stuberg, W.A., Koehler, A., Witicha, M., Temme, J., & Kaplan, P. (1989). Comparison of femoral torsion assessment using goniometry and computerized tomography. *Pediatric Physical Therapy, 1,* 115–118.

Stuberg, W.A., & Metcalf, W.K. (1988). Reliability of quantitative muscle testing in healthy children and in children with Duchenne muscular dystrophy using a hand-held dynamometer. *Physical Therapy, 68,* 977–982.

Sutherland, D.H. (1997). The development of mature gait. *Gait & Posture, 6,* 163–170.

Sutherland, D.H., Olshen, R.A., Biden, E.N., & Wyatt, M.P. (1988). *The Development of Mature Walking.* Oxford: Mac Keith Press.

Sutherland, D.H., Olshen, R., Cooper, & Woo, S.L.Y. (1980). The development of mature gait. *The Journal of Bone and Joint Surgery, 62-A,* 336–353.

Tolo, V. (1996). The lower extremity. In R.T. Morrissey & S.L. Weinstein (Eds.), *Lovell and Winter's pediatric orthopedics* (pp. 1047–1075). Philadelphia, PA: Lippincott Raven Publishers.

Trueta, J. (1968). *Studies of the development and decay of the human frame* (p. 37). Philadelphia: W.B. Saunders.

Tudor, A., Ruzic, L., Sestan, B., Sirola, L., & Prpic, T., (2009). Flat-footedness is not a disadvantage for athletic performance in children aged 11 to 15 years. *Pediatrics,* 123(3), e386–392.

Van Den Berg-Emons, R.J., Van Baak, M.A., Speth, L., & Saris, W.H. (1998). Physical training of school children with spastic cerebral palsy: Effects on daily activity, fat mass and fitness. *International Journal of Rehabilitation Research, 21,* 179–194.

Walker, J. (1991). Musculoskeletal development: A review. *Physical Therapy, 71*(12), 878–889.

Wearing, S.C., Hills, A.P., Nuala, M., Byrne, N.M., Hennig, E.M., & McDonald, M. (2004). The arch index: A measure of fat or flat feet? *Foot & Ankle International.* 25(8), 575–581.

Weinstein, S.L. (2001). Developmental hip dysplasia and dislocation. In R.T. Morrissey & S.L. Weinstein (Eds.), *Lovell and Winter's pediatric orthopedics* (pp. 905–956). Philadelphia: Lippincott-Raven.

Wenger, D.R. (1993a). Calcaneovarus and metatarsus varus. In D.R. Wenger & M. Rang (Eds.), *The art and practice of children's orthopedics* (pp. 103–136). New York: Raven Press.

Wenger, D.R. (1993b). Flat foot and children's shoes. In D.R. Wenger & M. Rang (Eds.), *The art and practice of children's orthopedics* (pp. 77–102). New York: Raven Press.

Wenger, D.R., Mauldin, D., Speck, G., Morgan, D., & Lieber, R.L. (1989). Corrective shoes and inserts as treatment for flexible flat foot in infants and children. *Journal of Bone and Joint Surgery (American), 71*(6), 800–810.

Wessel, J., Kaup, C., Fan, J., Ehalt, R., Ellsworth, J., Speer, C., Tenove, P., & Dombrosky, A. (1999). Isometric strength measurements in children with arthritis: Reliability and relation to function. *Arthritis Care Resource, 12*(4), 238–246.

Widhe, T. (2001). Spine: posture, mobility and pain. A longitudinal study from childhood to adolescence. *European Spine Journal, 10*, 118–123.

Wiley, M.W., & Damiano, D.L. (1998) Lower-extremity strength profiles in spastic cerebral palsy. *Developmental Medicine & Child Neurology, 40*, 100–107.

Wilkins, K. (1986). Bowlegs. *The Pediatric Clinics of North America, 33*(6), 1429–1438.

Williams, P.F. (1982). *Orthopedic management in childhood.* London: Blackwell Scientific Publications.

Wright, J.C., & Bell, D. (1991). Lumbosacral joint angles in children. *Journal of Pediatric Orthopedics, 11*, 748–751.

Zaleske, D.J. (2001). Metabolic and endocrine abnormalities. In R.T. Morrissey & S.L. Weinstein (Eds.), *Lovell and Winter's pediatric orthopedics* (pp. 177–214). Philadelphia: Lippincott Williams and Wilkins.

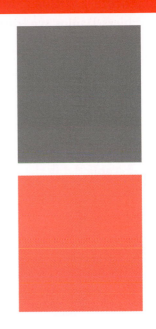

CHAPTER 6

Musculoskeletal System: Considerations and Interventions for Specific Pediatric Pathologies

—LINDA PAX LOWES, PT, PhD

—LINDSAY ALFANO, DPT, PCS

—MARGO ORLIN, PT, PhD

This chapter applies principles of musculoskeletal development to common pediatric conditions and discusses intervention strategies. For educational purposes, this book is divided into systems. The human body, however, operates through an interaction of all of the systems. Individuals with neurological impairment are affected by the musculoskeletal system, and in contrast, individuals with musculoskeletal impairment can make improvements through refinements in the nervous system. For example, someone who repeatedly injures a joint may alleviate the problem by educating the nervous system to move in a new pattern. Likewise, functional abilities of an individual with neurological impairment can be enhanced through improvements in ROM or force production. In this chapter, only the musculoskeletal aspects of disease will be addressed. For information on the neurological components, please refer to Chapters 7 and 8. The end of the chapter provides more in-depth information and intervention suggestions for two common pediatric conditions with significant musculoskeletal concerns: cerebral palsy and Down syndrome.

Musculoskeletal Pathologies of Connective Tissue

The first diseases to be discussed are those that affect a child's connective tissue, which includes ligaments, tendons, and cartilage (Table 6.1). Ehlers-Danlos syndrome, juvenile idiopathic arthritis (JIA), and hemophilia are the three pediatric connective tissue disorders that will be discussed in this chapter. Osteogenesis imperfecta is also a collagen disorder but will be discussed in the section on bone due to the significant bone pathology that accompanies it. Lupus erythematosus is another condition affecting the connective tissue, primarily of women between the ages of 15 and 45. Although less common, pediatric systematic and neonatal lupus erythematosus affect children. Detailed information about lupus is not discussed in this text, but some general information is presented in Table 6.1.

Ehlers-Danlos syndrome (EDS)

Ehlers-Danlos syndrome (EDS) is a heterogeneous group of connective tissue disorders that affects 1 out every 5,000 people. There is no difference in the incidence rate among gender or race. Abnormal collagen synthesis associated with EDS can lead to skin hyperextensibility, ligamentous laxity, tissue fragility, delayed wound healing, atrophic scarring, and easy bruising and bleeding (Parapia & Jackson, 2008). See Table 6.1 for information on the etiology, pathology, impairment, and functional limitation associated with the six subclassifications of EDS.

Intervention, duration, and frequency for a child with EDS are based on the severity of the disease and needs of the child and family. The child and family will need information about the disease and assistance developing a preventative health plan to optimize the child's functional skills, fitness, peer interactions, and independence. Recreational choices should be based on the child's interests but must also be evaluated for the potential for joint injury due to the ligamentous laxity and the system's heightened reaction to trauma (i.e., excessive bleeding, bruising, and poor healing). Recommended activities might include swimming, cycling,

Table 6.1 Pediatric Diseases Affecting Connective Tissue

Diagnosis	Etiology	Pathology	Body Functions and Structure Impairments	Potential Activity Limitations and Participation Restrictions
Classic Ehlers-Danlos Syndrome (EDS)(Parapia & Jackson, 2008)	Autosomal dominant inheritance	Abnormal Collagen Type V	Developmental delay, hyperextensibility of the skin and joints, scarring, hernias, easy bruising, muscle hypotonia, structural cardiac anomalies	• Need to avoid physical activities that put bones and joints at risk • May encounter social stigma • May limit choice of hobby or activities as isometric and strenuous weight-bearing exercise must be avoided
Hypermobility EDS	Autosomal dominant inheritance	Unknown	Skin laxity, velvet skin, joint hypermobility with frequent dislocations	
Vascular EDS	Autosomal dominant	Abnormal Collagen Type III	Arterial rupture, varicose veins, easy bruising, hypermobility of small joints	
Kyphoscoliosis EDS	Autosomal recessive	Deficiency of an enzyme that provides stability to collagen (lysyl-hydroxylase)	Joint laxity (b715)*, scoliosis from birth, sclera fragility, hypotonia in infants	

Table 6.1 Pediatric Diseases Affecting Connective Tissue—cont'd

Diagnosis	Etiology	Pathology	Body Functions and Structure Impairments	Potential Activity Limitations and Participation Restrictions
Arthroclasia EDS	Autosomal dominant	Abnormal Collagen Type I	Joint hypermobility and frequent dislocations, kyphoscoliosis, skin fragility, easy bruising, hypotonia	
Dermatosparaxis EDS	Autosomal recessive	Abnormal Collagen Type I	Sagging, redundant skin with soft doughy feeling, easy bruising, hernia, premature rupture of fetal membranes	
Pediatric lupus erythematosus (Hiraki et al., 2008)	Cause unknown	Multi-system immune dysregulation	Primary symptom is inflammation. Other symptoms are variable but may include arthritis, oral and nasal rash or ulcers, kidney dysfunction, headaches, cerebral-vascular injury, cognitive dysfunction, cardiac or lung infection, Raynaud's, fatigue, fever or weight loss	• Multi-system problems often lead to hospitalizations • Pain (b280), fatigue, and other discomfort may impact physical abilities and limit social interaction • Diminished social interaction and cognitive difficulties may lead to depression
Juvenile idiopathic arthritis (JIA)—systemic onset (Ravelli & Martini, 2007)	• Uncertain; believed to have a genetic and environmental component. • Auto-immune dysfunction related to increased interleukin 1 (IL-1) • (Finckh et al., 2006; Finckh & Gabay, 2008)	• Joint inflammation involving few or many joints • Joint synovium proliferates causing a massive overgrowth (pannus), which can erode the adjacent cartilage and bone	• ROM limitations (b710) • Joint space narrowing and/or destruction • Significant pain (b280)	• May limit mobility (d455) and self-care activities (d599) • May impair handwriting (d345)

Continued

Table 6.1 Pediatric Diseases Affecting Connective Tissue—cont'd

Diagnosis	Etiology	Pathology	Body Functions and Structure Impairments	Potential Activity Limitations and Participation Restrictions
		• Joint adhesions and osteophytes (bony spurs) possible		
JIA—oligoarthritis	• Cause unknown • Early childhood; peaks 2–4 years • Almost always female	• Joint inflammation involving four or fewer joints • Pannus can erode the adjacent cartilage and bone • Joint adhesions and osteophytes possible	• ROM limitations (b710)—most commonly the knee, ankle, and fingers • Joint space narrowing and/or destruction • 20% have chronic iritis, which may lead to blindness	• May limit mobility (d455) and self-care activities (d599) • May impair handwriting (d345)
JIA—rheumatoid-factor-negative polyarticular onset	• Cause unknown • Peaks between 2–4 years and again between 6–12 years • Females more common than males	• Joint inflammation involving five or more joints • Pannus can erode the adjacent cartilage and bone • Joint adhesions and osteophytes possible	• ROM limitations generally of bilateral knees, wrists, and ankles (b710) • Joint space narrowing and/or destruction	• May limit mobility (d455) and self-care activities (d599) • May impair handwriting if finger involvement (d345)
JIA—rheumatoid-factor-positive polyarticular onset	• Same as adult rheumatoid-factor-positive rheumatoid arthritis • Mostly teen girls	• Typically symmetric polyarthritis affecting small joints or hands and feet, sometimes including knees and ankles		

Table 6.1 Pediatric Diseases Affecting Connective Tissue—cont'd

Diagnosis	Etiology	Pathology	Body Functions and Structure Impairments	Potential Activity Limitations and Participation Restrictions
		• 30% have rheumatoid nodules on the forearm or elbow		
Hemophilia	• Defect in gene on X chromosome • Incidence 1 per 5,000 live male births	Missing protein (clotting factor) required for blood clotting.	• Joint destruction, leading to premature arthritis and chronic pain (b280) • Muscle disuse atrophy (b730) • ROM limitations (b710) • Potential nerve compression • If bleeding occurs in the brain, sensory, motor, or cognitive impairments may develop; if the bleeding is severe, death may result	• Pain may lead to diminished interaction with peers and absence from school/work • Functional limitations due to pain (b280) and joint swelling

*Numbers in parentheses refer to ICF-CY classification.

dance, tennis, or golf. Roughhouse play or contact sports should be avoided.

Juvenile Idiopathic Arthritis

Juvenile idiopathic arthritis (JIA), previously known as juvenile rheumatoid arthritis, is not a single disease but rather an exclusion classification for all types of arthritis of unknown origin occurring before the age of 16 years. Scientists believe that cytokines, which are signaling proteins used in cellular communication, play a role in the pathophysiology of this disease. Poor regulation of the cytokine interleukin 1 (IL-1) is believed to play a major role, but cytokines IL 15, 18, and 21 are also implicated.

There are seven main categories of JIA based on characteristics seen in the first 6 months of the illness. The three types most often seen by physical therapists—systemic, oligoarthritis, and rheumatoid-factor-positive polyarthritis—are discussed below and the less common rheumatoid-factor-negative polyarthritis, enthesitis-related, psoriatic, and undifferentiated arthritis will not be discussed. **Systemic onset JIA** accounts for around 15% of all reported cases and is generally the most painful form of the disease (Adams & Lehman, 2005). Its onset is accompanied or preceded by a fever for 2 weeks or longer. Frequently, a rash is also present. Other systemic manifestations can include heart infections, swollen glands, an enlarged spleen, abdominal pain, anemia, and growth retardation (Rhodes, 1991). Joint involvement is generally symmetrical and polyarticular (involving more than four joints). It occurs in boys and girls equally, generally between the ages of 5 and 15 years. The high number of joints involved, long duration of disease, and resulting orthopedic changes make this type of JIA one of the most debilitating.

Another complication that affects approximately 5% of children with systemic JIA is a life-threatening disease called **macrophage activation syndrome**. Signs of this condition include sustained fever and neurological changes (Ravelli & Martini, 2007). A child should seek medical attention immediately if macrophage activation is suspected.

The next two types of JIA do not involve fever and are classified by the distribution of the disease. **Oligoarthritis** is the most common of all JIA subtypes and is defined as asymmetrically affecting four or fewer joints after the first 6 months of the disease. Girls are four times more likely to have oligoarthritis, with onset typically occurring before 6 years of age (Ravelli & Martini, 2007).

This subtype has the best prognosis of all varieties of JIA, with 23%–47% of children in remission after 6–10 years of onset. Permanent joint space narrowing is frequently seen following remission, but this causes severe chronic disability in less than 15% of the children (Calabro, Holgerson, Sonpal, & Khoury, 1976).

Involvement of an upper extremity joint is a poor prognostic factor in oligoarthritis as it typically signals progression into **extended oligoarthritis,** a more severe form with a higher joint count and longer duration. About 30% of children with oligoarthritis develop iridocyclitis within the first 5–7 years of the disease, which can cause significant visual deterioration (Ravelli & Martini, 2007). The American Academy of Pediatrics recommends regular eye exams every 3–6 months, depending on the other risk factors present (American Academy of Pediatrics, 1993)

Rheumatoid-factor-positive polyarticular arthritis is defined as involvement in five or more joints. It is the same as adult rheumatoid arthritis and almost exclusively occurs in adolescent females. There is symmetric involvement of the small hand and feet joints. Less frequently, the knees or ankles will also be involved. This is the only type of JIA in which rheumatoid nodules are found. They are present on the forearms or elbows of about 30% of children. The prognosis for rheumatoid-factor-positive polyarticular arthritis is not favorable, with up to 50% developing severe deforming arthritis within 5 years (Ravelli & Martini, 2007).

In any type of JIA, early detection is very important to avoid secondary pathology that can decrease optimal long-term outcomes (Finckh, Liang, van Herckenrode, & de Pablo, 2006). Joints present as painful, swollen, warm, and inflamed. Inflammation can lead to capsular hypertrophy, irregular bone growth, or osteoporosis and small stature (Okumus, Erguven, Deveci, Yilmaz,

& Okumus, 2008; Thorton, Ashcroft, & O'Neill, 2008). Prolonged inflammation and swelling can stretch the surrounding ligaments and lead to chronic joint instability when the swelling subsides. Painful inflammation of muscles and tendons can cause the child to move less or to adapt an abnormal movement pattern. Over time decreased motion can lead to joint contractures. All of these changes can alter the normal skeletal alignment and lead to further destructive forces on the body.

Inflammation can also change the growth rate of bones. **Inflammatory hyperemia** can stimulate adjacent growth plates and cause overgrowth or cause early physeal closure and subsequent limb shortening (Sherry & Mosca, 1996). If just part of the growth plate is affected, the bone can grow asymmetrically and cause angular postural deformities. This growth alteration will lead to a limb length discrepancy.

Leg length discrepancy (LLD) is a common complication of oligoarthritis due to disease of the knee. Intraarticular cortisone injections have been shown to decrease the severity of the discrepancy (Schneider & Passo, 2002). If the disease onsets earlier than 9 years of age, overgrowth of the involved knee and premature growth arrest of the acetabulum and femoral head are most often noted. Generally the overgrowth in the knee does not exceed 3 centimeters. Conversely, if the disease onsets after 9 years of age, premature closure of the growth plate with subsequent shortening of the involved extremity is most common. Early growth plate closure can result in more severe deformity, with a discrepancy of up to 6 centimeters (Simon, Whiffen, & Shapiro, 1981).

Foot deformities are prevalent in children with JIA. A sample of 144 consecutive JIA clinic patients was evaluated, and over 80% had some degree of foot dysfunction. The most common problems were pronated rearfoot (73%) or midfoot (72%), and toe valgus and ankle range of motion (ROM) limitations (35%) (Spraul & Koenning, 1994). Abnormal pressure distribution under the foot when walking can be indicative of pathology. Analysis has shown that children with JIA do not sufficiently load the great toe during terminal stance. This is likely due to joint stiffening at the metatarsalphalangeal joint and can impact the effectiveness of push off (Dhanendran, Hutton, Klennerman, Witemeyer, & Ansell, 1980).

Subluxations or ankylosing (fusing) of the cervical spine can lead to limited neck extension ROM. Temporomandibular joint disease is also more prevalent in this population than in typical youth (Weiss, Arabshahi, & Johnson, 2008).

Examination of a child with JIA must include assessment of physical disability, functional skills, and quality of life. A thorough examination will include measuring strength (Wessel et al., 1999), skeletal alignment, ROM, fatigue, endurance, edema, and pain. The 6-minute walk test is a reliable measure of walking endurance in this population (Lelieveld, Takken, van der Net, & van Weert, 2005; Paap, van der Net, Helders, & Takken, 2005). Normal values for distance and heart rate response in children under the age of 12 years without disability are reported by Lammers and colleagues (Lammers, Hislop, Flynn, & Haworth, 2008).

The Childhood Health Assessment Questionnaire (CHAQ), Juvenile Arthritis Quality of Life Questionnaire (JAQQ), and the Childhood Arthritis Health Profile are frequently used to measure disability in children with JIA. Many preschool and elementary school children have been shown to have a developmental delay on the Bayley II Scales of Infant Development and the Pediatric Evaluation of Disability Index (van der Net et al., 2008). Developmental screening and stimulation, if required, should be included in a JIA assessment.

Getting a clear picture of child complaints can be difficult as they vary within one day, week, or year. For example, children often report increased pain and stiffness in the morning and with cold temperatures, while functional skills may decline at the end of the day due to fatigue. A thorough examiner should inquire into a typical day, week, and even year to assess the patterns of impairment.

Intervention objectives for children with JIA would include pain relief; prevention/remediation of ROM, strength, and deformity; and maintenance or improvement of functional abilities. This is best accomplished through an interdisciplinary team with the child and the family as the center. Team members may include a pediatric rheumatologist, orthopedic surgeon, physical therapist, occupational therapist, case manager, nurse specialist, educator, psychologist, and nutritionist. Due to the chronic and variable nature of the disease, the selection of team members will need to change in order to meet the ongoing needs of the child as the disease changes and progresses over time.

Therapy intervention should include child and family education, pain management, deformity prevention, ROM maintenance or improvement, strengthening, promotion of functional abilities, and physical fitness. The child should be given information about the disease and allowed to participate in determining the plan of care. A program of joint protection and therapeutic exercise can help to prevent or reduce pain. Self-ROM activities spaced throughout the day can prevent stiffening from prolonged lack of movement. Movement and stretching can be painful at first, but most children report that regular gentle movement helps alleviate pain.

Modalities can also be used for short-term relief of pain. Heat can increase flexibility and reduce pain and muscle spasms, but must be used with caution on acutely swollen joints (Cakmak & Bolukbas, 2005). Depending on the size of the area to be treated and the desired penetration, this can be accomplished through the use of a hot shower or bath, hot packs, or ultrasound. Remain cognizant that ultrasound over growth plates is not advised. Paraffin treatments are often very soothing to the painful hands and feet of a child with rheumatoid-factor-positive polyarticular JIA.

Although many children do not tolerate ice, it can be a useful aid in combating the effects of acute inflammation by providing vasoconstriction and analgesia. Massage is a more tolerable method of pain relief. Its effectiveness is documented by a study that showed that when a family member provided daily 15-minute massages for 1 month, the patient reported decreased pain, and both the patient and family member reported decreased anxiety levels, which was substantiated by a decrease in cortisol levels in their saliva (Field, Hernandez-Reif, Diego, Schanberg, & Kuhn, 2005).

Living With JIA

Poor fitness is a common finding in almost all children with JIA, both during an exacerbation and while in remission. One study documented deficits in both aerobic and anaerobic exercise capabilities in 95% of children tested (van Brussel et al., 2007). Poor fitness can contribute to poor functional skills. Lelieveld et al. (2007) showed a strong correlation between anaerobic capacity and functional abilities. Community-based exercise programs have been shown to improve endurance and decrease joint symptoms (Klepper, 1999). Eighty percent of the children with polyarticular JIA who participated in an eight-week program of low-impact aerobics, strengthening, and flexibility exercises reported a significant improvement in joint pain and all had improved endurance. High-impact weight-bearing exercises performed over a sustained period have been shown to improve density (Gannotti et al., 2007). Caution must be exercised when children with joint involvement participate in high-impact exercise to ensure that the benefits outweigh the risk of joint damage. A review article (Klepper, 2008) reported modest improvement in fitness and overall quality of life improvements with regular exercise. It is important to note that none of the programs reported any detrimental changes to the child.

Selection of lifelong fitness activities should be based on the child's interest, while minimizing risk to the joints and maximizing therapeutic benefit. An activity that provides ROM, strengthening and cardiovascular endurance would be optimal. The level of stress the activity puts on the joints must be evaluated prior to initiating a program. The child should also be advised of the need to include pre- and postactivity stretching. Aquatic therapeutic exercise has been shown to improve ROM (Bacon, Nicholson, Binder, & White, 1991) and can be performed in a group setting. Tepid pool water can help motion and minimize fatigue. Additional activities such as tai chi, low-impact aerobics, and cycling may be good choices. Contact sports or sports such as basketball or gymnastics, which stress joints, should be avoided.

Preventative Measures

Education about **joint protection** may also help minimize the stress on the joints by avoiding end-range positions and high-torque movements. The use of aides to help with activities of daily living (ADL) is one way to limit joint stress. Large-handled items can improve grip strength while reducing joint stress. When selecting assistive devices, it is important to remember that compliance is often low in children unless they are included in the decision-making process and value the device. In order for children to value a device it must enhance performance of an important task, or they must understand the importance of preventative medicine. The concept of preventative medicine may be difficult for children, as many go through a natural period of feeling invincible or are unable to project themselves several decades into the future. Devices that are prescribed for preventative health but that ultimately diminish performance or speed are frequently discarded. For example, a child is unlikely to continue to use a walker or cane to improve movement patterns and reduce stress on joints if he can walk faster unaided.

School-age children should avoid carrying heavy stacks of books through school. Frequent lifting and carrying of books and backpacks may cause added stress to the joints of the spine and upper extremities in children and adolescents with JIA, resulting in exacerbation of symptoms. If the child is given two sets of books, one could be left in each classroom and the other set could remain at home for homework. Items that need to go with the child from room to room could be kept in a backpack for ambulatory children or in a bag attached to a walker or wheelchair.

Splinting is also an important consideration in children with JIA. A splint can provide stability, maintain the extremity in an optimal position for function, and reduce degenerative deformity. An ankle-foot orthosis provides stability for ambulation while maintaining ankle integrity. A wrist extension splint increases grip force by utilizing the tenodesis effect. Night splints are used to increase or maintain ROM.

Hemophilia

Hemophilia is a chronic bleeding disorder but will be discussed in this chapter because it has a significant impact on a child's joints. In general, hemophilia is an X-linked condition in which one or more clotting proteins are not produced by the body (see Table 6.1), which results in excessive bleeding, both internally and externally. Being an X-linked disorder, males are more likely to have the disease and females are often carriers. If both parents have the hemophilia gene, however, a female offspring can be born with hemophilia. The three most common types of hemophilia are labeled A, B, and C.

Type A is considered classic hemophilia and accounts for 80% of all cases. Clotting factor VIII is deficient in this subtype and results in severe bleeding in about 60% of those affected. Hemophilia B, also known as Christmas disease, involves a factor IX deficiency and is less common. About 50% of people with type B have severe symptoms. Hemophilia C is a very rare autosomal recessive type of hemophilia that is most commonly seen in the Ashkenazi Jewish community.

A fourth bleeding disorder, von Willebrand disease (VWD), is a deficiency or defect in the von Willebrand factor. Bleeding in individuals with VWD tends to be limited to the mucous membranes and is most often expressed as frequent nosebleeds, heavy menstrual flow, and excessive bleeding after surgery, dental work, or childbirth. Joint bleeds are less common with von Willebrand disease.

Recombinant (genetically engineered) clotting factor is available as either a prophylactic measure in severe forms of hemophilia or to treat an acute bleeding episode. Physical therapy intervention for managing ROM and strength and promoting functional skill plays a large role in the overall well-being of children with this disorder. The National Hemophilia Foundation (http://www.hemophilia.org) has a physical therapy working group that produces best practice resources.

Examination of a child with hemophilia will include recording the child's history, tracking the number and frequency of joint bleeds, ROM and strength assessment, measurement of edema, and level of functional skills. Pain is almost universally present, and a referral to a pain specialist may be needed. The use of nonsteroidal anti-inflammatories can cause platelet damage, so other options such as narcotics, massage, or relaxation techniques may need to be incorporated.

Joints that have recurrent bleeding episodes are referred to as "target joints." The most frequent target joints and the resulting sequelae are listed in Table 6.2. Prevention of joint bleeds, and immediate management of bleeds that do occur, is essential for preventing permanent destructive changes such as thickening of the synovial tissue, breakdown of cartilage in the

joint, narrowing of the joint space, and contractures of the muscles surrounding the joint. Splints, orthoses, and other assistive devices are often needed to immobilize a bleeding or painful joint, prevent deformity, improve ROM and function, or support an unstable or weak joint.

Promoting physical health and development is also important. Young children may need kneepads or helmets when gaining crawling and walking skills. Suggestions for minimizing risk, while still allowing the child the opportunity to develop new skills, should be provided. Installing baby gates, padding sharp edges on furniture, and removing furniture that might tip over easily are some examples of ways to minimize injury. Parents should be reminded that some bleeding during the infant and toddler years is unavoidable, and overprotecting the child can limit the child's gross motor, cognitive, and emotional growth. As the child matures, a regular program of safe exercise should be encouraged. The National Hemophilia Foundation has a booklet for patients rating the perceived safety of various sports (Anderson & Forsyth, 2005). For example, a partial list of the activities deemed least likely to cause injury includes archery, aquatics, and elliptical trainers. On the more dangerous end of the spectrum, examples include lacrosse, power lifting, snowmobiling, trampolines, hockey, and karate as sports that are likely to cause injury. The booklet also contains training principles.

Conditions Affecting Bone

Bone health is affected by many factors. The development of an upright posture and subsequent stress on the bones contributes to the normal postnatal developmental changes in bony alignment. If the normal developmental sequence of upright activities is absent, delayed, or performed in atypical ways, the stresses to the bone will be different and can lead to atypical postural alignment. Lower extremity rotation abnormalities are common in ambulatory children with JIA or CP and dramatically increase the force across the knee (Gannotti et al., 2007). Children with JIA typically externally rotate their legs into a position of greater comfort, while children with CP have an internally rotated gait and do not experience the normal derotation of the neonatal antetorsion.

Disuse also adversely affects bone by delaying secondary ossification centers and causing the bone to reabsorb. Therefore, children with significant movement impairments, such as those seen with severe CP, spina bifida, or arthrogryposis multiplex congenital,

■ **Table 6.2** Typical Changes in Hemophilia Target Joints

Joint	Changes with Recurrent Bleeds
Knee	Flexion deformity with quadriceps atrophy
	Posterior subluxation, valgus, and external rotation of the tibia
	Hypertrophy of the medial femoral condyle
	Squaring of the patella
	Widening of the intracondylar notch
Elbow	Enlarged olecranon fossa with decreased flexion and extension
	Enlarged radial head resulting in decreased forearm rotation
	Subchondral bone cysts, especially on proximal ulna
Ankle	Flattening of talus
	Valgus deformity
	Osteophyte formation
	Calf atrophy
	Loss of dorsiflexion
Hip	Avascular necrosis similar to Legg-Calvé-Perthes disease
	Cystic changes in superior weight-bearing area of femoral head
	Osteophyte formation
Shoulder	Pronounced osteophyte formation
	Atrophy of head of humerus, resulting in varus deformity

Source: National Hemophilia Foundation. (2004). *Physical therapist's guide to bleeding disorders.*

are at greater risk for fractures due to disuse atrophy of the bones. Demineralization occurs quickly. One study found a 34% decrease in bone mineralization after being placed in non-weight-bearing immobilization following a fracture or surgery in only 4–6 weeks (Szalay et al., 2008). Poor bone mineralization also accompanies chronic conditions such as hemophilia (Barnes et al., 2004), leukemia (White et al., 2005), symptomatic epilepsy (Sheth & Hermann, 2008), long-term glucocorticoids (Sochett & Makitie, 2005), growth hormone deficiency and idiopathic scoliosis (Hunt et al., 2005). Likewise, conditions involving the digestive system, such as Crohn's disease (Harpavat et al., 2005) and irritable bowel disorder (Sylvester, 2005), have associated bone density deficiencies.

Although not commonly seen in the United States today due to improved knowledge and dietary supplements, both **scurvy** and **rickets** are diseases caused by dietary insufficiency, which can lead to bone abnormalities (see Table 6.3).

Fortunately, there are documented methods to promote healthy bone mineralization. Evidence suggests that calcium supplements can increase bone mineralization in healthy children (Vatanparast & Whiting, 2006) and in children with growth hormone deficiency (Zamboni, Antoniazzi, Lauriola, Bertold, & Tató, 2006). Impact exercise such as running and jumping can increase bone mineral density. Numerous studies demonstrate an increase in bone density in typically developing children with a consistent

Table 6.3 Bony Disorders

Diagnosis	Etiology	Pathology	Body Functions and Structure Impairments	Potential Activity Limitations and Participation Restrictions
Arthrogryposis multiplex congenital (Bevan et al., 2007)	• Unclear • Congenital disorder • Suspect teratogens • Lack of in utero movements may contribute • In utero muscular atrophy caused by muscle disease, virus, or maternal fever • Insufficient room due to lack of amniotic fluid or abnormally shaped uterus	• Deficit in the motor unit leads to severe fetal weakness • Fetal immobility leads to hypoplastic joint development and contractures	• Although contractures can vary between patients, the following presentation is most typical: shoulder adduction and internal rotation, elbow extension, wrist flexion and ulnar deviation, finger flexion, thumb in palm, hip flexion, abduction and external rotation, knee flexion, clubfeet (b710)* • Hip dislocation/subluxation • Jaw and tongue ROM limitations • Limbs appear tubular and lack normal joint creases • Diminished muscle mass and strength • Atypical fibrotic and lipid deposits • Fewer anterior horn cells in spinal cord	• Mobility difficulties (d455) • Diminished ADL skills such as dressing (d540) • Poor grasp (d4401) and handwriting (d345) • Feeding (d550) or speech difficulties (d330)

Table 6.3 Bony Disorders—cont'd

Diagnosis	Etiology	Pathology	Body Functions and Structure Impairments	Potential Activity Limitations and Participation Restrictions
Blount disease (Tibia vara)	• Two onset patterns • Infantile: obese children who walked before 1 year of age • Juvenile: most common in obese African American teenagers	• Compression of medial portion of proximal tibial physes that inhibits normal endochondral growth	• Lateral bowing of the tibia • Medial knee instability (b715)	• Pain (b280) • Knee instability may limit physical activities (d920) • Progressive joint degeneration • Cosmesis
Legg-Calvé-Perthes	• Unclear • Numerous associated factors include maternal smoking, low birth weight, and cesarean delivery • Higher incidence in lower socioeconomic, urban areas leads to hypothesis of nutritional deficit	• Unclear • Current theory; vascular disruption leading to aseptic necrosis (Weinstein, 1996) • Systemic component suspected because epiphyseal changes have been noted in the nonproblematic joints; blood content abnormalities	• Limp due to pain (b280) or weak abductor muscles • Frequently positive Trendelenburg sign • Limited ROM in hip abduction and internal rotation (b710) • Pain in hip or groin with activity (b280) • May see referred knee pain (b280)	• Pain can limit play (d9200) and ADL (d599) • Limp
Slipped capital femoral epiphysis	• Unclear; • 2.5:1 male to female ratio • Higher incidence in African Americans	• Posterior displacement of the capital femoral epiphysis from femoral neck	• Antalgic limp • Pain in groin or referred to anteriomedial thigh and knee (b280) • External rotation posturing	• Pain may limit activities • Long-term degenerative changes

Continued

Table 6.3 Bony Disorders—cont'd

Diagnosis	Etiology	Pathology	Body Functions and Structure Impairments	Potential Activity Limitations and Participation Restrictions
	• Local trauma associated with about 25% of cases • Decreased anteversion • Inflammation may weaken physeal plate • Endocrine imbalance • Delayed skeletal maturity • Obesity • Hormone levels; generally prepubescent onset (ages 10–15 years) • Hereditary contribution	through a weakened physis	• Decreased hip flexion, abduction and internal rotation (b710) • Leg moves into external rotation when flexed	
Scurvy	Dietary insufficiency of vitamin C (ascorbic acid)	• Decreased thickness of bone cortex and epiphyseal plates Decreased bone available for calcification	Fragile bones predisposed to fractures	Propensity for fractures limits play (d9200)
Rickets	Deficiency of vitamin D/lack of exposure to sunlight (sunlight converts body substance into vitamin D)	Deficiency interferes with bone calcification	Long bones bend under body weight resulting in abnormalities such as genu varum or valgum	• Cosmesis • May interfere with play (d9200) and ADL (d599)

Table 6.3 Bony Disorders—cont'd

Diagnosis	Etiology	Pathology	Body Functions and Structure Impairments	Potential Activity Limitations and Participation Restrictions
Osteogenesis imperfecta (Burnei et al., 2008)	OI is a heritable disease that is distinguished by four features that present in the following causal relationship: genetic disorder, collagen defect, bone fragility, and frequent fracture.	• Defects in type I collagen, which is the primary component of the protein matrix in bone, tissues, and organs • Increased bone turnover • Sequelae vary but often include short stature, scoliosis, poor tooth formation, hearing loss, blue sclera, translucent skin, triangular shaped face, osteoporosis, and ligamentous laxity	• Propensity for fractures and deformities • Severe scoliosis may impair cardio-respiratory status	• Fragility interferes with play (d9200) and ADL (d599) • Deformities may diminish ADL skills (d599) and mobility (d455)

*Numbers in parentheses refer to ICF-CY classification.

program of impact exercise (Hind & Burrows, 2007; Vicente-Rodriguez et al., 2007; McKay et al., 2005). Improvements in bone mineralization were not seen in children who participated in non-weight-bearing exercise such as swimming (Grimston, Willows, & Hanley, 1993).

Weight-bearing programs also improve bone mineral density and promote hip modeling in children with CP. Children with CP increased bone density by participating in 60 minutes of lower extremity weight bearing 3 or more days per week (Stuberg, 1992). The benefits were not maintained when only 30 minutes of weight bearing was provided. It was also suggested that intermittent weight bearing with movement was most beneficial to hip joint modeling (Stuberg, 1992). Intermittent weight bearing with movement can be accomplished by partial weight bearing ambulation through a use of a treadmill or gait trainer. Also, selecting an upright standing frame that allows some weight shifting would provide movement. Weight bearing is an important part of physical therapy intervention with young children with neuromuscular diseases that delay the development of stance.

Just as weight bearing is important for postnatal bone health, studies have shown that movement is important for prenatal joint development in birds and is believed to be important in humans as well. Inadequate in utero movement may impede the initial breakdown of the mesenchyme that forms the precursor to the joint space (Murray & Drachman, 1969). The formation of human joints proceeds rapidly from onset of mesenchymal breakdown to formation of a structure resembling an adult joint. The process is generally completed within a 4- to 7-week period. This rapid progress is beneficial to the fetus as the joints are most susceptible to deformation from teratogens during this period (Walker, 1991)

Disorders Involving Bone

Osteogenesis Imperfecta

Osteogenesis imperfecta (OI) is a genetic collagen mutation that manifests with fragile bones (see Table 6.3). Multiple fractures at birth are seen in severe forms of the disease. Mild forms of OI, however, may not be detected until later in childhood, after the child begins walking and presents to the emergency room with a fracture resulting from an insignificant injury. Examination of type I collagen and DNA may be necessary to differentiate between OI and abuse (Burnei, Vlad, Georgescu, Gavriliu & Dan, 2008).

Medical management is symptomatic, not curative. Bisphosphonates are prescribed to help improve bone density. Although it frequently takes weeks to months to see an effect of the bisphosphonates, they are generally successful at reducing bone pain, improving ambulation potential, and improving bone density. The most frequent surgical procedure is internal fixation of long bones. The goal of surgery is to minimize the incidence of fracture and avoid bone bowing, which compounds bone stress. This procedure is especially beneficial in children with marked bowing of bones and frequent fractures (Burnei et al., 2008).

Physical therapy plays an important role in the management of children with OI. Child and caregiver information is necessary to minimize recurrent fractures. Although roughhouse play and contact sports should be avoided, an aggressive yet safe exercise and standing program will help the child develop strength and endurance, maintain or increase ROM, and promote mineralization through weight bearing. Additionally, the physical therapist provides consultation for bracing and adaptive equipment selection. Developmental stimulation may also be needed to compensate for weakness and delayed skill acquisition caused by immobilization for fractures.

Although typically developing children also break bones, it is not the norm for healthy children to sustain a fracture. Fracture rates for healthy children do peak in early adolescence when bone turnover is high and mineralization often lags behind height and weight (Goulding, 2007). Some children have a predisposition to fracture. After a child has one fracture, the risk of subsequent fractures increases 2–3 times (Goulding, 2007). Repeat fractures account for the majority of reported pediatric fractures. A typical profile of a "fracture-prone" child would include having a first fracture before age 5 years, an aversion or allergy to cow's milk, low dietary calcium intake, and obesity (Goulding, Grant, & Williams, 2005). Low calcium intake leads to poor bone mineral content and smaller bone size.

Even though fracture-prone children may have a broken bone at an early age, children younger than 3 years should be evaluated for possible child abuse. Statistics suggest that first-born children, premature infants, stepchildren, children from families with low socioeconomic status, and those with a physical or learning difficulty are at higher risk for abuse (Lyden, 2009). It is a healthcare provider's legal responsibility to report suspected child abuse to the social work department or the police.

Epiphyseal Fracture

Epiphyseal fracture, a fracture that goes through the growth plate, can cause growth arrest in a child's bone. Epiphyseal fracture accounts for around 20% of pediatric fractures, most often in boys in the early adolescent period (Eiff, Hatch, & Calmbach, 2002).

The Salter-Harris classification system (Salter & Harris, 1963) is used to describe the extent of growth plate damage (see Fig. 6.1). If the fracture does not completely cross the epiphysis (Salter-Harris I or II), healing is generally good. If the fracture extends through the epiphyseal border (Salter-Harris III or IV), either complete or asymmetric growth arrest is more likely (Wattenbarger, Gruber, & Phieffer, 2002). Similarly, a crushing injury (Salter-Harris V) can have poor resolution. A complete arrest can lead to a significant limb length inequality, while asymmetrical arrest may result in angular deformities as one portion of the bone continues growing. The extent of the abnormality that develops is dependent on the type of fracture, age of the child, and stage of skeletal maturity.

Greenstick fractures are also specific to pediatrics (see Fig. 6.2). Greenstick fractures can occur in long

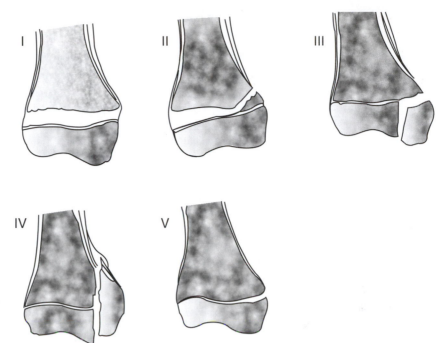

Figure 6.1 Schematic drawing of Salter-Harris classification of fractures of the growth plate.

bones when a force applied to one side of the bone breaks the cortex on the side of the impact and bends the other. This type of fracture frequently causes angular deformity and requires examination by an orthopedic physician (Goulding, 2007).

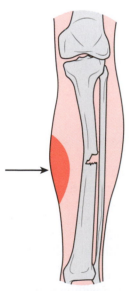

Figure 6.2 Greenstick fractures can occur in long bones when a force applied to one side of the bone breaks the cortex on the side of the impact and bends the other.

Following a fracture, weight bearing is commonly limited. The physical therapist will need to teach crutch or walker ambulation on both level surfaces and stairs. The age, cognitive ability, amount of pain, general physical health, family support, and environmental challenges must all be considered before dispensing a walking aid. Children 6 years or older, with typical intelligence, can generally learn how to use crutches. If the young child also sustained additional injuries or is not coping with the pain well, a walker should be considered. Children around 2 1/2 years can be taught how to use a walker. Time should be spent with the child to make sure the weight-bearing status is understood and followed.

Strengthening, ROM, and transfer skills should also be taught to anyone with compromised mobility. Typically the joints directly above and below the fracture are most susceptible to contracture because the child avoids moving the affected area to avoid pain. Ankle pumps and knee flexion and extension exercises are commonly needed.

Acquired Limb Length Discrepancy

There are three general classifications of acquired limb length discrepancy: direct, though growth retardation, and indirect through growth stimulation (see Table 6.4). An epiphyseal fracture, which causes growth arrest, eventually results in an indirect limb length inequality. A direct discrepancy can result if overriding bone segments are not corrected in a fracture. Elevated

Table 6.4 Causes of Indirect Limb Length Discrepancy

Classification	By Growth Retardation	By Growth Stimulation
Congenital	• Congenital hemiatrophy • Developmental hip dysplasia • Club foot	• Syndromes associated with partial giantism such as Klippel-Trénaunay, Parkes Weber • Hemophilia-induced hemarthrosis
Infection/ Inflammation	Epiphyseal plate destruction due to osteomyelitis, tuberculosis, or septic arthritis	• Increased blood flow associated with diaphyseal osteomyelitis, JIA (particularly in children under 3 years of age) and in chronic knee synovitis seen in children with hemophilia may cause overgrowth • Metaphyseal tuberculosis • Septic arthritis
Mechanical	Long-term weight relieving immobilization	Traumatic arteriovenous aneurysms
Neurologic	Paralysis or movement dysfunction such as poliomyelitis, spina bifida, or CP	
Trauma	• Damage to epiphyseal plate • Marked overriding of diaphyseal fragments • Severe burns	• Femur or tibia fractures can lead to osteosynthesis, particularly in young children • Diaphyseal operations; bone graft removal, osteotomy
Tumors	Tumor may invade growth plate Irradiation may damage growth plate Tumor may originate in cartilage cells; Ollier disease or enchondromatosis	Tumors may cause vascular malformations and stimulate growth through excessive circulation; hemangiomatosis, Klippel-Trénaunay-Weber syndrome Stimulation in nonvascular tumors; neurofibromatosis, Wilms tumor
Others	• Legg-Calvé-Perthes disease • Slipped capital femoral epiphysis	

Source: Adapted from Moseley, C.F. (1996). Leg length discrepancy and angular deformity of the lower limbs. In R.T. Morrissey & S.L. Weinstein (Eds.), *Lovell and Winter's pediatric orthopedics* (pp. 849–901). Philadelphia: Lippincott-Raven.

blood flow to a bone due to a tumor or hemophilia can cause an indirect inequality due to bone overgrowth or retardation.

When evaluating a limb length discrepancy, the examiner must also consider **"apparent" limb length discrepancies** caused by joint contractures, angular deformities, hip subluxation or dislocation, pelvic obliquity or spinal alignment, etc. A thorough limb length examination, therefore, must incorporate examination of the muscle length, the joints above and below the bone in question, and the child's posture.

If it is determined that a true limb length discrepancy is present, treatment is planned based on:

• The amount of the discrepancy
• The preferences of the child and family

• Age of the child
• Skeletal maturity
• Neuromuscular status
• Child's general health
• Motivation/compliance
• Family support
• Intelligence
• Emotional stability
• Presence of additional pathology

General guidelines for treatment of leg length discrepancy in children without a neurological condition are provided in Table 6.5. These guidelines do not take into account the individual characteristics of each child, so they should be considered only as general guidelines, not treatment recommendations.

■ **Table 6.5** Leg Length Inequality General
■ Treatment Guidelines

0–2 cm: No treatment
2–4 cm: Shoe lift
2–6 cm: Epiphyseodesis, shortening
6–20 cm: Lengthening that may or may not be combined with other procedures
>20 cm: Prosthetic fitting

Even mild leg length discrepancies can increase energy expenditure, and a discrepancy as small as 1 centimeter alters the amount of postural sway seen in a child (Mahar, Kirby, & MacLeod, 1985; Moseley, 1991). The most obvious sequelae of a moderate to severe limb length discrepancy is cosmesis. Functional limitations, pain, and secondary degenerative changes may also be present. The child will need to make gait pattern changes to accommodate the inequality that can result in secondary impairments. For example, if the child toe walks on the short side, dorsiflexion ROM will be lost in this ankle. Additionally, the altered gait pattern may put atypical stress on the knees or back resulting in pain or long-term degenerative changes. In the upper extremity, moderate or severe limb length discrepancies can interfere with bimanual activities.

Congenital limb loss accounts for the majority of pediatric amputations in the western world. It is estimated that 60% of limb deficiencies in children are congenital in nature, followed by trauma, tumors, and other infections (Nelson et al., 2006). Limb buds form between 2 and 6 weeks gestation. It is believed that congenital limb deletions occur between 3 and 8 weeks of gestation. The International Society for Prosthetics and Orthotics (ISO-ISPO) has established a standardized classification system for congenital amputations. A **transverse deficiency** has been defined as the level at which the limb terminates. In **longitudinal deficiencies**, the deficient bones are named in sequence from proximal to distal, and it is specified as to whether the deficit is partial or total. Bones that are not named are considered present and healthy (Krajbich, 1998). The clinical spectrum of limb deficiencies can be extremely complex from diagnosis to treatment.

Hemimelia

Hemimelia refers to an absence or gross shortening of a bone. Fibular hemimelia is considered the most common of the lower limb deficiencies, with an incidence of 1–2 per 100,000 live births (Ghanem, 2008). The clinical presentation can range from a missing toe or tarsal coalition to the absence of the entire fibular bone. Associated impairments can include hypoplasia, instability of the patella, anterior/posterior knee instability, limb length inequality, tibial deformity, disruption of the ankle morphology, and possible forefoot defects (Stanitski & Stanitski, 2003). Treatment recommendations are based on a detailed evaluation of the limb and will be discussed in detail for all deficiencies.

Tibial hemimelia was first described by Billroth (cited in Weber, 2008). Tibial hemimelias are considered extremely rare, with an incidence of approximately 1 per 1,000,000 live births (Ghanem, 2008). Treatment for this deficiency is based on an extensive evaluation of the exact malformations of the limb. As with fibular deficiencies, tibial deficiencies can range from tibial hypoplasia with no other tissue malformations to complete absence of the tibia with other deformities in the femur, patella, fibula, and foot (Weber, 2008).

Proximal femoral focal deficiency (PFFD) is specifically characterized by deformity of the proximal portion of the femur. Classifications of femur abnormalities have been described by Aitken (1959) and Amstutz and Wilson (1962) (cited in Westberry & Davids, 2009). There is a wide variety of clinical features in the PFFD population, including a mild minimal shortening of the femur with normal hip development to a more severe complete absence of the femur with possible associated problems of acetabular dysplasia, smaller thigh musculature, knee joint deformity, and other possible impairments throughout the lower limb (Gillespie & Torode, 1983).

Treatment Options

Treatment for all limb deficiencies is based on the extent of the deficiency and associated limb inequality. The primary goal of treatment is maximizing function. If there is greater than 50% shortening of the limb, surgeries such as a Symes or Boyd amputation, rotation plasty, knee fusion, and femoropelvic arthodesis is typically performed followed by a prosthetic fitting. Limb lengthening is an option if the final predicted discrepancy is less than 20 cm but is a complex and lengthy treatment that may be financially and emotionally taxing on the child and family (Walker et al., 2009). This procedure is discussed in more detail later in the chapter. There are other available ancillary surgeries for correction of knee joint deficiencies, including instability, patellofemoral problems, or genu valgum (Walker et al., 2009).

Epiphysiodesis

An epiphysiodesis can equalize limb length by slowing growth in the longer leg. An epiphysiodesis completely stops the growth at the epiphysis of the bone but only slows the growth of the entire limb due to contributions of the other growth plates in the limb. The shorter leg continues to grow at its normal rate until it reaches skeletal maturity.

Successful planning is necessary so that the shorter limb will grow until approximate symmetry is obtained. This is accomplished by estimating growth velocity and skeletal maturity. Growth velocity is estimated by plotting growth every 6 months for 2 or more years (Herring, 2002). Skeletal maturity, an indicator of the amount of growth remaining, cannot be determined by the child's age alone, due to varying maturation rates. Estimates of skeletal maturity can be determined by comparing ossification levels seen on a radiograph to documented standards. Radiographs of the left hand and wrist are compared to standards in either the **Greulich-Pyle Atlas** (Greulich & Pyle, 1959) or **Tanner-Whitehouse Atlas** (Tanner & Buckler, 1997). The **Risser sign** can also estimate skeletal maturity by using iliac crest radiographs to grade the appearance of the secondary ossification centers. Grades between 0 (no appearance) and 4 (completed ossification) are assigned. Estimation of skeletal maturity is still imprecise and subjective, which contributes to the difficulty in accurately treating a leg length inequality. Maturity estimations and growth velocity are then used to project how quickly and for how long the child will grow. Based on the proposed timeline, the longer bone is cauterized to stop growth while the shorter limb continues to grow.

Leg Lengthening

If the discrepancy is too large for a shortening procedure, lengthening of the shorter limb can be done in isolation or in combination with an epiphysiodesis of the longer limb. Leg lengthening, however, can be an expensive, prolonged process with risks of serious complications including infection, malunion, contractures, possible fractures, scarring, and decreased bone strength. The procedure involves performing an osteotomy to remove the bone cortex and then applying a device to distract the bone while providing external stability. A monolateral or circumferential device can be used to distract the leg, provide stability, and correct angular deformities (see Figs. 6.3 and 6.4.)

Regardless of the type of device, physical therapy is critical to ensuring a functional outcome. Intervention goals include performing and instructing the family in pin site wound care to prevent infection, ROM, strengthening, and progressive ambulation.

ROM limitations can develop quickly during leg lengthening procedures for several reasons. Initially, pain and anxiety associated with the surgery limit movement. Additionally, the pins or wires that attach the fixator go through the muscle and can cause pain or physically limit movement. Finally, as the bone is lengthened, muscles and nerves must also stretch to accommodate the new distance. ROM is commonly lost in hip extension, knee flexion and extension, and ankle dorsiflexion. Knee flexion limitations tend to resolve over time when the device is removed; however, knee extension deficits have been associated with more chronic functional limitations (Moseley, 1991). The therapist should carefully monitor all joint motion as the type of apparatus, previous

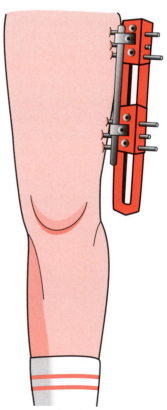

Figure 6.3 A monolateral lengthening device.

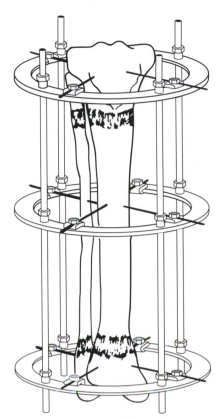

Figure 6.4 A circumferential lengthening device.

deformity, and child activities can all contribute to ROM complications.

Children who have a leg lengthened are encouraged to be active. Although children with fixators are typically hesitant to ambulate, children are encouraged to ambulate as much as possible. This promotes ROM, strength, and bone consolidation, as well as helps with the psychosocial aspects of the extended intervention. Temporary lifts for the child's short leg may need to be fabricated to allow weight bearing as the limb length changes.

Upper Extremity Deletions

Upper extremity deletions are more common than lower (2:1), with 40% of all deletions being a transverse left radial deletion (Nelson et al., 2006) Expert recommendations suggest that an active prosthetic device can be considered by age 12 to 15 months. Children typically use upper extremity prostheses for specific tasks but prefer using their residual limb for daily activities if the prosthesis does not improve their function. They report that upper extremity prostheses can be bulky and uncomfortable. Additionally, the use

of a prosthesis eliminates sensory input that using a residual limb provides (Biddiss & Chau, 2007; James et al., 2006).

The Prosthetic Upper Extremity Functional Index (PUFI) (James et al., 2006) and the University of New Brunswick (UNB) Test of Prosthetic Function (Wright, Hubbard, Naumann, & Jutai, 2003) (http://www.unb.ca/biomed/unb_test_of_prosthetics_function.pdf) are two assessments that can evaluate the child's functional abilities while wearing the prosthesis.

The decision to lengthen a bone or amputate the extremity at an optimal level for a prosthesis is based on many factors. Severity of the abnormality is obviously the most important factor. Lengthening can be a painful and arduous procedure. If the bone is significantly involved, an amputation and prosthesis can be a more functional solution. Frequently this is a hard option for parents to choose.

Because children grow, adjustments to the prosthesis harness or socket may be necessary every 3 to 6 months. Replacement of the prosthesis will be needed about every year for children less than 5 years of age and every other year for children age 5–12 years. Ten to thirty percent of children will need a socket adjustment or surgical correction of their stump because the bone continues to grow and causes pain if it is too close to the surface (Nelson et al., 2006). Physical therapy care for children with amputations has similarities to adult treatment in that it must include proper donning and doffing of the prosthesis, stump management, assistance in functional problem solving, strengthening and maintaining/achieving optimal ROM. Pediatric care may also include teaching developmental milestones if the amputation occurs early in life. Growth also creates challenges because new prosthetics are needed on a regular basis. Table 6.6 lists common gait deviations and possible solution for a child using a prosthesis for a transtibial amputation.

Disorders Involving the Spine
Adolescent Idiopathic Idiosis (AIS)

Scoliosis is a curvature of the spine that can have a structural or nonstructural origin. A structural curve is fixed without the typical spinal flexibility and is caused by an abnormality of the shape or structure of the vertebrae. A nonstructural curve is flexible and caused by positioning, muscular weakness/imbalance, or a neuropathy.

There are several types of idiopathic scoliosis that are classified by the age of appearance. **Infantile**

Table 6.6 Common Transtibial Amputation Gait Deviations

Gait Cycle Phase	Deviation	Possible Causes
Initial contact (heel strike)	Knee is fully extended	• Suspension is faulty (does not maintain knee in 5°–10° of flexion) • Preflexion of the socket is insufficient • Foot is too anterior
	Knee is excessively flexed (>10°)	• Suspension is faulty (maintains knee in >10° of flexion) • Possible flexion contracture is present
	Length is unequal stride	• Suspension is faulty (may limit knee range of motion) • Poor gait pattern is present
Heel strike to foot flat (loading response)	Knee flexion is not smooth or controlled, may look "jerky"	• Quadriceps are weak
	Knee flexion is abrupt and uncontrolled	• Foot is too posterior • Socket is too flexed (foot is excessively dorsiflexed) • Heel on shoe is too high • Plantarflexion bumper or heel wedge in foot is too firm • Shoe does not allow heel cushion to compress sufficiently
	Knee remains extended and patient "rides" the heel through to mid-stance	• Foot is too anterior • Socket flexion is insufficient (foot plantarflexed) • SACH heel is too soft (if > 0.95 cm [³⁄₈ in]) • Heel on shoe is too low • Poor gait pattern is present (excessive use of knee extensors)
	Piston action occurs. Patient may be dropping too deeply into the socket (best viewed in the coronal plane as patient walks away from observer)	• Suspension is too loose • Not enough prosthetic socks are used • Socket modifications are faulty (not enough support under mediotibial flare or patellar tendon)
Midstance	Pylon leans medially	• The socket has too much adduction • Foot may be outset
	Pylon leans laterally	• The socket has too little adduction • Foot may be inset
	1.27-cm (¹⁄₂-in) varus moment is not apparent (for some patients this may be desirable to reduce torque)	• Foot is relatively outset
	Varus moment is excessive (>1.27 cm [¹⁄₂ in] is never desirable)	• Foot is too inset • Mediolateral socket dimension is too wide
	There are <5.08 cm (2 in) between feet at midstance	• Foot is inset (narrow base gait)
	There are >10.16 cm (4 in) between feet at midstance	• Foot is too outset

Table 6.6 Common Transtibial Amputation Gait Deviations—cont'd

Gait Cycle Phase	Deviation	Possible Causes
	Lateral trunk bends to the prosthetic side at midstance	• Prosthesis is too short • Because of residual limb pain, patient leans laterally to reduce torque • Prosthesis is too long • Foot is too outset
Terminal stance (heel-off)	Heel-off occurs early and abruptly. The patient appears to "drop off" the foot at the end of stance phase Heel-off is delayed. The patient's knee may tend to hyperextend. The patient may describe a feeling of "walking uphill"	• Because of excessive posterior position of the foot, toe lever arm is too short • Foot may be excessively dorsiflexed (sockets in too much flexion) • Because of excessive anterior placement of the foot, toe lever arm is too long • The foot may be plantarflexed (insufficient socket flexion)
Preswing (toe-off)	"Drop off" occurs. The patient appears to fall too quickly to the sound side Socket drops away from residual limb (evident when the anterior socket gaps or the posterior proximal socket rim drops distally in relation to the popliteal region)	• Foot is too posterior • Foot is too dorsiflexed (excessive socket flexion) • Suspension is too loose (for supracondylar sockets) or indentation is located too high above the femoral condyles (for patellar tendon–bearing supracondylar-suprapatellar sockets) • Patient may not be wearing enough prosthetic socks
Swing	Foot "whips" medially or laterally during initial swing Prosthetic foot touches the floor during midswing	• Cuff suspension tabs are not aligned evenly • Prosthetic socket is rotated medially or laterally with respect to the line of progression • Prosthesis is too long • Suspension is too loose • Knee flexion may be limited by the socket or suspension system • Patient may have muscle weakness or lack of gait training

Source: Adapted with permission from Kapp, S.L. (2004). Visual analysis of prosthetic gait. In D.G. Smith, J.W. Michael, J.H. Bowker (Eds.), *Atlas of amputations and limb deficiencies: Surgical, prosthetic, and rehabilitation principles* (3rd ed., pp. 385–394). Rosemont: American Academy of Orthopaedic Surgeons.

scoliosis is seen in children less than 3 years of age and **juvenile scoliosis** appears between the ages of 3 and 10 years. **Adolescent scoliosis** (the focus of this section) is diagnosed between age 10 years and skeletal maturity. The etiology of adolescent idiopathic scoliosis is unclear but is believed to have a hereditary component (Wynn-Davies, 1968). It has an incidence of 2%–3% (Scoliosis Research Society, 2003). Small curves of about 10° affect boys and girls equally. Incidence changes dramatically if the curve is greater than 20°, where a 10:1 female dominance is seen (Bunnell, 2005). This suggests that curve progression is greater in girls than boys.

The Cobb method is the standard way to quantify curve size using an anterior-posterior x-ray view. Figure 6.5 shows the Cobb method for measuring the amount of curvature.

To calculate a Cobb angle from an x-ray, the vertebrae that are at the greatest tilt on either end of the curve are identified. A line is drawn parallel to the top

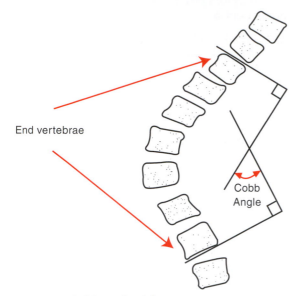

End vertebrae

Cobb
Angle

Figure 6.5 Cobb method for measuring curve.

end plate of the top vertebra and the bottom end plate of the bottom vertebra. Perpendicular lines are then drawn from each of these. The angle formed where these two perpendicular lines intersect is the amount of curvature (Tolo & Wood, 1993). The Cobb method is a good estimate of curvature magnitude but should not be used to quantify small changes, as the angle measurement can change based on the position of the child during the x-ray or the examiner's lines. Additionally, the Cobb method assesses only the lateral aspect of the major curvature. Scoliotic curves frequently have a major curve and a compensatory, opposite smaller curve. In addition, a rotational component and lordosis are typically present.

The rotational component of scoliosis is termed a **"rib hump"** and is produced by a rotation of the spine and subsequent protrusion of one side of the ribs. The **Adam's Forward Bend Test** (described in Chapter 5) is used to check for a rip hump by looking at the child's back when the child bends forward with arms hanging down freely. Lordosis is another component of scoliosis and is typically most pronounced at the curve apex (center) (Dickson, 1999).

School screening for scoliosis is commonly done in many states, but there is some controversy regarding its value. Critics are concerned about subjecting incorrectly identified children to unnecessary follow-up radiographs. Large radiographs expose the child to radiation, which in high amounts may result in a small but significant increase in cancer risk (Côté, Kreitz,

Cassidy, Dzus, & Martel, 1998). Studies have reported the ability of the Adam's Forward Bend Test to accurately detect a 10° to 40° curve (sensitivity) at between 77% and 83% (Goldberg, Dowling, Fogarty, & More, 1995; Karachalios et al., 1999). Karachalios and colleagues found the specificity of detecting a 10° curve to be 93% in a sample of 2,700 students, which suggests that a small number of students were incorrectly referred for follow-up.

Other screening tools are available, but these also have limitations. A scoliometer can be used to determine the angle of trunk rotation. A scoliometer is a level that is used with the individual in the same forward bend position as the Adam's bend test (see Fig. 5.18). The scoliometer is placed perpendicularly on the apex of the curve, with the center of the level placed on the most prominent spinous process. The angle of trunk rotation is then measured.

Despite the limitations of the screening tools and the risk of over-referral, recent evidence suggests that routine school screenings are useful in optimizing scoliosis intervention. In a Canadian study performed after national screening was discontinued, one clinic reported that 42% of all new patients were inappropriately referred. This is a higher rate of error than the reported sensitivity of the Adam's Forward Bend Test (Goldberg et al., 1995; Karachalios et al., 1999). Additionally, of the new patients with scoliosis, 32% presented too late for optimal bracing (Beauséjour, Roy-Beaudry, Goulet, & Labelle, 2007). Similar results were reported by Bunge and colleagues (2007), where the average curve of the patients referred to the orthopedist through a routine screening program was 24° in contrast to an average curve of 40° if the child was referred by a primary care doctor.

Bunnell (2005) and colleagues have developed guidelines for maximizing the efficiency of routine screening based on sex, age, type, and magnitude of the curve and skeletal maturity. These guidelines are presented in Table 6.7. Guidelines for follow up screening were also developed and are presented in Table 6.8 (Bunnell, 2005).

Treatment guidelines for idiopathic scoliosis vary among physicians. Intervention can be conservative or by surgical correction through spinal fusion. There is consensus that curves over 35° with a significant rotational component require surgical correction (Lenssinck et al., 2005). During the postsurgical inpatient stay, the physical therapist teaches log rolling, bed mobility, ROM exercises, transfers, and other ADL skills using movement patterns that avoid spinal

■ Table 6.7 Scoliosis Screening Guidelines

Girls
3 female :1 male
Females have 10× risk of progression and fusion

10 years old
<12 years have 3× risk of progression
Pre-menarche risk of progression is reduced 2/3 after menarche

Thoracic and double-major curves
3× risk of progression of nonthoracic curves

Growth potential
Greatest increase during growth spurt

Curve magnitude
20% for 20° curves
60% for 30° curves
90% for 50° curves

Risser stage/skeletal maturity
Risk reduced 2/3 if iliac crest more than 50% capped

Source: Bunnell, W.P. (2005). Selective screening for scoliosis. *Clinical Orthopaedics and Related Research, 434,* 40–45.

■ Table 6.8 Guidelines for Scoliosis Referral

- If no rib hump at 10 years of age, none of the children's curves progressed.
- 5° scoliometer trunk rotation angle does not need rescreening; significant scoliosis is not present nor likely to develop.
- 10° or > scoliometer trunk rotation angle should be referred to physician
- 5° to 9° scoliometer trunk rotation angle should be rescreened every 6 months until 1 year after the occurrence of menarche.

Source: Bunnell, W.P. (2005). Selective screening for scoliosis. *Clinical Orthopaedics and Related Research, 434,* 40–45.

rotation. The child can learn to don and doff the orthoses while lying in bed to avoid trunk rotation. Strengthening exercises without resistance, such as quadriceps and gluteal sets, can also be beneficial.

When initiating ambulation postsurgery, the therapist must watch for orthostatic hypotension. Orthostatic hypotension is a rapid drop in blood pressure when moving into a standing position and can cause the child to become dizzy or faint. Postoperative bed rest following a major surgery puts the child at risk for orthostatic hypotension. To minimize the risk of this happening, the child should be instructed to perform ankle pumps to promote blood circulation. To improve compliance, a gimmick such as asking the child to do 10 ankle pumps during each commercial while watching television can be used. When ambulation training is commenced, it is important to make the transition from lying to standing slowly. If necessary, a tilt table can be used to raise the child to an upright position at tolerable increments.

Bracing, exercise, or a combination of the two are possible conservative treatments for lesser curves. The reported efficacy of conservative treatment varies widely in scientific literature. Recent evidence suggests that an intense program of exercise can be effective (Lenssinck et al., 2005). Exercise programs reported include the Schroth method (Lehnert-Schroth, 2007), postural training, and hitch and slide exercises. In children with large thoracic level curves, exercises for respiratory capability may also be needed as the curve may impede thoracic expansion and limit breathing (Shepard, 1995).

An orthosis is often prescribed for children with curves between 20° and 35°. Orthotic intervention has been shown to stop the progression of 90% of 20°–35° curves, if the brace is worn 23 hours/day (Nicholson, Ferguson-Pell, Smith, Edgar, & Morley, 2003). Twenty-three hours each day is a substantial commitment. Nicholson and colleagues (2003) investigated wearing compliance. In their study sample, compliance ranged from 8% to 90% (M = 65%). More striking is the finding that reported compliance was overestimated by an average of 150% (SD = 50%) (Nicholson et al., 2003).

Physical therapists must also encourage the child to remain physically active during brace intervention. Cardiopulmonary fitness is an important component of the child's health plan and can be achieved through community-based fitness activities such as dancing, cycling, swimming, and various types of physical education classes. Being involved in community activities can also assist with the poor self-image that may accompany wearing a brace.

If a scoliosis is detected but is flexible, the therapist should also assess leg length asymmetry, uneven hip or shoulder heights during standing, increased space between the elbow and the trunk on the concave side of the curve, and muscular or neurological abnormalities. These signs may indicate that the adolescent's scoliosis is not idiopathic, but rather occurring due to another condition or pathology (e.g., leg length discrepancy, pelvic obliquity). To optimize outcomes, the physical therapist must perform a differential diagnosis to ensure that the treatment plan addresses the cause of the scoliosis, if known.

Arthrogryposis Multiplex Congenita

Arthrogryposis multiplex congenita (AMC) is a collection of syndromes characterized by multiple contractures and joint deformities at birth believed to be a result of a decreased fetal movement (see Table 6.3). The most common form of arthrogryposis is referred to as **amyoplasia**, where there is deficient formation of the muscle tissue. The etiology of the decreased fetal movement is unclear but is theorized to be due to patch damage of the anterior horn cells in the spinal column (Mennen, van Heest, Ezaki, Tonkin, & Gericke, 2005). Arthrogryposis is fatal in the neonatal period in about 50% of newborns (Bevan et al., 2007). In 90% of surviving children, all four extremities are involved with a symmetrical distribution of multiple joints (Bevan et al., 2007). Because of the damage to the spinal cord anterior horn cells, the muscles of children with AMC are underdeveloped. Extremities often have a tubular appearance without the normal skin folds over joints (see Fig. 6.6).

Disorders of the Hip

Developmental Dysplasia of the Hip

During gestation, the initial limb bud undergoes a remarkable process of growth and modeling in response

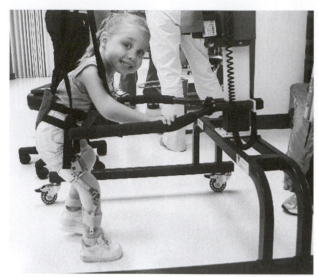

Figure 6.6B Child with arthrogryposis taking steps in a partial weight-bearing harness. Note standing pattern due to hip and knee contractures.

to in utero movement and stresses. This process is clearly illustrated in the hip joint. Early in gestation, the fetal femoral head is almost completely surrounded by a deep acetabulum. With fetal growth, the diameter of the acetabulum surpasses the increase in acetabular depth, resulting in a shallower acetabulum. Additionally, the femoral head is initially spherical but becomes more flattened due to constriction in the uterus as the fetus grows. It is hypothesized that the unstable hip joint facilitates the passage of the fetus through the birth canal; however, it also may lead to a dislocated or subluxed hip (Walker, 1991). Postnatally, the depth of the acetabulum increases with growth, and the femoral head returns to a more spherical shape to form a congruent stable joint.

Developmental dysplasia of the hip (DDH) is a condition of pathological hip instability. It is diagnosed in 1 to 1.5 out of 1,000 neonates, with the left hip most often involved (Song, McCarthy, MacEwen, Fuchs, & Dulka, 2008) (see Table 6.9). Ultrasound is the gold standard for confirming hip dislocation; however, hip abduction limitation or asymmetry is the most consistent clinical sign of hip dysplasia in neonates (Senaran, Ozdemir, Ogun, & Kapicioglu, 2004). A hip abduction limitation is reported to be present in 41% of children later diagnosed with developmental hip dysplasia (Senaran et al., 2004). Typically, a neonate will have between 75° and 90° of abduction in each hip. If a significant limitation or

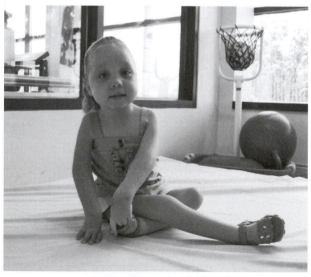

Figure 6.6A Child with arthrogryposis. Note tubular appearance of extremities.

■ **Table 6.9** Congenital Joint Anomalies

Diagnosis	Etiology	Pathology	Body Functions and Structure Impairments	Potential Activity Limitations and Participation Restrictions
Talipes Equinovarus	• Unknown • Speculated multifactorial: genetic component, arrested embryonic development, neuromuscular abnormalities, mechanical uterine constriction	Displacement of the navicular, calcaneus, and cuboid bones around the talus	Hindfoot equinus with varus of the forefoot and heel and adducted forefoot	• Interferes with standing (d4154),* ambulation (d450), and other upright activities • Difficulty fitting shoes • Cosmesis
Developmental Dysplasia of the Hip (DDH)	• Multifactorial: • Genetic predisposition; first born; 80% female • Ethnic: higher incidence in Native Americans, lower incidence in Chinese and Africans • Mechanical: breech position, oligohydramnios (insufficient amniotic fluid) • Neuromuscular: myelomeningocele	• Subluxation, dislocation or dysplasia of the hip • Hypertrophied ridge of cartilage in the superior, posterior and inferior aspects of the acetabulum called a neolimbus	• Unstable hip joint • Limited hip abduction (b710) • Poor weight-bearing surface • Apparent leg length discrepancy if femur not residing in the acetabulum • Poor hip socket development	• Can interfere with motor milestone acquisition • Impedes ambulation (d450) and other upright activities • Leg length inequality may be cosmetically displeasing and require increased energy expenditure for ambulation • Painful degenerative changes over time

*Numbers in parentheses refer to ICF-CY classification.

even a small asymmetry (5°–10°) exists, developmental hip dysplasia should be considered. Other clinical signs can include skin fold asymmetry, pistoning, or an apparent leg length discrepancy, as examined using Galeazzi sign (see Fig. 6.7)

Examination of the Hip

The **Ortolani** and **Barlow signs** are the two primary clinical tests used to assess hip stability in neonates less than 1 month of age. The Ortolani sign (Fig. 6.8) is the palpable sensation of the femoral head gliding over the neolimbus (cartilaginous ridge) as it moves back into the acetabulum. The infant's hips and knees are flexed 90°. The thigh is gently abducted, which brings the femoral head from its dislocated posterior position forward into the acetabulum, hence reducing the femoral head back into the acetabulum. In a positive finding, there is a palpable and audible clunk as hip reduces.

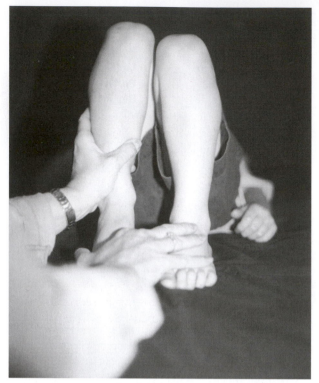

Figure 6.7 Example of Galeazzi sign. Note differences in knee height. The lower knee indicates a hip dislocation.

The Barlow maneuver (Fig. 6.9) is a more aggressive maneuver in which the hip is flexed and adducted while the examiner palpates the femoral head as it exits the acetabulum (Wenger, 1993). The hip is flexed and the thigh adducted, while pushing posteriorly in the line of the shaft of femur, causing the femoral head to dislocate posteriorly from the acetabulum. Dislocation is palpable as femoral head slips out of the acetabulum.

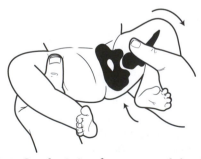

Figure 6.8 Ortolani sign for suspected developmental dysplasia of the hip.

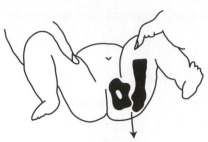

Figure 6.9 Barlow maneuver for suspected developmental dysplasia of the hip.

Both the Ortolani and the Barlow tests must be performed on one leg at a time, when the infant is completely relaxed, as muscle contractions can hide the instability. During both tests the examiner's thumb is on the anterior surface of the thigh while the fingers are palpating the posterior joint space. Both the Ortolani and Barlow signs require training with an experienced mentor to ensure reliability. A physical therapist working with neonates in a neonatal ICU, nursery, or outpatient program should be able to perform the tests accurately and reliably.

Treatment of Developmental Dysplasia of the Hip

The unstable hip joint should be a consideration when positioning or performing ROM with all neonates, not just those showing clinical signs of joint instability. Positions of extreme or forceful extension should be avoided as it may lead to dislocation (Salter, 1968). Additionally, a relationship has been reported between sleeping position preferences and hip dysplasia. In a sample of 41 infants with a preferred side-lying position, hip dysplasia was seen in the upper hip of 19 of the children (Heikkila, Ryoppy, & Louhimo, 1985). It was hypothesized that the position of adduction and internal rotation of the upper hip reduced the remolding stimulus of the acetabulum.

The Agency for Healthcare Research and Quality (http://www.ahrq.gov) suggests that 60%–80% of clinically diagnosed hips and 90% of hips diagnosed with ultrasound will resolve spontaneously. Although this suggests this population is likely being overtreated, unresolved DDH can lead to devastating disability later in life. Fortunately, the most common intervention for DDH in a neonate or infant, the **Pavlik harness,** shown in Figure 6.10, has very few detrimental side effects.

The harness maintains the hip in a position of flexion and abduction that can promote acetabular

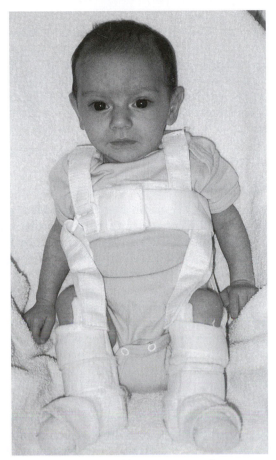

Figure 6.10 The Pavlik harness is used to maintain the hip in flexion and abduction to promote acetabular development and prevent hip subluxation in infants with developmental dysplasia of the hip.

development, while avoiding the subluxing positions of extension and adduction. The harness is preferable over casting because it allows spontaneous movement; however, hip spica casts are sometimes used if adequate containment cannot be achieved using the harness. The Pavlik harness has a success rate of approximately 95% for subluxed hips and 85% for dislocations if used correctly (Cashman, Round, Taylor, & Clarke, 2002). Although complications associated with the use of the Pavlik harness are infrequent, periodic monitoring of the hips is required to avoid avascular necrosis (bone death due to inadequate blood supply), femoral nerve palsy, or inferior dislocations. If the dysplastic hip is not detected in the neonatal or infancy period, the prognosis is less favorable. Infants over 9 months of age may need to have a closed hip reduction and then be placed in a hip spica cast. Often the cast can be fabricated to allow weight

bearing and ambulation. If the closed reduction is unsuccessful, an open reduction and containment may be warranted (Guille, Pizzutillo, & MacEwen, 2000). Surgical reduction is preceded by 2–3 weeks of traction to avoid avascular necrosis. Generally, home traction can be used to avoid a lengthy hospital stay.

Legg-Calvé-Perthes

Legg-Calvé-Perthes (LCP) syndrome is a bone abnormality that predominantly affects boys' hips (4:1 male: female ratio) between the ages of 4 and 8 years of age. The boys are typically of shorter stature due to delayed bone growth and tend to be active and athletic (Bahmanyar, Montgomery, Weiss, & Ekbom, 2008). The cause of LCP is believed to be multi-factorial but results in avascular necrosis of the femoral head. A recent report suggests that heavy maternal smoking during pregnancy increases the risk of the child having LCP by 100% (Bahmanyar et al., 2008). Another theory also links second-hand smoke to an increased incidence of LCP (Mehta, Conybeare, Hinves, & Winter, 2006). The proximal femur receives its blood supply from three sources: the extracapsular arterial ring made up of the medial and lateral femoral circumflex vessels, the ascending cervical vessels, and the vessel of the ligamentum teres. Interruption of the blood flow from the medial femoral circumflex artery is suspected to lead to aseptic avascular necrosis of the femoral head and bone reabsorption.

Children with LCP often present with a limp of insidious onset (Weinstein, 1996). The limp is commonly a drop in the pelvis of the swinging leg and trunk leaning toward the stance side (Westhoff, Petermann, Hirsch, Willers, & Krauspe, 2006). The child may not complain of much pain unless prompted, and usually reports it is aggravated by activity, relieved by rest, and may be referred to the anteriomedial thigh or knee. Parents may initially dismiss the child's complaints due to the inconsistent presentation of pain.

Treatment decisions are based on the age of the child and extent of femoral head involvement. The Salter-Thompson classification system categorizes hips into two groups. In group A, less than 50% of the head is involved; in group B, more than 50% of the head is involved. Obviously, if less than 50% of the head is involved, the prognosis is better; whereas if more than 50% is involved, the prognosis is potentially poor.

Conservative treatment, most often prescribed for Salter-Thompson group A, can include observation, ROM exercises, traction, use of a wheelchair to limit weightbearing, bilateral long leg casts with a fixed abduction bar (called Petrie casts), or braces. The goal of intervention is to optimize containment of the femoral head within the acetabulum. Hip abduction puts the head of the femur deepest into the acetabulum, thus preventing further flattening of the femoral head and encouraging remodeling back into a spherical shape. The necrotic tissue is gradually replaced with new bone and the compression encourages congruent shaping.

Surgical treatment for LCP disease can be a tenotomy to lengthen shortened muscles, a proximal varus osteotomy of the femur to reposition the femoral head securely in the acetabulum, or a shelf osteoplasty to deepen the acetabulum and provide better coverage of the femoral head. Consensus on the best treatment, or even if treatment is needed, has not been reached. A study by Canavese and Dimeglio (2008) suggests that group A LCP disease in children 6 years old or younger is most often a self-limiting condition and responds well to conservative treatment. Two studies of children between the ages of 4 and 6 years with group B disease (combined N = 352) reported no difference in outcome between the conservative and surgical treatment groups. Interestingly, one-third of children with a diagnosis of LCP also present with a diagnosis of ADHD (Loder, Schwartz, & Hensinger, 1993).

Optimal long-term outcome is dependent on the shape and congruency of the femoral head and acetabulum at skeletal maturity. Flattened femoral heads presented few problems, but irregularly shaped heads were a chronic source of problems (Lecuire, 2002). An irregular shaped femoral head or incongruence can lead to long-term degenerative osteoarthritis.

Physical therapy helps encourage optimal outcome by addressing pain, ROM, and strength issues. Hip abduction and external rotation are the best positions for placing the femoral head into the acetabulum. Frequent muscle spasms, pain or an altered gait pattern have led to decreases in hip abduction ROM. Aquatics can be a great resource for exercise in maintaining ROM and strength. Home exercise programs to increase abduction and external ROM and strength can remediate this impairment. Reduction in weight bearing might be necessary if pain is severe. Instructions in crutch walking will allow the child to be active while keeping weight off of the leg. Education about activity choices should also be provided. Distance running and football are two examples of activities that are likely to increase pain.

Slipped Capital Femoral Epiphysis

Slipped capital femoral epiphysis (SCFE) is a hip problem that affects both sexes, but is more common in adolescent males (Loder et al., 2008; Gomez-Bento et al., 2007). The incidence of SCFE has risen dramatically over the past 20 years from around 4 cases per 100,000 children in 1981 to 10 cases per 100,000 children in 2000 (Murray & Wilson, 2008). It is also affecting younger children. The mean age of diagnosis has dropped almost a year and is now 12.6 years for boys and 11.6 for girls (Murray & Wilson, 2008). These changes are attributed to the growing pediatric obesity rate.

In SCFE, the femoral epiphysis slides posterior in relation to the femoral neck. On radiographs, this has been compared to ice cream slipping off of the cone. A child with a SCFE presents with mild to moderate hip or anterior thigh pain with activity (Greene & Ross, 2006). A limp may be present and ROM is frequently limited in flexion, abduction, and internal rotation (Pellecchia, Lugo-Larchevegue, & Deluca, 1996). When the hip is passively flexed, it tends to fall into an externally rotated position. If a SCFE is suspected, the child should see an orthopedic surgeon immediately, as progression of the slip can lead to permanent deformation and disability.

SCFE can affect one or both hips. Treatment is surgical screw fixation of the displaced bone back on the acetabulum. Although there is not complete consensus, many surgeons will perform prophylactic pinning of the uninvolved hip of girls younger than 10 years and boys younger than 12 years due to the high incidence of developing bilateral disease.

Following surgery, the child will likely have weight-bearing restrictions. A physical therapist will provide crutch walking instruction. The PT will also instruct the patient in hip ROM and strengthening exercises. The child's hip will be very sore, so gravity-eliminated exercise in bed is often the first step. Quad sets, ankle pumps (dorsiflexion/plantarflexion), hip abduction/adduction slides across the bed, and sliding the heel up the bed so the knee moves into flexion are good starting exercises.

Disorders of the Leg and Foot

Blount Disease or Tibia Vara

Blount disease or **tibia vara** is an example of bones deformed by mechanical stress (see Table 6.3). The excess weight from obesity repeatedly overloads immature bones, resulting in abnormal growth slowing at the medial aspect of the proximal tibia (bowlegs). Blount disease can have an infantile or juvenile onset. Obese children who walk before 1 year of age are most likely to have the infantile type. Children normally have some degree of bowlegs until age 2 years; however, if it persists beyond 3 years of age, Blount disease should be considered (Do, 2001). A knee-ankle-foot orthosis worn during ambulation can be prescribed to attempt correction of the angulation in children under the age of 3 years (Do, 2001).

Late-onset Blount disease occurs primarily in obese teenage boys (Wills, 2004). Late-onset Blount disease requires surgical correction through a tibial osteotomy or progressive realignment by an external fixation device (Laville, Chau, Willemen, Kohler, & Garin, 1999). Counseling on lifestyle choices should be part of best-practice care. Obesity can lead to numerous long-term medical complications such as diabetes, heart disease, arthritis, and sleep apnea. Children do not typically snore. Obese children who snore may have sleep apnea and should be referred to a pediatrician to see if a sleep study is warranted (Gordon et al., 2006).

Congenital Talipes Equinovarus

Congenital talipes equinovarus (clubfoot) is a bone anomaly that results in a cavus (high arch), adductus (metatarsals), varus, and equines (calcaneus) (CAVE) deformity. Pathological positioning of the navicular, talus, cuboid, calcaneous, os calcis navicular cuboid, and metatarsal bones all contribute to the deformity (see Fig. 6.11).

Clubfoot occurs in approximately 1–1.2 of every 1,000 live births in Caucasian populations but can be much higher in other ethnic groups (Gurnett, Boehm, Connolly, Reimschisel, & Dobbs, 2008; Roye & Roye, 2002). It occurs more frequently in males (2:1 ratio) and

the cause is most often unclear (Gurnett et al., 2008; Roye & Roye, 2002). Historically, clubfoot was attributed to prolonged foot positioning associated with breech positioning or fetal/placenta size imbalance. More recently, it is thought that genetic and environmental factors play an important role (Gurnett et al., 2008).

Without intervention, a clubfoot deformity is not self-correcting. Children in underdeveloped countries that are unable to access treatment for congenital clubfoot walk on the lateral border of their affected foot and develop callus formation, arthritis, and subtalar and midfoot stiffness (Gurnett et al., 2008; Roye & Roye, 2002). Pain is not typically associated with this fixed deformity.

Treatment options for children born with clubfoot include serial casting and surgical intervention. Serial casting, if initiated within the first month of life, is the first intervention implemented despite the severity of the deformity (Roye & Roye, 2002). Ignacio Ponseti identified a sequential casting procedure for optimal biomechanical results that addresses distal deformities before proximal ones. Full descriptions of this method are readily available in the medical literature (Noonan & Richards, 2003; Roye & Roye, 2002). Taping with a nonelastic tape is also used in some settings to correct these minor deformities. In this technique, a physical therapist provides stretching and manipulation interventions to the affected foot. The foot and ankle are then taped to maintain the foot in the new position and provide a prolonged stretch to the tissues (Noonan & Richards, 2003).

In some cases, when conservative methods are unable to effectively reduce the deformity, surgical intervention may be implemented. The goal of surgical intervention is to return to the foot to the proper anatomical position (Roye & Roye, 2002). After surgery, the physical therapist may need to address any areas of resulting muscle weakness and promote acquisition of gross motor skills.

Conditions Affecting Muscle
Congenital Muscular Torticollis

Congenital muscular torticollis (CMT) is a nonprogressive unilateral contracture of the sternocleidomastoid muscle (see Table 6.10). The incidence of CMT has skyrocketed recently due to the "back to sleep program," which encourages parents to put infants supine when sleeping to minimize the risk of Sudden Infant Death Syndrome (Losee & Mason, 2005). To help

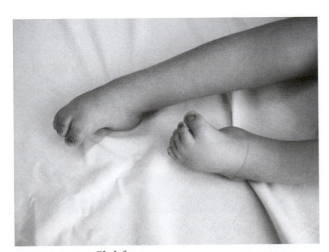

Figure 6.11 Clubfoot.

counteract this epidemic, parents should make a concerted effort to give the baby sufficient "tummy time" while the child is awake. Tummy time places the child's head in the end range of rotation on the side of the face that is on the surface. It also encourages neck strengthening when the baby lifts his head to turn it. In the supine position, the child is more likely to allow his head to fall into a preferred position. Neck strengthening is also minimal in supine.

Typical neonates should have 100° or more neck rotation and lateral flexion of at least 65° (Ohman & Beckung, 2008). Children with CMT hold their heads in lateral flexion with rotation to the opposite side and have limited ROM in the other direction (see Fig. 6.12).

Prior to initiating physical therapy for CMT, numerous other, more serious conditions that can manifest as torticollis must be ruled out. A posterior fossa tumor, which can be fatal if not treated, can present as torticollis. Sandifer's syndrome is a gastrointestinal condition that also mimics torticollis (Kabakuş & Kurt, 2006). Putting a child with Sandifer's syndrome in prone, a typical treatment for CMT, can increase reflux and make the child more irritable and reinforce the child's posture of apparent left torticollis.

When dealing with a true CMT or positionally acquired torticollis, resolution of symptoms is as high as 95%, if physical therapy is initiated in the first 3 months of life, and remains high if initiated in the first year of life (Do, 2006; Tatli et al., 2006). Infants with mild contracture (<10°) respond well to active home exercises. This would include environmental changes such as arranging the child's crib and changing table to promote turning the head to look at caregivers and stimulating active head turning in response to toys or sounds. Towel rolls or small soft collars can be used to prevent the child's head from falling passively into the shortened direction. Encouraging symmetrical head lifting from a prone position can also stretch and strengthen muscles. This can be accomplished by placing the infant prone on elbows over a small towel roll on the caregiver's chest and encouraging the infant to look up at the caregiver.

For children with more severe contracture, controlled manual stretching is added to ensure a good outcome (Cheng et al., 2001). The sternocleidomastoid performs both lateral flexion toward the same side and rotation toward the opposite side. Stretching should be performed when the child is relaxed. Toys, sounds, music, or pictures can be used to distract the child. Stretching can be performed in two parts (see Figs. 6.13 and 6.14).For lateral flexion, stabilization is provided over the shoulder girdle to prevent elevation. Using an open flat hand and avoiding the ear, the caregiver moves the head into opposite side lateral flexion. For rotation, stabilization is moved anterior to prevent both elevation and protraction of

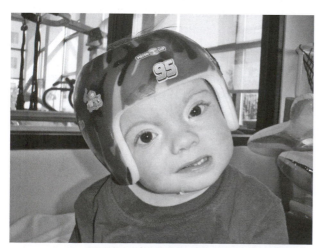

Figure 6.12 Picture of a child with torticollis wearing a helmet to correct plagiocephaly. Note posture of neck rotation and lateral flexion.

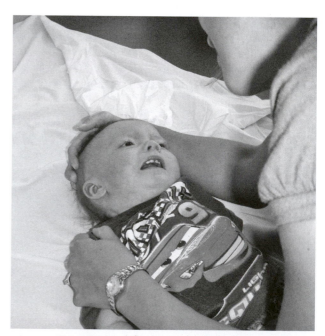

Figure 6.13 Lateral flexion stretch for congenital muscular torticollis. Note open hand, avoidance of ear, and stabilization of opposite shoulder.

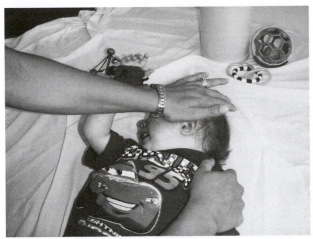

Figure 6.14 Neck rotation stretch for congenital muscular torticollis. Note open hand, avoidance of ear, and stabilization of shoulder opposite of rotation.

the shoulder. Again using an open flat hand and avoiding the child's ear, the head is turned toward the involved muscle. Even with the addition of a stretching program, a small percentage of children (5%) will require surgical intervention, especially if physical therapy is not initiated early.

Torticollis is frequently accompanied by **plagiocephaly** (misshapen head) or facial asymmetries. A physician should rule out craniosynostosis, which is a potentially life-threatening premature closing of the cranial sutures as a cause of a misshapen head before physical therapy is initiated. When the child has medical clearance, a hierarchy of treatment options is available. A parent resource fact sheet entitled "Deformational Plagiocephaly and Cranial Remolding in Infants" is available through the Pediatric Section of the APTA.

Head repositioning is the first option and should be included for every child. The child is kept off the flattened part of the head by sleeping on his or her side or using a gel pad to position the head, and spending more awake time in prone. More moderate asymmetries may require a repositioning helmet (see Fig. 6.12) (Bialocerkowski, Vladusic, & Howell, 2005). Both repositioning and wearing a helmet work best when initiated early. Surgical correction is also an option for correcting the head shape. A lack of reliable and valid clinical assessment measures makes it difficult to determine when a referral back to the physician is necessary for more aggressive measures (Mortenson & Steinbok, 2006).

Comprehensive treatment of CMT would also include a screening for hip instability, as associations between developmental dysplasia of the hip (DDH) and CMT have been observed. In a study of 102 patients with CMT, there was a 12.5% coexistence of DDH. Infants who were less than 1 month old when diagnosed with DDH had a 9% risk of subsequent development of CMT. Boys with DDH were 4.97 times more likely than girls to have both DDH and CMT regardless of which diagnosis preceded the other. It is recommended that all children with CMT be screened for DDH, and infants, especially boys, treated for DDH should be watched for the development of CMT (von Heideken et al., 2006).

Duchenne Muscular Dystrophy

Duchenne muscular dystrophy (DMD) is the most common muscular dystrophy and is a fatal disease of progressive weakness of the skeletal and respiratory muscles (Table 6.10). The typical life expectancy of a child with DMD is between 20 and 30 years (Yiu & Kornberg, 2008). DMD is caused by an X-linked recessive defect on the Xp21 portion of the X chromosome and is present in 1 of every 3,500 live births. This gene encodes the production of a protein called dystrophin that is linked to muscle function (Deconinck & Dan, 2007). With X-linked recessive disease, males will have the disease, while females will be carriers and can pass the disease on and may exhibit muscle weakness or cardiomyopathy (Bushby et al., 2010). In addition to muscle changes, genetic and blood composition abnormalities are present. A language delay is also frequently seen in boys with DMD and is related to later cognitive difficulties (Cyrulnik, Fee, De Vivo, Goldstein, & Hinton, 2007). A case study describing the evaluation and intervention of a child with DMD is presented in Chapter 23.

Boys with DMD are generally clumsy, may walk up on their toes, and show gross motor regression over time. For some boys with DMD, the first sign of the disease is delayed walking, beginning around 18 months of age. **Pseudohypertrophy** (enlargement without increased strength) of the calf muscles presents later in development due to the accumulation of fat and connective tissue in the muscle. This may give the appearance of a strong muscle, but examination will reveal a pattern of weakness that affects proximal musculature greater than distal. To compensate for the proximal weakness, the boys may use their upper extremities to manually assist knee extension by "walking" the hands up the lower extremities when moving

Table 6.10 Muscular Disorders

Diagnosis	Etiology	Pathology	Body Functions and Structure Impairments	Potential Activity Limitations and Participation Restrictions
Duchenne muscular dystrophy	• X-linked recessive trait • Defect on the Xp21 portion of the X chromosome	• Muscle composition abnormalities • Progressive degeneration of the muscle fibers and variation in fiber size • Connective and adipose tissue deposits	• Progressive muscle weakness; proximal >distal (b730)* • Plantarflexion, hip flexion, and iliotibial band contractures (b710) • Progressive scoliosis	• Fatal • Motor skill regression • Loss of ambulation (d450)
Spinal muscular atrophy (Nicole, Diaz, Frugier, & Melki, 2002)	• Autosomal recessive defect of chromosome 5	• Unclear • Includes non-progressive loss of anterior horn cells	• Muscular weakness (b730)	• Progressive difficulty with physical activities eventually ending in death
Congenital muscular torticollis (Davids, Wenger, & Mubarak, 1993)	• Unclear • Current theory is intrauterine or perinatal compartment syndrome	• Unilateral contracture of the sternocleidomastoid muscle • May lead to plagiocephaly if untreated.	• Head is tilted toward involved side and chin is rotated toward opposite side • Limited ROM in lateral flexion towards uninvolved side and rotation toward involved side (b710) • Skewed vertical and midline orientation	• Cosmesis • Distorted orientation may interfere with play (d9200) • Limited ROM may impede dressing (d540)

*Numbers in parentheses refer to ICF-CY classification.

from the floor to standing. This is referred to as **Gower's sign** (Fig. 6.15).

The initial proximal muscular weakness seen in DMD also results in other atypical movement patterns that can lead to soft tissue contractures. The boys adopt a wide base of support to maximize balance and use biomechanical alignment to maintain an upright position with the least muscular effort. For example, knee hyperextension and increased lumbar lordosis move the child's center of gravity in front of the knee joint to reduce the need for active quadriceps contraction. Toe walking is used to take advantage of joint end range as a means of stability. These alignment changes lead to equinus contractures of the ankles, hip flexion contractures, and iliotibial band contracture. One of the gold standards of treatment that can prolong function is steroids. The use of either prednisone or deflazacort has been shown to prolong ambulation for up to 3 years (King et al., 2007). Physical therapy intervention changes dramatically over the course of DMD due to the progressive, degenerative nature of the disease. Although the primary impairment in DMD is weakness,

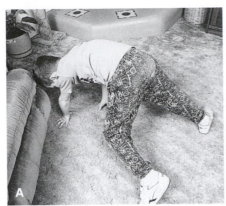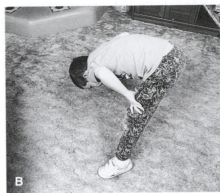

Figure 6.15 Gower's sign used by children with muscular dystrophy to compensate for proximal weakness. *(From Porr, S.M., & Rainville, E.B. [1999]. Pediatric therapy: A systems approach. Philadelphia: F.A. Davis, with permission. Photo courtesy of MDA, Tucson, AZ.)*

aggressive strengthening should be avoided. In particular, eccentric contractions are detrimental, as the mechanically induced damage puts a high stress on fragile membranes and provokes microlesions that could eventually lead to loss of calcium homeostasis and cell death (Deconinck & Dan, 2007). Typically, daily activities and a modest, regular fitness routine of stretching is all that is recommended for children with DMD. Aquatic programs can provide an enjoyable source of exercise in children with DMD; however, they need to be monitored for overexertion. Children with DMD should be allowed to be active and play with their peers, but should be encouraged to stop when they are tired.

ROM helps maintain optimal alignment and is particularly important early in the disease. Boys with DMD develop atypical compensatory movements to compensate for weakness. These atypical movements can lead to ROM limitations that can interfere with ambulation. Prolonged ambulation can help reduce further contractures and promote cardiopulmonary fitness and is associated with a lower risk of developing scoliosis (Kinali, Main, & Eliahoo, 2007). Despite an appropriate physical therapy program, ambulation skills are often lost by 12 years of age and the child uses a wheelchair (Yiu & Kornberg, 2008). Hip and knee flexion contractures are common once the child is wheelchair dependent but can be addressed through standing programs, prone lying, and night splints. Ankle-foot-orthoses (AFOs) are rarely prescribed as they often prevent children from utilizing compensatory mechanisms and thus prevent the child from being able to walk. Maintaining ROM in late-stage DMD, however, provides sufficient flexibility to optimize caregiver handling and child comfort.

Surgeries are occasionally needed to increase ROM or to stabilize the spine to stop scoliosis progression. These procedures are used judiciously, however, because children with DMD are prone to developing weakness and pneumonia with bed rest. Scoliosis affects 75%–90% of nonambulatory children with DMD (Kinali, Messina & Mercuri, 2006; Kinali et al., 2007). Surgical intervention is considered when the curve of the spine reaches 20°–30°, especially if the child is under the age of 14 years (Cervellati, Bettini, & Moscato, 2004; Eagle et al., 2007; Kinali et al., 2006). Most experts agree that bracing is ineffective at stopping curve progression and therefore advocate early surgery (Driscoll & Skinner, 2008; Kinali et al., 2007; Kinali et al., 2006). Early surgery is recommended due to the likely possibility that progressive pulmonary function decline will make surgery impossible when the child is older.

Although bracing cannot stop scoliosis progression in children with DMD, it can help improve postural control and breathing in adolescents with significant weakness. Rigid bracing may not be appropriate as it is not well tolerated and can result in skin breakdown. A soft brace may provide sufficient postural control to assist pulmonary function. Maintenance of respiratory muscle function can also be promoted through the use of spirometers. Respiratory function decline is inevitable, however, and nighttime ventilation is needed in late adolescence or early adulthood (Eagle et al., 2007). Aggressive postop physical therapy is important to minimize the debilitating effects of bed rest. ROM, gentle isometric or concentric strengthening, and spirometry may limit deterioration due to bed rest. Additionally, children with DMD are encouraged to resume ambulation quickly to avoid developing muscle atrophy or pneumonia. The progressive nature of DMD puts the child at increased risk for rapid decline with immobility.

Equipment selection also helps prolong functional skills. As the disease progresses, a wheelchair will be needed for mobility and positioning. In the late stages, equipment to aid in caregiving may be needed such as hospital beds, transfer lifts, power mobility.

Education regarding energy conservation is important for children with DMD. For some children in the late stages of ambulation, most of their energy will be expended walking to and from activities. This will leave little energy left for participation in school or interaction with friends. Providing the child with a scooter or wheelchair for long distances can conserve energy and allow the child to actively participate in recreation activities with his peers. Clustering the classrooms the child attends will also help reduce energy expenditure.

Spinal Muscular Atrophy

Spinal muscular atrophy (SMA) also manifests in muscular weakness. SMA is a group of autosomal recessive disorders caused by mutation or deletion of the survival motor neuron 1 (SMN1) gene (Kostova et al., 2007; Lunn & Want, 2008). This genetic disruption is characterized by degeneration of the anterior horn cells of the spinal cord, muscle atrophy and widespread weakness, and absent deep tendon reflexes (Nicole et al., 2002; Lunn & Want, 2008). Sensation and cognition are not typically impaired. It occurs in one of every 10,000 live births (Lunn & Want, 2008).

Three classifications of SMA are used, which reflect the severity, rate of decline, and age of onset of the disease (Nicole et al., 2002) (see Table 6.11). Acute **Werdnig-Hoffman disease** (type I disease) is the most severe form with the earliest onset and most rapid demise. Acute Werdnig-Hoffman disease comprises 50% of all children diagnosed with SMA and manifests before 6 months of age and results in death by age

2 years (Lunn & Want, 2008). The intermediate form of SMA is chronic Werdnig-Hoffman disease (type II disease), while Kugelberg-Welander disease (type III disease) has the latest onset. Symptoms of type II SMA typically occur between the ages of 7 and 18 months; most children are able to sit independently and some may walk short distances with assistive devices. Children with SMA type II may live into adulthood with proper treatment and monitoring of pulmonary function. Children with Kugelberg-Welander disease have the mildest form of SMA and typically develop the ability to walk independently. Onset of type III SMA occurs after 18 months of age. Children may walk independently or with an assistive device into late adolescence or early adulthood before transitioning into a wheelchair. Children with type III SMA may have a typical lifespan.

Clinical features of all three classifications include limb and trunk weakness, with muscle atrophy more pronounced proximally and in the lower extremities. There will be hypotonia and areflexia (absence of reflexes) (Iannaconne, 2007). The musculoskeletal system of children with SMA undergoes progressive deformities due to muscle weakness and immobility that include soft tissue contractures, hip subluxation, and scoliosis. A higher incidence of talipes equino varus (club foot) is also reported (Thompson, 1996).

In addition to the musculoskeletal system, the gastrointestinal and respiratory systems are also impaired in SMA. Children with SMA have difficulty with their gastrointestinal tract and typically develop dysphagia and constipation. Dysphagia can result in failure to thrive in infants, especially with type I SMA. Constipation results from hypotonia of the abdominal muscles and immobility and is most severe in children with type I SMA. Constipation can be improved with increased activity, water, and fiber intake.

Restrictive lung disease is common in SMA. It affects children with type I severely and may be very mild or nonexistent in children with type III. At this point, there is no successful treatment for SMA. However, understanding of the underlying genetics of the condition has grown substantially in past years. This has led to many clinical trials involving gene therapy that increase SMN2 expression in experimental models (Lunn & Want, 2008). Further research will continue to advance the knowledge and understanding of the molecular pathogenesis of this disease and implications for future treatments.

Although there is no cure for SMA, physical therapy can help enhance the quality of life of the child. The focus of physical therapy intervention for children with

Table 6.11 Onset and Prognosis of SMA Classifications

Type of SMA	Onset	Death	Motor Limits
I	0-6 months	<2 years	Doesn't sit
II	7-18 months	>2 years	Usually doesn't stand
III	> 18 months	adult	Stands and walks alone

SMA differs based on the type of SMA; however, common goals include maintenance of ROM, strength, and improving or maintaining development and function.

For children with type I SMA, most therapeutic treatments are designed to improve or maintain respiratory function, encourage developmental milestones, minimize ROM limitations, and improve feeding and swallowing mechanics. Exercise has been shown to be beneficial in mouse models of SMA, but there is little evidence in children (Biondi et al., 2008). Children with type II SMA typically benefit from interventions that prolong ambulation. Scoliosis progresses rapidly as children with neuromuscular diseases become nonambulatory (Kinali et al., 2006). As the spinal curve progresses, it can cause a decline in respiratory function and thus require surgical intervention.

Preventing contractures in children with type II or III SMA is very difficult, if not impossible (Wang, Ju, Chen, Lo, & Jong, 2004). Parents should be instructed in a reasonable program of positioning and ROM but be reminded that despite the most diligent program, some decline in ROM is inevitable. As children with type III SMA grow, they can outgrow their muscles' capacity and begin to lose function. Therefore, strengthening, nutrition, and weight management education are important interventions for these children. Traditional growth charts may be inappropriate due to the decrease in lean muscle mass (Messina et al., 2008). Education in energy conservation techniques to prevent fatigue and falls in these children is another critical aspect of their care.

Physical therapists, as a part of the multidisciplinary team coordinating the child's care, have an integral role in obtaining power mobility for a child with SMA. Independent mobility is important in cognitive, social, and emotional development in all children (Campos et al., 2000; Jones, McEwen, & Hansen, 2003). Obtaining a means of independent mobility for children with SMA is a crucial aspect of their care. Encouraging participation in recreation and leisure activities can improve social development and self esteem in children. Physical therapists can educate families on the importance of leisure activities in quality of life and help families find available resources in their area.

Idiopathic Toe Walking

Idiopathic toe walking (ITW) is a diagnosis of exclusion. This means that the child walks on his or her toes without a discernable neurological or sensory cause. The toe walking can be intermittent or constant. Current literature varies on the incidence of familial toe walking with estimates of a genetic component ranging between 30% and 70% of children with ITW (Hemo, Macdessi, Pierce, Aiona, & Sussman 2006; Sala, Shulman, Kennedy, Grant, & Chu 1999; Stricker & Angulo, 1998).

Intermittent periods of toe walking can be a normal component of development up to age 3 (Alvarez, De Vera, Beauchamp, Ward, & Black, 2006; Hemo et al., 2006). Therefore, to have the diagnosis of ITW, a child must be over the age of 3 years. Typical gait is characterized by heel strike at initial contact and in the three rockers of gait. The term "rocker" is used to describe a point during the gait cycle when the foot is transitioning between phases as described by Perry (1992). The first rocker occurs after heel strike at initial contact when the foot progresses into plantarflexion. The second rocker is present during the midstance phase of gait when the tibia advances over the foot and pushes the ankle into dorsiflexion. The third rocker occurs in late stance and the push-off phase as the foot moves from dorsiflexion into plantarflexion for push-off. A child who uses a toe walking gait pattern typically has a toe touch initial contact, which leads to a loss of the first and second rockers of gait. The third rocker tends to occur early, causing an early heel rise and decreased force production during push-off (Alvarez et al., 2006). Children who use a toe walking pattern frequently have shorter step lengths than typical peers.

When performing an evaluation of a child with a diagnosis of ITW, it is important to check ROM, muscle tone, leg length, deep tendon reflexes, clonus, Babinski reflex, gait pattern, ankle/foot alignment, dorsiflexion, and plantar flexion strength. A quick screen of speech, and fine and gross motor skill is also important, as research has found a correlation between ITW and developmental delays. Shulman and colleagues (1997) found as many as 77% of children who walked on their toes had a speech delay, 33% had a fine motor delay, 40% showed a visuomotor delay, and 27% had a gross motor delay. There is also a correlation between the severity of toe walking and speech delay. These statistics might suggest that there is more to ITW than an isolated, benign condition. More research is needed to investigate whether ITW is part of a constellation of developmental delay symptoms.

Physical therapy interventions for ITW consist of increasing ankle ROM, frequently through the use of serial casting, strengthening ankle dorsiflexors and plantarflexors, and the use of orthoses. An evidence-based algorithm for treating a child with ITW has been developed at Nationwide Children's Hospital and can be found in Figure 6.16. For children who have mildly

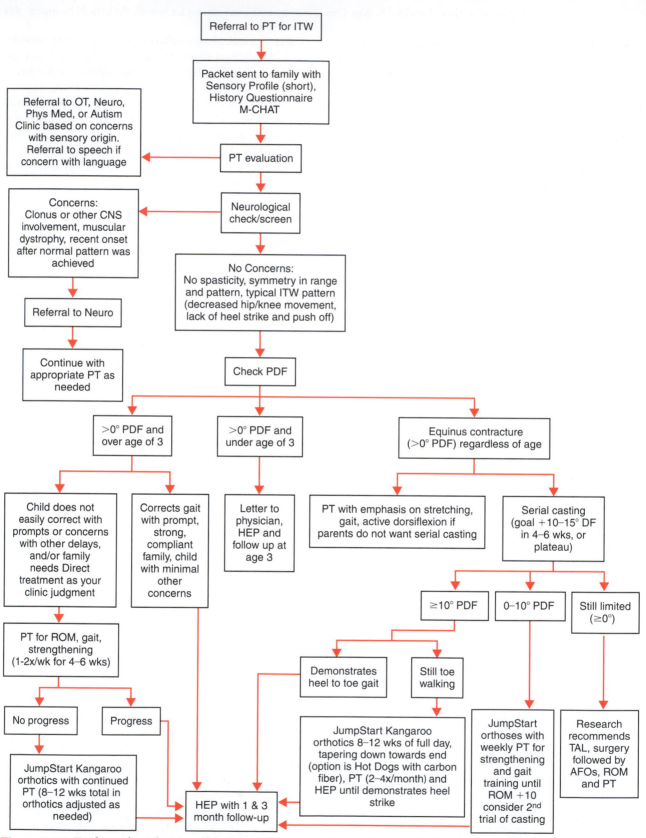

Figure 6.16 Evidence-based protocol for idiopathic toe walking. AFO = ankle foot orthosis; HEP = home exercise program; ITW = idiopathic toe walking; PDF = passive dorsiflexion PT = physical therapy; ROM = range of motion; TAL = tendo Achillis lengthening

decreased ankle dorsiflexion ROM (0°–10°), a stretching program should be implemented. If the child has ROM less than or equal to 0° traditional stretching, and strengthening protocols may not be effective in increasing ROM (Stott, Walt, Lobb, Reynolds, & Nicol, 2004), then serial casting may be the best option to improve ankle ROM (Brouwer, Davidson, & Olney 2000; Stott et al., 2004).

When performing serial casting, the goal is to achieve at least 10° of ankle dorsiflexion with the knee extended. This is the ROM required in typical gait pattern (Stott et al., 2004). Casting protocols are individualized, but tend to be 4–6 weeks in length and involve reapplication of a cast every 7 days until the child reaches the ROM goal or plateaus. After a casting protocol is finished, a strengthening program should be initiated. It is a common misconception that children who toe walk have strong plantarflexors. Research has shown that these children tend to have weaker plantarflexors than typical peers (Alvarez et al., 2006; Brouwer et al., 2000). Children who toe walk are not using the full ROM at the ankle and therefore are not strengthening the muscle through its full range. Periods of immobilization while in serial casts can compound this weakness. Weakness is more pronounced in older children than in younger children who toe walk.

If children have the necessary ROM and are still toe walking, orthotic intervention may be required. Rigid shoe inserts or off-the-shelf AFOs may be beneficial in helping to break the pattern of toe walking in some children. Children with ITW will likely only need an orthosis for a short period of time (6–12 months);

therefore, Tidball and colleagues (2009) recommend an off-the-shelf model rather than more expensive custom orthoses, if an appropriate size and style is available.

In cases where serial casting is ineffective, surgical intervention may be indicated. In these cases, a percutaneous tendon lengthening or a tendo-Achilles lengthening is typically performed (Hemo et al., 2006; Stott et al., 2004). Scientific literature supporting the use of botulinum toxin as an effective treatment for ITW is currently not available.

Brachial Plexus Injuries

The brachial plexus is made up of spinal nerve roots C5, C6, C7, C8, and T1 (see Fig. 6.17). A **brachial plexus injury (BPI)** occurs when these nerve roots are stretched, causing transient or permanent nerve damage and interrupting muscle innervations and diminishing sensation. BPI can be caused in neonates during a vaginal delivery or in older children as a result of a sports injury or other trauma. Several factors can increase a neonate's risk of BPI. Gestational weight over 8 pounds, breech presentation (transverse orientation rather than head down in pelvis) during delivery, and the use of a forceps or evacuation pump to deliver the baby all increase the risk of BPI. The dysfunction seen in the infant depends upon which nerves are stretched. For a description of the motor and sensory changes seen with injury to each nerve, please see Table 6.12.

Erb's Palsy and Klumpke's Palsy

The two most common constellations of injury are Erb's palsy (C5 and C6) and Klumpke's palsy (C8 and T1).

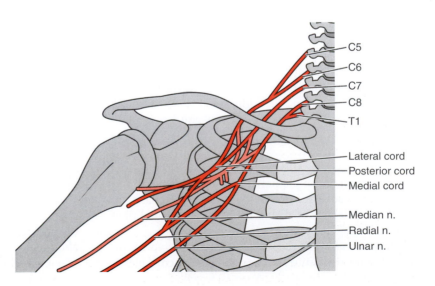

Figure 6.17 Schematic drawing of brachial plexus. Damage to C5 and C6 results in Erb's and C8 and T1 result in Klumpke's palsy.

Table 6.12 Common Brachial Plexus Lesions

Lesion	Motor Deficits/Muscle	Sensory Deficits	Nerves
Erb's Palsy (C5, C6)	Abduction, flexion, and rotation at shoulder; weak shoulder extension—*deltoid, rotator cuff*	Posterior and lateral aspect of arm	Axillary, suprascapular, upper and lower subscapular
	Very weak elbow flexion and supination of radioulnar joint—*biceps brachii and brachialis*	Radial side of forearm—thumb and first finger	Musculocutaneous; radial nerve to supinator and brachioradialis muscles
	Susceptible to shoulder dislocation—loss of *rotator cuff muscles* "Waiter's tip" position		Suprascapular, upper and lower subscapular
Klumpke's Palsy (C8, T1)	Loss of thumb opposition—*thenar muscles*	Ulnar side of forearm, hand, half of fourth finger, and all of fifth—*ulnar and medial antebrachial cutaneous*	Thenar branch of median nerve
	Loss of adduction of thumb—*adductor pollicis*		Ulnar nerve
	Loss of abduction and adduction of metacarpophalangeal joints; flexion at metacarpophalangeal joints and extension of interphalangeal joints—*lumbricals and interossei*		Deep branch of ulnar and median
	Very weak flexion of proximal interphalangeal and distal interphalangeal joints—*flexor digitorum superficialis and flexor digitorum profundus*		Ulnar and median

A child with Erb's palsy has a characteristic appearance that has been named the "waiter's tip." The shoulder is in internal rotation and adduction, the wrist flexed, and the fingers extended as if the child is waiting for someone to slip a tip into their hand from behind (see Fig. 6.18)

Klumpke's palsy affects the muscles of the hand and the sensation of the medial arm. The hand is held in a claw position of extension of the metacarpal phalangeal joints and flexion of distal, intra, and proximal phalangeal joint. The thumb is in abduction.

Prognosis for full recovery varies on the type of injury. Infants with injury to the complete brachial plexus (C1–C5 and T1) have a poor prognosis with traditional therapy and should be referred to a neurosurgeon for possible surgical reconstruction. Infants with Erb's palsy have a very good prognosis, if therapy is initiated at birth. The majority of infants have recovered tricep, bicep, deltoid, and wrist extensor by 6 months of age. If significant improvement is not seen by 6 months of age, long-term disability is likely (DiTaranto, Campagna, Price, & Grossman, 2004).

Successful outcome is dependent on treatment beginning at birth. The family will need information about positioning the arm so that it is not left hanging when the child is being held. They will also need to

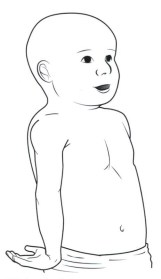

Figure 6.18 Waiter's tip.

remember that the perception of pain is not present in the involved arm, so injury can occur without the child crying. Incorporating frequent ROM into the daily routine will help prevent potential contractures due to the static positioning caused by muscle imbalances. Strengthening of the involved muscles through play activities and weight bearing will improve function. In the initial period, activities that minimize the effects of gravity on the movement will be helpful. For example, trying to have the child extend and abduct the shoulder to reach a toy may be too difficult. However, if the child is held on the caregiver's lap with the arm supported on a table, this movement is simplified by eliminating the need for shoulder flexion and reduces the effects of gravity.

Cerebral Palsy

Although cerebral palsy (CP) is primarily a neurologic condition, it is accompanied by characteristic bone and muscle impairments of varying severity. Research suggests that muscles of children with CP have more variability in the size of the muscle fibers, altered muscle fiber type composition, atrophy, decreased vascularization, increased extracellular space, and an increase in fatty and connective tissue deposits in the muscle (Foran, Steinman, Barash, Chambers, & Lieber, 2005). All of these differences are believed to contribute to the weakness seen in children with CP.

To understand the implications of these changes, one must have an understanding of myosin-based muscle fiber classification. Myosin is a muscle fiber protein that regulates the muscle's elastic and contractile properties. (More information on muscle histology can be found in Chapter 5.) Myosin heavy chain (MyHC) determines the speed and force of the contraction. Slow MyHC I have a large oxidative capacity and fatigue resistance. Fast MyHC IIa and especially fast MyHC IIx (known to be expressed in type 2B fibers) have a lower oxidative capacity and low fatigue resistance (Pontén & Stål, 2007).

Muscles in children with CP have a proportionally higher number of MyHC IIx fibers. Pontén and Stål (2007) suggest that the low oxidative capacity and fewer capillaries (MyHC IIx) intensify the weakness and fatigability seen in children with CP. They also suggest that disuse is a likely cause of this switch. This led them to deduce that decreased voluntary motor unit recruitment is a predominating factor for the fiber type changes seen in CP. This premise is based on the fact that exercise increases capillary networks and causes a shift from faster to slower fiber type composition. This would suggest that exercise could play a large role in improving muscle performance.

Other researchers place more emphasis on a child's inability to activate agonist muscles volitionally, or excessive antagonist muscle coactivation, reducing force or torque-generating capacity (Tedroff, Knutson, & Soderberg, 2008). Studies have demonstrated a higher level of coactivation in children with CP compared to typically developing children (Givon, 2009; Poon & Hui-Chan, 2009; Tedroff et al., 2008).

Children with CP also have lower bone mineralization and delayed bone maturation (Ihkkhan& Yalçin, 2001). This can predispose a child to fracture (Stevenson, Conaway, Barrington, Cuthill, Worley, & Henderson, 2006). The risk of fracture in a child with CP is greatest if the child is a Gross Motor Functional Classification level 3 or 4 (see Chapter 7 for a description of these levels), has greater body fat, and is on a feeding gastrostomy tube (Henderson, Kairalla, Abbas, & Stevenson, 2004; Stevenson et al., 2006).

The characteristic musculoskeletal abnormalities of CP will be presented for each body segment. For information on the neurologic sequelae of CP, refer to Chapters 7 and 19.

Spine

Children with CP are more likely to develop scoliosis or other curvatures of the spine, such as a thoracic kyphosis. The overall incidence of scoliosis in children with CP is about 25% but increases with increased severity (Renshaw, Green, Griffin, & Root, 1996). The lack of stability combined with a decreased amount of movement places the child's spine in atypical postures for prolonged periods of time. Over time this can result in either a flexible or fixed deformity. Additional contributing factors to spinal deformity can be atypical muscle pull or muscle imbalances. Finally, leg length inequality, which is frequently seen in children with hemiplegic CP, will disrupt pelvic symmetry, and the spine compensates with a scoliosis.

Pelvis and Hip

Problems at the pelvis and hip result from bony abnormalities, alignment, and shape and muscle abnormalities, length, and function. The distribution of hypertonicity around the hip, commonly seen in children with spastic types of CP, of hip flexion, adduction, and internal rotation can lead to atypical posture, bone alignment, and ROM limitations. Movement into hip extension, abduction, and external rotation are almost universally limited.

Pelvic alignment abnormalities include obliquity and posterior or anterior tilts. As mentioned previously, pelvic obliquity is most often associated with leg length discrepancy. A posterior pelvic tilt is typically attributable to limited hamstring range. The hamstrings are composed of a two-joint muscle crossing both the hip and knee joints. In sitting, especially if the knees are extended, the hamstrings in children with CP do not have sufficient range to accommodate a neutral pelvis. The pelvis rotates in a posterior direction to reduce the stretch on the hamstrings, and the child will sit with the knees flexed, the pelvis rotated posterior and the back rounded. One way to reduce the pull on the hamstrings is to have the child use the **"W" sitting position** (Fig. 6.19).

The child flexes both the hips and the knees and in doing so places the short hamstrings on slack. In standing, hip flexor tightness will frequently pull the pelvis into an anterior pelvic tilt. If the hamstring length is significantly limited, the child will bend the knees to reduce the strain caused by the anterior pelvic tilt.

Another common problem in children with CP is **hip subluxation** or **dislocation**. Both bony and muscular factors contribute to hip instability. Neonates are born with a shallow acetabulum, flat femoral head, high femoral neck-shaft angle, and femoral antetorsion, all of which contribute to hip instability. In typically developing children, bony remodeling deepens the acetabulum, makes the femoral head more spherical, reduces anteversion, and decreases the femoral neck-shaft inclination through weight bearing and the normal pull of muscles. Children with CP, however,

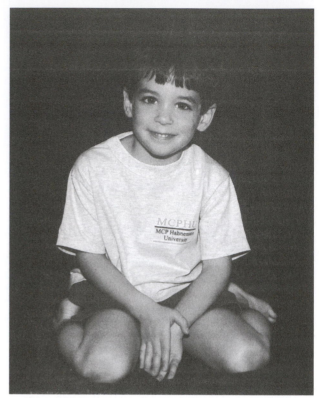

Figure 6.19 Picture of child in "W" sitting posture. The knees are flexed and the hips are flexed and internally rotated. Children with hip anteversion, limited hamstring length, and/or limited hip external rotation use this position.

have delayed motor milestones; therefore, the bones are not subjected to normal weight-bearing forces at an early age.

The instability of the hip is compounded by ROM limitations and atypical muscular pull/spasticity. Adequate ROM allows the hip to move into a stable, well-covered position in the acetabulum. Children with CP tend to lose abduction range and develop hip flexion contractures, both of which are detrimental to hip stability. Critical ROM values for hip stability include maintaining at least 30° of abduction and avoiding a hip flexion contracture of 20°–25° or more (Renshaw et al., 1996).

Foot and Ankle

The most common impairment of the foot and ankle is reduced dorsiflexion ROM due to a shortened gastrocnemius. Hypertonicity of the gastrocnemius, combined with an inability to generate sufficient stability around the ankle, result in the child assuming a plantarflexed position during weight bearing. Over time, this can result in severe limitations in dorsiflexion ROM. This will limit the child's ability to fit into orthoses or shoes and significantly reduces their base of support in standing.

The inability to maintain a stable foot also contributes to a breakdown of the longitudinal arch, resulting in an **equinovalgus** (flatfoot) position. This further impairs the child's ability to perform balance reactions with the feet. Orthoses are used both to control the plantarflexion and to maintain the longitudinal arch. Unfortunately, they also eliminate movement of the ankle, which leads to significant weakness of the ankle musculature. When orthoses are necessary for ROM or stability, it is essential to include strengthening activities and time out of the orthoses. When the child reaches skeletal maturity, a subtalar or triple arthrodesis procedure can be performed for a permanent correction. In a triple arthrodesis, the orthopedic surgeon will fuse the talocalcaneal, talonavicular, and calcaneocuboid joints, resulting in a rigid foot but in a more anatomically correct position.

Posture

The musculoskeletal and neurologic impairments seen in children with spastic CP culminate in characteristic postures. In standing, young children tend to stand on their toes with their knees extended, hips adducted and internally rotated, and the pelvis in an anterior tilt. As the child gets larger, the weight of the body, inadequate muscle power, and surgical lengthening of the muscles can result in the crouched posture of ankle dorsiflexion and knee flexion. The hips will generally remain in adduction, flexion, and internal rotation.

The hamstrings are one of the major influences in sitting postures of children with spastic CP. The limited range makes long sitting virtually impossible. When the child attempts this position, the knees are kept in partial flexion and the pelvis rotates posteriorly to accommodate the shortened hamstrings. The pelvic tilt, in turn, results in compensating postures in the spine. The lumbar and thoracic spine is in a compensatory kyphotic position while the child hyperextends the neck to maintain the head in a neutral position. This position makes using the hands and playing difficult.

Intervention

CP is a complex manifestation of a nonprogressive brain injury resulting in a varied combination of impairments and limitations in activities and participation. Detailed intervention options are provided in Chapter 8 on the neuromuscular system and plan of care. The interventions targeted at musculoskeletal impairment are discussed here. Due to the complexity of CP, these impairment level interventions would not be used in isolation without addressing the functional, activity, and participation limitations of the child.

In children with CP, maintaining or increasing ROM is a high priority. Deficits in ROM change the normal skeletal alignment and decrease fluency and efficiency of movement. Stretching before and after exercise is a good way to warm up and may prevent injury in children with or without a disability. Unfortunately, passive stretching is not effective in increasing ROM, reducing spasticity, or improving walking efficiency in children with spasticity (Cadenhead, McEwen, & Thompson, 2002; Pin, Dyke, & Chan, 2006; Wiart, Darrah, & Kembhavi, 2008). Even maintaining current muscle length requires the muscles to be in an elongated state for 6 hours or more (Lespargot, Renaudin, Khouri, & Robert, 1994; Tardieu, Lespargot, Tabary, & Bret, 1988). Clearly, this cannot be done by a parental program of passive ROM.

If the child is not using the range during ADL, splinting should be considered. Resting splints worn while the child sleeps can provide the required time without interfering with muscle exercise during the day. Additionally, including periods of prone lying while watching television, playing, reading, or sleeping can assist in maintaining hip extension. The decision to use braces such as an AFO should be carefully evaluated. The brace can help reduce gastroc-soleus shortening and may provide a stable base of support, but it prevents the child from using ankle movements as a balance strategy and may lead to disuse atrophy. It is recommended that the child continue to spend time without the braces to determine whether the braces are indeed beneficial (Kott & Held, 2002), to allow for continued unrestricted motor learning, and to promote ankle strength. If braces or splints are needed during the day, it is imperative that the problem of disuse atrophy be considered and a strengthening program be included in the child's intervention plan. This strengthening program may include activities to strengthen all movements at the ankle (i.e., dorsiflexion, plantarflexion, eversion, and inversion), as well as balance activities to improve activation of the muscles that support the ankle and foot.

If ROM and splinting are not successful, the child may need tendon lengthening or transfers. Tendon lengthening is a surgical procedure that uses a cut in the tendon to allow it to elongate. Frequently, several tendons are lengthened during the same procedure. The gastrocnemius, hamstrings, and hip adductors are the most commonly lengthened and can be performed in isolation as needed or all in a single surgery. A tendon transfer moves the tendon to a new attachment on the bone, allowing a more relaxed position and may encourage a more efficient pull of the muscle. The procedure is especially beneficial in the upper extremity to help the child extend the fingers, thumb, and wrist if a strong flexion synergy is present.

Bone surgery is also sometimes indicated. A femoral derotational osteotomy is used to better position the head of the femur in the acetabulum to maximize hip stability. The femur is cut distal to the greater trochanter and the head is realigned. Aggressive postop care by the physical therapist can minimize the disability associated with a major surgery. One study reported that encouraging weight bearing as tolerated following surgery resulted in an earlier return to standing (M = 26 days sooner) and a return to baseline walking almost 4 months sooner than the group of children who were initially non–weight bearing. Pain at 8 days postop was also significantly less for the weight bearing as tolerated group, but pain at the time of initial standing and walking was not significantly different between groups (Schaefer, McCarthy, & Josephic, 2007).

Strength training can also make a significant positive impact on children with CP. Damiano and Abel (1998) and others have laid the groundwork to demonstrate that a strengthening program can provide many positive benefits in gait characteristics, endurance, and functional activities (Blundell, Shepherd, Dean, Adams, & Cahill, 2003; Eagleton, Iams, McDowell, Morrison, & Evans, 2004; Morton, Brownlee, & McFayden, 2005). The early concerns that increasing strength would increase spasticity have been refuted, and the impact weakness has on function has been demonstrated (Eagleton et al., 2004). A recent systematic review concluded that strength training with progressive resistive exercise and/or electrical stimulation in school-aged children with CP who are walking may not be beneficial (Scianni, Butler, Ada, & Teixeira-Salmela, 2009). Further research is needed to determine what strengthening interventions are beneficial in children with CP and also whether there are specific points in development when these interventions would be most effective. One example of the role of strength in functional skills is the residual weakness and disability seen following spasticity-reducing procedures such as selective dorsal rhizotomy and oral or intrathecal medication (Poon & Hui-Chan, 2009). Strengthening in children with CP is discussed in Chapters 8 and 19.

Down Syndrome

Children with Down syndrome have a higher incidence of a number of health problems, including cardiac, hearing, endocrine, developmental, dental, and others (Davidson, 2008; van Cleve & Cohen, 2006). Neuromuscular impairments and limitations of children with Down syndrome are discussed in Chapters 7, 8, and 21. Typical short stature and low metabolic rate predispose a child to being overweight (Davidson, 2008). People with Down syndrome have decreased muscle tone (hypotonia) and lax ligaments that may account for some of the orthopedic abnormalities.

Many musculoskeletal problems also occur with higher frequency in people with Down syndrome and may require intervention from physical therapists, occupational therapists, or orthopedic surgeons. The most common orthopedic problem is a flexible flatfoot or pes planus (Mik, Gholve, Scher, Widmann, & Green, 2008).

Rigid flatfeet or pes valgus, caused by a medially tilted superior aspect of the talus, may also be seen but is less common. Evidence suggests that the use of flexible supramalleolar orthoses (SMO) improves gross motor skills in young children (3–8 years) with Down syndrome by improving foot stability (Martin, 2004; Selby-Silverstein, Hillstrom, & Palisano, 2001).

Developmental dysplasia of the hip and acetabular dysplasia may be present at birth or develop with age. Older children and adolescents who develop a limp may have an acquired hip dislocation due to ligamentous laxity. This laxity also contributes to chronic patellar dislocation, pes planus, and ankle pronation. Ligamentous laxity in combination with obesity can easily result in premature arthritis and chronic pain in adults with Down syndrome.

Atlantoaxial instability, an enlarged space between the first and second vertebrae, is present in approximately 15% of all individuals with Down syndrome (Tassone & Duey-Holtz, 2008). A schematic drawing of atlantoaxial instability is shown in Figure 6.20.

This presents a risk that excessive motion of the atlas on the axis will cause the spinal cord to become compressed. Theoretically, sports with a higher risk for neck compression, such as boxing, diving, horseback riding, gymnastics, and jumping on the trampoline, could cause spinal cord injury. It is estimated that 1%–2% of people with atlantoaxial instability will develop complications

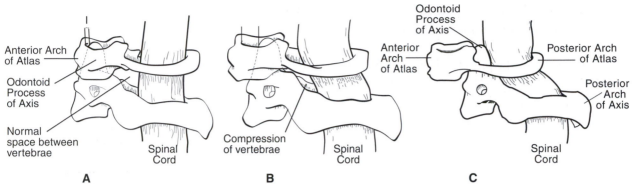

Figure 6.20 Atlantoaxial instability. *(A)* Normal relationship. *(B)* Atlantoaxial subluxation without spinal cord impingement. *(C)* Impingement on the spinal cord by the ondontoid process and posterior arch of the atlas. *(Adapted from Gajdosik, C.G., & Ostertag, S. [1996]. Cervical instability and Down syndrome: Review of the literature and implications for physical therapists.* Pediatric Physical Therapy, 8, *31–36. Original source: Martich, V., Ben-Ami, T., Yousefzaden, D.K.,& Roizen, N.J. (1992). Hypoplastic posterior of arch C-1 in children with Down syndrome: A double jeopardy.* Radiology, 183, *[127].)*

(Tassone & Duey-Holtz, 2008). Currently, Special Olympics requires athletes to be screened before participating. Evidence of instability would prohibit athletes from activities that place undue stress on neck structures. There is controversy, however, over the benefit of routine screening. Some professionals question the value of screening due to reliability problems with the radiographs, uncertainty as to whether an asymptomatic instability precedes symptomatic instability, and the low incidence of sports injuries causing neurological symptoms. Most professionals agree that initial radiographs should be taken between 3 and 5 years of age but no longer suggest obtaining repeated routine screening x-rays other than those that are required for participation by the Special Olympics (van Cleve & Cohen, 2006).

Therapists should know the status of a child's neck prior to selecting activities that may put stress on the neck. Children with normal neck x-rays do not need activity restrictions; however, those who have atlantoaxial instability should have restrictions (Cohen, 1999; Committee on Sports Medicine, 1984). In these children, it is important to avoid exercises that may place excessive pressure on the head and neck, such as tumbling and excessive neck flexion or extension. The therapist will also be a resource to the family regarding the risks of extracurricular activities and facilitate appropriate medical follow up if the child is symptomatic.

Summary

The human body operates through a complex interaction of many body systems. The musculoskeletal system is an integral component of a healthy and efficient system. Interventions made on the musculoskeletal system can improve the functional abilities of many children. An understanding of the development and potential pathologies of children will allow the physical therapist to design effective interventions that meet the needs of the child and family. Compliance at home will be maximized if the activities are fun and incorporated into the family's normal routine, and if the child and family are included in the planning. If the child and family have helped identify the problems and solutions, they will value the information and are more likely to comply with the program. Lastly, the therapist must remember that therapy interventions are only one component of the child's and family's life. Realistic expectations will allow the family to succeed and feel empowered.

DISCUSSION QUESTIONS

1. Discuss the implications for strength training in children with cerebral palsy.

2. Describe atlantoaxial instability and the symptoms you should be aware of when working with children with Down syndrome. How would its presence change your therapy program?

3. What are the important components of a musculoskeletal examination for a child with Down syndrome?

4. List the components of a therapy intervention program for a child with systemic juvenile idiopathic arthritis.

5. Discuss the factors that are considered when determining intervention for an adolescent with scoliosis.

6. What is the role of the physical therapist when working with an adolescent with scoliosis?

Recommended Readings

Klepper, S.E. (2008). Exercise in pediatric rheumatoid diseases. *Current Opinion in Rheumatology*, *20*(5), 619–624.

Mik, G., Gholve, P., Scher, D., Widmann, R., & Green, D. (2008). Down syndrome: Orthopedic issues. *Current Opinion in Pediatrics*, *20*, 30–36.

Verschuren, O., Ada, L., Maltais, D.B., Gorter, J.W., Scianni, A., & Ketelaar, M. (2011). Muscle strengthening in children and adolescents with spastic cerebral palsy: Considerations for future resistance training protocols. *Physical Therapy*, *91*(7), 1130–1139.

Wiart, L., Darrah, J., & Kembhavi, G. (2008). Stretching with children with cerebral palsy: What do we know and where are we going? *Pediatric Physical Therapy*, *20*(2), 173–178.

References

Adams, A.,& Lehman, T.J. (2005). Update on the pathogenesis and treatment of systemic onset juvenile rheumatoid arthritis. *Current Opinion in Rheumatol*ogy, *17*(5), 612–615.

Alvarez, C., De Vera, M., Beauchamp, R., Ward, V., & Black, A. (2006). Classification of idiopathic toe walking based on gait analysis: Development and application of the ITW severity classification. *Gait Posture, 26*, 428–435.

American Academy of Pediatrics, Section on Rheumatology and Section on Ophthalmology. (1993). Guidelines for ophthalmologic examinations in children with juvenile rheumatoid arthritis. *Pediatrics*, *92*(2), 295–296.

Anderson, A., & Forsyth, A. (2005). *Play it safe: Bleeding disorders, sports and exercise.* National Hemophilia Foundation.

Bacon, M.C., Nicholson, C., Binder, H., & White, P.H. (1991). Juvenile rheumatoid arthritis: Aquatic exercise and lower-extremity function. *Arthritis Care Resource, 4*(2), 102–105.

Bahmanyar, S., Montgomery, S.M., Weiss, R.J., & Ekbom, A. (2008). Maternal smoking during pregnancy, other prenatal and perinatal factors, and the risk of Legg-Calvé-Perthes disease. *Pediatrics*, *122*(2), e459–464.

Barnes, C., Wong, P., Egan, B., et al. (2004). Reduced bone density among children with severe hemiplegia. *Pediatrics*, *114*(2), e177–181.

Beauséjour, M., Roy-Beaudry, M., Goulet, L., & Labelle, H. (2007). Patient characteristics at the initial visit to a scoliosis clinic: A cross-sectional study in a community without school screening. *Spine*, *32*(12), 1349–1354.

Bevan, W.P., Hall, J.G., Bamshad, M., Staheli, L.T., Jaffe, K.M., & Song, K. (2007). Arthrogryposis multiform congenital (amyoplasia): An orthopedic perspective. *Journal of Pediatric Orthopedics*, *27*(5), 594–600.

Bialocerkowski, A.E., Vladusic, S.L., & Howell, S.M. (2005). Conservative interventions for positional plagiocephaly: A systemic review. *Developmental Medicine and Child Neurology, 47*(8), 563–570.

Biddiss, E., & Chau, T. (2007). Upper-limb prosthetics: Critical factors in device abandonment. *American Journal of Physical Medicine and Rehabilitation*, *86*, 977–987.

Biondi, O., Grondard, C., Lécolle, S., Deforges, S., Pariset, C., Lopes, P., & Charbonnier, F. (2008). Exercise-induced activation of NMDA receptor promotes motor unit development and survival in a type 2 spinal muscular atrophy model mouse. *Journal of Neuroscience, 28*(4), 953–962.

Blundell, S.W., Shepherd, R.B., Dean, C.M., Adams, R.D., & Cahill, B.M. (2003). Functional strength training in cerebral palsy: A pilot study of a group circuit training class for children aged 4–8 years. *Clinical Rehabilitation, 17*(1), 48–57.

Brouwer, B., Davidson, L.K., & Olney, S.J. (2000).Serial casting in idiopathic toe-walkers and children with spastic cerebral palsy. *Journal of Pediatric Orthopedics, 20*, 221–225.

Bunge, E.M., Juttman, R.E., de Kleuver, M., van Beizen, F.C., de Koning, J.H., & NESCIO group. (2007). Health-related quality of life in patients with adolescent idiopathic scoliosis after treatment: Short-term effects after brace or surgical treatment. *European Spine Journal, 16*(6), 83–89.

Bunnell, W.P. (2005). Selective screening for scoliosis. *Clinical Orthopaedics and Related Research, 434*, 40–45.

Burnei, G., Vlad, C., Georgescu, I., & Gavriliu, T.S., & Dan, D. (2008). Osteogenesis imperfecta: Diagnosis and treatment. *Journal of American Academy of Orthopedic Surgery, 16*(6), 356–366.

Bushby, K., Finkel, R., Birnkrant, D.J., Case, L.E., Clemens, P.R. Cripe, L., & Constantin, C. (2010). Diagnosis and management of Duchenne muscular dystrophy, part 1: Diagnosis, and pharmacological and psychosocial management. *Lancet Neurology, 9*(1), 77–93.

Cadenhead, S.L., McEwen, I.R., & Thompson, D.M. (2002). Effect of passive range of motion exercises on lower-extremity goniometric measurements of adults with cerebral palsy: A single-subject design. *Physical Therapy, 82*(7), 658–669.

Cakmak, A., & Bolukbas, N. (2005). Juvenile rheumatoid arthritis: physical therapy and rehabilitation. *Southern Medical Journal, 98*(2), 212–216.

Calabro, J.J., Holgerson, W.B., Sonpal, G.M., & Khoury, M.I. (1976). Juvenile rheumatoid arthritis:A general review and report of 100 patients observed for 15 years. *Seminars in Arthritis and Rheumatism, 5*(3), 257–298.

Campos, J.J., Anderson, D.I., Barbu-Roth, M.A., Hubbard, E.M., Hertenstein, M.J., & Witherington, D. (2000). Travel broadens the mind. *Infancy, 1*(2), 149–219.

Canavese, F., & Dimeglio, A. (2008). Perthes' disease: Prognosis in children under six years of age. *Journal of Bone Joint Surgery British, 90*(7), 940–945.

Cashman, J.P., Round, J., Taylor, G. & Clarke, N.M. (2002). The natural history of developmental dysplasia of the hip after early supervised treatment in the Pavlik harness: A prospective, longitudinal follow-up. *Journal of Bone and Joint Surgery British, 84*(3), 418–425.

Cervellati, S., Bettini, N., Moscato, M., et al. (2004). Surgical treatment of spinal deformities in Duchenne muscular dystrophy: A long term follow-up study. *European Spine Journal, 13*, 441–448.

Cheng, J.C., Wong, M.W., Tang, S.P., Chen, T.M., Shum, S.L., & Wong, E.M. (2001). Clinical determinants of the outcome of manual stretching in the treatment of congenital muscular torticollis in infants: A prospective study of eight hundred and twenty-one cases. *Journal of Bone and Joint Surgery American, 83*-A(5), 679–687.

Cohen, W.I. (1999). Health care guidelines for individuals with Down Syndrome: 1999 revision. *Down Syndrome Quarterly, 3*(4), 1–15.

Committee on Sports Medicine.(1984). Atlantoaxial instability in Down syndrome. *Pediatrics, 74*(1), 152–154.

Côté, P., Kreitz, B.G., Cassidy, S.D., Dzus, A.K., & Martel, J. (1998). A study of the diagnostic accuracy and reliability of the scoliometer and Adam's forward bend test. *Spine, 23*(7), 796–802.

Cyrulnik, S.E., Fee, R.J., De Vivo, D.C., Goldstein, E., & Hinton, V.J. (2007). Delayed developmental language milestones in children with Duchenne muscular dystrophy. *Journal of Pediatrics, 150*(5), 474–478.

Damiano, D.L., & Abel, M.F. (1998). Functional outcomes of strength training in spastic cerebral palsy. *Archives of Physical Medicine and Rehabilitation, 79*(2), 119–125.

Davids, J.R., Wenger, D.R., & Mubarak, S.J. (1993). Congenital muscular torticollis: Sequella of intrauterine or perinatal compartment syndrome. *Journal of Pediatric Orthopedics, 13*(2), 141–147.

Davidson, M.A. (2008). Primary care for children and adolescents with Down syndrome. *Pediatric Clinics North America, 55*(5), 1099–111.

Deconinck, N., & Dan, B. (2007). Pathophysiology of Duchenne muscular dystrophy. Current hypotheses. *Pediatric Neurology, 36*(1), 1–7.

Dhanendran, M., Hutton, W.C., Klennerman, L., Witemeyer, S., & Ansell, B.M. (1980). Foot function in juvenile chronic arthritis. *Rheumatology and Rehabilitation, 19*, 20–24.

DiTaranto, P., Campagna, L., Price, A.E., & Grossman, J.A. (2004). Outcome following postoperative treatment of brachial plexus birth injuries. *Journal of Child Neurology, 19*(2), 87–90.

Do, T.T. (2001). Clinical and radiographic evaluation of bowlegs. *Current Opinions in Pediatrics, 13*(1), 424–426.

Do, T.T. (2006). Congenital muscular torticollis: Current concepts and review of treatment. *Current Opinion in Pediatrics, 18*(1), 26–29.

Driscoll, S.W., & Skinner, J. (2008). Musculoskeletal complications of neuromuscular disease in children. *Physical Medicine and Rehabilitation Clinics of North America, 19*, 163–194.

Eagle, M., Bourke, J., Bullock, R., Gibson, M., Mehta, J., Giddlings, D., Straub, V., & Bushby, K. (2007). Managing Duchenne muscular dystrophy: The additive effect of spinal surgery and home nocturnal ventilation on improving survival. *Neuromuscular Disorders, 17*, 470–475.

Eagleton, M., Iams, A., McDowell, J., Morrison, R., & Evans, C.L. (2004). The effects of strength training on gait in adolescents with cerebral palsy. *Pediatric Physical Therapy, 16*(1), 22–30.

Eiff, M. P., Hatch, R. L., & Calmbach, W. L. (2002). *Fracture management for primary care* (2nd ed.). Philadelphia: Saunders.

Field, T., Hernandez-Reif, M., Diego, M., Schanberg, S., & Kuhn, C. (2005). Cortisol decreases and serotonin and dopamine increase following massage therapy. *International Journal of Neuroscience, 115*(10), 1397–1413.

Finckh, A., & Gabay, C. (2008). At the horizon of innovative therapy in rheumatology: New biologic agents. *Current Opinion in Rheumatology, 20*(3), 269–275.

Finckh, A., Liang, M.H., van Herckenrode, C.M., & de Pablo, P. (2006). Long term impact of early treatment on radiographic progression in rheumatoid arthritis: A meta-analysis. *Rheumatology, 55*(6), 864–872.

Foran, J.R., Steinman, S., Barash, I., Chambers, H.G., & Lieber, R.L. (2005). Structural and mechanical alterations in spastic skeletal muscle. *Developmental Medicine and Child Neurology, 47*(10), 713–717.

Gajdosik, C.G., & Ostertag, S. (1996). Cervical instability and Down syndrome: Review of the literature and implications for physical therapists. *Pediatric Physical Therapy, 8*, 31–36.

Gannotti, M.E., Nahorniak, M., Gorton, G.E., Sciascia, K., Sueltenfuss, M., Synder, M., & Zaniewski, A. (2007). Can exercise influence low bone mineral density in children with juvenile rheumatoid arthritis? *Pediatric Physical Therapy, 19*(2), 128–139.

Ghanem, I. (2008). Epidemiology, etiology, and genetic aspects of reduction deficiencies of the lower limb. *Journal of Child Orthopedics, 2*, 329–332.

Gillespie, R., & Torode, I.P. (1983). Classification and management of congenital abnormalities of the femur. *The Journal of Bone and Joint Surgery, 65*, 557–568.

Givon, U. (2009). Muscle weakness in cerebral palsy. *Acta Orthopaedica et Traumatologica Turcica, 43*, 87–93.

Goldberg, C.J., Dowling, F.E., Fogarty, E.E., & More, D.P. (1995). School scoliosis screening and the United States Preventative Services Task Force: An examination of long-term results. *Spine, 20*(12), 1368–1374.

Gomez-Benito, M.J., Moreo, P., Pérez, M.A., Paseta, O., García-Aznar, J.M., Barrios, C., & Doblaré, M. (2007). A damage model for the growth plate: Application to the prediction of slipped capital epiphysis. *Journal of Biomechanics, 40*(15), 3305–3313.

Gordon, J.E., Hughes, M.S., Shepherd, K., Szymanski, D., Schoenecker, P., Parker, L., Uong, E.C. (2006). Obstructive sleep apnoea syndrome in morbidly obese children with tibia vara. *Journal of Bone Joint Surgery British, 88*(1), 100–203.

Goulding, A., Grant, A.M., & Williams, S.M. (2005). Bone and body composition of children and adolescents with repeated forearm fractures. *Journal of Bone and Mineral Research, 20*(12), 2090–2096.

Goulding, A. (2007). Risk factors for fractures in normally active children and adolescents. *Med Sport Science, 51*, 102–120.

Greene, K.A., & Ross, M.D. (2008). Slipped capital femoral epiphysis in a patient referred to physical therapy for knee pain. *Journal of Orthopedic Sports Physical Therapy, 38*(1), 26.

Greulich, W., & Pyle, S. (1959). *Radiographic atlas of the skeletal development of the hand and wrist* (2nd ed.). Stanford, CA: Stanford University Press.

Grimston, S.K., Willows, N.D., & Hanley, D.A. (1993). Mechanical loading regime and its relationship to bone mineral density in children. *Medicine and Science in Sports and Exercise, 25*(11), 1203–1207.

Guille, J.T., Pizzutillo, P.D., & MacEwen, G.D. (2000). Development dysplasia of the hip from birth to six months. *Journal of American Academy of Orthopedic Surgeons, 8*(4), 232–242.

Gurnett, C.A., Boehm, S., Connolly, A., Reimschisel, T., & Dobbs, M.B. (2008). Impact of congenital alipes equinovarus etiology on treatment outcomes. *Developmental Medicine and Child Neurology, 50*, 498–502.

Harvapat, M., Greenspan, S.L., O'Brien, C., et al. (2005). Altered bone mass in children at diagnosis of Crohn disease: A pilot study. *Journal of Pediatric Gastroenterology Nutrition, 40*(3), 295–300.

Heikkila, E., Ryoppy, S., & Louhimo, I. (1985).The management of primary acetabular dysplasia: Its association with habitual side-lying. *Journal of Bone and Joint Surgery British, 67*(1), 25–28.

Hemo, Y., Macdessi, S.J., Pierce, R.A., Aiona, M.D., & Sussman, M.D. (2006). Outcome of patients alter achilles tendon lengthening for treatment of idiopathic toe walking. *Journal of Pediatric Orthopedics, 26*, 336–340.

Henderson, R.C., Kairalla, J., Abbas, A., & Stevenson, R.D. (2004). Predicting low bone density in children and young adults with quadriplegic cerebral palsy. *Developmental Medicine and Child Neurology, 46*(6), 416–419.

Herring, J.A. (2002). Scoliosis. In J.S. Herring (Ed.). *Tachdjian's pediatric orthopedics, 213*–321. Philadelphia: W.B. Saunders Co.

Hind, K., & Burrows, M. (2007). Weight-bearing exercise and bone mineral accrual in children and adolescents: A review of controlled trials. *Bone, 40*(1), 14–27.

Hiraki, L.T., Benseler, S.M., Tyrrell, P.N., Hebert, D., Harvey, E., & Silverman, E.D. (2008). Clinical and laboratory characteristics and long-term outcome of pediatric systemic lupus erythematosus: A longitudinal study. *Journal of Pediatrics, 152*(4), 550–556.

Hunt, V.W., Qin, L., Cheung, C.S., et al. (2005). Osteopenia: Anew prognostic factor of curve progression in adolescent idiopathic scoliosis. *Journal of Bone Joint Surgery American, 87*(12), 2709–2716.

Iannaconne, S.T. (2007). Modern management of spinal muscular atrophy. *Journal of Child Neurology, 22*(8), 974–978.

Ihkkhan, D.Y., & Yalçin, F. (2001). Changes in skeletal maturation and mineralization in children with cerebral palsy and evaluation of related factors. *Journal of Child Neurology, 16*(6), 425–430.

James, M.J., Bagley, A.M., Brasington, K., Lutz, C., McConnell, S., & Molitor, F. (2006). Impact of prostheses on function and quality of life for children with unilateral congenital below-the-elbow deficiency. *Journal of Bone and Joint Surgery American, 88*, 2356–2365.

Jones, M.A., McEwen, I.R., & Hansen, L. (2003).Use of power mobility for a young child with spinal muscular atrophy. *Physical Therapy, 83*, 253–262.

Kabakuş, N., & Kurt, A. (2006). Sandifer syndrome: A continuing problem of misdiagnosis. *Pediatrics International, 48*(6), 622–625.

Kapp, S.L. (2004). Visual analysis of prosthetic gait. In D.G. Smith, J.W. Michael, & J.H. Bowker (Eds.), *Atlas of amputations and limb deficiencies: surgical, prosthetic, and rehabilitation principles.* (3rd ed., pp. 385–394). Rosemont: American Academy of Orthopaedic Surgeons.

Karachalios, T., Sofianos, J., Roidis, N., Sapkas, G., Korres, D., & Nikolopoulos, K. (1999). Ten-year follow-up evaluation of a school screening program for scoliosis: Is the forward-bending test an accurate diagnostic criterion for the screening of scoliosis? *Spine, 24*(22), 2318–2324.

Kinali, M., Main, M., Eliahoo, J., et al. (2007). Predictive factors for the development of scoliosis in Duchenne muscular dystrophy. *European Journal of Pediatric Neurology, 11*, 160–166.

Kinali, M., Messina, S., & Mercuri, E. (2006). Management of scoliosis in Duchenne muscular dystrophy: A large 10-year retrospective study. *Developmental Medicine and Child Neurology, 48*, 513–518.

King, W.M., Ruttencutter, R., Nagaraja, H.N., Matkovic, V., Landoll, J., Hoyle, C., Mendell, J.R., & Kissel, J.T. (2007). Orthopedic outcomes of long-term daily corticosteroid treatment in Duchenne muscular dystrophy. *Neurology, 68*, 1607–1613.

Klepper, S.E. (1999). Effects of an eight-week physical conditioning program on disease signs and symptoms in children with chronic arthritis. *Arthritis Care Research, 12*(1), 52–60.

Klepper, S.E. (2008). Exercise in pediatric rheumatoid diseases. *Current Opinion in Rheumatology, 20*(5), 619–624.

Kostova, F.V., Williams, V.C., Heemskerk, J., et al. (2007). Spinal muscular atrophy: Classification, diagnosis, management, pathogenesis, and future research directions. *Journal of Child Neurology, 22*(8), 926–945.

Kott, K.M., Held, S.L. (2002). Effects of orthoses on upright functional skills of children and adolescents with cerebral palsy. *Pediatric Physical Therapy, 14*(4), 199–207.

Krajbich, J.I. (1998). Lower-limb deficiencies and amputation in children. *Journal of the American Academy of Orthopedic Surgery, 6*, 358–367.

Lammers, A.E., Hislop, A.A., Flynn, Y., & Haworth, S.G. (2008). The 6-minute walk test: Normal values for children of 4–11 years of age. *Archives of Disease in Childhood, 93*(6), 464–468.

Laville, J.M., Chau, E.,Willemen, L., Kohler, R., & Garin, C. (1999). Blount's disease: Classification and treatment. *Journal of Pediatric Orthopedics B, 8*(1), 19–25.

Lecuire, F. (2002).The long-term outcome of primary osteochondritis of the hip (Legg-Calva-Perthes' disease). *Journal of Bone and Joint Surgery British, 84*(5), 636–640.

Lehnert-Schroth, C. (2007). *Three-dimensional treatment for scoliosis: A physiotherapeutic method for deformities of the spine.* Palo Alto, CA: Martindale Press.

Lelieveld, O.T., Takken, T., van der Net, J., & van Weert, E. (2005). Validity of the 6-minute walking test in juvenile idiopathic arthritis. *Arthritis and Rheumatism, 53*(2), 304–307.

Lelieveld, O.T., van Brussel, M., Takken, T., et al. (2007). Aerobic and anaerobic exercise capacity in adolescents with juvenile idiopathic arthritis. *Arthritis and Rheumatism, 57*(6), 898–904.

Lenssinck, M.L., Frijlink, A.C., Berger, M.Y., Bierman-Seinstra, S.M., Verkerk, K., & Verhagen, A.P. (2005). Effect of bracing and other conservative interventions in the treatment of idiopathic scoliosis in adolescents: A systematic review of clinical trials. *Physical Therapy, 85*(12), 1329–1339.

Lespargot, A., Renaudin, E., Khouri, N., & Robert, M. (1994). Extensibility of hip adductors in children with cerebral palsy. *Developmental Medicine and Child Neurology, 36*(11), 980–988.

Loder, R.T., Aronsson, D.D., Weinstein, S.L., Breur, G.J., Ganz, R., & Leunig, M. (2008). Slipped capital femoral epiphysis. *Instructional Course Lectures, 57,* 473–498.

Loder, R.T., Schwartz, E.M., & Hensinger, R.N. (1993). Behavioral characteristics of children with Legg-Calve-Perthes. *Journal of Pediatric Orthopedics, 5,* 598–601.

Losee, J.E., & Mason, A.C. (2005). Deformational plagiocephaly: Diagnosis, prevention, and treatment. *Clinical Plastic Surgery, 150*(5), 474–478.

Lunn, M.R., & Want, C.H. (2008). Spinal muscular atrophy. *Lancet, 371,* 2120–2133.

Lyden, C. (2009). Caring for the victim of child abuse in the pediatric intensive care unit. *Dimensions of Critical Care Nursing, 28*(2), 61–66.

Mahar, R.K., Kirby, R.L., & MacLeod, D.A. (1985). Simulated leg-length discrepancy: Its effect on mean center-of-pressure position and postural sway. *Archives of Physical Medicine and Rehabilitation, 66,* 822–824.

Martin, K. (2004). Effects of supramalleolar orthoses on postural stability in children with Down Syndrome. *Developmental Medicine and Child Neurology, 46*(6), 406–411.

McKay, H., MacLean, L., Petit, M., et al. (2005). "Bounce at the Bell": A novel program of short bouts of exercise improves proximal femur bone mass in early pubertal children. *British Journal of Sports Medicine, 39*(8), 521–526.

Mehta, J.S., Conybeare, M.E., Hinves, B.L., & Winter, J.B. (2006). Protein C levels in patients with Legg-Calve-Perthes disease: Is it a true deficiency? *Journal of Pediatric Orthopedics, 26*(2), 200–203.

Mennen, U., van Heest, A., Ezaki, M.B., Tonkin, M., & Gericke, G. (2005). Arthrogryposis multiplex congenital. *Journal Hand Surgery British, 30*(5), 468–474.

Messina, S., Pane, M., De Rose, P., Vasta, I., Sorleti, D., Aloysius, A., & Mercuri, E. (2008). Feeding problems and malnutrition in spinal muscular atrophy type II. *Neuromuscular Disorders: NMD, 18*(5), 389–393.

Mik, G., Gholve, P., Scher, D., Widmann, R., & Green, D. (2008). Down syndrome: Orthopedic issues. *Current Opinion in Pediatrics, 20,* 30–36.

Mortenson, P.A., & Steinbok, P. (2006). Quantifying positional plagiocephaly: Reliability and validity of anthropometric measurements. *Journal Craniofacial Surgery, 17*(3), 413–419.

Morton, J.F., Brownlee, M., & McFadyen, A.K. (2005).The effects of progressive resistive training for children with cerebral palsy. *Clinical Rehabilitation, 19,* 283–289.

Moseley, C.F. (1991). Leg lengthening: the historical perspective. *Orthopedic Clinics of North America, 22*(4), 555–561.

Moseley, C.F. (1996). Leg length discrepancy and angular deformity of the lower limbs. In R.T. Morrissey & S.L. Weinstein (Eds.), *Lovell and Winter's pediatric orthopedics* (pp. 849–901). Philadelphia: Lippincott-Raven.

Murray, A.W., & Wilson, N.I. (2008). Changing incidence of slipped capital femoral epiphysis: A relationship with obesity? *Journal of Bone Joint Surgery British, 90*(1), 92–94.

Murray, P.D., & Drachman, D.B. (1969). The role of movement in the development of joints and related structures: The head and neck in the chick embryo. *Journal of Embryology and Experimental Morphology, 22*(3), 349–371.

Nelson, V.S., Flood, K.M., Bryant, P.R., Huang, M.E., Pasquina, P.R., & Roberts, R.L. (2006). Limb deficiency and prosthetic management. 1. Decision making in prosthetic prescription and management. *Archives of Physical Medicine and Rehabilitation*, 87(3 Suppl), S3–9.

Nicholson, G.P., Ferguson-Pell, M.W., Smith, K., Edgar, M., & Morley, T. (2003). The objective measurement of a spinal orthoses use for the treatment of adolescent idiopathic scoliosis. *Spine, 28*(19), 2243–2250.

Nicole, S., Diaz, C., Frugier, T., & Melki, J. (2002). Spinal muscular atrophy: Recent advances and future prospects. *Muscle and Nerve, 26*(1), 4–13.

Noonan, K., Richards, B.S. (2003). Nonsurgical management of idiopathic clubfoot. *Journal of American Academy of Orthopedic Surgery, 11,* 392–402.

Ohman, A.M., & Beckung, E.R. (2008). Reference values for range of motion and muscle function of the neck in infants. *Pediatric Physical Therapy, 20*(1), 53–58.

Okumus, O., Erguven, M., Deveci, M., Yilmaz, O., & Okumus, M. (2008). Growth and bone mineralization in patients with juvenile idiopathic arthritis. *Indian Journal of Pediatrics, 75*(3), 239–243.

Paap, E., van der Net, J., Helders, P.J.M., & Takken, T. (2005). Physiologic response of the six-minute walk test in children with juvenile idiopathic arthritis. *Arthritis and Rheumatism, 53*(3), 351–356.

Parapia, L.A., & Jackson, C. (2008). Ehlers-Danlos syndrome: A historical review. *British Journal of Haematology, 141*(1), 32–35.

Pellecchia, G.L., Lugo-Larchevegue, N., & Deluca, P.A. (1996). Differential diagnosis in physical therapy evaluation of thigh pain in an adolescent boy. *Journal of Orthopedic Sports Physical Therapy, 23*(1), 51–55.

Perry J. (1992). *Gait analysis normal and pathological function.* Thorofare, NJ: Slack.

Pin, T., Dyke, P., & Chan, M. (2006). The effectiveness of passive stretching in children with cerebral palsy. *Developmental Medicine and Child Neurology, 48*(10), 855–862.

Pontén, E.M., & Stål, P.S. (2007). Decreased capillarization and a shift to fast myosin heavy chain IIx in the biceps brachii muscle from young adults with spastic paresis. *Journal of the Neurological Sciences, 253*(1–2), 25–33.

Poon, D.M.Y., & Hui-Chan, C.W.Y. (2009). Hyperactive stretch reflexes, co-contraction, and muscle weakness in children with cerebral palsy. *Developmental Medicine and Child Neurology, 51,* 128–135.

Ravelli, A., & Martini, A. (2007). Juvenile idiopathic arthritis. *Lancet, 369*(9563), 767–778.

Renshaw, T.S., Green, N.E., Griffin, P.P., & Root, L. (1996) Cerebral palsy: Orthopaedic management. *Instructional Course Lecture, 45,* 475–490.

Rhodes, V.J. (1991). Physical therapy management of patients with juvenile rheumatoid arthritis. *Physical Therapy, 71,* 910–919.

Roye, D.P., & Roye, B.D. (2002). Idiopathic congenital talipes equinovarus. *Journal of the American Academy of Orthopedic Surgery, 10*(4), 239–248.

Sala, D.A., Shulman, L.H., Kennedy, R.F., Grant, A.D., & Chu, M.L.Y. (1999). Idiopathic toe walking: A review. *Developmental Medicine and Child Neurology, 41,* 846–848.

Salter, R.B. (1968). Etiology, pathogenesis and possible prevention of congenital dislocation of the hip. *Canadian Medical Association Journal, 98*(20), 933–945.

Salter, R.B., & Harris, W.R. (1963). Injuries involving the epiphyseal plate. *Journal of Bone and Joint Surgery American, 45*, 587–622.

Schaefer, M.K., McCarthy, J.J., & Josephic, K. (2007). Effects of early weight bearing on the functional recovery of ambulatory children with cerebral palsy after bilateral proximal femoral osteotomy. *Journal of Pediatric Orthopedics, 27*(6), 668–670.

Schneider, R., & Passo, M.H. (2002). Juvenile rheumatoid arthritis. *Rheumatic Diseases Clinics of North America, 28*(3), 503–530.

Scianni, A., Butler, J.M., Ada, L., & Teixeira-Salmeda, L.F. (2009). Muscle strengthening is not effective in children and adolescents with cerebral palsy: A systematic review. *Australian Journal of Physiotherapy, 55*(2), 81–87.

Scoliosis Research Society. (March 31, 2003). Retrieved from http://www.srs.org

Selby-Silverstein, L., Hillstrom, H.J., & Palisano, R.J. (2001). The effect of foot orthoses on standing foot posture and gait of young children with Down syndrome. *Neurorehabilitation, 16*(3), 183–193.

Senaran, H., Ozdemir, H.M., Ogun, T.C., & Kapicioglu, M.I. (2004). Value of limited hip abduction in developmental dysplasia of the hip. *Pediatrics International, 46*(4), 456–458.

Shepard, J.A. (1995). The bronchi: An imaging perspective. *Journal of Thoracic Imaging, 10*(4), 236–254.

Sherry, D.D., & Mosca, V.S. (1996). Juvenile rheumatoid arthritis and seronegative spondyloarthropathies. In R.T. Morrissey & S.L. Weinstein (Eds.), *Lovell and Winter's pediatric orthopedics* (pp. 537–577). Philadelphia: Lippincott-Raven.

Sheth, R.D., & Hermann, B.P. (2008). Bone in idiopathic and symptomatic epilepsy. *Epilepsy Research, 78*(1), 71–76.

Shulman, L.H., Sala, D.A., Chu, M.L.Y., McCaul, P.R., & Sandler, B.J. (1997). Developmental implications of idiopathic toe walking. *Journal of Pediatrics, 130*, 541–546.

Simon, S., Whiffen, J., & Shapiro, F. (1981). Leg-length discrepancy in monarticular and pauciarticular oligoarthritis juvenile rheumatoid arthritis. *Journal of Bone and Joint Surgery [Am], 63*, 209.

Sochett, E.B,. & Makitie, O. (2005). Osteoporosis in chronically ill children. *Annals of Medicine, 37*(4), 286–294.

Song, F.S., McCarthy, J.J., MacEwen, G.D., Fuchs, K.E., & Dulka, S.E. (2008). The incidence of occult dysplasia of the contralateral hip in children with unilateral hip dysplasia. *Journal of Pediatric Orthopaedics, 28*(2), 173–176.

Spraul, G., & Koenning, G. (1994). A descriptive study of foot problems in children with juvenile rheumatoid arthritis (JRAJIA). *Arthritis Care Resource, 7*(3), 144–150.

Stanitski, D.F., & Stanitski, C.L. (2003). Fibular hemimelia: A new classification system. *Journal of Pediatric Orthopaedics, 23*, 30–34.

Stevenson, R.D., Conaway, M., Barrington, J.W., Cuthill, S.L., Worley, G., & Henderson, R.C. (2006). Fracture rate in children with cerebral palsy. *Pediatric Rehabilitation, 9*(4), 396–403.

Stott, N.S., Walt, S.E., Lobb, G.A., Reynolds, N., & Nicol, R.O. (2004). Treatment for idiopathic toe-walking: Results at skeletal maturity. *Journal of Pediatric Orthopedics, 24*, 63–69.

Stricker, S.J., & Angulo, J.C. (1998). Idiopathic toe walking: A comparison of treatment methods. *Journal of Pediatric Orthopedics, 18*, 289–293.

Stuberg, W.A. (1992). Considerations related to weight bearing programs in children with developmental disabilities. *Physical Therapy, 72*, 35–40.

Sylvester, F.A. (2005). IBD and skeletal health: Children are not small adults! *Inflammatory Bowel Disease, 11*(11), 1020–1023.

Szalay, E.A., Bosch, P., Schwend, R.M., et al. (2008). Adolescents with idiopathic scoliosis are not osteoporotic. *Spine, 33*(7), 802–806.

Tanner, J.M., & Buckler, J.M. (1997). Revision and update of Tanner-Whitehouse clinical longitudinal charts for height and weight. *European Journal of Pediatrics, 156* (3), 248–249.

Tardieu, C., Lespargot, A., Tabary, C., & Bret, M.D. (1988). For how long must the soleus muscle be stretched each day to prevent contracture? *Developmental Medicine and Child Neurology, 30*(1), 3–10.

Tassone, J.C., & Duey-Holtz, A. (2008). Spine concerns in the Special Olympian with Down syndrome. *Sports Medicine and Arthroscopy Review, 16*(1), 55–60.

Tatli, B., Aydinli, N., Caliskan, M., Ozmen, M., Bilir, F., & Acar, G. (2006). Congenital muscular torticollis: Evaluation and classification. *Pediatric Neurology, 34*(1), 41–44.

Tedroff, K., Knutson, L.M., & Soderberg, G.L. (2008). Co-activity during maximum voluntary contraction: A study of four lower-extremity muscles in children with and without cerebral palsy. *Developmental Medicine and Child Neurology, 50*, 377–381.

Thompson, G.H. (1996). Neuromuscular disorders. In R.T. Morrissey & S.L. Weinstein (Eds.), *Lovell and Winter's pediatric orthopaedics* (pp. 537–577). Philadelphia: Lippincott-Raven.

Thorton, J., Ashcroft, D., O'Neill, T., et al. (2008).A systemic review of the effectiveness of strategies for reducing fracture risk in children with juvenile idiopathic arthritis with additional data on long-term risk of fracture and cost of disease management. *Health Technology Assessment, 12*(3), iii–ix,xi–xiv, 1–208.

Tidball, A., Alexander, H., & Lowes, L.P. (2009). Personal communication.

Tolo, V.T., & Wood, B. (1993). *Pediatric orthopedics in primary care* (pp. 83–102). Baltimore: Williams & Wilkins.

van Brussel, M., Lelieveld, O.T., van der Net, J., et al. (2007). Aerobic and anaerobic exercise capacity in children with juvenile idiopathic arthritis. *Arthritis and Rheumatism, 57*(6), 891–897.

van Cleve, S.N., & Cohen, W.I. (2006). Part I: Clinical practice guidelines for children with Down syndrome from birth to 12 years. *Journal of Pediatric Health Care, 20*(1), 47–54.

van der Net, J., van der Torre, P., Engelbert, R.H., et al. (2008). Motor performance and functional ability in preschool and early school-aged children with juvenile idiopathic arthritis: A cross-sectional study. *Pediatric Rheumatology Online Journal, 2*.

Vatanparast, H., & Whiting, S.J. (2006). Calcium supplementation trials and bone mass development in children, adolescents, and young adults. *Nutrition Review, 64*(4), 204–209.

Vicente-Rodriguez, G., Dorado, C., Ara, I., et al. (2007). Artistic versus rhythmic gymnastics: effects on bone and muscle mass ion young girls. *Internal Journal of Sports Medicine, 28*(5), 386–393.

von Heideken, J., Green, D.W., Burke, S.W., Sindle, K., Denneen, J., Haglund-Akerlind, Y., & Widmann, R.F. (2006). The relationship between developmental dysplasia of the hip and congenital muscular torticollis. *Journal of Pediatric Orthopaedics, 26*(6), 805–808.

Walker, J. (1991). Musculoskeletal development: A review. *Physical Therapy, 71*(12), 878–889.

Walker, J.L., Knapp, D., Minter, C., Boakes, J.L., Salazar, J.C., Sanders, J.O., Lubicky, J.P., Drvaric, D.M., & David, J.R. (2009). Adult outcomes following amputation or lengthening for fibular deficiency. *Journal of Bone and Joint Surgery American, 91*, 797–804.

Wang, H.Y., Ju, Y.H., Chen, S.M., Lo, S.K., & Jong, Y.J. (2004).Joint range of motion limitations in children and young adults with spinal muscular atrophy. *Archives of Physical Medicine and Rehabilitation, 85*, 1689–1693.

Wattenbarger, J.M., Gruber, H.E., & Phieffer, L.S. (2002). Physeal fractures, part I: Histologic features of bone, cartilage and bar formation in a small animal model. *Journal of Pediatric Orthopedics, 22*(6), 703–709.

Weber, M. (2008). New classification and score for tibial hemimelia. *Journal of Child Orthopedics, 2*, 169–175.

Weinstein, S.L. (1996). Developmental hip dysplasia and dislocation. In R.T. Morrissey & S.L. Weinstein (Eds.). *Lovell and Winter's pediatric orthopedics.* Philadelphia: Lippincott Raven.

Weiss, P.F., Arabshahi, B., Johnson, A., et al. (2008). High prevalence of temporomandibular joint arthritis at disease onset in children with juvenile idiopathic arthritis, as detected by magnetic resonance imaging, but not by ultrasound. *Arthritis and Rheumatism, 58*(4), 1189–1196.

Wenger, D.R. (1993). Developmental dysplasia of the hip. In D.R. Wenger & M. Rang (Eds.), *The art and practice of children's orthopedics* (pp. 256–296). New York: Raven.

Wessel, J., Kaup, C., Fan, J., Ehalt, R., Ellsworth, J., Speer, C., Tenove, P., & Dombrosky, A. (1999). Isometric strength measurements in children with arthritis: Reliability and relation to function. *Arthritis Care Resource, 12*(4), 238–246.

Westberry, D.E., & Davids, J.R. (2009). Proximal focal femoral deficiency (PFFD) management options and controversies. *Hip International, 19*(6), 18–25.

Westhoff, B., Petermann, A., Hirsch, M.A., Willers, R., & Krauspe, R. (2006). Computerized gait analysis in Legg Calvé Perthes disease: Analysis of the frontal plane. *Gait Posture, 24*(2), 196–202.

White, J., Flohr, J.A., Winter, S.S., Vener, J., Feinauer, L.R., & Ransdell, L.B. (2005). Potential benefits of physical activity for children with acute lymphoblastic leukemia. *Pediatric Rehabilitation, 8*(1), 53–58.

Wiart, L., Darrah, J., & Kembhavi, G. (2008). Stretching with children with cerebral palsy: What do we know and where are we going? *Pediatric Physical Therapy, 20*(2), 173–178.

Wills, M. (2004). Orthopedic complications of childhood obesity. *Pediatric Physical Therapy, 16*(4), 230–235.

Wright, F.V., Hubbard, S., Naumann, S., & Jutai, J. (2003). Evaluation of the validity of the prosthetic upper extremity functional index for children. *Archives of Physical Medicine and Rehabilitation, 84*(4), 518–527.

Wynn-Davies, R. (1968). Familial (idiopathic) scoliosis: A family survey. *Journal of Bone and Joint Surgery, British Edition, 50*, 24–30.

Yiu, E.M., & Kornberg, A.J. (2008). Duchenne muscular dystrophy. *Neurology India, 56*(3), 236–247.

Zamboni, G., Antoniazzi, F., Lauriola, S., Bertold, F., & Tató, L. (2006). Calcium supplementation increases bone mass in GH-deficient prepubertal children during GH replacement. *Hormone Research, 65*(5), 223–230.

CHAPTER 7

Neuromuscular System: Examination, Evaluation, and Diagnoses

—Caroline Goulet, PT, PhD

—Jennifer Furze, PT, DPT, PCS

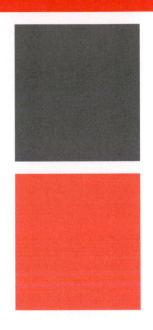

The human nervous system is a fascinating system that includes all of the neural and support cells located within the central nervous system (CNS) and the neural axons that enter or exit the brain and spinal cord. This complex system has a built-in innate organization that simplifies the control of movement. Redundancy exists at most levels within the system to allow a safety net when there is damage of neural structures. The capacity for neural plasticity can assist with recovery from injury or disease, with the most recovery occurring based on how the individual uses the system. Evidence in the fields of neuroscience, psychology, education, and sports has contributed to our current knowledge of how movement is controlled by the interaction of the neuromuscular system with the other systems and within the constraints of the task environment. Physical therapists need a functional knowledge of these neuroscience essentials to apply clinical reasoning skills to the examination, evaluation, and intervention of children with neuromuscular disorders.

This chapter will first discuss the evolution of neurorehabilitation practices in relationship to the theoretical underpinning of movement control. Following the American Physical Therapy Association, *Guide to Physical Therapist Practice* (APTA, 2001) (hereafter referred to as the *Guide*), examination and evaluation strategies for the neuromuscular system will be described using the structure and nomenclature of the International Classification of Functioning, Disability and Health (ICF) (World Health Organization [WHO], 2001). The clinical management of common pediatric neuromuscular disorders related to the Physical Therapy Practice Patterns 5B (Impaired Neuromotor Development) and 5C (Impaired Motor Function and Sensory Integrity Associated with Nonprogressive

Disorders of the Central Nervous System) will then be presented, followed by a discussion about prognosis and recovery as it relates to neuroplasticity in children.

Theoretical Background of Movement Control

Rehabilitation practices develop in parallel with scientific theories. From new knowledge in basic sciences emerge new theories or new viewpoints about how the brain controls movement and the relative influence of, and organization among, the different systems involved. A theory of motor control provides clinicians with a set of assumptions about how movement is controlled. These assumptions are then translated into clinical applications. Theories of motor control are used as the conceptual framework for hypothesis-oriented clinical practice. The application of specific theories to practice will influence a therapist's clinical decision-making process through the sets of assumptions underlying the hypotheses formulated from the examination findings and through the prioritizing of problems to be addressed.

With this brief introduction to motor control theories, it is hoped that how physical therapy practice has been shaped in the past and how acceptance of one or more of these theories would lead the therapist to different examinations and interventions can begin to be understood. This is important for a beginning understanding of the nature of problems in some children with neuromuscular deficits and to comprehend current research on motor control. None of these theories hold the complete theoretical position to explain how humans control and learn movement. Each theory builds on, and borrows from, the previous ones, as it should, based on support or lack thereof from scientific evidence. The process will continue as more is learned, and you will need to periodically update your basis for examination and intervention.

Early theories of motor control—reflex and hierarchical theories—had a major impact on physical therapy practice in the late 1950s to early 1970s. The main neurofacilitation approaches such as Bobath's Neurodevelopmental Treatment (NDT) (Bobath, 1964, 1985; Bobath & Bobath, 1984), Brunnstrom's (1992) and Rood's (Stockmeyer, 1967) approaches, Kabat and Knott's Proprioceptive Neuromuscular Facilitation (PNF) (Knott & Voss, 1968), and Ayres's Sensory Integration Therapy (SI) (Ayres, 1979) originated from these theories.

The abnormal reflexes and muscle tone observed after damage to the cortex in children with cerebral palsy (CP), or in individuals after a cerebrovascular accident or a traumatic brain injury (TBI), were believed to be the origin of abnormal movements. Therapists thought that if they could inhibit primitive reflexes and normalize tone, neural plasticity could be induced through facilitation of residual higher brain regions to assume functions of damaged brain regions. However, although perhaps effective to improve quality of movement, the treatment effects were not long lasting, and did not appear to transfer from one setting or environment to another (Horak, 1992; Shumway-Cook & Woollacott, 2001). Over the last 30 years, new theories of motor control have gradually emerged from advances in neuroscience as well as from an overture to look at other disciplines' perspective on movement (Sweeney, Heriza, & Markowitz, 1994).

Reflex Theory

At the turn of the 20th century, Sir Charles Sherrington, an English neurophysiologist, mapped basic spinal cord reflexes in animal models (Sherrington, 1906, 1947). The reflex loop (sensory receptor–afferent sensory input–efferent motor output–muscle effector) was thought to be the basic unit of movement. Sherrington suggested that activation of one reflex triggered the activation of another reflex and that movement was the result of a series of reflex-triggered events. The Reflex Theory of motor control proposed that sensory inputs are responsible for triggering all movement, thus essential to movement generation. In those days of poliomyelitis epidemics, facilitation of reflexes was used to generate movement and compensate for the muscle weakness observed in individuals with poliomyelitis, since polio selectively destroyed the alpha motor neurons.

Much has been learned about spinal cord circuitry since Sherrington, and it is now clear that movement is possible in the absence of sensory inputs. Sensory-deprived animals have been shown to learn and develop functional movements (Taub, 1976), and ballistic movements occur too quickly for timely transmission of sensory input into the CNS to activate the movement. However, it is important to note that deafferented (no sensory inputs from skin, joints, or muscle after dorsal roots lesion) monkeys deprived of visual inputs from birth took longer to learn new movements, and that these movements were not as smooth or coordinated (Taub, Goldberg, & Taub, 1975). So, although sensory inputs are undeniably important for motor learning and motor control, they are not obligatory as originally suggested by Sherrington.

Hierarchical Theory

Reflexes triggered by specific sensory input were then described as the simplest form of movement, whereas voluntary movements were more complex movements (Fig. 7.1). The Hierarchical Theory considered the reflex a "primitive behavior" rather than the basic unit of movement as suggested by the Reflex Theory, suggesting that motor control was achieved in a top-down fashion from the cerebral cortex to the spinal cord (Jackson & Taylor, 1932; Phillips & Porter, 1977; Reed, 1982; Walsche, 1961).

The so-called primitive reflexes were thought to be suppressed with the development of higher control. Behaviors such as sucking, grasping, or neonatal walking observed in infants were described as primitive reflexes occurring at the spinal level. It was believed that as the infant matured, further neural differentiation and myelination of neurons occurred, leading to the emergence of head- and trunk-righting abilities. The cortex eventually matured to initiate and control all lower levels, allowing the development of more complex and skillful movements, such as reaching to grasp an object, or crawling. These observations were correlated to the reappearance of certain "primitive" behaviors after acquired brain injury. Reflex testing was therefore used to detect problems with the development of the nervous system. Motor control was thought of as a relatively fixed predefined series of steps.

It would, however, be most inefficient for the brain to control and generate muscle activation for every movement, and this would not substantiate our ability to execute complex movements in the absence of feedback. Furthermore, reflex testing may not correlate as highly as previously thought with the degree of motor disorder (Bartlett, 1997). It is now acknowledged that reflex responses are not simple stereotyped movements but can vary based on the person's internal state and on the external environment without any influence from cortical input (Wolpaw & Tennisen, 2001) and that some lower-level reflexes, such as the pain withdrawal reflex, sometimes appropriately dominate movement. Finally, development does not occur in a stepwise manner. Reaching and walking have been shown to be self-generated movements responsive to ongoing sensory feedback and not requiring cortical control (Lee, von Hofsten, & Cotton, 1997; Ulrich, Ulrich, Angulo-Kinzler, & Chapman, 1997). Automatic postural movements, which are also not under cortical control, are influenced by the task and environment (Burleigh, Horak, & Malouin, 1994; Burleigh & Horak, 1996).

Motor Programming Theory

The Motor Programming Theory, a contemporary version of the Hierarchical Theory, suggested that the cortex would generate a desired motor outcome and not be involved with the details for how the outcome was achieved. Specific muscle activations would be coordinated at lower levels (Rothwell, 1994). Reflexes were viewed as less flexible motor programs with a faster response time rather than as "primitive behaviors." Networks of neurons within the spinal cord—central pattern generators (CPGs)—work together as a whole to produce rhythmic, patterned motor commands, such as the commands for repetitive stepping (locomotion). More complex programs developed at the cortex level result from motor learning and are used to simplify the production of movement.

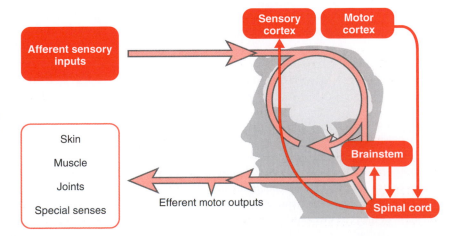

Figure 7.1 Reflex theory of motor control. Sensory (afferent) input causes motor (efferent) output between the peripheral nervous system and the spinal cord, as well as between the spinal cord and the brainstem and cortex. (*Redrawn from Horak, F.B. [1991]. Assumptions underlying motor control for neurological rehabilitation. In M.J. Lister [Ed.], Contemporary management of motor problems: Proceedings of the II STEP Conference [p. 13]. Alexandria, VA: Foundation for Physical Therapy.*)

Given a specific task, environment, and expected sensory consequences for evaluating the accuracy of response, these motor programs specify the relationships between past movement experiences (conditions, execution parameters, outcomes, and sensory consequences) and the required movement parameters—force, velocity, and amplitude, among others. Your signature pattern is similar whether you sign your name in small script on a piece of paper using finger movement or in larger script on a blackboard using the whole arm and shoulder, the motor program being the same.

Systems Theories

The Systems Theory, originally known as the Distributive Theory, was first introduced in the 1930s by Nicolai Bernstein, a Russian physiologist (Bernstein, 1967; Latash, 1998a), although his research was not translated until 1967. Bernstein hypothesized that movements emerged from the interaction of many systems, each contributing to different aspects of motor control, with no single focus of control, rather than being either peripherally or centrally driven (Fig. 7.2).

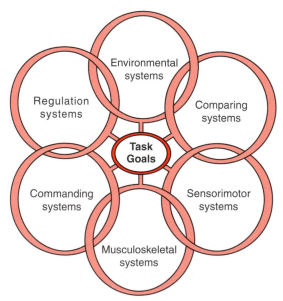

SYSTEMS THEORY OF MOTOR CONTROL

Figure 7.2 Systems theory of motor control. The interlocking circles depict the circular motor control with the task goals as the central outcome desired. *(Redrawn from Horak, F.B. [1991]. Assumptions underlying motor control for neurological rehabilitation. In M.J. Lister [Ed.], Contemporary management of motor problems: Proceedings of the II STEP Conference [pp. 11–28]. Alexandria, VA: Foundation for Physical Therapy.)*

The "control" shifts among systems depending on the individual's internal state, the specific motor task, and the environmental conditions (Latash, Latash, & Meijer, 1999, 2000).

Bernstein (1967) also suggested that "patterns of movement" or motor synergies emerged from the interaction between systems to resolve a degrees-of-freedom problem created from the intrinsic redundancy within the systems involved in the performance of voluntary movement. Given a specific environment and task, movements were produced by neurons and muscles working together as units. For example, consistent movement strategies are used to maintain balance in standing (Horak & Nashner, 1986; Nashner, 1982). When standing on a platform, a sudden backward motion of the surface will result in the sequential activation of the gastroc-soleus, hamstrings, and paraspinal muscles in a coordinated distal to proximal pattern named the **ankle strategy** (Fig. 7.3A). If the environmental conditions are changed, a different and more adaptive response will appear; for example, when standing crosswise on a narrow balance beam, a more challenging task, the strategies used to maintain balance change. A proximal to distal sequential activation of the abdominals, quadriceps, and tibialis anterior muscles will be used (Fig. 7.3B). This **hip strategy** is used in response to bigger threats to balance.

The timing and amplitude of these postural responses to perturbation have been shown to vary with the amplitude and speed of the perturbation (Horak, 1991; Inglis, Horak, Shupert, & Jones-Rycewicz, 1994; Shumway-Cook & Woollacott, 2001). These responses occur within 80 to 100 milliseconds from the perturbation, as opposed to a simple spinal reflex response that would occur within 30 milliseconds of the stimulus, or a consciously driven movement where transmission to and from the cortex requires greater than 100 milliseconds. Terms such as *long latency reflex responses* (transmission to and from the brainstem), *automatic postural responses, motor programs,* or *synergies* have been used to describe these strategies believed to be ways to simplify the control of standing balance.

Finally, Bernstein (1967) emphasized the constraints of the musculoskeletal system and environment (e.g., inertia and gravity) on movement. These could influence physical therapy interventions designed to improve movement. For example, if joint contracture prevented movement, the focus of interventions would be on increasing the range of motion (ROM).

The **Uncontrolled Manifold Theory** (UCM) is a systems theory based on a refined concept of motor synergies emphasizing the *stability* of important

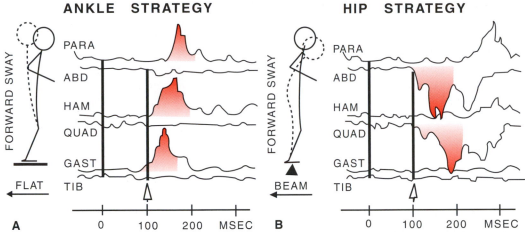

Figure 7.3 Automatic postural muscle responses to backward perturbations of the floor surface. *(A)* An "ankle strategy" is used when falling forward on the flat surface. A finely sequenced group of contractions begins around 80 to 100 milliseconds after the floor moves, in the posterior muscles as shown by the onset of the gastrocnemius, followed by hamstrings, followed by paraspinals. *(B)* When the threat to balance is greater, a different strategy to control posture is triggered. A "hip strategy," abdominals first, followed by the quadriceps and anterior tibialis muscles, is selected to maintain postural control. *(Adapted from Horak, F.B., & Nashner, L.M. [1986]. Central programming of postural movements: Adaptation to altered support configurations.* Journal of Neurophysiology, 55, *1372. Copyright 1986 by American Physiology Society. Reprinted with permission.)*

performance variables and the *flexibility* of motor patterns to address unexpected events. It offers a refined concept of task-specific motor synergies that allows for the adaptability and flexibility inherent to voluntary movement (Latash, Scholz, & Schoner, 2007; Scholz & Schoner, 1999).

From the Systems Theory evolved the **Task-Oriented Theory** of motor control, in which all systems interact to control movement in the context of a functional task in a meaningful environment (Horak, 1991). For instance, when thirsty you perform the task of getting a drink without thinking about activating a specific reaching movement.

Implications for examination and intervention focusing on functional movement, rather than movements without a purpose, follow from this variation of the theory. Therapists first identify the critical systems involved in carrying out a task (e.g., visual, somatosensory, and vestibular systems are all involved in balance), evaluate and treat those impairments amenable to modification (e.g., ROM, muscle weakness, and cardiopulmonary deconditioning), and identify tasks and activities important to the child. These activities or tasks may be used to structure the physical therapy examination and intervention.

The **Dynamic Systems Theory** supports a systems-like theory of motor control that assumes that control

of movement shifts among systems following a principle of self-organization between the components that make up the individual and the surrounding environment (Thelen & Smith, 1993). In this approach, variability within and between individuals is considered an essential component of motor development (Helders, 2010).

A common example in the inanimate world is the organization that occurs in flowing water particles when the speed of the stream of water is increased. At first, if the flow of water is slow, the water organizes into drops. As the flow increases, the water forms into a stream. This "organization" is dependent on the controlling variable of the velocity/volume of water flow. An example related to movement is the switch made by a horse from walking to a canter and to a gallop, which simply occurs as a result of an increased speed of movement and a greater change in the angle of hip extension (Bernstein, 1967; Heriza, 1991a). Experiments involving oscillating finger movements have shown that the mathematical methods, as well as principles of change from one pattern to another, can be applied to transitions in movement behavior in humans. When moving slowly, it is possible for you to alternate abduction-adduction of your right and left index fingers respectively; if asked to increase the speed of the movements, the right and left fingers will eventually automatically adduct-abduct simultaneously (Kelso, 1995).

Consider a young child with CP creeping on hands and knees. Under certain conditions, the child is able to use a reciprocal creeping pattern (opposite side arm and leg moving together). Under other conditions, however, the organization of the motor behavior changes or transitions to another pattern, moving both legs together symmetrically to advance forward, commonly referred to as bunny hopping (Scholz, 1990). The variable, internal or external to the individual, that influences the system to transition is considered the control parameter. When the child is creeping, the control parameter could be the speed of movement or the frequency of the hip movements in different directions. As the rate of hip movements increases, the tendency to keep a controlled reciprocal pattern becomes unstable or likely to change, and the locomotor pattern transitions to a bunny hop. The degree of stiffness at the hip and pelvic girdle could also qualify as a control parameter because, as the stiffness increases, the reciprocal pattern becomes less stable (likely to change) until eventually the pattern changes to the bunny hop.

The concept of a control parameter can be very important for clinical interventions because it suggests that therapists identify what factors, internal or external, are likely to promote change in the movements produced. These control parameters can be intrinsic to the individual, or extrinsic, such as in the environment or motor task to be accomplished. This idea of a triad of constraints consisting of the person, the environment, and the task—and the spontaneous interaction of systems affecting motor control—has greatly influenced current examination and intervention ideas (Fig. 7.4). For example, following this theory, a movement would be observed and measured to determine the control parameters so that these parameters could be influenced, and perhaps cause a shift of the movement to a more efficient or optimal coordinated pattern. Use of this concept for intervention is discussed in Chapter 8.

Neuronal Group Selection Theory

One drawback of the Systems Theories is the little emphasis placed on the CNS. A more recent theory, the **Neuronal Group Selection Theory (NGST),** offers a balance between a pure systems approach and one that recognizes the powerful role of the CNS in movement (Hadders-Algra, 2000). This theory proposes that infant motor development includes two periods of increasing variability caused by the dynamic organization of cells, and two periods of decreasing variability due to the selection of the most effective response patterns for a particular situation (Siegler, 2002; Helders, 2010).

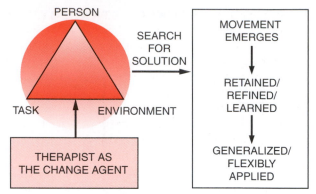

Figure 7.4 Triad of constraints to movement. Considering the individual, the environment, and the task to be accomplished, a movement solution is initiated. A first movement attempt emerges. After practice, the movement can be retained, refined, and learned. Once the movement plan is learned, it is stored in memory. This theory suggests that it can be generalized and applied to other similar tasks and/or environments. The therapist can act as a change agent in this process by altering the person's state or experience level, the task, and/or the environment, causing the solution and learning process to lead to a different outcome. *(Adapted from Newell, K.M., & Valvano, J. [1998]. Therapeutic intervention as a constraint in learning and relearning movement skills.* Scandinavian Journal of Occupational Therapy, 5, *53, with permission.)*

According to this theory, cortical and subcortical systems dynamically organize into variable neural networks. The neural networks are collections of interconnected neurons that act as functional units dealing with a specific type of motor behavior or information from a specific sensory system (Siegler, 2002). The structure and function of these groups are created by the infant's development (genetic coding) and behavioral experience (environmental exposure and active movement).

Early in the development, there is a set of primary neuronal groups determined by evolution, which has been termed the *primary repertoire.* For example, in the development of postural stability in sitting, 4- to 6-month-old infants show crude anterior and posterior trunk muscle contraction patterns to maintain the sitting position (Hadders-Algra, Brogren, & Forssberg, 1996). After environmental experiences, the afferent information induces modifications in the strength of synaptic connections within and between the neuronal groups; those more adaptable to the environmental factor create a secondary repertoire of neuronal groups.

These secondary repertoires allow for situation-specific selection of neuronal groups based, for example, on the environment or task to generate the most efficient postural adjustment in sitting (Hadders-Algra, Brogren, & Forssberg, 1998) or a well-coordinated reaching pattern (Konczak & Dichgans, 1997; Konczak, Borutta, & Dichgans, 1997).

During the primary phase, motor activity is variable and not strictly tuned to the environmental conditions. This variable movement gives rise to self-generated, variable afferent information. The afferent inputs contribute to motor behaviors that are functional in diverse situations. After the transient phase of selection, variability of movement responses are reduced at first and then increased because of the barrage of sensory input from continued experience. The phase of secondary or adaptive variability starts, leading to a variable movement repertoire, with efficient motor function for each specific situation. Individuals can adapt movements to task-specific constraints or generate a repertoire of motor solutions for a single motor task.

Therapists would try to judge the stage of development that the child is in—primary versus secondary variability—and then design intervention to assist the child in developing success with efficient and variable movement for a motor skill. For example, a child with severe motor disability related to CNS damage may not have basic primary neuronal networks. To increase the child's primary repertoire for movement, a therapist might provide the child with variable practice in different postures: supine, prone, sitting, and so on. The therapist would then provide frequent experience with trial and error movement to facilitate selection of the secondary repertoire of neuronal groups. To date, there is evolving, but insufficient, evidence supporting these intervention methods (Vereijken, 2010; Vereijken & Thelen, 1997.

Examination and Evaluation

The information provided in this section augments that presented in several other chapters regarding a Pediatric Physical Therapy Examination and Plan of Care (see Table 1.3). Details of testing procedures and standardized tests of function and development commonly used for children with neuromuscular disabilities are described in this chapter. In Chapter 3, the use of reliable and valid tests and measures is presented, as well as a more extensive list of tests and measures (see Table 3.12 and Appendix 3.B). A discussion of issues to consider in developing the examination of motor problems in children with neuromuscular disease or disability follows.

Examination of children with neuromuscular disabilities is complex and requires testing of different domains. There is a need for the development of reliable, valid tests and measures for many areas related to children with neuromuscular disease or disability, including satisfaction with services and quality of life measures (refer to Chapter 3). Therapists should be diligent in following research that describes new tests and measures. The therapist might be required to refer children to designated testing centers for complex measurement if specific and complicated decisions are necessary (e.g., gait laboratory assessments to make surgery determinations). It is important, however, not to get lost in high-technology information and lose sight of improving the outcome of personal functional activity and participation in the home, school, and community.

Knowledge of normal motor development is critical for pediatric physical therapists. Normal development of motor skills is fascinating and beautiful. With motivation and persistence, typically developing children seem to flow through acquisition, fluency, and generalization of motor behaviors. Without struggle, new motor skills emerge. Most examination and intervention techniques for children were based on a developmental model.

Historically, it was hypothesized that children must be taken through a normal developmental sequence to appropriately learn basic motor skills (Bobath, 1964; Stockmeyer, 1967; Voss, 1972). For example, it was believed that a child needed to learn to crawl before walking. Based on new hypotheses related to normal motor development and theories on motor control and motor learning, this model has largely been replaced by the idea that intervention should focus on teaching age-appropriate functional motor behaviors. So if independent mobility is the objective for a 12-year-old, the child should be encouraged to either walk with assistive devices or learn to propel a wheelchair rather than to crawl. For a child with milder neurological deficits, the typical patterns seen in children with normal development may function as the gold standard for the most effective and efficient movements (Atwater, 1991).

The major goal of interventions for a child should be to improve the child's motor ability for activity and participation in the home, school, and community. Functional movements required for daily activities and community participation (e.g., gait and locomotion, balance, reach and grasp, transfers) that are important to the child and caregiver must be evaluated first. After examining how the child moves and the quality of movement, then the causes of the restrictions in activity and participation can be determined by assessing impairments of body structures and functions (e.g., ROM, strength, coordination).

Testing Considerations

Testing can be difficult in children with neuromuscular disability because of the variable nature of their motor behaviors. The variability can be attributed to fluctuating abnormal muscle tone, poor motor coordination, medications or factors related to fatigue, age, behavior, pain, and attention, among others. Variability in motor coordination can occur because of immaturity of development, where the child is trying different patterns of motor activity in an attempt to arrive at the most efficient pattern. Variability could be a result of specific neuromuscular differences causing impaired control of descending input to the motor neuronal pools or integration of sensory inputs. Most likely, it is a combination of many factors. The important point is that test items may need to be repeated across time in a single session, and again at a later session to determine both the best and most common behavior.

The setting for the examination is important because children perform differently in different environments. Some tests are completed by observation in the child's natural environment or by interview of the parent or child about the child's abilities in natural settings. These evaluations may provide a more accurate view of the child's ability to use his or her motor capabilities within the day-to-day environment.

The child with neuromuscular disorders may have concomitant cognitive deficits and/or emotional/behavioral problems. Although it is difficult to determine how much these affect the child's motor performance, these issues should be monitored and measured in simple but reliable ways so that their extraneous effect on motor outcomes may be estimated. For example, short behavioral checklists have been created to accompany some developmental tests. Alternatively, a standard three-point behavioral rating indicating simply that the child (1) appears to understand and comply to best of ability, (2) appears to understand and comply some of the time with testing procedures, or (3) frequently appears to not understand or comply with testing can be used. By using this scale to estimate the validity of the examination results, interpretation of the findings can be done in a more consistent manner.

Tests and measures that rely more heavily on observation of typical motor behaviors, rather than on asking the child to perform specific motor skills, may reduce the child's problems with understanding and complying with testing procedures. Observational measurements also help with evaluation of infants or young children who are not developmentally ready to follow directions. Observations at different times of the day and in different settings also provide insight into either internal biorhythms or environmental effects on motor behaviors.

The *Guide* (APTA, 2001), Parts One and Two, lists many constructs that should be evaluated through use of tests and measures, the basic tools for gathering this data, and the type of data that can be generated for documentation of motor behaviors in children who have neuromuscular disability. Table 7.1 lists the most commonly used tests and measures specific to children and adolescents with neuromuscular disability (Patterns 5B, 5C, and 5D) organized by the *Guide*'s testing categories, including the age range for the tests and their recommended use based on the three major testing purposes (discriminative, predictive, evaluative). Specific testing considerations and descriptions of some of these tests follow. Refer to the references and other chapters for more details related to all tests.

Examination of Body Functions: Neuromusculoskeletal and Movement-Related Functions

Impairment of body structures and functions within diagnoses varies greatly, dependent on the location and severity of injury, age at the time of injury, motor behaviors that the child learns to use and practice in his or her regular environment, and available supports. One commonality among diagnoses is that the neuromuscular system is disrupted, causing the child to have difficulty with movement that often, in the long term, leads to low fitness levels. Although examination and intervention need to be individualized to the child's specific motor disability, a focus should be on developing meaningful functional movement and promoting general long-term health and fitness.

Muscle Tone Functions

Even when not voluntarily moving, there is an active state of muscle contraction, a resting "readiness to move." This state is often referred to as *muscle tone*. Children with Impaired Neuromotor Development (Pattern 5B) or with Acquired Nonprogressive Neuromuscular

Table 7.1 Common Tests and Measures for Children with Neuromuscular Disability*

Categories	Tests and Measures	Age	Level of Measurement	Recommended Use
Gait, Locomotion, and Balance	• Laboratory analysis/ posturography (kinematic, kinetic, EMG)	Any age	Body function	Discriminative Predictive Evaluative
	Infant Tests			
	• Test of Infant Motor Performance (TIMP)	34 weeks postconceptual age to 16 weeks postterm		Discriminative Predictive Evaluative
	• Movement Assessment of Infant (MAI)	0–12 months	Body function	
	• Harris Infant Neuromotor Test (HINT)	3–12 months	Activity	
	• Alberta Infant Motor Scale (AIMS)	0–18 months		
	Developmental Tests			
	• Bayley Scales of Infant Development, 2nd ed. (BSID2)	0–2 years		
	• Peabody Developmental Motor Scales, 2nd ed. (PDMS-2)	0–6 years	Activity	Discriminative
	• Bruininks-Oseretsky Test of Motor Proficiency, 2nd ed. (BOT-2)	4.5–14.5 years		
	Single-Item Tests			
	• Functional Reach Test (FRT)/Modified FRT			
	• Pediatric FRT			
	• Fisher Reach Test			
	• Timed Up-and-Go (TUG)	4–12 years	Activity	Discriminative
	• Timed Up and Down Stairs (TUDS)			
	• Timed Obstacle Ambulation Test (TOAT)			
	• Pediatric Clinical Test for Sensory Interaction in Balance (P-CTSIB)	4–12 years	Body function	Discriminative
	• Clinical Observation of Motor and Postural Skills (COMPS)	5–9 years	Body function	Discriminative Evaluative
Neuromotor and Sensory Integration	• Miller Assessment of Preschoolers (MAP)	2–5 years	Body function Activity	Discriminative Evaluative
	• Southern California Sensory Integration Tests (SCSIT)	6–16 years	Body function	

Continued

Table 7.1 Common Tests and Measures for Children with Neuromuscular Disability—cont'd

Categories	Tests and Measures	Age	Level of Measurement	Recommended Use
	Developmental Tests			
	• BSID2	0–2 years	Activity	Discriminative
	• PDMS-2	0–5 years		Evaluative
	• BOT-2	5–14 years		
	Objectives			
	• Goal Attainment Scaling (GAS)	Any age		Evaluative
	• Gross Motor Function Measure (GMFM)	2–5 years	Activity	Discriminative Evaluative
Motor Function (motor control and learning)	• MAI • TIMP • HINT • AIMS	Infants	Body function Activity	Discriminative Predictive Evaluative
	• GMFM	2–5 years		
	• Gross Motor Performance Measure (GMPM)	Any age		
	• Videography			
	• Laboratory tests (kinematics, kinetics, EMG, endurance)	Any age	Body function	
	• Pediatric Evaluation of Disability Inventory (PEDI)	6 months– 7.5 years	Activity Participation	Discriminative Evaluative
	• School Function Assessment (SFA)	5–14 years		
	• Childhood Health Assessment Questionnaire (CHAQ)	1–19 years		
	• Pediatric PT Outcome Measure System (PPT-OMS)	0–21 years		
Reflex Integrity	• MAI • TIMP	Infants	Body function Activity	Discriminative Predictive Evaluative
Muscle Tone	• Modified Ashworth Scale • Spasticity Measurement System (SMS)	Any age	Body function	Discriminative Discriminative Evaluative

*For further information on these tests and measures, see Chapter 3, Appendix 3.A.

Sources: Finch, E., Brooks, D., Stratford, P.W., & Mayo, N.E. (2002). *Physical Rehabilitation Outcome Measures: A Guide to Enhanced Clinical Decision Making.* (2nd ed.). Philadelphia: Lippincott Williams & Wilkins; American Physical Therapy Association (2002). *Interactive Guide to Physical Therapist Practice: With catalog of tests and measures,* Version 1.0. Alexandria, VA: Author.

Disorders (Patterns 5C and 5D) will frequently show aberrant states of resting and active muscle tone, from too high (hypertonicity) to too low (hypotonicity). Fluctuating tone will result in involuntary movements, such as athetosis and ataxia. Many interventions have been designed to alter aberrant muscle tone to help children with neuromuscular disability produce more typical motor behaviors.

Hypertonicity is defined as an abnormal increase in resistance to passive movement about a joint (Sanger et al., 2003). It can appear after damage to supraspinal areas of the brain, such as occur in CP, or after a traumatic brain injury (TBI), spinal cord injury, or various other neurological damage. Neurological and musculoskeletal changes occur as hypertonicity develops. Three terms are commonly associated with different forms of hypertonia in children: spasticity, dystonia, and rigidity (Sanger et al., 2003).

Spasticity is defined as resistance to passive movement, which increases with increasing speed of stretch (velocity-dependent) and varies with the direction of joint movement, and/or increases rapidly above a threshold speed or joint angle (Sanger et al., 2003). It is hypothesized to be caused by a lack of normal presynaptic inhibition (Rothwell, 1994). The basic circuitry diagrammed in Figure 7.5 depicts an increased afferent activation (attributable to decreased presynaptic inhibition) of interneurons that triggers an increased activation of both alpha and gamma motor neurons. Irradiation of this excessive input also causes overactivation of neighboring agonists and antagonists (i.e., cocontraction of muscles). As a result, the child appears stiff and unable to relax enough to move.

A large amount of the stiffness appear to be accounted for by intrinsic changes in the musculoskeletal system, such as contracture of the collagen tissue, decrease in the viscoelastic properties of the muscle tissue, collagen accumulation in the muscles, changes in muscle fibers (atrophy especially of type 2 fibers, predominance of type 1 fibers), and decreased force production of muscle cells (Booth, Cortina-Borja, & Theologis, 2001; Dietz & Berger, 1995; Dietz, 1999). A child may thus present with stiffness without exaggerated stretch reflex activity (Berger, Horstmann, & Dietz, 1984). Since spasticity, unlike rigidity, is velocity-dependent, the therapist will want to alter the speed when moving the extremity to determine whether spasticity is present. During intervention and functional positioning, it will be important to move the joint and extremity slowly to reduce the amount of spasticity that is exhibited if spasticity interferes with the child's ability to perform activities such as rolling and

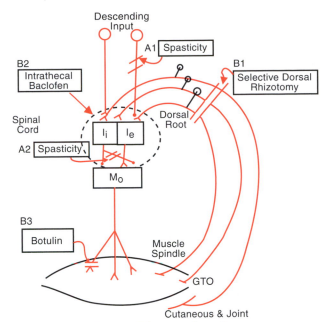

Figure 7.5 Schema of the spinal cord circuitry to demonstrate spasticity mechanisms and treatment. Sensory neurons from the muscle, skin, and joints traverse through the dorsal roots into the spinal cord to synapse on inhibitory interneurons (I_i) excitatory interneurons (I_e), and motor neurons (M_o). Descending input from higher levels of the spinal cord and brain also synapse on interneurons and motor neurons in the spinal cord. A balance of inhibitory and excitatory input regulates activation of motor neurons, which in turn activate muscle fibers. Spasticity is hypothesized to be caused by (A1) a reduction in descending inhibitory input or (A2) a reduction in presynaptic inhibitory input. Methods to reduce spasticity include (B1) selective dorsal rhizotomy or cutting some of the sensory afferents to decrease excitatory input into the spinal cord; (B2) intrathecal pump titrations of baclofen, a chemical that acts as an inhibitory neurotransmitter similar to gamma-aminobutyric acid, into the spinal cord to increase the inhibitory influence on the interneurons and motor neurons; and (B3) botulin (Botox) injections into the muscle to temporarily block transmission of the motor neuron to the muscles at the neuromuscular synapse. GTO = Golgi tendon organ.

transfers. Joint contractures can also develop as a result of the limited movement across joints.

Decreased facilitation of polysynaptic reflexes may result in weakness and paresis during movement in individuals with hypertonicity (Damiano & Abel, 1998; Dietz & Berger, 1995; Dietz, 1999; Wiley & Damiano,

1998). To compensate for this weakness, the child may use cocontraction to create sufficient tension for postural control and movement. Normal modulation of reflex activity that should occur during movements such as gait can also be disrupted (Stein, Yang, Belanger, & Pearson, 1993).

Today there are effective surgical and drug interventions aimed at decreasing spasticity by lowering excitation into the motor neuron pools:

- *Selective dorsal rhizotomy* is a surgical procedure that selectively cuts the problematic nerve roots in the spinal cord (Albright, 2003; Engsberg, Ross, Collins, & Park, 2006, 2007; Kan et al., 2008; Langerak et al., 2008; McLaughlin et al., 2002; Park & Johnston, 2006; Trost, Schwartz, Krach, Dunn, & Novacheck, 2008).
- *Intrathecal or oral baclofen* is prescribed to inhibit the motor neuron pools (Albright, 2007; Albright & Ferson, 2009; Borowski, Shah, Littleton, Dabney, & Miller, 2008; Borowski et al., 2010; Brochard, Lempereur, Filipetti, & Rémy-Néris, 2009; Dan et al., 2010; Delgado et al., 2010; Motta, Stignani, & Antonello, 2008; van Doornik et al., 2008; Ward, Hayden, Dexter, & Scheinberg, 2009).
- *Botulin injections* are used to interrupt muscle contraction (Dai, Wasay, & Awan, 2008; Goldstein, 2006; Guettard et al., 2009; Hoare et al., 2010; Mackey, Miller, Walt, Waugh, & Stott, 2008; Pascual-Pascual & Pascual-Castroviejo, 2009; Py, Zein Addeen, Perrier, Carlier & Picard, 2009).

Figure 7.5B demonstrates the activation site for each of these interventions to decrease spasticity. These therapies may be used for a nonambulatory child with severe involvement to reduce muscle tone so that adequate personal care, ROM, and position changes can be performed. They may also be used for the child who is ambulatory, to improve the child's gait and functional mobility.

Although studies have definitely reported reductions in spasticity with use of these three techniques, it is clear that once spasticity is altered through medication or surgery, normal movement does not just emerge (Giuliani, 1991; McLaughlin et al., 2002). The underlying secondary musculoskeletal changes, i.e., weakness and contractures, can still impede movement. The child has also learned motor patterns that are different because of the previous presence of spasticity. When the spasticity is decreased, those learned motor patterns do not just disappear, and they are potentially not effective for the new lower tone situation (Olree, Engsberg, Ross, &

Park, 2000). For example, the child with hypertonicity in the legs may walk with excessive hip adduction, hip internal rotation, knee flexion, and plantar flexion. Once muscle tone is reduced, he or she may be unable to walk because he or she still attempts to use all or part of this pattern. Functional movement improvements demonstrated through research studies vary and have not always been shown to be better than aggressive strength and exercise programs routinely administered by physical therapists (Graubert, Song, McLaughlin, & Bjornson, 2000; McLaughlin et al., 2002). Research on the ideal criteria under which to use these drug and surgical techniques in the ambulatory child should continue.

The relationship between hypertonicity and motor function continues to be debated. It was commonly believed that intervention to reduce hypertonicity would improve motor function (Bly 1991; Bobath & Bobath, 1984). The theory was that if the abnormal muscle tone could be prevented or normalized, then the child would move appropriately and the subsequent musculoskeletal changes would not occur to further hinder movement. This theory then made sense in that there were secondary musculoskeletal and neurological changes that made "normal" movement impossible. Consequently, alteration of muscle tone was originally a main focus of treatment for neurodevelopmental treatment (NDT) for children with hypertonicity (Bobath & Bobath, 1984). However, NDT has not been shown to change long-term motor learning (Barry, 1996; Butler & Darrah, 2001).

On the other hand, hypertonicity could be used for optimal motor function (Landau, 1974; Sahrmann & Norton, 1977). There is evidence that, during gait, a given level of tension developed by a spastic muscle during stretch would produce less electromyographic (EMG) activity than a healthy muscle. Consequently, the regulation of muscle tension at the spinal level may need to be increased to have optimal ability for independent ambulation (Dietz, 1999; Latash & Anson, 1996). This pattern for development of muscle tension controlled completely at the spinal level (as opposed to from the supraspinal level) and an increased use of cocontraction of agonist and antagonist muscles may be the most efficient way for these individuals to move (Crenna, 1998; Damiano, 1993). The cocontraction may be a useful strategy to increase joint stability, to limit the degrees of freedom while learning a movement, or to allow the motor system to respond with more stability to perturbations (Damiano, Martellotta, Sullivan, Granata, & Abel,

2000; Vereijken, van Emmerik, Whiting, & Newell, 1992; Latash & Anson, 1996).

Research in a small number of children with CP (n = 10; mean age, 9.2 years) has shown that those who use more cocontraction muscle activity show better energy efficiency for overground ambulation (Damiano et al., 2000). So there may come a time where the use of hypertonic patterns of movement, to a certain extent, is optimal for functional movement and therapy to reduce it may be detrimental to the individual (Latash & Nicholas, 1996).

Dystonia is a movement disorder in which involuntary sustained or intermittent muscle contractions cause twisting and repetitive movements and/or abnormal postures (Sanger et al., 2003). It is commonly triggered by attempts of voluntary movement and may fluctuate over time. Although dystonia may be a cause of hypertonia when there is muscle activity at rest or when muscle activity begins before the onset of the passive movement, hypertonia is not always present in dystonia (Sanger et al., 2003).

Rigidity is the more extreme type of hypertonicity, postulated to be caused by changes in the transcortical long latency reflex activity or disruption of the basal ganglia's normal interaction with the motor cortex anterior to the central sulcus (Rothwell, 1994). The 2003 Task Force on Childhood Motor Disorders (Sanger et al. 2003) defined rigidity as a resistance to passive joint movement present at very low speeds of movement, independent of the imposed speed, with no speed or angle threshold. Simultaneous cocontraction of agonist and antagonist muscles may occur. After being moved, the limb does not tend to return toward a particular position or extreme joint angle. Finally, voluntary movement in distal muscle groups does not lead to involuntary movements, although rigidity may worsen (Sanger et al., 2003). The resistance can be uniform through the ROM—*leadpipe rigidity*—or cause a series of jerks throughout the movement—*cogwheel rigidity* (Iyer, Mitz, & Winstein, 1999; Rothwell, 1994). Rigidity is not velocity dependent, so as the therapist moves the extremity either quickly or slowly, the amount of resistance that is felt does not increase or decrease.

Hypotonicity is an excessively low resistance to passive stretch. In clinical practice, probably more children receiving physical therapy services demonstrate low muscle tone, especially in the trunk and neck, than high muscle tone. It is hypothesized that hypotonicity results from a loss of efferent or afferent activity to lower motor neurons and subsequent changes in the

musculoskeletal tissue. This can be caused by injuries to lower motor neurons, muscular or connective tissue diseases (e.g., spinal muscular atrophy and congenital malformation of connective tissue), or reduction in descending input from the brain to activate the alpha and gamma motor neurons (Lundy-Ekman, 1998). Childhood neuromuscular disorders such as CP and Down syndrome display hypotonicity stemming from decreased descending inputs. Infants born at full term, without birth trauma or specific diagnoses, can also demonstrate hypotonicity. Although this may have some effect on early development, it has not been related to long-term delay in motor development (Parush et al., 1998; Pilon, Sadler, & Bartlett, 2000).

The loss of descending excitatory input may be related to cerebellar or vestibular disorders. The vestibulospinal descending pathway is important in the regulation of muscle tone, particularly in relation to control of posture and balance (Nashner, 1982; Lundy-Ekman, 1998). Input from the vestibular apparatus, which provides us with information about gravitational forces, exerts excitatory influences on the extensor motor neurons, particularly those innervating postural muscles. With lower muscle tone, the child tends to hold stationary postures by extending the joints completely and "hanging" on ligaments. The shoulders may slope forward and the arms hang, excessive kyphosis or lordosis may be apparent, and the legs may be locked into full extension to hyperextension. Children with hypotonicity tend to have large ROMs in their joints, perhaps caused by lower muscle tone (Pilon et al., 2000). The continual strategy of "hanging" on the ligaments may further stretch the joint structures to extremes.

Furthermore, reduction of gamma input will upset the regulation of the state of the muscle spindle. This sensor specifically gives us information on the length of the muscle and the velocity of change in length (Latash, 1998b; Rothwell, 1994). More important, the spindle afferent activity provides the primary information for our kinesthetic sense (Proske & Gandevia, 2009). Knowing the position of your body in space has a powerful effect on movement ability. Coordinated movement is difficult without adequately sensing your changing position in space. Accordingly, children with low muscle tone tend to move less and demonstrate less coordination in the mid-ranges of movement. For example, when standing still, the child with hypotonicity may appear to be steady, but when asked to lower to the floor, he or she will just drop down, going from one static position to another without smooth control. For movement transitions, the objective is to control the speed of movement without allowing the antagonist to completely relax. Instead, the antagonist should be maintained in a state of controlled cocontraction with the agonist. The balance between the activation of the agonist and antagonist may also be disrupted in children with hypotonicity.

Tone Assessment Objectively assessing muscle tone is difficult because of the variety of factors (spasticity, muscle weakness or poor power production, morphological changes in muscle and connective tissue, and cocontraction of antagonistic muscle groups) influencing muscle tone. The most commonly used way to quantify muscle tone is to evaluate resistance to passive movement at different speeds of movement using a *mild, moderate, severe* scale.

The more descriptive modified Ashworth scale is a structured method for assessing spasticity (Table 7.2) (Clopton et al., 2005; Craven, & Morris, 2010; Platz, Eickhof, Nuyens, & Vuadens, 2005). This is a six-point rating scale that can help to objectify the amount of spasticity that is present in a specific muscle group or groups (Bohannon & Smith, 1987). While this information about body structure and function is important, it will be essential to document how spasticity limits the child from engaging in activities, including moving from the floor to standing and gait, as well as participation restrictions that may include playing with peers. Although the modified Ashworth scale is commonly used to measure spasticity in children, it is important

for clinicians to be aware that its reliability remains questionable (Blackburn, van Vliet, & Mockett, 2002; Damiano et al., 2002; Mutlu, Livanelioglu, & Gunel, 2008). When using the modified Ashworth scale, care should be taken to document specifically how tone was measured to improve reliability on retesting.

Because of the complex nature of muscle tone, which varies during voluntary movement, measurements of muscle tone during passive movement is not a valid estimate of the influence of muscle tone on active movement (Crenna, 1999; Dietz, 1999; Holt, Butcher, & Fonseca, 2000; Rothwell, 1994). Levels of spasticity per the Ashworth scale show little correlation with functional ability (Fellows, Kaus, & Thilmann, 1994). Damiano, Dodd, and Taylor (2002) suggested that the measurement of resistance torque during passive joint movement using an isokinetic dynamometer correlated better to function than the modified Ashworth scale.

Newer techniques to assess muscle tone or stiffness during voluntary movement are currently under development for laboratory (Crenna, 1999) and clinical use (Holt et al., 2000). The Pendulum test has been shown to be more sensitive to differentiate children with mild to moderate quadriceps spasticity (Bohannon, Harrison, & Kinsella-Shaw, 2009; Fowler, Nwigwe, & Ho, 2000; Graham, 2000; Syczewska, Lebiedowska, & Pandyan, 2009; White, Uhl, Augsburger, & Tylkowski, 2007). In this test, the lower leg is dropped and allowed to oscillate like a pendulum; an electrogoniometer positioned on the knee is used to record the amplitude of the first swing from full knee extension to full knee flexion (Graham, 2000).

Holt and colleagues (2000) used clinical measurements of leg length, body weight, and swing cycle (seconds) during leg swinging in supported standing to quantify stiffness based on the movement for a hybrid mass-spring pendulum. This measure was shown to correlate highly with a high-technology motion systems analysis of the leg swinging, and to show validity and reliability in a small group of children with and without CP (Holt et al., 2000). Muscle tone tests of this nature will likely become the preferred measure in the future. Clinical use of the Pendulum test or quantification of resistance torque during passive motion can improve the ability to show subtle change in spasticity across time or with intervention.

It is important to remember that although it is helpful to describe muscle tone and understand its impact on function, it may not be appropriate or effective to focus physical therapy intervention on altering muscle tone. Intervention to change motor

■ **Table 7.2** Modified Ashworth Scale

Score	Definition
0	No increase in muscle tone (MT)
1	Slight increase in MT, catch/release, increase at end of range
2	Slight increase in MT, catch and minimal resistance through rest of range
3	More marked increase in MT through most of range
4	Considerable increase in MT, passive movement difficult
5	Affected parts rigid in flexion or extension

Source: Bohannon, R.W., & Smith, M.B. (1987). Interrater reliability of a modified Ashworth scale of muscle spasticity: Suggestion from the field. *Physical Therapy, 65,* 46–47, with permission.

coordination through practice and use of additional sensory cues may be more appropriate, with longer lasting impact, as discussed in Chapter 8.

Movement Functions

Motor Reflexes Reflex testing is integrated in the *Guide* (APTA, 2001) under the categories of Neuromotor and Sensory Integration, and Motor Function, as noted in Table 7.1.

Involuntary Movement Reactions: Balance Reactions The control of posture is hypothesized to be a "missing link" in the ability to produce coordinated and efficient functional movements in many children with neuromuscular disability. If one cannot maintain or regain balance, then it becomes very difficult to move with purposeful intent. To comprehend problems in development, versus those caused by disease or insult, clinicians need to understand the typical development of postural control.

Postural and movement control has historically been described as developing in a cephalocaudal manner, meaning that head control develops before trunk and lower extremity control. Proximal control (at the trunk) was also thought to develop before distal control (at the hands and feet) (Gesell, 1945). However, more recently, motor control has been described as having regional and intertwining circles of development with no areas of the body developing in isolation from other areas (Adolph & Eppler, 2002; Thelen & Spencer, 1998). Infants are always developing movements and postural control throughout the body. As the infant moves against gravity in sitting, and then in standing, the postural control components become more important because they balance more mass farther from a smaller base of support (BOS). Interventions to improve postural control are commonly used when working with children with neuromuscular dysfunction, because problems with postural control can potentially limit further development of movement and exploration.

Table 7.3 summarizes the development of postural control system by system, including the musculoskeletal system (muscles, connective tissue, and joints for actual movement), the sensory system (visual, vestibular, and somatosensory cues for postural adjustments),

▪ Table 7.3 Typical Development of Postural Control

System	Components	Age of Maturation to Adultlike Capacity and Related Issues
Musculoskeletal	Force production	Developing through life; under one year of age, low force production capability is a constraint for sitting and standing
	Range of motion	Developing through the teen years; should not be a constraint until elderly
	Body geometry	• Infants have large heads in relation to body size • Changes rapidly during growth spurts at different ages dependent on gender and hormonal development
Sensory	Vision	Sensory receptors mature at birth • Acuity improves for distance vision over first year of life • Preference for reliance on visual input for postural orientation corrections (from birth to 1 year for sitting balance; until 3 years for standing balance) • From birth to death, vision used as primary information when first learning a task or in a novel environment
	Somatosensory (cutaneous and proprioceptive)	Sensory receptor mature at birth • Infants 6 months or older can use somatosensory inputs for maintenance of sitting balance • 4–6 years: emerging use of somatosensory input for sensory conflict resolution • 7–10 years: adultlike ability to use somatosensory input for sensory conflict resolution
	Vestibular	Sensory receptor mature at birth • 7–10 years: use vestibular input as the reference system in an adultlike manner for resolution of sensory conflict

Continued

Table 7.3 Typical Development of Postural Control—cont'd

System	Components	Age of Maturation to Adultlike Capacity and Related Issues
	Sensory integration	• 7–10 years: accurate selection of sensory information for maintenance of postural control.
Neuromuscular	Reactive postural control—SITTING	5–6 months (presitting) • Activation of directionally specific muscle coordination patterns (MCPs)—agonists opposite to the side to which the child is falling • With variable timing (cocontractions and reversals of proximal to distal patterns) • Poor adaptation to task-specific conditions 7–10 months (sitting): • Decreased timing variability of directionally specific MCPs (activations of leg, trunk, neck muscles) 9 months–3 years (transient toddling phase): • Invariant use of directionally specific MCPs, some use of cocontractions • Good modulation of pelvic muscles at BOS for adaptations to task-specific conditions 3 years–adulthood • Variability in directionally specific MCPs • less cocontraction and use of neck muscles to improve variability of postural control
	Reactive postural control—STANDING	• At about 1 year of age (independent standing): *grossly* directionally specific (distal to proximal) MCPs • 1½–3 years: directionally specific MCPs *consistent* • 4–6 years: *variability* of MCPs occurs (may be due to growth spurts or sensory integration changes) • 7–10 years: adultlike use of directionally specific MCPs Factors influencing the choice of reactive MCP for maintenance of postural control: surface; availability of sensory cues; instructions for task
	Anticipatory postural activations (APAs)	APAs observed in some tasks at about 1 year of age 4–6 years: APAs in lever pull task 6–8 years: variable APAs in stand and reach tasks 9–12 years: more consistent APAs in stand and reach task • Task-dependent—mature after reactive MCPs in a specific posture and after practice/experience with movement in the posture • 1st APA response in a new movement: cocontraction (freezing the degrees of freedom); after practice, more variability in postural control and movement occurs (Vereijken et al., 1992)

and the neuromuscular system (neural coordination and activation of motor neurons). Development of the **musculoskeletal system** is important primarily in the first year of life, as the development of muscle strength can limit postural control ability. After the first year, adequate muscle strength and joint ROM are available for control of stationary postures, such as sitting and standing, and during movement. This system does affect postural control during growth spurts where the child needs to adjust muscle activations for changes in body size. The **sensory system organization** for postural control proceeds from being primarily visually dependent to one where somatosensory inputs can trigger motor output to control balance. At transition stages (e.g., beginning to sit, beginning to stand), visual dependence reemerges until the child learns more stability. The ability to resolve sensory conflicts (mismatched input from the three senses) matures gradually to an adultlike state by adolescence (Nolan, Grigorenko, & Thorstensson, 2005).

For reactive postural control (when responding to an external sensory cue) within the neuromuscular system, there appear to be innate patterns of muscle coordination (postural strategies), loosely organized for sitting balance and, perhaps, more tightly organized for standing balance. These patterns show a stagelike development, with disorganization in standing postural motor coordination patterns at 4 to 6 years of age, which may be attributed to growth spurts or lack of maturation of the sensory organization necessary for postural control. Adultlike reactive postural control appears evident at 7 to 10 years of age.

Anticipatory postural control (feedforward postural commands that actually precede the primary movement) ensures that posture is adequately controlled before the coordinated movement starts (Thelen & Spencer, 1998). For example, when you reach out for an object, before the arm muscles contract and the arm begins to move, muscles in your legs contract to stabilize your balance in anticipation of the balance perturbation with arm movement. This contributes to smooth and coordinated movements. Development of anticipatory postural control seems to follow a similar sequence to reactive control; however, the patterns of motor coordination depend more on practice and learning of different tasks and activities in different environments (Hodges, Hayes, Horn, & Williams,

2005). There also appear to be periods in development when infants and children use cocontraction to reduce the degrees of freedom to be controlled (Hodges et al., 2005; Vereijken et al., 1992). With practice, the use of these cocontraction strategies gradually decreases, which allows more flexible and adaptable control of posture.

Control of Voluntary Movement Functions Most movements are probably a combination of "feedforward" or open-loop mechanisms triggered by a motor command from the cerebral cortex or brainstem structures, and "feedback" or closed-loop mechanisms triggered by sensory input. Figure 7.6 depicts the pathways for both feedback and feedforward movements. With the exception of the monosynaptic reflexes, feedback movements are generally slower than feedforward movements because of the added transmission time for the sensory information to initially trigger or modify the motor output.

In feedforward movements, two things happen simultaneously. A motor plan to produce the appropriate muscle activations for the motor task is sent to the spinal cord. In addition, a copy of the plan, the **efference copy** or corollary discharge, is hypothesized to be stored elsewhere in the brain. As the person moves, the sensory systems provide feedback information, an **afference copy**, on how the movement is progressing and on the potential success of the movement (Burleigh & Horak, 1996; Burleigh et al., 1994; Fuchs, Anderson,

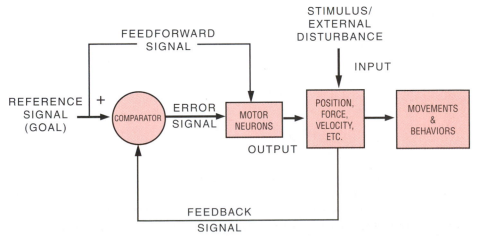

Figure 7.6 Feedback and feedforward movement. A closed-loop negative feedback system for control of movements (lighter arrows) is depicted for slower movements with ongoing adjustment caused by feedback. Feedforward signals (darker arrows) allow quicker and preplanned movement in anticipation of sensory input. *(From Horak, F.B. [1991]. Assumptions underlying motor control for neurological rehabilitation. In M.J. Lister [Ed.],* Contemporary management of motor problems: Proceedings of the II STEP Conference *[p. 14]. Alexandria, VA: Foundation for Physical Therapy.)*

Binder, & Fetz, 1989). This allows for alterations to occur during the movement to improve the final outcome. Based on the final outcome, the feedforward plan can also be modified for future use by comparing the afference copy with the efference copy and making the necessary modifications. These learned or stored plans for movement have been called **motor programs** (Schmidt, 1991; Shumway-Cook & Woollacott, 2001). Motor programs related to postural control have been referred to as central set (Hay & Redon, 1999; Horak & Diener, 1994; Horak, Diener, & Nashner, 1989). The CNS triggers a specific sequence of muscle activity to counteract the expected postural perturbations and adapts the postural adjustments to the changes in postural demands based on experience. It could thus be useful for the therapist to determine whether there are motor problems in situation when movement is driven by sensory feedback or when the child has to call up previously learned programs for fast movements. In these cases, intervention may focus on triggering movements with sensory input or designing the therapy to practice movements that require use of previously learned motor programs.

Coordination of Voluntary Movements Integration of sensorimotor signals at several levels within the CNS is necessary for the control of a coordinated voluntary

movement (Nielsen, 2004). Testing of impairments in movement coordination, agility, initiation, modification, and control is difficult and generally requires a laboratory with complex computerized equipment that measures kinematics, kinetics, and EMG during movements such as gait (Graubert et al., 2000) and reaching (Fetters & Kluzik, 1996).

In a slightly less complicated manner, single joints can be characterized during movement using only kinematic data. An example of this testing method is the quantification of leg-kicking coordination (Geerdink, Hopkins, Beek, & Heriza, 1996; Heriza, 1991b). Markers were placed on the lower extremity joints of infants to record the kinematics during spontaneous voluntary leg kicking. The joint angle data were then plotted in angle-time diagrams. Differences in the amount and velocity of movement in the joint of a full-term infant at 40 weeks' gestational age and a high-risk premature infant at the same gestational age are illustrated in Figure 7.7. Differences in coordination can be noted visually or quantified via measurements, such as maximal joint angle movement or velocity. Using this technique, subtle coordination differences can be used in a discriminative manner to compare across children with typical and atypical movement capability and in an evaluative manner for examining intervention effectiveness. Direct

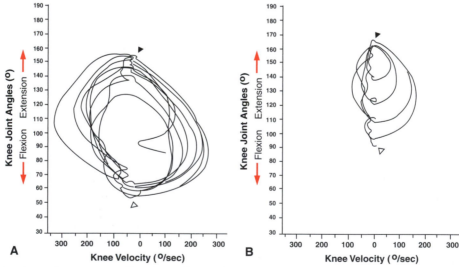

Figure 7.7 Evaluation of motor coordination. Phase-plane trajectories of knee joint angle to knee velocity during spontaneous kicking behavior of two infants: *(A)* Low-risk premature infant at 40 weeks gestation; *(B)* High-risk infant at 40 weeks gestation. Note that the low-risk infant shows greater range of knee joint movement at a greater variety of velocities compared to the high-risk infant. The difference in the coordination pattern can be visualized and quantified. *(Adapted from Heriza, C.B. [1991]. Implications of a dynamical systems approach to understanding infant kicking behavior.* Physical Therapy, 71, *222–235, Fig. 2 A&B.)*

examination of dexterity, agility, and coordination can be completed through the administration of the Movement Assessment Battery for Children, 2nd edition (Henderson & Sugden, 2007), or the Gubbay Tests of Motor Proficiency standardized for children between 8 and 12 years of age (Gubbay, 1975).

To specifically examine the neuromuscular system for motor coordination problems during balancing, EMG recording of muscle activity, ground force reaction recordings via use of force plates to calculate center of pressure (COP) movement, and recording of three-dimensional (3-D) kinematics to either document movement at the joints or to calculate center of mass (COM) movement have been used in laboratory settings (Liu, 2001; Zaino, 1999; Moe-Nilssen, 1998). This type of examination allows determination of actual selection, timing, sequencing, and amplitude of muscle activity; estimations of the COP (under the feet); and COM (whole body) movement and control during the motor activity. These sophisticated, labor-intensive, and expensive types of testing may be necessary for children when important decisions are being made regarding invasive surgical procedures or during research studies of procedural interventions. This equipment will probably not be available for routine use; however, the ability to interpret results from this testing is necessary because of its widespread use in hospitals and in research studies.

Clinical testing of the neuromuscular system usually involves methods of observational analysis of motor coordination during balancing. For example, therapists can place the child on a moveable surface (e.g., tilt boards, balls), move the surface under the child, and subjectively grade the motor response caused by the perturbation. This information is reported as "clinical observations" under Tests and Measures and is intended to document whether the child has the appropriate balancing motor strategies of head and trunk righting, arm and leg counterbalancing, and protective extension. Although these tests are informative, their reliability is questionable.

Videotapes have been made during testing of children's balancing strategies (Lowes, 1996). The videotapes were later coded for the child's predominant motor coordination pattern used to balance during the testing, for example, use of ankle strategy, hip strategy, or crouching strategy. Inter- and intra-rater reliabilities were moderate among three raters (Luyt et al., 1996). Although repeated viewing of the videotapes might improve reliability, a more detailed analysis of the strategy through use of EMG may be

necessary. Further modification and testing of this system of coding motor coordination responses need to be done before this can be a viable measurement system.

Involuntary Movement Functions

Hyperkinetic or unwanted excess movements are commonly seen in children with neuromuscular disorders (Sanger et al., 2010). These involuntary movements, including dystonia, chorea, athetosis, tremor, and ataxia, can significantly impact on motor functions.

Involuntary Contractions of Muscles As mentioned earlier in the chapter with reference to hypertonia, increased tone is not always present in dystonia, a movement disorder in which involuntary sustained or intermittent muscle contractions cause twisting and repetitive movements and/or abnormal postures (Sanger et al., 2003). Although dystonia has commonly been associated with damage to the basal ganglia, in many cases of dystonia, no injury to the basal ganglia can be identified. Other brain areas like the cerebellum, brainstem, or sensory cortex can be causes of dystonia (Sanger et al., 2010).

Chorea, described as "an on-going, random-appearing sequence of one or more discrete movements or movement fragments" varying in timing, duration, direction, and body location, can be distinguished from dystonia by the unpredictable and continuous nature of movements and from athetosis by the presence of discrete movements within the continuing sequence of movements (Sanger et al., 2010, p. 1542).

Athetosis is described as a "slow, continuous, involuntary writhing movement that prevents maintenance of a stable posture" (Sanger et al., 2010, p. 1542). It is characterized by smooth continuous random movements not composed of identifiable fragments of movement. Because of the extra movement that occurs, individual with diskinetic CP have been shown to have a higher resting metabolic rate (Johnson, Goran, Ferrara, & Poehlman, 1996).

Tremor is "a rhythmic back-and-forth or oscillating involuntary movement about a joint axis," or a rhythmic alternating movement with relative symmetry in speed (Sanger et al., 2010, p. 1544). Related to the trigger of the involuntary movement, tremor is labeled resting tremor, postural tremor, or action tremor. Intention tremor refers to a cerebellar dysfunction characterized by worsening of tremor when reaching for a target, which can resemble dysmetria, inaccurate movements leading to repeated overcorrective attempts (Sanger et al., 2010).

The term **ataxia** refers to a gross lack of coordinated movements that generally originates from damage to the cerebellum (Bastian, 1997). A child with ataxia has normal strength with no hypertonia; however, the movements are jerky and inaccurate (Montgomery, 2000). Depending on where the cerebellar lesion occurs, the child may have limb ataxia, truncal ataxia, or gait ataxia (Lundy-Ekman, 1998). Children with gait ataxia have poor balance and can be described as demonstrating movement similar to that of a person who is intoxicated.

Standardized Assessment of Movement Functions

As discussed in Chapter 3, there are several standardized screening and developmental tests for infants and young children that are based on the typical sequence of motor skill acquisition. Each presents a scheme for observational and handling examinations of children's motor function, reflexes, and postural patterns. Rating of the quality of postural control, presence of reflex movements, and coordination in static positions of lying, sitting, and standing, and during movements is described. Examples of these tests include the Harris Infant Neuromotor Test (HINT) (Harris & Daniels, 2001), Test of Infant Motor Performance (TIMP) (Campbell, Kolobe, Wright, & Linacre, 2002), Movement Assessment of Infant (MAI) (Chandler, Andrews, & Swanson, 1980), Gross Motor Performance Measure (GMPM) (Boyce et al., 1995), and the Alberta Infant Motor Scale (AIMS) (Piper & Darrah, 1994).

Developmental tests for young children include items related to complex balance and coordination, such as balance on one foot, hopping, galloping, jumping patterns, and skipping, as well as gross and fine motor skills. Examples of these are the Bayley Scales of Infant Development (2nd ed.) (BSID2) (Bayley, 1993), the Gross Motor Function Measure (Russell et al., 1993), and the Peabody Developmental Motor Scales (2nd ed.) (PDMS-2) (Fewell & Folio, 2000). The Bruininks-Oseretsky Test of Motor Proficiency (2nd ed.) (BOT-2) (Bruininks & Bruininks, 2005) is one of the few tests of motor performance for older children aged 4 to 21 years. These tests have moderate to good reliability and validity and therefore might be used for discriminative, evaluative, and predictive purposes.

Examination of Activities and Participation: Mobility

There are several standardized functional tests that either directly or indirectly examine the child's activity and participation levels including the Pediatric Evaluation of Disability Inventory (PEDI) (Haley, Coster, Ludlow, Haltiwanger, & Andrellas, 1992; Coster, Haley, & Baryza, 1994), Childhood Health Assessment Questionnaire (CHAQ) (Feldman et al., 1995; Singh, Athreya, Fries, & Goldsmith, 1994), and School Function Assessment (SFA) (Coster, Deeney, Haltiwanger, & Haley, 1998).

Additionally, there are two minimal datasets designed to measure population-based outcomes of children receiving either physical therapy care as outpatients—the Pediatric Physical Therapy Outcome Management System (PPT-OMS) (Palisano, Haley, Westcott, & Hess, 1999; McEwen, Arnold, Hansen, & Johnson, 2003)—or students with disabilities in elementary school or high school receiving school-based occupational therapy and physical therapy services—the School Outcomes Measure (SOM) (School Outcomes Measure Administrative Guide, 2007). All are examples of tools to measure children's participation in home, school, and community activities and their personal activity and participation in society. Reliability and validity have been shown to be appropriate for the PEDI and the SFA (Coster et al., 1994, 1998; Haley et al., 1992; Hwang, Davies, Taylor, & Gavin, 2002).

These developmentally and functionally based tests measure many aspects of movement. By focusing on specific items within the scales, the physical therapist can use them as discriminative tests to document general problems with postural stability or coordination. They are also useful as evaluative measures to document functional movement outcomes related to intervention to improve postural control or other impairments.

Care should be taken regarding the test used and population being examined because of problems with the responsivity (ability of a test to reflect meaningful change across time) of some of these tests (Coster et al., 1994; Palisano, Kolobe, Haley, Lowes, & Jones, 1995). These tests were designed specifically to document development of motor behaviors. Many of these tests are normed on large groups of children, allowing the tests to function well in a discriminative manner. Appropriate reliability and validity have also been established for most, so the tests can also be used for evaluative purposes. In children with severe neuromuscular disability, or when examining very specific motor behaviors, use of a developmental motor test is often not responsive to the small changes the child may make with time or procedural interventions. Tests that are individualized and sensitive to the specific motor objectives of the intervention may be unavailable.

Furthermore, in children with neuromuscular involvement, sometimes the intervention is focused on educating the caregiver to influence the child's motor skill and practice. Standardized tests that document specific caregiver positioning and handling behaviors are currently nonexistent, with the exception of the PEDI, which includes a scale to rate the amount of caregiver assistance needed for several activities of daily living. New tests need to be developed in this area.

Balance: Changing and Maintaining Body Position

The ability to maintain balance (postural control) may be assessed by examining the systems that contribute to our ability to balance (musculoskeletal, sensory, and neuromuscular) or by examining functional tasks (activity level) that stress one's ability to maintain balance (Westcott, Lowes, & Richardson, 1997).

Musculoskeletal System   Examination of the musculoskeletal system's contribution to postural control—for example, ROM and muscle force production—can be completed following the methods discussed in Chapter 5. Adaptations of these tests for use with children with neuromuscular disability may be necessary because of the presence of contractures, abnormal muscle tone, sensory deficits, and cognitive disorders. The therapist should try to follow the standardized procedures and, if changes in procedures are made, record the changes. Retesting, using the same procedures, will ensure better reliability.

Sensory System   To assess the sensory system's contribution to postural control, the impact of changes in visual, vestibular and/or somatosensory information available to the child on balance can be systematically observed and measured. By testing under different conditions, a particular sensory system or combinations of systems causing problems with postural control in standing can be estimated. Procedural interventions focused on practice using the impaired sensory system and/or education about safety precautions can be prescribed based on the test results. The Pediatric Clinical Test of Sensory Interaction for Balance (P-CTSIB) and the platform computerized posturography protocol Sensory Organization Test (SOT) are age-related tests used to quantify the ability of children to maintain standing balance in the presence of sensory conflicts, each providing different and complementary information (Gagnon, Swaine, & Forget, 2006). Table 7.4 describes the sensory conditions for the P-CTSIB and SOT.

The P-CTSIB was developed as a low-cost clinical method to test sensory organization for maintenance of static standing balance (Crowe, Deitz, Richardson, & Atwater, 1990); it is an inexpensive clinical alternative to platform posturography (Fig. 7.8). The P-CTSIB uses the same six sensory conditions as platform posturography. Visual conflict is provided by use of a hatlike apparatus made up of a lightweight dome that, although allowing some diffuse light to come through, impedes the peripheral vision. As the child sways, the dome moves in synchrony with the head to simulate

■ Table 7.4 Sensory Organization Test

Conditions		Sensory Systems Available and Providing Accurate Information
Surface	Vision	
Stable surface	**1.** Eyes open	All sensory systems—vision, somatosensory, and vestibular—available and providing accurate information about body position
	2. Eyes closed	No vision; must use accurate somatosensory and vestibular information
	3. Visual conflict	Sensory conflict caused by inaccurate visual information; must ignore vision and use accurate somatosensory and vestibular information
Moving/ compliant surface	**4.** Eyes open	Sensory conflict caused by inaccurate somatosensory information from moving/compliant platform; must ignore somatosensory and use accurate visual and vestibular information
	5. Eyes closed	No vision; sensory conflict caused by inaccurate somatosensory information; must ignore somatosensory and use accurate vestibular information
	6. Visual conflict	Sensory conflict caused by inaccurate somatosensory and visual information; must ignore both and use accurate vestibular information

Source: Shumway-Cook, A., & Horak, F.B. (1986). Assessing the influence of sensory interaction on balance: Suggestion from the field. *Physical Therapy*, 66, 1548–1550.

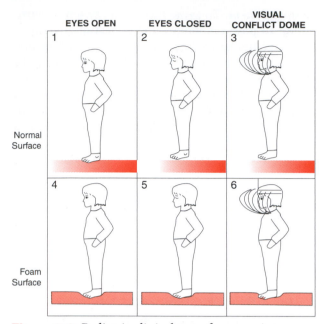

EYES OPEN   **EYES CLOSED**   **VISUAL CONFLICT DOME**

Normal Surface

Foam Surface

Figure 7.8 Pediatric clinical test of sensory interaction for balance (P-CTSIB). Testing conditions for the P-CTSIB include (1) eyes open, normal surface: vision, somatosensory, and vestibular available; (2) eyes closed, normal surface: no vision, somatosensory and vestibular available; (3) dome, normal surface: vision compromised, somatosensory and vestibular available; (4) eyes open, foam surface: somatosensory compromised, vision and vestibular available; (5) eyes closed, foam surface: no vision, somatosensory compromised, vestibular available; and (6) dome, foam surface: vision and somatosensory compromised, vestibular available. *(From Crowe, T.K., Deitz, J.C., Richardson, P.K., & Atwater, S.W. [1990]. Interrater reliability of the Clinical Test of Sensory Interaction for Balance. Physical and Occupational Therapy in Pediatrics, 10, 9, with permission.)*

the moving visual surround of the platform posturography tests. Somatosensory conflict is provided by having the child stand on a piece of medium-density closed-cell foam, which dampens somatosensory input during somatosensory conflict conditions. Both the amount of time the child can stand in a feet-together position and the visual measure of anterior-posterior sway are recorded. These raw measurements are then combined for each of the six conditions and transformed into an ordinal scale spanning the inability to balance in the condition to the ability to balance for a maximum of 30 seconds with less than 5° of sway. These ordinal scores are then summed across sensory

conditions to yield sensory system scores, which provide the tester with information about whether the child can process and use each of the three sensory systems: vision, somatosensory, and vestibular (Deitz, Richardson, Westcott, & Crowe, 1996).

Interrater reliability (Crowe et al., 1990) and test-retest reliability (Pelligrino, Buelow, Krause, Loucks, & Westcott, 1995; Westcott, Crowe, Deitz, & Richardson, 1994) of the P-CTSIB have been established for children both with and without disability. Although interrater reliability for sway measurements is moderate, test-retest reliability is lower. Pilot norms have been established for typically developing children (Deitz, Richardson, Atwater, & Crowe, 1991; Richardson, Atwater, Crowe, & Deitz, 1992). This was an easy test for the children with typical development, ages 4 to 9 years. The children were able to stand for 30 seconds with less than 5° of sway in all conditions except the last two, where the time dropped by a few seconds, and the sway increased by several degrees, especially in the younger children.

The P-CTSIB has been used to identify sensory organization differences between children who are typically developing and subsets of children with learning disability (Deitz et al., 1996), CP (Lowes, 1996), and DS (Westcott, Lowes, Richardson, Crowe, & Deitz, 1997), which demonstrates some construct validity for the test. Scores on the P-CTSIB also correlate with functional activities related to postural stability; therefore, performance on the test to some extent reflects functional ability (Lowes, 1996). Because of the level of interrater reliability, the beginning normative, and validity information, this test could be useful for discriminative purposes. However, because of the moderate test-retest reliability, it is less appropriate for evaluative purposes without further research.

Platform computerized posturography measurement of sensory organization is being used with increasing frequency in clinics despite the high cost of the apparatus (Rine, Rubish, & Feeney, 1998). For the posturography test, the child stands on a computer-controlled, movable force platform facing the center of a three-sided movable visual enclosure. A computer-driven Sensory Organization Test (SOT) protocol provides information about the interaction of the three sensory systems—somatosensory, visual and vestibular—contributing to postural control. During the assessment, inaccurate visual and somatosensory information about the orientation of the body is delivered to the child's feet, joints, and vision through controlled, calibrated tilt of the support surface and rotation of the visual surroundings in proportion to body sway. Body sway in standing is measured under six sensory conditions detailed in Table 7.4.

The protocol determines the ability of the child to use vision, somatosensation (cutaneous and proprioceptive information), and vestibular information to maintain an upright position. The modified SOT (mSOT) protocol excludes the use of the visual surround and simply measures how well an individual can maintain postural stability under the other four sensory conditions. The mSOT does not provide information on visual-vestibular conflict resolution. Computerized posturography has been reported to have fair to good reliability for most postural parameters in typically developing 9- to 10-year-old children (Geldhof et al., 2006).

Functional Tasks

There are a few functional tests related to postural control that were developed for older adults but have been adapted for children. These tests are relatively simple to administer and score; thus, they are used easily in clinical practice. The Berg Balance Scale is a functional balance test composed of movements and positions used by people throughout the day, such as moving from sit to stand, picking up objects from the floor, reaching, and turning in standing (Berg & Norman, 1996). Although originally developed for older adults, the directions, encouragement given, and safety procedures have been modified for use in pediatrics and renamed the Pediatric Balance Scale (Blair, 1999; Franjoine, Gunther, & Taylor, 2003). Test-retest and interrater reliability were high when reviewing videotapes of children performing the items, so this test could be used for evaluative purposes.

The Functional Reach Test (FRT) (Duncan, Weiner, Chandler, & Studenski, 1990), a test for the limits of stability (LOS), has been shown to be reliable to assess dynamic standing balance in children older than 4 years and should be used with caution with children younger than 3 years of age. Normative reach data are for 3-year-old children, 11.4 +/− 2.6 cm (mean +/− SD); 4-year-old children, 13.6 +/− 3.0 cm; and 5-year-old children, 15.7 +/− 4.4 cm (Norris, Wilder, & Norton, 2008). Functional Reach Test scores are affected by both method of reach (one-arm versus two-arm) and method of measurement (finger-to-finger versus toe-to-finger). Toe-to-finger measurements have been shown to be more reliable than finger-to-finger measures, with the two-arm toe-to-finger being the best method. When using this method, a change of 5 cm or more is likely to represent a true clinical difference

(Volkman, Stergiou, Stuberg, Blanke, & Stoner, 2007). As scores increase with height, height categories may be useful when using the test for discriminative purposes (Volkman, Stergiou, Stuberg, Blanke, & Stoner, 2009).

Because standing can be quite difficult for some children with disabilities, the Modified Functional Reach Test (MFRT) measures the distance an individual can reach forward in sitting or standing positions (Donahoe, Turner, & Worrell, 1994; Wheeler, Shall, Lewis, & Shepherd, 1996). The pediatric version of the FRT, the Pediatric Reach Test (PRT), modified to include side reaching in both sitting and standing positions, has been shown to be a valid and reliable measure of balance for typically developing children and children with CP (Bartlett & Birmingham, 2003).

Walking and Moving Around

Testing procedures for gait and locomotion at the impairment level are discussed in detail in Chapter 5. At the activity level, the "Timed Up-and-Go" (TUG) Test (Podsiadlo & Richardson, 1991) consists of recording the amount of time required to rise from a chair, walk 3 m, turn around, return to the chair, and sit down again (Habib & Westcott, 1998; Habib, Westcott, & Valvano, 1999). The Timed Obstacle Ambulation Test (TOAT) is currently being developed. It consists of an obstacle course that requires the child to move across different floor surfaces; step up, down, and over; duck under obstacles; and negotiate through turns and a narrow path (Benedetto et al., 1999). Interrater, intrarater, and test-retest reliability on these single-item tests, as examined in small research studies, are generally high, making them good tests for evaluative purposes. More research is needed using larger pediatric populations to determine whether they can also be used for discriminative or predictive purposes.

Diagnosis

After performing the chosen tests and measures, the therapist needs to evaluate all of the examination findings, weighing all issues related to the child as well as the family, school, and community. This evaluation will lead to a physical therapy diagnosis or the diagnostic classification as delineated in the *Guide* (APTA, 2001). Based on the evaluation of findings, physical therapists should be able to differentiate between various neuromuscular conditions. For example, after screening a toddler who is toe walking, the physical therapist needs to decipher whether to treat or to refer back to the physician based on the **differential diagnosis** of idiopathic toe walking, tightness of the gastroc-soleus muscles caused by increased tone, or suspicion of fatty tissue in the muscles, among others.

Children with neuromuscular disability will likely fall into one of the three Preferred Practice Patterns discussed in the *Guide* (APTA, 2001): 5B: Impaired Neuromotor Development; 5C: Impaired Motor Function and Sensory Integrity Associated with Nonprogressive Disorders of the Central Nervous System— Acquired in Infancy or Childhood; or 5D: Impaired Motor Function and Sensory Integrity Associated with Nonprogressive Disorders of the Central Nervous System—Acquired in Adolescence or Adulthood. After a concise review of the neuroscience related to common pediatric neuromuscular disorders, a description of the most common diagnoses encountered in pediatric practice within each of the three Preferred Practice Patterns will highlight the major neuromuscular issues. Table 7.5 presents a synopsis of definition, etiology, alterations in body functions and structures, and

Table 7.5 Neuromuscular Conditions

Diagnosis	Definition	Etiology	Alterations in Body Functions and Structures	Potential Activity Limitations and Participation Restrictions	Potential Management
Autism	Developmental disability significantly affecting verbal and nonverbal communication and social interaction, generally evident before 3 years of age, that adversely affects a child's educational performance. Other characteristics often associated with autism are engagement in repetitive activities and stereotyped movements, resistance to environmental change or change in daily routines, and unusual responses to sensory experiences.	While the exact cause of autism is unknown, evidence suggests a multifactorial cause, with a strong genetic component. In addition, an infectious disease and toxic insult to the brain may play a role.	• Failure of language and communication development • Possible intellectual impairments • Sensitivity to touch and abnormal responses to sensory stimuli • Apraxia • Restricted, repetitive behaviors • Impaired motor imitation and coordination • Poor eye contact • Decreased muscle tone	• Difficulty with interpersonal relationships (d710)* • Decreased capacity for social relationships (d750) • Delay of developmental milestones and moving around (d455) • Decreased ability to maintain sustained active play (d9200) with peers or family • Decreased walking long distances (d4501) • Decreased participation in organized sports (d9201) and active recreation activities (d920)	• Comprehensive behavioral therapy utilizing various forms of positive and negative reinforcements • Sensory integration and sensory-based interventions • Social skill interventions • Early intervention and educational programs reinforcing consistency and structure • Physical therapy focusing on improving motor planning and sensory integration during gross motor activities • Family support and education

Table 7.5 Neuromuscular Conditions—cont'd

Diagnosis	Definition	Etiology	Alterations in Body Functions and Structures	Potential Activity Limitations and Participation Restrictions	Potential Management
Developmental Coordination Disorder (DCD)	Motor skills disorder with "marked impairment in motor coordination interfering with academic achievement or activities of daily living." DCD is not caused by a general medical condition or pervasive developmental disorder (PDD). Frequently occurs with learning disabilities and attention deficit disorders.	Unclear; however, problems may occur with the final "wiring" during the neural migration and organization of the CNS during last trimester of pregnancy This may be accentuated by other environmental issues after birth	• Decreased muscle tone, • Muscle weakness, • Motor incoordination, particularly hands	• Difficulty with handwriting, dressing—tying shoes and buttoning, grooming, and eating • Decreased participation in organized sports (d9201) and active recreation activities (d920)	• Task-specific intervention based • Perceptual motor training • Sensory integration training • Cognitive orientation to daily occupational performance
Down Syndrome (DS)	Genetic disorder in which the majority (approximately 90%) of individuals have an extra 21st chromosome	Nondysjunction of two homologous chromosomes during 1st or 2nd meiotic division	• Generalized low muscle tone • Muscle weakness • Slow postural reactions • Joint laxity • Intellectual impairments	• Delay of developmental milestones • Decreased ability to maintain sustained active play (d9200) with peers or family • Decreased participation in organized sports (d9201) and active recreation activities (d920)	• Surgery to correct any congenital heart defects • Physical therapy intervention initially focuses on attainment of developmental milestones, family education related to developmental activities, motor learning principles of changing environment • Lifelong focus on fitness

Continued

Table 7.5 Neuromuscular Conditions—cont'd

Diagnosis	Definition	Etiology	Alterations in Body Functions and Structures	Potential Activity Limitations and Participation Restrictions	Potential Management
Cerebral Palsy (CP)	Motor disability related to early damage of the brain in areas controlling motor behaviors	Early brain damage occurring in utero or during or shortly after birth	• Muscle weakness • Dysfunction in motor recruitment • Decreased balance • Decreased endurance • Dysfunction in integration of proprioception, vision, and vestibular input • Possible intellectual impairments	• Difficulty with activities of daily living including dressing, grooming, eating, mobility, including walking and running • Delay of developmental milestones • Decreased walking long distances (d4501) • Decreased activity tolerance, for example, running (d4552) • Decreased ability to maintain sustained active play (d9200) with peers or family • Decreased participation in organized sports (d9201) and active recreation activities (d920)	• Orthopedic management including surgical intervention, Botox injections, or oral medication to improve alignment, posture and reduce spasticity • Nutritional management including use of gastric tube if necessary • Physical therapy intervention may include intervention to improve posture, alignment, range of motion, strength, and activity and participation • Family education
Traumatic Brain Injury (TBI)	Physical external force to the head	Injuries caused by falls, motor vehicle accidents, sports injuries, and other accidental or intentional blows to the head	• Spasticity • Ataxia • Muscle contractures • Muscle weakness • Balance dysfunction • Intellectual behavioral, emotional, and speech deficits	• Decreased walking long distances (d4501) • Decreased activity tolerance, for example, running (d4552) • Decreased ability to maintain sustained active play (d9200) with peers or family	• Initial medical management can include stabilizing the child in the intensive care unit until no longer "medically fragile" • Orthopedic intervention may be

Table 7.5 Neuromuscular Conditions—cont'd

Diagnosis	Definition	Etiology	Alterations in Body Functions and Structures	Potential Activity Limitations and Participation Restrictions	Potential Management
				• Decreased participation in organized sports (d9201) and active recreation activities (d920)	indicated if the child sustained fractures • Physical therapy intervention focuses on initially preventing secondary complications including contractures, pressure ulcers, and pneumonia • Following this phase, focus shifts to a more active approach of mobility utilizing inter-professional approach to intervention due to complexity of systems involved
Myelomeningocele (MM)	Sac containing spinal fluid, meninges, and neural tissue protrudes through a posterior opening of spinal vertebra	Exact cause unknown; a combination of genetics and environment may contribute There appears to be a relationship between inadequate vitamin and folic acid intake and neural tube defects	• Diminished or absent trunk/LE sensation • Decreased or absent trunk/LE strength • Impaired bowel and bladder control • Changes in posture and alignment • Decreased balance • Possible poor motor control	• Decreased mobility (d455) and transfers (d420) • Decreased walking long distances (d4501) • Decreased activity tolerance, for example, running (d4552) • Decreased ability to maintain sustained active play (d9200) with peers or family	• Initial medical management following birth will include closure of neural sac followed by observation and assessment of hydrocephalus with implantation of VP shunt if appropriate. • As the child grows, a bowel and

Continued

Table 7.5 Neuromuscular Conditions—cont'd

Diagnosis	Definition	Etiology	Alterations in Body Functions and Structures	Potential Activity Limitations and Participation Restrictions	Potential Management
Myelomeningocele MM (continued)				• Decreased participation in organized sports (d9201) and active recreation activities (d920)	bladder program will be necessary • Physical therapy intervention may focus on strengthening innervated muscles, teaching compensatory patterns of movement, functional exercise and electrical stimulation, and providing the child with assistive/ adaptive equipment for mobility • Preventing secondary complications including contractures, scoliosis, and pressure ulcers will be important • Lifelong fitness and family education
Fetal Alcohol Syndrome (FAS)	Pattern of neurological and physical defects that can develop in a fetus when a woman drinks alcohol during pregnancy Criteria for diagnosis	Consumption of alcohol during pregnancy and fetal development Amount and length of consumption needed to produce FAS is unclear	• Intellectual impairments • Learning disabilities • Deficits in attention and memory • Communication deficits • Fine motor deficits	• Difficulty with handwriting (d345), dressing—tying shoes and buttoning (d540) • Delay of developmental milestones and moving around (d455)	• Comprehensive behavioral therapy • Sensory integration and sensory-based interventions • Physical therapy intervention may focus on

Table 7.5 Neuromuscular Conditions—cont'd

Diagnosis	Definition	Etiology	Alterations in Body Functions and Structures	Potential Activity Limitations and Participation Restrictions	Potential Management
	includes: • Pre- and postnatal growth retardation • CNS abnormalities • Craniofacial abnormalities		• Sensory integration deficits • Decreased perceptual motor skills	• Decreased ability to maintain sustained active play (d9200) with peers or family • Decreased participation in organized sports (d9201) and active recreation activities (d920)	improving perceptual motor training and gross motor skills incorporating a behavioral approach
Traumatic Spinal Cord Injury	Acute *traumatic* lesion of the spinal cord or cauda equina resulting in temporary or permanent sensory and/or motor deficits	Spinal cord injury caused by an external event (ICD-10 codes V01–Y98; ICD-9-CM codes E800–E999) rather than disease or degeneration	• Impaired sensory functions in UE/trunk/LE including touch and proprioception (b260–b270) • Impaired muscle functions (b730–b749) including tone and power in UE/trunk/LE strength • Impaired movement functions including control of voluntary movement and gait pattern functions (b750–b789) • Impaired functions of the respiratory system (b440–449) • Impaired bowel and bladder control • Impaired skin functions (b8)	• Impaired mobility (d4) including transfers (d420) and walking (d450) • Decreased ability to maintain sustained active play (d9200) with peers or family • Decreased participation in recreation and leisure (d920) such as active play (b9200) or organized sports (d9201)	• Medical emergency that requires immediate intervention to save life and reduce the long-term effects. • Corticosteroids are often used to reduce swelling that may further damage the spinal cord. • Surgery to remove tissues or bone that compresses the spinal cord and to stabilize fracture. • Physical therapy intervention may focus on strengthening innervated muscles, teaching compensatory patterns of movement, functional

Continued

Table 7.5 Neuromuscular Conditions—cont'd

Diagnosis	Definition	Etiology	Alterations in Body Functions and Structures	Potential Activity Limitations and Participation Restrictions	Potential Management
Traumatic Spinal Cord Injury *(continued)*					exercise and electrical stimulation, and providing the child with assistive/adaptive equipment for mobility • Preventing secondary complications including contractures, scoliosis, and pressure ulcers will be important • Lifelong fitness and family education
Asperger Syndrome	An autism spectrum disorder characterized by significant difficulties in social interaction, along with restricted and repetitive patterns of behavior and interests; differs from other disorders by its relative preservation of linguistic and cognitive development.	Exact cause unknown; likelihood of a genetic basis	• Impaired thought functions and higher-level cognitive functions— limited interests or an unusual preoccupation with a particular subject to the exclusion of other activities (b160) • Impaired control of voluntary movements— clumsy and uncoordinated motor movements (b7601–b7602)	• Peculiarities in speech and language, such as speaking in an overly formal manner or in a monotone, or taking figures of speech literally (d350) • Socially and emotionally inappropriate behaviors and inability to interact successfully with peers (d710–d779) • Problems with nonverbal communication, including the restricted use of gestures, limited or inappropriate facial expressions, or a peculiar, stiff gaze (d335)	• Interventions that address the three core symptoms of the disorder: poor communication skills, obsessive or repetitive routines, and physical clumsiness, building on the child's interests, offering a predictable schedule, teaching tasks as a series of simple steps, actively engaging the child's attention in highly structured activities, and provide regular reinforcement of behavior. The earlier the

Table 7.5 Neuromuscular Conditions—cont'd

Diagnosis	Definition	Etiology	Alterations in Body Functions and Structures	Potential Activity Limitations and Participation Restrictions	Potential Management
					intervention, the better. • Social skills training • Cognitive behavioral therapy • Medication, for coexisting conditions such as depression and anxiety • OT/PT for children with sensory integration problems or poor motor coordination • Specialized speech/language therapy • Parent training and support
Neurofibromatoses	• Genetic disorders that cause tumors to grow in the nervous system, beginning in the supporting cells that make up the nerves and the myelin sheath. The tumors grow on nerves and produce other abnormalities such as skin changes and	Genetic 30%–50% of new cases arise spontaneously through genetic mutation; once this change has taken place, the mutant gene can be passed on to succeeding generations.	• Impaired functions of the joints and bones (b710–b729) • Impaired functions of the skin (b810–b849)	• Potential impaired mobility including changing and maintaining body positions (d410–d429) or walking and moving (d450–d469) • Potential self care problems (d5) • Potential impaired interpersonal interactions and relationships (d710–d729)	• Surgery is often recommended to remove the tumors. If cancerous, treatment may include radiation or chemotherapy. • Interventions to prevent secondary impairment and optimize activity and participation.

Continued

Table 7.5 Neuromuscular Conditions—cont'd

Diagnosis	Definition	Etiology	Alterations in Body Functions and Structures	Potential Activity Limitations and Participation Restrictions	Potential Management
Neurofibromatoses *(continued)*	bone deformities. Neurofibromatosis type 1 (NF1) is the most common type Neurofibromatosis type 2 (NF2) Schwannomatosis—a variation of NF2				
STORCH Infections • Syphilis • Toxoplasmosis • Other agents (HIV, Lime disease, etc.) • Rubella • Cytomegalovirus • Herpes Simplex	From mother to infant— intrauterine infections	Maternal hematogenous infection (transplacental) more common than through the birth canal (transcervical)	• Intrauterine growth retardation • Impaired functions of the skin (b810–b849) • Possible impaired functions of the digestive, metabolic, and endocrine systems • Impaired functions of the joints and bones (b710–b729) • Possible impaired global mental function (b110–b139) • Possible impaired seeing and related functions (b210–b229) • Possible impaired hearing and vestibular functions (b230–b249)	• Variable depending upon extent of body structure/ function impairments • Decreased mobility (d455) and transfers (d420) • Delay of developmental milestones and moving around (d455) • Decreased ability to maintain sustained active play (d9200) with peers or family • Potential self-care problems (d5) • Problems with nonverbal communication, including the restricted use of gestures, limited or inappropriate facial expressions, or a peculiar, stiff gaze (d335) • Problems with speaking (d330)	Prevention: • Rubella: vaccine • HSV: no vaccine or screening; C-section in women who have history and active lesions • Syphilis: screened in 1st and 3rd trimester • Toxoplasmosis: transmitted by exposure to cat litter box or eating uncooked meat • HIV: use of antiretroviral drugs during pregnancy and C-section Management: • Infection-specific drugs

*Numbers in parentheses refer to ICF-CY classification.

activity limitations and participation restrictions, as well as potential management for common neuromuscular diagnoses.

Neuroscience Related to Common Pediatric Neuromuscular Disorders

A review of specific issues related to neuromotor development should help in understanding the origins of some impairments in body structures and functions and predict, with some accuracy, restrictions in activities and participation that may develop. The knowledge of what type of motor disability may develop allows the therapist to modify examination and intervention approaches to improve effectiveness and prevention of further disability. For example, based on knowledge of the specific CNS injury, it can be predicted that a child will develop hemiplegia, and early intervention can be focused on encouraging bilateral movement. It is important to remember that the prediction of functional outcomes based on the initial CNS lesion

remains difficult as one cannot predict the amount of neuroplasticity that might occur, and outcomes are based on a combination of the individual's genetic makeup, "nature and nurture" issues, and the effects of environmental experience, which cannot always be controlled (Penn, Rose, & Johnson, 2009; Wells, Minnes, & Phillips, 2009).

In the embryonic stages of development, growth of the CNS can be broken down into several processes: (1) neurulation, (2) ventral induction, (3) neuronal proliferation, (4) neuronal migration, (5) neural organization, and (6) myelination (Nieuwenhuys, Voogd, & van Huijzen, 2008; Volpe, 2008). Each process and examples of the outcome for the infant if neuromuscular development is disturbed during these stages are summarized in Table 7.6.

Insults to the CNS of a fetus can preferentially damage different structures based on the timing of the injury. Gestational age of 22 to 25 weeks is described as approximately the youngest survival age in babies

Table 7.6 Development of the Central Nervous System and Consequences of Disruption

Developmental Process	Timing from Conception	Definition of Process	Disorders Associated with Disruption of Process	Definition of Disorder	Outcome of Disorders (dependent on the extent and level of lesion)
Neurulation	3–4 weeks	Formation of neural tube	Encephalocele	Defects in neural tube closure in brain	Motor and/or cognitive impairments
			Myelomeningocele	Defects in neural tube closure in spinal cord	
Ventral induction	5–6 weeks	Formation of basic structures and brain subdivisions	Holoprosencephaly Agenesis of the corpus callosum	Failure of cleavage of prosencephalon leaving deficit in midline facial development Lack of development of corpus callosum (where fibers cross between left and right side of brain)	Facial structure, feeding, and cognitive impairment, ranging from mild developmental delay to severe mental retardation (MR) and cerebral palsy (CP) Bilateral coordination, visual perception, motor control, motor learning, and cognitive impairments, ranging from mild developmental delay to severe MR and CP

Continued

Table 7.6 Development of the Central Nervous System and Consequences of Disruption—cont'd

Developmental Process	Timing from Conception	Definition of Process	Disorders Associated with Disruption of Process	Definition of Disorder	Outcome of Disorders (dependent on the extent and level of lesion)
Neuronal proliferation	8–16 weeks	Neural and glial cells form and proliferate	Microencephaly	Reduced brain size and weight	Cognitive and motor impairments including abnormal muscle tone, postural control, and motor coordination, ranging from mild developmental delay to severe MR and CP
			Macroencephaly	Increased brain size and weight	
Neuronal migration	12–20 weeks	Neurons move from ventricular and subventricular zones to final destination	Generalized or focal seizures	Abnormal excessive electrical activity in the brain	Cognitive, sensory, and motor control impairments, ranging from mild to severe developmental delay to CP
			Lissencephaly	Abnormalities in gyral development and cortical surface area	
			Schizencephaly	Abnormal cavities or cysts in the brain	
			Focal cerebral dysgenesis	Lack of development of specific cortical sites	
Neuronal organization	24 weeks to 2–3 years	• Establishment and differentiation of subplate neurons • Alignment, orientation, and layering of neurons • Growth of axons and dendrites • Synaptogenesis	Frequently associated with other earlier neural development abnormalities	Lack of organization and extensive network of circuits intrinsic and extrinsic to cerebral cortex	Cognitive, sensory or motor control impairment ranging from mild coordination and learning disorders (DCD) to CP

Table 7.6 Development of the Central Nervous System and Consequences of Disruption—cont'd

Developmental Process	Timing from Conception	Definition of Process	Disorders Associated with Disruption of Process	Definition of Disorder	Outcome of Disorders (dependent on the extent and level of lesion)
		• Selective elimination of neurons, neuronal processes, and synapses • Glial cell proliferation and differentiation			
Myelination	23 weeks to adulthood	Development of myelin membrane around axons	Cerebral white matter hypoplasia	Deficient or absent myelin production, decreased number of tracts between brain and spinal cord, slow transmission along tracts	Mild to severe postural and motor control and coordination problems; difficulty producing quick movements

Source: Unanue, R., & Westcott, S.L. (2001). Neonatal asphyxia. *Infants and Young Children, 13*(3), 13–24, with permission.

born prematurely (Chan et al., 2001). By gestation week 24, the major structures of the brain are present. A lack of oxygen to the tissue in the brain can result from relatively minor stress to the infant's system; therefore, the neonatal intensive care unit environment needs to be carefully controlled.

Several terms are used to describe changes in oxygen to the brain. **Hypoxemia** is a decrease in the amount of oxygen in the blood. **Ischemia** is decreased perfusion to a tissue bed such as the brain. Often, hypoxemia and ischemia occur simultaneously or follow one another in premature infants. **Asphyxia** is the most severe lack of oxygen and by definition means "without pulse" (Volpe, 2008). Prolonged asphyxia generally results in hypotension and ischemia causing cellular death, which usually leads to permanent disability (Okereafor et al., 2008). Infants born prematurely as a result of maternal problems are also at great

risk for postbirth brain damage attributable to an immature cardiopulmonary system (Volpe, 2008).

Selective neuronal necrosis in the full-term infant is a neuronal injury with a characteristic pattern in the CNS (Volpe, 2008). Early neuronal changes occur within 24 to 36 hours, with signs of cell necrosis within several days. Over the next several weeks, macrophages consume the necrotic cells. With severe lesions, a cavity may form in the cerebral cortex that becomes a fluid-filled cyst. The neurons in the cerebral cortex and the hippocampus are vulnerable to hypoxic ischemic insults. With severe injury, there is diffuse involvement of the cerebral cortex. Additional areas of the CNS commonly affected by selective neuronal necrosis are the basal ganglia, thalamus, brainstem, cerebellum, and spinal cord. All of these can lead to motor disorders, and the degree of impairment will depend on the exact location of the lesion. Long-term neurological sequelae include cognitive impairments, spastic motor deficits, seizure disorders, visual impairments, and impairments of sucking, swallowing, and facial movements (Volpe, 2008).

Abnormal development of brain structures, unknown genetic alterations causing neurological malformations, lack of oxygen at or around birth or during early development, or insults and trauma to the head can all lead to a diagnosis of CP (Stanley, Blair, & Alberman, 2000). Lesions are generally not well defined. The cortex, subcortical nuclei, cerebellum, and basal ganglia are the major areas of the brain involved in movement generation and control. The importance of these areas is summarized in Table 7.7.

Periventricular leukomalacia (PVL) is the primary ischemic lesion of the preterm infant (Volpe, 2008). The highest incidence of cystic PVL (cysts form where neural tissue should be) occurs in infants born at 27 to 30 weeks' gestational age. PVL is located in the white matter and is usually more likely to injure the motor tracts of the lower extremities than those of the upper extremities at the border zones, or the watershed areas of the arterial circulation (Volpe, 2008). **Watershed regions** or **border zones** are terms used to describe the location between the end fields of the anterior, middle, and posterior cerebral arteries. The degree of ischemia needed to cause PVL varies as a function of gestational age and the development of the arterial circulation. The

Table 7.7 Major Motor Control Functions of the Cerebellum, Basal Ganglia, and Cerebral Cortex

Area of the Brain	Inputs to Area	Outputs to Other Areas	Disorders in Humans with Lesions/Diseases	Motor Control and Learning Function
Cerebellum • Vestibulocerebellum: fastigial nuclei • Spinocerebellum: interpositus nuclei and dentate nuclei	*Vestibular nuclei* • *Mossy fibers*— ascending and descending information • *Climbing fibers*— inferior olive nuclei	Via Purkinje cell to cerebellar nuclei to: • *Vestibular nuclei* to vestibulospinal tract and vestibuloocular tract • *Reticular formation* to reticulospinal tract • *Red nucleus* to rubrospinal tract and olive • *VPL thalamus* to cortex to corticospinal tract	• *Dysmetria* (over-/ undershoot target) • *Dysdiadochokinesia* (inability to move with a constant rhythm) • *Hypotonia* • *Asynergia* (impairment in interjoint coordination) • *Kinetic tremors* (during voluntary movement) • *Intentional tremors* (on approach to target) • *Postural tremors* (in maintaining constant position)	• Postural control • Eye-head and eye-body control • Integration of sensory input to affect descending systems for smooth volitional multijoint movements • Planning and preparation for movement • Possible role in motor learning and storage of motor program*s*
Basal Ganglia • Paleostriatum: globus pallidus • Striatum: caudate and putamen • Subthalamic: substantia nigra	*Cerebral cortex*: primary motor, premotor, supplementary motor, superior parietal, somatosensory *Limbic structures*: hypothalamus,	Inhibition from globus pallidus and excitation from substantia nigra to *VL of thalamus* to premotor and supplementary motor cerebral cortex to motor	Decreased thalamic output to cortex: • *Hypokinesias*: bradykinesia (slow movement, prolonged reaction time); involuntary tremor; rigidity; postural deficits	• *Oculomotor control* • *Movement initiation*: disinhibit areas of motor cortex and turn off postural activity allowing movement to occur • *Movement coordination*: sequencing movement fragments;

■ **Table 7.7** Major Motor Control Functions of the Cerebellum, Basal Ganglia, and Cerebral
■ Cortex—cont'd

Area of the Brain	Inputs to Area	Outputs to Other Areas	Disorders in Humans with Lesions/Diseases	Motor Control and Learning Function
	fornix, hippocampus, amygdaloid, cingulate gyrus of cerebral cortex	cortex to corticospinal tract and other descending tracts *Superior colliculi* to ocular areas	• *Dystonia*: sustained postures of neck, trunk, and limbs Increased thalamic output to cortex: • *Hyperkinesias*: chorea, ballism (excessive movement)	coordinate movements in parallel
Cerebral Cortex • Primary motor cortex (Brodmann's area 4) • Somatosensory cortex (area 3) • Premotor cortex (area 6): premotor and supplementary motor areas	Via thalamus from: *Spinal cord; basal ganglia; cerebellum Other cerebral cortex areas:* (particularly parietal and frontal)	*Cerebral cortex*: ipsilateral and contralateral sensory, motor, and other cortical areas *Basal ganglia Cerebellum* via pons *Red nuclei Reticular formation Spinal cord* via corticospinal tract	Paralysis Spasticity	Perceiving and interpreting sensory information Making conscious decisions and generation of movements Controlling voluntary movement; encoding direction of movement; control of movements in opposite directions, control of cocontraction (joint stiffness)

Source: Cohen, H. (1999). *Neuroscience for rehabilitation* (2nd ed.). Philadelphia: Lippincott Williams
& Wilkins; Latash, M.L. (1998a). *Neurophysiological basis of movement* (pp. 98–105). Champaign, IL:
Human Kinetics; Leonard, C.T. (1998). *The neuroscience of human movement* (pp. 124–128). St. Louis:
Mosby-Year Book; Lundy-Ekman, L. (1998). *Neuroscience: Fundamentals for rehabilitation* (pp. 69–84).
Philadelphia: W.B. Saunders.

most common long-term motor outcome of PVL is spastic (hypertonic) diplegic (primarily lower extremities) CP (Volpe, 2008).

Impaired Neuromotor Development
Autism

Autism, as defined by the Code of Federal Regulations (34 C.F.R. § 300.7) definitions of children with disabilities (Code of Federal Regulations, 2006), is a "developmental disability significantly affecting verbal and nonverbal communication and social interaction, generally evident before 3 years of age, that adversely affects a child's educational performance. Other characteristics often associated with autism are engagement in repetitive activities and stereotyped movements, resistance to environmental change or change in daily routines, and unusual responses to sensory experiences." There is wide variation in the manifestation of these characteristics.

The terms "autism spectrum disorder" (ASD) or "pervasive developmental disorder" (PDD) are used to indicate behavior conditions that exist on a continuum ranging from mildly to severely involved in the areas of socialization, communication, and behavior. According to the Diagnostic and Statistical Manual of Mental Disorders, 4th ed., Text Revision (DSM-IV-TR) (American Psychiatric Association, 2000), five major diagnoses fall under ASDs: (1) autism, (2) Asperger syndrome, (3) pervasive developmental disorder—not otherwise specified (PDD-NOS), (4) Rett syndrome, and (5) childhood disintegrative disorder.

Children having **autism** have qualitative impairment in social interactions and communication and restricted, repetitive, and stereotyped patterns of behaviors, interests, and activities. Over half of the children with autism are not considered to be intellectually impaired. Children with **Asperger syndrome** have social interaction deficits and restricted interests, but no deficits in cognition, speech, and language formation. They, and children with **PDD-NOS** who have a later onset, have fewer diagnostic symptoms and typically milder impairments than children with autism or Rett syndrome.

Rett syndrome is an x-linked genetic mutation where infant girls have an apparent period of normal development until age 6–18 months, followed by progressive neurological impairment, including ataxia, apraxia, hypotonia leading to hypertonia, stereotypic hand movements, and loss of acquired skills. Rett syndrome is the most severe and life-altering of the ASDs (National Autism Center, 2009). Childhood disintegrative disorder is extremely rare. The children appear to develop normally for the first 2 years of life and then begin to regress in their communication, social, and behavioral skills. They develop problems with adaptive skills such as independent walking or toileting (National Autism Center, 2009).

While the exact cause of autism is unknown, evidence suggests a multifactorial cause, with a strong genetic component (Abrahams & Geschwind, 2008). The genetic risk for autism is reported to be between 70% and 90%; however, no single genetic mutation is responsible for more than about 1% of ASDs (Geschwind, 2009). ASDs are becoming increasingly more prevalent or identified more often in today's society. In a recent publication from the Centers for Disease Control and Prevention, an average of 1 out of every 110 children, boys > girls (4:1), were diagnosed with ASDs in the United States (CDC, 2009). The U.S. Government Accountability Office (2005) reports a 500% increase in autism over the last decade.

Impairments of Body Structures and Functions Related to Motor Performance Sensory abnormalities are observed in over 90% of the children with autism (Geschwind, 2009), and sensory processing impairments have been demonstrated in 95% of children with ASDs (Tomchek & Dunn, 2007). The children may be overly responsive to typical sensory input (hypersensitive) or might be underresponsive to input (hyposensitive). Hypersensitive responses to tactile stimuli are common and hyposensitive responses are common to auditory and vestibular stimuli (Tomchek

& Case-Smith, 2009, p. 32). Some children have both hypersensitivity and hyposensitivity and their responses fluctuate, complicating intervention. Of particular interest to the physical therapist is the percentage of children with ASDs who have impairments in motor function. Approximately 10% have gross motor delay, and 60%–80% demonstrate hypotonia, gait problems, toe walking, or apraxia (Geschwind, 2009). In one study hypotonia was the most prevalent symptom, though it appears to improve over time, as does apraxia (Ming, Brimacombe, & Wagner, 2007).

Given the increasing incidence of children with ASDs, physical therapists should be involved in screening children for ASDs, especially since therapists are likely to be serving these children in early intervention programs because of their early motor delays and impairments. Any of the following signs could indicate potential ASDs:

- No babbling or gesturing by 12 months of age
- Inability to speak 1 word by 12 months of age
- Inability to combine 2 words by 2 years of age
- Any loss of language or social skills (Filipek et al., 1999)

In addition to these clinical signs, specific screening tools to assist in the identification of children with the potential to have ASDs exist. These tools include, among others, the Modified Checklist for Autism in Toddlers (M-CHAT), the Social Communication Questionnaire (SCQ) (Landa, 2008), and the various tests included in the Sensory Profile (Dunn, 1999). If either clinical signs or a positive test on a screening tool is noted, a referral to a comprehensive diagnostic team for evaluation is warranted. This team includes a psychologist, neurologist, psychiatrist, speech-language pathologist, and at times an occupational or physical therapist. Early identification and diagnosis is important so intervention and services can be provided. Currently, many children are not diagnosed with ASDs until they enter elementary school at 5 years of age; however, parents notice signs as early as 18 months.

Restrictions in Activities and Participation Children with ASDs demonstrate limitations in social and communication skills, which makes peer relationships and involvement in school and recreational activities challenging. As language and social skills begin to emerge, the delay or absence of these interactive skills becomes more evident. Children with ASDs may initially reach gross motor milestones, although age-appropriate attainment may be delayed

(Provost, Heimerl, & Lopez, 2007). Problems with muscle tone, motor abilities and coordination, and motor planning will impact their ability to play with others and participate in age-appropriate activities (Baranek, Parham, & Bodfish, 2005; Geschwind, 2009).

Staples and Reid (2010) found that children with ASDs were able to perform the skills on the Test of Gross Motor Development (Ulrich, 2000); however, they scored lower than typically developing age-matched peers and the quality of movement was poorer (Staples & Reid, 2010). In addition, these children had difficulty coordinating movements involving both arms and legs on the horizontal jump. During hopping activities, the children with ASDs did not use their arms in a coordinated fashion to help them generate force or assist with balance (Staples & Reid, 2010). Boys with high-functioning autism and Asperger syndrome have greater problems with balance and gait, slower speed and more dysrhythmia and timed movements of hands and feet, and an overflow of movements during a performance of time movements and stressed walking (Jansiewicz et al., 2006).

Performance on the Physical and Neurological Exam for Subtle Signs (PANESS) (Denekla, 1974) allowed for detection of subtle neurological signs and to discriminate boys 6 to 17 years of age with autism from those without (Jansiewicz et al., 2006). These motor problems can lead to activity and participation restrictions including limitations in gait, ball playing skills, and an inability to participate with peers in physical education activities or recreational sports, which can lead to further social isolation (Geschwind, 2009).

Potential Interventions Typically, intervention has focused on increasing quality of life and ability to participate in society. Interventions included in the *Occupational Therapy Practice Guidelines,* which have varying degrees of evidence to support them, include sensory integration and sensory-based interventions, relationship-based interactive interventions, school-based programs, social skills interventions, and comprehensive behavioral interventions (Tomchek & Case-Smith, 2009). They note four overall themes consistently linked to positive outcomes:

1. Effective intervention programs are developed from individualized analysis that includes assessment of the physiological basis for behaviors and the environment's influence on behavior.
2. The child's family is central to the intervention program and services should include family support and education.
3. Intervention services need to be intensive and comprehensive.
4. Facilitating active engagement of the child is the essential priority for all interventions (Tomchek & Case-Smith, 2009).

The National Autism Center (2009) notes that there are established treatments, many of which have a strong behavioral component, that have sufficient evidence of their effectiveness for them to be recommended. They note that a collaborative and carefully planned strategy is necessary once an intervention has been selected.

Physical therapists can address the motor components of ASDs, including poor motor planning and activity limitations associated with low muscle tone and sensory impairments. Evidenced-based practice guidelines are now available from the National Autism Center (2009) and the American Occupational Therapy Association (Tomchek & Case-Smith, 2009). Physical therapists should play a larger role in the intervention of children with ASDs since there is serious concern that motor deficits are not being well recognized by the school community, where most of the children with ASDs receive their services (Ming et al., 2007).

Developmental Coordination Disorder

The DSM-IV defines developmental coordination disorder (DCD) as a motor skills disorder in which a child shows "marked impairment in the development of motor coordination that significantly interferes with academic achievement or activities of daily living" not caused by a general medical condition or pervasive developmental disorder (PDD) (American Psychiatric Association, 1994). In 2000, the *DSM-IV* was updated to include "If mental retardation is present, the motor difficulties are in excess of those usually associated with mental retardation" (American Psychiatric Association, 2000).

The DSM-IV estimates that approximately 6% of children between 5 and 11 years of age have DCD. Children with DCD do not show specific signs of neuropathology or neurological insults. Clumsiness or motor incoordination may also be present in children with attention deficit hyperactivity disorder (ADHD) and specific learning disability (SLD) (Dewey, Kaplan, Crawford, & Wilson, 2002; Cermak & Larkin, 2002; Miller, Missiuna, Macnab, Malloy-Miller, & Polatajko, 2001). Imaging performed during activity (positron emission tomography [PET] scans and functional magnetic resonance imaging [MRI]) can now be used to diagnose ADHD and SLD. Findings suggest problems in the basal ganglia and cerebellum (Born & Lou, 1999; Krageloh-Mann et al., 1999). Based on the function of these areas for motor control, problems with appropriate force production, timing of muscle activity, forming perceptions based on sensory input, and motor learning could be expected. Studies of children born prematurely suggest that damage to the CNS leading to DCD most likely occurs in the last trimester. Problems may occur with the final "wiring" during the neural migration and organization of the CNS, and may be accentuated by other environmental issues after birth (Hadders-Algra & Lindahl, 1999).

Children with DCD are varied in terms of the specific motor skill problems they manifest and the severity of the disorder. Motor performance in daily activities is clumsy and below age expectations (Dewey & Wilson, 2001). Often there is poor performance in sports and handwriting. Many other labels have been given to children presenting with this disorder, such as apraxia, minimal brain dysfunction, clumsy child, developmental dyspraxia, motor coordination or learning problems, motor-perception dysfunction, physically awkward child, sensory integrative dysfunction, deficits in attention–motor control–perception (DAMP), and visuomotor disabilities (Kadesjö & Gillberg, 2001; Christiansen, 2000). These motor skill differences need to be differentiated from the maturational delay and normal variances that exist in the development of children's motor skill ability, which would not lead to a diagnosis of DCD (Davies & Rose, 2000).

Identifying children with DCD can be difficult, and the therapist needs to use clinical reasoning in conjunction with results from standardized tests (Crawford, Wilson, & Dewey, 2001). A diagnosis of DCD suggests that there is a specific motor disorder, and professional intervention may be of assistance to the child (Dewey & Wilson, 2001). Sometimes the motor problems are accompanied by SLD and/or ADHD. Comorbidity of DCD with SLD is reported to be as high as 70%, and 75% of children with SLD also have ADHD. A number of children show symptoms of all three disorders (Polatajko, 1999).

Associated Medical Issues Hyperactivity and problems focusing attention are common in children with DCD. Stimulant medications, such as Ritalin and Concerta, are often prescribed to increase attention span and thus improve learning. These medications can influence motor behavior by increasing the awareness of obstacles, therefore decreasing tripping and falling. Abnormalities in sensory modulation capability have been found in a subgroup of children with ADHD, and these sensory problems correlated with problems in emotional and attentional behavior (Mangeot et al., 2001). Specifically, children might have problems following directions and with behavioral control, leading to excessive frustration, low self-esteem, and depression (Missiuna, Gaines, Soucie, & McLean, 2006). As the child ages, these emotional issues may become more apparent and interfere with learning and function (Christiansen, 2000).

Impairments of Body Structures and Functions Related to Motor Performance Children with DCD may show soft neurologic signs such as low muscle tone, muscle weakness, and motor incoordination, especially in the hands; poor postural control; and delayed acquisition of motor milestones (Missiuna et al., 2006; Christiansen, 2000) (Fig. 7.9). Problems with muscle weakness, decreased energy expenditure, and decreased cardiorespiratory fitness in children with DCD have been identified as contributing factors to poor body awareness, decreased motor skill development, and diminished participation in leisure-time physical activities (Cairney, Hay, Faught, Flouis, & Klentou, 2007; Poulsen, Ziviani, & Cuskelly, 2008; Raynor, 2001).

Identification of the underlying neurological processes purportedly involved has been inconclusive. Theories for the postural and motor coordination problems have revolved around (1) poor processing of sensory systems, specifically the visual, somatosensory (proprioceptive and cutaneous), and vestibular systems (Horak, Shumway-Cook, Crowe, & Black, 1988; Rosblad & Von Hofsten, 1994; Willoughby & Polatajko, 1995); (2) poor integration and modulation of these sensory inputs for coordinating motor output (Mangeot et al., 2001; Willoughby & Polatajko, 1995); (3) poor force control (less precise), rhythm and timing control (Missiuna et al., 2006; Henderson, Rose, & Henderson, 1992); and (4) other CNS information-processing problems related to motor planning and memory (Horak et al., 1988; Skorji & McKenzie, 1997; van Dellen & Geuze, 1988; Wilson & McKenzie, 1998). The limited support from research studies for these theories may be because the diagnosis and etiology of DCD are poorly understood and appear so variable.

Restrictions in Activities and Participation Functionally, children with DCD reach all of the typical motor milestones and complete most activities independently. However, tasks that are sometimes delayed in acquisition include (1) fine motor sequencing tasks, such as handwriting and tying shoelaces; (2) complex coordination tasks, such as skipping, and performing two different gross motor tasks in close succession,

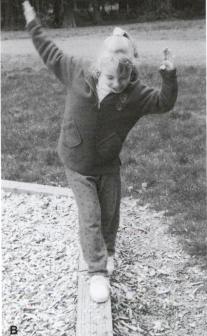
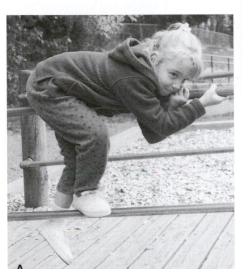
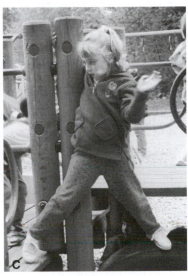

Figure 7.9 Child with developmental coordination disorder. *(A)* This 5-year-old child was asked to climb up on the railing and take sidesteps along it. Note that the child stays as low as possible and wraps herself around the bar because of poor postural control and perceptual problems affecting motor planning for achieving the task. *(B)* When asked to walk along a 6-inch-wide board that is approximately 4 inches off the ground, she has problems maintaining her balance. *(C)* When the child is attempting to move from one level of the climber to another over the tire, a task requiring motor planning and postural control, you note an awkward position because of her need to continue to hold onto the structure for balance, and a protruding tongue in her cheek.

such as dribbling a soccer ball and then transitioning to kick for the goal; and (3) learning new tasks that require integration of sensory input and motor planning, such as climbing on playground structures. Standardized pediatric examinations can assist in the identification of coordination disorders, specifically DCD in children. The Movement Assessment Battery for Children (M-ABC) (Henderson & Sugden, 2007) is a norm-referenced test for children aged 3 to 12 years old to determine whether the child is at risk for movement problems. This examination is divided into manual dexterity, ball skills, and static and dynamic balance categories and can be administered by teachers or parents. The M-ABC has been shown to identify characteristic features including gross motor performance consistent with DCD and thus might be an appropriate standardized tool in recognizing children with DCD (Missiuna, Rivard, & Bartlett, 2006; Slater, Hillier, & Civetta, 2010).

This test has been used recently in research as a tool to determine the effectiveness of physical therapy intervention with children diagnosed with DCD (Niemeijer, Schoemaker, & Smits-Engelsman, 2006; Niemeijer, Smits-Engelsman, & Schoemaker, 2007; Watemberg, Waiserberg, Zuk, & Lerman-Sagie, 2007). Other standardized measures, including the Peabody Developmental Motor Scales, 2nd ed., the Test of Gross Motor Development, and the BOT-2, are designed to identify motor delay in children. Although the BOT-2 has been used to identify probable cases of DCD, it is important to remember that it was designed to measure gross and fine motor control skills and motor delay, which can identify a different subset of children (Dewey & Wilson, 2001).

In addition to diagnostic tests that identify children with DCD, screening tests that are less time consuming and are valid for DCD also exist. Some of these screening tests include the Developmental Coordination

Disorder Questionnaire and the Children's Self-Perceptions of Adequacy in and Predilection for Physical Activity (CSAPPA). These screening tools identify children that should be further evaluated with a diagnostic test (Cairney, Veldhuizen, et al., 2007; Schoemaker et al., 2006; Hay, Hawes, & Faught, 2004). The Canadian Occupational Performance Measure is another outcome measure that should be considered when working with children with DCD, as this is a measure at the participation level and can be used for goal setting (Carswell et al., 2004). Participation can also be determined using the Children's Assessment of Participation and Enjoyment (CAPE), a measure of a child's participation in everyday activities outside of school, and the Preferences for Activities of Children (PAC), a measure of activity preferences used with children 6 to 21 years (King et al., 2004).

Longitudinal studies of children with DCD suggest that some problems may decrease, although they usually do not disappear totally (Christiansen, 2000; Fox & Lent, 1996; Gillberg, 1999). Personal factors related to participation restriction observed in children with DCD are depression, lack of motivation, low self-esteem, poor fitness level, and task-related anxiety. Some adolescents with DCD continue to have low academic achievement, few hobbies, poor self-esteem, poor athletic competence, less participation in community sports, and low aspirations for future endeavors, which can lead to decreased physical activity levels and increased risks associated with sedentary lifestyles (Kane & Bell, 2009). The main participation restriction identified by parents of children with DCD was related to problems with participation during grooming, dressing, and eating, especially when reaching middle-school age (Segal, Mandich, Polotajko, & Cook, 2002).

Potential Interventions Task-specific intervention based on motor learning principles, such as neuromotor task training, which accentuate the use of augmented feedback for learning, memory cues, and practice in varied environments, may assist with improving functional and sports motor behaviors (Hillier, 2007; Mandich, Polatajko, Macnab, & Miller, 2001a; Mandich, Polatajko, Missiuna, & Miller, 2001b; Missiuna, 2001; Niemeijer et al., 2006; Niemeijer et al., 2007; Polatajko, Mandich, Miller, & Macnab, 2001). In addition, perceptual motor training, sensory integration therapy, and motor learning principles improved the motor performance of children with DCD and ADHD (Watemberg et al., 2007). Motor imagery training has also been shown to improve performance in children with DCD (Wilson, Thomas, & Maruff, 2002). Another intervention approach used with

children diagnosed with DCD is Cognitive Orientation to Daily Occupational Performance (CO-OP). This approach focuses on increasing performance of the child using a problem-solving approach with task-specific strategies (Polatajko et al., 2001). CO-OP has demonstrated effectiveness as a treatment approach when compared with other treatment approaches, including multisensory, biomechanical, and neuromuscular (Miller et al., 2001). Recommended fitness activities include swimming and karate (Hillier, McIntyre, & Plummer, 2010; Hung & Pang, 2010). Assistance to make the child more successful and happy should include collaboration and consultation with the child, family, and other team members to (1) explain the nature of the disorder, (2) provide strategies for controlling sensory input to make learning more successful, and (3) devise appropriate consistent behavioral consequences to support the child in trying activities (Hillier, 2007).

Down Syndrome

Down syndrome (DS) is a genetic disorder in which the majority (approximately 90%) of individuals have an extra chromosome on chromosome pair 21. This usually occurs because of the nondysjunction of two homologous chromosomes during the first or second meiotic division. In a small percentage (3% to 4%), a translocation occurs in which, after breakage of homologous chromosomes, the pieces reattach to other intact chromosome pairs. The remaining individuals (2% to 4%) with DS have a mosaic disorder, in which some cells are normal and others are trisomy 21 (Stoll, Alembik, Dott, & Roth, 1998). Neuropathological differences as a result of the chromosomal abnormality include small, smooth (less convolutions) brain (similar to 76% of normal), especially in the frontal lobes; small (similar to 66%) cerebellum and brainstem (Aylward et al., 1997); structural differences in the dendritic spines of the pyramidal neurons; lack of myelination of neurons in the cortex and cerebellum; and decrease of neurons in the hippocampus and an increase in Alzheimer neurofibrillary tangles with age (Harris & Shea, 1991).

Associated Medical Issues Children with DS have varying degrees of intellectual disability, which lowers their drive or curiosity about the world and their motivation to try new things (Hayes & Batshaw, 1993; Pueschel, 1990). In 2007, the American Association on Mental Retardation changed its name to the American Association on Intellectual and Developmental Disabilities (AAIDD) to more accurately and positively represent individuals with intellectual disabilities. Specifically, the

AAIDD utilizes "intellectual disability" as the preferred term instead of "mental retardation" to focus on the participation abilities of individuals with intellectual disabilities and reduce the negative social stigma that is associated with mental retardation. A revised definition of intellectual disability consistent with the International Classification of Function, Disability, and Health model requires both an intelligence component (intelligence quotient of 70–75 or below), and an adaptive behavior component (deficits in conceptual, practical, and social skills) (AAIDD, 2010). When working with a child with intellectual limitations, the therapist is challenged to find ways to communicate with the child, to understand his or her expressive communication, and to determine what will motivate the child to try different movements (Kokubun, 1999). Often this is the missing link in motor learning; the child may not be motivated to practice movement because it is difficult and not reinforcing.

Congenital heart defects are a commonly (about 40% to 60%) associated medical disorder with DS that can affect exercise tolerance (Freeman et al., 1998). The most common defects are atrioventricular canal and ventriculoseptal defects, which can usually be surgically repaired. The therapist should understand the cardiac disorder and whether exercise needs to be modified to control effects on the heart.

Binaural hearing loss is also common in children with DS (Roizen, Wolters, Nicol, & Blondis, 1993), which is compounded by frequent otitis media. In addition to decreased response to sounds, there may be associated problems in the vestibular apparatus, which is located next to the sensory end organ for hearing. Vestibular impairment and cerebellar changes may combine to be the etiology of the muscle tone abnormalities. Eye conditions, including nearsightedness and farsightedness, lazy eye, astigmatism, nystagmus, and cataracts, are also common (Tsiaras, Pueschel, Keller, Curran, & Giesswein, 1999). Both the visual and vestibular deficits may account for part of the etiology of the postural control problems.

Impairments of Body Structures and Functions Related to Motor Performance Children with DS usually present with overall hypotonicity, muscle weakness, slow postural reactions and reaction time, and hyperflexible joints (Carvalho & Almeida, 2009; Cowley et al., 2010; Dellavia, Pallavera, Orlando, & Sforza, 2009; Mercer & Lewis, 2001; Tsimaras & Fotiadou, 2004) (Fig. 7.10).

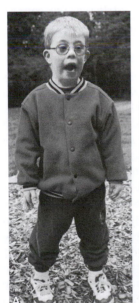
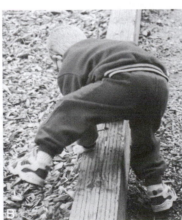
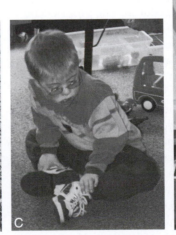
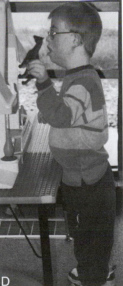

Figure 7.10 Child with Down syndrome. *(A)* When looking at the child's posture from the front, note his open mouth, sloping shoulders, and wide base of support, depicting lower muscle tone and poor postural control. *(B)* When asked to step over the low (4-inch) beam to enter the playground, he squats to support himself with his arms and sidesteps over the obstacle. *(C)* Note the wide base of support in sitting and the need to lean forward on his arms for assisted support to stay upright. *(D)* When looking at the child's posture from the side, note the open mouth, the choice to lean on the table for postural support, and the positioning of the legs locked into full knee extension, again to help maintain postural control and decrease the need for strength to maintain the position.

Because of the joint laxity, some children (about 15%) with DS show specific joint instability in the cervical atlantoaxial joint (Roizen & Patterson, 2003). This is verified by radiography, and the warning signs include gait changes, urinary retention, torticollis, reluctance to move the neck, and increased deep tendon reflexes. If instability exists, the therapist must be careful to not cause excessive end range of motion movements at the neck during any activity because slippage of this joint could cause a spinal cord injury. Contact sports and tumbling should be avoided. Precautions should be understood by the family and others who engage the child in physical activity.

Because of the hypotonia, ligamentous laxity, and intellectual disabilities, reaction times and movements of children with DS are generally slow and lack coordination (Inui, Yamanishi, & Tada, 1995). These findings have been demonstrated by studies of EMG activity patterns during reaching in adults with DS. Individuals with DS tend to use more cocontraction of antagonistic muscle pairs than do individuals without DS (Aruin, Almeida, & Latash, 1996). This is thought to develop as a compensatory pattern for improved control of the movement and protection from external perturbations.

To maintain a reaching movement to a target during a perturbation, there are four lines of defense (Gottlieb, Corcos, & Agarwal, 1989; Houk, 1979; Latash, 1998c). In individuals with DS, the connective tissue is hypoextensible, so the rebound effect of the connective tissue, the first line of defense, is reduced. The proprioceptors are not at a high state of readiness to respond (low muscle tone), and the brainstem areas may be slow to respond because of differences in cerebellum development. Therefore, the effectiveness of the second (stretch reflex) and third lines of defense (long-latency reflex) is reduced. The fourth line of defense, voluntary redirection, must then be used. Fast voluntary responses to incoming feedback are generally not seen in individuals with DS, leaving the accuracy of the movement at great risk for not being redirected quickly enough to hit the target. To combat these problems, it is hypothesized that the individual cocontracts to produce better sensory feedback and limb stability. Excessive cocontraction causes movements to be slow. Moving more slowly also allows more time to receive and integrate feedback from proprioceptors.

The infant or child with DS takes a longer time to develop antigravity postures, and the postural alignment is different from typically developing children, because the child tends to "hang" on his or her ligaments (Haley,

1986; Kokubun et al., 1997; Lauteslager, Vermeer, & Helders 1998; Shumway-Cook & Woollacott, 1985). As a result of the delay in postural development and hypotonicity, the child will also widen the base of support and cocontract agonists and antagonists, or decrease the degrees of freedom for movement to develop stability (Aruin & Almeida, 1997). Therefore the movement experiences of a child with DS become limited, which causes further delay of the development of feedforward postural control and variable free movements. The small cerebellum of an individual with DS may have implications related to poor proprioception, difficulty using sensory input to learn motor behaviors, and problems using the vestibular system for postural control. This may explain why these children are visually dependent for postural control (Shumway-Cook & Woollacott, 1985).

The presence of hypotonicity, joint laxity, and decreased muscle strength will, over time, cause excessive wear and tear on the joints. Adults with DS develop early musculoskeletal changes, including patellofemoral instability, genu valgus, pes planus, and hip instability (Hresko, McCarthy, & Goldberg, 1993; Merrick et al., 2000; Prasher, Robinson, Krishnan, & Chung, 1995).

Restrictions in Activities and Participation   The child with DS shows delay in early motor and intellectual development. Standardized pediatric tests may assist the physical therapist in identifying the degree of delay and help with goal setting. The tests that may be appropriate to consider with this population include the Alberta Infant Motor Scale (Piper & Darrah, 1994) for infants up to 18 months of age, the PDMS-2 (Fewell & Folio, 2000) for children 1 month to 6 years of age), the PEDI (Coster et al., 1994; Haley et al., 1992) for children 6 months to 7.5 years, and the Gross Motor Function Measure (GMFM) (Russell et al., 1993), which has been validated on children with DS (Russell et al., 1998). The CAPE and the PAC might also be used to measure participation and activity preferences with children 6 to 21 years (King et al., 2004).

Development of antigravity postures of sitting and standing and of the early mobility skills of crawling and walking can be quite delayed (Lloyd, Burghardt, Ulrich, & Angulo-Barroso, 2010). Use of high-intensity treadmill training to facilitate earlier walking and reduce walking delay has demonstrated success with walking, occurring 90 days earlier than children in a control group (Ulrich, Lloyd, Tiernan, Looper, & Angulo-Barroso, 2008; Ulrich, Ulrich, Angulo-Kinzler, & Yun, 2001; Wu, Looper, Ulrich, Ulrich, &

Angulo-Barroso, 2007). Walking allows the child to better explore the environment and advance in cognitive and language skills. Gait efficiency may be reduced due to the cocontraction around joints as a result of compensating for hypotonia, ligamentous laxity, and decreased balance. Research has demonstrated that preadolescents with DS are able to reduce their stiffness and impulse values to significantly improve their walking behavior on the treadmill following active task-specific practice (Smith, Kubo, Black, Holt, & Ulrich, 2007).

As children with DS grow, they may continue to have difficulty with eye-hand control and speed of movement required for ball skills, with the strength and speed needed for ballistic movements, such as jumping; and with the postural control needed for one-foot functional movement to negotiate stairs and kick a ball (Palisano et al., 2001; Spano et al., 1999).

Children with DS may require more time to learn complex movements; the severity of impairments affects the rate but not the upper limit of motor function (Palisano et al., 2001). In a study to develop motor growth curves for children with DS, Palisano and colleagues determined that children with DS will attain developmentally appropriate gross motor skills; however, it will take more time for them to learn these skills compared to their typically developing aged-matched peers (Palisano et al., 2001). Once the child has achieved the basic motor skills such as running and stair climbing, unless there are other medical issues, higher motor behaviors can eventually be addressed through adapted physical education or community recreation programs such as the Special Olympics.

Potential Interventions The physical therapist must coordinate and communicate with all other service providers as a member of an interdisciplinary team serving the needs of the infant and child with DS and the family. Collaboration is beneficial to learn ways to structure communication and the play environment for better participation. Generally, a structured environment, a small number of choices, and practice followed by rewards are successful strategies (McEwen, 2000). Special behavior management plans should be formulated, agreed on by the family and other professionals, and integrated into the plans of the entire team involved with the child.

A vital part of the intervention program is family education. The family is instructed in how to encourage appropriate developmental activities using the intervention strategies discussed in Chapter 8. Practice in different environments, which forces a change

of critical factors about the movement, may teach the child new methods of postural and prime movement control (Dichter, DeCicco, Flanagan, Hyun, & Mongrain, 2000). The options for movement can be varied, which allows for greater exploration and learning. For example, in an attempt to change the cocontracted EMG activation patterns during reaching, researchers asked adults with DS to practice a reaching movement repetitively (1,100 times per subject) at increasingly faster paces. The results showed that the subjects began to reach using a typical triphasic reaching pattern rather than the cocontraction pattern (Almeida, Corcos, & Latash, 1994). Use of group intervention with young children with DS in early intervention to facilitate peer modeling and socialization may also be an effective treatment strategy (LaForme Fiss, Effgen, Page, & Shasby, 2009). Use of variations in the environment, the components of the task, and practice are discussed in greater detail in Chapter 8.

Regular exercise programs should be incorporated into the child's routine for the health and fitness benefits, because it is common for children with DS to become sedentary and obese as they age (Fernhall & Pitetti, 2001; Graham & Reid, 2000; Rubin, Rimmer, Chicoine, Braddock, & McGuire, 1998). Because children with DS are typically more sedentary and less physically active, they are at increased risk for secondary health conditions, including type II diabetes, cardiovascular disease, and osteoporosis (Rimmer, Heller, Wang, & Valerio, 2004). Cardiovascular exercise programs and community programs to keep children physically active have been shown to improve peak oxygen consumption and maximum workload (Dodd & Shields, 2005). Intervention to improve strength and coordination and to decrease wear and tear on the weight-bearing joint structures should be implemented as preventive practice. Upper extremity resistance training has demonstrated effectiveness in improving muscle endurance in this population (Shields, Taylor, & Dodd, 2008).

Orthotics, particularly supramalleolar orthotics, may be used as a tool to improve postural stability, lower extremity alignment and prevent secondary deformities that can result from malalignment and overuse (Martin, 2004; Selby-Silverstein, Hillstrom, & Palisano, 2001). When considering orthotics as a potential intervention for children, the physical therapist should utilize clinical reasoning skills to determine when in the developmental motor process these orthotics should be implemented. Recent evidence suggests that utilizing orthotics with children with DS prior to the child's ability to independently ambulate could have a negative impact on their motor skill development (Looper & Ulrich, 2010). For more information on DS, see the case study from birth to young adulthood of an individual with DS presented in Chapter 21.

Impaired Motor Function and Sensory Integrity Associated With Nonprogressive Disorders of the Central Nervous System

Cerebral Palsy

Children with CP have motor disability related to early damage of the brain in areas controlling motor behaviors. Different patterns of dyscontrol can be observed dependent on the etiology, location, and extent of the insult. Although the lesion does not progress, the sequelae may vary as the child ages as a result of the development of atypical motor habits used by the children to compensate for poor motor and postural control, and motor learning deficits. Because movement is difficult, these children also tend to move less and develop poor cardiovascular fitness.

Classification of children with CP is very complex. Historically, children with CP were classified by the *distribution* of the motor disability. Quadriplegia signified that all limbs were involved; hemiplegia, one side was involved; and diplegia, when primarily the lower extremities were involved, as seen in Figure 7.11. The figure legend notes the subtle differences that can be

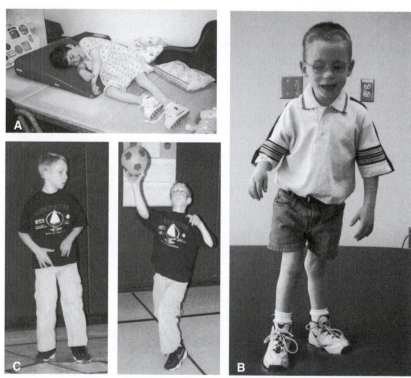

Figure 7.11 Children with cerebral palsy. *(A)* Child with spastic quadriplegia. Note the flexion at the head, shoulders, elbows, wrists, fingers, and trunk, and the positioning of the legs into extension on one side and flexion on the other. The child recently had adductor and hamstring muscle release surgery. This child has no voluntary movement. Bilateral ankle-foot orthoses (AFOs) hold her feet in a neutral position. *(B)* Child with spastic diplegia. Although the legs are more involved than the arms, the right upper extremity is also involved. Note the slight arm flexion greater on the right, the slight forward lean of the trunk, the hyperextension in both legs, and increased weight bearing on the left. Feet are flat on the surface with the use of AFOs. Another typical posture of a child with spastic diplegia would be with bilateral knee flexion, hip internal rotation, and weight bearing on toes bilaterally. *(C left)* Child with a mild left spastic hemiplegia. Left arm and leg show increased muscle tone through posturing of the left arm in greater elbow flexion than the right, and the thumb abducted into the palm of the hand; the left leg is also slightly flexed at the knee; and weight is borne on the ball of the foot only, the heel held off the surface. *(C right)* This weight-bearing posture is exaggerated when he exerts himself to catch a ball.

observed even from a still photograph. Differences in the body areas affected by CP become more apparent when the child is moving or stressed. The distributions can indicate the location of the lesion and sometimes the time the lesion occurred. This is based on the changing vulnerability of tissues in the developing fetus and infant. Although this classification system sounds simple, the actual determination of classification is controversial. Frequently, there are subtle motor problems in all extremities and definite asymmetrical distributions of movement dysfunction.

A second classification method indicates the *type of muscle tone* or motor control disorder. Categories include (1) spastic (exaggerated reflexes with abnormal patterns of posture and movement), (2) dyskinetic (atypical patterns of posture and involuntary, uncontrolled, recurring, and sometimes stereotyped movements) including subtypes of dystonic (involuntary, sustained or intermittent muscle contraction with repetitive movements and abnormal postures) and athetosis (slow, continuous, writhing movements), (3) ataxic (inability to generate normal or expected voluntary movement trajectories not due to weakness or involuntary muscle activity) and (4) mixed (spasticity and dyskinesia) (Wright & Wallman, 2012). Children with CP have also been classified based on the subjective degree of movement disorder, such as mild, moderate, or severe. Fluctuations in the behavioral state of the child (i.e., whether happy or sad, excited, or disinterested) can affect muscle tone. Children also generally present with a mixture of tonal symptoms depending on the location of the original neurological insult.

It is very common to find children with hypotonic trunk muscles and hypertonic extremity muscles. Muscle tone in different body areas can vary depending on the position in which the child is tested; for example, generally there is higher extensor tone when the child is in supine compared with prone, perhaps because of the additional muscle activation caused by one of the primitive reflex pathways (tonic labyrinthine reflex) (Bobath, 1985). Research has also shown that measurements of muscle tone through examination of passive movement do not necessarily reflect what is observed during active movement by the child (Crenna, 1998, 1999; Holt et al., 2000). This difference is hypothesized to be caused by neurological differences and to the child actively cocontracting or "fixing" muscles to compensate for muscle weakness and poor postural control. This compensatory technique, "fixing," is also used by the typically developing child when learning new

movements. A child will cocontract agonist and antagonist muscles to freeze or decrease the degrees of freedom to be controlled during early attempts to perform a motor skill (Damiano, 1993; Vereijken et al., 1992). After practice, the child will learn to release the cocontractions to allow more free or variable, and thus more adaptive, movement. The child with CP may learn to use this technique exclusively and become fixed at this learning stage. Adaptive changes from using only this movement method can further exacerbate muscle weakness, joint contractures, and poor postural and prime movement control. New ways to document active muscle tone are currently being developed and are described under the Examination section.

A newer and more widely accepted system to classify children with CP from birth to 18 years old is the **Gross Motor Function Classification System—Expanded and Revised (GMFCS E&R)**, a classification system of the gross motor function of children and youth with CP (Palisano, Rosenbaum, Bartlett, & Livingston, 2007). The severity of motor disability is rated on a 5-point scale that describes functional abilities in sitting, walking, and wheeled mobility (Table 7.8). This classification system characterizes motor abilities for children based on child's age: before 2nd birthday, between 2nd and 4th, 4th and 6th, 6th and 12th, and 12th and 18th birthdays. The descriptions for the 6 to 12 and 12 to 18 age range reflect the potential impact of environmental and personal factors on mobility. The GMFCS E&R may be more reliable and valid than other systems because the rater is making a judgment on functional ability rather than trying to classify by neurological symptoms (Beckung & Hagberg, 2000; Bodkin, Robinson, & Perales, 2003; Palisano, Rosenbaum, Bartlett, & Livingston, 2008; Wood & Rosenbaum, 2000).

In addition to the classification systems described above, two other classification systems have been developed to parallel the GMFCS in the areas of hand function and communication. The Manual Ability Classification System (MACS) depicts how children with cerebral palsy utilize their hands in daily activities. The MACS was developed to highlight the importance of hand function for independence in children with CP. The five levels of this scale are based upon the child's need for assistance to perform manual activities in school, leisure, and every day activities. Classificiation Level I indicates the child handles objects easily and successfully and Level V indicates the child does not handle objects and has severely limited ability to perform even simple actions (Eliasson et al., 2006). The Communication Function Classification System (CFCS)

■ **Table 7.8** Gross Motor Function Classification System (GMFCS) Expanded and Revised for Children with Cerebral Palsy. Descriptions and Illustrations for Children Between 6th and 12th Birthday.

Level	Abilities
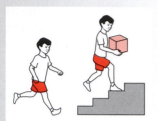	**Level I – Walks without Limitations** Children walk at home, school, outdoors, and in the community. Children are able to walk up and down curbs without physical assistance and stairs without the use of a railing. Children perform gross motor skills such as running and jumping but speed, balance, and coordination are limited. Children may participate in physical activities and sports depending on personal choices and environmental factors.
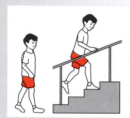	**Level II – Walks with Limitations** Children walk in most settings. Children may experience difficulty walking long distances and balancing on uneven terrain, inclines, in crowded areas, confined spaces or when carrying objects. Children walk up and down stairs holding onto a railing or with physical assistance if there is no railing. Outdoors and in the community, children may walk with physical assistance, a hand-held mobility device, or use wheeled mobility when traveling long distances. Children have at best only minimal ability to perform gross motor skills such as running and jumping. Limitations in performance of gross motor skills may necessitate adaptations to enable participation in physical activities and sports.
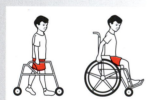	**Level III – Walks Using a Hand-Held Mobility Device** Children walk using a hand-held mobility device in most indoor settings. When seated, children may require a seat belt for pelvic alignment and balance. Sit-to-stand and floor-to-stand transfers require physical assistance of a person or support surface. When traveling long distances, children use some form of wheeled mobility. Children may walk up and down stairs holding onto a railing with supervision or physical assistance. Limitations in walking may necessitate adaptations to enable participation in physical activities and sports.
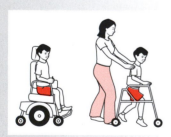	**Level IV – Self-Mobility with Limitations: May Use Power Mobility** Children use methods of mobility that require physical assistance or powered mobility in most settings. Children require adaptive seating for trunk and pelvic control and physical assistance for most transfers. At home, children use floor mobility (roll, creep, or crawl), walk short distances with physical assistance, or use powered mobility. When positioned, children may use a body support walker at home or school. At school, outdoors, and in the community, children are transported in a manual wheelchair or use powered mobility. Limitations in mobility necessitate adaptations to enable participation in physical activities and sports.

Table 7.8 Gross Motor Function Classification System (GMFCS) Expanded and Revised for Children with Cerebral Palsy. Descriptions and Illustrations for Children Between 6th and 12th Birthday.—cont'd

Level	Abilities
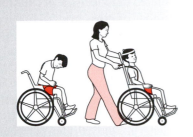	**Level V – Transported in Manual Wheelchair** Children use methods of mobility that require physical assistance or powered mobility in most settings. Children require adaptive seating for trunk and pelvic control and physical assistance for most transfers. At home, children use floor mobility (roll, creep, or crawl), walk short distances with physical assistance, or use powered mobility. When positioned, children may use a body support walker at home or school. At school, outdoors, and in the community, children are transported in a manual wheelchair or use powered mobility. Limitations in mobility necessitate adaptations to enable participation in physical activities and sports.

Source: Palisano, R.J., Rosenbaum, P., Bartlett, D., & Livingston, M. (2007). GMFCS E&R © CanChild Centre for Childhood Disability Research, McMaster University. Expanded version for children before 2nd birthday to 18th birthday available at: http://motorgrowth.canchild.ca/en/GMFCS/resources/GMFCS-ER.pdf Figures adapted from http://motorgrowth.canchild.ca/en/GMFCS/resources/GMFCS6-12-DescriptorsIllustrations.pdf

was developed to determine the communication abilities of children with CP. The five level classification system identifies the following communication roles: sender, receiver, pace of communication, and the degree of familiarity with the communication partner (Hidecker et al., 2011. Classification Level I indicates the child is an effective sender and receiver of communication with unfamiliar and familiar partners and Level V indicates the child is seldom an effective sender and receiver of communication even with familiar partners.

Associated Medical Issues Because of the brain insult, children with CP often have a range of associated issues, including cognitive impairments, behavioral and psychological problems, visual impairments, hearing impairments, sensory impairments, and seizure disorders in addition to the neuromuscular impairments related to motor performance (Imms & Dobb, 2010). The severity and impact of these medical conditions on the child vary depending upon the location and the extent of the injury to the brain. The physical therapist should screen the child for visual, hearing, and cognitive issues during the physical therapy examination and make referrals to appropriate health care professionals for diagnostic testing to determine the extent of these conditions. Visual deficits can influence motor output and can result in activity limitations, so the physical therapist should be aware of this impact.

Therapists need to monitor the occurrences of seizures, protect the child from external injury caused by the involuntary movement associated with the seizure, and watch for respiratory or cardiac problems during the seizure. If seizures are increasing, the child's family and physician should be contacted, because increased brain damage might occur with every seizure. Most seizure disorders are pharmacologically controlled by medications such as Dilantin and Tegretol. Some medications cause the child to appear sedated. Caution should be taken with vestibular stimulation (e.g., swinging, spinning) in children with seizure disorders as this movement might trigger a seizure.

Impairments of Body Structures and Functions Related to Motor Performance The specific motor control impairments of children with CP are variable and correlate to the classification and type of CP. The child may demonstrate timing errors in motor recruitment, including the inability to isolate the activation of specific muscles in a pattern according to postural or voluntary movement demands, called selective voluntary motor control (Sanger, 2006). Children with CP recruit both agonist and antagonist muscle groups at the same time, which limits limb movement and speed (Tedroff, Knutson, Soderberg, 2006). This cocontraction can also be caused by impaired reciprocal inhibition (Damiano, Dodd, & Taylor, 2002). In addition to the inability to isolate certain muscles for activation, the recruitment of motor units is disorderly and slower than normal (Stackhouse, Binder-Macleod, & Lee, 2005; Tammik et al., 2008). Thus, the muscle is not completely activated, which results in decreased force production and weakness. Reinforcement of abnormal neural circuits can occur in children with CP due to the repetitive abnormal movement patterns that exist from birth. This repetitive process influences myelination and, in children with CP who have less movements, can cause a decrease in myelination (Farmer, 2003). Because of some or all of these differences in motor control, the child with CP has abnormal timing and muscle activation patterns. This can cause the (1) initiation of movement to be delayed, (2) rate of force development to be slowed down, (3) muscle contraction time to be prolonged, and (4) timing of agonist to antagonist activation to be disrupted. Extremity movements appear slow and stiff and are coarse. That is, when trying to perform the primary movement, the child might move in mass flexion or extension patterns without being able to dissociate individual limb or joint movements (Sanger, 2006).

Development and use of reactive and anticipatory postural control and postural sway also appear to be delayed and not integrated with the prime movement (Donker, Ledebt, Roerdink, Savelsbergh, & Beek, 2008; Hadders-Algra, Brogen, Katz-Salamon, & Forssberg, 1999). In standing, children with CP may lower their center of gravity by flexing the knees, with the feet in either excessive dorsiflexion or plantar flexion (Lowes, 1996). Children with CP may demonstrate cocontraction or lack of selective voluntary motor control of the lower extremity muscles, particularly in uncoupled patterns such as hip flexion with knee extension, during the gait cycle leading to deficits in gait pattern and speed (Fowler & Goldberg, 2009). The use of ankle and hip strategies depends on the environmental situation, with a preponderance to use proximal muscles first or just show mass cocontraction when perturbed (Hadders-Algra et al., 1999). The biomechanical position alone influences the postural control activity of the child. Children without disability who position themselves in the crouched position will show postural muscle activity similar to that of children with CP when perturbed (Woollacott et al., 1998). Use of ankle-foot orthoses that control the foot position but allow some movement at the ankle (e.g., hinged ankle-foot orthosis) seems to help the child with CP to establish more adaptable coordination patterns for postural control (Figueiredo, Ferreira, Moreira, Kirkwood, & Fetters, 2008; Morris, 2002; Rogozinski, Davids, Davis, Jameson, & Blackhurst, 2009).

Evidence now suggests that weakness, or the inability to produce adequate muscle force, seen in children with CP is attributed both to neural and muscle tissue changes (Lieber et al., 2004; Mockford & Caulton,

2010). These altered muscle tissue changes include loss of type 2 high-force producing fibers with slower twitch type 1 fibers that lead to muscles that produce prolonged low-grade force but can't create fast, high-velocity force (Ito et al., 1996; Mockford & Caulton, 2010). Lengthened sacromeres in the altered muscle tissue of children with CP reduces the number of cross bridges formed and thus decreases the force output (Lieber & Friden, 2002). In addition, shortened muscle bellies contain fewer sacromeres, which limits the force-generating capacity of these spastic muscles (Malaiya et al., 2007). Finally, a reduced muscle cross-sectional area and tightness in the collagen tissues of spastic muscles reduces the force generation (Elder et al., 2003; Friden & Lieber, 2003). These secondary changes further limit movement ability and endurance for activity (Bjornson, Belza, Kartin, Logsdon, & McLaughlin, 2007; Law et al., 2006). Less movement sets up the child for problems with osteoporosis caused by less weight bearing and decreased endurance caused by little activity (Fowler et al., 2007).

These motor issues can be compounded by problems with sensory systems. Proprioception, vision, and vestibular information and the integration of this information to guide movement are often compromised in the child with CP. Therefore, the feedback the child is getting from the movement may be inaccurate, delayed, and/or insufficient for assisting with learning more coordinated movement.

Restrictions in Activities and Participation Since movement control is a problem for children with CP, utilizing a standardized test can help to objectify the child's motor capabilities. Tests to consider when working with children with CP include the Test of Infant Motor Performance (Campbell et al., 2002) for infants 32 weeks' gestation to 4 months corrected age, the Alberta Infant Motor Scale (Piper & Darrah, 1994) for infants up to 18 months of age, the PDMS-2 (Fewell & Folio, 2000) for children 1 month to 6 years of age, the GMFM (Russell et al., 1993), the PEDI (Coster et al., 1994; Haley et al., 1992) for children 6 months to 7.5 years, and the SFA (Coster et al., 1998) for children in grades K–6. The CAPE and the PAC might also be used to measure participation and activity preferences with children 6 to 21 years (King et al., 2004). Refer to the Standardized Assessment of Movement Functions in the beginning of this chapter and in Chapter 3 for a more detailed description of the purpose of each of these tests. Due to immobility and decreased physical activity levels, children with CP also have decreased levels of endurance that can lead to activity and participation restrictions. The 6-minute walk test has been shown to be a valid and reliable measure in assessing the endurance of ambulatory children with CP (Maher, Williams, & Olds, 2008).

Functionally, children with CP have difficulty with maintaining postural control in stationary postures, such as sitting and standing; transitional movements between supine, prone, sit, and stand; functional mobility; and more complex movement and athletic skills. Because balance can be an issue for children with CP, assessment tools that evaluate balance should be considered. The TUG, Berg Balance Scale (BBS), and the PRT have all demonstrated reliability and validity for children with CP; however, only the PRT was able to differentiate between Gross Motor Function Classification Levels (Gan, Tung, Tang, & Wang, 2008).

Children with CP may have oral motor control problems resulting in feeding and speech disorders, which require close collaboration with occupational therapists and speech-language pathologists. Lack of practice with movement can decrease the child's movement experiences and learning opportunities. Because of the diffuse nature of the original lesion, difficulty with motor development may be compounded by the coexistence of intellectual impairments and sensory disorders (visual and/or hearing impairments). Intellectual impairments may affect the child's ability to understand the purpose of intervention and motivation to practice movement. Visual and hearing impairments limit the avenues for communication and community participation.

Potential Interventions The limitations and restrictions that a child with CP might have include the mildest of minor gait deviations to the total inability to move and perform any activity of daily living (ADLs). Therefore, the range of interventions is equally diverse. As always, the physical therapist must coordinate and communicate with all other service providers as a member of an interdisciplinary team serving the needs of the child and family. The therapist will document that communication and the results of interventions. The parents and child will be instructed in an intervention program as appropriate. The family will frequently be instructed in how to maintain ROM, increase strength, and encourage activities and participation within the child's ability levels. The specific procedural interventions to alter the child's motor control, to prevent or improve secondary impairments, to provide adequate sensory feedback to enhance motor learning, and to teach

more flexible and functional motor patterns and skills are discussed in Chapter 8. Because many children with CP also have musculoskeletal and cardiopulmonary limitations, these areas must also be addressed, as presented in Chapters 5, 6, and 9.

Promising interventions, such as strength training in children with CP, have proven to be effective in increasing the strength of the targeted muscle groups and improving the gait and functional capability of the child (Dodd, Taylor, & Graham, 2003; Eagleton, Iams, McDowell, Morrison, & Evans, 2004; Unger, Faure, & Frieg, 2006). In a systematic review of strength training, Mockford and Caulton (2008) found isotonic training to be more effective than isokinetic, with greatest gait and functional improvements in younger rather than older children. However, a recent systematic review of only six studies cautions that muscle strengthening might not be that effective in adolescents with CP who are walking (Scianni, Butler, Ada, & Teixeira-Salmela, 2009).

There are now studies to support the use of constraint-induced movement therapy (CIT) in children having hemiplegic CP. Improvements have been noted in the affected upper extremity function (Charles & Gordon, 2005; Sutcliffe, Gaetz, Logan, Cheyne, & Fehlings, 2007) and gait (Coker, Karakostas, Dodds, & Hsiang, 2010). Intensive treadmill training to improve gross motor function, gait speed, and endurance has also demonstrated some effectiveness in children with CP (Cherng, Liu, Lau, & Hong, 2007; Dodd & Foley, 2007; Mattern-Baxter, Bellamy, & Mansoor, 2009). This may be an important first step in helping children with limited movement abilities learn to stay active and maintain higher levels of fitness to reduce secondary complications of obesity and cardiovascular and pulmonary compromise as they age.

Many children with CP need to use assistive devices for mobility and other aids for ADLs, which are included in Chapters 17 and 18. In addition to assistive and adaptive equipment, the physical therapist may want to consider orthotics as a potential intervention to improve gait kinematics including control of equinus, improved heel-strike at initial contact, reduced knee hyperextension during stance, and increased stride length (Abel, Juhl, Vaughan, & Damiano, 1998; Brunner, Meier, & Ruepp, 1998; Carlson et al., 1997). Although orthotics have shown to improve gait parameters at the body structure level, there are mixed results about the effects at the activity level (Knott & Held, 2002). Interventions are discussed in more detail in Chapter 8, and a case study of a child with

CP from birth to young adulthood is presented in Chapter 19.

Traumatic Brain Injury

Traumatic brain injury (TBI) occurs in more than 1.7 million people every year in the United States, with almost 500,000 visits to emergency rooms a year made by children 0 to 14 years (CDC, 2010). Children (0–4 years) and adolescents (15–19 years) are among the individuals most likely to sustain a TBI (CDC, 2010; Faul, Xu, Wald, & Coronado, 2010). Males were also more likely to be injured than were females, with boys between the ages of 0 to 4 years having the highest rates of TBI-related injuries and deaths (CDC, 2010). About 75% of TBIs are concussions or other forms of mild TBI (CDC, 2003). The injuries can be caused by falls, motor vehicle accidents, sports injuries, and other accidental or intentional blows to the head. The child can receive many musculoskeletal and vital organ injuries concomitant with the blow to the head. No head injury is exactly the same as another. Thus, examination and intervention for children with TBI are variable and complex.

Damage to the brain in closed-head TBI occurs focally, from the point of impact, and diffusely, through the reverberations that occur to the brain within the cranium or shearing forces caused after the initial blow (Geddes, Hackshaw, Vowles, Nickols, & Whitwell, 2001). Ischemic damage can also occur after the initial trauma if the child stops breathing (Geddes et al., 2001). Cerebral edema occurs, caused by biological products leaking from the dead cells, and normal immune system products sent by the body to combat the damage aggregates at the area of injury and can destroy remaining unharmed brain tissue if left uncontrolled. Shunting procedures to relieve intracranial pressure can be used to improve outcomes for the child (De Luca et al., 2000; Downard et al., 2000; Munch et al., 2000).

Pharmacological agents are also used to control postinjury trauma caused by increased intracranial pressure, and later inflammation of tissues. Drug therapies given soon after the injury may reduce swelling and accumulation of toxic products, thus reducing cell damage and ultimately the functional deficit (Hall, Vaishnav, & Mustafa, 2010; Perel et al., 2010). To date, these drug therapies have primarily been used in adults after stroke and TBI (Pradeep, Narotam, & Narendra, 2009; Vink & van den Heuvel, 2010), but use in children is being explored (Natale et al., 2007). Careful monitoring to keep intracranial pressure at a normal level after CNS injury in the premature infant or after TBI in a child is also being shown to promote better functional motor and cognitive outcomes (Wiegand & Richards, 2007).

Associated Medical Issues Because of inactivity during the initial comatose state after the injury, children with TBI can show problems with hypertension. The blood pressure level generally will return to normal with neurological improvement. Brainstem disturbances from the injury may also potentially cause circulatory and ventilatory inefficiency even after the child is mobile. These cardiopulmonary issues should be monitored and controlled for during examination and intervention.

Most children with TBI show some cognitive, emotional, and behavioral control problems during rehabilitation, attributed to the susceptibility of the frontal and temporal lobes to shearing force damage (Kirkwood et al., 2000; Vargha-Khadem, 2001). These problems can include hyperactivity; distractibility, involving poor ability to filter out unimportant sensory stimuli in the environment; and difficulty with auditory and visual perception (Fay et al., 1994). Personality changes may include poor control of frustration and anger and difficulty with social judgment. Some of these problems may be reduced with drug therapies (Hornyak, Nelson, & Hurvitz, 1997). Overall, intellectual levels and memory ability of the child may also decrease from preinjury status (Bowen et al., 1997; Ewing-Cobs et al., 1997), and the child often requires referral for special education programs on return to school.

Impairments of Body Structures and Functions Related to Motor Performance As a result of the injury, the child is generally comatose for a period of time. In general, the longer the child is in a comatose state, the worse the final outcome. A commonly used scale to rate the degree of coma is the Glasgow Coma Scale for adults and children. This scale is easy to administer, is reliable, and a good predictor of outcome (Kirkham, Newton, & Whitehouse, 2006). It measures eye opening, verbal response, and motor response. The eight or ten level adult Rancho Levels of Cognitive Functioning (Hagen, Malkmus, Durham & Bowman, 1979; Hagen, 1998) is a comprehensive scale of cognitive functioning as outlined in Table 7.9.

After the child gains consciousness, varying signs of motor and cognitive problems will be present, depending on the location of focal or diffuse brain damage. Within a relatively short period of time, on average 3 weeks, most, but not all, children with TBI can recover to preinjury functional motor status (Chaplin, Deitz, & Jaffe, 1993). However, cognitive and behavioral

Table 7.9 Rancho Levels of Cognitive Functioning

I	**No Response: Total Assistance** • Complete absence of observable change in behavior when presented with visual, auditory, tactile, proprioceptive, vestibular, or painful stimuli.
II	**Generalized Response: Total Assistance** • Demonstrates generalized reflex response to painful stimuli. • Responds to repeated auditory stimuli with increased or decreased activity. • Responds to external stimuli with physiological changes generalized, gross body movement, and/or not purposeful vocalization. • Responses noted above may be same regardless of type and location of stimulation. • Responses may be significantly delayed.
III	**Localized Response: Total Assistance** • Demonstrates withdrawal or vocalization to painful stimuli; responds to discomfort by pulling tubes or restraints. • Responses directly related to type of stimulus—turns toward or away from auditory stimuli, blinks when strong light crosses visual field, follows moving object passed within visual field. • Responds inconsistently to simple commands, may respond to some persons (especially family and friends) but not to others.
IV	**Confused/Agitated: Maximal Assistance** • Alert and in heightened state of activity. • Purposeful attempts to remove restraints or tubes or crawl out of bed. • May perform motor activities such as sitting, reaching, and walking but without any apparent purpose or upon another's request. • Very brief and usually nonpurposeful moments of sustained alternatives and divided attention. • Absent short-term memory. • May cry out or scream out of proportion to stimulus even after its removal, may exhibit aggressive or flight behavior. • Mood may swing from euphoric to hostile with no apparent relationship to environmental events. • Unable to cooperate with treatment efforts. • Verbalizations are frequently incoherent and/or inappropriate to activity or environment.
V	**Confused, Inappropriate Nonagitated: Maximal Assistance** • Alert, not agitated, but may wander randomly or with a vague intention of going home. • May become agitated in response to external stimulation and/or lack of environmental structure. • Not oriented to person, place, or time. • Frequent brief periods of nonpurposeful sustained attention. • Severely impaired recent memory, with confusion of past and present in reaction to ongoing activity. • Absent goal-directed problem solving, self-monitoring behavior; often demonstrates inappropriate use of objects without external direction. • May be able to perform previously learned tasks when structured and cues provided; unable to learn new information. • Able to respond appropriately to simple commands fairly consistently with external structures and cues. • Responses to simple commands without external structure are random and nonpurposeful in relation to command. • Able to converse on a social, automatic level for brief periods of time when provided external structure and cues. • Verbalizations about present events become inappropriate and confabulatory when external structure and cues are not provided.

Continued

Table 7.9 Rancho Levels of Cognitive Functioning—cont'd

VI	Confused, Appropriate: Moderate Assistance • Inconsistently oriented to person, time, and place. • Able to attend to highly familiar tasks in nondistracting environment for 30 minutes with moderate redirection. • Remote memory has more depth and detail than recent memory. • Vague recognition of some staff. • Able to use assistive memory aide with maximum assistance. • Emerging awareness of appropriate response to self, family, and basic needs. • Moderate assist to problem solve barriers to task completion. • Supervised for old learning (e.g., self care); shows carryover for relearned familiar tasks (e.g., self care). • Maximum assistance for new learning with little or no carryover. • Unaware of impairments, disabilities and safety risks. • Consistently follows simple directions. • Verbal expressions are appropriate in highly familiar and structured situations.
VII	Automatic, Appropriate: Minimal Assistance for Daily Living Skills • Consistently oriented to person and place, within highly familiar environments. Moderate assistance for orientation to time. • Able to attend to highly familiar tasks in a nondistraction environment for at least 30 minutes with minimal assist to complete tasks. • Minimal supervision for new learning; demonstrates carryover of new learning. • Initiates and carries out steps to complete familiar personal and household routine but has shallow recall of what he/she has been doing. • Able to monitor accuracy and completeness of each step in routine personal and household ADLs and modify plan with minimal assistance. • Superficial awareness of his/her condition but unaware of specific impairments and disabilities and the limits they place on his/her ability to safely, accurately and completely carry out his/her household, community, work, and leisure ADLs. • Minimal supervision for safety in routine home and community activities. • Unrealistic planning for the future, unable to think about consequences of a decision or action, overestimates abilities. • Unaware of others' needs and feelings. • Oppositional/uncooperative. • Unable to recognize inappropriate social interaction behavior.
VIII	Purposeful, Appropriate: Stand-By Assistance • Consistently oriented to person, place, and time. • Independently attends to and completes familiar tasks for 1 hour in distracting environments. • Able to recall and integrate past and recent events. • Uses assistive memory devices to recall daily schedule, "to do" lists and record critical information for later use with stand-by assistance. • Initiates and carries out steps to complete familiar personal, household, community, work, and leisure routines with stand-by assistance and can modify the plan when needed with minimal assistance. • Requires no assistance once new tasks/activities are learned. • Aware of and acknowledges impairments and disabilities when they interfere with task completion but requires stand-by assistance to take appropriate corrective action. • Thinks about consequences of a decision or action with minimal assistance. • Overestimates or underestimates abilities.

Table 7.9 Rancho Levels of Cognitive Functioning—cont'd

	• Acknowledges others' needs and feelings and responds appropriately with minimal assistance. • Depressed, irritable, low frustration tolerance/easily angered, argumentative, self-centered. • Uncharacteristically dependent/independent. • Able to recognize and acknowledge inappropriate social interaction behavior while it is occurring and takes corrective action with minimal assistance.
IX	Purposeful, Appropriate: Stand-By Assistance on Request • Independently shifts back and forth between tasks and completes them accurately for at least two consecutive hours. • Uses assistive memory devices to recall daily schedule, "to do" lists and record critical information for later use with assistance when requested. • Initiates and carries out steps to complete familiar personal, household, work, and leisure tasks independently and unfamiliar personal, household, work and leisure tasks with assistance when requested. • Aware of and acknowledges impairments and disabilities when they interfere with task completion and takes appropriate corrective action but requires stand-by assist to anticipate a problem before it occurs and take action to avoid it. • Able to think about consequences of decisions or actions with assistance when requested. • Accurately estimates abilities but requires stand-by assistance to adjust to task demands. • Acknowledges others' needs and feelings and responds appropriately with stand-by assistance. • Depression may continue; may be easily irritable; may have low frustration tolerance. • Able to self-monitor appropriateness of social interaction with stand-by assistance.
X	Purposeful, Appropriate: Modified Independent • Able to handle multiple tasks simultaneously in all environments but may require periodic breaks. • Able to independently procure, create, and maintain own assistive memory devices. • Independently initiates and carries out steps to complete familiar and unfamiliar personal, household, community, work, and leisure tasks but may require more than usual amount of time and/or compensatory strategies to complete them. • Anticipates impact of impairments and disabilities on ability to complete daily living tasks and takes action to avoid problems before they occur but may require more than usual amount of time and/or compensatory strategies. • Able to independently think about consequences of decisions or actions but may require more than usual amount of time and/or compensatory strategies to select the appropriate decision or action. • Accurately estimates abilities and independently adjusts to task demands. • Able to recognize the needs and feelings of others and automatically respond in appropriate manner. • Periodic periods of depression may occur; irritability and low frustration tolerance when sick, fatigued, and/or under emotional stress. • Social interaction behavior is consistently appropriate.

Sources: Hagen, C., Malkmus, D., Durham, P., & Bowman, K. (1979). Levels of cognitive functioning. In Professional Staff Association of Rancho Los Amigos Hospital (Eds.). *Rehabilitation of the Head Injured Adults: Comprehensive Physical Management.* Downey, CA: Rancho Los Amigos Hospital, Inc. Revised 1997; Head Trauma Resources. Retrieved from http://www.head-trauma-resource.com/rancho-los-amigos.htm

differences from the preinjury state often persist throughout the child's life (Barlow, Thomson, Johnson, & Minns, 2005; Gerrard-Morris et al., 2010).

Common impairments of body structures and functions related to movements that the child with TBI may show include spasticity, ataxia, musculoskeletal contractures, paralysis or muscle weakness, and difficulty with increasing speed of movement. These problems affect speech movements as well as other general movements (Chaplin et al., 1993; Haley, Cioffi, Lewin, & Baryza, 1990). Examination and intervention for these impairments can be the same as those used for similar impairments in children with DS and CP.

Postural control problems, specifically ataxia, are common in children with TBI (Haley et al., 1990). The children demonstrate difficulty grading their postural control to the task and environmental constraints. Both sensory and motor systems for postural control are compromised. Specifically, children with TBI who show ataxia generally have slow responses to perturbations, which are potentially caused by vestibular and sensory organization problems (Vatovec, Velikovic, Smid, Brenk, & Zargi, 2001) and the use of too much force (higher amplitude of EMG activity) when they respond. They also show abnormal spatial and temporal coordination of the postural synergies. These coordination problems are hypothesized to be caused by damage of the stored synergy motor programs, possibly in the cerebellum, and secondary musculoskeletal constraints, such as contractures that change the biomechanics of the child's movements.

Restrictions in Activities and Participation Children with TBI can have a variety of limitations in movement that influence activities. These are dependent on concomitant injuries, but in general, they show relatively rapid improvements in ambulation and motor ability to complete ADLs (Chaplin et al., 1993; Haley et al., 1990). Subtle problems with functional movement may be affected by sensory and cognitive problems. Specifically, the child may have difficulty with the cognitive components related to movement, such as focusing attention, understanding verbal directions, and planning motor responses. For example, an automatic motor response of arm movement could be invoked by throwing a ball to the child, causing a functional catching response. The same movement cannot be invoked with a verbal command to reach out. Hypothetically, this occurs because the cognitive planning of the volitional movement is disrupted as a result of frontal lobe damage. However, the lower motor centers (rubrospinal, reticulospinal, and vestibulospinal) can still invoke a normal motor reaction. Higher-level sports-related activities requiring complex motor planning, coordination, and postural control, such as jump-rope games or basketball, may continue to be difficult. Children with TBI also run the risk of becoming sedentary, causing lower levels of fitness. Encouragement to find an activity that the child enjoys will assist in maintenance and improvement of fitness levels.

To assist the therapist in identifying the activity and participation limitations of the child with a TBI, standardized pediatric tests including the PEDI (Coster et al., 1994; Haley et al., 1992) and the WeeFIM (Uniform Data System for Medical Rehabilitation, 2000) may be appropriate. The WeeFIM is a pediatric version of the Functional Independent Measure (FIM) used for adult patients in rehabilitation settings. This test measures a child's ability to perform self-care, sphincter control, transfers, locomotion, communication, and social function. If the physical therapist wants to assess the child's motor development, then the PDMS-2 (Fewell & Folio, 2000) for children 1 month to 6 years of age or the BOT-2 (Bruininks & Bruininks, 2005) for older children ages 4 to 21 years may be appropriate tests, recognizing that these specific tools were developed to evaluate a child's gross and fine motor development as opposed to functional abilities. The CAPE and the PAC might also be used to measure participation and activity preferences with children 6 to 21 years (King et al., 2004).

Potential Interventions The focus of physical therapy interventions when the child is in a comatose state is on prevention of secondary impairments such as contractures. As the child is coming out of the coma, the therapist should request active movement by the child in response to the passive ROM and sensory stimuli. It is commonly believed that sensory stimulation—cutaneous (brushing and tapping), auditory (talking and music), visual (use of lights and bright-colored objects), gustatory (introduction of different tastes—bitter, sweet—to the tongue), and olfactory (introduction of different odors—spices, flower scents—to the nose)—might trigger the child to come out of the coma. However, despite numerous studies showing some promise of sensory stimulation interventions for individuals in coma, more rigorous study is needed to support its effectiveness (Lombardi et al., 2002; Meyer et al., 2010).

Although neurorehabilitation for children after TBI can be rewarding because of the changes in functional ability, the challenges are great, reflecting the complexity of neurological problems related to cognitive ability and behavioral control. The physical therapist must work with the child and family as a team to determine and employ appropriate behavior management strategies.

A structured environment, cues for improving functional memory, and consistency in responses to behavioral outbursts all facilitate the rehabilitation process (Sullivan, 1998). For example, a consistent daily routine should be developed that can be learned by the child. The younger child can have a schedule of activities depicted via pictures. The older child who can read can be given, or be taught to create, a written schedule to improve independent adherence to daily activities. When the child becomes frustrated or angry, consistent consequences should be used by everyone involved with the child. The consequences may range from warnings and then loss of rewards (such as recess or television privileges) to removal of the child from the activity in a "time out" for recomposure and then completion of the task that initially provoked the child.

The social and emotional trauma to the family related to the suddenness and cause of the injury can be a challenge for the therapist in providing family-centered care. The children and their families may suffer from depression and guilt over the accident, making motivation for functional progress difficult. A family's behavior may range from ignoring the differences in the child's ability by requesting behaviors that are too difficult for the child, to overprotecting the child and not allowing him or her to work toward independence. These attitudes can vary day to day as acceptance of the child's new situation develops. Counselors and psychologists can assist when the children or families have continued difficulty moving through the stages of acceptance.

The specific procedural interventions used with the child will depend on the extent of limitations in body structures and functions and restrictions in activities and participation. Children with a TBI have decreased balance capabilities and gait speed as well as increased step length variability compared to typically developing age-matched peers (Katz-Leurer, Rotem, Lewitus, Keren, & Meyer, 2008). Thus, the interventions used for these children might be similar to those used for children with CP or DS. Interventions using motor learning concepts, detailed in Chapter 8, may assist the child to develop better coordination patterns. In addition to considering the type of intervention, the intensity of physical therapy should also be evaluated. Physical therapy intensity in an in-patient rehabilitation hospital was positively correlated to improved scores and minimal clinically important difference on the PEDI (Dumas, Haley, Carey, & Shen, 2004).

Myelodysplasia

Spina bifida, or "split spine," indicates that bony structures of the spinal vertebra fail to close over the posterior aspect of the spinal cord at some level or levels during neurulation, around week 3 or 4 of gestation. **Myelodysplasia** is defined as a displacement of some tissue in a sac that protrudes through this posterior opening of the spinal vertebra. The degree to which neural elements are involved in this protrusion and the level of the spinal cord affected define the severity of the loss of motor and sensory function around and below that level. In meningocele, a sac protrudes at the spinal opening containing spinal fluid and meninges but no neural tissues; thus, lower motor neuron damage is unlikely.

Myelomeningocele (MM) is a condition in which the protruding sac contains spinal fluid, meninges, and neural tissue (Fig. 7.12). Either in utero, or very shortly after birth, the protruding tissue is excised and the spinal opening is surgically closed. The etiology of these defects is unknown but is thought to be a combination of genetics and environment. There appears to be a relationship between inadequate vitamin and folic acid intake and neural tube defects such as MM (Bowman,

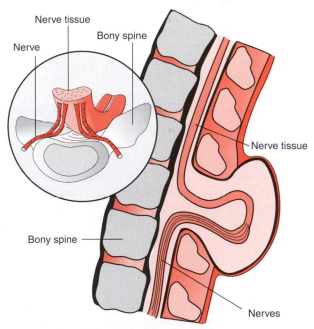

Figure 7.12 Schematic drawing of the myelomeningocele deformity. In this form of myelodysplasia, the sac protruding from the spinal cord contains meninges, spinal fluid, and neural elements, resulting in loss of neural innervation of structures below the level of the sac. *(Redrawn from Gram M.C. [1999]. Myelodysplasia (spina bifida). In S.K. Campbell [Ed.], Decision making in pediatric neurologic physical therapy [p. 201]. Philadelphia: Churchill Livingstone. Redrawn from Meyers, G.J., Cerone, S.B., & Olson, A.L. [1981]. A guide for helping the child with spina bifida [p. 115]. Springfield, IL: Charles C Thomas.)*

Boshnjaku, & McLone, 2009). The open lesions of MM in the fetus can be detected before birth by measurement of the mother's serum alpha-fetoprotein levels, by ultrasound, or more invasively by amniocentesis. This information is used to counsel families. There is a worldwide decline in the prevalence of MM secondary to several factors including folic acid fortification, prenatal diagnosis, and unknown factors (Bowman et al., 2009).

Children with MM have a mixture of lower motor neuron and brain dysfunction that affects motor control, learning, and functional motor ability. The severity of these neuromuscular deficits varies depending on the type and amount of tissue involved in the congenital lesion and on complications such as hydrocephalus. *Associated Medical Issues* In addition to the impairments of the spinal cord, the brain and other internal structures can also be affected in MM. Approximately 51% to 65% of children with myelodysplasia develop **hydrocephalus**, an excessive accumulation of fluid dilating the cerebral ventricles after the primary spinal site is closed, and require shunt placement (Bowman et al., 2009). The main cause of hydrocephalus is a congenital brain malformation known as Arnold-Chiari or Chiari II malformation, where the brainstem is displaced inferiorly beyond the foramen magnum, causing partial blockage of the passage of cerebrospinal fluid (CSF) from the brain to the spinal cord. Excessive CSF then builds up in the ventricles, causing pressure on the CNS tissue that can further compromise brain tissue and development. Hydrocephalus is controlled via placement of a ventricular-peritoneal (VP) shunt, which is a plastic catheter that routes the excess CSF from the ventricles into the peritoneal cavity where it is harmlessly reabsorbed. The VP shunt can become clogged, shift, or become dysfunctional because of growth of the child. Children must be monitored closely for shunt failure and, if it is noted, referred immediately to their physician, since in one group of children the most common cause of death was unrecognized shunt malfunction (Bowman et al., 2009). Signs of shunt failure are described in Table 7.10. Hydrocephalus is the main cause of cognitive deficits in children with MM (Lindquist, Uvebrant, Rehn, & Carlsson, 2009).

Latex allergies are more prevalent in children with myelodysplasia than other pediatric neurologic conditions. Rates of latex allergy in children with myelodysplasia range from 0%–22% (Meeropol, Frost, Puch, Roberts, & Ogden, 1993) or 18%–40% (Majed et al., 2009; Zsolt et al., 1999). This is of significant concern to physical therapists, as some of the equipment that may

---

Table 7.10 Signs of Shunt Malfunction in Children

- Headache
- Irritability
- Fever unrelated to illness
- Nausea
- Increased spasticity in innervated muscles
- Problems with vision
- Problems with speech
- Increased difficulty with postural control
- Decreased performance in school
- Decreased level of consciousness

Sources: Garton, H., Kestle, J., & Drake, J. (2001). Predicting shunt failure on the basis of clinical symptoms and signs in children. *Journal of Neurosurgery, 94*(2), 202–210; Kim, T., Stewart, G., Voth, M., Moynihan, J., & Brown, L. (2006). Signs and symptoms of cerebrospinal fluid shunt malfunction in the pediatric emergency department. *Pediatric Emergency Care, 22*(1), 28–34.

---

be used—balls, wheelchair seats and tires, and braces—contain some type of latex. The biggest concern with latex allergy is the life-threatening condition of anaphylaxis. The physical therapist should educate families to avoid exposure to latex products in the community.

Increased pressure of the CSF over the spinal cord, called hydromyelia, can also occur as a result of the Arnold-Chiari malformation. Increased weakness in the upper extremity muscles, particularly the hands, is common in hydromyelia. For example, the child will not have the strength to button and unbutton clothes. Also, as the child grows and develops, the spinal cord may tether as a result of the development of adhesions or bony spurs at the lesion closure site that do no allow the spinal cord to slide normally. Excessive stretch to the spinal cord can cause metabolic changes and ischemia of neural tissue with degeneration of muscle function (Samuels et al., 2009). Possible signs of tethering might include a change in sensation or continence, inability to perform or difficulty performing tasks that the child was previously capable of performing, spasticity in muscles with sacral nerve roots, development of scoliosis at a young age, and reduced activity level tolerance. Both of these conditions can cause changes in muscle tone and further paralysis of previously innervated muscles. Therefore, innervation levels and other signs of changes in status must be routinely monitored, and the child's physician informed so that surgical treatment can be instituted to prevent further damage and impairment.

Impairments in bowel and bladder control are common because the innervations to these areas are at the sacral level of the spinal cord. Kidney problems may arise from difficulty emptying the bladder. Hydronephrosis occurs as a result of a spastic bladder wall and/or a spastic urethral sphincter. The pressure from this spasticity causes urine to reflux toward the kidney. Earlier in the 20th century, this damage was a major cause of death.

Management of bowel and bladder secretions is critical to prevent the social problems associated with incontinence. Therapists need to assist the child and family with the transfer and fine motor skills needed to manage daily bowel and bladder care. If toileting is not an option, which it may not be for many children, then clean intermittent catheterization (CIC) may be required. This involves inserting a small plastic tube into the bladder to drain urine. Usually CIC is performed every 3 to 4 hours to completely empty the bladder. Predictors of independence for CIC for children between the ages of 5 to 18 years are the ability to remain focused and to walk (Donlau et al., 2010). Socially acceptable continence is achieved by 74% of individuals with MM (Kessler, Lackner, Kiss, Rehder, & Madersbacher, 2006).

Intellectual and visual perceptual deficits may occur in children with MM, especially in children with hydrocephalus. Impairments may be noted in speed of processing, immediate registration (encoding and consolidating of information), learning and memory, organization, and high-level language, with more problems with more complex and less structured tasks. The decrease in cognitive abilities noted over time may reflect difficulty with acquisition of cognitive skills in the expected period. The cumulative pattern of cognitive deficits over time become apparent as the child is expected to be more functionally independent or becomes more challenged with schoolwork (Jacobs, Northam, & Anderson, 2001). Children with MM may also show different verbal abilities with deficits in discourse, characterization, and high frequency of irrelevant utterance in which they tend to "chatter," giving the appearance of understanding (Vachha & Adams, 2009). Therapists need to be aware of these issues to best modify the environment for better learning of motor skills and to provide appropriate exercise programs based on the child's abilities. A robust positive link has been noted between family focus on intellectually and culturally enhancing activities and language performance among children with MM and shunted hydrocephalus (Vachha & Adams, 2009).

Impairments of Body Structures and Functions Related to Motor Performance Depending on the location and severity of the lesion, children with MM may present with impairments in posture, balance and gait, with loss of trunk and leg sensation, decreased upper and lower extremity strength with partial to full paralysis of leg muscles, and orthopedic malalignment caused by muscle imbalances, as well as impairment of bowel and bladder control (Hetherington & Dennis, 1999; Hinderer, Hinderer, & Shurtleff, 2006; Kessler et al., 2006). Motor function in individuals with MM is disordered in a manner similar to cerebellar lesions, and they have similar deficits in predictive cerebellar motor control (Dennis, Salman, Juranek, & Fletcher, 2010).

Lower extremity movements, possible orthotics, and potential for ambulation for children with MM at various spinal levels are summarized in Table 7.11. Some children with thoracic and high-lumbar-level lesions might start walking; less than 20% are still walking by age 9 years. Children with mid-lumbar-level lesions are more likely to start walking, and between 40% and 70% are still walking at 9 years (Williams, Broughton, & Menelaus, 1999). Most children with sacral lesions will reach and maintain functional ambulation with assistive devices and/or orthotics (Antonelli-Greco, Bozovich, & Drnach, 2008; Williams et al., 1999).

Restrictions in Activities and Participation Functional motor limitations include problems with development of independent mobility. The degree of limitation is dependent on the spinal lesion level, cognitive ability of the child, and presence of associated medical issues.

To assist the therapist in identifying the activity and participation limitations of the child with MM, standardized pediatric tests, including the PEDI (Coster et al., 1994; Haley et al., 1992), the WeeFIM (Uniform Data System for Medical Rehabilitation, 2000), and the SFA (Coster et al., 1998) may be appropriate. The CAPE and the PAC might also be used to measure participation and activity preferences with children 6 to 21 years (King et al., 2004). Physical therapists should assess the child's endurance, as ambulation with an assistive device or propulsion with a manual wheelchair will be the child's primary mode of locomotion. The 6-minute walk test or bicycle ergometry are objective endurance tests that may be appropriate.

The social outcomes in adults with MM directly correlate with the level of the lesion. Those with lesions below L3 are more likely to have IQs over 80, walk, be independent, drive, and be employed than those with higher-level lesions (Woodhouse, 2008).

Table 7.11 Orthoses and Mobility Expectations for Children With Myelomeningocele

Spinal Segment	Lower Extremity Movement	Possible Orthotic	Indications	Ambulation
Thoracic	Absent	Trunk-hip-knee-ankle-foot orthosis (THKAF), parapodium	• Upright positioning	Exercise walking only
L1–3	Hip flexion, adduction	Hip-knee-ankle-foot orthosis (HKAFO) Reciprocal gait orthosis RGO	• Unable to maintain an upright posture with hips extended • RGO indicated to facilitate hip extension and swing phase	Short distances in house
L3–4	Knee extension	Knee-ankle-foot orthosis (KAFO)	• Medial and lateral knee instability • Weak quads (grade 4 or less)	Household with limited community
L4–5	Hip abduction Knee flexion Ankle dorsiflexion/inversion Toe extension	Ankle-foot-orthosis (AFO)	• Medial and lateral knee or ankle instability • Insufficient knee extension moment • Lack of or ineffective push-off • Inadequate toe clearance • Crouched gait	Household with limited community
S1–S3	Hip extension Knee flexion Ankle plantar flexion/evertion Toe flexion	Supramalleolar orthosis (SMA) Shoe orthotic	• Prevention of foot deformities or skin breakdown caused by unequal weight distribution • Medial and lateral ankle instability • Poor alignment of subtalar joint, forefoot, or rear foot	Community

Sources: Hinderer, K.A., Hinderer, S.R., Shurtleff, D.B. (2006). Myelodysplasia. In: S.K. Campbell, D.W. Vander Linden, R.J. Palisano (Eds.), *Physical therapy for children* (3rd ed., p. 778). St. Louis: Saunders Elsevier; Antonelli-Greco, C., Bozovich, M.S., Drnach, M. (2008). Practice patterns and pediatrics. In M. Drnach (Ed.), *The clinical practice of pediatric physical therapy* (p. 92). Baltimore: Lippincott Williams & Wilkins.

Potential Interventions Children with MM will have a number of complex surgeries during their first few years of life. During this time, the physical therapist will collaborate with the team of professionals serving the child and family. Based on the extent of neural damage, overall goals for intervention would focus on (1) strengthening innervated muscles and teaching the compensatory patterns of movements and postural control necessary for the child to achieve functional movement, (2) prevention of further musculoskeletal problems (lower extremity contractures, osteoarthritis, scoliosis, kyphosis) or pain, and

(3) prevention of skin breakdown (decubitus ulcers) caused by excessive pressure over bony protuberances as a result of loss of sensation below the level of the lesion. A systematic review of six studies has shown that electrical stimulation, exercise training, and motor skills training lead to improvements in strength in children with MM without adverse effects (Dagenais et al., 2009).

The type of mobility encouraged must be individualized according to the child's and/or family's desires, social issues, the child's energy consumption for different types of mobility, and the child's cognitive development (Franks, Palisano, & Darbee, 1991; Knutson & Clark, 1991; Liptak, Shurtleff, Bloss, Baltus-Hebert, & Manitta, 1992; McDonald, Jaffe, Mosca, & Shurtleff, 1991; Park, Song, Vankoski, Moore, & Dias, 1997). Assistance with early mobility should be encouraged, as studies of children have linked early mobility to development of some cognitive abilities (Katz-Leurer, Weber, Smerling-Kerem, Rottem, & Meyer, 2004). Studies including children with MM have shown that certain cognitive abilities, such as depth perception, cause-and-effect links, and object permanence (in which objects are understood to continue to exist even when out of sight), are learned by infants only if they are able to move around in their environment (Campos, Bertenthal, & Kermoian, 1992).

Based on experience and knowledge of the spinal levels of muscle innervation, basic rules for the type of mobility to recommend for children with MM have been developed (Gram, 1999) (see Table 7.10). Generally, children with lumbar-level lesions should be encouraged to ambulate with appropriate orthoses and assistive devices. Children with higher-level lesions may find this very difficult and rely on wheelchair mobility. Changes in body size, energy expenditure for mobility, postural control, and other needs of children as they grow may also affect the type of mobility needed (Bartonek & Saraste, 2001; Cuddeford et al., 1997). For instance, a child who was able to ambulate with crutches may opt to use a wheelchair when moving into high school to negotiate quickly between classes. Because of the difficulty with mobility, children with MM have a tendency toward being sedentary, becoming obese, and having poor physical fitness. These issues should be addressed by the therapist through general counseling and planning for lifelong fitness programs.

Fewer children with MM now die in infancy and the first few years of life, and the overall outcomes have improved (Bowman et al., 2009). Of children born with MM between 1975 and 1979 and treated at a single U.S. institution, 74% survived into young adulthood (Bowman et al., 2009). The major challenge for these individuals is transitioning to appropriate care in the adult medical community.

Prognosis and Recovery

After the examination of the child and evaluation of the findings, as part of the plan of care, the physical therapist predicts a prognosis for the child in terms of motor function, foreseeing the level of improvement by the end of treatment as well as how long it might take to reach that level of function. For an accurate prognosis, the physical therapist needs to take into account the potential for neuroplasticity and its influence on the overall recovery of the child.

Neural Plasticity

A compelling body of evidence from the basic sciences strongly supports the notion that after injury the CNS is plastic and can change, challenging the original assumption of an irreparable CNS, supporting a paradigm shift from compensation to recovery. Functional outcomes following functional hemispherectomy to control progressive seizure disorders are strong evidence of brain plasticity. This surgical procedure leaves part of the frontal and occipital lobes of the affected hemisphere to support the unaffected hemisphere. All major pathways are cut, with portions of the supporting structures remaining intact.

Hemispherectomy is indicated only when an individual has a seizure disorder uncontrolled by medical intervention. Reported patients' functional recovery posthemispherectomy is convincing (Bates & Zadai, 2003). There is a plethora of information from scientific studies about neural plasticity, and a proper discussion of this important topic is beyond the scope of this chapter and text. A few key principles will be highlighted, and the reader is encouraged to read Johnston (2009), Kleim and Jones (2008), and Levin, Kleim, and Wolf (2009) for a review of the implications of neural plasticity in rehabilitation. As physical therapists, efforts are directed toward capitalizing on neural plasticity, defined as any change in the nervous system that is not periodic and lasts more than a few seconds (Bach-y-Rita, 1990; Held, 1998; Leonard, 1998), to improve motor function.

Habituation is a very short-term change in neurotransmitter release and postsynaptic receptor sensitivity, causing a decreased response to a specific repetitive stimulus. In physical therapy intervention, therapists provide continued activation of sensory pathways to cause habituation. For example, if a child is overly sensitive to touch, the therapist may use a brushing program (continued pressure and light touch activation) to decrease touch sensitivity. Long-term potentiation (LTP) includes a synthesis of proteins to improve synaptic transmission and growth of new synaptic connections. It results in a more easily activated and maintained response of the neural pathways potentiated and is thought to explain learning and memory at the neural level. Therapists try to provoke LTP in children with neuromuscular dysfunction by using practice of motor skills. The potential for recovery of the neural system after injury is the underpinnings of intervention for children with neuromuscular dysfunction. Physical therapy intervention programs, such as focused repetitive practice, constraint-induced therapy, and body weight-supported treadmill training, which incorporate long-term motor learning techniques, have been shown to be effective in altering motor patterns, and possibly reducing secondary effects of hypertonicity (Barry, 1996; Dietz, 1999; Sutcliffe et al., 2007; Pidcock, Garcia, Trovato, Schultz, & Brady, 2009).

Denervation hypersensitivity, synaptic hypereffectiveness, unmasking of silent synapses, and cortical map reorganization all appear to be related to use after the original damage (Held & Pay, 1999; Jenkins & Merzinich, 1992; Liepert, Bauder, Miltner, Taub, & Weiller, 2000; Merzenich & Jenkins, 1993; Morris, Crago, DeLuca, Pidikiti, & Taub, 1997; Nudo, Wise, SiFuentes, & Milliken, 1996; Segal, 1998) and experience in a variety of environments (Held, 1998). This knowledge is transferred to clinical practice by having patients practice motor tasks in different environments to enhance positive changes after damage to the CNS.

The clinical evidence related to forced-use paradigm or constraint-induced movement therapy (CIMT) to improve movement control of the affected limbs can be summarized by the saying "use it or lose it" (Charles, Lavinder, & Gordon, 2001; Coker et al., 2010; DeLuca, Echols, Ramey, & Taub, 2003; Freed, Catlin, Bobo, Fagan, & Moebes, 1999; Sutcliffe et al., 2007; Taub & Wolf, 1997). This intervention approach also supports early intervention for children with brain damage. In contrast with adults, children are not necessarily relearning a motor skill but instead may be learning it for the first time. Therefore, the earliest assistance, guidance, and encouragement to move and experience a variety of environments may be very important for shaping the quality and quantity of later movements (Dobkin, 1998; Guralnick, 1998; Harris, 1998; Majnemer, 1998; Pakula & Palmer, 1998). The

use of virtual environment stimulation to specifically match the sensory and motor capacities of the child to provide the best environmental stimulation promotes cortical reorganization (Latash, 1998c; Rose, Johnson, & Attree, 1997; You et al., 2005). The evidence related to neuroplasticity and walking recovery after a spinal cord injury is also compelling (Behrman, Bowden, & Nair, 2006; Edgerton, 1997).

Finally, it is important to keep in mind that other deficits related to decrease normal function of the areas that assisted with the early recovery may appear later in development, as well as secondary changes in the musculoskeletal tissues. Lack of movement or repetition of specific patterns of movement can alter the developing muscle and skeletal tissue.

Neural plasticity is the basis for learning in the intact brain and relearning after brain damage. It is driven by changes in behavioral, sensory and cognitive experiences (Kleim & Jones, 2008). Restoration and compensation of compromised functions result from brain reorganization (Levin, Kleim, & Wolf, 2009). It is now well accepted that motor training can induce structural and functional adaptation within the brain and spinal cord and that the nature and localization of this plasticity is directly related to the specific motor experience (Adkins, Boychuk, Remple, & Kleim, 2006).

Kleim and Jones (2008) very effectively synthesized principles of plasticity derived from decades of basic neuroscience research that are most relevant to rehabilitation (see Table 7.12):

1. *Use it or lose it*: The lack of use may lead to further deterioration of functions.
2. *Use it and improve it*: Training can improve function and promote plasticity.
3. *Specificity*: The nature of the training dictates the nature of the plasticity; for example, skill training induces synaptogenesis (formation of new synapses and sprouting of new axons terminal, synaptic potentiation), strengthening of existing synapses, and reorganization of movement representations with the motor cortex (cortical remapping), whereas endurance training induces angiogenesis (formation of new blood vessels in the motor cortex), and strength training alters spinal motoneurons excitability and induces synaptogenesis within the spinal cord without altering motor map organization (Adkins et al., 2006).
4. *Repetition* and 5) *Training Intensity*: Matters to induce plasticity.

Table 7.12 Principles of Experience-Dependent Plasticity

Principle	Description
Use it or lose it	Failure to drive specific brain functions can lead to functional degradation.
Use it and improve it	Training that drives a specific brain function can lead to an enhancement of that function.
Specificity	The nature of the training experience dictates the nature of the plasticity.
Repetition matters	Induction of plasticity requires sufficient repetition.
Intensity matters	Induction of plasticity requires sufficient training intensity.
Time matters	Different forms of plasticity occur at different times during training.
Salience matters	The training experience must be sufficiently salient to induce plasticity.
Age matters	Training induced plasticity occurs more readily in younger brains.
Transference	Plasticity in response to one training experience can enhance the acquisition of similar behaviors.
Interference	Plasticity in response to one experience can interfere with the acquisition of other behaviors.

Source: Kleim, J.A., & Jones, T.A. (2008). Principles of experience-dependent neural plasticity: Implications for rehabilitation after brain damage. *Journal of Speech, Language, and Hearing Research, 51*(1), S225–S239.

6. *Time*: Neural plasticity is time-dependent as different forms of plasticity occur at different times.

7. *Salience*: The training must be meaningful to the individual as motivation and attention promote plasticity.

8. *Age*: Although the loss of a few neurons usually does not significantly change functional abilities, the CNS utilizes the inherent redundancy built in the system to accommodate for more severe damage. The fetus initially has an overabundance of neurons. During fetal periods of cellular overabundance, damage from an injury to the nervous system may be reduced. Although it is not the general rule that early brain damage results in greater recovery (Rose et al., 1997), damage to neural tissues during uterine development may have an advantage over similar damage in the infant or adult (Kolb, 1999; Kolb, Forgie, Gibb, Gorny, & Rowntree, 1998; Kolb, Gibb, & Gorny, 2000; Kolb & Whishaw, 1998; Kujala, Alho, & Naatanen, 2000). From birth through adulthood, there are usually several sensory and motor pathways to record similar sensations and generate similar movements. As these neurons synapse with other neurons, there is replication in neuronal projections that are later pruned for increased specificity of neuronal activity (Leonard, 1998).

9. *Transference* and 10) *Interference*: While neural plasticity in response to a specific training experience can enhance the acquisition of similar movement, it may also interfere with learning other tasks (Kleim & Jones, 2008).

Plan of Care

The evaluation, diagnosis, and prognosis should lead to the plan of care and the components of the intervention for children with neuromuscular disorders, as discussed in Chapter 8. Because functional changes in activities and participation are the overall goal of intervention, the intervention should be child-centered and reflect meaningful functional activities for the child or caregiver (Randall & McEwen, 2000).

Summary

The neurological system, from conception, includes some redundancy of neurons and pathways to decrease the effect of injury. Although the neural tissue does not regenerate after injury, there are many ways that functional recovery can occur through maintaining or expanding the capacity of the uninjured neurons and support cells. The primary way to influence the recovery of motor behaviors appears to be through continued use and practice of movements. This represents the basis for early intervention with infants and children immediately after injury or at high risk for later disability. It is recommended that therapists think through the rationale for their examination and intervention and be clear about the perspective that is driving the interventions selected.

DISCUSSION QUESTIONS

1. Which motor control theory is more likely to influence your examination approach to a 5-year-old with a traumatic brain injury? Explain why.

2. What are some ways of preventing neuromuscular disabilities?

3. For a 3-year-old child with DS, CP, TBI, and MM, construct a table to compare and contrast gross motor and social/cognitive/communication expectations with those expected for a typically developing child, and consider what would be appropriate child/family goals, activity goals, motor requirements to accomplish those goals, motor requirements that the child may already demonstrate, and motor requirements that may be missing from the child's movement repertoire.

4. How would your physical therapy examination of a 2-year-old boy with spastic diplegic CP differ from your examination of a 7-year-old girl with DCD?

5. Your employer has decided to do a regular pediatric balance clinic. Draft a thorough intake form that would include testing of all systems involved in postural control.

Recommended Readings

Bhat, A.N., Landa, R.J., Galloway. J.C. (2011). Current perspectives on motor functioning in infants, children, and adults with autism spectrum disorders. *Physical Therapy, 91*(7), 1116-1129.

Kleim, J.A., & Jones, T.A. (2008). Principles of experience-dependent neural plasticity: Implications for rehabilitation after brain damage *Journal of Speech, Language, and Hearing Research, 51*, S225–S239.

Ulrich, B.D. (2010). Opportunities for early intervention based on theory, basic neuroscience, and clinical science. *Physical Therapy, 90*, 1868–1880.

References

Abel, M.F., Juhl, G.A., Vaughan, C.L., & Damiano, D.L. (1998). Gait assessment of fixed ankle-foot orthoses in children with spastic diplegia. *Archives of Physical Medicine and Rehabilitation, 79*, 126–133.

Abrahams, B.S., & Geschwind, D.H. (2008). Advances in autism genetics: On the threshold of a new neurobiology. *Nature Reviews Genetics, 9*(5), 341–55.

Adkins, D.L., Boychuk, J., Remple, M.S., & Kleim, J.A. (2006). Motor training induces experience-specific patterns of plasticity across motor cortex and spinal cord. *Journal of Applied Physiology, 101*, 1776–1782.

Adolph, K.E., & Eppler, M.A. (2002). Flexibility and specificity in infant motor skill acquisition. *Progress in Infancy Research, 2*, 121–167.

Albright, A.L. (2003). Neurosurgical treatment of spasticity and other pediatric movement disorders. *Journal of Child Neurology, 18*(Suppl. 1), S67–S78.

Albright, A.L. (2007). Intrathecal baclofen for childhood hypertonia. *Child's Nervous System, 23*, 971–979.

Albright, A.L., & Ferson, S.S. (2009). Intraventricular baclofen for dystonia: Techniques and outcomes. *Journal of Neurosurgery: Pediatrics, 3*(1), 11–14.

Almeida, G., Corcos, D.M., & Latash, M.L. (1994). Practice and transfer effects during fast single-joint elbow movements in individuals with Down syndrome. *Physical Therapy, 74*, 1000–1016.

American Association on Intellectual and Developmental Disabilities (AAIDD). (2010). *Intellectual disability: Definition, classification, and systems of supports* (11th ed.). Washington, DC: Author.

American Physical Therapy Association (APTA). (2001). Guide to physical therapist practice (2nd ed.). *Physical Therapy, 81*, 1–768.

	Typically Developing	DS	CP	TBI	MM
Gross motor expectations					
Social/cognitive/ communication expectations					
Examples of child/ family goals					
Activity goals					
What abilities does a child need to accomplish these goals? *e.g., strength, ROM, weight shifting, etc.*					
What are the components of the goals that the child may already demonstrate?					
What components of the goals may be missing from the child's movement repertoire?					

American Physical Therapy Association (APTA). (2002). *Interactive Guide to Physical Therapist Practice: With catalog of tests and measures*, Version 1.0. Alexandria, VA: Author.

American Psychiatric Association. (1994). *Diagnostic and statistical manual of mental disorders.* Washington, DC: Author.

American Psychiatric Association. (2000) *Diagnostic and statistical manual of mental disorders (DSM-IV).* Washington, DC: Author.

Antonelli-Greco, C., Bozovich, M.S., & Drnach, M. (2008). Practice patterns and pediatrics. In M. Drnach (Ed.), *The clinical practice of pediatric physical therapy* (p. 92). Baltimore: Lippincott Williams & Wilkins.

Aruin, A.S., & Almeida, G.L. (1997). A coactivation strategy in anticipatory postural adjustments in persons with Down syndrome. *Motor Control, 1,* 178–191.

Aruin, A.S., Almeida, G.L., & Latash, M.L. (1996). Organization of a simple two-joint synergy in individuals with Down syndrome. *American Journal of Mental Retardation, 101,* 256–268.

Atwater, S.W. (1991). Should the normal motor developmental sequence be used as a theoretical model in pediatric physical therapy? In M.J. Lister (Ed.), *Contemporary management of motor problems: Proceedings of the II STEP Conference* (pp. 89–93). Alexandria, VA: Foundation for Physical Therapy.

Aylward, E.H., Habbak, R., Warren, A.C., Pulsifer, M.B., Barta, P.E., Jerram, M., & Pearlson, G.D. (1997). Cerebellar volume in adults with Down syndrome. *Archives of Neurology, 54,* 209–212.

Ayres, A.J. (1979). *Sensory integration and the child.* Los Angeles: Western Psychological Services.

Bach-y-Rita, P. (1990). Brain plasticity as a basis for recovery of function in humans. *Neuropsychologia, 28*(6), 547–554.

Baranek, G.T., Parham, D., & Bodfish, J.W. (2005). Sensory and motor features in autism: Assessment and intervention. In F.R. Volkmar, R. Paul, A. Klin, & D. Cohen (Eds.), *Handbook of autism and pervasive developmental disorders* (Vol. 2, pp. 831–857). Hoboken, NJ: Wiley.

Barlow, K.M., Thomson, E., Johnson, D., & Minns, R.A. (2005). Late neurologic and cognitive sequelae of inflicted traumatic brain injury in infancy. *Pediatrics, 116*(2), e174–e185.

Barry, M.J. (1996). Physical therapy interventions for patients with movement disorders due to cerebral palsy. *Journal of Child Neurology, 11*(Suppl. 1), S51–S60.

Bartlett, D. (1997). Primitive reflexes and early motor development. *Developmental and Behavioral Pediatrics, 18,* 151–157.

Bartlett, D., & Birmingham, T. (2003). Validity and reliability of a Pediatric Reach Test. *Pediatric Physical Therapy, 15,* 84–92.

Bartonek, A., & Saraste, H. (2001). Factors influencing ambulation in myelomeningocele: A cross-sectional study. *Developmental Medicine and Child Neurology, 43,* 253–260.

Bastian, A.J. (1997). Mechanisms of ataxia. *Physical Therapy, 77,* 672–675.

Bates, A.L., & Zadai, C.C. (2003). Acute care physical therapist evaluation and intervention for an adult after right hemispherectomy. *Physical Therapy, 83,* 567–580.

Bayley, N. (1993). *Bayley scales of infant development* (2nd ed.). San Antonio, TX: Psychological Corporation.

Beckung, E., & Hagberg, G. (2000). Correlation between ICIDH handicap code and Gross Motor Classification System in children with cerebral palsy. *Developmental Medicine and Child Neurology, 42,* 669–673.

Behrman, A.L., Bowden, M.G., & Nair, P.M. (2006). Neuroplasticity after spinal cord injury and training: An emerging paradigm shift in rehabilitation and walking recovery. *Physical Therapy, 86,* 1406–1425.

Benedetto, M., Thawinchai, N., Prasertsukdee, S., Tieman, B., O'Brien, M., & Westcott, S. (1999). Reliability and validity of a new assessment tool to measure pediatric functional mobility: A pilot study. *Pediatric Physical Therapy, 11,* 214–215.

Berg, K.O., & Norman, K.E. (1996). Functional assessment of balance and gait. *Clinics in Geriatric Medicine, 12,* 705–723.

Berger, W., Horstmann, G., & Dietz, V. (1984). Tension development and muscle activation in the leg during gait in spastic hemiparesis: Independence of muscle hypertonia and exaggerated stretch reflexes. *Journal of Neurology, Neurosurgery, and Psychiatry, 47,* 1029–1033.

Bernstein, N. (1967). *The coordination and regulation of movement.* London, England: Pergamon Press.

Bjornson, K., Belza, B., Kartin, D., Logsdon, R., & McLaughlin, J.F. (2007). Ambulatory physical activity performance in youth with cerebral palsy and youth who are developing typically. *Physical Therapy, 87,* 248–257.

Blackburn, M., van Vliet, P., & Mockett, S.P. (2002). Reliability of measurements obtained with the Modified Ashworth Scale in the lower extremities of people with stroke. *Physical Therapy, 82,* 25–34.

Blair, L.C. (1999). Assessment of functional balance of a pediatric client using the Berg Balance Test. *Pediatric Physical Therapy, 11,* 225.

Bly, L. (1991). A historical and current view of the basis of neurodevelopmental therapy. *Pediatric Physical Therapy, 3,* 131–135.

Bobath, B. (1964). Facilitation of normal postural reactions and movement in the treatment of cerebral palsy. *Physiotherapy, 50,* 246–262.

Bobath, B. (1985). *Abnormal postural reflex activity caused by brain lesions.* Rockville, MD: Aspen Publishers.

Bobath, K., & Bobath, B. (1984). The neuro-developmental treatment. In D. Scrutton (Ed.), *Management of the motor disorders of children with cerebral palsy* (pp. 6–17). Philadelphia: Lippincott.

Bodkin, A.W., Robinson, C., & Perales, F.P. (2003). Reliability and validity of the gross motor function classification system for cerebral palsy. *Pediatric Physical Therapy, 15*(4), 247–252.

Bohannon, R.W., Harrison, S., & Kinsella-Shaw, J. (2009). Reliability and validity of pendulum test measures of spasticity obtained with the Polhemus tracking system from patients with chronic stroke. *Journal of Neuro Engineering and Rehabilitation, 6,* 30.

Bohannon, R.W., & Smith, M.B. (1987). Interrater reliability of a modified Ashworth scale of muscle spasticity: Suggestion from the field. *Physical Therapy, 65,* 46–47.

Booth, C.M., Cortina-Borja, M.J.F., & Theologis, T.N. (2001). Collagen accumulation in muscles of children with cerebral palsy and correlation with severity of spasticity. *Developmental Medicine and Child Neurology, 43,* 314–320.

Born, P., & Lou, H.C. (1999). Imaging in learning disorders. In K. Whitmore, H. Hart, & G. Willems (Eds.), *A neurodevelopmental approach to specific learning disorders* (pp. 247–258). London: Mac Keith.

Borowski, A., Littleton, A.G., Borkhuu, B., Presedo, A., Shah, S., Dabney, K.W., Lyons, S., McMannus, M., & Miller, F. (2010). Complications of intrathecal baclofen pump therapy in pediatric patients. *Journal of Pediatric Orthopedics, 30*(1), 76–81.

Borowski, A., Shah, S.A., Littleton, A.G., Dabney, K.W., & Miller, F. (2008). Baclofen pump implantation and spinal fusion in children: Techniques and complications. *Spine, 33*(18), 1995–2000.

Bowen, J.M., Clark, E., Bigler, E.D., Gardner, M., Nilsson, D., Gooch, J., & Pompa, J. (1997). Childhood traumatic brain injury: Neuropsychological status at the time of hospital discharge. *Developmental Medicine and Child Neurology, 39*(1), 17–25.

Bowman, R.M., Boshnjaku, V., & McLone, D.G. (2009). The changing incidence of myelomeningocele and its impact on pediatric neurosurgery: A review from the Children's Memorial Hospital. *Child's Nervous System, 25*(7), 801–806.

Boyce, W.F., Gowland, C., Rosenbaum, P.L., Lane, M., Plews, N., Goldsmith, C.H., Russell, D.J., Wright, V., Potter, S., & Harding, D. (1995). The Gross Motor Performance Measure: Validity and responsiveness of a measure of quality of movement. *Physical Therapy, 75*(7), 603–13.

Brochard, S., Lempereur, M., Filipetti, P., & Rémy-Néris, O. (2009). Changes in gait following continuous intrathecal baclofen infusion in ambulant children and young adults with cerebral palsy. *Developmental Neurorehabilitation, 12*(6), 397-405.

Bruininks, R., & Bruininks, D. (2005). *Bruininks-Oseretsky test of motor proficiency* (2nd ed.). Circle Pines, MN: American Guidance Service.

Brunner, R., Meier, G., & Ruepp, T. (1998). Comparison of a stiff and spring-type ankle-foot orthoses to improve gait in spastic hemiplegic children. *Journal of Pediatric Orthopedics, 18*, 719–726.

Brunnstrom, S. (1992). *Movement therapy in hemiplegia* (2nd ed.). Philadelphia: Lippincott.

Burleigh, A., & Horak, F. (1996). Influence of instruction, prediction, and afferent sensory information on the postural organization of step initiation. *Journal of Neurophysiology, 75*, 1619–1627.

Burleigh, A.L., Horak, F.B., & Malouin, F. (1994). Modification of postural responses and step initiation: Evidence for goal-directed postural interactions. *Journal of Neurophysiology, 72*, 2892–2902.

Butler, C., & Darrah, J. (2001). Effects of neurodevelopmental treatment (NDT) for cerebral palsy: An AACPDM evidence report. *Developmental Medicine and Child Neurology, 43*, 778–790.

Cairney, J., Hay, J.A., Faught, B.E., Flouis, A., & Klentou, P. (2007). Developmental coordination disorder and cardiorespiratory fitness in children. *Pediatric Exercise Science, 19*, 20–28.

Cairney, J., Veldhuizen, S., Kurdyak, P., Missiuna, C., Faught, B., & Hay, J. (2007). Evaluating the CSAPPA subscales as potential screening instruments for developmental coordination disorder. *Archives of Diseases in Children, 92*, 987–991.

Campbell, S.K., Kolobe, T.H.A., Wright, B., & Linacre, J.M. (2002). Validity of the Test of Infant Motor Performance for prediction of 6-, 9-, and 12-month scores on the Alberta Infant Motor Scale. *Developmental Medicine and Child Neurology, 44*, 263–272.

Campos, J.J., Bertenthal, B.I., & Kermoian, R. (1992). Early experience and emotional development: The emergence of wariness of heights. *Psychological Science, 3*, 61–64.

Carlson, W.E., Vaughan, C.L., Damiano, D.L., et al. (1997). Orthotic management of gait in spastic diplegia. *American Journal of Physical Medicine and Rehabilitation, 76*, 219–225.

Carswell, A., McColl, M.A., Baptise, S., Law, M., Polatajko, H., & Pollock, M. (2004). The Canadian Occupational Performance Measure: A research and clinical literature review. *Canadian Journal of Occupational Therapy, 71*(4), 210–222.

Carvalho, R.L., & Almeida, G.L. (2009). Assessment of postural adjustments in persons with intellectual disability during balance on the seesaw. *Journal of Intellectual Disability Research, 53*(4), 389–395.

Centers for Disease Control and Prevention (CDC), National Center for Injury Prevention and Control. (2003). *Report to Congress on mild traumatic brain injury in the United States: steps to prevent a serious public health problem.* Atlanta: Author.

Centers for Disease Control and Prevention (CDC). (2009). Prevalence of autism spectrum disorders: Autism and Developmental Disabilities Monitoring Network, United States, 2006. In *Surveillance Summaries,* December 18, 2009. MMWR 2009;58(No. SS-10):1–20.

Centers for Disease Control and Prevention (CDC). (2010). *Injury prevention and control: Traumatic brain injury.* Retrieved from http://www.cdc.gov/traumaticbraininjury/statistics.html

Cermak, S.A., & Larkin, D. (2002). *Developmental coordination disorder.* Albany: Delmar.

Chan, K., Ohlsson, A., Synnes, A., Lee, D.S., Chien, L.Y., & Lee, S.K. (2001). Survival, morbidity, and resource use of infants of 25 weeks' gestational age or less. *American Journal of Obstetrics and Gynecology, 185*(1), 220–226.

Chandler, L., Andrews, M., & Swanson, M. (1980). *Movement assessment of infants.* Rolling Bay, WA: Rolling Bay Press.

Chaplin, D., Deitz, J., & Jaffe, K.M. (1993). Motor performance in children after traumatic brain injury. *Archives of Physical Medicine and Rehabilitation, 74*, 161–164.

Charles, J., & Gordon, A.M. (2005). A critical review of constraint-induced movement therapy and forced use in children with hemiplegia. *Neural Plasticity, 12*(2–3), 245–261.

Charles, J., Lavinder, G., & Gordon, A.M. (2001). Effects of constraint-induced therapy on hand function in children with hemiplegic cerebral palsy. *Pediatric Physical Therapy, 13*, 68–76.

Cherng, R., Liu, C., Lau, T., & Hong, R. (2007). Effect of treadmill training with body weight support on gait and gross motor function in children with spastic cerebral palsy. *American Journal of Rehabilitation and Physical Medicine, 86*, 548–555.

Christiansen, A.S. (2000). Persisting motor control problems in 11- to 12-year-old boys previously diagnosed with deficits in attention, motor control, and perception (DAMP). *Developmental Medicine and Child Neurology, 42*, 4–7.

Clopton, N., Dutton, J., Featherston, T., Grigsby, A., Mobley, J., & Melvin, J. (2005). Interrater and intrarater reliability of the modified Ashworth scale in children with hypertonia. *Pediatric Physical Therapy, 17*(4), 268–274.

Code of Federal Regulations. Title 34: Education. 34 CFR §300.7(b), (c). U.S.C. 1401(3)(A) and (B); 1401(26). Available at http://cfr.vlex.com/vid/300-7-child-with-disability-19761359

Cohen, H. (1999). *Neuroscience for rehabilitation* (2nd ed.). Philadelphia: Lippincott Williams & Wilkins.

Coker, P., Karakostas, T., Dodds, C., & Hsiang, S. (2010). Gait characteristics of children with hemiplegic cerebral palsy before and after modified constraint-induced movement therapy. *Disability and Rehabilitation, 32*(5), 402–408.

Coster, W., Deeney, T., Haltiwanger, J., & Haley, S. (1998). *School function assessment.* San Antonio, TX: Psychological Corporation.

Coster, W.J., Haley, S., & Baryza, M.J. (1994). Functional performance of young children after traumatic brain injury: A 6-month follow-up study. *American Journal of Occupational Therapy, 48*(3), 211–218.

Cowley, P.M., Ploutz-Snyder, L., Baynard, T., Heffernan, K., Jae, S.Y., Hsu, S., Lee, M., Pitetti, K.H., Reiman, M.P., & Fernhall, B. (2010). Physical fitness predicts functional tasks in individuals with Down syndrome. *Medicine and Science in Sports and Exercise, 42*(2), 388–393.

Craven, B.C., & Morris, A.R. (2010). Modified Ashworth scale reliability for measurement of lower extremity spasticity among patients with SCI. *Spinal Cord, 48*(3), 207–213.

Crawford, S.G., Wilson, B.N., & Dewey, D. (2001). Identifying developmental coordination disorder: Consistency between tests. *Physical and Occupational Therapy in Pediatrics, 20*(2–3), 29–50.

Crenna, P. (1998). Spasticity and spastic gait in children with cerebral palsy. *Neuroscience and Biobehavioral Reviews, 22,* 571–578.

Crenna, P. (1999). Pathophysiology of lengthening contractions in human spasticity: A study of the hamstring muscles during locomotion. *Pathophysiology, 5,* 283–297.

Crowe, T.K., Deitz, J.C., Richardson, P.K., & Atwater, S.W. (1990). Interrater reliability of the Clinical Test of Sensory Interaction for Balance. *Physical and Occupational Therapy in Pediatrics, 10,* 1–27.

Cuddeford, T.J., Freeling, R.P., Thomas, S.S., Aiona, M.D., Rex, D., Sirolli, H., Elliott, J., & Magnusson, M. (1997). Energy consumption in children with myelomeningocele: A comparison between reciprocating gait orthosis and hip-knee-ankle-foot orthosis ambulators. *Developmental Medicine and Child Neurology, 39,* 239–242.

Dagenais, L.M., Lahay, E.R., Stueck, K.A., White, E., Williams, L., & Harris, S.R. (2009). Effects of electrical stimulation, exercise training and motor skills training on strength of children with meningomyelocele: A systematic review. *Physical & Occupational Therapy in Pediatrics, 29*(4), 445–463. doi: 10.3109/01942630903246018

Dai, A.I., Wasay, M., & Awan, S. (2008). Botulinum toxin type A with oral baclofen versus oral tizanidine: A nonrandomized pilot comparison in patients with cerebral palsy and spastic equinus foot deformity. *Journal of Child Neurology, 23*(12), 1464–1466.

Damiano, D.L. (1993). Reviewing muscle cocontraction: Is it a developmental, pathological, or motor control issue? *Physical and Occupational Therapy in Pediatrics, 12,* 3–20.

Damiano, D.L., & Abel, M.F. (1998). Functional outcomes of strength training in spastic cerebral palsy. *Archives of Physical Medicine and Rehabilitation, 79,* 119–125.

Damiano, D.L., Dodd, K., & Taylor, N.F. (2002). Should we be testing and training muscle strength in cerebral palsy? *Developmental Medicine and Child Neurology, 44*(1), 68–72.

Damiano, D.L., Martellotta, M.S., Sullivan, D.J., Granata, K.P., & Abel, M.F. (2000). Muscle force production and functional performance in spastic cerebral palsy: Relationship of co-contraction. *Archives of Physical Medicine and Rehabilitation, 81,* 895–900.

Damiano, D.L., Quinlivan, J.M., Owen, B.F., Payne, P., Nelson, K.C., & Abel, M.F. (2002). What does the Ashworth scale really measure and are instrumented measures more valid and precise? *Developmental Medicine and Child Neurology, 44*(2), 112–118.

Dan, B., Motta, F., Vles, J.S.H., Vloeberghs, M., Becher, J.G., Eunson, P., Gautheron, V., Lütjen, S., Mall, V., Pascual-Pascual, S., Pauwels, P., & Røste, G.K. (2010). Consensus on the appropriate use of intrathecal baclofen (ITB) therapy in paediatric spasticity. *European Journal of Paediatric Neurology, 14*(1), 19–28.

Davies, P.L., & Rose, J.D. (2000). Motor skills of typically developing adolescents: Awkwardness or improvement? *Physical and Occupational Therapy in Pediatrics, 20*(1), 19–42.

Deitz, J., Richardson, P.K., Westcott, S.L., & Crowe, T.K. (1996). Performance of children with learning disabilities on the Pediatric Clinical Test of Sensory Interaction for Balance. *Physical and Occupational Therapy in Pediatrics, 16,* 1–21.

Deitz, J.C., Richardson, P.K., Atwater, S.W., & Crowe, T.K. (1991). Performance of normal children on the Pediatric Clinical Test of Sensory Interaction for Balance. *Occupational Therapy Journal of Research, 11,* 336–356.

Delgado, M.R., Hirtz, D., Aisen, M., Ashwal, S., Fehlings, D.L., McLaughlin, J., Morrison, L.A., Shrader, M.W., Tilton, A., & Vargus-Adams, J. (2010). Practice parameter: Pharmacologic treatment of spasticity in children and adolescents with cerebral palsy (an evidence-based review): Report of the Quality Standards Subcommittee of the American Academy of Neurology and the Practice Committee of the Child Neurology Society. *Neurology, 74*(4), 336–343.

Dellavia, C., Pallavera, A., Orlando, F., & Sforza, C. (2009). Postural stability of athletes in Special Olympics. *Perceptual and Motor Skills, 108*(2), 608–622.

De Luca, G.P., Volpin, L., Fornezza, U., Cervellini, P., Zanusso, M., Casentini, L., Curri, D., Piacentino, M., Bozzato, G., & Colombo, F. (2000). The role of decompressive craniectomy in the treatment of uncontrollable post-traumatic intracranial hypertension. *Acta Neurochirurgica, Supplementum, 76,* 401–404.

DeLuca, S.C., Echols, K., Ramey, S.L. & Taub, E. (2003). Pediatric constraint-induced movement therapy for a young child with cerebral palsy: Two episodes of care. *Physical Therapy, 83,* 1003–1013.

Denekla, M. (1974). Development of motor coordination in normal children. *Developmental. Medicine and Child Neurology, 16,* 729–741.

Dennis, M., Salman, M.S., Juranek, J., & Fletcher, J.M. (2010). Cerebellar motor function in spina bifida meningomyelocele. *Cerebellum,* July 22. doi: 10.1007/s12311-010-0191-8.

Dewey, D., Kaplan, B.J., Crawford, S.G., & Wilson, B.N. (2002). Developmental coordination disorder: Associated problems inattention, learning, and psychosocial adjustment. *Human Movement Science, 21*, 905–918.

Dewey, D., & Wilson, B.N. (2001). Developmental coordination disorder: What is it? *Physical and Occupational Therapy in Pediatrics, 20*(2–3), 5–27.

Dichter, C.G., DeCicco, J., Flanagan, S., Hyun, J., & Mongrain, C. (2000). Acquiring skill through intervention in adolescents with Down syndrome. *Pediatric Physical Therapy, 12*, 209.

Dietz, V. (1999). Supraspinal pathways and the development of muscle-tone dysregulation. *Developmental Medicine and Child Neurology, 41*, 708–715.

Dietz, V., & Berger, W. (1995). Cerebral palsy and muscle transformation. *Developmental Medicine and Child Neurology, 37*, 180–184.

Dobkin, B.H. (1998). Activity-dependent learning contributes to motor recovery. *Annals of Neurology, 44*, 158–160.

Dodd, J.D., Taylor, N.F., & Graham, H.K. (2003). A randomized clinical trial of strength training in young people with cerebral palsy. *Developmental Medicine and Child Neurology, 45*, 652–657.

Dodd, K.J., & Foley, S. (2007). Partial body-weight supported treadmill training can improve walking in children with cerebral palsy: A clinical controlled trial. *Developmental Medicine and Child Neurology, 49*, 1010–105.

Dodd, K.J., & Shields, N. (2005). A systematic review of the outcomes of cardiovascular exercise programs for people with Down syndrome. *Archive of Physical Medicine and Rehabilitation, 86*(10), 2051–2058.

Donahoe, B., Turner, D., & Worrell, T. (1994). The use of functional reach as a measurement of balance in boys and girls without disabilities ages 5 to 15 years. *Pediatric Physical Therapy, 6*, 189–193.

Donker, D.F., Ledebt, A., Roerdink, M., Savelsbergh G., & Beek, P.J. (2008). Children with cerebral palsy exhibit greater and more regular postural sway than typically developing children. *Experimental Brain Research, 184*(3), 363–370.

Donlau, M., Imms, C., Mattsson, G.G., Mattsson, S., Sjörs, A., & Falkmer, T. (2010). Children and youth with myelomeningocele's independence in managing clean intermittent catheterization in familiar settings. *Acta Paediatrica*, doi: 10.1111/j.1651-2227.2010. 02044.x. [Epub ahead of print]

Downard, C., Hulka, F., Mullins, R.J., Piatt, J., Chesnut, R., Quint, P., & Mann, N.C. (2000). Relationship of cerebral perfusion pressure and survival in pediatric brain-injured patients. *Journal of Trauma, 49*(4), 654–658.

Dumas, H.M., Haley, S.M., Carey, T.M., & Shen, P. (2004). The relationship between functional mobility and the intensity of physical therapy intervention in children with traumatic brain injury. *Pediatric Physical Therapy, 16*, 157–164.

Duncan, P.W., Weiner, D.K., Chandler, J., & Studenski, S. (1990). Functional reach: A new clinical measure of balance. *Journal of Gerontology, 45*, M192–M197.

Dunn, W. (1999). *Sensory profile*. San Antonio, TX: Pearson.

Eagleton, M., Iams, A., McDowell, J., Morrison, R., & Evans, C. (2004). The effects of strength training on gait in adolescents with cerebral palsy. *Pediatric Physical Therapy, 16*, 22–30.

Edgerton, V.R. (1997). Use-dependent plasticity in spinal stepping and standing. *Advances in Neurology: Neuronal Regeneration, Reorganization, and Repair, 72*, 233–247.

Elder, G.C., Kirk, J., Stewart, G., Cook, K., Weir, D., Marshall, A., & Leahey, L. (2003). Contributing factors to muscle weakness in children with cerebral palsy. *Developmental Medicine Child Neurology, 45*, 542–550.

Eliasson, A.C., Krumlinde-Sundholm, L., Rösblad, B., Beckung, E., Arner, M., Öhrvall, A.M., & Rosenbaum, P. (2006). The Manual Ability Classification System (MACS) for children with cerebral palsy: Scale development and evidence of validity and reliability. *Developmental Medicine Child Neurology, 48*, 549–554.

Engsberg, J.R., Ross, S.A., Collins, D.R., & Park, T.S. (2006). Effect of selective dorsal rhizotomy in the treatment of children with cerebral palsy. *Journal of Neurosurgery: Pediatrics, 105*(Suppl. 1), 8–15.

Engsberg, J.R., Ross, S.A., Collins, D.R., & Park, T.S. (2007). Predicting functional change from preintervention measures in selective dorsal rhizotomy. *Journal of Neurosurgery: Pediatrics, 106*(4), 282–287.

Ewing-Cobbs, L., Fletcher, J.M., Levin, H.S., Francis, D.J., Davidson, K., & Miner, M.E. (1997). Longitudinal neuropsychological outcome in infants and preschoolers with traumatic brain injury. *Journal of the International Neuropsychological Society, 3*, 581–591.

Farmer, S. (2003). Key factors in the development of lower limb coordination: Implications for the acquisition of walking in children with cerebral palsy. *Disability Rehabilitation, 25*, 807–816.

Faul, M., Xu, L., Wald, M.M., & Coronado, V.G. (2010). *Traumatic brain injury in the United States: Emergency department visits, hospitalizations, and deaths.* Atlanta: Centers for Disease Control and Prevention, National Center for Injury Prevention and Control.

Fay, G.C., Jaffe, K.M., Polissar, N.L., Liao, S., Rivara, J.B., & Martin, K.M. (1994). Outcome of pediatric traumatic brain injury at three years: A cohort study. *Archives of Physical Medicine and Rehabilitation, 75*, 733–741.

Feldman, B.M., Ayling-Campos, A., Luy, L., Stevens, D., Silverman, E.D., & Laxer, R.M. (1995). Measuring disability in juvenile dermatomyositis: Validity of the Childhood Health Assessment Questionnaire. *Journal of Rheumatology, 22*, 326–331.

Fellows, S.J., Kaus, C., & Thilmann, A.F. (1994). Voluntary movement at the elbow in spastic hemiparesis. *Annals of Neurology, 36*, 397–407.

Fernhall, B., & Pitetti, K.H. (2001). Limitations to physical work capacity in individuals with mental retardation. *Clinical Exercise Physiology, 3*, 76–85.

Fetters, L., & Kluzik, J. (1996). The effects of neurodevelopmental treatment versus practice on the reaching of children with spastic cerebral palsy. *Physical Therapy, 76*(4), 346–358.

Fewell, R., & Folio, R. (2000). *Peabody Developmental Motor Scale* (2nd ed.). Austin, TX: Pro-Ed.

Figueiredo, E.M., Ferreira, G.B., Moreira, R., Kirkwood, R.N., & Fetters, L. (2008) Efficacy of ankle-foot orthoses on gait of children with cerebral palsy: Systematic review of literature. *Pediatric Physical Therapy, 20*(3), 207–223.

Filipek, P.A., Accardo, P.J., Baranek, G.T. et al. (1999). The screening and diagnosis of autistic spectrum disorders. *Journal of Autism and Developmental Disorders, 29*(6), 439–84.

Finch, E., Brooks, D., Stratford, P.W., & Mayo, N.E. (2002). *Physical rehabilitation outcome measures: A guide to enhanced clinical decision making*. (2nd ed.). Philadelphia: Lippincott Williams & Wilkins.

Fowler, E.G., & Goldberg, E.J. (2009). The effect of lower extremity selective voluntary motor control on interjoint coordination during gait in children with spastic diplegic cerebral palsy. *Gait Posture, 29*(1), 102–107.

Fowler, E., Kolobe, T., Damiano, D., Thorpe, D.E., Morgan, D.W., Brunstrom, J.E., Coster, W.J., Henderson, R.C., Ptetti, K.H., Rimmer, J.H., Rose, J., & Stevenson, R.T. (2007). Promotion of physical fitness and prevention of secondary conditions for children with cerebral palsy: Section on pediatrics research summit proceedings. *Physical Therapy, 87*, 1495–1510.

Fowler, E.G., Nwigwe, A.I., & Ho, T.W. (2000). Sensitivity of the pendulum test for assessing spasticity in persons with cerebral palsy. *Developmental Medicine and Child Neurology, 42*(3), 182–189.

Fox, A.M., & Lent, B. (1996). Clumsy children. Primer on developmental coordination disorder. *Canadian Family Physician, 42*, 1965–1971.

Franjoine, M.R., Gunther, J.S., & Taylor, M.J. (2003). The pediatric balance scale: A modified version of the Berg Scale for children with mild to moderate motor impairment. *Pediatric Physical Therapy, 15*(2), 114–128.

Franks, C.A., Palisano, R.J., & Darbee, J.C. (1991). The effect of walking with an assistive device and using a wheelchair on school performance in students with myelomeningocele. *Physical Therapy, 71*, 570–578.

Freed, S.S., Catlin, P.A., Bobo, L.M., Fagan, E.L., & Moebes, M.N. (1999). The effect of constraint-induced movement on upper extremity function in children with hemiplegia. *Pediatric Physical Therapy, 11*, 226–227.

Freeman, S.B., Taft, L.F., Dooley, K.J., Allran, K., Sherman, S.L., Hassold, T.J., Khoury, M.J., & Saker, D.M. (1998). Population-based study of congenital heart defects in Down syndrome. *American Journal of Medical Genetics, 80*(3), 213–217.

Friden, J., Lieber, R. (2003). Spastic muscle cells are shorter and stiffer than normal cells. *Muscle Nerve, 26*, 157–164.

Fuchs, A.F., Anderson, M.E., Binder, M.D., & Fetz, E.E. (1989). The neural control of movement. In H.D. Patton, A.F. Fuchs, B. Hille, A.M. Scher, & R. Steiner (Eds.), *Textbook of physiology: Excitable cells and neurophysiology,* (Vol. 1, pp. 503–509). Philadelphia: W.B. Saunders.

Gagnon, I., Swaine, B., & Forget, R. (2006). Exploring the comparability of the Sensory Organization Test and the Pediatric Clinical Test of Sensory Interaction for Balance in children. *Physical and Occupational Therapy in Pediatrics, 26*(1–2), 23–41.

Gan, S., Tung, L., Tang, Y., & Wang, C. (2008). Psychometric properties of functional balance assessment in children with cerebral palsy. *Neurorehabilitation & Neural Repair, 22*(6), 745–753.

Garton, H., Kestle, J., & Drake, J. (2001). Predicting shunt failure on the basis of clinical symptoms and signs in children. *Journal of Neurosurgery, 94*(2), 202–210.

Geddes, J.F., Hackshaw, A.K., Vowles, G.H., Nickols, C.D., & Whitwell, H.L. (2001). Neuropathology of inflicted head injury in children. I. Patterns of brain damage. *Brain, 124*(7), 1290–1298.

Geerdink, J.J., Hopkins, B., Beek, W.J., & Heriza, C.B. (1996). The organization of leg movements in preterm and full-term infants after term age. *Developmental Psychobiology, 29*(4), 335–351.

Geldhof, E., Cardon, G., De Bourdeaudhuij, I., Danneels, L., Coorevits, P., Vanderstraeten, G., & De Clercq, D. (2006). Static and dynamic standing balance: test-retest reliability and reference values in 9 to 10 year old children. *European Journal of Pediatrics, 165*(11), 779–786.

Gerrard-Morris, A., Taylor, H.G., Yeates, K.O., Walz, N.C., Stancin, T., Minich, N., & Wade, S.L. (2010). Cognitive development after traumatic brain injury in young children. *Journal of the International Neuropsychological Society, 16*, 157–168.

Geschwind, D.H. (2009). Advances in autism. *Annual Review of Medicine, 60*, 367–80.

Gesell, A. (1945). *The embryology of behavior* (p. 169). New York: Harper.

Gillberg, C. (1999). Management of behavioral problems in specific learning disorders. In K. Whitmore, H. Hart, & G. Willems (Eds.), *A Neurodevelopmental approach to specific learning disorders* (pp. 270–279). London: Mac Keith.

Giuliani, C.A. (1991). Dorsal rhizotomy for children with cerebral palsy: Support for concepts of motor control. *Physical Therapy, 71*, 248–259.

Goldstein, E.M. (2006). Safety of high-dose botulinum toxin type A therapy for the treatment of pediatric spasticity. *Journal of Child Neurology, 21*(3), 189–192. doi: 10.2310/7010.2006.00041

Gottlieb, G.L., Corcos, D.M., & Agarwal, G.C. (1989). Strategies for the control of voluntary movements with one mechanical degree of freedom. *Behavior and Brain Science, 12*, 189–250.

Graham, A., & Reid, G. (2000). Physical fitness of adults with an intellectual disability: A 13-year follow-up study. *Research Quarterly for Exercise and Sport, 71*, 152–161.

Graham, H.K. (2000). Pendulum test in cerebral palsy. *The Lancet, 355*, 2184.

Gram, M.C. (1999). Myelodysplasia (spina bifida). In S.K. Campbell (Ed.), *Decision making in pediatric neurologic physical therapy* (pp. 198–234). Philadelphia: Churchill Livingstone.

Graubert, C., Song, K.M., McLaughlin, J.F., & Bjornson, K. (2000). Changes in gait at 1-year post-selective dorsal rhizotomy: Results of a prospective randomized study. *Journal of Pediatric Orthopaedics, 20*(4), 496–500.

Gubbay, S.S. (1975). *The clumsy child: A study of developmental apraxia and agnosticataxia*. London: W.B. Saunders.

Guettard, E., Roze, E., Abada, G., Lemesle, C., Vidailhet, M., Laurent-Vannier, A., & Chevignard, M.P. (2009). Management of spasticity and dystonia in children with acquired brain injury with rehabilitation and botulinum toxin A. *Developmental Neurorehabilitation, 12*(3), 128–138.

Guralnick, M.J. (1998). Effectiveness of early intervention for vulnerable children: A developmental perspective. *American Journal of Mental Retardation, 102*(4), 319–345.

Habib, Z., & Westcott, S. (1998). Assessment of anthropometric factors on balance tests in children. *Pediatric Physical Therapy, 10*, 101–109.

Habib, Z., Westcott, S.L., & Valvano, J. (1999). Assessment of dynamic balance abilities in Pakistani children age 5–13 years. *Pediatric Physical Therapy, 11*, 73–82.

Hadders-Algra, M. (2000). The neuronal group selection theory: Promising principles for understanding and treating developmental motor disorders. *Developmental Medicine and Child Neurology, 42,* 707–715.

Hadders-Algra, M., Brogren, E., & Forssberg, H. (1996). Ontogeny of postural adjustments during sitting in infancy: Variation, selection, and modulation. *Journal of Physiology (London), 493,* 273–288.

Hadders-Algra, M., Brogren, E., & Forssberg, H. (1998). Postural adjustments during sitting at preschool age: Presence of a transient toddling phase. *Developmental Medicine and Child Neurology, 40,* 436–447.

Hadders-Algra, M., Brogren, E., Katz-Salamon, M., & Forssberg, H. (1999). Periventricular leukomalacia and preterm birth have different detrimental effects on postural adjustments. *Brain, 122,* 727–740.

Hadders-Algra, M., & Lindahl, E. (1999). Pre- and perinatal precursors of specific learning disorders. In K. Whitmore, H. Hart, & G. Willems (Eds.), *A neurodevelopmental approach to specific learning disorders* (pp. 166–190). London: Mac Keith.

Hagen, C. (1998). *Revised Rancho Levels of Cognitive Functioning.* Downey, CA: Rancho Los Amigos Hospital.

Hagen, C., Malkmus, D., Durham, P., & Bowman, K. (1979). Levels of cognitive functioning. In Professional Staff Association of Rancho Los Amigos Hospital (Eds.), *Rehabilitation of the head injured adults: Comprehensive physical management.* Downey, CA: Rancho Los Amigos Hospital.

Haley, S.M. (1986). Postural reactions in infants with Down syndrome: Relationship to motor milestone development and age. *Physical Therapy, 66,* 17–22.

Haley, S.M., Cioffi, M.I., Lewin, J.E., & Baryza, M.J. (1990). Motor dysfunction in children and adolescents after traumatic brain injury. *Journal of Head Trauma Rehabilitation, 5,* 77–90.

Haley, S.M., Coster, W.J., Ludlow, L.H., Haltiwanger, J.T., & Andrellas, P.J. (1992). *Pediatric Evaluation of Disability Inventory.* Boston: PEDI Research Group.

Hall, E.D., Vaishnav, R., & Mustafa, A.G. (2010). Antioxidant therapies for traumatic brain injury. *Neurotherapeutics, 7*(1), 1–61.

Harris, S.R. (1998). The effectiveness of early intervention for children with cerebral palsy and related motor disorders. In M.J. Guralnick (Ed.), *The effectiveness of early intervention* (pp. 327–347). Baltimore: Paul H. Brookes.

Harris, S.R., & Daniels, L.E. (2001). Reliability and validity of the Harris Infant Neuromotor Test. *Journal of Pediatrics, 139*(2), 249–253.

Harris, S.R., & Shea, A.M. (1991). Down syndrome. In S.K. Campbell (Ed.), *Pediatric neurologic physical therapy* (2nd ed., pp. 131–168). New York: Churchill Livingstone.

Hay, J.A., Hawes, R., & Faught, B.E. (2004). Evaluation of a screening instrument for developmental coordination disorder. *Journal of Adolescent Health, 34,* 308–313.

Hay, L., & Redon, C. (1999). Feedforward versus feedback control in children and adults subjected to a postural disturbance. *Experimental Brain Research, 125,* 153–162.

Hayes, A., & Batshaw, M.L. (1993). Down syndrome. *Pediatric Clinics of North America, 40*(3), 523–535.

Held, J.M. (1998). Environmental enrichment enhances sparing and recovery of function following brain damage. *Neurology Report, 22,* 74–78.

Held, J.M., & Pay, T. (1999). Recovery of function after brain damage. In H. Cohen (Ed.), *Neuroscience for rehabilitation* (2nd ed., pp. 419–439). Philadelphia: Lippincott Williams & Wilkins.

Helders, P.J.M. (2010). Variability in childhood development. *Physical Therapy, 90*(12), 1708–1709.

Henderson, S.E., Rose, P., & Henderson, S. (1992). Reaction time and movement time in children with developmental coordination disorder. *Journal of Child Psychology and Psychiatry, 33,* 895–905.

Henderson, S.E., & Sugden, D. (2007). *Movement assessment battery for children* (2nd ed.). San Antonio, TX: Pearson.

Heriza, C. (1991a). Motor development: Traditional and contemporary theories. In M.J. Lister (Ed.), *Contemporary management of motor problems: Proceedings of the II STEP Conference* (pp. 99–126). Alexandria, VA: Foundation for Physical Therapy.

Heriza, C.B. (1991b). Implications of a dynamical systems approach to understanding infant kicking behavior. *Physical Therapy, 71*(3), 222–235.

Hetherington, R., & Dennis, M. (1999). Motor function profile in children with early onset hydrocephalus. *Developmental Neuropsychology, 15*(1), 25–51.

Hidecker, M., Paneth, N., Rosenbaum, P, Kent, R., Lillie, J., Eulenberg, J, Chester, K., Johnson, B., Michalsen, L., Evatt, M., & Taylor, K. (2011). Developing and validating the Communication Function Classification System (CFCS) for individuals with cerebral palsy. *Developmental Medicine and Child Neurology, 53*(8), 704–710.

Hillier, S. (2007). Intervention for children with developmental coordination disorder: A systematic review. *Internet Journal of Allied Health Sciences and Practice, 5*(3), 1–11.

Hillier, S., McIntyre, A., & Plummer, L. (2010). Aquatic physical therapy for children with developmental coordination disorder: A pilot randomized controlled trial. *Physical & Occupational Therapy in Pediatrics, 30*(2), 111–124.

Hinderer, K.A., Hinderer, S.R., & Shurtleff, D.B. (2006). Myelodysplasia. In S.K. Campbell, D.W. Vander Linden, & R.J. Palisano (Eds.), *Physical therapy for children* (3rd ed., pp. 735–789). St. Louis: Saunders Elsevier.

Hoare, B.J., Wallen, M.A., Imms, C., Villanueva, E., Rawicki, H.B., & Carey, L. (2010). Botulinum toxin A as an adjunct to treatment in the management of the upper limb in children with spastic cerebral palsy (UPDATE). *Cochrane Database of Systematic Reviews (Online),* (1), CD003469.

Hodges, N.J., Hayes, S., Horn, R., Williams, A.M. (2005). Changes in coordination, control and outcome as a result of extended practice on a novel motor skill. *Ergonomics, 48,* 1672–1685.

Holt, K.G., Butcher, R., & Fonseca, S. (2000). Limb stiffness in active leg swinging of children with spastic hemiplegic cerebral palsy. *Pediatric Physical Therapy, 12,* 50–61.

Horak, F.B. (1991). Assumptions underlying motor control for neurological rehabilitation. In M.J. Lister (Ed.), *Contemporary management of motor problems: Proceedings of the II STEP Conference* (pp. 11–28). Alexandria, VA: Foundation for Physical Therapy.

Horak, F.B. (1992). Motor control models underlying neurologic rehabilitation of posture in children. In H. Forssberg & H. Hirschfeld (Eds.), *Movement disorders in children* (pp. 21–30). Basel: Karger.

Horak, F.B., & Diener, H.C. (1994). Cerebellar control of postural scaling and central set in stance. *Journal of Neurophysiology, 72*, 479–493.

Horak, F.B., Diener, H.C., & Nashner, L.M. (1989). Influence of central set on human postural responses. *Journal of Neurophysiology, 62*, 841–853.

Horak, F.B., & Nashner, L.M. (1986). Central programming of postural movements: Adaptation to altered support configurations. *Journal of Neurophysiology, 55*, 1369–1381.

Horak, F.B., Shumway-Cook, A., Crowe, T.K., & Black, F.O. (1988). Vestibular function and motor proficiency of children with impaired hearing, or with learning disability and motor impairments. *Developmental Medicine and Child Neurology, 30*, 64–79.

Hornyak, J.E., Nelson, V.S., & Hurvitz, E.A. (1997). The use of methylphenidate in paediatric traumatic brain injury. *Pediatric Rehabilitation, 1*, 15–17.

Houk, J.C. (1979). Regulation of stiffness by skeletomotor reflexes. *Annual Reviews in Physiology, 41*, 99–114.

Hresko, M.T., McCarthy, J.C., & Goldberg, M.J. (1993). Hip disease in adults with Down syndrome. *Journal of Bone and Joint Surgery, British Volume, 75*(4), 604–607.

Hung, W.W. & Pang, M.Y. (2010). Effects of group-based versus individual-based exercise training on motor performance in children with developmental coordination disorder: A randomized controlled study. *Journal of Rehabilitation Medicine, 42*(2): 122–128.

Hwang, J., Davies, P.L., Taylor, M.P., & Gavin, W.J. (2002). Validation of School Function Assessment with elementary school children. *Occupational Therapy Research Journal: Occupation, Participation & Health, 22*(2), 48–58.

Imms, C., & Dodd, K.J. (2010). What is cerebral palsy? In K.J. Dodd, C. Imms, & N.F. Taylor (Eds.), *Physiotherapy and occupational therapy for people with cerebral palsy: A problem-based approach to assessment and management* (pp. 7–29). London: Mac Keith.

Inglis, J.T., Horak, F.B., Shupert, C.L., & Jones-Rycewicz, C. (1994). The importance of somatosensory information in triggering and scaling automatic postural responses in humans. *Experimental Brain Research, 101*(1), 159–164.

Inui, N., Yamanishi, M., & Tada, S. (1995). Simple reaction times and timing of serial reactions of adolescents with mental retardation, autism, and Down syndrome. *Perceptual Motor Skills, 81*(3 Pt 1), 739–745.

Ito, J., Araki, A., Tanaka, H., Tasaki, T., Cho, K., & Yamazaki, R. (1996). Muscle histopathology in spastic cerebral palsy. *Brain Development, 18*, 299–303.

Iyer, M.B., Mitz, A.R., & Winstein, C. (1999). Motor 1: Lower centers. In H. Cohen (Ed.), *Neuroscience for rehabilitation* (2nd ed., pp. 209–242). Philadelphia: Lippincott Williams & Wilkins.

Jackson, J.H., & Taylor J. (1932). *Selected writings of John B. Hughlings, I and II.* London: Hodder & Stoughter.

Jacobs, R., Northam, E., & Anderson, V. (2001). Cognitive outcome in children with myelomeningocele and perinatal hydrocephalus: a longitudinal perspective. *Journal of Developmental and Physical Disability, 13*(4), 389–405.

Jansiewicz, E.M., Goldberg, M.C., Newschaffer, C.J., Denckla, M.B., Landa, R., & Mostfsky, S.H. (2006). Motor signs distinguish children with high functioning autism and Asperger's syndrome from controls. *Journal of Autism and Developmental Disorders, 36*, 613–621.

Jenkins, W.M., & Merzinich, M.M. (1992). Cortical representational plasticity: Some implications for the bases of recovery from brain damage. In N. von Steinibuchel, D.Y. von Cramon, & E. Poppel (Eds.), *Neuropsychological rehabilitation* (pp. 20–35). Berlin: Springer-Verlag.

Johnson, R.K., Goran, M.I., Ferrara, M.S., & Poehlman, E.T. (1996). Athetosis increases resting metabolic rate in adults with cerebral palsy. *Journal of the American Dietetic Association, 96*(2), 145–148.

Johnston, M.W. (2009). Plasticity in the developing brain: Implications for rehabilitation. *Developmental Disabilities Research Reviews, 15*, 94–101.

Kadesjö, B., & Gillberg, C. (2001). The comorbidity of ADHD in the general population of Swedish school-age children. *Journal of Child Psychology and Psychiatry, 42*, 487–492.

Kan, P., Gooch, J., Amini, A., Ploeger, D., Grams, B., Oberg, W., Simonsen, S., Walker, M., & Kestle, J. (2008). Surgical treatment of spasticity in children: Comparison of selective dorsal rhizotomy and intrathecal baclofen pump implantation. *Child's Nervous System, 24*(2), 239–243.

Kane, K., & Bell, A. (2009). A core stability group program for children with developmental coordination disorder: 3 clinical case reports. *Pediatric Physical Therapy, 21*(4), 375–382.

Katz-Leurer, M., Rotem, H., Lewitus, H., Keren, O., & Meyer, S. (2008). Relationship between balance abilities and gait characteristics in children with post-traumatic brain injury. *Brain Injury, 22*(2), 153–159.

Katz-Leurer, M., Weber, C., Smerling-Kerem, Rottem, H., & Meyer, S. (2004). Prescribing the reciprocal gait orthosis for myelomeningocele children: A different approach and clinical outcome. *Pediatric Rehabilitation, 7*(2), 105–109.

Kelso, J.A.S. (1995). *Dynamic patterns: The self-organization of brain and behavior.* Cambridge, MA: MIT Press.

Kessler, T.M., Lackner, J., Kiss, G., Rehder, P., & Madersbacher, H. (2006). Predictive value of initial urodynamic pattern on urinary continence in patients with myelomeningocele. *Neurourology and Urodynamics, 25*(4), 361–367.

Kim, T., Stewart, G., Voth, M., Moynihan, J., & Brown, L. (2006). Signs and symptoms of cerebrospinal fluid shunt malfunction in the pediatric emergency department. *Pediatric Emergency Care, 22*(1), 28–34.

King, G., Law, M., King, S., Hurley, P., Rosenbaum, P., Hanna, S., Kertoy, M., & Young, N. (2004). *Children's Assessment of Participation and Enjoyment & Preferences for Activities of Children manual.* San Antonio, TX: Pearson.

Kirkham, F.J., Newton, C.R.J.C., & Whitehouse, W. (2008). Paediatric coma scales. *Developmental Medicine and Child Neurology, 50*(4), 267–274.

Kirkwood, M., Janusz, J., Yeates, K.O., Taylor, H.G., Wade, S.L., Stancin, T., & Drotar, D. (2000). Prevalence and correlates of depressive symptoms following traumatic brain injuries in children. *Child Neuropsychology* (*Neuropsychology, Development and Cognition: Section C*), *6*(3), 195–208.

Kleim, J.A., & Jones, T.A. (2008*).* Principles of experience-dependent neural plasticity: Implications for rehabilitation after brain damage *Journal of Speech, Language, and Hearing Research, 51*, S225–S239.

Knott, K.M., & Held, S.L. (2002). Effects of orthoses on upright functional skills of children and adolescents with cerebral palsy. *Pediatric Physical Therapy*, 14, 199–207.

Knott, M., & Voss, D. (1968). *Proprioceptive neuromuscular facilitation*. New York: Harper & Row.

Knutson, L.M., & Clark, D.E. (1991). Orthotic devices for ambulation in children with cerebral palsy and myelomeningocele. *Physical Therapy*, 71, 947–960.

Kokubun, M. (1999). The relationship between the effect of setting a goal on standing broad jump performance and behaviour regulation ability in children with intellectual disability. *Journal of Intellectual Disability Research*, 43(Pt 1), 13–18.

Kokubun, M., Shinmyo, T., Ogita, M., Morita, K., Furuta, M., Haishi, K., Okuzumi, H., & Koike, T. (1997). Comparison of postural control of children with Down syndrome and those with other forms of mental retardation. *Perceptual Motor Skills*, 84(2), 499–504.

Kolb, B. (1999). Synaptic plasticity and the organization of behaviour after early and late brain injury. *Canadian Journal of Experimental Psychology*, 53(1), 62–76.

Kolb, B., Forgie, M., Gibb, R., Gorny, G., & Rowntree, S. (1998). Age, experience and the changing brain. *Neuroscience and Biobehavioral Reviews*, 22(2), 143–159.

Kolb, B., Gibb, R., & Gorny, G. (2000). Cortical plasticity and the development of behavior after early frontal cortical injury. *Developmental Neuropsychology*, 18(3), 423–444.

Kolb, B., & Whishaw, I.Q. (1998). Brain plasticity and behavior. *Annual Review of Psychology*, 49, 43–64.

Konczak, J., Borutta, M., & Dichgans, J. (1997). The development of goal-directed reaching in infants. II. Learning to produce task-adequate patterns of joint torque. *Experimental Brain Research*, 113(3), 465–474.

Konczak, J., & Dichgans, J. (1997). The development toward stereotypic arm kinematics during reaching in the first 3 years of life. *Experimental Brain Research*, 117(2), 346–354.

Krageloh-Mann, I., Toft, P., Lunding, J., Andresen, J., Pryds, O., & Lou, H.C. (1999). Brain lesions in preterms: Origin, consequences and compensation. *Acta Paediatrica*, 88(8), 897–908.

Kujala, T., Alho, K., & Naatanen, R. (2000). Cross-modal reorganization of human cortical functions. *Trends in Neuroscience*, 23(3), 115–120.

LaForme Fiss, A.C., Effgen, S.K., Page, J., & Shasby, S. (2009). Effect of sensorimotor groups on gross motor acquisition for young children with Down syndrome. *Pediatric Physical Therapy*. 21(2), 158–166.

Landa, R.J. (2008). Diagnosis of autism spectrum disorders in the first 3 years of life. *Nature Clinical Practice Neurology*, 4(3), 138–47.

Landau, W.M. (1974). Spasticity: The fable of a neurological demon and the emperor's new therapy. *Archives of Neurology*, 31, 217–219.

Langerak, N.G., Lamberts, R.P., Fieggen, G., Peter, J.C., van der Merwe, L., Peacock, W.J., & Vaughan, C.L. (2008). A prospective gait analysis study in patients with diplegic cerebral palsy 20 years after selective dorsal rhizotomy. *Journal of Neurosurgery: Pediatrics*, 1(3), 180–186.

Latash, M.L. (1998a). Virtual reality: A fascinating tool for motor rehabilitation (to be used with caution). *Disability and Rehabilitation*, 20(3), 104–105.

Latash, M.L. (1998b). *Progress in motor control: Bernstein's traditions in movement studies*. Champaign, IL: Human Kinetics.

Latash, M.L. (1998c). *Neurophysiological basis of movement* (pp. 98–105). Champaign, IL: Human Kinetics.

Latash, M.L., & Anson, G. (1996). What are "normal" movements in atypical populations? *Behavioral Brain Science, 19*, 55–106.

Latash, L.P., Latash, M.L., & Meijer, O.G. (1999). 30 years later: The relation between structure and function in the brain from a contemporary point of view (1996), part I. *Motor Control*, 3(4), 329–332, 342–345.

Latash, L.P., Latash, M.L., & Meijer, O.G. (2000). 30 years later: On the problem of the relation between structure and function in the brain from a contemporary viewpoint (1996), part II. *Motor Control*, 4(2), 125–149.

Latash, M.L., & Nicholas, J.J. (1996). Motor control research in rehabilitation medicine. *Disability and Rehabilitation*, 18(6), 293–299.

Latash, M.L., Scholz, J.P., & Schoner, G. (2007). Toward a new theory of motor synergies. *Motor Control*, 11, 276–308.

Lauteslager, P.E.M., Vermeer, A., & Helders, P.J.M. (1998). Disturbances in the motor behavior of children with Down's syndrome: The need for a theoretical framework. *Physiotherapy*, 84, 5–13.

Law M, King G, King S, et al. (2006). Patterns of participation in recreational and leisure activities among children with complex physical disabilities. *Developmental Medicine and Child Neurology*, 48, 337–342.

Lee, D.N., von Hofsten, C., & Cotton, E. (1997). Perception in action approach to cerebral palsy. In K.J. Connolly & H. Forssberg (Eds.), *Neurophysiology and neuropsychology motor development* (pp. 257–258). London: Mac Keith.

Leonard, C.T. (1998). *The neuroscience of human movement* (pp. 124–128). St. Louis: Mosby–Year Book.

Levin, M.F., Kleim, J.A., Wolf, S.L. (2009). What do motor "recovery" and "compensation" mean in patients following a stroke? *Neurorehabilitation and Neural Repair, 23*, 313319.

Lieber, R., & Friden, J. (2002) Spasticity causes a fundamental rearrangement of muscle-joint interaction. *Muscle Nerve*, 25, 265–270.

Lieber, R., Steinman, S., Barash, I., et al. (2004). Structural and functional changes in spastic skeletal muscle. *Muscle Nerve*, 29, 615–627.

Liepert, J., Bauder, H., Miltner, W.H.R., Taub, E., & Weiller, C. (2000). Treatment-induced cortical reorganization after stroke in humans. *Stroke*, 31, 1210–1216.

Lindquist, B., Uvebrant, P., Rehn, E., & Carlsson, G. (2009). Cognitive functions in children with myelomeningocele without hydrocephalus. *Child's Nervous System*, 25(8), 969–975.

Liptak, G.S., Shurtleff, D.B., Bloss, J.W., Baltus-Hebert, E., & Manitta, P. (1992). Mobility aids for children with high-level myelomeningocele: Parapodium versus wheelchair. *Developmental Medicine and Child Neurology, 34*, 787–796.

Liu, W. (2001). *Anticipatory postural adjustments in children with cerebral palsy and children with typical development during forward reach tasks in standing*. Unpublished doctoral dissertation, MCP Hahnemann University, Philadelphia.

Lloyd, M., Burghardt, A., Ulrich, D.A., & Angulo-Barroso, R. (2010). Physical activity and walking onset in infants with Down syndrome. *Adapted Physical Activity Quarterly, 27*(1), 1–16.

Lombardi, F., Emilia, R., Taricco, M., De Tanti, A., Telaro, E., Liberati, A. (2002). Sensory stimulation of brain-injured individuals in coma or vegetative state: Results of a Cochrane systematic review. *Clinical Rehabilitation, 16*, 464–472.

Looper, J., & Ulrich, D.A. (2010). Effect of treadmill training and supramalleolar orthosis use on motor skill development in infants with Down syndrome: A randomized clinical trial. *Physical Therapy, 90*(3), 382–390.

Lowes, L.P. (1996). An evaluation of the standing balance of children with cerebral palsy and the tools for assessment. Unpublished doctoral dissertation, MCP Hahnemann University, Philadelphia.

Lundy-Ekman, L. (1998). *Neuroscience: Fundamentals for rehabilitation* (pp. 69–84). Philadelphia: W.B. Saunders.

Luyt, L., Bodney, S., Keller, J., et al. (1996). Reliability of determining motor strategy used by children with cerebral palsy during the Pediatric Clinical Test of Sensory Interaction for Balance. *Pediatric Physical Therapy, 8*, 180.

Mackey, A.H., Miller, F., Walt, S.E., Waugh, M. & Stott, N.S. (2008). Use of three-dimensional kinematic analysis following upper limb botulinum toxin A for children with hemiplegia. *European Journal of Neurology, 15*(11), 1191–1198. doi: 10.1111/j.1468-1331.2008.02271.x

Maher, C.A., Williams, M.T., & Olds, T.S. (2008). The 6 minute walk test for children with cerebral palsy. *International Journal of Rehabilitation Research, 31*(2), 185–188.

Majed, M., Nejat, F., Khashab, M.E., Tajik, P., Gharagozloo, M., Baghban, M., & Sajjadnia A. (2009). Risk factors for latex sensitization in young children with myelomeningocele. *Journal of Neurosurgery: Pediatrics, 4*(3), 285–288.

Majnemer, A. (1998). Benefits of early intervention for children with developmental disabilities. *Seminars in Pediatric Neurology, 5*(1), 62–69.

Malaiya, R., McNee, A., Fry, N., et al. (2007). The morphology of the medial gastrocnemius in typically developing children and children with spastic hemiplegic cerebral palsy. *Journal of Electromyography & Kinesiology, 17*, 657–663.

Mandich, A.D., Polatajko, H.J., Macnab, J.J., & Miller, L.T. (2001a). Treatment of children with developmental coordination disorder: What is the evidence? *Physical and Occupational Therapy in Pediatrics, 20*(2–3), 51–68.

Mandich, A.D., Polatajko, H.J., Missiuna, C., & Miller, L.T. (2001b). Cognitive strategies and motor performance in children with developmental coordination disorder. *Physical and Occupational Therapy in Pediatrics, 20*(2–3), 125–143.

Mangeot, S.D., Miller, L.J., McIntosh, D.N., McGrath-Clarke, J., Simon, J., Hagerman, R.J., & Goldson, E. (2001). Sensory modulation in children with attention-deficit-hyperactivity disorder. *Developmental Medicine and Child Neurology, 43*, 399–406.

Martin, K. (2004) Effects of supramalleolar orthoses on postural stability in children with Down syndrome. *Developmental Medicine and Child Neurology, 46*, 406–411.

Mattern-Baxter, K., Bellamy, S., & Mansoor, J. (2009). Effects of intensive locomotor treadmill training on young children with cerebral palsy. *Pediatric Physical Therapy, 21*, 308–319.

McDonald, C.M., Jaffe, K.M., Mosca, V.S., & Shurtleff, D.B. (1991). Ambulatory outcome of children with myelomeningocele: Effect of lower-extremity muscle strength. *Developmental Medicine and Child Neurology, 33*, 482–490.

McEwen, I. (2000). Children with cognitive impairments. In S.K. Campbell, D.W. Vander Linden, & R.J. Palisano (Eds.), *Physical therapy for children* (2nd ed., pp. 502–532). Philadelphia: W.B. Saunders.

McEwen, I.R., Arnold, S.H., Hansen, L.H., & Johnson, D. (2003). Interrater reliability and content validity of a minimal data set to measure outcomes of students receiving school-based occupational therapy and physical therapy. *Physical and Occupational Therapy in Pediatrics, 23*(2), 77–95.

McLaughlin, J.F., Bjornson, K., Temkin, N., Steinbok, P., Wright, V., Reiner, A., Roberts, T., Drake, J., O'Donnell, M., Rosenbaum, P., Barber, J., & Ferrel, A. (2002). Selective dorsal rhizotomy: Meta-analysis of three randomized controlled trials. *Developmental Medicine and Child Neurology, 44*(1), 17–25.

Meeropol, E., Frost, J., Puch, L., Roberts, J., & Ogden J.A. (1993). Latex allergy in children with myelodysplasia: A survey of Shriners Hospitals. *Journal of Pediatric Orthopedics, 13*(1), 1–4.

Mercer, V.S., & Lewis, C.L. (2001). Hip abductor and knee extensor muscle strength of children with and without Down syndrome. *Pediatric Physical Therapy, 13*(1), 18–26.

Merrick, J., Ezra, E., Josef, B., Hendel, D., Steinberg, D.M., & Wientroub, S. (2000). Musculoskeletal problems in Down syndrome. European Paediatric Orthopaedic Society survey: The Israeli sample. *Journal of Pediatric Orthopedics, 9*(3), 185–192.

Merzenich, M.M., & Jenkins, W.M. (1993). Reorganization of cortical representations of the hand following alterations of skill inputs induced by nerve injury, skin island, transfers, and experience. *Journal of Hand Therapy, 18*, 89–104.

Meyer, M.J., Megyesi, J., Meythaler, J., Murie-Fernandez, M., Aubut, J., Foley, N., Salter, K., Bayley, M., Marshall, S., & Teasell, R. (2010). Acute management of acquired brain injury Part III: An evidence-based review of interventions used to promote arousal from coma. *Brain Injury, 24*(5), 722–729.

Meyers, G.J., Cerone, S.B., & Olson, A.L. (1981). *A guide for helping the child with spina bifida.* Springfield, IL: Charles C. Thomas.

Miller, L.T., Missiuna, C.A., Macnab, J.J., Malloy-Miller, T., & Polatajko, H.J. (2001). Clinical description of children with developmental coordination disorder. *Canadian Journal of Occupational Therapy, 68*, 5–15.

Ming, X., Brimacombe, M., & Wagner, G.C. (2007). Prevalence of motor impairment in autism spectrum disorders. *Brain and Development, 29*, 565–570.

Missiuna, C. (2001). Strategies for success: Working with children with developmental coordination disorder. *Physical and Occupational Therapy in Pediatrics, 20*(2–3), 1–4.

Missiuna, C., Gaines, B.R., Soucie, H., & McLean, J. (2006). Parental questions about developmental coordination disorder: A synopsis of current evidence. *Paediatrics and Child Health, 11*(8), 507–512.

Missiuna, C., Rivard, L., & Bartlett, D. (2006) Exploring assessment tools and the target of intervention for children with developmental coordination disorder. *Physical and Occupational Therapy in Pediatrics, 26*(1), 71–89.

Mockford, M., & Caulton, J.M. (2008). Systematic review of progressive strength training in children and adolescents with cerebral palsy who are ambulatory. *Pediatric Physical Therapy, 20*, 318–333.

Mockford, M., & Caulton, J.M. (2010). The pathophysiological basis of weakness in children with cerebral palsy. *Pediatric Physical Therapy, 22*, 222–233.

Moe-Nilssen, R. (1998). A new method for evaluating motor control in gait under real-life environmental conditions. Part 2: Gait analysis. *Clinical Biomechanics, 13*, 328–335.

Montgomery, P.C. (2000). Achievement of gross motor skills in two children with cerebellar hypoplasia: Longitudinal case reports. *Pediatric Physical Therapy, 12*, 68–76.

Morris, C. (2002). A review of the efficacy of lower-limb orthoses used for cerebral palsy. *Developmental Medicine and Child Neurology, 44*, 205–211.

Morris, D., Crago, J., DeLuca, S., Pidikiti, R., & Taub, E. (1997). Constraint induced movement therapy for recovery after stroke. *Neurorehabilitation, 9*, 29–43.

Motta, F., Stignani, C., & Antonello, C.E. (2008). Effect of intrathecal baclofen on dystonia in children with cerebral palsy and the use of functional scales. *Journal of Pediatric Orthopedics, 28*(2), 213–217.

Munch, E., Horn, P., Schurer, L., Piepgras, A., Paul, T., & Schmiedek, P. (2000). Management of severe traumatic brain injury by decompressive craniectomy. *Neurosurgery, 47*(2), 315–322.

Mutlu, A., Livanelioglu, A., & Gunel, M.K. (2008). Reliability of Ashworth and modified Ashworth scales in children with spastic cerebral palsy. *BioMed Central Musculoskeletal Disorders, 9*, 44.

Nashner, L.M. (1982). Adaptation of human movement to altered environments. *Trends in Neuroscience, 10*, 358–361.

Natale, J.E., Guerguerian, A.M., Joseph J.G., et al. (2007). Pilot study to determine the hemodynamic safety and feasibility of magnesium sulfate infusion in children with severe traumatic brain injury. *Pediatric Critical Care in Medicine, 8*(1), 1–9.

National Autism Center (2009). *Evidence-based practice and autism in schools: A guide to providing appropriate interventions to students with autism spectrum disorders.* Randolph, MA: Author. Available at http://www.nationalautismcenter.org

Newell, K.M., & Valvano, J. (1998). Therapeutic intervention as a constraint in learning and relearning movement skills. *Scandinavian Journal of Occupational Therapy, 5*, 51–57.

Nielsen, J.B. (2004). Sensorimotor integration at spinal level as a basis for muscle coordination during voluntary movement in humans. *Journal of Applied Physiology, 96*, 1961–1967.

Niemeijer, A.S., Schoemaker, M.M., & Smits-Engelsman, B.M. (2006). Are teaching principles associated with improved motor performance in children with developmental coordination disorder: A pilot study. *Physical Therapy, 86*(9), 221–230.

Niemeijer, A.S., Smits-Engelsman, B.M., & Schoemaker, M.M. (2007). Neuromotor task training for children with developmental coordination disorder: A controlled trial. *Developmental Medicine and Child Neurology, 49*, 406–411.

Nieuwenhuys, R., Voogd, J., & van Huijzen, C. (2008). *The human central nervous system* (4th ed.). Berlin: Springer.

Nolan, L., Grigorenko, A., & Thorstensson, A. (2005). Balance control: Sex and age differences in 9- to 16-year-olds. *Developmental Medicine and Child Neurology, 47*, 449–454.

Norris, R.A., Wilder, E., & Norton, J. (2008). The Functional Reach Test in 3–5-year-old children without disabilities. *Pediatric Physical Therapy, 20*, 47–52.

Nudo, R.J., Wise, B.M., SiFuentes, F., & Milliken, G.M. (1996). Neural substrates for the effects of rehabilitative training on motor recovery after ischemic infarct. *Science, 272*, 1791–1794.

Okereafor, A., Allsop, J., Counsell, S.J., Fitzpatrick, J., Azzopardi, D., Rutherford, M.A, & Cowan, F.M. (2008). Patterns of brain injury in neonates exposed to perinatal sentinel events. *Pediatrics, 121*, 906–914.

Olree, K.S., Engsberg, J.R., Ross, S.A., & Park, T.S. (2000). Changes in synergistic movement patterns after selective dorsal rhizotomy. *Developmental Medicine and Child Neurology, 42*, 297–303.

Pakula, A.L., & Palmer, F.B. (1998). Early intervention for children at risk for neuromotor problems. In M.J. Guralnick (Ed.), *The effectiveness of early intervention* (pp. 99–108). Baltimore: Paul H. Brookes.

Palisano, R.J., Haley, S.M., Westcott, S., & Hess, A. (1999). Pediatric Physical Therapy Outcome Management System. *Pediatric Physical Therapy, 11*, 220.

Palisano, R.J., Kolobe, T.H., Haley, S.M., Lowes, L.P., & Jones, S.L. (1995). Validity of the Peabody Developmental Gross Motor Scale as an evaluative measure of infants receiving physical therapy. *Physical Therapy, 75*, 939–948.

Palisano, R.J., Rosenbaum, P., Bartlett, D., Livingston, M. (2007). *GMFCS – E&R*. Hamilton, Ontario, Canada: CanChild Centre for Childhood Disability Research, McMaster University. Available at http://motorgrowth.canchild.ca/en/GMFCS/resources/GMFCS-ER.pdf

Palisano, R., Rosenbaum, P., Bartlett, D., & Livingston, M. (2008). Content validity of the expanded and revised Gross Motor Function Classification System. *Developmental Medicine and Child Neurology, 50*(10), 744–750.

Palisano, R.J., Walter, S.D., Russell, D.J., Rosenbaum, P.L., Gemus, M., Galuppi, B.E., & Cunningham, L. (2001). Gross motor function of children with Down syndrome: Creation of motor growth curves. *Archives of Physical Medicine and Rehabilitation, 82*(4), 494–500.

Park, B.K., Song, H.R., Vankoski, M.S., Moore, C.A., & Dias, L.S. (1997). Gait electromyography in children with myelomeningocele at the sacral level. *Archives of Physical Medicine and Rehabilitation, 78*, 471–475.

Park, T.S., & Johnston, J.M (2006). Surgical techniques of selective dorsal rhizotomy for spastic cerebral palsy: Technical note. *Neurosurgical FOCUS, 21*(2), E7.

Parush, S., Yehezkehel, I., Tenenbaum, A., Tekuzener, E., Bar-Efrat/Hirsch, I., Jessel, A., & Ornoy, A. (1998). Developmental correlates of school-age children with a history of benign congenital hypotonia. *Developmental Medicine and Child Neurology, 40*(7), 448–452.

Pascual-Pascual, S., & Pascual-Castroviejo, I. (2009). Safety of botulinum toxin type A in children younger than 2 years. *European Journal of Paediatric Neurology, 13*(6), 511–515.

Pelligrino, T.T., Buelow, B., Krause, M., Loucks, L.C., & Westcott, S.L. (1995). Test-retest reliability of the Pediatric Clinical Test of Sensory Interactions for Balance and the Functional Reach Test in children with standing balance dysfunction. *Pediatric Physical Therapy, 7,* 197.

Penn, P.R., Rose, F.D., & Johnson, D.A. (2009). Virtual enriched environments in paediatric neuropsychological rehabilitation following traumatic brain injury: Feasibility, benefits and challenges. *Developmental Neurorehabilitation, 12*(1), 32–43.

Perel, P., Roberts, I., Shakur, H., Thinkhamrop, B., Phuenpathom, N., & Yutthakasemsunt, S. (2010) Haemostatic drugs for traumatic brain injury. *Cochrane Database Systematic Review,* (1), CD007877.

Phillips, C.G., & Porter, R. (1977). *Corticospinal neurones: Their role in movement.* New York: Academic Press.

Pidcock, F.S., Garcia, T., Trovato, M.K., Schultz, S., & Brady, K.D. (2009). Pediatric constraint-induced movement therapy: A promising intervention for childhood hemiparesis. *Topics in Stroke Rehabilitation, 16*(5), 339–345.

Pilon, J.M., Sadler, G.T., & Bartlett, D.J. (2000). Relationship of hypotonia and joint laxity to motor development during infancy. *Pediatric Physical Therapy, 12,* 10–15.

Piper, M., & Darrah, J. (1994). *Motor assessment of the developing infant.* Philadelphia: W.B. Saunders.

Platz, T., Eickhof, C., Nuyens, G., & Vuadens, P. (2005). Clinical scales for the assessment of spasticity, associated phenomena, and function: A systematic review of the literature. *Disability and Rehabilitation, 27*(1–2), 7–18.

Podsiadlo, D., & Richardson, S. (1991). The timed "up and go": A basic functional mobility test for frail elderly persons. *Journal of the American Geriatric Society, 39,* 142–148.

Polatajko, H.J. (1999). Developmental coordination disorder (DCD): Alias the clumsy child syndrome. In K. Whitmore, H. Hart, & G. Willems (Eds.), *A neurodevelopmental approach to specific learning disorders* (pp. 119–133). London: Mac Keith.

Polatajko, H.J., Mandich, A.D., Miller, L.T., & Macnab, J.J. (2001). Cognitive Orientation to Daily Occupational Performance (CO-OP)—Part II: The evidence. *Physical and Occupational Therapy in Pediatrics, 20*(2–3), 83–106.

Poulsen, A.A., Ziviani, J.M., & Cuskelly, M. (2008). Leisure time physical activity energy expenditure in boys with developmental coordination disorder: The role of peer relations self-concept perceptions. *OTJR: Occupation, Participation and Health, 28*(1), 30–39.

Pradeep, K., Narotam, J.F., & Narendra, N. (2009) Brain tissue oxygen monitoring in traumatic brain injury and major trauma: outcome analysis of a brain tissue oxygen-directed therapy. *Journal of Neurosurgery, 111*(4), 72–682.

Prasher, V.P., Robinson, L., Krishnan, V.H., & Chung, M.C. (1995). Podiatric disorders among children with Down syndrome and learning disability. *Developmental Medicine and Child Neurology, 37*(2), 131–134.

Professional Staff Association of Rancho Los Amigos Hospital (1982). *Rancho Los Amigos Pediatric Levels of Consciousness for Infants, Preschoolers, and School-Age children scale. Rehabilitation of the head injured adult: Comprehensive physical management.* Downey, CA: Author.

Proske, U., & Gandevia, S.C. (2009). The kinaesthetic senses. *The Journal of Physiology, 587,* 4139–4146.

Provost, B., Heimerl, S., & Lopez, B.R. (2007). Levels of gross and fine motor development in young children with autism spectrum disorder. *Physical and Occupational Therapy in Pediatrics, 27*(3), 21–36.

Pueschel, S.M. (1990). Clinical aspects of Down syndrome from infancy to adulthood. *American Journal of Medical Genetics Suppl., 7,* 52–56.

Py, A., Zein Addeen, G., Perrier, Y., Carlier, R., & Picard, A. (2009). Evaluation of the effectiveness of botulinum toxin injections in the lower limb muscles of children with cerebral palsy. Preliminary prospective study of the advantages of ultrasound guidance. *Annals of Physical and Rehabilitation Medicine, 52*(3), 215–223.

Randall, K.E., & McEwen, I.R. (2000). Writing patient-centered functional goals. *Physical Therapy, 80,* 1197–1203.

Raynor, A.J. (2001). Strength, power, and coactivation in children with developmental coordination disorder. *Developmental Medicine and Child Neurology, 43,* 676–684.

Reed, E.S. (1982). An outline of a theory of action systems. *Journal of Motor Behavior, 14,* 98–134.

Richardson, P.K., Atwater, S.W., Crowe, T.K., & Deitz, J.C. (1992). Performance of preschoolers on the Pediatric Clinical Test of Sensory Interaction for Balance. *American Journal of Occupational Therapy, 46,* 793–800.

Rimmer, J.H., Heller, T., Wang, E., & Valerio, I. (2004). Improvements in physical fitness in adults with Down syndrome. *American Journal of Mental Retardation, 109,* 165–74.

Rine, R.M., Rubish, K., & Feeney, C. (1998). Measurement of sensory system effectiveness and maturational changes in postural control in young children. *Pediatric Physical Therapy, 10,* 16–22.

Rogozinski, B.M., Davids, J.R., Davis, R.B., Jameson, G.J., & Blackhurst, D.W. (2009) The efficacy of the floor-reaction ankle-foot orthosis in children with cerebral palsy. *The Journal of Bone and Joint Surgery. American, 91*(10), 2440–2447.

Roizen, N.J., & Patterson, D. (2003). Down's syndrome. *The Lancet, 361,* 1281–1289.

Roizen, N.J., Wolters, C., Nicol, T., & Blondis, T.A. (1993). Hearing loss in children with Down syndrome. *Journal of Pediatrics, 123*(1), S9–S12.

Rosblad, B., & Von Hofsten, C. (1994). Repetitive goal-directed arm movements in children with developmental coordination disorders: Role of visual information. *Adapted Physical Activity Quarterly, 11,* 190–202.

Rose, F.D., Johnson, D.A., & Attree, E.A. (1997). Rehabilitation of the head-injured child: Basic research and new technology. *Pediatric Rehabilitation, 1,* 3–7.

Rothwell, J.D. (1994). *Control of human voluntary movement.* Cambridge, England: Cambridge University Press.

Rubin, S.S., Rimmer, J.H., Chicoine, B., Braddock, D., & McGuire, D.E. (1998). Overweight prevalence in persons with Down syndrome. *American Journal of Mental Retardation, 36,* 175–181.

Russell, D., Palisano, R., Walter, S., Rosenbaum, P., Gemus, M., Gowland, C., Galuppi, B., & Lane, M. (1998). Evaluating motor function in children with Down syndrome: Validity of the GMFM. *Developmental Medicine and Child Neurology, 40,* 693–701.

Russell, D., Rosenbaum, P., Gowland, C., Hardy, S., Lane, M., Plews, N., McGavin, H., Cadman, D., & Jarvis, S. (1993).

Gross motor function measure (2nd ed.). Hamilton, Ontario, Canada: Gross Motor Measure Group.

Sahrmann, S.A., & Norton B.J. (1977). The relationship of voluntary movement to spasticity in the upper motor neuron syndrome. *Annals of Neurology, 2*, 460–465.

Samuels, R., McGirt, M.J., Attenello, F.J., Garcés Ambrossi, G.L., Singh, N., Solakoglu, C., Weingart, J.D., Carson, B.S., & Jallo, G.I. (2009). Incidence of symptomatic retethering after surgical management of pediatric tethered cord syndrome with or without duraplasty. *Child's Nervous System, 25*(9), 1085–1089.

Sanger T.D. (2006). Arm trajectories in dyskinetic cerebral palsy have increased random variability. *Journal of Child Neurology, 21*, 551–557.

Sanger, T.D., Chen, D., Fehlings, D.L., et al. (2010). Definition and classification of hyperkinetic movements in childhood. *Movement Disorders, 25*(11), 1538–1549.

Sanger, T.D., Delgado, M.R., Gaebler-Spira, D., et al. (2003). Task force on childhood motor: classification and definition of disorders causing hypertonia in childhood. *Pediatrics, 111*, e89–e97.

Schmidt, R.A. (1991). *Motor performance and learning: Principles for practitioners.* Champaign, IL: Human Kinetics.

Schoemaker, M.M., Flapper, B., Verheij, N.P., et al. (2006). Evaluation of the Developmental Coordination Disorder Questionnaire as a screening instrument. *Developmental Medicine and Child Neurology, 48*, 668–73.

Scholz, J.P. (1990). Dynamic pattern theory: Some implications for therapeutics. *Physical Therapy, 70*(12), 827–843.

Scholz, J.P., & Schoner, G. (1999). The uncontrolled manifold concept: identifying control variables for a functional task. *Experimental Brain Research, 126*, 289–306.

School Outcomes Measure Administrative Guide. (2007). The University of Oklahoma Health Sciences Center, Department of Rehabilitation Science, Oklahoma City, OK. Retrieved from http://www.ah.ouhsc.edu/somresearch/adminGuide.pdf

Scianni, A., Butler, J.M., Ada, L., & Teixeira-Salmela, L.F. (2009). Muscle strengthening is not effective in children and adolescents with cerebral palsy: a systematic review. *The Australian Journal of Physiotherapy, 55*(2), 81–87.

Segal, R.L. (1998). Spinal cord plasticity is a possible tool for rehabilitation. *Neurology Report, 22*, 54–60.

Segal, R., Mandich, A, Polotajko, H., & Cook, J.V. (2002). Stigma and its management: A pilot study of parental perceptions of the experiences of children with developmental coordination disorder. *American Journal of Occupational Therapy, 56*, 422–428.

Selby-Silverstein, L., Hillstrom, H.J., & Palisano, R.J. (2001). The effect of foot orthoses on standing foot posture and gait of young children with Down syndrome. *NeuroRehabilitation, 16*, 183–193.

Sherrington, C.S. (1906). *The integrative action of the nervous system.* Silliman Lectures. New Haven, CT: Yale University Press.

Sherrington, C.S. (1947). *The integrative action of the nervous system.* Cambridge, MA: Cambridge University Press.

Shields, N., Taylor, N.F., & Dodd, J. (2008) Effects of a community-based progressive resistance training program on muscle performance and physical function in adults with down syndrome: A randomized controlled trial. *Archives of Physical Medicine and Rehabilitation, 89*(7), 1215–1220.

Shumway-Cook, A., & Horak, F.B. (1986). Assessing the influence of sensory interaction on balance: Suggestion from the field. *Physical Therapy, 66*, 1548–1550.

Shumway-Cook, A., & Woollacott, M.H. (1985). Dynamics of postural control in the child with Down syndrome. *Physical Therapy, 65*, 1315–1322.

Shumway-Cook, A., & Woollacott, M.H. (Eds.). (2001). *Motor control: Theory and practical applications* (2nd ed.). Philadelphia: Lippincott Williams & Wilkins.

Siegler, R.S. (2002). Variability and infant development. *Infant Behaviour and Development, 25*, 550–557.

Singh, G., Athreya, B.H., Fries, J.F., & Goldsmith, D.P. (1994). Measurement of health status in children with juvenile rheumatoid arthritis. *Arthritis and Rheumatology, 37*, 1761–1769.

Skorji, V., & McKenzie, B. (1997). How do children who are clumsy remember modeled movements? *Developmental Medicine and Child Neurology, 39*(6), 404–408.

Slater, L.M., Hillier, S.L., & Civetta, L.R. (2010). The clinimetric properties of performance-based gross motor tests used for children with developmental coordination disorder: A systematic review. *Pediatric Physical Therapy, 22*, 170–179.

Smith, B.A., Kubo, M., Black, D.P., Holt, K.G., & Ulrich, B.D. (2007) Effect of practice on a novel task: Walking on a treadmill: Preadolescents with and without Down syndrome. *Physical Therapy, 87*(6), 766–777.

Spano, M., Mercuri, E., Rando, T., Panto, T., Gagliano, A., Henderson, S., & Guzzetta, F. (1999). Motor and perceptual-motor competence in children with Down syndrome: Variation in performance with age. *European Journal of Paediatric Neurology, 3*(1), 7–13.

Stackhouse, S., Binder-Macleod, S., & Lee, S. (2005). Voluntary muscle activation, contractile properties, and fatigability in children with and without cerebral palsy. *Muscle Nerve, 31*, 594–601.

Stanley, F., Blair, E.M., & Alberman, E. (2000). *Cerebral palsies: Epidemiology and causal pathways.* London: Mac Keith.

Staples, K.L, & Reid, G. (2010). Fundamental movement skills and autism spectrum disorders. *Journal of Autism Developmental Disorder, 40*, 209–217.

Stein, R.B., Yang, J.F., Belanger, M., & Pearson, K.G. (1993). Modification of reflexes in normal and abnormal movements. *Progress in Brain Research, 97*, 189–196.

Stockmeyer, S.A. (1967). An interpretation of the approach of Rood to the treatment of neuromuscular dysfunction. *American Journal of Physical Medicine, 46*, 901–956.

Stoll, C., Alembik, Y., Dott, B., & Roth, M.P. (1998). Study of Down syndrome in 238,942 consecutive births. *Annals of Genetics, 41*(1), 44–51.

Sullivan, K.J. (1998). Functionally distinct learning systems of the brain: Implications for brain injury rehabilitation. *Neurology Report, 22*, 126–131.

Sutcliffe, T.L., Gaetz, W.C., Logan, W.J., Cheyne, D.O., & Fehlings, D.L. (2007). Cortical reorganization after modified constraint-induced movement therapy in pediatric hemiplegic cerebral palsy. *Journal of Child Neurology, 22*, 1281–1287.

Sweeney, J.K., Heriza, C.B., & Markowitz, R. (1994). The changing profile of pediatric physical therapy: A 10-year analysis of clinical practice. *Pediatric Physical Therapy, 6*, 113–118.

Syczewska, M., Lebiedowska, M.K., & Pandyan, A.D. (2009). Quantifying repeatability of the Wartenberg pendulum test parameters in children with spasticity. *Journal of Neuroscience Methods, 178*(2), 340–344.

Tammik, K., Matlep, M., Ereline, J., et al. (2008). Quadriceps femoris muscle voluntary force and relaxation capacity in children with spastic diplegic cerebral palsy. *Pediatric Exercise Science, 20*, 18–28.

Taub, E. (1976). Motor behavior following deafferentation in the developing and motorically mature monkey. *Advances in Behavioral Biology, 18*, 675–705.

Taub, E., Goldberg, I., & Taub, P. (1975). Deafferentation on monkeys: Pointing at a target without visual feedback. *Experimental Neurology, 46*, 178–186.

Taub, E., & Wolf, S. (1997). Constraint induced movement techniques to facilitate upper extremity use in stroke patients. *Topics in Stroke Rehabilitation, 3*, 38–61.

Teasdale, G., & Jennett, B. (1974). Assessment of coma and impaired consciousness: A practical scale. *The Lancet, 2*, 81–84.

Tedroff, K., Knutson, L.M., & Soderberg, G.L. (2006). Synergistic muscle activation during maximum voluntary contractions in children with and without spastic cerebral palsy. *Developmental Medicine and Child Neurology, 48*, 789–96.

Thelen, E., & Smith, L.B. (1993). *A dynamic systems approach to the development of cognition and action.* Cambridge, MA: MIT Press.

Thelen, E., & Spencer, J. (1998). Postural control during reaching in young infants: A dynamic systems approach. *Neuroscience Biobehavioral Reviews, 22*, 507–514.

Tomchek, S.D., & Case-Smith, J. (2009). *Occupational therapy practice guidelines for children and adolescents with autism.* Bethesda, MD: American Occupational Therapy Association.

Tomchek, S.D., & Dunn, W. (2007). Sensory processing in children with and without autism: a comparative study using the Short Sensory Profile. *American Journal of Occupational Therapy, 61*(2), 190–200.

Trost, J.P., Schwartz, M.H., Krach, L.E., Dunn, M.E., & Novacheck, T.F. (2008). Comprehensive short-term outcome assessment of selective dorsal rhizotomy. *Developmental Medicine and Child Neurology, 50*(10), 765–771.

Tsiaras, W.G., Pueschel, S., Keller, C., Curran, R., & Giesswein, S. (1999). Amblyopia and visual acuity in children with Down's syndrome. *British Journal of Ophthalmology, 83*(10), 1112–1114.

Tsimaras, V.K., & Fotiadou, E.G. (2004). Effect of training on the muscle strength and dynamic balance ability of adults with Down syndrome. *Journal of Strength and Conditioning Research/National Strength & Conditioning Association, 18*(2), 343–347.

Ulrich, D.A. (2000). *Test of gross motor development* (2nd ed.). Austin, TX: Pro-Ed.

Ulrich, D.A., Lloyd, M.C., Tiernan, C.W., Looper, J.E., & Angulo-Barroso, R.M. (2008) Effects of intensity of Treadmill training on developmental outcomes and stepping in infants with Down syndrome: A randomized trial. *Physical Therapy, 88*(1), 114–122.

Ulrich, B.D., Ulrich, D.A., Angulo-Kinzler, R., & Chapman, D.D. (1997). Sensitivity of infants with and without Down syndrome to intrinsic dynamics. *Research Quarterly for Exercise and Sport, 68*(1), 10–19.

Ulrich, D.A., Ulrich, B.D., Angulo-Kinzler, R.M., & Yun, J. (2001). Treadmill training of infants with Down syndrome: Evidence-based developmental outcomes. *Pediatrics, 108*(5), E84.

Unanue, R., & Westcott, S.L. (2001). Neonatal asphyxia. *Infants and Young Children, 13*(3), 13–24.

Unger, M., Faure, M., & Frieg, A. (2006). A strength training in adolescent learners with cerebral palsy a randomized controlled trial. *Clinical Rehabilitation, 20*, 469–477.

Uniform Data System for Medical Rehabilitation (2000). *The WeeFIM System Clinical Guide*, Version 5.01. Buffalo, NY: UDSMR.

U.S. Government Accountability Office (2005). *Education of children with autism* (GOA-05-220 Special Education). Washington, DC: Author.

Vachha, B., & Adams, R. (2009). Implications of family environment and language development: comparing typically developing children to those with spina bifida. *Child: Care, Health and Development, 35*, 709–716.

Van Dellen, T., & Geuze, R.H. (1988). Motor response processing in clumsy children. *Journal of Child Psychology and Psychiatry, 29*, 489–500.

van Doornik, J., Kukke, S., McGill, K., Rose, J., Sherman-Levine, S., & Sanger, T.D. (2008). Oral baclofen increases maximal voluntary neuromuscular activation of ankle plantar flexors in children with spasticity due to cerebral palsy. *Journal of Child Neurology, 23*(6), 635–639.

Vargha-Khadem, F. (2001). Generalized versus selective cognitive impairments resulting from brain damage sustained in childhood. *Epilepsia, 42*(Suppl. 1), 37–40; discussion, 50–51.

Vatovec, J., Velikovic, M., Smid, L., Brenk, K., & Zargi, M. (2001). Impairments of vestibular system in infants at risk of early brain damage. *Scandinavian Audiology Supplement, 52*, 191–193.

Vereijken, B. (2010). The complexity of childhood development: Variability in perspective. *Physical Therapy, 90*(12), 1850–1859.

Vereijken, B., & Thelen, E. (1997). Training infant treadmill stepping: The role of individual pattern stability. *Developmental Psychobiology, 30*(2), 89–102.

Vereijken, B., van Emmerik, R.E.A., Whiting, H.T.A., & Newell, K.M. (1992). Freezing degrees of freedom in skill acquisition. *Journal of Motor Behavior, 24*, 133–142.

Vink, R. & van den Heuvel, C. (2010) Substance P antagonists as a therapeutic approach to improving outcome following traumatic brain injury. *Neurotherapeutics, 7*(1), 74–80.

Volkman, K.G., Stergiou, N., Stuberg, W., Blanke, D., & Stoner, J. (2007). Methods to improve the reliability of the Functional Reach Test in children and adolescents with typical development. *Pediatric Physical Therapy, 19*, 20–27.

Volkman, K.G., Stergiou, N., Stuberg, W., Blanke, D., & Stoner, J. (2009). Factors affecting functional reach scores in youth with typical development. *Pediatric Physical Therapy, 21*(1), 38–44.

Volpe, J.J. (2008). *Neurology of the newborn* (5th ed.). Philadelphia, PA: Saunders Elsevier.

Voss, D.E. (1972). Proprioceptive neuromuscular facilitation: The PNF method. In P.H. Pearson & C.E. Williams (Eds.), *Physical therapy services in the developmental disabilities* (pp. 223–282). Springfield, IL: Charles C Thomas.

Walsche, F.M.P. (1961). Contribution of John Hughlings Jackson to neurology. *Archives of Neurology, 5*, 99–133.

Ward, A., Hayden, S., Dexter, M., & Scheinberg, A. (2009). Continuous intrathecal baclofen for children with spasticity and/or dystonia: Goal attainment and complications associated with treatment. *Journal of Paediatrics and Child Health, 45*(12), 720–726.

Watemberg, N., Waiserberg, N., Zuk, L., & Lerman-Sagie, T. (2007). Developmental coordination disorder in children with attention-deficit-hyperactivity disorder and physical therapy intervention. *Developmental Medicine and Child Neurology, 49*, 920–925.

Wells, R., Minnes, P., & Phillips, M. (2009). Predicting social and functional outcomes for individuals sustaining paediatric traumatic brain injury. *Developmental Neurorehabilitation, 12*(1): 12–23.

Westcott, S.L., Crowe, T.K., Deitz, J.C., & Richardson, P.K. (1994). Test-retest reliability of the Pediatric Clinical Test of Sensory Interaction for Balance (P-CTSIB). *Physical and Occupational Therapy in Pediatrics, 14*, 1–22.

Westcott, S.L., Lowes, L.P., & Richardson, P.K. (1997). Evaluation of postural stability in children: Current theories and assessment tools. *Physical Therapy, 77*, 629–645.

Westcott, S.L., Lowes, L.P., Richardson, P.K., Crowe, T.K., & Deitz, J. (1997). Difference in the use of sensory information for maintenance of standing balance in children with different motor disabilities. *Developmental Medicine and Child Neurology, 39* (Suppl. 75), 32–33.

Wheeler, A., Shall, M., Lewis, A., & Shepherd, J. (1996). The reliability of measurements obtained using the Functional Reach Test in children with cerebral palsy. *Pediatric Physical Therapy, 8*, 182.

White, H., Uhl, T.L., Augsburger, S., & Tylkowski, C. (2007). Reliability of the three-dimensional pendulum test for able-bodied children and children diagnosed with cerebral palsy. *Gait & Posture, 26*(1), 97–105.

Wiegand, C., Richards, P. (2007). Measurements of intracranial pressure in children: a critical review of current methods. *Developmental Medicine & Child Neurology, 49*, 935–941.

Wiley, M.E., & Damiano, D.L. (1998). Lower extremity strength profiles in spastic cerebral palsy. *Developmental Medicine and Child Neurology, 40*, 100–107.

Williams, E.N., Broughton, N.S., Menelaus, M.B. (1999) Age related walking in children with spina bifida. *Developmental Medicine and Child Neurology, 41*, 446–449.

Willoughby, C., & Polatajko, H.J. (1995). Motor problems in children with developmental coordination disorder: A review of the literature. *American Journal of Occupational Therapy, 49*, 787–797.

Wilson, P.H., & McKenzie, B.E. (1998). Information processing deficits associated with developmental coordination disorder: A meta-analysis of research findings. *Journal of Child Psychiatry, 6*, 829–840.

Wilson, P.H, Thomas, P.R., & Maruff, P. (2002). Motor imagery training ameliorates motor clumsiness in children. *Journal of Child Neurology, 17*, 491–498.

Wolpaw, J.R., & Tennissen, A.M. (2001). Activity-dependent spinal cord plasticity in health and disease. *Annual Review of Neuroscience, 24*, 807–843.

Wood, E., & Rosenbaum, P. (2000). The Gross Motor Function Classification System for cerebral palsy: A study of reliability and stability over time. *Developmental Medicine and Child Neurology, 42*, 292–296.

Woodhouse, C.R.J. (2008). Myelomeningocele: Neglected aspects. *Pediatric Nephrology, 23*(8), 1223–1231.

Woollacott, M.H., Burtner, P., Jensen, J., Jasiewicz, J., Roncesvalles, N., & Sveistrup, H. (1998). Development of postural responses during standing in healthy children and children with spastic diplegia. *Neuroscience and Biobehavioral Reviews, 22*, 583–589.

World Health Organization (2001). *International classification of functioning, disability and health.* Geneva: Author.

Wright, M., & Wallman, L. (2012). Cerebral palsy. In S.K. Campbell, R.J. Palisano, & M. N. Orlin, (Eds.), *Physical therapy for children* (4th ed., pp. 577–625). St. Louis: Elsevier Saunders.

Wu, K., Looper, J., Ulrich, B.D., Ulrich, D.A., & Angulo-Barroso, R.M. (2007). Exploring effects of different treadmill interventions on walking onset and gait patterns in infants with Down syndrome. *Developmental Medicine and Child Neurology. 49*(11), 839–845.

You, S.H., Jang, S.H., Kim, Y.H., Kwon, Y.H., Barrow, I., & Hallett, M. (2005). Cortical reorganization induced by virtual reality therapy in a child with hemiparetic cerebral palsy. *Developmental Medicine and Child Neurology, 47*, 628–635.

Zaino, C.A. (1999). Motor control of a functional reaching task in children with cerebral palsy and children with typical development: A comparison of electromyographic and kinetic measurements. Unpublished doctoral dissertation, MCP Hahnemann University, Philadelphia.

Zsolt, S., Seidl, R., Bernert, G., Dietrich, W., Spitzauer, S. & Urbanek, R. (1999). Latex sensitization in spina bifida appears disease-associated. *Journal of Pediatrics, 134*, 344–348.

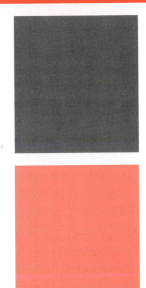

CHAPTER 8

Neuromuscular System: The Plan of Care

—Joanne Valvano, PT, PhD

—Alyssa LaForme Fiss, PT, PhD, PCS

A well-developed plan of care is the vehicle to greater functional independence and participation for children with neurological disorders. The processes of examination and evaluation outlined by the *Guide to Physical Therapist Practice* (American Physical Therapy Association [APTA], 2001: hereafter referred to as the *Guide*) lead to the plan of care. In developing such a plan, therapists integrate fundamental principles of pediatric physical therapy, such as family-centered care, a focus on individualized functional outcomes, and a commitment to the interdisciplinary process. Therapists rely on a working knowledge of (1) limitations in body structures and functions and restrictions in activities and participation associated with each child's specific diagnosis, (2) principles of motor development, motor control, and motor learning, and (3) the extant evidence for pediatric neurological interventions.

Chapter 7 addresses limitations in body structures and functions and restrictions in activities and participation associated with neurological conditions. This chapter will apply principles of motor development, learning, and control to a framework for activity-focused interventions and will review the evidence for pediatric neurological interventions addressed in the framework. This content will follow these guidelines based on principles of pediatric physical practice:

1. The intervention plan should ultimately focus on the child's participation in life's roles through the preservation and enhancement of function as well as prevention of secondary impairments. The intervention plan follows a top-down approach (P.H. Campbell, 1991) in which desired functional outcomes are determined first, and then components that limit these outcomes are assessed.

347

2. While the plan of care focuses on functional abilities that enhance independence in daily routines, the physical therapist should be aware that the relationship between function and quality of life is complex. In addition to functional abilities, other factors such as social networks, the child's understanding of the disability, and reciprocal relationships may determine quality of life (Shelly et al., 2008).

3. To increase quality of life across the life span, intervention should foster the family's development as advocates and decision makers who can be proactive about their child's needs. It is also important to foster independence in the children with whom therapists work, so that they can learn to take responsibility and advocate for their own needs as they approach adulthood.

4. The plan of care should focus on individualized, meaningful goals that the child or family have identified as important. Furthermore, the child's collaboration should be encouraged in developing the plan of care and setting goals, when developmentally appropriate. Child-centered, functional goals may be associated with greater gains when parents identify them as meaningful and relevant to their situation (Randall & McEwen, 2000).

5. The goals and objectives that structure the plan of care should be well written and measurable. Efforts by physical therapists to refine their goal writing will be rewarded time and again in practice. Goals and objectives are necessary for fulfilling administrative requirements for the Individualized Education Program (IEP) and the Individualized Family Service Plan (IFSP), or for reimbursement. Furthermore, the outcomes related to the intervention will be enhanced by goals that are well thought out, clearly stated, and measurable (Bower, McLellan, Arney, & Campbell, 1996).

6. To the greatest extent possible, the plan for physical therapy intervention should be integrated into an interdisciplinary plan for the child that is focused on the endpoint of enhanced performance and participation in school, home, and community.

7. The plan of care should effectively integrate three components of intervention outlined by the *Guide* (2001). The first component includes communication and coordination with parents, other members of the interdisciplinary team, and community agencies. For example, a physical therapist might communicate with an orthotist regarding an ankle-foot orthosis or with an adaptive physical education teacher regarding a child's readiness for a particular gym activity. The second component involves instruction to family, classroom staff, and child in many areas, including safety, assistive technology, and adaptations to the home or classroom environment. The third component includes procedural interventions, which are "hands-on" procedures individualized to each child's plan of care.

8. When developing a plan of care, the physical therapist should develop a systematic method to evaluate the therapeutic effect of the interventions provided to each child.

Intervention Strategies

Although all three components of intervention outlined in the *Guide* (2001) are fundamental to the plan of care, the discussion in this chapter will emphasize direct therapeutic interventions, or procedural interventions, provided by the physical therapist, family members, or other members of the intervention team. With the goals and objectives delineated, the physical therapist is faced with the practical challenge of planning intervention activities that will achieve these goals and objectives. Because of the complexity of neuromuscular impairments, there are many approaches or intervention strategies (Adams & Snyder, 1998) that can be implemented. Optimally, therapists should seek out the strongest evidence available that supports a wide array of interventions. However, high-level evidence is limited for many pediatric neurological interventions.

Evidence-based practice integrates the best research evidence with the therapist's clinical expertise and the individual circumstances of the patient (Straus, Richardson, Glasziou, & Haynes, 2005). The readers are referred to the levels of evidence used by the American Academy for Cerebral Palsy and Developmental Medicine (Butler & Darrah, 2001). In this framework, the highest level of evidence is achieved through the randomized controlled trial (RCT), which studies an intervention by randomly assigning study participants to an intervention group or a control group.

There is currently a paucity of studies in pediatric physical therapy that report significant treatment effects structured by the randomized controlled design. For example, many studies report pre-post intervention changes in one cohort of children. Over the years, methodological issues have constrained research on pediatric neurological interventions. The individual expression of most pediatric neurological diagnoses and ethical concerns makes it difficult to have a control group. This variability among participants requires a large sample size to detect a significant effect of the intervention.

Furthermore, in the past, outcome measures may not have been adequately sensitive to change. Rosenbaum

(2010) questions whether the rigors of the RCT, which focus on one specific intervention while controlling as many elements of the clinical situation as possible, may limit our understanding of the life-course perspective that is increasingly a priority in neurodisability. He proposed that identifying and understanding sources of variation such as age, level of function, and outcomes to be evaluated in children with neurodisability may lead to valuable insights into the complex issues that affect participation.

In recent years, the emphasis on evidence-based practice has encouraged more rigorous standards among researchers. Methodological challenges are being addressed through interagency collaboration to increase sample size, advanced statistical methods, and improved measures of change. Commitment to evidence-based practice has also encouraged strategies to help therapists evaluate and make the best use of the extant evidence.

One important resource is the systematic review. In a systematic review, the research on the specific topic is gathered, and each component study is critically appraised for the level of evidence. Then, a conclusion is made regarding the cumulative weight of the evidence (Jewell, 2011). The reader is encouraged to seek

out multiple systematic reviews on pediatric interventions that have been published recently in journals commonly accessed by pediatric physical therapists. Table 8.1 lists systematic reviews that address intervention strategies discussed later in this chapter. Another effort to improve evidence-based practice is the development of clinical management guidelines (APTA, Section on Pediatrics, 2004), which outline the sequence and timing of interventions that should achieve the best outcome for children with specific diagnoses using the best evidence (O'Neil et al., 2006).

Until a solid evidence-based consensus about a pediatric neurological intervention is available, physical therapists are challenged to make judgments by seeking a broad base of knowledge about possible approaches and critically evaluating the scientific merit, as well as the practical merit. In this chapter, information on multiple intervention strategies for children with neurological impairments is presented, with the most current evidence available. The authors expect that the reader will contemplate the information, read the research cited for interventions of interest, update the ever-changing literature on topics of interest, communicate with colleagues, and develop personal guidelines for intervention.

Table 8.1 Evidence-Based Interventions for Children With Neurological Disorders: Systematic Reviews (SR)

Intervention	Author (date)	# articles (SR)	Question	Findings
Ankle-Foot Orthoses (AFO)	Figueiredo, Ferreira, Moreira, Kirkwood, & Fetters (2008)	20 articles	What is the quality of current research on the influence of AFOs on gait in children with cerebral palsy (CP)?	Stronger research is needed to support use of AFOs for children with CP.
Aquatics	Getz, Hutzler, & Vermeer (2006)	11 articles	Are aquatic interventions effective for children with neuromotor impairments?	There is a lack of evidence evaluating effects of aquatic interventions in children with neuromotor impairments. No negative findings were reported in the research.
Body Weight–Supported Treadmill Training (BWSTT)	Damiano & DeJong, (2009)	29 articles	What are the strength, quality, and conclusiveness of evidence supporting use of treadmill training and body weight support in children with motor disabilities? Are protocol guidelines for BWSTT available?	The use of BWSTT with children with Down syndrome is supported, but additional research is needed to support the use of BWSTT with other pediatric populations. Current guidelines are not available.

Continued

Table 8.1 Evidence-Based Interventions for Children With Neurological Disorders: Systematic Reviews (SR)—cont'd

Intervention	Author (date)	# articles (SR)	Question	Findings
BWSTT *(continued)*	Mattern-Baxter (2009)	10 articles	What is the effect of BWSTT on gross motor function, balance, gait speed, and endurance in children with CP?	Current evidence suggests BWSTT may be effective to improve gait, endurance, and walking function in children with CP. Additional research is needed to confirm the efficacy of BWSTT.
	Mutlu, Krosschell, & Spira (2009)	8 articles	What is the effect of BWSTT on functional outcomes and ambulation for children with CP?	There is not enough evidence to support improved functional outcomes and ambulation effects with BWSTT for children with CP. Additional controlled trials are needed to determine benefits and efficacy of BWSTT for children with CP.
	LaForme Fiss & Effgen (2006)	15 articles	What is the effectiveness of BWSTT for children with disabilities?	The effectiveness of BWSTT cannot be supported because of low levels of evidence available. Additional research is needed to confirm seemingly positive results of beginning research.
Conductive Education (CE)	Darrah, Watkins, Chen, & Bonin (2004)	15 articles	What is the effectiveness of CE for children with cerebral palsy?	Effectiveness of CE for children with CP cannot be supported or refuted because of limited research and low levels of evidence.
Constraint-Induced Movement Therapy (CIMT)	Charles & Gordon (2005)	15 articles	What does the research say regarding forced use and CIMT for children with hemiplegia?	Forced use and CI therapy appear to be promising for improving hand function in children with hemiplegia, but available research represents lower levels of evidence. Additional research is needed to confirm these findings for clinical practice.
Functional Electrical Stimulation (FES)/ Neuromuscular Electrical Stimulation (NMES)	Kerr, McDowell, & McDonough (2004)	18 articles	What is the effect of electrical stimulation on strength and motor function for children with CP?	There is more evidence to support the use of NMES over transcutaneous electrical nerve stimulation (TENS). Additional research is needed to confirm these findings.

Table 8.1 Evidence-Based Interventions for Children With Neurological Disorders: Systematic Reviews (SR)—cont'd

Intervention	Author (date)	# articles (SR)	Question	Findings
	Seifart, Unger, & Burger (2009)	5 articles	What is the effect of lower limb FES in children with CP?	Stimulation of the gastrocnemius with or without tibialis anterior muscle may lead to greater gait improvements than stimulation of the anterior tibialis muscle alone. More research differentiating between FES and NMES protocols are needed.
Hippotherapy	Snider, Korner-Bitensky, Kammann, Warner, & Saleh (2007)	9 articles	What is the effect of horseback riding therapy for children with CP?	Evidence to support hippotherapy as an effective intervention to improve muscle symmetry in trunk and hip and to improving muscle tone in children with CP is of fair strength. Additional controlled trials should be conducted to confirm these results and to address participation outcomes.
	Sterba (2007)	11 articles	Does horseback riding used as therapy improve gross motor function in children with CP?	Horseback riding therapy and hippotherapy are supported as gross motor rehabilitation for children with CP. Additional research should be completed.
Neurodevelopmental Treatment (NDT)	Brown & Burns (2001)	15 articles	Is NDT an effective intervention for children with CP?	Efficacy of NDT is inconclusive, with 6 published studies supporting benefits of NDT and 9 with no benefit.
	Butler & Darrah (2001)	21 articles	Is NDT an effective intervention for children with CP?	There is no advantage of NDT over alternative forms of physical therapy for children with CP. Additional research needs to be completed to provide a more comprehensive view of NDT.
Postural Control	Harris & Roxborough (2005)	12 studies	What research exists about the effectiveness and efficacy of postural control interventions for children with CP?	There is not enough evidence to support that postural control interventions for children with CP are effective because of lower levels of evidence. Additional studies with stronger designs are needed.

Continued

Table 8.1 Evidence-Based Interventions for Children With Neurological Disorders: Systematic Reviews (SR)—cont'd

Intervention	Author (date)	# articles (SR)	Question	Findings
Sensory Integration (SI)	Vargas & Camilli (1999)	16 studies	Do existing studies support the efficacy of SI?	SI treatments are as effective as other treatment methods. Larger effects were found in psychoeducational and motor categories.
Serial Casting	Blackmore, Boettcher-Hunt, Jordan, & Chan (2007)	22 articles	What is the effect of casting alone or in combination with botulinum toxin type A on equinus in children with CP?	There is not enough evidence to support casting over no casting, to support casting in combination with botox over either intervention alone, or to support that order of casting and botox affects the outcome. Additional research is needed.
Strengthening	Scianni, Butler, Ada, & Teixeira-Salmela (2009)	5 articles	Do strengthening exercises increase strength without increasing spasticity and improve activity, and is there any carryover after cessation in children and adolescents with CP?	Strengthening exercises have not shown a significant effect in improving strengthening or walking speed for children with CP. Based on the available evidence, strengthening exercises are not effective for children with CP who are ambulatory. Further research is needed.
	Mockford & Caulton (2008)	13 articles	Is progressive strength training on function and gait effective for children with CP who are ambulatory?	No significant adverse effects were found. Function and gait improvements were greater in preadolescents.
	Dodd, Taylor, & Damiano (2002)	11 articles	Is strength training beneficial for people with CP?	Training can increase strength and may improve motor activity in people with CP without adverse effects. More research is needed.
	Darrah, Fan, Chen, Nunweiler, & Watkins (1997)	7 articles	What is the effect of progressive resistive muscle strengthening for children with CP?	Progressive resistive exercise of isolated muscle groups increased muscle performance in children with CP. Additional research is needed to clarify the relationship between strength training and functional abilities.

Table 8.1 Evidence-Based Interventions for Children With Neurological Disorders: Systematic Reviews (SR)—cont'd

Intervention	Author (date)	# articles (SR)	Question	Findings
Stretching	Wiart, Darrah, & Kembhavi (2008)	7 articles	What is the current research regarding mechanisms of muscle contracture in CP and the effectiveness of stretching?	Additional research on structural changes that occur in the shortened muscles of children with CP and effects of stretching interventions is needed.
	Pin, Dyke, & Chan (2006)	4 articles	What is the effectiveness of passive stretching for children with spastic CP?	Limited evidence supports the effectiveness of passive stretching to increase range of motion, reduce spasticity, or improve walking efficiency in children with CP. Sustained stretching of longer duration was more effective in improving range of movements and to reduce spasticity. Further research is needed to more effectively address this topic.
	Leong (2002)	17 articles	Are passive muscle stretches effective for children in vegetative or minimally conscious states?	No conclusive evidence supports effectiveness of passive range of motion exercises.
Weight bearing	Pin (2007)	10 articles	What is the evidence for the effectiveness of static weight bearing activities for children with CP?	There is some evidence to support the use of static weight bearing to increase bone mineral density and to temporarily reduce spasticity. However, evidence supporting the effectiveness of static weight-bearing exercises in children with CP is limited because of lower level of evidence.

Activity-Focused Intervention

Specific intervention activities or procedures that therapists use to execute the plan of care are usually derived from a recognized intervention approach. Current approaches to physical therapy for children with neurological conditions are characterized as task-oriented (or activity-focused) (Darrah, Wiart, & Magill-Evans, 2008). These approaches focus on practice of meaningful functional tasks and assume that the child is an active participant in a learning process, motivated by the goal to accomplish a specific task. Changes in multiple systems, including motor, perceptual, and cognitive, are driven by the active participation in the functional activity. These approaches are supported by advances in neuroscience that stress repetition and problem solving associated with practice to foster brain reorganization associated with neural plasticity (Fisher & Sullivan, 2001). Over the past two decades, task-oriented approaches have emerged as an alternative to traditional impairment-focused physical therapy approaches, which emphasize skillful handling and sensory inputs provided by the therapist as a means to facilitate normal patterns of movement and improve function.

In this chapter, a specific task-oriented model called activity-focused interventions (Valvano, 2004) is presented. First, motor learning theories, which provide the framework for activity-focused interventions, are reviewed. Next, the elements of the activity-focused model of intervention are discussed. Then, strategies to enhance the active motor learning experience are discussed, and finally, impairments in body structures and functions that place limits on motor performance and learning are addressed.

Active Process of Motor Learning: Theoretical Perspectives

Information-Processing Perspective

Two major perspectives that have guided the research on motor learning and development are the information-processing perspective and dynamic systems perspectives. Understanding the fundamental concepts from these perspectives is helpful in understanding the theory that supports motor learning strategies. Recommended readings on the conceptual framework of each of these perspectives are provided at the end of the chapter.

The information-processing perspective emphasizes the cognitive processes associated with learning motor skills. Understanding these cognitive processes should help therapists to structure practice for children with special needs. The information-processing perspective views the learner as an active processor of information. Information processing is essential to motor learning, which is defined as "a set of internal processes associated with practice or experience leading to a relatively permanent change in the capability for a motor skill" (Schmidt, 1988, p. 375). Repeated motor activity without active participation and information processing would yield very little gain in terms of motor learning. How could a baseball player perfect his batting if he were passively moved through each hit in practice? How could an infant learn visually guided reaching if his or her hand were passively directed to the object? How could a child with cerebral palsy (CP) learn to complete a transfer if he or she were passively moved on each repetitive trial?

Stages of Information Processing The information processing that occurs before the actual production of the movement commences contributes to the process of motor learning (Light, 2003). According to the model proposed by Schmidt (1988), the processing that occurs before movement execution includes (1) stimulus identification, which involves selectively attending to and integrating relevant stimuli from the environment, (2) response selection, which involves choosing a suitable motor response, and (3) response programming, which structures or prepares the appropriate response in the central nervous system (CNS) (see Fig. 8.1). These hypothetical processing steps affect reaction time, which is the duration in time between the presentation of an environmental stimulus, or the impetus to move, and the actual initiation of the movement response. The stages of information processing interact with two other elements of the information-processing perspective: memory and attention. These hypothetical processing stages provide a framework to explain the information processing deficits, which contribute to the slow, awkward quality of movement seen in children with neurological impairments.

Specifically, this framework has been used to explain the slow information processing times, poor visual and spatial ability, and timing deficits typical of developmental coordination disorder (DCD) (David, 1995, 2000; Maruff, Wilson, Trebilcock, & Currie, 1998; Missiuna, Rivard, & Bartlett, 2003; Wilson & McKenzie, 1998). David (2000) suggests that deficits in stimulus identification explain difficulty with spatial organization and with judging distances. These children might bump into objects or have difficulty with spatial judgments on the playground. David also describes how memory functions could affect the response selection in children with DCD. A child playing baseball might not recall the best orientation relative to the plate when hitting the baseball or the best way to hold the bat. In soccer, the child may not remember the best kick, based on the configuration of his opponents on the field. Moreover, David (2000) proposed that difficulties with timing of responses and with grading the level of force may also relate to deficits in response selection. Impairments in response programming might affect the ability to remember the sequence of elements of a functional action. Children with DCD may not effectively use anticipatory control, developed from prior experience, and consequently depend heavily on visual feedback (Missiuna et al., 2003). If the sequence of a movement response, such as tying a shoelace or getting onto a tricycle, cannot be taken from memory and executed, the child must rely on the feedback provided in the

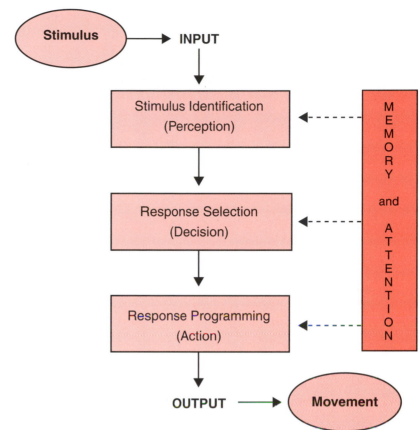

Figure 8.1 Information-processing model. *(Adapted, by permission, from Schmidt, R.A., & Lee, T.D. [1999]. Motor control and learning: A behavioral emphasis [3rd ed., p. 45]. Champaign, IL: Human Kinetics.)*

course of performance, thereby making the movement slow and laborious. Production deficits may also contribute to the inefficient movement in DCD.

Developmental aspects of information processing have been addressed in the literature. The time to process information is age related. It takes younger children longer to process feedback information, especially complex information. The precision of information that can be used for feedback also varies with age (Gallagher & Thomas, 1989; Newell & Carlton, 1980; Newell & Kennedy, 1978; Sullivan, Kantak, & Burtner, 2008).

The stages of information processing could help therapists plan activities for motor learning. For example, the stages of information processing can be applied to the practice of walking with a cane by a child with traumatic brain injury (TBI). Because of perceptual, cognitive, and attention constraints, as well as frustration levels during the course of recovery, the child's physical therapist might grade the challenge in terms of the information-processing demands. The child's therapist might begin working in a very quiet part of a gym with very little equipment and no other children. This would reduce demands on attention and make it easier to identify and process relevant stimuli.

The therapist might even help the child to focus on salient visual cues. Gradually a more complex stimulus array could be introduced. Selective attention is a critical element to motor learning, and attention processes should be a focus of effective learning interventions.

After the basic ability to walk with a cane is acquired, the therapist might decide to teach the child to walk around obstacles. To grade the challenge for stimulus identification, the obstacles should initially be large, brightly colored, and contrasting with the floor. Eventually the obstacles might be more subtle and challenging to detect. The placement of obstacles in the child's way could also be graded in terms of the complexity of their pattern. When the therapist conducts the practice in the hallway, the number of response options might also increase the challenge. In addition to obstacles to step around, the therapist might present additional movement challenges, such as a broom to step over, an unexpected person to walk around, or a small box that has to be moved out of the path, until the child can walk in numerous natural environments.

Finally, response-programming challenges can be modified by the complexity of the response that has to be organized for execution. The number of response elements, one index of complexity, would be minimal if the walking were initiated on cue from a standing position with the cane already placed in the child's hand. The programming requirements (and reaction time) would be increased if the child were required, on cue, to grasp the cane and move from sitting to standing and then initiate a step. Programming requirements could also be graded by the degree of accuracy required in the movement response. The programming requirements should be adjusted to the stage of learning, with the ultimate focus on the requirements in the child's functional environment.

Memory The second important concept from the information-processing perspective is **memory**. Memory functions are important to enable the learner to benefit from prior experience. There are many elaborate models to depict the functions of memory in motor learning in the literature. The fundamental components of memory are depicted in Figure 8.2. Two basic concepts relevant to therapeutic practice by children are **short-term** and **long-term memory** (Schmidt, 1988; Schmidt & Wrisberg, 2008). Children are constantly bombarded by environmental stimuli that are held very briefly in what is referred to as the short-term sensory store. Only relevant stimuli are selectively attended to and processed in a theoretical structure called short-term memory. This short-term memory is also called the working memory because it is the theoretical structure where information about the goal-oriented movement and the sensory cues associated with the movement are processed. Information resides in short-term memory only for seconds. If there is adequate active mental processing in the short-term memory, information can

be encoded or packaged for storage into the long-term memory. Examples of an active mental processing are allocating attention to focus on the movement, mentally rehearsing a movement, evaluating the outcome of the movement, or making comparisons with previous movement trials. Encoding into long-term memory is critical in the information-processing perspective because information "stored" in the long-term memory can be retrieved when it is needed again for a functional movement response. Active practice and processing are very important for encoding information into long-term memory, or "making memories," that can be retrieved and adapted for future performance.

Motor Program The memory representation of a movement that can be retrieved when needed for a functional action is called the **motor program**. A motor program can be viewed as a pre-structured motor command, which defines and shapes the essential details of a skilled action (Schmidt & Wrisberg, 2008). The motor program is responsible for determining the major events in the movement pattern.

However, there is often considerable interaction with sensory processes to refine the movement and adapt it to environmental demands (Schmidt & Wrisberg, 2008). There cannot be a motor program for all of the possible variations of a movement class (e.g., throwing at different velocities, at different intensities, and in different directions). The concept of the **generalized motor program** was described by Schmidt (1988) to address this limitation. Although some fundamental assumptions of the generalized motor program are under theoretical debate, it provides the practical distinction between basic invariant features of the motor

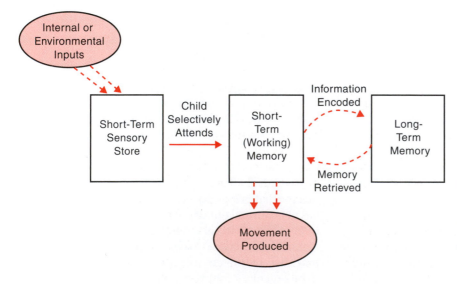

Figure 8.2 Model of memory structures.(*Adapted, by permission, from Schmidt, R.A. [1988]. Motor control and learning: A behavioral emphasis [2nd ed., p. 91]. Champaign, IL: Human Kinetics.*)

program related to the spatiotemporal structure of the movement and the changeable or variant features, which modify the movement to meet task requirements (Schmidt & Wrisberg, 2008).

For example, the generalized motor program for kicking a soccer ball has invariant features that define kicking, including the relative time it takes to complete each component of the movement. Variant or changeable features of the motor program, such as the overall force with which the ball is kicked, or the direction of the kick, are called **parameters** of the motor program. Variable practice of multiple parameters of an action class theoretically makes the mental representation (motor program) more flexible, and therefore should promote generalization of the skill to many new situations (Schmidt & Wrisberg, 2008). A physical therapist might provide variable practice by working on the transition from chairs of varied heights and with different seat surfaces.

A fundamental principle in motor learning is the difference between performance and learning. Changes in **performance** immediately seen during the practice of a task may not be permanent. **Learning** is a relatively permanent effect of practice or experience, and it is measured by retention of the practiced motor task (Schmidt, 1988; Winstein, 1991). Certain practice strategies may be associated with great benefits in performance but are detrimental long-term learning. For example, high amounts of guidance or feedback may encourage fast and essentially error-free motor performance. However, the effect on long-term learning is quite the opposite. Too much dependence on guidance and feedback during practice may limit the information processing and memory functions required to develop the mental representation that is required for long-term learning, or retention (Schmidt & Wrisberg, 2008).

Attention The final construct of information processing discussed here is attention. **Attention** can be defined as the allocation and focusing of information-processing resources (McDowd, 2007). Selective attention involves focusing on the relevant stimuli for interaction with the environment. This concept has relevance for young children with neurological immaturity, who have difficulty focusing attention. It also has implications for motor learning by children who have attention deficit disorder, for whom filtering out irrelevant environmental stimuli may be difficult.

Of great clinical relevance is the general assumption that there is a limited capacity of attention. Basically, children can concentrate on a limited amount of information at one time. For well-learned tasks, the performer does not have to direct as much attention to generating the movement response. If a movement is well learned, the child can execute the response quickly (e.g., kicking a soccer ball), with relatively little attention. For complex tasks, if some components are performed without attention demands, information processing resources can be available for other parts of the movement. For example if the kicking action is automatic, the soccer player can direct his or her attention to the actions of the opponents and the configuration of the players on the field. In natural environments, such as the classroom, children are often required to focus on many things at once.

Researchers have learned about attention limitations by using dual task or divided attention paradigms. In these paradigms, a competing, or dual, task is introduced as the child performs a primary task. The effects of performance on the primary and secondary tasks are observed. Basically, the interference that one task has with another depends on how well learned or automatic the primary task is. If it is well learned, it does not require much attention, and other processes can be conducted in parallel (Huang & Mercer, 2001; Schmidt & Lee, 2005).

The concept of divided attention has applications to balance and gait in children. Although postural control is an automatic process, it draws from the overall information-processing resource. In general, balance and/or gait patterns in children can be affected by dual tasks (e.g., walking and carrying lunch on a tray while monitoring to keep the contents from falling off) or cognitive tasks in children. The extent of the decrement in balance is influenced by the child's age, the complexity or difficulty of the competing task, how well learned each competing task is, and the demands for postural control. The decrement in performance associated with dual tasks is significantly greater for children with neurological conditions, such as DCD and CP (Laufer, Ashkenazi, & Josman, 2008; Reilly, Woollacott, van Donkelaar, & Saavedra, 2008).

Strategies that might be used to address the role of attention include (1) taking the child to a high level of primary task performance before introducing interference of competing tasks, (2) using dual tasks to evaluate level of learning of a primary task or development of postural control, and (3) practicing functional tasks in the natural environment, where attention is divided among competing tasks.

In summary, the information-processing framework emphasizes the cognitive aspects of motor learning. It embodies constructs, such as attention, memory, and mental representations, that are established and refined through experience and practice. This framework has been the basis for much of the research on practice variables that enhance motor learning, including augmented information and structure of practice.

Constructs from the information-processing perspective, especially memory and attention, have been applied to developmental research with young infants and can be applied to models of early intervention strategies for infants at risk for neurological impairments (Valvano & Rapport, 2006). However, information-processing theory in this chapter will be applied only to intentional motor skill learning in school-aged children.

Motor Learning Principles

Dynamic Systems Perspective

While the information-processing perspective addresses cognitive systems and their role in motor learning, the dynamic systems perspective on motor learning provides more of a theoretical framework for how movement behavior is organized and how it changes with activity-focused interventions.

There have been two major influences on the dynamic systems perspective: the writings of Nikolai Bernstein (1967) and the science of nonlinear dynamics applied to organization and nonlinear change in complex physical and biological systems. According to Bernstein, motor learning involves problem solving, or actively finding a coordination strategy that will enable a functional motor task to be executed. The process of learning does not merely involve repetition of the movement; it involves going through the process of solving the problem again and again (Bernstein, 1967). This is apparent in the school-aged child who spends hours trying to master a computer game and in early walkers who practice upright balance. Adolph, Vereijken, and Shrout (2003) report that infant walkers practice balance walking for more than 6 accumulated hours per day and average between 500 and 1,500 steps per hour! That is 29 football fields per day (Adolph & Berger, 2006).

Complex Movement Systems With Many Component Systems Bernstein emphasized the multiple systems that cooperate in the performance of functional movement. The dynamic systems theory views the learner as a complex biological system composed of many independent but interacting subsystems. The interaction of multiple systems, reiterated several times in Chapter 7, is the foundation for the systems model of motor control, which has had great influence on task-oriented

models of intervention for adults and children with neurological impairments. The interaction of these multiple systems promotes a movement organization that is preferred, or "natural," as the learner performs a task under specific task and environmental conditions (Davids, Button, & Bennet, 2008). Shumway-Cook and Woollacott (2012) compare this self-organization of the elements of the movement system with the cells in the heart, which work collectively to make the heart beat.

The concept of a complex self-organizing movement system is applied to the classic example of the development of independent stepping by infants (Heriza & Sweeney, 1994; Thelen, 1986). Thelen proposed that each of the multiple systems (including cognition, motivation, strength, tonus control, and body characteristics) associated with locomotion has its own developmental timetable and progresses at its own rate. Changes in these interacting systems create opportunities for the emergence of the new, preferred locomotor behaviors (Heriza, 1991; Spencer & Schoner, 2003). If all of the subsystems are at a specified state or level of organization, walking emerges as the preferred pattern of locomotion. If one of the participating systems were not at the proper state (e.g., hip extension strength not developed), independent stepping would not emerge as the preferred behavior. The self-organizing movement system intrinsic to the infant also interacts with the task and the context of the action, which drive the motor behavior. Stepping behaviors will not emerge unless the infant perceives the action goal, such as moving toward a parent or favorite toy.

Movement Versus Action In the dynamic systems perspective, the difference between action and movement is critical. Action involves the accomplishment of a task, the intention to realize a functional goal, and a strategy to achieve the goal (Gentile, 1987; Majsak, 1996; Newell & Valvano, 1998; Van der Weel, van der Meer, & Lee, 1991). Change at the movement level involves the coordination of movement patterns, which allows the action goal to be achieved. Change at the movement level is not sufficient for action. The emphasis on action in the dynamic systems perspective is compatible with current models of motor control, which focus on purposeful activity rather than the achievement of movement components for their own sake. The task is required to give meaning and a goal structure to the movement pattern.

Degrees of Freedom Bernstein suggested that finding the coordination to achieve a functional action involved controlling all of the redundant **degrees of freedom** (DFs), or all of the possible independent planes of motion in the joints in the body to coordinate an efficient movement (Newell & McDonald, 1994). The DFs are redundant in that there are more available options for movement than the child needs to perform the task. According to Bernstein, this coordination of the DFs of the joints, which exceed 100, is accomplished by organizing these DFs into functional groups or synergies that constrain the muscles or joints to act as functional units. The hip and knee in walking, or the elbow and shoulder in reaching, are linked together as functional units or synergies. That is, the movement of one segment can be easily predicted by the movement of the other. However, in the case of walking and reaching, the linkage of the distal segments may be more variable to adapt the movement to the task demands.

Likewise, in the process of learning complex motor skills that require discrete movement at all segments, basic synergies are differentiated and refined, so the movement can be more flexibly adapted to task demands. This process of differentiation is illustrated in the novice compared to the expert skier. The novice skier appears "stiff" as he skis down the hill. The movement is stiff because he "freezes" the DFs by either holding the joints stiff in cocontraction or using simple, undifferentiated synergies of the trunk and leg segments. It is too challenging for the novice to control muscular forces of all of the segments and coordinate them with passive forces such as the force of gravity. Over time, the skier learns to differentiate the joints and adapt to subtle challenges on the hill. The advanced skier is able to use the physical effects of gravity and the motion-dependent forces from the leg and trunk movements to make smooth, fast movements down the hill.

Note that in skilled performance, the internal forces generated by muscle activation patterns (theoretically directed by the motor program) are coordinated with external or physical forces including gravity, inertia, and motion-dependent forces. **Motion-dependent forces** are forces that act on one segment as a result of movement from adjacent segments in the body. Try shaking your hand vigorously and note that there are forces that are apparently acting on the humerus. Also, think of the forces generated by a countermovement, such as when a pitcher winds up and twists before pitching the baseball. The contribution of these physical forces challenges the traditional notion of a motor program, which can, theoretically, be retrieved to organize a movement response.

Consider again the classic case of infant kicking. The motor program that organizes a single muscle activation pattern for kicking would be an inadequate description. Additional nonneural forces such as gravity, inertia,

and motion-dependent forces complement the forces that contribute to the kick from neural activation. The interaction of these forces is different when the baby kicks in supine position from when the baby kicks while supported in a semireclining position (Jensen, Ulrich, Thelen, Schneider, & Zernicke, 1994). Therefore, from the dynamic systems perspective, the motor program is considered to be "softly assembled" to account for environmental contributions to the motor response.

The flexible control of DFs and the integration of non-neural forces are depicted in the throwing task of the 7-year old boy in Figure 8.3A. Note the differentiation at the spine, the intuitive use of a countermovement

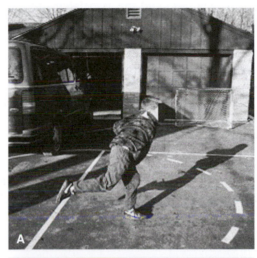

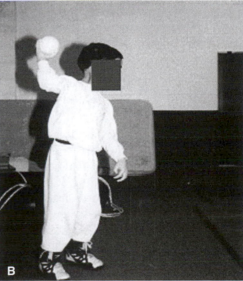

Figure 8.3 Coordination of the degrees of freedom during throwing tasks by (*A*) a boy with typical development and (*B*) a boy with spastic diplegia.

(which uses the elastic properties of muscle and connective tissue to contribute to the force generation), and the weight shift (motion-dependent forces) that characterize this movement. Contrast this to the throwing behaviors of a child with CP (Fig. 8.3B), who limits the DFs by holding the trunk stiffly, minimizing the motion-dependent forces and forces of gravity and inertia. The expected difference in functional outcome between the two children is obvious. This intuitive sequence of freezing, then flexibly freeing the DF, explains the limitations in two-handed catching in children with DCD (Utley, Steenbergen, & Astill, 2007). Likewise, Bly suggests that children with neurological conditions may adaptively "freeze the DF" when attempting a challenging or new task, and the associated stiffness and cocontraction is mistakenly attributed to spasticity (Bly, 1991).

The coordination of the DF during functional activity is individual for each child. This may explain why it is often difficult to change the form or quality of the movement in children with neurological impairments (Valvano & Newell, 1998). Latash and Anson (1996) argue that the atypical quality of movement of children with disability represents the best solution for achieving a functional goal given the impairments in the component systems that contribute to the movement. However, certain "preferred" patterns of movement may be inefficient or lead to secondary impairments. For example, sitting in an asymmetrical manner might lead to scoliosis; sitting in a "W-sit" pattern may affect the integrity of the hip joint and soft tissue. The judgment of the physical therapist, as the change agent, is critical here in determining the efficacy of intervention goals at the movement level. When practicing functional tasks, such as ascending or descending stairs, the therapist might try to differentiate between components of movement that are critical for safely executing the task and those that relate more to style and aesthetics.

Concepts About Change In the past decades, movement scientists have applied mathematical principles to develop a dynamic pattern theory that addresses Bernstein's questions about organization of movement and changes that occur during motor learning (Haken, Kelso, & Bunz, 1985; Kelso, 1984; Scholz, 1990). This section will focus on a few practical concepts from dynamic pattern theory that can be useful in conducting activity-focused interventions.

Dynamic systems are systems that change. For motor behaviors to change, with intentional skill learning or during development, the intrinsic coordination tendencies of the child must change (Kelso, 1984; Newell,

1996; Newell & Valvano, 1998; Scholz, 1990; Zanone, Kelso, & Jeka, 1993). The term **coordination**, from a dynamic systems framework, refers to the organization of the body segments into a behavioral unit, which clinicians might call a pattern of movement. There can be qualitative change in the coordination, which defines the relationship of segments to one another (e.g., palmar grasp versus pincer grasp). There can also be quantitative change, such as changes in speed, timing, or magnitude of the movement. The latter refine or scale the basic pattern to meet task demands. According to dynamic pattern theory, changes in motor behavior are induced by variables called **control parameters.** Control parameters take on different values and, when they reach a critical value, provide the necessary conditions to induce a change in motor behavior.

The metaphor of the control parameter can be applied to clinical interventions. The physical therapist, through careful task analysis and analysis of the child's movement characteristics, can identify factors that will support the desired change during the practice of functional tasks. Control parameters can reside in one or many of the multiple subsystems that contribute to the complex movement system. They can also be external to the performer.

Consider the common clinical example of toe walking by a child with CP. Often, if the child walks very slowly, he or she may demonstrate heel strike at initial contact. However, as the speed of the walking increases, the child may contact with the forefoot. The increased velocity of the stepping may be a control parameter related to the task that influences the transition from heel contact to forefoot contact. The degree of muscle stiffness, selective muscle control, or the postural control challenge in the increased velocity condition could be control parameters internal to the child that influence the transition to toe walking.

An ankle-foot orthosis may also be a control parameter because it changes the degree of stiffness in the ankle, resulting in heel contact during gait. Another example of the control parameter is the systematic change in grip patterns used for functional grasp and release. Grip pattern changes in a systematic way so that the number of fingers (2 to 10) used to grip can be predicted by the size of the object relative to the thumb span (Newell, Scully, McDonald, & Baillargeon, 1989). Here, the size of the object is a control parameter.

The concept of **stability** in the dynamic systems perspective describes the resistance to change or transition to another motor behavior. The stability of a certain movement pattern or coordination used to achieve an action is determined by the intrinsic characteristics of the child's movement system under certain task and environmental conditions. The behavior that is stable is called the **preferred behavior**. The loss of stability of one motor behavior supports a pattern switch or transition. Transitions or pattern shifts occur in development because change in the component systems of the infant makes the current pattern unstable or less "natural." These component systems self-organize, and new motor patterns emerge as the preferred ones to achieve an action (e.g., belly crawling transitions to creeping on hands and knees for locomotion). These periods of instability are critical for progression to new motor behaviors.

In the previous examples of change, the control parameters provided the necessary conditions for the systems to reorganize (or transition) to an alternative behavior that was available to the child. Often the coordination (or patterns of movement) required to perform functional activities, such as serving a tennis ball or walking with crutches, is not available to the child. In these cases, the acquisition of a new coordination option must be acquired through focused, intentional effort.

With practice, a new motor coordination can emerge (Wenderoth, Bock, & Krohn, 2002; Zanone & Kelso, 1994). From a dynamic systems perspective, practice creates instability in stable movement behaviors just as changes in component systems in development create instability. With practice, newly learned solutions replace the original ones (Scholz & Kelso, 1990; Zanone & Kelso, 1994). In the example of an adult learning a new golf swing, many contributing systems determine the individual's preferred golf swing. Practice of an alternative golf swing creates instability in the previous behavior and a new preferred behavior (golf swing) emerges from practice. The practice encourages changes in systems that support this new coordination, such as flexibility in the trunk, strength in the arms, and neural reorganization. In a similar way, practicing a functional task by children with neurological conditions can support changes in motor behavior.

Experiments that examine the concept of stability suggest that, for intentional learning, the coordination of to-be-learned motor behavior is in competition with the intrinsic existing tendencies of the mover. If the existing movement pattern is very stable, practice may have diminished effects. If the existing pattern is not stable, goal-directed practice results in further destabilization of the existing movement pattern and a

transition to the desired behavior. Furthermore, the likelihood of change is affected by the degree to which the requirements of the to-be-learned behavior are different from those of the current behavior (Scholz & Kelso, 1990; Schoner, Zanone, & Kelso, 1992; Wenderoth, Bock, & Krohn, 2002; Zanone & Kelso, 1994). Concepts about stability and the likelihood of change can be applied to the process of prognosis in the *Guide* (2001), which requires therapists to anticipate the potential for change in the child.

Constraints on Action   The idea of the control parameter has been applied to practical learning situations through the construct of **constraints on action** (Davids et al., 2008; Newell, 1986). Constraints can be multiple factors related to the performer, the task, and the environment (or context of learning) that interact with each other to influence the preferred behavior that will emerge. This concept has been applied to interventions with varied clinical populations (Clark; 1995; Majsak, 1996; Newell, 1986; Newell & Valvano, 1998; Shumway-Cook & Woollacott, 2012). These factors are called constraints because they limit or constrain the possible movement outcomes that might emerge as the child attempts to achieve an action. Constraints can be enablers or positive influences to learning (because they restrict the possible outcomes to positive ones) or limiters to learning (because they inhibit change or support the outcome that is not desired).

Task constraints relate to the goal of the task or the rules of the activity, which may be implicit or explicit. The environmental constraints involve physical manipulations, such as the support medium, as well as physical supports, such as adaptive equipment. The environment also includes the psychosocial environment and the performance environment. The performance environment includes augmented information, such as feedback and guidance, that is provided to the child to enhance learning.

Newell and Valvano (1998) propose that the physical therapist, along with parents and other professionals on the intervention team, are change agents as the child learns functional motor activities. The change agents support and foster change to meet the action goals in the plan of care. The physical therapist interacts with constraints related to the task, the environment, and the characteristics of the infant or child to support the transition, which embodies the achievement of the action goal. In that way, the input from the physical therapist can be considered a constraint on the action that emerges with practice.

Activity-Focused Interventions

This section discusses a model called **activity-focused intervention** (Fig. 8.4) that focuses on goal-oriented practice of functional activities. The physical therapist is a change agent who plans and adapts activity-focused interventions, which will lead to the desired activity and participation changes outlined in the plan of care. Activity-focused interventions involve structured practice and repetition of functional actions with consideration of the constraints of the task, the environment, and the individual that influence motor behaviors. The physical therapist, as a change agent, also integrates activity-focused interventions with interventions that address impairments in body functions and structures.

There is a growing body of empirical evidence for the benefits of interventions that focus on practice of functional motor activity. One important intervention that emphasizes functional practice is constraint-induced movement therapy to improve function in the affected upper extremity of children with hemiplegic CP. Repetition and practice with the affected upper extremity in functional activity is encouraged by "constraining" the dominant hand with a cast or mitt (DeLuca, Echols, Ramey, & Taub, 2003; Naylor & Bower, 2005; Taub, Ramey, DeLuca, & Echols, 2004). More recent studies suggest that forced bimanual practice may have similar benefits (Gordon, Schneider, Chinnan, & Charles, 2007).

The concept of constraint therapy has also been applied to gait (Coker, Karakostas, Dodds, & Hsiang, 2010). Functional gains associated with interventions that inherently require intensive repetitions, such as body weight-supported treadmill training (Damiano & DeJong, 2009) and balance practice (Shumway-Cook, Hutchinson, Kartin, Price, & Woollacott, 2003), also support task-oriented approaches. Furthermore, there are also documented changes with practice of functional tasks individualized to children with CP and developmental delay (Ketelaar, Vermer, Hart, van Petegem-van Beek, & Helders, 2001) and children with DCD (Shoemaker, Niemeijer, Reynderes, & Smits-Englesman, 2003).

An important feature of the activity-focused model is the integration of impairment-focused interventions with the functional practice. These impairments may be viewed as constraints of the learner that limit the process of motor learning and may cause secondary impairments (see Valvano, 2004, for details of the model).

The understanding of how impairments in body functions and structures impact motor skill learning is a unique contribution of the physical therapist in teaching children functional movement skills for home and community activities and participation. For children with neurological impairments, it is important to reflect on the impact of impairments on function, not only for the short term but also for the lifetime of the child (Campbell, 1999).

There are three practical steps for activity-focused interventions:

1. Develop **activity-related goals and objectives** that will increase function and enhance activities and participation, especially in daily routines, based on priorities of the child and family, in collaboration with the intervention team.

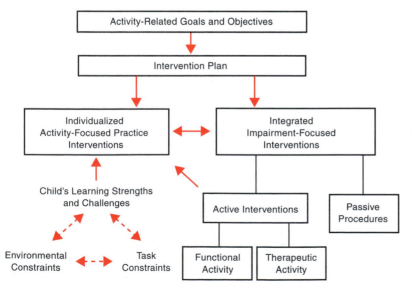

Figure 8.4 Model of interventions for children with neurological impairments, which integrates activity-focused interventions with impairment-focused interventions by physical therapist or occupational therapist as change agent. *(Reprinted from Valvano, J. [2004]. Activity-focused motor interventions for children with neurological conditions. Physical and Occupational Therapy in Pediatrics, 24, with permission.)*

2. Plan **activity-focused interventions** that empha-size practice of functional tasks by (a) using motor learning guidelines from the literature as a foundation for planning therapeutic practice, with focus on environment and task variables, and (b) adapting these practice guidelines, when necessary, to address the child's individual learning strengths and needs.

3. Integrate **impairment-focused interventions** with activity-focused interventions. These are optimally executed in the context of goal-related functional activity but may also be executed outside the context of functional activity.

Although this model of activity-focused interventions can be applied to motor development in infants and young children (Valvano & Rapport, 2006), the description that follows will be most applicable to children of school age.

Guidelines for Conducting Activity-Focused Practice
Developing Goals for Practice

Goals that structure the plan of care are achieved after (1) careful consideration of the examination findings, (2) development of a clinical impression that links impairments in body functions and structures with restrictions in activities and participation, and (3) consideration of the prognosis for meaningful change. Long-term goals of the intervention plan are developed in collaboration with the child and family or educational and medical team. The first part of this chapter discussed concepts that should be integrated into goals and objectives. From the long-term goals established in the intervention plan of care (usually every 6 months for an IFSP, every school year for an IEP, and more frequently in the hospital setting), short-term objectives are developed. Short-term objectives can be directed toward (1) acquiring a new motor task, (2) increasing skill or fluency of a motor task or generalizing it to natural environments, or (3) in some cases, reducing an impairment to prevent secondary disability. It is recommended that the physical therapist also develop practice objectives, which guide the development of practice strategies for a single or group of practice sessions. These practice goals should eventually lead to the achievement of the long-term functional goal. The physical therapist should consider the stability of the current behavior to develop expectations for change or the prognosis.

Model for Activity-Focused Interventions

The model for intervention depicted in Figure 8.4 illustrates the interaction of the constraints related to the task, environment, and the person. It suggests that the physical therapist intervene with practice strategies directed toward the task and the environment to promote learning. The broken lines from the child to the task and environment signify the importance of individualizing these practice strategies to meet the individual learning strengths and limitations of the child.

Many practice variables from the motor learning literature have been studied in adults or children with no disability. These practice variables provide an important foundation for conducting practice, based on processes of learning common to all learners. Unfortunately, empirical data to verify that these motor-learning principles apply to children with neurological impairments are just emerging. Therefore, the physical therapist should personalize interventions for each learner and consider how developmental factors and characteristics of the child, including strengths and limitations, might affect the process of motor learning. In some cases motor learning principles may have to be adapted to address these individual limitations (Valvano, 2004).

Neurological impairments in body functions and structures may challenge motor learning processes in children with neurological conditions. Selective attention may be impaired (Hood & Atkinson, 1990), and sensory deficits, including visual, perceptual, proprioceptive, and tactile could affect information processing and judgments important for motor learning (Lee & Cook, 1990; Stiers et al., 2002). Slow information processing has been documented in children with CP (Parks, Rose, & Dunn, 1989). Because children with neurological diagnoses have limited experience, they also have a limited repertoire of movements to draw on for development of a movement plan for novel tasks (Goodgold-Edwards & Gianutsos, 1991). They may have difficulty developing memory representations of movements and may rely on sensory feedback for performance (Eliasson, Gordon, & Forssberg, 1992, 1995).

Limitations in motor learning processes may be compounded by motor control impairments. There are deficits in force production, in terms of strength (Damiano, Dodd, & Taylor, 2002) as well as in selective control. The latter affects reliable motor performance during practice due to impaired timing and sequencing of muscle activation, phasing of agonist and antagonist, and coordination of movement (Olney & Wright, 2006). There is also greatly increased trial-to-trial variability when children with neurological impairments practice a skill (Eliasson et al., 1992; Thorpe & Valvano, 2002; Valvano & Newell, 1998). These limitations in motor control cause the process of motor learning to be more effortful and complex. The increased complexity increases the requirement for practice. These findings may also increase the requirement for guidance and feedback. (See Valvano, 2004, for details.)

This approach of adapting practice variables to the child's individual learning characteristics can be linked to the concept of the "**challenge point**" (Guadagnoli & Lee, 2004). The challenge point hypothesis indicates that, when teaching a motor task, the instructor should select practice conditions that present an optimum level of challenge to the learner. This optimum level elicits active cognitive processes critical for learning, but does not exceed the capability of the learner. If the instructor sets the challenge point too high or low, the level of learning can be affected.

Sullivan and colleagues (2008) applied this concept to explain the different effects of reduced frequency of verbal feedback in a group of young adults compared with a group of children between 8 and 14 years old. Adults who practiced an experimental arm movement task with feedback provided after 50% of the trials performed with better consistency during the retention test compared to the group provided with feedback on 100% of the practice trials. In contrast, children with 100% feedback demonstrated greater accuracy and consistency on retention than those who received 50% feedback. Sullivan and colleagues (2008) propose that the benefits of reduced frequency of feedback that are heavily substantiated in adults do not carry over to children because of different information-processing capabilities.

The concept of the challenge point may also be applied to the findings of Lin and colleagues (Lin, Sullivan, Wu, Kantak, & Winstein, 2007), which showed an advantage of blocked practice for the retention of three movement tasks in adults with Parkinson's disease. This is contrary to the robust advantage for random practice that has been well established in typical adults. Limitations in memory functions important for task shifting could affect the learning processes that are exploited by random practice in healthy adults.

In the following section, the guidelines for practice that can increase the efficiency of practice are reviewed. These guidelines are intuitive applications from the motor learning literature and from discussions of pediatric applications provided by, but not limited to, Duff and Quinn (2002), Heriza (1991), Gentile (1992),

Howle (2003), and Larin (2006). Not all of the proposed guidelines have been empirically tested. The reader is encouraged to reflect on the applications, remain current in the literature, and test these guidelines in clinical settings.

Planning Activity-Focused Interventions: Practice

Guideline No. 1: Practice! Practice! Practice! From a dynamic systems perspective, multiple trials are required to develop the stable, preferred movement patterns necessary for performing functional actions. Furthermore, flexibility in practice, which enables the learner to explore many movement variations, is recommended (Dusing & Harbourne, 2010; Harbourne & Stergiou (2009); Vereijken, 2010). As children practice, their learning should not be expected to be error-free. The development of error detection and problem-solving capabilities is an important part of motor learning. Remember that active learning is not restricted to the practice session. Help the parents and classroom personnel challenge the child with movement problems throughout the course of the day and to reinforce and generalize learning to different environments (Damiano, 2006).

The literature does not provide optimal guidelines for the frequency, duration of practice, and timing of rests during practice sessions. The motor learning literature evaluates the relative benefits of massed practice (duration of practice greater than duration of rest) versus distributed practice (rest greater than practice) (Schmidt & Wrisberg, 2008). However, these findings are difficult to generalize to the type of practice, the learning context, and the characteristics of children with neurological impairments during practice. Issues of fatigue and attention in children, as well as external factors relating to type of setting, academic schedule, and travel by the therapist set constraints on frequency and scheduling.

Studies of the effectiveness of increased frequency of intervention in children with CP are beginning to demonstrate positive outcomes. Studies examining increasing intensity of intervention have noted improved motor development (Mayo, 1991), and specific functional goals (Bower & McLellen, 1992, 1994), improved Gross Motor Function Measure (GMFM) scores (Bower, Michell, Burnett, Campbell, & McLellan, 2001; Stiller, Marcoux, & Olson, 2003; Trahan & Malouin, 2002), and improved Pediatric Evaluation of Disability Inventory (PEDI) scores (Dumas, Haley, Carey & Ni, 2004; Stiller et al., 2003) as compared to less frequent intervention for young children with disabilities.

Optimally, the frequency and schedule of practice sessions should be focused around the learning goal, the phase of practice, and the rate of learning of the child. For example, a child may be scheduled for weekly sessions of physical therapy. For this child, short-term high-frequency sessions might support learning of the emergent skill. A reduced frequency might be adequate as the child solidifies and practices the new skill. Integrating the practice into the natural environment for fluency and generalization may be influenced by the creativity and involvement of parents and school personnel.

The stage of learning has implications for many practice strategies. Gentile (1992) proposed two very practical stages of learning: early and late. During the early stage of learning, the learner discovers (1) the conditions that must be met in order to be successful with the task and (2) a possible coordination strategy to achieve the task. In the later stage of practice, the learner develops skill, the coordination is refined, and the movement becomes efficient (Gentile, 1992). Remember that the sensory motor and motor production deficits demonstrated by children with neurological impairments may prolong the early phases of practice and have implications for variables discussed later in this section.

Planning Activity-Focused Interventions: Task

Task constraints are those that relate to the actual content of practice and the goal of the task or the rules of the activity, which may be implicit or explicit. Task constraints also include implements used during practice, including toys. There is much discussion of the task-related variables in the motor-learning literature, and the reader is encouraged to pursue the recommended readings.

Guideline No. 2: Make Practice Fun and Motivating

Because repeated trials are required to learn a motor skill, the challenge for the physical therapist is to balance the rigors of therapeutic practice with a learning environment that is fun and motivating. Remember that play is the work of children (Parham & Fazio, 2008). Often, motor learning goals can be incorporated into playful games, and physical therapists are challenged to plan motivating activities that are developmentally appropriate. Selective attention to the task should be obtained when the task is presented. Allowing children who are developmentally capable to set the goals in the intervention plan enhances the motivation to practice. As a complement to individual intervention, the use of sensorimotor playgroups can also provide an enjoyable and motivating environment, providing opportunities to increased practice of developmental skills (LaForme Fiss, Effgen, Page, & Shasby, 2009).

Guideline No. 3: Thoughtfully Plan the Practice Activities

Thoughtful planning of composition and the nature of the tasks that are practiced is critical to effective activity-focused interventions. The task practiced may be the identical task specified in the activity goal of the intervention plan, such as eating solids with a fork, ascending stairs with no railing, driving a power chair, or kicking a soccer ball. On the other hand, the activity structured for the practice session may be a related task or developmental play activity that addresses a component of movement that is required for the target activity.

This practice strategy is depicted by a kindergarten student working toward the functional goal of ascending or descending a standard set of stairs without assistance. Impairments in antigravity force generation and impaired selective control of lower extremity muscles limit her ability to advance the leg and accurately place the foot onto the step. Her physical therapist complements the practice of the target task of ascending the steps with an alternate task, such as climbing on the jungle gym, to address the component of flexing the advancing leg against gravity. The strategy of planning related tasks that address critical movement components can help to vary practice and address the challenges of having young children perform repeated practice trials of the same task. The therapist should always carefully evaluate whether the achievement of the component practiced in a related task will transfer to the activity outlined in the intervention plan of care.

In general, motor learning theory predicts a small amount of transfer between tasks, so practice of the target skill is recommended (Larin, 2006; Schmidt & Lee, 2005; Winstein, Gardner, McNeal, Barto, & Nicholson, 1989). However, practice of related tasks that focus on shared movement components may play an increased role in motor learning by children with neurological impairments, who must develop the movement patterns required for the targeted activity. The extent to which components of movement practiced in a related activity transfer to the targeted activity requires empirical study. Transfer generally depends on the degree to which common elements of the movement are shared. Horne and colleagues (1995) reported on interventions that involved six or seven activities specifically designed to facilitate acquisition of specific movement components. Practice of these activities increased performance in children from 21 to 34 months of age. The children also demonstrated generalization of each movement component to untreated exemplar activities. Gains in hip extension from practice on a specially designed tricycle were found to transfer to improvements in gait in children with CP (King et al., 1993). For children with cognitive limitations, practice of prerequisite skills may not be advisable because of difficulty with transfer to the targeted activity (McEwen & Hansen, 2006).

Guideline No. 4: Use Toys to Promote Desired Functional Outcomes

Toys should meet the developmental needs of the child and the objective of the practice session. The features of the objects drive the motor behavior that emerges, so the perceptual and physical features of the toys should be carefully evaluated. They should be age and developmentally appropriate. Research has shown that physical toys, such as slides, tricycles, and climbing materials, promote improved interaction with peers as compared to manipulative toys, such as puzzles or play dough, which tend to promote parallel play (Fontaine, 2005). In general, toys may be used as motivators for a child to participate, but should not detract the child's selective attention from the primary focus of the practice.

Guideline No. 5: Adjust Task Complexity and Difficulty

The task difficulty and complexity should be at the appropriate level and should be carefully individualized for the child. Physical therapists should try to plan activities with just the right amount of challenge relative to the child's skills (Campbell, 1999). They should develop a plan regarding where to start and where to progress with the course of practice. The complexity of the task can be graded on the number of elements, because additional elements increase the information-processing requirements as well as the movement production requirements.

The complexity of a task also depends on whether it is a closed or open task. For a closed task, the environment (e.g., a staircase, the hole on a putting green) remains the same from one practice trial to another. In an open task, the environmental conditions (e.g., a busy hallway, the configuration of opponents in a tennis match) change on each trial, so many solutions are possible (Gentile, 1987; Schmidt & Wrisberg, 2008).

Adaptations to practice may provide a less difficult version of the task to be learned. A gradual transition to a more difficult version of the task is made as the child progresses. Motor learning literature cautions that transfer to the target task may not be guaranteed. However, adapting the task for difficulty may be applicable to children with limits in strength and endurance. Safety is another reason for grading the difficulty of the task. Adaptations can be made by reducing the task requirements or by giving physical support for safety. An example of an adapted practice is working on gait in the parallel bars, with the intention of progressing to independent walking. Repeated practice trials in the parallel bars may increase skill in the parallel bars but teaches a different dynamic and coordination than what is needed for independent walking. Although safety and skill level may require task adaptations, the therapist should reflect on the transfer of learning to the goal in the plan of care.

Assistive aids, such as walkers, crutches, or a parapodium, can be used in functional mobility tasks. The optimal features of assistive aids can significantly affect function for children with disability. For example, posterior walkers enhance locomotor function of certain children with CP (Logan, Byers-Hinkley, & Ciccone, 1990). Assistive devices have also been found to improve mobility and decrease the amount of required caregiver assistance as measured on the PEDI (Ostensjo, Carlberg & Vollestad, 2005). Guidelines for selecting assistive aids are covered in Chapters 6, 17, and 18.

Part-task training is another practice adaptation. It is generally defined as practice on some component of the whole task as pretraining for performance of the whole task. The motor learning literature suggests using part-task training for complex skills when practicing the whole task is too difficult for the learner (Schmidt & Wrisberg, 2008). One common type of part-practice is segmentation or progressive part practice, in which one part is practiced and then another part is added until, finally, the parts are all practiced together (Schmidt & Lee, 2005).

An example of segmentation is starting with practice of dribbling a basketball and then combining it with passing to a team member or shooting it into the hoop. The effectiveness of part-practice depends on the nature of the target skill and how intricately the component parts are related (Schmidt & Wrisberg, 2008; Shumway-Cook & Woollacott, 2012). Part-practice is not effective if separating the components changes the way in which the individual parts are performed. For example, practicing the back swing component of a golf swing separately from the forward swing could change the dynamics of the forward swing, because the sequence of muscle activity and the momentum for the forward swing depend on continuity with the back swing (Schmidt & Wrisberg, 2008). Also, for part-task practice to be effective, it must transfer to the whole task learning. Part-practice is especially effective with tasks having many parts, such as most activities of daily living.

Part-practice is most useful when the practiced component is a subaction or small whole contained within the functional complex task (Schmidt & Lee, 2005; Schmidt & Wrisberg, 2008; Winstein, Pohl, & Lewthwaite, 1994). This principle was demonstrated in a study by Winstein and colleagues (1994) that examined the effects of part-practice, which focused on shifting weight in standing onto the leg affected by a stroke. These adult subjects demonstrated improved weight shifting in standing with feet in line after part-practice, but there was no improvement in functional gait measures. In this case, the lateral weight shift was not a naturally occurring unit of the task of walking, which involves more forward shift of the center of mass.

As with many motor learning variables, general guidelines for part-task practice may have to be adapted to address limitations in neurological functions. Part-task training may be beneficial when children show sequencing deficits or difficulty with components of movement critical to bilateral task performance (Valvano & Rapport, 2006). The advantage of part-task practice may also be task-dependent in children. Recent research demonstrated faster learning of multi-component visual motor task with whole-task practice (Yakut, 2003).

Guideline No. 6: Schedule Practice to Enhance Retention and Transfer The motor learning literature provides research on two practice variables that apply here: variable versus specific practice, and random versus blocked practice. Specific, or nonvaried, practice involves repetitive trials of one task variation of an action class (e.g. throwing a ball from the desired distance, ascending steps on one staircase, standing from sitting in one chair). Variable practice involves many variations of the action class (throwing different balls from different positions, ascending multiple staircases with different riser heights, standing from chairs with different seat heights). Recall that motor programming theory predicts that **variable practice** would improve generalization of the motor skill because it involves many parameters of the motor program. From a dynamic systems perspective, part-task practice increases stability of the coordination strategy across environmental and task constraints. The advantages of variable practice in learning an experimental task by typically developing children have been demonstrated (Granda-Vera & Montilla, 2003; Wulf, 1991). The effects of variable practice have not been studied specifically in children with neurological physical impairments.

When two or more tasks are performed in a practice session, they can be scheduled in a drill-like fashion where trials of one task are repeated before moving to the next. This is called **blocked practice**. **Random practice** involves practice of all of the task variations with no predictable (random) order. Research with adult subjects shows a very robust effect for random practice because random practice encourages more active processing that makes a more well-developed memory representation. However, the effect for children is somewhat equivocal. The decision to schedule practice according to a blocked or random fashion may relate to the characteristics of the task and the child learner.

Taylor (1999) conducted a pilot study to evaluate the relative effects of blocked versus random practice on the learning of three variations of crutch tasks by 7-year-olds with no disability. The advantage of random practice was not demonstrated. The multiple effects of the child's learning style, the degree of difficulty of the task variations, and prior experience were noted. A combination of blocked practice utilized early on until the learner gets the basic idea of the movement, followed by random practice later has been suggested to be optimal for children for variations of certain tasks (Gentile, 1987, 1992; Pigott & Shapiro, 1984). It is possible that the increased trial-to-trial variability in children with neurological diagnoses may increase the requirement for blocked practice. Furthermore, the complexity of the movement may prolong the early stage of practice. Issues of memory and attention should also be considered. In children with hemiplegic CP, blocked practice demonstrated improved differentiation of force rates during initial skill attainment and similar retention of grasp control as compared to random practice (Duff & Gordon, 2003). On the other hand, for some children, random practice may enhance learning because it reduces the boredom associated with drill practice of one task.

Planning Activity-Focused Interventions: Environment

The environment-related interventions will be discussed in terms of the physical environment, the psychosocial environment, and the performance environment. The **performance environment** involves the augmented information provided by the change agent.

Guideline No. 7: Adapt the Physical Environment to Support Desired Motor Behaviors The **physical environment** includes objects (including assistive technology) and persons, as well as sensory features of the environment. The perception-action framework (Fetters & Ellis, 2006; Gibson, 1979), which has been integrated into dynamic systems approaches, stresses that the movement behaviors that emerge during activity are intricately tied to information in the environment. Likewise, functional action facilitates perception. This perception-action match is typified by the tendency of adults to select a strategy of stepping or climbing onto a step, based on the ratio of the stair riser height to the leg length (Warren, 1984) and extensor strength in the legs (Konczak, 1990).

There is some evidence that infants and young children also perceive actions according to their own movement capabilities (Adolph, Eppler, & Gibson, 1993). This perception-action concept is illustrated in Figure 8.5. The young boy, at 2 years of age, was challenged by the action goal of ascending the stairs. A four-point movement solution naturally emerged when the stair riser height was relative to his size and movement capabilities. The two-point solution (upright) naturally emerged when the riser height relative to his leg length decreased. Note that he naturally sought assistance to descend the stairs because the task and the environmental features did not match his perceived motor capabilities as he tried to perform the action.

Objects in the environment that provide opportunities for movement are called **affordances**. According to the perception-action framework, these affordances depict the reciprocal relationship between the person and the environment. As tasks and the environment are adapted for therapeutic practice, the therapist should evaluate the affordances available to the child for movement. Affordances, such as the steps in the case of the toddler, can be control parameters or constraints that affect action. Fetters and Ellis (2006) describe affordances in the case of a 4-year old trying to shoot a basketball into a hoop. The young basketball player's successful action (sinking the ball into the basket) emerges with the "appropriate person-environment fit." Changes in the size and weight of the basketball and the size and height of the basket afford shooting the ball into the hoop and are linked to his successful action.

For children with neurological impairments, sensory stimuli in the environment can influence the learning experience, especially if selective attention is impaired. Children who have difficulty with automatic performance of one task may find it difficult to perform multiple tasks. The physical environment is especially important for infants and children for whom sensory inputs can be disorganizing. Children with DCD may have associated sensory integration disorders. Factors such as ambient temperature, lighting, noise level, or even odors can significantly affect the ability to selectively attend to and participate in practice activities. The physical environment might be modified to reduce fear and increase security for the child. Knowing the child's special needs will help to maximize the sensory aspects of the physical environment.

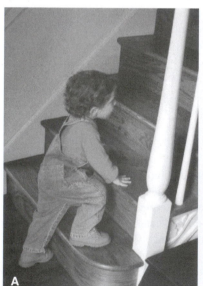
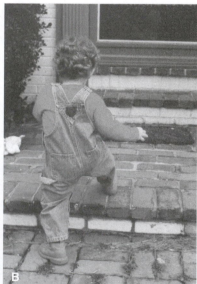
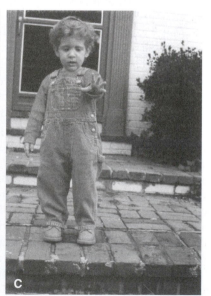

Figure 8.5 Variations of stair tasks by a 2-year-old boy with typical development, influenced by the features of the environment relative to his movement capabilities. (*A*) Four-point movement for high step. (*B*) Two-point solution when riser height is reduced. (*C*) Seeking assistance to descend step.

Other features of the physical environment include equipment and the floor surface for locomotor activities. Therapeutic equipment, such as balls and bolsters, is often used during practice to support the emergence of a certain movement skill. The physical therapist might use the movable surface of an exercise ball to elicit transition from prone to sit. The buoyancy of the water is an environmental adaptation that enhances motor behavior in aquatic therapy.

The success of activity-focused behaviors is often dependent on appropriate use of adapted equipment. McEwen (1992) suggests that adaptive equipment could be a constraint (a control parameter) on the social interactions that a child performs in the classroom. Children perform better when they feel comfortable and secure in their environment. They do poorly when they perceive a threat to balance or posture, such as sitting in a chair, which is not optimal. Well-planned seating and mobility aids are "enabling technology" that enhance function (Wilson Howle, 1999). Adapted seats, sidelyers, and supportive standers can also improve participation in classroom and home. The issues relating to adaptive equipment are discussed in Chapters 17 and 18.

Guideline No. 8: _Conduct Practice in the Natural Environment When Practical_ There is evidence that optimal learning and generalization of learning for children with neurological impairments occurs in the **natural environment** where the skill will be used (Karnish, Bruder, & Rainforth, 1995; Roper & Dunst, 2003). The natural environment provides constant opportunities for motor learning. Therefore, it is the role of the change agent not only to teach motor activities but also to help families and classrooms create environments that support and promote opportunities for learning. This is especially the case for children with cognitive limitations, for whom transfer from the clinical to natural environment is difficult (Brown, Effgen & Palisano, 1998; McEwen & Hansen, 2006).

Guideline No. 9: _Consider the Influence of the Psychosocial Environment_ Psychosocial issues that influence motor learning, including motivation, expectations, and encouragement, constitute the **psychosocial environment**. Therapists should support the psychosocial environment through sound family-centered practice and integration of physical therapy into the classroom and the community for full participation. This aspect of intervention is a critical element of current models of intervention. Strategies for supporting the family are elaborated in Chapter 4 and throughout the text. Strategies for early intervention are discussed in Chapter 11; for the classroom, in Chapter 12; and for other settings, in Chapters 13 to 16. The therapist should be in tune with the child's needs and flexibly adapt practice. Children should be given choices and participate in decision making (Larin, 2006).

Guideline No. 10: _Thoughtfully Provide Augmented Information_ The performance environment refers to the augmented information provided during the learning situation. Recall that **augmented information** involves information provided by an external source to complement the intrinsic information available to the learner through problem solving and performance of the task. According to the dynamic systems perspective, the change agent provides augmented information to guide the child's search for the motor coordination that will enable the functional action to be achieved. The change agent can dramatically affect the outcome of practice by carefully choosing and executing augmented information.

Recall that there are many sources of augmented information besides feedback. Although much of the literature focuses on feedback, in terms of the opportunities for augmented information, the options are numerous. The planning of augmented information involves three dimensions: the type of augmented information characterized by the mode of presentation, the content, and the timing. It is difficult to give hard and fast rules regarding augmented information during therapeutic practice because of the lack of empirical data. Theoretically, it is important to integrate the augmented information with modifications of the task and the environment and how they interact with the special learning needs of the child.

INSTRUCTION. Instruction may be presented verbally or through visual demonstration or modeling. Verbal instructions provide information about the task requirements and may enhance selective attention to the relevant aspects of the task. Generally, instructions should be brief and to the point (Schmidt & Wrisberg, 2008).

DEMONSTRATION AND MODELING. Instruction provided through the visual mode is effective for young children, who rely heavily on visual cues (Bradley & Westcott, 2006; Hatzitaki, Zisi, Kollias, & Kioumourtzoglou, 2002; Shumway-Cook & Woollacott, 1985). For example, children with Down syndrome demonstrate less skill with verbal processing relative to visual processing (Iarocci & Burack, 1998). Modeling of the motor task, from a video or live model, can enhance motor learning and self-confidence in children (Larin, 2006). When providing live or video demonstrations, it is advisable to cue the child to the features of the movement to which they should attend (Kernodle & Carlton, 1992). KNOWLEDGE OF RESULTS AND KNOWLEDGE OF PERFORMANCE. **Knowledge of results** provides information about how well the outcome of the child's practice trial met the task goal (Schmidt & Lee, 2005). Consider the child's developmental level in terms of how much time the child needs to process the information and the complexity of the information. This would be especially pertinent for children with cognitive delays or impaired information processing. The requirement for feedback should be evaluated for each child, relative to the task that is practiced. Verbal feedback is often critical in adult motor learning studies, in which the goal is to improve accuracy or timing of a simple experimental task and the increments of change are not perceptible by the learner (Magill, 1992; Salmoni, Schmidt, & Walter, 1984). However, in the clinical environment, the outcome of a practice trial for many tasks (such as throwing a beanbag into a box) may be obvious to the child, making knowledge of results redundant and not necessary. On the other hand, for certain tasks, impaired proprioceptive or visual integration may increase the requirement for feedback about the outcome of the movement.

Knowledge of performance provides feedback information about the movement patterns that the child uses to perform movements. Intuitively, this would seem to be more valuable in teaching children with physical impairments. However, it may be difficult for some children with neurological deficits to process information about their movement patterns as they focus on the performance of difficult movements (Thorpe & Valvano, 2002). A more external focus directed toward the task goal in the environment may be more appropriate (Thorpe et al., 2003; Wulf, Shea, & Park, 2001).

Because children with neurological impairments may have difficulty with developing a plan of action, feedback alone may not be sufficient. It may be more practical to provide cues about what to do on future trials to improve performance, based on prior performance (Kernodle & Carlton, 1992; Newell & Valvano, 1998). These cues may be especially important when the task is unfamiliar to the child and when the child must develop a new pattern of coordination to achieve the functional activity goal.

COGNITIVE STRATEGIES. **Cognitive strategies** are learning tools or techniques that facilitate learning by addressing cognitive systems, such as attention and memory. They are tools that help the learner to organize, store, or retrieve information (Alley & Deshler, 1979).

Examples of cognitive strategies are methods to improve attention, mental rehearsal of the movement, use of labels to enhance memory, use of rhymes or rhythms to remember a sequence, and strategies for comparing one trial with another for accuracy. Although children with typical development usually develop these cognitive strategies intuitively and use them to aid performance (David, 1985), children with cognitive and learning impairments often do not use cognitive strategies during practice of a motor skill. There is some evidence that helping children to use strategies improves their learning (Dawson, Hallahan, Reeve, & Ball, 1980; Horgan, 1985). For children with neurological diagnoses, teaching them to mentally rehearse the skill or to use visual imagery might enhance motor skill learning (Thorpe & Valvano, 2002). Cognitive strategies may also focus on metacognitive skills such as problem solving and strategic processes required to accomplish action goals (Polatajko, Mandich, & Missiuna, 2001).

PHYSICAL GUIDANCE. An important mode of augmented information for the physical therapist is **physical guidance**. From the motor learning perspective, physical guidance provides a general "feel" of the movement that will achieve a function (Wulf, Shea, & Whitacre, 1998). These physical guidance cues are similar to those provided by a coach in guiding a golf swing or a gymnastic maneuver. Physical guidance may be called **manual guidance** when the cueing is provided manually by the instructor. Facilitation techniques from the neurodevelopmental treatment (NDT) approach (discussed in the sections that follow provide manual guidance because they give information about the target movement pattern; they also have therapeutic goals such as muscle elongation, joint stability, and increased range of motion (ROM) (Bly & Whiteside, 1997; Bobath & Bobath, 1984; Howle, 2003). From a motor learning perspective, the informational properties of the guidance are emphasized.

In a series of single-case studies, physical guidance was found to be beneficial in the early phases of learning a novel, complex motor skill by children with CP for whom the task presented a reasonable challenge. After getting the general idea of the movement, these children continued to improve performance, even when the guidance was withdrawn (Valvano, Heriza, & Carollo, 2002). Furthermore, kinematic analysis provides preliminary evidence that the physical guidance encouraged the development of task-specific patterns of movement required to perform the task. Physical guidance, for some children, can be beneficial in the early phases of practice because it is difficult for the child with neurological impairments to develop a coordination plan.

Physical guidance may save effort and frustration in the early phase of learning for children with special needs. However, the learner may become dependent on the physical guidance, at the expense of developing an internal reference for the correct movement (Sidaway et al., 2008). Therefore, the guidance should be phased out and withdrawn after the child gets the general idea of the movement solution. Then, the child should be given the opportunity to problem solve and self-correct as he or she refines the movement strategy.

When teaching a motor skill, it is advisable to determine, for the individual child, the amount and type of information that will be useful for error detection and skill development. The amount of information should allow active exploration and trial and error and not allow the child to become overly dependent on the guidance.

The requirement for guidance may be increased, especially early in practice, for children with sensory and motor impairments who may have a limited repertoire of movement patterns to draw on and who demonstrate difficulty developing a "feel" for the functional movement pattern required to achieve the task goal. For these children, the movement challenge is more complex. It has been demonstrated in adults that the complexity of a gross motor skill affects the requirement for augmented information (Wulf et al., 1998). The responsible clinician, therefore, should monitor the effects of augmented information and be sensitive to the learning style and personal characteristics of the learners engaging in therapeutic practice.

The logic for practice guidelines related to feedback and guidance is based on the cognitive processes associated with intentional explicit motor learning. Therefore, the distinction between explicit and implicit memory processes is relevant. In **explicit learning**, the performer is aware of goals and features of the task critical for performance. In **implicit learning**, although there is active involvement in the task performance, the emphasis is on repetition of the task and not on conscious attention to the rules (Schmidt & Wrisberg, 2008; Shumway-Cook & Woollacott, 2012). The role of instruction is diminished in implicit learning. It is often difficult to categorize the type of learning processes involved with skill learning. There may be a combination of implicit and explicit learning in all motor skills. *Guideline No. 11: Apply Behavioral Strategies for Children Unable to Benefit From Verbally Mediated Guidance and Feedback* The type of feedback, instruction, and guidance provided depends on the nature of

the learning required for the skill. For children with cognitive impairments, learning may depend more on visual cues and repetition (McEwen & Hansen, 2006). Because of this, therapeutic interventions may need to be modified to promote optimal learning. Children with cognitive impairments may benefit from interventions that increase opportunities to practice functional tasks in the natural environment to promote generalization and maintenance of skills.

For some children, especially those with challenging behaviors or TBI, **behavioral programming**, commonly referred to as *applied behavior analysis* or *behavior modification*, is an appropriate methodology to assist in achieving goals. Behavioral programming maintains that much of human behavior is functional and the product of learning. Therefore, a change in targeted behaviors is quite obtainable. Behavioral programming emphasizes functional assessment of behaviors and evaluation of environments where the behaviors are noted, and uses a variety of change strategies based on these assessments to achieve team and family determined goals. Strategies such as positive reinforcement of desired behaviors, fading supports, ignoring of challenging behaviors, and scheduled teaching are often used (Alberto & Troutman, 2009). Concepts about behavioral programming are discussed briefly in Chapter 1.

Integrating Interventions for Impairments in Body Functions and Structures With Activity-Focused Interventions for Participation

According to the model in Figure 8.4, focus on the characteristics of the child also involves integration of interventions that focus on impairments in body functions and structures with the activity-focused interventions seeking to reduce restrictions in activities and participation. From a "top down" perspective (P.H. Campbell, 1991; Heriza & Sweeney, 1994), problem solving about impairments of body function and structures begins after the specified functional goals are established. Impairment-level interventions are important, not only to support activities and participation, but also to reduce the risk of secondary impairments. Because impairments in body structures and functions associated with neurological diagnoses are numerous and have a unique expression in each child, the interventions should be individualized. According to Figure 8.4, impairment-focused interventions are divided into two major categories: active and passive. In the sections that follow, the evidence on these two categories of impairment-focused interventions is presented. Readers are encouraged to review the studies of interest and judge their clinical importance. To aid in this process, Table 8.1 lists systematic reviews of intervention topics addressed in the sections that follow.

Activity-Based Impairment Focused Interventions
Active impairment-focused interventions attempt to ameliorate the effects of impairments (or limitations in body functions and structures) through practice of a meaningful functional task or developmental activity. The logic for addressing impairments in the context of activity is based on the assumption that changes in motor control emerge as the child engages in active practice and problem solving. Therefore, the benefits of practicing the activity are twofold: improved performance of the functional activity and amelioration of impairments that limit functional movement components. The impairment-focused activity may be the target activity specified in the goal, or an alternative activity that addresses the impairment. Figure 8.6 depicts functional play activities enjoyed by Joey, a kindergarten student with hemiplegic CP, who demonstrates impairments in selective control and hypertonicity expressed in a flexion pattern in the right upper extremity. The limitation in active elbow extension limits the use of the affected hand as an assist in bimanual activities. Therapy goals for Joey included improved functioning of the affected upper extremity as an assist in bimanual

activity, specifically the class of actions that require active reaching for and supporting objects with the right hand as the left hand performs more complex functions (e.g. reaching for a cup and holding it with the right as the left hand pours; reaching for a tube of toothpaste with the right and holding it as the left hand unscrews the lid). Play activities depicted in Figure 8.6 address the impairments in selective motor control by encouraging the active elbow extension that is required for reaching with the affected hand in bimanual activity.

The therapist makes a judgment about the expected transfer of impairment-level gains to the target activity. Dichter and colleagues (2001) demonstrated that play activities by children with Down syndrome geared toward impairments in balance, visual motor control, and strength did transfer to functional tasks for Special Olympics competition. Physical education programs, adapted swimming, modified aerobics, and dancing (including wheelchair dancing) are all activities that are helpful in increasing strength, as well as stamina and endurance (Eckersley & King, 1993).

Activities directed toward impairments in body functions and structures can be enhanced by motor learning strategies described previously in this chapter. A commonly used strategy is manual guidance. Figure 8.7A depicts the use of manual guidance by Joey's physical therapist in the early phase of practice

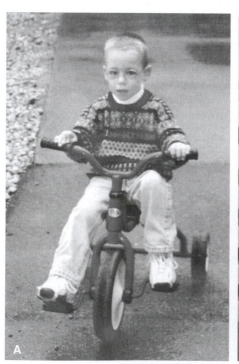
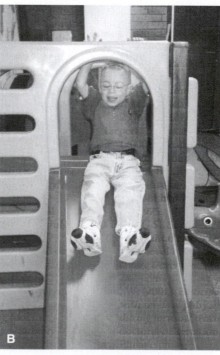

Figure 8.6 Functional activities that address impairments in selective motor control in the right upper extremity of a kindergarten student. *(A)* Riding tricycle. *(B)* Sliding down sliding board.

of a stepping task. The guidance gives him a "feel" for the advancement of the tibia over the right plantargrade foot, which are limited by hypoextensible plantar flexor muscles and reduced selective control of lower extremity muscles, and limited weight bearing. This reduction in impairments eventually carries over into performance of a stepping task in the context of play (Fig. 8.7B).

Activities that address impairments can also be enhanced by therapeutic modalities. These adaptations might include assistive technology or mechanical aids used to enhance the performance of the activity. These include the application of tone-inhibiting casts, which are used as adjuncts to therapy to stabilize the foot and improve the alignment, and ankle-foot orthoses to provide support (Figueiredo et al., 2008; Knutson & Clark, 1991) and perhaps to reduce energy expenditure in gait (Mossberg, Linton, & Friske, 1990).

Functional electrical stimulation (FES) provided during gait (Seifart et al., 2010) or upper extremity tasks (Ozer, Chesher, & Scheker, 2006) is another example of therapeutic modalities that can be used in functional activity to enhance impairment-level changes. FES involves stimulation of intact peripheral nerves to activate their target muscles in a functional manner. The term FES is often interchanged with neuromuscular electrical stimulation (NMES), which is aimed at muscle strengthening or spasticity reduction.

Electrical stimulation complements active practice by addressing limitations in force production, selective control, and timing of muscle activity. In most cases, an electrical current is delivered to the skin with a portable battery-operated device. A particular muscle or group of muscles is stimulated as the child actively performs functional movement (e.g., gait or reaching). The timing of the stimulation provides a sensory cue and assists the muscle activation patterns that will help to achieve the goal. One example is electrical stimulation to the triceps surae to improve foot contact in children with CP (Carmick, 1997). Stimulation of the gastrocnemius alone or in combination was found to be more effective at improving gait in children with CP than stimulating the tibialis anterior alone (Seifart et al., 2009). Two published systematic reviews suggest that more rigorous research designs are required to study the effect of NMES and FES (Kerr et al., 2004; Seifart et al., 2009). One precaution with NMES is a history of seizures, because some systemic absorption of the electric current might occur (Reed, 1997).

Biofeedback has also been used to improve muscle activation, selective control, and timing in the context of functional tasks. With biofeedback, the motor output is displayed to reflect muscle activity measured by electromyography or force production. A visual or auditory signal helps to focus attention to the motor response and supplement that with information not naturally available to the learner. Augmented biofeedback can be effective in increasing head and neck posture, reducing hypertonia, improving weight bearing, and reducing

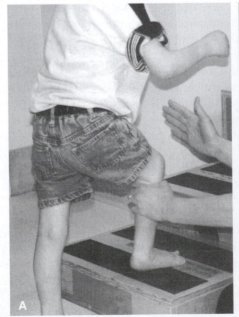
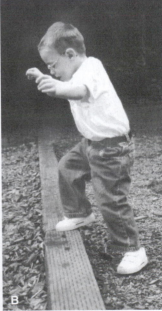

Figure 8.7 (*A*) Use of physical guidance during practice of a stepping task performed by a child with cerebral palsy, addressing impairments in lower extremity tone and selective control. (*B*) Carryover of impairment-level gains to a stepping task in the play environment.

drooling. Dursun and colleagues (2004) used EMG biofeedback treatment to address gait in children with CP and found improvements in tonus of plantar flexor muscles, active ROM of the ankle joints, and improved gait function. However, carryover without feedback is limited. Furthermore, generalization of muscle control or components of movement to real-life tasks has not been consistent (Bertoti & Gross, 1988; Floodmark, 1986; Seeger, Caudrey, & Scholes, 1981).

Modifications of the task or environment also help to focus on impairments of body structure and function during activity. In **aquatic therapy**, the purposeful activities performed by children in the water might address impairments such as increased stiffness and weakness. The aquatic environment provides weight relief to the body, warmth, buoyancy, antigravity positioning, and increased resistance. This medium allows greater ease of movement, relaxation of spastic muscles, and strengthening (Dumas & Francesconi, 2002; Fragala-Pinkham, Dumas, Barlow, & Pasternak, 2009).

Hippotherapy is an example of purposeful activity by the child, during which the rhythmical movements of the horse are directed to reduce limitations in posture, balance, and mobility (Snider et al., 2007). Gains in strength and postural control associated with hippotherapy can transfer to improved gross motor function, improved functional gait performance, and reduced energy expenditure during gait (McGibbon, Andrade, Widener, & Cintas, 1998). While riding the horse, the child practices active postural and balance strategies under functional, motivating, and changing environmental conditions. A systematic review of hippotherapy and therapeutic riding completed by Snider and colleagues (2007) reported emerging evidence that hippotherapy has positive therapeutic effects on impairments of body structure and function for children with CP. However, the authors caution that the studies reviewed had small sample sizes and limited diagnoses of study participants. A second review by MacKinnon and colleagues (1995) identifies favorable effects of therapeutic riding for children with CP, learning disability (LD), mental retardation, and language disorders.

Partial weight-bearing treadmill training is an activity that adapts the task and environment to work on goals of increased functional mobility (Damiano & DeJong, 2009; Mutlu et al., 2009; Zwicker & Mayson, 2010). The treadmill adapts the task by adjusting the requirement for weight bearing and guiding the timing and direction of the steps.

The activity-based impairment-focused interventions addressed above involve performance of a *functional* task or *developmental play*. As depicted in Figure 8.4, another category of activity-based impairment-focused interventions involve *therapeutic* tasks. **Resistive exercise** with free weights or isokinetic devices by children is a primary example of this category. Resistive exercise addresses force production deficits very common in neurological diagnoses. In recent years, considerable evidence has been put forth in support of resistive exercise for increasing strength in children with CP.

In the past, vigorous strengthening was considered contraindicated in children who demonstrated increased tone because of the fear that resistive work would increase spasticity in children with CP. In fact, over the past few years, there have been many studies that have demonstrated major gains in strength and function without detrimental effects on spasticity (Darrah et al., 1997; Damiano & Abel, 1998; Damiano et al., 2002; Harvey & Russell, 2009). Although Scianni and colleagues (2009) raise some questions regarding the effectiveness of strengthening programs to improve gait for children and adolescents with CP, O'Connell and Barnhart (1995) reported gains associated with resistive exercise in subjects with spasticity as well as subjects with myelomeningocele (MM).

It is important that the effects of strengthening programs be investigated in children who demonstrate functional weakness associated with hypotonia, such as children with Down syndrome (Dichter, 1994; Mercer & Lewis, 2001). Additionally, strengthening programs need to be considered for children who are not ambulatory. Williams and Pountney (2007) developed a static bicycle strengthening program for children with CP who were not ambulatory. Participants demonstrated significant improvements in GMFM scores, indicating improved functional performance after strengthening.

Proprioceptive neuromuscular facilitation (PNF) (Eckersley & King, 1993) is an alternative to traditional resistive strengthening with weights that has been applied to children with neurological impairments. This technique integrates neural concepts into strengthening activities. The premise is that muscle actions are more efficient when working in patterns in which movements are diagonal and rotational and when the movement goes from distal to proximal. The active movements in PNF are guided by the physical therapist. Hand placement is carefully planned to provide an appropriate level of resistance, guidance, or sensory feedback. Stretch and traction make use of the elastic properties of the muscle. Verbal prompts serve a motivating function. The efficacy of PNF has not been studied systematically in children with neurological impairments. Eckersley and King (1993) report a clinical impression of increased strength after using PNF in children with MM.

Passive Impairment-Focused Interventions **Passive procedures** do not involve purposeful activities and participation on the part of the child. Passive procedures are usually directed toward musculoskeletal limitations associated with abnormal muscle tone. Included in this category are interventions directed toward reducing joint limitations or soft tissue contractures. Examples are passive ROM exercises or application of night splints. Therapists intuitively incorporate passive ROM exercises to maintain or increase flexibility; however, there is limited evidence to guide this intervention (Cadenhead, McEwen, & Thompson, 2002; Harris, 1990).

Pin and colleagues (2006) published a systematic review of passive stretching with children with CP, and this review was updated by Wiart and colleagues (2008) to include active stretching. Both reviews stated that current research in the area of stretching was inconclusive due to methodological issues, small sample sizes, and few available studies. They suggest alternatives such as flexibility and fitness goals. Two studies reported only limited advantages of passive ROM exercises (McPherson, Arends, Michaels, & Trettin, 1984; Miedaner & Renander, 1987). Miedaner and Renander (1987) demonstrated an advantage of passive ROM provided twice weekly compared with lower frequency. However, there were limitations to the design of this study, which lacked a control group. Fragala and colleagues (2003) suggest that the effects of passive ROM exercises vary and may depend on many factors, including child-related factors (growth, underlying motor control, and capability for active movement) and external factors (frequency of passive exercise, positioning, and use of orthoses). They propose that the evidence favors prolonged stretching over brief and intermittent passive stretching. The findings of a study by Tardieu, Lespargot, Tabary, and Bret (1988) demonstrate that to prevent contracture of the soleus muscles for children with CP, prolonged stretch for several hours per day is necessary. In their study, the effects of stretch on contractures were not apparent in those for whom the muscle was elongated 2 hours per day. There was a positive effect on muscles elongated for at least 6 hours per day.

Serial casting or splinting is a method of applying sustained stretch to a muscle. A systematic review of serial casting by Blackmore and colleagues (2007) concluded that weak evidence existed to support the efficacy of serial casting in children with CP. The effects of serial casting may be enhanced by botulinum toxin A injections, which effect a transient chemical denervation by disturbing the actions of acetylcholine at the neuromuscular junction (Booth, Yates, Edgar, & Bandy, 2003).

The findings of Tardieu and colleagues (1988) support the use of splints and casts (Phillips & Audet, 1990) for prolonged stretch. For children with TBI, splints and serial casting are commonly used to effect a prolonged static stretch (Blaskey & Jennings, 1999; Conine, Sullivan, Mackie, & Goodman, 1990). Limitations in ROM are also addressed by positioning devices such as standing frames (Gudjonsdottir & Stemmons-Mercer, 2002; Stuberg, 1992). Use of a sidelyer or seating devices also provides some passive input to preserve biomechanical integrity (McEwen, 1992).

Manual therapy techniques, including soft tissue mobilization, joint mobilization, massage, and myofascial release, are procedures administered to reduce biomechanical or musculoskeletal impairments, but there is little research to support their use. The use of these manual techniques should be guarded, with consideration of developmental factors and risks of injury and fracture (Harris & Lundgren, 1991).

Passive procedures may be preparatory to practice of a functional activity and administered by a therapist or caregiver to create a more optimal readiness for a motor learning experience. Activities that provide tactile, vestibular, or proprioceptive input in a playful manner might be used before functional activity, to regulate sensory reactivity and improve behavioral organization (Miller & Summers, 2001). The effectiveness of these preparatory procedures has not been studied systematically.

Passive preparatory procedures are used in the Neurodevelopmental Treatment perspective. These procedures, which elongate or increase mobility of spastic muscles, theoretically improve the ease and quality of voluntary movement that follow (Boehme, 1988; Howle, 2003). For the young student in Figure 8.7, elongation of the ankle plantar flexors is a passive procedure that could prepare him for better active movement of the tibia over the foot during the task of ascending stairs. Figure 8.8A depicts a preparatory activity provided to increase flexibility in the hand to enhance weight bearing during a functional play activity (Fig.8.B). According to current models of intervention, the need for these preparatory procedures should be evaluated on a case-by-case basis, and the therapist should not create a long-term dependence on them. The important question is, "Will the child be able to perform the task in the natural environment when the preparatory passive procedures are not available?"

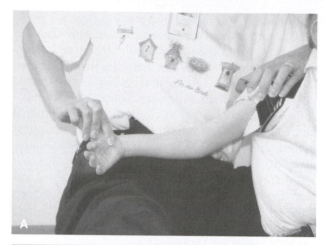

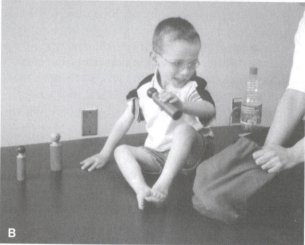

Figure 8.8 (*A*) Preparatory passive procedure and (*B*) functional play activity by a boy with cerebral palsy.

Established Approaches to Intervention

This section will review established approaches to pediatric neurological interventions that have significantly influenced physical therapy practice. Current evidence for these established approaches will also be reported.

Neurodevelopmental Treatment (NDT)

NDT, originated in the 1940s by Karl and Berta Bobath, has had enormous impact on the treatment of children with neurological disorders. The change in focus from an orthopedic to a neurological perspective was the hallmark of this approach. Sensory and motor impairments including abnormal tone were interpreted as release phenomena controlled by lower centers of the hierarchical nervous system. The Bobaths emphasized skillful handling by the therapist to reduce the effects of abnormal tone and encourage the emergence of normal postural components as the basis for normal movement. The output, or movement response of the child, was directly related to the input provided by the therapist, which, if properly executed, would produce immediate positive changes during a treatment session (Bobath & Bobath, 1984).

Through the years, NDT has been an empirical approach with management techniques developed by Berta Bobath and other master clinicians who followed. There have been many advances in neuroscience and pediatric physical therapy since NDT began, and the theoretical basis has evolved. In the 1990s, the NDT Association instructor group responded to the changes in neurosciences and in pediatric physical therapy that challenged the initial assumptions of the Bobaths. This led to a publication that updates the assumptions about NDT and the intervention strategies (Howle, 2003).

According to Howle (2003), NDT is family centered and is focused on functional outcomes. Assumptions about treatment are consistent with current movement science. Handling techniques that direct movement to the best possible solution are still integral to NDT. According to Howle, therapeutic handling is necessary to (1) regulate sensory inputs, (2) direct the intention of the movement, (3) encourage more effective synergies, (4) guide force levels and the speed and direction of movement, and (5) constrain or increase flexibility in the DF. Facilitation techniques establish postures and movement components that carry over into function. Inhibition techniques suppress abnormal patterns of movement and provide the opportunity for more efficient movement adaptations (Bly & Whiteside, 1997; Boehme, 1988; Howle, 2003). NDT attempts to integrate current motor learning principles and emphasizes the goal of gradually reducing the reliance on passive handling techniques.

This current model of NDT is compatible with the activity-focused model presented in this chapter, because it uses procedures to address impairments in body functions and structures in the context of therapeutic practice. An NDT perspective includes adjunct interventions to manage symptoms of spasticity, such as orthoses, splints, and tone-inhibiting casts intended to maintain ROM and prevent deformity. NDT includes many preparatory interventions to reduce the effects of impairments in muscle tone and some soft tissue restrictions, to allow movement components to occur (Boehme, 1988; Nelson, 2001).

Despite the popularity of the NDT approach, there is very little formal evidence of its efficacy (Brown & Burns, 2001). A review sponsored by the American Academy of Cerebral Palsy and Developmental Medicine examined the evidence for NDT and concluded that the preponderance of results did not confer any advantage to NDT over the alternatives with which it was compared (Butler & Darrah, 2001). Additional research about NDT, with operationally defined treatment techniques, clearly defined outcome measures, and samples large enough to provide sufficiently credible evidence would be beneficial. Editorials by Damiano (2007) and Van Sant (2008) encourage therapists to rely on evidence-based approaches to pediatric physical therapy and avoid clinging to NDT and continuing to alter its fundamental principles to make it consistent with current research. It may be time to progress away from NDT and develop more current evidenced-based interventions.

Research on the efficacy of NDT presents many challenges, including the facts that there are no standard treatments delivered in a standardized manner, the skill levels and aims of therapists vary, and family influences are difficult to standardize (Butler & Darrah, 2001). Benefits of an NDT-oriented program to improve dynamic coactivation of the trunk in infants were demonstrated in a controlled study that did attempt to delineate and standardize the intervention approach (Arndt, Chandler, Sweeney, Sharkey, & McElroy, 2008). The clinician's individual evaluation of NDT strategies can be difficult because NDT is often combined with other therapy techniques, medical treatments, and motor learning strategies common to all task-oriented approaches.

Sensorimotor Approach

The sensorimotor approach is another facilitation approach, less well known than NDT. Certain concepts from this framework are still in use, and activities from this framework are often used in combination with NDT (Harris, 1990; Heriza & Sweeney, 1995). The sensorimotor approach was developed by Margaret Rood, who relied very heavily on a neuroanatomical basis for the treatment. She outlined four stages of development of motor control as a basis for normal movement: (1) reciprocal innervation (which involves flexion and extension patterns), (2) cocontraction, (3) stability superimposed on mobility (when there is movement of a segment over a distal stability point, such as the weight-bearing phase in walking and creeping), and (4) mobility superimposed on stability (which involves a free distal part moving on a stabilizing proximal part, such as reaching to grasp an object). The final component, in which phasic movement of a segment, such as the arm in reach or the leg in stepping, is stabilized by tonic contraction of the trunk and limb girdles, represents the high level of control required for advanced movement.

These stages of development of motor control occur in key patterns of posture and movement: supine flexion, prone extension (pivot prone), prone on elbows, prone on hands, all fours, semisquat, and walking. Proximal-to-distal and cephalocaudal development are emphasized in the approach (Stockmeyer, 1972). This approach is based on a hierarchical model of motor control and assumes that lesions in the CNS result in lack of higher-level control over movements. Although the rigid adherence to the developmental progression emphasized in the approach is not consistent with current models of motor control and motor learning, therapists may find the categories of movement, such as mobility superimposed on stability, useful in planning activities for children with impairments in strength or postural control.

Rood also formulated treatment techniques using specific sensory stimuli to elicit desired movement and postural responses on an automatic level. These stimulation techniques include icing and brushing, which are mediated through the tactile system, and stretch, resistance, vibration, pressure, and joint compression, which are mediated through the proprioceptive sense (Eckersley & King, 1993; Harris, 1990). There is no systematic study of the effectiveness or contraindications to these techniques.

Sensory Integration Approach

Sensory integration (SI) theory and therapy were developed by A. Jean Ayres in the 1960s to address the sensory processing and the motor and perceptual impairments of children with learning disabilities. According to SI theory, motor learning is dependent on the ability to take in sensory information derived from the environment and from movement of the body, process and integrate these sensory inputs within the CNS, and use this information to plan and produce organized behavior (Ayres, 1972, 1979; Spitzer & Roley, 2001). SI theory has undergone considerable development since it was first proposed by Ayres, and SI therapy has expanded to address a wide variety of diagnoses characterized by difficulty with detecting, regulating, interpreting, and responding to sensory input.

Miller & colleagues (2007) propose three subgroups of sensory processing disorder that can be addressed with SI therapy. The first subgroup is sensory modulation disorder, which is characterized by "difficulty responding to sensory input with behavior that is graded relative to the degree, nature or intensity of the sensory information" (Miller, Anzalone, Lane, Cermak, & Osten, 2007, p. 136). This results in a child's difficulty adapting to sensory challenges encountered in daily routines. Sensory modulation disorder may be characterized by sensory overresponsivity (for example, tactile defensiveness) or, sensory underresponsivity (lack of awareness of sensory information), or sensory seeking/craving (varied behaviors to seek sensory input). The second subgroup is sensory discrimination disorder, characterized by difficulty with accurately perceiving sensory stimuli (for example, auditory or visual discrimination disorders). The third subgroup is sensory-based motor disorder, which includes postural disorder (difficulty stabilizing the body to meet environmental demands) and dyspraxia (impaired ability to plan, sequence, or execute novel actions).

For children with neurological disorders, SI therapy can address: (1) motor dysfunction linked to impairments in motor planning, postural control, or sensory discrimination (Bundy, Lane, Murray, & Fisher, 2002; Parham & Mailloux, 1996) or (2) related behavioral problems with attention (distractibility, impulsivity, disorganization) or emotions (anxiety, aggression, tantrum behaviors) that can be linked to sensory modulation dysfunction (Miller & Summers, 2001).

In the motor function domain, SI therapy is most well known for its application to children with mild motor involvement typically seen in children with DCD. However, therapists apply interventions from an SI approach to children with multiple neurological disorders, including CP. (See Roley, Blanche, and Schaaf [2001] for a review of applications of SI to diverse populations.) SI has also been associated with positive outcomes in children with severe and profound cognitive delays (Lunnen, 1999; Montgomery & Richter, 1980). SI interventions facilitate the child's ability to make adaptive motor responses to specific sensory stimulation (including tactile, vestibular, proprioceptive), while engaging in purposeful motor activity. This purposeful motor activity is essential to the intervention process (Bundy et al., 2002).

SI is directed not toward the mastery of specific tasks or skills but rather toward improving the brain's capacity to perceive, remember, and plan motor activity (Lunnen, 1999). SI therapy frequently uses activities that provide vestibular stimulation to influence balance, muscle tone, ocular-motor responses, movements against gravity, postural adjustments, and arousal or activity level. Suspended equipment, such as hammocks, tire swings, and trapeze bars, is often used to provide controlled vestibular challenges. Linear movement and low-to-ground vestibular activities are sometimes used with children who are hypersensitive to movement. Inputs, such as weight bearing, resistance, movement against gravity, traction, vibration, and weighted objects, are also used to encourage adaptive postural and movement responses. Evidence for the efficacy of SI for improving motor function in children with DCD is equivocal. Critics of this approach argue that the use of behavioral or cognitive strategies in the context of actual functional tasks may be associated with better outcomes in terms of functional motor behaviors (David, 2000; Mandich, Polatajko, Missiuna, & Miller, 2001; Polatajko, Mandich, Miller, & Macnab, 2001).

In the behavioral domain, SI interventions are commonly used for children having tactile defensiveness or abnormally increased sensitivity to tactile input. This hypersensitivity is a phenomenon of the tactile system that results in feelings of discomfort from certain types of tactile stimulation. Sensitivity to touch may be environmental (e.g., a child experiencing discomfort with equipment or clothing, such as socks) or people-related (e.g., a child avoiding other children). Limited motor activity may render children with significant physical limitations unable to engage in normal sensory activities that tend to normalize sensory responses.

Children with neuromuscular dysfunction, such as CP or TBI, may display tactile defensiveness by fisting hands and arching away from the stimulus. In some cases, tactile defensiveness may contribute to toe walking. SI focuses on techniques, such the use of tactile deep-pressure, and graded exposure to tactile stimuli in the context of adaptive play activities, to normalize responses to environmental tactile stimulation (DeGangi, 1990).

Conductive Education

Another approach serving children with CP and similar movement dysfunction is Conductive Education (CE). It is not considered a physical therapy intervention, but pediatric physical therapists may be involved. A Hungarian neurologist, Andras Peto, developed this approach in the 1940s. CE is a holistic approach to development and education of children with neurological dysfunction. It is not a therapy system, but a system of education that aims to teach children to be active and self-reliant participants in the world. Emphasis is on motivation, developing self-esteem, and emotional and cognitive growth along with motor function (Hari & Tillemans, 1984; Kozma & Balogh, 1995).

CE is an intensive, integrated curriculum that includes cognitive, motor, personal care, and communication learning in real life contexts. Motor skills are integrated into everyday tasks. The close relationship between language and movement is recognized, so rhythmical intention, the use of conscious vocalization with repetitive, dynamic words or rhythmical song, is used before and during movement. Children must learn to mentally prepare for action. The children learn to move their bodies, constantly transitioning from one position to the next. Basic wooden equipment, ladder frames, and slatted tables (see Fig. 8.9) are used almost exclusively. Individuals trained in this approach are called "conductors." There is evidence that children with CP achieve their motor goals when participating in a CE program (Effgen & Chan, 2010). There is no evidence, however, to suggest that CE is any more effective than special education and therapy, as practiced in most parts of the developed world, in meeting the developmental needs of children with CP (Darrah et al., 2004). In fact, although CE was doing integrated therapeutic programs in the natural environment long before it was standard practice in the United States, today there is remarkable similarity between CE and integrative, interdisciplinary, special education and therapeutic intervention (Bourke-Taylor, O'Shea, & Gaebler-Spira, 2007; Effgen, 2001). If therapists are doing interdisciplinary intervention with a functional focus, in natural environments using extensive repetition and practice for motor learning, they are doing CE, just perhaps without wooden equipment and singing. Research suggests that children with CP develop further under an intensive therapy program than when receiving CE or just special education (Stiller et al., 2001).

This approach obviously focuses on active learning in the context of a functional environment. It emphasizes motor leaning strategies such as observational learning from the group, cognitive strategies from rhymes, rhymes and songs, and practice. The focus is not on impairment level interventions, and the assumption is that they will be ameliorated in the context of functional activity.

Summary

This chapter offered guiding principles for developing and applying the intervention plan for children with a range of neurological impairments causing limitations in body structures and functions and restrictions in activity and participation. It outlined the theoretical perspectives from which current motor learning principles are derived. An activity-focused model of intervention, based on concepts of change from a dynamic systems perspective, was introduced to structure the intervention of physical therapists. The model stresses practice of functional motor skills by children with neurological diagnoses. Readers are challenged to develop personal guidelines for best practice by reviewing the information presented in this chapter, investigating the evidence, and integrating personal experience and communication with other therapists and families of children with neurological impairments.

DISCUSSION QUESTIONS

1. How do cognitive aspects of motor learning (information processing, memory, and attention) contribute to the learning of functional motor activities by children with neurological impairments?

2. Discuss the role of the pediatric physical therapist as a "change agent" in the process of promoting functional goals in the intervention plan of care.

3. Discuss three practical ways in which a physical therapist can intervene with task constraints to promote the acquisition and learning of functional motor skills.

4. Discuss three practical ways in which a physical therapist can intervene with environmental

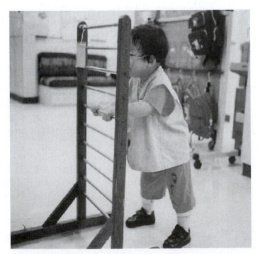

Figure 8.9 Child in Conductive Education program using ladder frame for walking.

constraints to promote the acquisition of functional motor skills. Refer to the physical environment as well as the performance environment.

5. Impairments in multiple body systems affect motor learning. Describe a strategy for addressing impairments of body functions and structures in the context of an intervention plan that focuses on improving functional activity.

Recommended Readings

Coker, C.A. (2009). *Motor learning and control for practitioners.* Scottsdale, AZ: Holcomb Hathaway.

Schmidt, R.A., & Wrisberg, C.A. (2008). *Motor performance and learning.* Champaign, IL: Human Kinetics.

Shumway-Cook A., & Woollacott, M.H. (2012). Motor learning and recovery of function. In A. Shumway-Cook & M.H. Woollacott (Eds.), *Motor control: Translating research into clinical practice* (4th ed.). Philadelphia: Lippincott Williams & Wilkins.

References

Adams, R.C., & Snyder, P. (1998). Treatments for cerebral palsy: Making choices of intervention from an expanding menu of options. *Infants and Young Children, 10*, 1–22.

Adolph, K.E., & Berger, S.E. (2006). Motor development. In W. Damon, R.M. Lerner, D. Kuhn, & R.S. Siegler (Eds.), *Handbook of child psychology, vol. 2: Cognition, perception, and language* (6th ed., pp. 161–213). Hoboken, NJ: John Wiley.

Adolph, K., Eppler, M., & Gibson, E. (1993). Development of perception of affordances. In C. Rovee-Collier & L. Lipsitt (Eds.), *Advances in infancy research,* Vol. 8 (pp. 51–98). Norwood, NJ: Ablex Publishing.

Adolph, K.E., Vereijken, B., & Shrout, P.E. (2003). What changes in infant walking and why. *Child Development, 74,* 475–497.

Alberto, P.A., & Troutman, A.C. (2009). *Applied behavior analysis for teachers* (8th ed.). Upper Saddle River, NJ: Pearson Education.

Alley, G.R., & Deshler, D.D. (1979). *Teaching the learning disabled adolescent: Strategies and methods.* Denver: Love Publishing.

American Physical Therapy Association (APTA) (2001). *Guide to physical therapist practice* (2nd ed.). *Physical Therapy, 81,* 1–768.

American Physical Therapy Association (APTA), Section on Pediatrics. (2004). *Physical therapy clinical management guideline for children with spastic diplegia* Working document submitted by M. Fragala & M. O'Neil, chairs of task force to develop a clinical management guideline. Alexandria, VA: Author.

Arndt, S.W., Chandler, L.S., Sweeney, J.K., Sharkey, M.A., & McElroy, J.J. (2008). Effects of a neurodevelopmental treatment–based trunk protocol for infants with posture and movement dysfunction. *Pediatric Physical Therapy, 20,* 11–22.

Ayres, A.J. (1972). *Sensory integration and learning disorders.* Los Angeles: Western Psychological Services.

Ayres, A.J. (1979). *Sensory integration and the child.* Los Angeles: Western Psychological Services.

Bernstein, N. (1967). *The co-ordination and regulation of movements.* New York: Pergamon.

Bertoti, D.B., & Gross, A.L. (1988). Evaluation of biofeedback seat insert for improving active sitting posture in children with cerebral palsy: A clinical report. *Physical Therapy, 68,* 1109–1113.

Blackmore, A.M., Boettcher-Hunt, E., Jordan, M., & Chan, M.D.Y. (2007). A systematic review of the effects of casting on equinus in children with cerebral palsy: An evidence report of the AACPDM. *Developmental Medicine & Child Neurology, 49,* 781–790.

Blaskey, J., & Jennings, M.C. (1999). Traumatic brain injury. In S.K. Campbell (Ed.), *Decision making in pediatric neurologic physical therapy* (pp. 84–140). Philadelphia: Churchill Livingstone.

Bly, L. (1991). A historical and current view of the basis of NDT. *Pediatric Physical Therapy, 3*(3), 131–135.

Bly, L., & Whiteside, A. (1997). *Facilitation techniques based on NDT principles.* San Antonio: Therapy Skill Builders.

Bobath, K., & Bobath, B. (1984). The neuro-developmental treatment. In D. Scrutton (Ed.), *Management of the motor disorders of children with cerebral palsy* (pp. 6–16). Philadelphia: J.B. Lippincott.

Boehme, R. (1988). *Improving upper body control.* Tucson: Therapy Skill Builders.

Booth, M.Y., Yates, C.C., Edgar, T.S., & Bandy, W.D. (2003). Serial casting vs. combined intervention with Botulinum toxin A and serial casting in the treatment of spastic equinus in children. *Pediatric Physical Therapy, 15*(4), 216–220.

Bourke-Taylor, H., O'Shea, R., & Gaebler-Spira, D. (2007). Conductive education: A functional skills program for children with cerebral palsy. *Physical and Occupational Therapy in Pediatrics, 27*(1), 45–62.

Bower, E., & McLellan, D.L. (1992). Effect of increased exposure to physiotherapy on skill acquisition of children with cerebral palsy. *Developmental Medicine and Child Neurology, 34,* 25–39.

Bower, E., & McLellan, D.L. (1994). Assessing motor-skill acquisition in four centers for the treatment of children with cerebral palsy. *Developmental Medicine and Child Neurology, 36,* 902–909.

Bower, E., McLellan, D.L., Arney, J., & Campbell, M.J. (1996). A randomized controlled trial of different intensities of physiotherapy and different goal-setting procedures in 44 children with cerebral palsy. *Developmental Medicine & Child Neurology, 38,* 226–237.

Bower, E., Mitchell, D., Burnett, M., Campbell, M.J., & McLellan, D.L. (2001). Randomized controlled trial of physiotherapy in 56 children with cerebral palsy followed for 18 months. *Developmental Medicine & Child Neurology, 43,* 4–15.

Bradley, N., & Westcott, S.L. (2006). Motor control: Developmental aspects of motor control in skill acquisition. In S.K. Campbell, D.W. Vander Linden, & R.J. Palisano (Eds.), *Physical therapy for children* (3rd ed., pp. 77–130). Philadelphia: Churchill Livingstone.

Brown, G.T., & Burns, S.A. (2001). The efficacy of neurodevelopmental treatment in paediatrics: A systematic review. *British Journal of Occupational Therapy, 64*(5), 235–244.

Brown, D.A., Effgen, S., & Palisano, R. (1998). Performance following ability-focused physical therapy intervention in individuals with severely limited physical and cognitive abilities. *Physical Therapy, 78*(9), 934.

Bundy, A.C., Lane, S., Murray, E.A., & Fisher, A.G. (2002). *Sensory integration: Theory and practice.* Philadelphia: F.A. Davis.

Butler, C., & Darrah, J. (2001). Effects of neurodevelopmental treatment (NDT) for cerebral palsy: An AACPDM evidence report. *Developmental Medicine and Child Neurology, 43,* 778–790.

Cadenhead, S.L., McEwen, I.R., & Thompson, D.M. (2002). Effects of passive range of motion exercises on lower extremity goniometric measurements of adults with cerebral palsy: A single-subject design. *Physical Therapy, 82,* 858–869.

Campbell, P.H. (1991). Evaluation and assessment in early intervention for infants and toddlers. *Journal of Early Intervention, 15,* 36–45.

Campbell, S.K. (1999). Models for decision making in pediatric neurologic physical therapy. In S.K. Campbell (Ed.), *Decision making in pediatric neurologic physical therapy.* Philadelphia: Churchill Livingstone.

Carmick, J. (1997). Use of neuromuscular electrical stimulation and dorsal wrist splint to improve the hand function of a child with spastic hemiparesis. *Physical Therapy, 77,* 661–671.

Charles, J., & Gordon, A.M. (2005). A critical review of constraint-induced movement therapy and forced use in children with hemiplegia. *Neural Plasticity, 12*(2–3), 245–261.

Clark, J.E. (1995). Dynamic systems perspective on the development of complex adaptive skill. In C. Dent-Read & P. Zukow-Goldring (Eds.), *Evolving explanations of development* (pp. 383-406). Washington, DC: American Physiological Association.

Coker, P., Karakostas, T., Dodds, C., & Hsiang, S. (2010). Gait characteristics of children with hemiplegic cerebral palsy before and after modified constraint-induced movement therapy. *Disability and Rehabilitation, 32*(5), 402–408.

Conine, T.A., Sullivan, T., Mackie, T., & Goodman, M. (1990). Effect of serial casting for the prevention of equinus in patients with acute head injury. *Archives of Physical Medicine and Rehabilitation, 71,* 310–312.

Damiano, D.L. (2006). Activity, activity, activity: Rethinking our physical therapy approach to cerebral palsy. *Physical Therapy, 86*(11), 1534–1540.

Damiano, D.L. (2007). Pass the torch, please! *Developmental Medicine & Child Neurology, 49,* 723.

Damiano, D.L., & Abel, M.F. (1998). Functional outcomes of strength training in spastic cerebral palsy. *Archives of Physical Medicine and Rehabilitation, 79,* 119–125.

Damiano, D.L., & DeJong, S.L., (2009). A systematic review of the effectiveness of treadmill training and body weight support in pediatric rehabilitation. *Journal of Neurological Physical Therapy, 33*(1), 27–44.

Damiano, D.L., Dodd, K., & Taylor, N.F. (2002). Should we be testing and training muscle strength in cerebral palsy? *Developmental Medicine and Child Neurology, 44,* 68–72.

Darrah, J., Fan, J.S., Chen, L., Nunweiler, J., & Watkins, B. (1997). Review of the effects of progressive resistive muscle strengthening in children with cerebral palsy: A clinical consensus. *Pediatric Physical Therapy, 9,* 12–17.

Darrah, J., Watkins, B., Chen, L., & Bonin, C. (2004). Effects of conductive education intervention for children with a diagnosis of cerebral palsy: An AACPDM evidence report. *Developmental Medicine & Child Neurology, 46,* 198–203.

Darrah, J., Wiart, L., & Magill-Evans, J. (2008). Do therapists' goals and interventions for children with cerebral palsy reflect principles in contemporary literature? *Pediatric Physical Therapy, 20*(4), 334–339.

David, K.S. (1985). Motor sequencing strategies in school-aged children. *Physical Therapy, 65,* 883–889.

David, K.S. (1995). Developmental coordination disorders. In S.K. Campbell, D.W. Vander Linden, & R.J. Palisano (Eds.), *Physical therapy for children* (pp. 425–458). Philadelphia: W.B. Saunders.

David, K.S. (2000). Developmental coordination disorders. In S.K. Campbell, D.W. Vander Linden, & R.J. Palisano (Eds.), *Physical therapy for children* (2nd ed., pp. 471–501). Philadelphia: W.B. Saunders.

Davids, K., Button, C., & Bennett, S. (2008). *Dynamics of skill acquisition: A constraints-led approach.* Champaign, IL: Human Kinetics.

Dawson, M.M., Hallahan, D.P., Reeve, R.E., & Ball, D.W. (1980). The effect of reinforcement and verbal rehearsal on selective attention in learning disabled children. *Journal of Abnormal Child Psychology, 8,* 133–144.

DeGangi, G. (1990). Perspectives on the integration of neurodevelopmental treatment sensory integrative therapy. *NDTA Newsletter,* March, pp. 1, 6.

DeLuca, S., Echols, K., Ramey, S.L., & Taub, E. (2003). Pediatric constraint-induced movement therapy for a young child with cerebral palsy: Two episodes of care. *Physical Therapy, 83,* 1003–1013.

Dichter, C.G. (1994). Relationship of muscle strength and joint range of motion to gross motor abilities in school-aged children with Down syndrome. Unpublished doctoral dissertation, Hahnemann University, Philadelphia.

Dichter, C.G., DeCicco, J., Flanagan, S., Hyun, J., & Mongrain, C. (2001). Acquiring skill through intervention in adolescents with Down syndrome. [Abstract]. *Pediatric Physical Therapy, 12,* 209.

Dodd, K.J., Taylor, N.F., & Damiano, D.L. (2002). A systematic review of the effectiveness of strength-training programs for people with cerebral palsy. *Archives of Physical Medicine & Rehabilitation, 83,* 1157–1164.

Duff, S.V., & Gordon, A.M. (2003). Learning of grasp control in children with hemiplegic cerebral palsy. *Developmental Medicine and Child Neurology, 45*(11), 746–757.

Duff, S., & Quinn, L. (2002). Motor learning and motor control. In D. Cech & S. Martin (Eds.), *Functional movement development across the life span* (2nd ed., pp. 86–117). Philadelphia: W.B. Saunders.

Dumas, H., & Francesconi, S. (2002). Aquatic therapy in pediatrics: Annotated bibliography. *Physical and Occupational Therapy in Pediatrics, 20*(4), 63–78.

Dumas, H.M., Haley, S.M., Carey, T.M., & Ni, P.S. (2004). The relationship between functional mobility and the intensity of physical therapy intervention in children with traumatic brain injury. *Pediatric Physical Therapy, 46,* 157–164.

Dursun, E., Dursun, N., & Alican, D. (2004). Effects of biofeedback treatment on gait in children with cerebral palsy. *Disability and Rehabilitation, 26*(2), 116–120.

Dusing, S.C. & Harbourne, R.T. (2010). Variability in postural control during infancy: implications for development, assessment, and intervention. *Pediatric Physical Therapy, 90*(12), 1838–1849.

Eckersley, P.M., & King, J. (1993). Principles of treatment. In P.M. Eckersley (Ed.), *Elements of paediatric physiotherapy* (pp. 323–341). New York: Churchill-Livingstone.

Effgen, S.K. (2001). Occurrence of gross motor behaviors in U.S. preschools and conductive education preschools in Hong Kong. [Abstract]. *Physical Therapy, 81,* A78.

Effgen, S.K., & Chan, L. (2010). Occurrence of gross motor behaviors and attainment of motor objectives in children with cerebral palsy participating in conductive education. *Physiotherapy Theory and Practice, 26*(1), 22–39.

Eliasson, A.C., Gordon, A.M., & Forssberg, H. (1992). Impaired anticipatory control of isometric forces during grasping by children with cerebral palsy. *Developmental Medicine and Child Neurology, 34,* 216–225.

Eliasson, A.C., Gordon, A.M., & Forssberg, H. (1995). Tactile control of isometric forces during grasping in children with cerebral palsy. *Developmental Medicine and Child Neurology, 33,* 661–670.

Fetters, L. & Ellis, T. (2006). A perception-action framework for physical therapy for persons with neurological dysfunction: Use of therapeutic affordances and unitless ratio. *Journal of Neurological Physical Therapy, 30*(3), 142–147.

Figueiredo, E.M., Ferreira, G.B., Moreira, R.C.M., Kirkwood, R.N, & Fetters, L. (2008). Efficacy of ankle-foot orthoses on gait of children with cerebral palsy: A systematic review of the literature. *Pediatric Physical Therapy, 20,* 207–223.

Fisher, B.E., & Sullivan, K.J. (2001). Activity-dependent factors affecting post-stroke functional outcomes. *Topics in Stroke Rehabilitation, 8*(3), 31–44.

Floodmark, A. (1986). Augmented auditory feedback as an aid in gait training of the cerebral palsied child. *Developmental Medicine and Child Neurology, 28,* 147–155.

Fontaine, A.M. (2005). Developmental ecology of early peer interactions: The role of play materials. *Enfrance, 57*(2), 137–154.

Fragala, M.A., Goodgold, S., & Dumas, H. (2003). Effects of lower extremity passive stretching: Pilot study of children and youth with severe limitations in self-mobility. *Pediatric Physical Therapy, 15,* 167–175.

Fragala-Pinkham, M.A., Dumas, H.M., Barlow, C.A., & Pasternak, A. (2009). An aquatic physical therapy program at a pediatric rehabilitation hospital: A case series. *Pediatric Physical Therapy, 21*(1), 68–78.

Gallagher, J.D., & Thomas, J.R. (1989). Effect of varying post-KR intervals upon children's motor performance. *Journal of Motor Behavior, 12,* 41–46.

Gentile, A.M. (1987). Skill acquisition: Action, movement, and neuromuscular processes. In J.A. Carr & R.B. Shepherd (Eds.), *Movement science: Foundation for physical therapy in rehabilitation* (pp. 93–154). Rockville, MD: Aspen Publications.

Gentile, A.M. (1992). The nature of skill acquisition: Therapeutic implications for children with movement disorders. In H. Forssberg & H. Hirschfeld (Eds.), *Movement disorders in children. Medical Sports Science, 36,* 31–40, Basel, Switzerland: Karger.

Getz, M., Hutzler, Y., & Vermeer, A. (2006). Effects of aquatic interventions in children with neuromotor impairments: A systematic review of the literature. *Clinical Rehabilitation, 20*(11), 927–936.

Gibson, J.J. (1979). *The ecological approach to visual perception.* Boston: Houghton-Mifflin.

Goodgold-Edwards, S., & Gianutsos, J.G. (1991). Coincidence anticipation performance of children with spastic cerebral palsy and nonhandicapped children. *Physical and Occupational Therapy in Pediatrics, 10,* 49–82.

Gordon, A.M., Schneider, J.A., Chinnan, A., & Charles, J.R. (2007). Efficacy of a hand-arm bimanual intensive therapy (HABIT) in children with hemiplegic cerebral palsy: A randomized control trial. *Developmental Medicine & Child Neurology, 49*(11), 830–838.

Granda-Vera, J., & Montilla, M.M. (2003). Practice schedule and acquisition, retention, and transfer of a throwing task in 6-year-old children. *Perceptual and Motor Skills, 96*(3pt1), 1015–1024.

Guadagnoli, M.A., & Lee, T.D. (2004). Challenge point: A framework for conceptualizing the effects of various practice conditions in motor learning. *Journal of Motor Behavior, 36,* 212–224.

Gudjonsdottir, B., & Stemmons-Mercer, V. (2002). Effects of a dynamic versus static prone stander on bone mineral density and behaviour in 4 children with severe cerebral palsy. *Pediatric Physical Therapy, 14,* 38–46.

Haken, H., Kelso, J.A.S., & Bunz, H. (1985). A theoretical model of phase transitions in human hand movements. *Biological Cybernetics, 51,* 347–356.

Harbourne, R.T., & Stergiou, N. (2009). Movement variability and the use of nonlinear tools: principles to guide physical therapist practice. *Physical Therapy, 89,* 267–282.

Hari, M., & Tillemans, T. (1984). Conductive education. In D. Scrutton (Ed.), Management of the motor disorders of children with cerebral palsy. *Clinics in Developmental Medicine, 90,* 19–35.

Harris, S.R. (1990). Therapeutic exercise for children with neurodevelopmental disabilities. In J. Basmajian (Ed.), *Therapeutic exercise* (5th ed., pp. 163–173). Baltimore: Williams & Wilkins.

Harris, S.R., & Lundgren, B.D. (1991). Joint mobilization in children with central nervous system disorders: Indications and precautions. *Physical Therapy, 71,* 890–896.

Harris, S. R., & Roxborough, L. (2005). Efficacy and effectiveness of physical therapy in enhancing postural control in children with cerebral palsy. *Neural-plasticity, 12*(2-3), 229–243.

Harvey, A., & Russell, D. (2009). What is the evidence of the effectiveness of strengthening for children with cerebral palsy aged 4–18 years? Retrieved from http://www.canchild.ca/en/canchildresources/StrengtheningforChildrenwithCP.asp

Hatzitaki, V., Zisi, V., Kollias, I., & Kioumourtzoglou, E. (2002). Perceptual-motor contributions to static and dynamic balance control in children. *Journal of Motor Behavior, 34,* 161–170.

Heriza, C.B. (1991). Motor development: Traditional and contemporary theories. In M.J. Lister (Ed.), *Contemporary management of motor control problems: Proceedings of the II STEP Conference* (pp. 99–126). Alexandria, VA: American Physical Therapy Association.

Heriza, C.B., & Sweeney, J.K. (1994). Pediatric physical therapy: Part I. Practice, scope, scientific basis, and theoretical foundation. *Infants and Young Children, 7,* 20–32.

Heriza, C.B., & Sweeney, J.K. (1995). Pediatric physical therapy: Part II. Approaches to movement dysfunction. *Infants and Young Children, 8,* 1–14.

Hood, B., & Atkinson, J. (1990). Sensory visual loss and cognitive deficits in selective attentional system of normal infants and neurologically impaired children. *Developmental Medicine and Child Neurology, 32,* 1067–1077.

Horgan, J. (1985). Mnemonic strategy instruction in coding, processing and recall of movement-related cues in mentally retarded children. *Perceptual and Motor Skills, 57,* 547–557.

Horne, E.M., Warren, S.F., & Jones, H.A. (1995). An experimental analysis of neurobehavioral motor intervention. *Developmental Medicine and Child Neurology, 37,* 697–714.

Howle, J.M. (2003). *Neuro-developmental treatment approach: Theoretical foundations and principles of clinical practice.* Laguna Beach, CA: Neurodevelopmental Treatment Association.

Huang, H., & Mercer, V. (2001). Dual task methodology: Application in studies of cognitive and motor performance in adults and children. *Pediatric Physical Therapy, 13,* 133–140.

Iarocci, G., & Burack, J.A. (1998). Understanding the development of attention in persons with mental retardation: Challenging the myths. In J.A. Burack, R.M. Hodapp, et al. (Eds.), *Handbook of mental retardation and development* (pp. 349–381). New York: Cambridge University Press.

Jensen, J.L., Ulrich, B.D., Thelen, E., Schneider, K., & Zernicke, R.F. (1994). Adaptive dynamics of leg movement patterns of human infants: 1. The effects of posture on spontaneous kicking. *Journal of Motor Behavior, 26,* 303–312.

Jewell, D.V. (2011). *Guide to evidence-based physical therapist practice.* Sudbury, MA: Jones & Bartlett Learning.

Karnish, K., Bruder, M.B., & Rainforth, B. (1995). A comparison of physical therapy in the school-based treatment contexts. *Physical and Occupational Therapy in Pediatrics, 15,* 1–25.

Kelso, J.S. (1984). Phase transitions and critical behavior in human bimanual coordination. *American Journal of Physiology, 15,* R10000–R10004.

Kernodle, M.W., & Carlton, L.G. (1992). Information feedback and the learning of multiple-degree of freedom activities. *Journal of Motor Behavior, 24,* 187–196.

Kerr, C., McDowell, B., & McDonough, S. (2004). Electrical stimulation in cerebral palsy: A review of effects on strength and motor function. *Developmental Medicine and Child Neurology, 46,* 205–213.

Ketelaar, M., Vermer, A., Hart, H., van Petegem-van Beek, E. & Helders, J.J. (2001). Effects of a functional therapy program on motor abilities of children with cerebral palsy. *Physical Therapy, 81,* 1534–1545.

King, E.M., Gooch, J.E., Howell, G.H., Peters, M.L., Bloswick, D.S., & Brown, D.R. (1993). Evaluation of the hip-extensor tricycle in improving gait in children with cerebral palsy. *Developmental Medicine and Child Neurology, 35,* 1048–1054.

Knutson, L.M., & Clark, J.E. (1991). Orthotic devices for ambulation in children with cerebral palsy and myelomeningocele. *Physical Therapy, 71*(12), 947–960.

Konczak, J. (1990). Toward an ecological theory of motor development: The relevance of the Gibsonian approach to vision for motor development research. In J.E. Clark & J.H. Humphrey (Eds.), *Advances in motor development research* (Vol. 3, pp. 201–223). New York: AMS Press.

Kozma, I., & Balogh, E. (1995). A brief introduction to conductive education and its application at an early age. *Infants and Young Children, 8,* 68–74.

LaForme Fiss, A.C., & Effgen, S.K. (2006). Outcomes for young children with disabilities associated with the use of partial body weight supported treadmill training: An evidence based review. *Physical Therapy Reviews, 11,* 179–189.

LaForme Fiss, A.C., Effgen, S.K., Page, J., & Shasby, S.B. (2009). Effect of sensorimotor groups on gross motor acquisition for young children with Down syndrome. *Pediatric Physical Therapy, 21*(2), 158–166.

Larin, H. (2006). Motor learning: Theories and strategies for the practitioner. In S.K. Campbell, D.W. Vander Linden, & R.J. Palisano (Eds.), *Physical therapy for children,* (3rd ed., pp. 131–160). Philadelphia: W.B. Saunders Publisher.

Latash, M.L., & Anson, J.G. (1996). What are "normal movements" in a typical population? *Behavior and Brain Sciences, 19,* 26.

Laufer, Y., Ashkenazi, T., & Josman, N. (2008). The effects of a concurrent cognitive task on the postural control of young children with and without developmental coordination disorder. *Gait & Posture, 27*(2), 347–351.

Lee, D.N., & Cook, M.L. (1990). Basic perceptuo-motor dysfunctions in cerebral palsy. In M. Jeannerod (Ed.), *Attention and performance XVIII: Motor representation and control* (pp. 583–602). Mahwah, NJ: Lawrence Erlbaum Associates.

Leong, B. (2002). Critical review of passive muscle stretch: Implications for the treatment of children in vegetative and minimally conscious states. *Brain Injury, 16,* 169–183.

Light, K.E. (2003). Issues of cognition for motor control. In P.C. Montgomery & B.H. Connolly (Eds.), *Clinical applications for motor control* (pp. 245–268). Thorofare, NJ: Slack.

Lin, C.H., Sullivan, K.J., Wu, A.D., Kantak, S. & Winstein, C.J. (2007). Effect of task practice order on motor skill learning in adults with Parkinson disease: A pilot study. *Physical Therapy, 87,* 1120–1131.

Logan, L., Byers-Hinkley, K., & Ciccone, C.D. (1990). Anterior vs. posterior walkers: A gait analysis study. *Developmental Medicine and Child Neurology, 32,* 1044–1048.

Lunnen, K.Y. (1999). Children with multiple disabilities. In S.K. Campbell (Ed.), *Clinical decision making in pediatric neurologic physical therapy* (pp. 141–197). New York: Churchill Livingstone.

MacKinnon, J.R., Noh, S., Laliberte, D., Lariviere, J., & Allan, D.E. (1995). Therapeutic horseback riding: A review of the literature. *Physical and Occupational Therapy in Pediatrics, 15*(1), 1–15.

Magill, R.A. (1992). Augmented feedback in skill acquisition. In R.N. Singer & L.K. Tennant (Eds.), *Handbook on research in sport psychology* (pp. 143–189). New York: Macmillan.

Majsak, M. (1996). Application of motor learning principles to the stroke population. *Topics in Stroke Rehabilitation, 3*(2), 27–59.

Mandich, A.D., Polatajko, H.J., Missiuna, C., & Miller, L.T. (2001). Cognitive strategies and motor performance in children with developmental coordination disorder. *Physical and Occupational Therapy in Pediatrics, 20*(2–3), 125–143.

Maruff, P., Wilson, P., Trebilcock, M., & Currie, J. (1998). Abnormalities of imagined motor sequences in children with developmental coordination disorder. *Neuropsychologia, 37*, 1317–1324.

Mattern-Baxter, K. (2009). Effects of partial body weight supported treadmill training on children with cerebral palsy. *Pediatric Physical Therapy, 21*(1), 12–22.

Mayo, N.E. (1991). The effect of physical therapy for children with motor delay and cerebral palsy: A randomized clinical trial. *American Journal of Physical Medicine and Rehabilitation, 70*(5), 258–267.

McDowd, J.M. (2007). An overview of attention: Behavior and brain. *Journal of Neurologic Physical Therapy, 31*, 98–103.

McEwen, I.R. (1992). Assistive positioning as a control parameter of social communicative interactions between students with profound multiple disabilities and classroom staff. *Physical Therapy, 72*, 634–647.

McEwen, I.R., & Hansen, L.H. (2006). Children with motor and cognitive impairments. In S.K. Campbell, D.W. Vander Linden, & R.J. Palisano (Eds.), *Physical therapy for children* (2nd ed., pp. 591–624). Philadelphia: W.B. Saunders.

McGibbon, H., Andrade, C., Widener, G., & Cintas, H.L. (1998). Effect of an equine-movement therapy program on gait, energy expenditure, and motor function in children with spastic cerebral palsy: A pilot study. *Developmental Medicine and Child Neurology, 40*, 754–762.

McPherson, J.J., Arends, T.G., Michaels, M.J., & Trettin, K. (1984). The range of motion of long-term knee contractures of four spastic cerebral palsied children: A pilot study. *Physical and Occupational Therapy in Pediatrics, 4*(1), 17–34.

Mercer, V.S., & Lewis, C.L. (2001). Hip abductor and knee extensor muscle strength of children with and without Down syndrome. *Pediatric Physical Therapy, 13*, 18–26.

Miedaner, J.A., & Renander, J. (1987). The effectiveness of classroom passive stretching programs for increasing or managing passive range of motion in nonambulatory children: An evaluation of frequency. *Physical and Occupational Therapy in Pediatrics, 7*(3), 35–43.

Miller, J.J., Anzalone, M.E., Lane, S.J., Cermak, S.A., & Osten, E.T. (2007). Concept evolution in sensory integration: A proposed nosology for diagnosis. *The American Journal of Occupational Therapy, 61*(2), 135–140.

Miller, L.J., & Summers, C. (2001). Clinical applications in sensory modulation dysfunction: Assessment and intervention considerations. In S.S. Roley, E.I. Blanche, & R. Schaaf (Eds.), *Sensory integration with diverse populations* (pp. 247–274). San Antonio: Therapy Skill Builders.

Missiuna, C., Rivard, L., & Bartlett, D. (2003). Early identification and risk management of children with developmental coordination disorder. *Pediatric Physical Therapy, 15*(1), 32–37.

Mockford, M., & Caulton, J.M. (2008). Systematic review of progressive strength training in children and adolescents with cerebral palsy who are ambulatory. *Pediatric Physical Therapy, 20*(4), 318–333.

Montgomery, P.C., & Richter, E. (1980). *Sensorimotor integration for the developmentally disabled child: A handbook.* Los Angeles: Western Psychological Services.

Mossberg, K.A., Linton, K.A., & Friske, K. (1990). Ankle-foot orthoses: Effect on energy expenditure of gait in spastic diplegic children. *Archives of Physical Medicine and Rehabilitation, 71*(7), 490–494.

Mutlu, A., Krosschell, K., & Spira, D.G. (2009). Treadmill training with partial body-weight support in children with cerebral palsy: a systematic review. *Developmental Medicine & Child Neurology, 51*(4), 268–275.

Naylor, C.E., & Bower, E. (2005). Modified constraint-induced movement therapy for young children with hemiplegic cerebral palsy. *Developmental Medicine & Child Neurology, 47*, 365–369.

Nelson, C.A. (2001). Cerebral palsy. In D.A. Umphred (Ed.), *Neurological rehabilitation* (4th ed., pp. 259–286). St. Louis: Mosby.

Newell, K.M. (1986). Constraints on the development of coordination. In M.G. Wade & H.T.A. Whiting (Eds.), *Motor development in children: Aspects of coordination and control.* Boston: Martinus Nijhoff.

Newell, K.M. (1996). Change in movement and skill: Learning, retention, and transfer. In M.L. Latash & M.T. Turvey (Eds.), *Dexterity and its development* (pp. 339–376). Mahwah, NJ: Lawrence Erlbaum Associates.

Newell, K.M., & Carlton, L.G. (1980). Developmental trends in motor response recognition. *Developmental Psychology, 16*, 550–554.

Newell, K.M., & Kennedy, J.A. (1978). Knowledge of results and children's motor learning. *Developmental Psychobiology, 14*, 531–536.

Newell, K.M., & McDonald, P.V. (1994). Learning to coordinate the redundant biomechanical degrees of freedom. In S. Swinnen, H. Heuer, J. Massion, & P. Casaer (Eds.), *Inter-limb coordination: Neural, dynamical and cognitive constraints* (pp. 515–536). San Diego: Academic Press.

Newell, K.M., Scully, D.M., McDonald, P.V., & Baillargeon, R. (1989). Task constraints and infant grip configurations. *Developmental Psychobiology, 22*, 817–832.

Newell, K.M., & Valvano, J. (1998). Therapeutic intervention as a constraint in the learning and relearning of movement skills. *Scandinavian Journal of Occupational Therapy, 5*, 51–57.

O'Connell, D.G., & Barnhart, R. (1995). Improvement in wheelchair propulsion in paediatric wheelchair users through resistance training: A pilot study. *Archives of Physical Medicine and Rehabilitation, 76*, 368–372.

Olney, S.J., & Wright, M.J. (2006). Cerebral palsy. In S.K. Campbell, D.W. Vander Linden, & R.J. Palisano (Eds.), *Physical therapy for children* (3rd ed., pp. 625–664). Philadelphia: W.B. Saunders.

O'Neil, M.E., Fragala-Pinkham, M.A., Westcott, S.L., Martin, K., Chiarello, L.A., Valvano, J., & Rose, R.U. (2006). Physical therapy clinical management recommendations for children with cerebral palsy—spastic diplegia: Achieving functional mobility outcomes. *Pediatric Physical Therapy, 18*(1), 49–72.

Ostensjo, S., Carlberg, E.B., & Vollestad, N.K. (2005). The use and impact of assistive devices and other environmental modifications on everyday activities and care in young children with cerebral palsy. *Disability and Rehabilitation, 27*(14), 849–861.

Ozer, K.O., Chesher, S.P., & Scheker, L.R. (2006). Neuromuscular electrical stimulation and dynamic bracing for the management of upper-extremity spasticity in children with cerebral palsy. *Developmental Medicine & Child Neurology, 48*(7), 559–563.

Parham, D., & Fazio, L. (2008). *Play in occupational therapy for children.* St. Louis: Mosby.

Parham, L.D., & Mailloux, Z. (1996). Sensory integration. In J. Case-Smith, A.S. Allen, & P. Nuse Pratt (Eds.), *Occupational therapy for children* (3rd ed., pp. 307–356). St. Louis: Mosby.

Parks, S., Rose, D.J., & Dunn, J.M. (1989). A comparison of fractionated reaction time between cerebral palsied and nonhandicapped youths. *Adapted Physical Activity Quarterly, 6,* 379–388.

Phillips, W.E., & Audet, M. (1990). Use of serial casting in the management of knee joint contractures in an adolescent with cerebral palsy. *Physical Therapy, 70,* 521–523.

Pigott, R., & Shapiro, D. (1984). Motor schema: The structure of the variability session. *Research Quarterly for Exercise and Sport, 55,* 41–55.

Pin, T. W. (2007). Effectiveness of static weight-bearing exercises in children with cerebral palsy. *Pediatric Physical Therapy, 19*(1), 62–73.

Pin, T., Dyke, P., & Chan, M. (2006). The effectiveness of passive stretching in children with cerebral palsy. *Developmental Medicine & Child Neurology, 48,* 855.

Polatajko, H.J., Mandich, A.D., Miller, L.T., & Macnab, J.J. (2001). Cognitive orientation to daily occupational performance: Part II. The evidence. *Physical and Occupational Therapy in Pediatrics, 20*(2–3), 125–143.

Randall, K.E., & McEwen, I.R. (2000). Writing patient-centered functional goals. *Physical Therapy, 80*(12), 1197–1203.

Reed, B. (1997). The physiology of neuromuscular electric stimulation. *Pediatric Physical Therapy, 9,* 96–102.

Reilly, D.S., Woollacott, M.H., van Donkelaar, P., & Saavedra, S. (2008). The interaction between executive attention and postural control in dual-task conditions: Children with cerebral palsy. *Archives of Physical Medicine and Rehabilitation, 89*(5), 834–842.

Roley, S., Blanche, E.I., & Schaaf, R.C. (2001). *Understanding the nature of sensory integration with diverse populations.* San Antonio: Therapy Skill Builders.

Roper, N., & Dunst, C.J. (2003). Communication intervention in natural learning environments: Guidelines for practice. *Infants and Young Children, 16,* 215–226.

Rosenbaum P. (2010). The randomized controlled trial: An excellent design, but can it address the big question of neurodisability? *Developmental Medicine and Child Neurology, 52*(11), 1066–1067.

Salmoni, A.W., Schmidt, R.A., & Walter, C.B. (1984). Knowledge of results and motor learning: A review and critical reappraisal. *Psychological Bulletin, 95,* 355–386.

Schmidt, R.A. (1988). *Motor control and learning: A behavioral emphasis* (2nd ed.). Champaign, IL: Human Kinetics.

Schmidt, R.A., & Lee, T.D. (1999). *Motor control and learning: A behavioral emphasis* (3rd ed.). Champaign, IL: Human Kinetics

Schmidt, R.A., & Lee, T.D. (2005). *Motor control and learning: A behavioral emphasis* (4th ed.). Champaign, IL: Human Kinetics.

Schmidt, R.A., & Wrisberg, C.A. (2008). *Motor performance and learning.* Champaign, IL: Human Kinetics.

Scholz, J.P. (1990). Dynamic pattern theory: Some implications for therapeutics. *Physical Therapy, 70,* 827–843.

Scholz, J.P., & Kelso, J.A.S. (1990). Intentional switching between patterns of bimanual coordination depends on the intrinsic dynamics of the patterns. *Journal of Motor Behavior, 22,* 98–124.

Schoner, G., Zanone, P.G., & Kelso, J.A.S. (1992). Learning as change of coordination dynamics: Theory and experiment. *Journal of Motor Behavior, 24,* 29–48.

Scianni, A., Butler, J.M., Ada, L., & Teixeira-Salmela, L.F. (2009). Muscle strengthening is not effective in children and adolescents with cerebral palsy: A systematic review. *The Australian Journal of Physiotherapy, 55*(2), 81–87.

Seeger, B.R., Caudrey, D.J., & Scholes, J.R. (1981). Biofeedback therapy to achieve symmetrical gait in hemiplegic cerebral palsied children. *Archives of Physical Medicine and Rehabilitation, 62,* 364–368.

Seifart, A., Unger, M., Burger, M. (2009). The effect of lower limb functional electric stimulation on gait of children with cerebral palsy. *Pediatric Physical Therapy, 21,* 23–30.

Shelly, A., Davis, E., Waters, E., Mackinnon, A., Reddihough, D., Boyd, R., Ried, S. & Graham, H.K. (2008). The relationship between quality of life and functioning for children with cerebral palsy. *Developmental Medicine and Child Neurology, 50,* 199–203.

Shoemaker, N.M., Niemeijer A.S., Reynderes, K., & Smits-Englesman, B.C. (2003). Effectiveness of neuromotor task training for children with developmental coordination disorder: A pilot study. *Neural Plasticity, 10,* 155–163.

Shumway-Cook, A., Hutchinson, S., Kartin, D., Price, R., & Woollacott, M.H. (2003). Effect of balance training on recovery of stability in children with cerebral palsy. *Developmental Medicine & Child Neurology, 45,* 591–602.

Shumway-Cook, A., & Woollacott, M.H. (1985). The growth of stability: Postural control from a developmental perspective. *Journal of Motor Behavior, 17,* 131–147.

Shumway-Cook, A., & Woollacott, M.H. (2012). *Motor control: Translating research into clinical practice* (4th ed.). Philadelphia: Lippincott Williams & Wilkins.

Sidaway, G., Ahn, S., Boldeau, P., Griffin, S., Noyes, B., & Pelletier, K. (2008). A comparison of manual guidance and knowledge of results in the learning of a weight bearing skill. *Journal of Neurologic Physical Therapy, 32*(1), 32–38.

Snider, L., Korner-Bitensky, N., Kammann, C., Warner, S., & Saleh, M. (2007). Horseback riding as therapy for children with cerebral palsy: Is there evidence of its effectiveness? *Physical and Occupational Therapy in Pediatrics, 27*(2), 5–23.

Spencer, J.P., & Schöner, G. (2003). Bridging the representational gap in the dynamic systems approach to development. *Developmental Science, 6,* 392–412.

Spitzer, S., & Roley, S.S. (2001). Sensory integration revisited: A philosophy of practice. In S. Roley, E.I. Blanche, & R.C. Schaaf (Eds.), *Understanding the nature of sensory integration with diverse populations* (pp. 3–27). San Antonio, TX: Therapy Skill Builders.

Sterba, J.A. (2007). Does horseback riding therapy or therapist-directed hippotherapy rehabilitate children with cerebral palsy? *Developmental Medicine and Child Neurology, 49*(1), 68–73.

Stiers, P., Vanderkelen, R., Vanneste, G., Colne, S., DeRamme-laere, M., & Vandenbussche, E. (2002). Visual-perceptual impairment in a random sample of children with cerebral palsy. *Developmental Medicine and Child Neurology, 44*(6), 370–382.

Stiller, C., Hall, H., Marcoux, B.C., & Olson, R.E. (2001). The effect of conductive education, intensive therapy, and special education services on motor skills in children with cerebral palsy. *Physical and Occupational Therapy in Pediatrics, 23*(3), 31–50.

Stiller, C., Marcoux, B.C., & Olson, R.E. (2003). The effect of conductive education, intensive therapy, and special education services on motor skills in children with cerebral palsy.

Stockmeyer, S.A. (1972). An interpretation of the approach of Rood to the treatment of neuromuscular dysfunction. *American Journal of Physical Medicine, 46*, 900–956.

Straus, S.E., Richardson, W.S., Glasziou, P., & Haynes, R.B. (2005). *Evidence based medicine: How to practice and teach EBM* (3rd ed.). New York: Churchill Livingstone.

Stuberg, W. (1992). Consideration related to weight bearing programs in children with developmental disability. *Physical Therapy, 72*, 35–40.

Sullivan, K.J., Kantak, S.S., & Burtner, P.A. (2008). Motor learning in children: Feedback effects on skill acquisition. *Physical Therapy, 88*(6), 721–732.

Tardieu, C., Lespargot, A., Tabary, C., & Bret, M.D. (1988). For how long must the soleus muscle be stretched each day to prevent contracture? *Developmental Medicine and Child Neurology, 30*, 3–10.

Taylor, J. (1999). Blocked and random practice of crutch walking skills in young children. Unpublished master's thesis, MCP Hahnemann University, Philadelphia.

Taub, E., Ramey, S., DeLuca, S., & Echols, K. (2004). Efficacy of constraint-induced movement therapy for children with cerebral palsy with asymmetric motor impairment. *Pediatrics, 113*(2), 305–312.

Thelen, E. (1986). Development of coordinated movement: Implication for early human development. In H.T.A. Whiting (Ed.), *Motor development in children: Aspects of coordination and control* (pp. 107–120). Boston: Martinus Nijhoff.

Thorpe, D.E., Shewokis, P.A., Kilby, J.M., Markham, J.R., Roberson, T.M., & Seymour, S.K. (2003). Does KP-driven internal or external focus of attention facilitate the learning of a novel tossing task in typically developing children? [Abstract]. *Journal of Sport and Exercise Psychology, 25*(Supp.), 132.

Thorpe, D.E., & Valvano, J. (2002). The effects of knowledge of results and cognitive strategies on motor skill learning by children with cerebral palsy. *Pediatric Physical Therapy, 14*, 2–15.

Trahan, J., & Malouin, F. (2002). Intermittent intensive physiotherapy in children with cerebral palsy: A pilot study. *Developmental Medicine and Child Neurology, 44*, 233–239.

Utley, A., Steenbergen, B., & Astill, S.L. (2007). Ball catching in children with developmental coordination disorder: Control of the degrees of freedom. *Developmental Medicine and Child Neurology, 49*, 34–38.

Valvano, J. (2004). Activity-focused motor interventions for children with neurological conditions. *Physical and Occupational Therapy in Pediatrics, 24*, 79–107.

Valvano, J., Heriza, C.B., & Carollo, J. (2002). The effects of physical and verbal guidance on the learning of a gross motor skill by children with cerebral palsy. Unpublished data.

Valvano, J., & Newell, K.M. (1998). Practice of a precision isometric grip force task by children with spastic cerebral palsy. *Developmental Medicine and Child Neurology, 40*, 464–473.

Valvano, J., & Rapport, M.J. (2006). Activity-focused interventions for infants and children with neurological conditions. *Infants and Young Children, 19*(4), 292–307.

Van der weel, F.R., van der Meer, A.L.H., & Lee, D.N. (1991). Effect of task on movement control in cerebral palsy: Implications for assessment and therapy. *Developmental Medicine and Child Neurology, 33*, 419–426.

Van Sant, A.F. (2008). Are we anchored to NDT? *Pediatric Physical Therapy, 20*(1), 1–2.

Vargas, S., & Camilli, G. (1999). A meta-analysis of research on sensory integration treatment. *The American Journal of Occupational Therapy, 53*, 189–198.

Vereijken, B. (2010). The complexity of childhood development: Variability in perspective. *Pediatric Physical Therapy, 90*(12), 1850–1859.

Warren, W.J. (1984). Perceiving affordances: The visual guidance of stair climbing. *Journal of Experimental Psychology: Human Learning and Memory, 10*, 683–704.

Wenderoth, N., Bock, O., & Krohn, R. (2002). Learning a new bimanual coordination pattern is influenced by existing attractors. *Motor Control, 26*, 166–182.

Wiart, L., Darrah, J., & Kembhavi, G. (2008). Stretching with children with cerebral palsy: what do we know and where are we going? *Pediatric Physical Therapy, 20*, 173–178.

Williams, H., & Pountney, T. (2007). Effects of a static bicycling programme on the functional ability of young people with cerebral palsy who are non-ambulant. *Developmental Medicine & Child Neurology, 49*, 522–527.

Wilson, P.H., & McKenzie, B.E. (1998). Information processing deficits associated with developmental coordination disorder: A meta-analysis of research findings. *Journal of Child Psychology and Psychiatry, 39*, 829–840.

Wilson Howle, J.M. (1999). Cerebral palsy. In S.K. Campbell (Ed.), *Decision making in pediatric neurologic physical therapy* (pp. 23–83). Philadelphia: Churchill Livingstone.

Winstein, C.J. (1991). Designing practice for motor learning: Clinical implications. In M.J. Lister (Ed.), *Contemporary management of motor problems: Proceedings of the II Step Conference* (pp. 65–76). Alexandria, VA: American Physical Therapy Association.

Winstein, C.J., Gardner, E.R., McNeal, D.R., Barto, P.S., & Nicholson, D.E. (1989). Standing balance training: Effects on balance and locomotion in hemiparetic adults. *Archives of Physical Medicine and Rehabilitation, 70*, 755–762.

Winstein, C.J., Pohl, P.S., & Lewthwaite, R. (1994). Effects of physical guidance and knowledge of results on motor learning: Support for the guidance hypothesis. *Research Quarterly for Exercise and Sport, 65*, 316–323.

Wulf, G. (1991). The effect of type of practice on motor learning in children. *Applied Cognitive Psychology, 5*, 123–134.

Wulf, G., Shea, C.H., & Matschiner, S. (1998). Frequent feedback enhances complex skill learning. *Journal of Motor Behavior, 30*, 180–192.

Wulf, G., Shea, C., & Park, J.H. (2001). Attention and motor performance: Preferences of an external focus. *Research Quarterly for Exercise & Sport, 72*(4), 335–344.

Wulf, G., Shea, C.H., & Whitacre, C.A. (1998). Physical guidance benefits in learning a complex motor skill. *Journal of Motor Behavior, 30*, 367–380.

Yakut, C. (2003). Effect of sequential versus simultaneous practice on learning a multi-component visual-motor task. Unpublished Doctoral Dissertation, University of Michigan.

Zanone, P.G., & Kelso, J.A.S. (1994). The coordination dynamics of learning: Theoretical structure and research agenda. In S. Swinnen, H. Heuer, J. Massion, & P. Casaer (Eds.), *Interlimb coordination*. San Diego: Academic Press.

Zanone, P.G., Kelso, J.A.S., & Jeka, J.J. (1993). Concepts and methods for a dynamical approach to behavioral coordination and change. In G.J.P. Savelsbergh (Ed.), *The development of coordination in infancy* (pp. 89–153). San Diego: Elsevier Science Publishers.

Zwicker, J.G., Mayson, T.A. (2010). Effectiveness of treadmill training in children with motor impairments: an overview of systematic reviews. *Pediatric Physical Therapy, 22*, 361–377.

CHAPTER 9

Cardiovascular and Pulmonary Systems

—CAROLE A. TUCKER, PT, PhD, PCS, RCEP

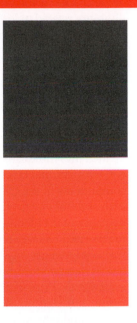

Cardiovascular and pulmonary (CVP) impairments of body structures and functions that occur during infancy and childhood can, in the short term, be life threatening. Medical and physical therapy intervention, in these cases, is focused primarily on acute-care issues.

However, the long-term effects of CVP conditions can alter the physical, social, and cognitive growth of a child, resulting in multifaceted restrictions on activities and participation. Physical therapists treating children with CVP conditions must not only focus on the evaluation and treatment of short-term CVP systems-related impairments, but also carefully consider issues related to long-term compliance, prevention of secondary impairments, and the effects of impairments and interventions on the maturing child's changing social, cognitive, and behavioral development, and eventual role in society.

In the past decade, the emergence of improved diagnostic procedures and interventions for CVP conditions has improved care and quality of life for these children and their families. Unfortunately, these improvements have been counterbalanced by increasingly sedentary lifestyles, lack of physical activity and fitness in children, and the impact of obesity-related childhood chronic health conditions. The role of physical therapists in providing care for children with CVP conditions is shifting. Physical therapists are uniquely prepared to improve and increase opportunities for physical activity for all children, including those with CVP and neuromuscular conditions.

The overall objective of this chapter is to provide the entry-level physical therapy practitioner with the necessary foundational knowledge to develop effective evaluation, examination, and procedural interventions for children with CVP conditions. In this chapter, a detailed overview is provided of the development and maturation of the CVP systems' structure and function, and the impact of common pediatric CVP conditions on the growth and development of children framed within the context of the International Classification of Functioning, Disability and Health for Children and Youth (ICF-CY) (World Health Organization, 2007). Clinical guidelines to assist the reader in determining appropriate examination and intervention techniques for children with CVP conditions and related impairments are presented. Physical fitness and the emerging issues concerning health promotion and wellness programs for all children are also addressed. The final focus of the chapter is the physical therapist's role in reducing disability related to long-term CVP effects of childhood obesity and physical inactivity.

Structure and Function

Overview of Cardiovascular and Pulmonary Function

The discussion of CVP function is organized according to "systems theory," with the systems' components subdivided into three categories: individual (or organismic), environment, and task (Fig. 9.1). Individual or organismic components of the CVP systems include characteristics such as the ability to generate muscle force of inspiration, diameter of the blood vessels, range of motion (ROM) of the thorax, or airway responsiveness. Environmental system components for CVP function include gravity, air quality, temperature, humidity, and oxygen content of the available air. Primary tasks of the CVP systems are ventilation, circulation, and respiration, which exchange, deliver, and remove gases to maintain the pH level of the body in a range that allows for cellular function. The magnitude of gas exchange must be sufficient to provide the body's tissues with enough oxygen and removal of end-product gases to sustain life, and to provide enough additional energy for growth and development in

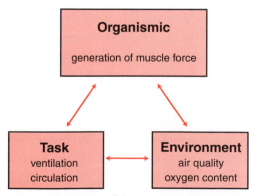

Figure 9.1 Schematic of the systems theory as it applies to the cardiovascular and pulmonary systems.

children. At any given time these CVP systems' tasks are performed in concert with the individual and environmental system components.

Constraints on ventilation, circulation, and respiration are often related to the basic forces and laws of physics (e.g., mechanical, fluid, chemical, and electrical laws). CVP systems activity is primarily controlled through the nervous system, which is basically constrained by electrical conduction properties, as well as chemical constraints locally.

Ventilation (the flow of gases between the lungs and the external environment) is dependent upon lung compliance, thoracic compliance, airway resistance, and the interplay of forces generated by the respiratory muscles. Ventilation, in particular, is "constrained" or affected by mechanical factors such as the shape and size of the thorax, the rigidity or flexibility of the ribcage, the forces generated by the muscles of respiration, the force-length relationship in muscles, the elastic recoil properties of the thorax, and effective airway diameter.

Circulation (the movement of blood throughout the body) is dependent on pressure gradients, blood flow, blood volume, and the sequence of forces generated by the cardiac muscle. Fluid forces and pressure gradients in the heart and vasculature affect circulation. In addition, muscle force-length properties and electrical activity of the heart muscle are responsible for many of the pressure changes that provide circulation.

For **respiration** (gas exchange at the alveolar and tissue level) to be effective, both ventilation and circulation must be accomplished. Respiration is dependent on pressure and chemical gradients, diffusion of chemicals across cell membranes, and capillary interfaces.

The dynamic interplay between ventilation, circulation, and respiration determines the overall level of functioning of the CVP systems at any given instant. Over a longer time frame, CVP system components are altered by growth and maturation, providing a dynamic set of system performance constraints that differ between infancy and adulthood. As a child grows and environmental exploration and societal involvement increase, CVP conditions will have different effects on the components of daily life and quality of life. In infancy, CVP conditions can interfere with feeding, growth, and wakefulness, thereby limiting environmental exploration. In a young child, community mobility, participation, and socialization with peers through play and school attendance can be affected.

During teenage years, socialization, employment, and concerns involving transition into an independent adulthood become increasingly important. Medical management and interventions for CVP conditions should consider the broader perspective and impact of care on activities, participation, and quality of life throughout maturation.

Although the structure and function of the CVP systems reflect the complex interaction between the cardiovascular and pulmonary systems, the maturation of each system follows a different sequence of events. The heart is one of the first functioning organs within the growing fetus, and it performs the task of circulation in utero. On the other hand, the pulmonary system does not perform its primary task of ventilation until after birth. An understanding of the maturation of the CVP systems provides an ability to gauge the effect of growth-related interdependence of the two systems and how a small change in one system component can, over time, have an effect on other parts of the system as they mature.

Maturation of the Cardiovascular System

The heart is derived from multiple cell lineages and must differentiate into unique regions, each possessing different physiological, electrical, and anatomical properties (Cordes & Srivastava, 2009; Buckingham, Meilhac, & Zaffran, 2005; Kirby & Waldo, 1995). Development of the heart's structure begins in the first days of embryonic life with the merging of two epithelial tubes to form the single cardiac tube. Contractions of the heart begin at about 17 days of gestation, although effective blood flow does not occur until the end of the first month. In this early embryonic heart, no intracardiac valves are present; rather, endocardial cushions prevent backflow into the atria with ventricle contraction. At approximately 3½ weeks of embryonic life, a process known as *cardiac looping* takes place. The single cardiac tube folds onto itself, effectively forming the right and left sides of the heart, and subsequently the endocardial cushions turn into the cardiac valves. This looping process is critical to ensure correct anatomical formation of the heart, and disruption of this process during the first few weeks of gestation can result in serious cardiac structural defects. Cardiac formation is also dependent on biomechanical forces, such as pressure, flows, and the resultant shearing forces present in the embryonic heart. Alterations in these forces in early gestation may result in atypical cardiac anatomy. As the embryonic heart continues to grow, coronary circulation is established. Fetal heart sounds can be detected by 8 to 10 weeks of gestation, indicating functioning of the circulatory system. In concert with the structural development, the cardiac conduction system is developing. This early, complex process influences the future emergence of arrhythmias in adulthood. (Jongbloed, Mahtab, Blom, Schalij, & Gittenberger-de Groot, 2008).

Despite the relatively early structural development of the heart, fetal circulation remains markedly different from adult circulation. In fetal circulation, only 12% of blood follows the pathway of adult circulation from the right atrium (RA) to the right ventricle (RV), through pulmonary circulation, to the left atrium (LA) and left ventricle (LV), and finally into the aorta for systemic circulation. Because the fetal blood is oxygenated by the placenta and maternal circulation, passing blood through the fetus's fluid-filled lungs is unnecessary and impractical.

Prenatal anatomical differences in the developing cardiac structure allow for two alternative circulation routes that effectively reduce blood flow through the nonfunctioning fetal pulmonary system. The first alternative route uses the **foramen ovale**, a one-way door in the atrial septum, which allows blood to flow from the RA into the LA (instead of into the pulmonary circulation), then to the LV, and eventually to the systemic circulation via the aorta. The second alternative route uses the **ductus arteriosus**, a vascular link outside the heart between the pulmonary artery and the aorta, allowing blood to exit the pulmonary artery and be delivered directly into the aorta for systemic circulation, effectively bypassing the lungs and the left heart entirely (Fig. 9.2). Within the first few hours of life, pressure changes within the cardiac chambers close the foramen ovale. Within a few weeks of life, the ductus arteriosus closes. There remains only one route for blood to flow through the body, that of adult circulation. (For further information, see the section on "Initiation of Breathing" in this chapter.)

A child continues to experience altered pressures and forces on the developing chest wall and within the cardiac system as musculoskeletal growth occurs. Transient alterations in pressures and flows within the heart and major vessels can occur. Some of these alterations, such as a transient heart murmur, are considered benign if there is no accompanying symptomatology. Other defects, such as a **coarctation of the aorta** (a stricture in the descending aorta), may become more serious and their effects become more pronounced with growth. Medical professionals routinely assess the

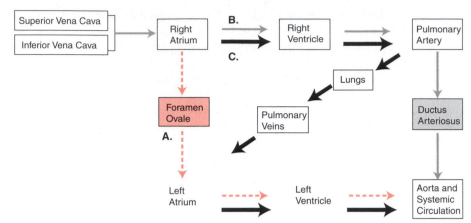

Figure 9.2 Potential routes of blood flow from right atrium to aorta in fetal circulation. (*A*) Right atrium through foramen ovale to left atrium to left ventricle to aorta (dashed arrows). (*B*) Right atrium to right ventricle to pulmonary artery through ductus arteriosus to aorta (thin arrows). (*C*) Right atrium to right ventricle to pulmonary artery to lungs to pulmonary veins to left atrium to left ventricle to aorta (thick arrows).

cardiac system throughout the child's growth, and any abnormalities noted in a child's cardiac exam deserve documentation and follow-up.

Maturation of the Pulmonary System

The pulmonary system begins to develop between 22 and 26 days of gestation with the formation of a lung bud, a node of endodermal tissue from which the trachea, bronchi, conducting airways, and alveoli arise. The mesodermal tissue surrounding the lung bud develops into the lungs' "support structures," such as pleura, smooth muscle, cartilage, collagen, and blood vessels (Kravitz, 1994). Pathophysiological processes (e.g., maternal and fetal infections) early in gestation can cause widespread systemic or multisystemic effects in both the developing pulmonary and cardiac systems. Between 8 and 16 weeks of gestational age, further branching of the conducting airways occurs down to the terminal bronchioles, and the pulmonary arterial system begins to form. By 17 weeks of gestation, the lung has lobes and the conducting airways have completed branching. In addition, the beginning of the alveolar capillary membranes is formed, providing the first possibility, albeit slight, for the survival of a preterm infant. During 17 to 24 weeks of gestation, the terminal bronchioles form buds, and some terminal bronchioles convert to respiratory bronchioles, allowing a potential site for gas exchange. The arterial system continues to grow, and the pulmonary capillary walls that are near to the respiratory bronchioles become thin, narrowing the diffusion distance for improved gas exchange possibilities. During this time, the support tissue becomes

more differentiated, with cartilage forming in the bronchi, collagen in the midsize airways, and elastin in the bronchioles. By the 23rd week, the type 2 alveolar cells that produce surfactant appear, and by 28 weeks of gestation, some surfactant is present, and the potential for some gas exchange is possible. Surfactant is a lipid-rich substance that allows adequate alveolar expansion by limiting surface tension across the alveolar membrane. Between 28 and 32 weeks gestation, the amount of surfactant increases in quantity, ensuring adequate lung inflation at birth. Infants who are born prematurely often experience respiratory complications secondary to the relative immaturity of the pulmonary system and limited surfactant production.

The pulmonary system is not functional until the first postnatal breath. In utero, the pulmonary system has been immersed in an aquatic environment, and aside from a few hiccups now and then, the respiratory system has not had to perform any function. The first postnatal breath is the initial test of the patency of the pulmonary system. During the first few breaths, the infant has to generate large inspiratory pressures to inflate the lungs and force the fluid within the airways and alveolar units into the lymphatic system. For the first few hours after birth, this diffusing process naturally occurs as the infant breathes. Transient newborn tachypnea, or mild respiratory distress, is not uncommon even in the healthiest of infants.

At birth, the full-term infant has a tracheobronchial tree with approximately 17 branches yet has a very limited number, only approximately 150 million, of primitive alveoli. During early childhood (until the age of approximately 4 years), the number of branches of the tracheobronchial tree increases to about 23, and the number of alveoli increases to approximately 300 million, similar to the adult lung. Alveolar size and diameter of the airways continue to increase as the child grows.

Important anatomical differences exist between the pulmonary system of an infant and that of an adult, which can predispose an infant to respiratory compromise (Table 9.1). Infants are born with a larynx that is structurally higher, enabling the infant to breathe better while feeding (sucking). It does, however, make the infant an obligatory nose breather, which may become problematic with nasal congestion or nasal obstruction. The diameter of the infant's airway is narrower from the nares all the way to the terminal bronchioles, making it more susceptible to obstruction (Decesare, Graybill-Tucker, & Gould, 1995). The decreased airway lumen also results in an increased resistance to airflow, increasing the work of breathing. In addition, the smooth muscle within the bronchioles is less developed, providing greater tendency for bronchiolar collapse, until approximately 5 years of age (Doershuk, Fischer, & Matthews, 1975). The alveolar walls of the infants are thicker, and the capillary beds are farther away from the alveolar membrane, impeding respiration by increasing

Table 9.1 Structural Differences in the CVP System of Children Compared With That of Adults

Airway	Higher larynx
	Smaller diameter of airways
	Increased resistance to airflow
	Increased work of breathing
	Less cartilage within the airway walls for support
Alveolar capillary membrane	Fewer alveoli
	Less developed collateral ventilation channels
	Thicker alveolar walls
	Capillary bed at a greater distance from alveolar wall
Bony thorax	Increased compliance of the ribcage
	Horizontal alignment of ribcage
Muscles of ventilation	Muscles perform as stabilizers rather than mobilizers
	Decreased length-tension relationship
	Diaphragm fibers have fewer fatigue-resistant fibers

the diffusion distance. Finally, there is less surface area for respiration because there are fewer alveoli.

The compliance, configuration, and muscle action of the chest wall of an infant also differ from those of older children. The healthy newborn's chest wall is primarily cartilaginous, making it extremely compliant (Gaultier, 1995). The cartilaginous ribs allow the distortion necessary for the infant's thorax to travel through the birth canal. However, this increased ribcage compliance results in decreased thoracic stability. The muscles of the infant's chest wall, not the ribs as in adults, are the primary stabilizers of the thorax to counteract the negative pleural pressure of the diaphragm during inspiration. The ribcage of an infant shows a more horizontal alignment of the ribs, rather than the elliptical shape of an older child. This configuration of the infant's ribcage alters the angle of insertion of the costal fibers of the diaphragm, with the orientation being more horizontal than vertical, decreasing the area of apposition (Gaultier, 1995). There is an increased tendency for the diaphragm muscle fibers to pull the lower ribs inward, thereby decreasing efficiency of ventilation and increasing distortion of the chest wall. The chest wall movement of an infant's thorax contributes very little to tidal breathing (Hershenson, Colin, Wohl, & Stark, 1990).

In addition to these differences in ribcage configuration and diaphragm alignment, muscular action associated with ventilation differs in infants. The diaphragm muscle in infants has different fiber-type composition. The diaphragm is the major muscle of respiration in infants as well as in adults. However, in the healthy newborn, only 20% of the muscle fibers of the diaphragm are fatigue-resistant fibers, compared with 50% in adults. This difference predisposes infants to earlier diaphragmatic fatigue. Accessory muscles of ventilation are at a mechanical disadvantage in the infant, secondary to the previously mentioned alterations in ribcage alignment and compliance. In addition, the infant uses some accessory muscles, such as the intercostal muscles, to stabilize, not mobilize, the chest wall during inspiration. The upper chest and neck accessory muscles are not well stabilized in young infants. Until the infant can elongate the cervical spine and stabilize the upper extremities, head, and spine, it is difficult for the accessory muscles to produce the reverse action needed to assist with ventilation. During times of respiratory distress, young infants without head and neck control may exhibit "head bobbing" as they attempt to use accessory muscles of ventilation. Elongation of the cervical spine during musculoskeletal growth will improve the length-tension relationship of some of the accessory muscles of respiration.

As a child grows and is exposed for longer durations to progressively more upright positions for mobility and activities, muscular and gravitational forces help mold the shape of the thorax and chest wall into a more typical adult configuration. The maturation of thoracic skeletal configuration, in turn, affects muscle mechanics by changing the length and alignment of the muscles. The anterior aspects of ribs begin to rotate downward, forming a more elliptical shape. The ribs begin to separate, creating larger intercostal spaces. Ossification of the thorax adds stability and reduces ribcage compliance. As the child gains head and neck control and purposeful upper extremity use, the muscles of the thorax, head, neck, and upper extremities are able to change roles from stabilizers to mobilizers and can better be used as accessory muscles of respiration. Greater ribcage motion becomes apparent during tidal breathing. The insertion alignment of the fibers of the diaphragm becomes more vertical with the changing shape of the thorax, resulting in a larger area of apposition. The interaction between trunk and abdominal control also increases the area of apposition, thereby increasing the efficiency of the diaphragm. Overall, the muscular and skeletal maturation occur simultaneously, providing a more adultlike thoracic mobility and stability.

Children who do not experience development of upright antigravity head, neck, and trunk control may not develop typical ribcage structure and function. Imbalances in muscle forces and support surfaces can lead to asymmetrical chest wall and ribcage formation and may result in eventual impairment in pulmonary function. Recent empirical evidence suggests that the complex interplay between thoracic and abdominal pressures impact feeding, digestion, and function, putting children with altered ribcage and abdominal musculature at risk for possible secondary gastrointestinal and movement impairments (Massery, 2006).

Postnatal Cardiovascular and Pulmonary Function

Immediately after birth, as the pulmonary system begins to function within the air-filled environment, volume and pressure shifts occur in the CVP systems. Within the first few minutes of ventilation, pulmonary vascular resistance decreases as the alveoli expand. Lower RV heart pressure is required to circulate pulmonary blood flow through the lungs. The umbilical blood flow to the RA stops, lowering the volume and the pressure in the RA. The LA blood volume and

pressure increase because of the increased pulmonary venous return. The LV now has more blood to pump from the LA to the systemic arterial system. All of these physiological changes cause a pressure shift within the cardiac chambers. The pressures within the left side of the heart become higher than the pressures within the right side of the heart; aortic pressure becomes higher than the pulmonary artery pressure. These alterations in atrial pressure cause the foramen ovale to close. Over a period of a few hours to a few weeks, the ductus arteriosus also closes because of physiological changes in the neonatal pulmonary and circulatory systems. Atypical persistence of these alternative fetal circulatory routes, that is, through the ductus arteriosus or foramen ovale, is detrimental to normal CVP function.

Functional Interaction of Cardiovascular and Pulmonary Systems

Thus far, the maturation of the structure and function of the cardiovascular and pulmonary systems have been addressed individually; however, the interaction between the two systems is intimately intertwined, and essentially the two systems function as one. Two examples illustrate the complex interaction between the cardiac and pulmonary systems.

In the first example, the effect of an isolated cardiac structural abnormality is considered. A **ventricular septal defect (VSD)** is an abnormal opening in the wall (septum) that separates the two ventricles of the heart. With a VSD, when the ventricles contract, there is a tendency for some LV blood to flow through the VSD into the RV instead of out to the systemic vascular system. This creates a higher-than-expected blood volume, and increases pressure in the RV of the heart as well as in the pulmonary circulation. The pulmonary capillaries respond to this higher blood flow by "leaking" fluid into the pulmonary interstitial spaces causing pulmonary edema. Lung compliance is reduced, ventilation becomes less efficient, and respiration is impaired. The lungs may respond to this chronic seepage of fluid from its vascular bed by becoming fibrotic over time, resulting in a more permanent pulmonary impairment. All of these secondary pulmonary effects are related directly to the primary structural cardiac defect of a VSD.

A second example of the interrelatedness of the cardiac and pulmonary systems function is found in the condition of **bronchopulmonary dysplasia (BPD)**. BPD refers to a chronic inflammation and destruction of airways, lung parenchyma, and the alveolar capillary membrane, resulting in a chronic obstructive pulmonary defect. Intrathoracic pressures are altered throughout the respiratory cycle in an obstructive pulmonary disease. These changes in intrathoracic pressures will alter cardiac preload and afterload. The destruction of the alveolar capillary membrane will result in an increased pulmonary vascular resistance. Finally, hypoxia in the pulmonary system causes vasoconstriction, increasing the pulmonary vascular resistance. The RV will have to work harder to push blood through the pulmonary vascular system and, over time, will hypertrophy and may eventually fail (Verklan, 1997). All of these secondary cardiac effects are related directly to the primary pulmonary defect of BPD.

Impairments in CVP systems function can significantly contribute to restrictions in activities within other aspects of a child's development. The social and cognitive developments of children rely on their ability to explore and interact with the environment. Impairments of the CVP systems in infants can affect endurance and activity tolerance, limiting environmental exploration. The ability to feed orally can be hampered in infants who have high respiratory rates or require mechanical ventilation. Language development, and therefore socialization, may be delayed in infants who require mechanical ventilation or who cannot adequately control ventilation to allow phonation. CVP impairments can also contribute to slowed physical growth, resulting in less muscle bulk and smaller stature because less oxygen is being delivered to the system and more calories are used to sustain the work of breathing. Therapists serving the needs of children must consider the wide-ranging effects of CVP conditions, particularly during infancy and early childhood, and provide physical therapy intervention for the whole child.

Cardiovascular and Pulmonary Conditions

Pediatric CVP conditions encompass a variety of diseases less often encountered in adults because (1) the defects may be surgically corrected by adulthood and no longer create impairment, (2) children may physically "outgrow" their symptoms, or (3) in unfortunate cases, children die from their disease before reaching adulthood. However, in recent years, with the increase in childhood obesity and sedentary lifestyles, children are exhibiting more "adultlike" CVP conditions. Risk factors for coronary heart disease (CHD) are already identifiable in overweight children with increases in asthma, sleep apnea, hypertension, hypercholestremia, and diabetes (Baker, 2007). Furthermore, overweight or obesity in childhood or adolescence increases the risk of CHD in adulthood.

Many different pathophysiological processes can cause similar patterns of impairments in body structures and functions and restrictions in activities and participation. Therefore, in this section, as is done in the American Physical Therapy Association (APTA)'s *Guide to physical therapist practice* (2001), conditions are grouped according to their resultant primary impairments to ventilation, circulation, and respiration. For the most common conditions, the definition, etiology, and pathophysiology for each diagnosis are described, followed by a brief discussion of diagnosis and management. Important but less common conditions are described in Tables 9.2 to 9.7.

Conditions That Impair Ventilation

Ventilation is dependent on airflow through the airways to the respiratory unit of the lung. Factors that affect ventilation include abnormalities of the airway and lung parenchyma, musculoskeletal abnormalities of the thoracic pump, neuromuscular abnormalities of the ventilatory muscles, conditions of central respiratory control, and integumentary conditions that affect the thorax.

Airway and Parenchymal Conditions

Ventilatory impairments resulting from pathophysiological processes that create airway narrowing cause increased airway secretions, effectively reducing the size of the airway, or cause changes in the pulmonary parenchyma. Asthma, cystic fibrosis (CF), infant respiratory distress syndrome (RDS), bronchopulmonary dysplasia (BPD), congenital pulmonary structural abnormalities, and immunological conditions are covered in this section.

Asthma

Asthma is an obstructive pulmonary disease characterized by episodic periods of reversible airway narrowing caused by airway inflammation, increased secretions, and smooth muscle bronchoconstriction. Even during periods of remission, some degree of airway inflammation is present. Asthma is the most common chronic childhood disease, affecting 5 million American children. The number of asthma cases increased by more than 160% in children under the age of 5 years, and by 74% in children 5 through 14 years of age, between 1980 and 1994 (Mannino et al., 1998). Asthma accounts for an estimated 11.8 million missed school days in the United States and is the third leading cause of preventable hospitalizations in the United States (Lara et al., 2002). Childhood asthma has an impact in later life, as

20% of children with asthma at 7 years of age had persistent asthma at 42 years of age (Henderson, 2008).

Exercise-induced bronchospasm (EIB), a subset of reversible airways disease, is classically defined by symptoms of shortness of breath, wheezing, cough, or tightness of the chest that occur 8 to 10 minutes into an exercise program with an exercise intensity of 70% to 85% of VO_{2max}. However, symptoms of airway narrowing that occur anytime during or immediately after exercise, and that resolve spontaneously within 20 to 30 minutes, are considered indicative of EIB. A 15% decrease from baseline pulmonary function testing (peak flow or forced expiratory volume in 1 second [FEV_1]) after exercise can confirm the diagnosis. Although some children have EIB without a diagnosis of asthma, many children who have mild asthma will demonstrate that exercise is one of their triggers for bronchospasm. Interestingly, EIB demonstrates refractory behavior in approximately 50% of individuals, meaning that a repeated bout of exercise within 2 hours of the initial episode will not exacerbate EIB (Bar-Or & Rowland, 2004). Exercise prescription in children with refractory EIB should take this into account as it could improve exercise performance in this group of children.

Etiology The exact etiology of asthma is unknown, although genetics, environment (air quality; indoor and outdoor air pollution; environmental allergens; cold, dry air), and infection have been implicated as possible causes. Asthma in school-age children is associated with immune system function, psychosocial factors, and frequency of respiratory infections in the first year of life (Klinnert et al., 2001). Recently it has been determined that the immune response at birth is a major determinant of responses to viral respiratory infections in the first year of life, implicating a potentially larger role of the immune system in asthma than previously appreciated (Henderson, 2008). For EIB, the most likely etiology is a response to the cooling and drying of the airway that occurs during exercise.

Pathophysiology Exacerbations of asthma occur in response to a trigger, whether an environmental irritant, a virus, cigarette smoke, or another factor. Physiologically, the bronchial mucosa becomes inflamed, decreasing the size of the airway lumen. The bronchial smooth muscle contracts, further decreasing the diameter of the airways. Mucus plugging narrows the airway even further. The result of these changes is an impaired ability to ventilate or move air through the airway.

During inspiration, the respiratory muscles pull open the chest wall, the attached pleurae, the lung parenchyma, and the airways. Therefore, during inspiration, the airways are as wide as they will be during the respiratory cycle, and inspiratory airflow may not be impaired. However, the lumen of the airways decreases in size throughout exhalation. Given the combined effects of bronchoconstriction, inflammation, and increased airway secretions, the airway lumen abnormally narrows during the exhalation phase of an asthma exacerbation. Clinically, the child with an exacerbation of asthma will present with a prolonged exhalation time. Wheezing at the end of exhalation may be present in a mild exacerbation. As the severity of exacerbation increases, wheezing occurs for a greater portion of the expiratory cycle. In severe airway constriction, the wheezing may occur during both inhalation and exhalation.

Diagnosis The diagnosis of asthma is clinically based on a history of episodic wheezing, shortness of breath, tightness in the chest, and/or coughing in the absence of any other obvious cause. Symptoms often worsen in the presence of aeroallergens, irritants, or exercise. Symptoms typically occur or worsen at night and/or upon awakening. There may be a family history of asthma, allergy, sinusitis or rhinitis, or allergic skin problems. Physical findings during an exacerbation include cough, hyperexpansion of the thorax, and wheezing during quiet or forced exhalation. Increased nasal secretions (e.g., sinusitis, rhinitis) and/or allergic skin problems (e.g., atopic dermatitis, eczema) may also be present. For older children who are able to participate in pulmonary function testing (PFT), an obstructive pattern will be demonstrated during periods of exacerbation. The FEV_1 will be less than 80% of the predicted value. With the use of a rescue drug (inhaled beta$_2$-agonist), an improvement in FEV_1 of at least 15% should be demonstrated.

Management Pharmacological management of airway inflammation is the most effective long-term management strategy for the control of the symptoms of asthma. Inhalation using metered-dose inhalers, dry powder inhalers, or nebulizers are the preferred methods of delivery for most asthma medications (Treatment Guidelines, 2008). Inhaled anti-inflammatory drugs, particularly corticosteroids, are the most effective long-term treatment and most commonly used drugs to achieve control of airway inflammation. In addition to corticosteroids, long-term management of moderate to severe asthma may include long-acting beta$_2$-agonists to improve control of leukotriene modifiers. These drugs need to be administered on a regular basis, regardless of the child's symptoms, for continued long-term pharmacological management. EIB without asthma does not demonstrate chronic inflammation of the airway; however, leukotriene modifiers are beneficial and approved by the Food and Drug Administration (FDA) for the control of EIB. Therefore, anti-inflammatory drugs are not used as maintenance drugs.

A "rescue" drug, usually a beta$_2$-adrenergic inhaled bronchodilator, may be added to the pharmacological management of reactive airway disease for the quick relief, generally within 3–5 minutes, of breakthrough symptoms such as cough, chest tightness, wheezing, or shortness of breath. These rescue drugs are used on an "as needed" basis. Anticholinergics, while used to treat chronic obstructive pulmonary disease, have not been approved for use by the FDA for the treatment of asthma. For children over the age of 12 years with moderate to severe asthma and specific allergens, the use of an anti-IgE antibody (e.g., Xolair) by subcutaneous injection every 2–4 weeks has been shown to be effective (Treatment Guidelines, 2008).

Physical therapy intervention includes secretion removal techniques and breathing exercises. In addition, individuals who have difficulty coordinating the movements and timing necessary for inhaling medications may benefit from physical therapy intervention to improve their techniques. Breathing exercises with emphasis on exhalation have been used to improve ventilatory patterns of those with an exacerbation of their symptoms. More scientific evidence is needed to support the use of varied breathing exercises for asthma treatment (Holloway & Ram, 2002). Aerobic conditioning should be encouraged in those with reactive airways disease. Special consideration should be given to (1) appropriate premedication with a short-acting beta$_2$-agonist before exercise, as needed, (2) temperature, humidity, and air quality of the exercise environment, and (3) a longer warm-up period that may decrease breakthrough symptoms. Aerobic exercise has been shown to be beneficial in children with asthma and EIB (Bar-Or & Rowland, 2004; Nixon, 1996).

Cystic Fibrosis

Cystic fibrosis (CF) affects the excretory glands of the body. Secretions made by these glands are thicker and more viscous and can obstruct various systems of the body: pulmonary, digestive, hepatic, and male reproductive. The enzymes of the gastrointestinal (GI) tract are often inadequate, causing malnutrition and a picture of "failure to thrive" in the face of adequate caloric intake. The pancreas can be affected, resulting in diabetes. Impairment of the pulmonary system is the most common cause of morbidity and mortality in children with CF. Thickened pulmonary secretions narrow or obstruct airways, leading to hyperinflation, infection, and tissue destruction.

Etiology   CF is an autosomal recessive, genetically inherited disease. Two gene-carrying parents statistically have a 25% chance of having a child with CF, a 50% chance of having a child who is a carrier of the disease, and a 25% chance of having a child who is genetically free of the disease. Both parents must be carriers of the defective gene to produce a child with the disease. The incidence of CF in the white population is 1:2,500 live births. There is a much lower incidence of CF in African American and Asian populations.

Pathophysiology   The prevailing defect in CF is within the chloride ion channels of the body. The chloride channels on the epithelial cells either are absent or fail to open appropriately (Aitken, 1996). There is increased sodium absorption of this membrane, causing a fluid imbalance within the tissues of the body. There is evidence that the altered epithelium in the airways also has a decreased ability to defend itself against bacterial pathogens, making it more susceptible to infection (Smith, Travis, Greenberg, & Welsh, 1996). Thickened and infected pulmonary secretions cause obstructive changes in the airways, hyperinflation of the lung parenchyma, and destruction of alveoli.

Diagnosis   The diagnosis of CF can be made by analyzing the amount of chloride found in the sweat of the child. A positive test for CF is a sweat chloride content over 60 mEq/L. The diagnosis of CF can also be made through genetic testing. Genetic testing is considered positive if mutations in the cystic fibrosis transmembrane conductance regulator (CFTR) gene are noted.

Often a diagnostic workup for CF will begin when a child presents with repeat pulmonary infections, especially if the causative agent is either *Staphylococcus aureus* or *Pseudomonas aeruginosa*. A newborn with meconium ileus, a small bowel obstruction indicating impairment of the digestive system, should also raise suspicions for the diagnosis of CF. The diagnosis of CF may also be considered in children with GI impairment and failure to thrive. If one child in a family is diagnosed with CF, all siblings should be tested for the disease.

Management   Improvements in the management of CF have resulted in a life expectancy of 32.5 years. The management of CF crosses many disciplines, including the physician, nutritionist, nurse, physical therapist, respiratory therapist, and social worker. Recent advances in gene-related therapy are offering better targeted treatment at the cellular level.

The primary goal of pulmonary care in children with CF is to prevent, or at least delay, any decline in lung function. Reducing bacterial load, improving secretion clearance, and treating airway inflammation are the mainstays of pulmonary care. Potent antibiotics, often using two or three different drugs to ensure success, may be necessary to treat the gram-negative pulmonary infections that commonly cause an exacerbation of CF. Resistance to antibiotics in the long term versus freedom from infections in the short term is a constant source of controversy concerning antibiotic coverage. Prophylactic anti-staphylococcal antibiotics have been shown to decrease the presence of *S. aureus* in young children, a positive finding, but more evidence is needed to confirm this finding in older children (Smyth & Walters, 2003). The use of aerosolized antibiotics has been successful in decreasing the number of acute exacerbations and improving lung function in children with CF, but there is an increase in resistant organisms to the antibiotics over time, limiting its widespread use (Mukhopadhyay et al., 1995). Aerosolized recombinant DNA (DNase, Pulmozyme) may be helpful in decreasing the viscoelastic properties of airway secretions, making them easier to clear from the tracheobronchial tree (Shah, Scott, Knight, & Hodson, 1996).

While evidence suggests that airway clearance techniques are efficacious before or after administration of dornase alfa, a longer duration of several hours before treatment appears to be of greater benefit than immediately following administration (Wilson, Robbins, Murphy, & Chang, 2007). Individuals colonized with *P. aeruginosa* may have more benefit if dornase alfa follows airway clearance techniques (Fitzgerald, Hilton, Jepson, & Smith, 2005). Aerosolized saline has also been used to enhance clearance of secretions (Eng et al., 1996). Direct treatment of airway inflammation with corticosteroids and ibuprofen has been studied. Although the use of prednisone, a corticosteroid, was shown to be beneficial by the measurement of FEV_1, there were significant growth retardation side effects in the children studied, limiting its incorporation into CF protocols (Nikolaizik & Schonl, 1996; Van Essen-Zandvliet et al., 1992). Inhaled steroids may have fewer systemic side effects and still help in controlling airway inflammation. Surprisingly, little scientific evidence supports the use of inhaled bronchodilators in individuals with CF, and additional research is needed to clarify the clinical role of bronchodilators. Individuals with significant pulmonary involvement may be candidates for lung or heart-lung transplants.

The pulmonary management of CF is critical, but the GI component must also be managed. Malabsorption of nutrients caused by pancreatic insufficiency can lead to malnutrition. Fifteen percent of adults with CF are insulin-dependent diabetics, and 75% have glucose intolerance. Individuals with CF-related diabetes have more severe pulmonary diseases, more frequent pulmonary exacerbations, poorer nutrition, and greater incidence of liver disease (Marshal et al., 2005). Poor nutrition has a negative impact on the pulmonary course of the disease (Borowitz, 1996). In fact, malnutrition has been shown to be an independent predictor of mortality (Corey & Farewell, 1996). Nutritional support, including a high-calorie diet and pancreatic enzyme replacement therapy, is often needed to maximize GI function. Recent reports also indicate that up to two-thirds of females with CF experience urinary incontinence to some degree, which is related to the increased intra-abdominal pressures generated for airway clearance through coughing (Nixon, Glazner, Martin, & Sawyer, 2002).

Physical therapy intervention for children with CF includes the performance and teaching of secretion removal techniques; an aerobic exercise program as an adjunct to secretion removal and for overall health and fitness; and education concerning medications, environmental controls, compliance with medical care, and benefits of aerobic conditioning. Recent evidence has highlighted the impact of various pharmacological and medical interventions on the quality of life of individuals with CF (Abbott & Gee, 2003; Goss & Quittner, 2007; Quittner, Modi, & Cruz, 2008). Given the complex and often burdensome nature of care of the individual with CF, the use of general and CF-specific outcome measures of quality of life should be incorporated within PT management. An example of a case study for a child with CF can be found in Chapter 20.

Infant Respiratory Distress Syndrome

Infant respiratory distress syndrome (RDS) is a restrictive pulmonary disease that results from inadequate levels of pulmonary surfactant and lung immaturity.

Etiology Type 2 alveolar cells begin to produce surfactant at about 20 weeks of gestation. Increasing amounts of surfactant are produced each week as gestational age progresses. Surfactant reaches adequate levels 2 weeks before birth. Therefore, the incidence of RDS is related to gestational age and birth weight. In the United States, RDS has been estimated to occur in 20,000–30,000 newborn infants each year and is a complication in about 1% of pregnancies. Approximately 50% of the neonates born at 26–28 weeks' gestation develop RDS, whereas fewer than 30% of premature neonates born at 30–31 weeks' gestation develop RDS. In one report, the incidence rate of respiratory distress syndrome was 42% in infants weighing 501–1500 g, with 71% reported in infants weighing 501–750 g, 54% reported in infants weighing 751–1,000 g, 36% reported in infants weighing 1,001–1,250 g, and 22% reported in infants weighing 1,251–1,500 g among the 12 university hospitals participating in the National Institute of Child Health and Human Development (NICHD) Neonatal Research Network (Hintz et al., 2007). Race, gender, and maternal health, especially maternal diabetes, are also contributing factors in the development of RDS.

Pathophysiology RDS is associated with inadequate amounts of surfactant in the lungs of a premature infant. Without adequate amounts of surfactant, there is a decrease in lung compliance, an increase in the work of breathing, collapse of airways and respiratory units, and mismatching of ventilation and perfusion. In premature infants, the alveolar wall is thicker and the pulmonary capillary is farther from the alveoli, making diffusion of gas all the more difficult. The resultant hypoxemia and hypoxia may lead to pulmonary vascular constriction and pulmonary hypertension.

Diagnosis Respiratory distress caused by alveolar collapse in a premature infant is the presenting sign of RDS. Typical signs of RDS include tachypnea, nasal flaring, intercostal and substernal retractions, and cyanosis within 4 hours of birth. Chest radiographs show a typical "ground glass" pattern, which indicates interstitial involvement.

Management Infants with RDS are provided with supplemental oxygen to avoid hypoxemia. Intubation and mechanical ventilation are necessary if oxygen therapy alone is not sufficient. Surfactant replacement therapy has been used to prevent and treat infants with RDS. Although surfactant replacement has had a significant positive impact on survival and quality of life for premature infants, chronic lung disease continues to develop in a significant number of premature infants (McColley, 1998). In recent years, a reduction in the morbidity and mortality of extremely premature infants with RDS has been noted and is related to improved management, including (1) the use of antenatal steroids to enhance pulmonary maturity, (2) appropriate resuscitation facilitated by placental transfusion and immediate use of continuous positive airway pressure (CPAP) for alveolar recruitment, (3) early administration of surfactant, (4) the use of gentler modes of ventilation, including early use of "bubble" nasal CPAP to minimize damage to the immature lungs, and (5) supportive therapies, such as diagnosis and management of patent ductus arteriosus (PDA), fluid and electrolyte management, trophic feeding and nutrition, and use of prophylactic fluconazole (Pramanik, 2010). Often these infants are placed on "stress precautions" to reduce environmental stimulation, including visual, auditory, and tactile stimulation, and perhaps even to mimic the in utero environment. Necessary procedures are often clustered to minimize the number of disturbances for the infant. Close coordination between nursing staff and other medical team members is helpful in reducing such stress. Physical therapy intervention includes direct care and consultation with nursing to provide positioning suggestions to optimize ventilation and pulmonary perfusion matching, enhance motor development, and improve secretion removal techniques if appropriate.

Bronchopulmonary Dysplasia

Bronchopulmonary dysplasia (BPD) is an obstructive pulmonary disease that is usually considered a sequela of RDS (Northway, Rosan, & Porter, 1967). The clinical definitions of BPD include (1) the need for ventilatory assistance for at least 3 days and the need for supplemental oxygen at 28 days of life (Bancalari, Abdenour, Feller, & Gannon, 1979), (2) the need for supplemental oxygen at 36 weeks gestational age (Bernstein, Heimler, & Sasidhara, 1998), and (3) radiographic abnormalities and chronic ventilation beyond the initial period of RDS (Korhonen, Tammela, Koivisto, Laippala, & Ikonen, 1999).

Etiology The exact etiology is not precisely understood, but it is related to exposure of immature lung tissue to high concentrations of oxygen, positive pressure mechanical ventilation, inadequate surfactant production, and infection. Preeclampsia, low birth weight, rapid birth weight recovery, packed red cell infusions, the presence of a patent ductus arteriosus, hyperoxia, and long duration of ventilator therapy have been correlated with an increased risk of developing BPD (Korhonen et al., 1999).

Pathophysiology BPD is characterized by inflammation (Hulsmann & van den Anker, 1997). Acutely, this results in persistent hyaline membranes, necrosis of the airway, and alveolar epithelium and inflammation. In the subacute phase, there is hypertrophy of bronchial smooth muscle and parenchymal fibrosis. In the chronic phase, airway remodeling occurs (Hulsmann & van den Anker, 1997). Infants with BPD may have chronic hypoxemia, often further exacerbated during feeding, crying, and activity. These children are more likely to have feeding disorders, with a resultant poor growth pattern, and are more likely to require rehospitalization within 2 years of discharge from the hospital compared with preterm infants without BPD. When they reach school age, children who had BPD as infants are more likely to have airway obstruction and airway reactivity than their counterparts without BPD (Gross, Iannuzzi, Kveselis, & Anbar, 1998). However, exercise capacity in long-term survivors of BPD did not differ from matched premature infants without BPD, although the children with BPD did use a greater percentage of their ventilatory reserve (Jacob et al., 1997). Children and adolescents with a history of BPD often exhibit decreased forced vital capacity, hyperinflation (high ratio of residual volume to total lung capacity), and airway hyperreactivity at rest. They may also show EIB, higher ventilatory costs and oxygen uptake at a given work rate, and arterial oxygen desaturation (Bar-Or & Rowland, 2004) during exercise.

Diagnosis The diagnosis is based on the infant's clinical course and radiographic evidence.

Management The medical management of BPD consists of surfactant replacement therapy, nutritional support, oxygen and ventilation support, diuretics, steroids, bronchodilators, and/or antibiotics. Physical therapy intervention may include positioning to optimize CVP function, secretion removal techniques, and provision of sensorimotor experiences to promote developmentally appropriate activities.

Congenital Structural Abnormalities

Congenital structural abnormalities of the pulmonary and associated systems are relatively uncommon, yet when they occur, they can cause significant respiratory compromise. Congenital thoracic malformations, including pulmonary sequestration, pulmonary agenesis or hypoplasia, diaphragmatic hernias, and tracheoesophageal fistulas, often have significant effects on pulmonary function. Detection of such malformations in the fetus provides opportunities for early decisions regarding surgical or conservative management, as well as family counseling. Most lesions require no antenatal intervention and shrink substantially in the third trimester. Symptomatic newborns generally require some form of surgical intervention, but evidence for either conservative or surgical management of newborns without symptoms remains controversial (Bush, 2009). See Table 9.2 for details of congenital structural abnormalities.

Table 9.2 Congenital Structural Abnormalities

Diagnosis	Definition	Etiology	Alterations in Body Functions and Structures	Potential Activity Limitations and Participation Restrictions	Potential Management
Pulmonary sequestration, pulmonary agenesis or hypoplasia	Pulmonary sequestration refers to a portion of the lung that is ventilated but not perfused. Pulmonary agenesis or hypoplasia refers to lack of or decreased development of pulmonary tissue.	Unknown etiology	• Altered structure and function of respiratory system (s430/b440)* • Recurrent infection in abnormal lung tissue • Poor growth • Poor feeding	• Decreased walking long distances (d4501) • Decreased activity tolerance—for example, running (d4552) • Delay of developmental milestones • Decreased ability to maintain sustained active play (d9200) with peers or family • Decreased participation in organized sports (d9201) and active recreation activities (d920)	• Majority require surgery to either remove abnormal tissue or repair defect in infancy. • Physical therapy may include preoperative and postoperative pulmonary care, breathing exercises, positioning for improved ventilation to the affected areas, early intervention to achieve developmental milestones, and parental instruction.

Table 9.2 Congenital Structural Abnormalities—cont'd

Diagnosis	Definition	Etiology	Alterations in Body Functions and Structures	Potential Activity Limitations and Participation Restrictions	Potential Management
Congenital diaphragmatic hernia (CDH)	Incomplete formation and closure of the diaphragm, resulting in herniation of abdominal contents into thorax	Unknown etiology Alteration in development between weeks 6–10 of gestation	• Altered structure and function of respiratory system (s430/b440) • Decreased pulmonary formation because thoracic space is occupied by abdominal contents • Poor growth • Poor feeding	• Delay of developmental milestones • Decreased ability to maintain sustained active play (d9200) with peers or family	• Surgical repair as fetus or neonate
Tracheoesophageal fistula (TEF)	Incomplete separation of the trachea and esophagus	Unknown etiology Alteration in development before 12 weeks gestation	• Altered structure and function of respiratory system (s430/b440) due to ventilatory impairments related to aspiration, airway narrowing, and secretions • Altered structure and function of digestive system—ingestion functions (b510) due to impairments in esophageal motility and impaired tracheal patency due to tracheomalacia or strictures • Difficulty feeding • Poor growth	• Delay of developmental milestones • Decreased ability to maintain sustained active play (d9200) with peers or family • Position restrictions (head elevated) to improve esophageal emptying and reduce risk of aspiration	• Surgical repair • Positioning to prevent aspiration and to improve gastric absorption • Physical therapy for bronchial hygiene and developmental intervention

*Numbers in parentheses refer to ICF-CY classification.

Immunological Conditions

Pediatric immunological conditions include (1) allergies, such as asthma, (2) autoimmune diseases, such as juvenile idiopathic arthritis (JIA) and systemic lupus erythematosus (SLE), and (3) immunodeficiency conditions, such as HIV/AIDS, and post-transplant immunosuppression. A discussion of asthma is given earlier in this chapter. JIA is a connective tissue condition more common in the peripheral extremities (ankles, knees, wrists, and elbows), but the shoulder, spine, and thoracic mobility may be affected, which in turn will affect the pulmonary system. SLE is an autoimmune disease that results in inflammation of joints, skin, kidneys, and the pleura, causing pain, poor breathing patterns, and atelectasis. Children with immunocompromise are often prone to opportunistic pulmonary infections, especially *Pneumocystis carinii* pneumonia.

Pathophysiology of Opportunistic Pulmonary Infections
The smaller airway diameter can predispose children to more significant ventilatory impairments during the pulmonary infectious process. Over the short term, acute pulmonary infections can result in increased airway secretions, hypoxemia, and airway inflammation. Chronic infection over the long term can result in destruction of the parenchyma or airway. Infectious and immune conditions can also cause interstitial lung disease, which is covered later in the section on respiration impairments.

Diagnosis of Opportunistic Pulmonary Infections
Signs and symptoms of respiratory distress (e.g., tachypnea, retractions) in combination with clinical signs of respiratory infections and immunocompromise are commonly used for diagnosis. The specific infectious agent can generally be isolated from sputum cultures or throat swabs. Tissue cultures from an open lung biopsy or washings from a bronchoalveolar lavage may need to be obtained to detect the causative agent.

Management
Antimicrobial or antiviral agents, in combination with supportive care as needed (e.g., oxygen, bronchodilators, mechanical ventilation), are the usual courses of treatment during acute infections. Physical therapy interventions may include provision of airway clearance techniques, frequent monitoring of the child's respiratory status, and instructing children in effective coughing and deep breathing exercises as appropriate for their age. Child and parent education concerning bronchial hygiene programs, environmental controls, and signs and symptoms of infection is important. Any reduction in activity tolerance or delays in development should warrant a physical therapy evaluation.

Musculoskeletal System Impairments

Optimal ventilation relies on a balance between the forces that act on the chest wall and abdomen— the compliance of the musculoskeletal thorax, the strength of the muscles of ventilation, and the compliance of the underlying lung tissue. Arthritis and arthrogryposis of the shoulders or spine can decrease joint ROM and restrict ribcage movement. Primary skeletal processes, such as achondroplasia or osteogenesis imperfecta, that alter the skeletal formation can affect muscle alignment, making the muscles less efficient at generating the necessary forces for ventilation. Children who have undergone surgical repair of congenital cardiac defects via a median sternotomy are at a much higher risk of developing scoliosis and/or kyphosis than their peers (Herrera-Soto, Vander Have, Barry-Lane, & Myers, 2007). The brief description given here illustrates how musculoskeletal abnormalities can impact CVP function.

Thoracic scoliosis, a lateral curvature of the thoracic spine, can alter ribcage movement, resulting in a ventilatory impairment. Thoracic scoliosis results in the rotation of the vertebral bodies. On the side of the concavity, there is decreased costovertebral motion and a decreased intercostal space. On the side of the convexity, the vertebral body rotation causes the ribs to move posteriorly, resulting in the classic posterior rib hump, decreased costovertebral motion, and widening of the intercostal spaces. Thoracic scoliosis, if severe enough, can restrict ventilation and decrease the efficiency of the ventilatory muscles. The lung tissue under a severe concavity is chronically underventilated and may become a source of infection. Changes in skeletal configuration may alter the force-length relationship of the attached muscles, often reducing their effectiveness of force generation.

Interestingly, sternal abnormalities, such as pectus excavatum or pectus carinatum, typically have minimal direct effects on ventilation (Fig. 9.3). CVP physical therapy intervention for these conditions may include thoracic mobility and breathing exercises, positioning to improve ventilation, preoperative and postoperative care, and secretion removal techniques as indicated. More in-depth discussions of musculoskeletal conditions can be found in Chapters 5 and 6.

Neuromuscular System Conditions

Ventilation requires a coordinated interplay between passive forces and active forces generated by muscle contractions. Alterations in the ability to generate the force of muscle contraction, from neuromuscular

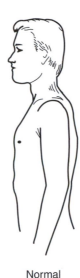
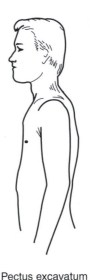
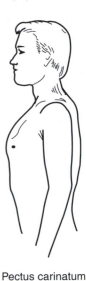

Normal   Pectus excavatum   Pectus carinatum

Figure 9.3 Structural abnormalities of the thoracic cage: Pectus excavatum and pectus carinatum. *(Adapted from Swartz, M.H. [1994]. Textbook of physical diagnoses: History and examination [2nd ed.]. Philadelphia: W.B. Saunders.)*

diseases such as muscular dystrophy, spinal cord injuries, or myelomeningocele, will affect the ability to ventilate. In addition to decreased ventilatory forces, atypical patterns of muscle strength caused by neuromuscular weaknesses can lead to alterations in ribcage and skeletal growth. Pathophysiological processes that result in decreased muscle coordination, such as cerebral palsy (CP) or upper motor neuron lesions, can affect not only extremity and trunk coordination but also respiratory coordination and coughing abilities. A child who has difficulty controlling respiratory muscle force generation and coordinating the timing of ventilatory muscle force may present with impaired ventilation, speech, and feeding. Localized and generalized muscle weakness can decrease ventilation in specific lobes or throughout the thorax, depending on the location and degree of weakness. Typically, infants with neuromuscular conditions have healthy pulmonary parenchyma. However, infectious processes, repeated aspiration in individuals with swallowing impairment, and atelectasis from hypoventilation can cause progressive ventilatory impairments. As the child with neuromuscular conditions grows and the disease progresses, movement may become less efficient, the child becomes less physically active, and decreased exercise and activity tolerance results.

The management of neuromuscular system impairments is discussed in greater depth in Chapters 7 and 8. CVP physical therapy intervention for these conditions may include thoracic mobility and breathing exercises, strengthening of the ventilatory muscles, adaptive seating that optimizes body and thoracic positioning to improve ventilation, providing and teaching assisted coughing techniques, and secretion removal techniques as indicated.

Conditions of Central Respiratory Control   Ventilation requires neural output from brainstem respiratory centers in response to increases in arterial carbon dioxide and decreases in arterial oxygenation. Congenital central hypoventilation syndrome (CCHS), and Arnold-Chiari malformation type II are the most commonly encountered conditions of central respiratory control (Pilmer, 1994). Table 9.3 provides details of conditions of central respiratory control.

Integumentary System Conditions   There are relatively few integumentary system impairments that result in significant CVP impairment in children. Worthy of brief mention is the effect of burns on the CVP systems. Acute complications from burns include infection, dehydration, a decreased ability to thermoregulate the body, decreased aerobic capacity, and issues related to smoke inhalation. Medical management, including skin grafting, skin substitutes, and cultured skin, may be used to close or cover the wounds to improve hydration and thermoregulation and prevent infection (see Chapter 10). Positioning to improve ventilation-perfusion and splinting to maintain joint mobility are appropriate. Ventilatory support, with the objective of keeping both airway pressure and oxygen support as low as possible, may be critical to the pulmonary parenchymal outcomes. Aerobic conditioning should begin as soon as the child is able to tolerate activity.

Long-term ventilatory impairments from thoracoabdominal burns may occur secondary to contraction of scar tissue or restrictions caused by the scar tissue during normal physical growth and development. Physical therapy

Table 9.3 Conditions of Central Respiratory Control

Diagnosis	Definition	Etiology	Alterations in Body Functions and Structures	Potential Activity Limitations and Participation Restrictions	Potential Management
Congenital central hypoventilation syndrome (CCHS) or "Ondine's curse"	Failure of autonomic control of respiration resulting in decreased output from the brainstem respiratory centers	Unknown, may have a genetic basis	• Altered function of respiratory system (b440)* due to probable defect in CO_2 and O_2 chemoreceptors	• Decreased participation in organized sports (d9201) and active recreation activities (d920) • Decreased ability to maintain sustained active play (d9200) with peers or family • Fatigue • Limitations in activity and environmental exploration	• Diaphragmatic pacing • Mechanical ventilation • Physical therapy to promote bronchial hygiene, developmental interventions, or exercise programs for those requiring 24-hour mechanical ventilation; parental instruction
Arnold-Chiari malformations (type 2)	Cerebellar tonsils descending through the foramen magnum causing brainstem and spinal cord compression	Often associated with myelomeningocele	• Altered structure and function of respiratory system (s430/b440) • Apnea, bradycardia, hypoventilation, cyanosis, and breath-holding spells • Altered structure and function of digestive system—ingestion functions (b510) due to swallowing or feeding difficulties	• Delay of developmental milestones • Decreased ability to maintain sustained active play (d9200) with peers or family	• Surgical decompression of malformation • Mechanical ventilation • Physical therapy may include monitoring respiratory status, and pulmonary hygiene

*Numbers in parentheses refer to ICF-CY classification.

intervention includes burn care and scar management, as well as thoracic mobility and breathing exercises.

Children with restrictive skin conditions such as juvenile scleroderma can have similar restrictions of their chest wall growth and mobility that may eventually result in ventilatory impairments.

Conditions That Impair Circulation

Circulation is dependent on blood flow, blood volume, vascular resistance, pressure gradients, and the force of muscle contraction of the heart. Circulatory defects in children are most often related to congenital cardiovascular structural defects. Congenital heart defects are the most common major birth defects, occurring in approximately 12–14:1,000 live births (Hoffman & Kaplan, 2002). Despite advances in detection and treatment, congenital heart disease accounts for 3% of all infant deaths and 46% of death from congenital malformations (Hoffman & Kaplan, 2002). The other significant conditions associated with circulatory impairment in children are pediatric myocardial disease, Kawasaki disease, and arrhythmias. Hypertensive conditions and dyslipidemias are becoming more common in children and adolescents. Related CVP impairments and principles of management, focusing on nutrition, physical activity, and pharmacological interventions, are similar to those for adults and are not addressed in this chapter.

Cardiovascular Structural Defects

Congenital cardiac defects are structural anomalies that either allow for an alternative route of blood through the CVP systems or obstruct the usual route of blood flow. The new routes for blood flow are called shunts. A shunt is termed either a right-to-left shunt or a left-to-right shunt, depending on which way blood is rerouted through the congenital cardiac structural defect. The direction of blood flow through the cardiac structural defect is dictated by the pressure gradient on either side of the defect. A cardiac defect is categorized as a left-to-right shunt when oxygenated blood (left heart blood) does not go out to the periphery but, rather, is returned to the lungs. A right-to-left shunt occurs when unoxygenated blood (right heart blood) bypasses the lungs and is sent directly out to the systemic circulation.

In this section congenital cardiac defects will be discussed based on three categories: left-to-right shunts, right-to-left shunts, and obstructions to the usual route of blood flow. A combination of several heart defects creates a more complex problem that can fall into more than one of these functional categories. Complex combinations of heart defects include hypoplastic left heart syndrome (HLHS), truncus arteriosus, and total anomalous pulmonary venous return (TAPVR).

Etiology The exact etiology of congenital cardiac defects is unknown. Genetic, environmental, and infectious factors play various roles in the disruption of the normal cardiac embryological formation. More severe defects are caused by disruption early in the cardiac formation process, whereas less severe defects generally occur later in gestation. Ten gene mutations have been identified that can cause isolated (not accompanied by other birth defects) heart defects (Pierpont et al., 2007).

Environmental factors can contribute to congenital heart defects. Women who contract rubella (German measles) during the first 3 months of pregnancy have a high risk of having a baby with a heart defect. Other viral infections, such as the flu, also may contribute, as may exposure to certain industrial chemicals (solvents). Some studies suggest that drinking alcohol or using cocaine in pregnancy may increase the risk of heart defects (American Heart Association Council on Cardiovascular Disease in the Young, 2007). Certain medications and chronic illnesses (e.g., poorly controlled diabetes) can also increase the risk. Congenital heart defects can be associated with syndromes resulting from chromosomal abnormalities (e.g., Down syndrome, Turner syndrome) as well as with a variety of inherited conditions (e.g., Noonan syndrome, Holt-Oram syndrome) (Pierpoint et al., 2007).

Pathophysiology of Left-to-Right Shunts Cardiac defects that cause too much blood to pass through the lungs create left-to-right shunts and are referred to as acyanotic defects. Such defects include patent ductus arteriosus (PDA), atrial septal defect (ASD), ventricular septal defect (VSD), and atrioventricular canal (AV canal or AVC). These defects allow oxygen-rich (red) blood that should be traveling to the body to recirculate through the lungs, causing increased pressure and stress in the lungs.

Ventricular septal defect (VSD) is the term used to describe an opening in the ventricular septum. VSDs are the most common form of congenital heart defects, accounting for 20% of congenital cardiac defects, and occurring in approximately 2.8:1,000 live births. A new route for blood to flow, from ventricle to ventricle, is now possible through the opening in the intraventricular septum (Fig. 9.4). Given that the pressures in the LVs are normally greater than the pressures in the RVs, blood flow through a VSD will be from the LV to the RV. This new route of blood will allow already oxygenated blood from the LV to flow back to the RV, back into the pulmonary arteries, and back into the lungs, bypassing the systemic circulation. The amount of blood shunted through a VSD is usually correlated to the severity of symptoms present in the child.

An **atrial septal defect (ASD)** is an opening in the atrial septum, the wall that separates the RA and LA. This defect also results in a left-to-right shunt attributable to the slightly higher pressure within the LA than the RA. The new route for this LA oxygenated blood will be as follows: LA to RA, to the RV, to the pulmonary artery, and back to the lungs. Typically, ASDs are less symptomatic than VSDs of similar size.

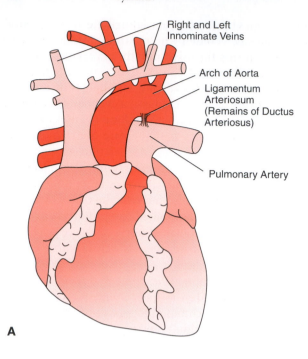

Right and Left
Innominate Veins

Arch of Aorta

Ligamentum
Arteriosum
(Remains of Ductus
Arteriosus)

Pulmonary Artery

A

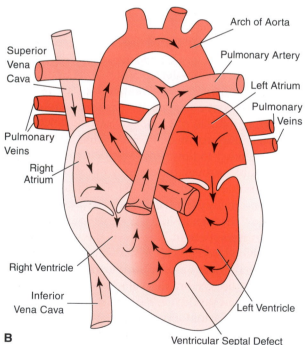

Arch of Aorta

Superior
Vena
Cava

Pulmonary Artery

Left Atrium

Pulmonary
Veins

Pulmonary
Veins

Right
Atrium

Right Ventricle

Inferior
Vena Cava

Left Ventricle

B

Ventricular Septal Defect

Figure 9.4 (*A*) Normal heart with typical anatomical features. (*B*) Ventricular septal defect. *(From Pryor, J., & Prasad, S. [2001]. Physiotherapy for respiratory and cardiac problems [3rd ed., p. 447]. Philadelphia: Churchill Livingstone, with permission.)*

Another common congenital cardiac defect is **patent ductus arteriosus (PDA),** which occurs in 799/million live births, primarily occurring in premature infants (Hoffman & Kaplan, 2002). The ductus arteriosus is the anatomical communication between the pulmonary artery and the aorta, which is present in fetal circulation. The ductus arteriosus typically closes within the first few days to weeks of a newborn's life, completely separating the aorta from the pulmonary artery. If this channel does not close, that is, the ductus arteriosus remains patent, there is an alternative route for blood flow. The direction of blood flow is dependent on the pressure difference between the ends of the ductus arteriosus. Within the first few minutes after the child's birth, the pressure changes within the heart chambers cause the left heart pressures (LA, LV, and aorta) to be greater than the right heart pressures (RA, RV, and pulmonary artery). Therefore the blood flow through a patent ductus arteriosus after birth will be from the aorta to the pulmonary artery, or from left to right, causing oxygenated blood to return to the lungs.

Diagnosis Prenatal ultrasounds and echocardiography can often detect cardiac and great vessel anatomical abnormalities. Postnatal echocardiography and radiological studies can also confirm congenital structural defects, and echocardiography has emerged as the standard diagnostic method. In infancy, suspicion of a cardiac defect may begin with a murmur, either systolic or diastolic, heard on cardiac auscultation. In some cases, when a cardiac murmur is the only sign of a cardiac defect, the physician may choose a "wait and see" approach, as some slight cardiac defects may close with time and with the child's growth. Other cardiac defects are more severe, and the auscultatory finding of a murmur is just one of many signs and symptoms being presented by the child. Infants with severe circulatory impairments are often poor feeders, acting uninterested or requiring prolonged feeding times. These children may also exhibit excessive fatigue, diaphoresis, tachypnea, and dyspnea. The severity of the signs and symptoms is directly related to the severity of the cardiac defect and the amount of blood being shunted.

A child with a left-to-right shunt will have an overwhelmed pulmonary vascular system because a portion of the systemic cardiac output will be returning to the pulmonary capillaries. The pressure within the pulmonary capillaries is increased, causing seepage of fluid out of the pulmonary capillaries into the interstitial space (i.e., congestive heart failure). Signs and symptoms of this increased pulmonary blood flow include crackles on auscultation of the lungs. Arterial oxygen saturation (SaO_2) values may be decreased depending on the extent of congestive heart failure present. Heart rates (HR) may be high. Depending on the extent of respiratory compromise, there may be nasal flaring, intercostal and substernal retractions, and rapid respiratory rate (RR). As a portion of the cardiac output returns to the pulmonary circulation, there is a decreased amount of blood flow systemically. Signs and symptoms of a decreased blood flow to the periphery will be decreased skin temperature; decreased muscle mass, especially in the extremities; decreased energy for crying or playing; decreased endurance for activity including feeding; mottled skin; and delayed motor milestones. The decrease in exercise tolerance is primarily related to the degree of associated hypertension (Bar-Or & Rowland, 2004).

Management The majority of symptomatic congenital cardiac defects require repair. Repair of cardiac defects is based on the amount of cardiac impairment and presenting symptoms. Interventional cardiology using cardiac catheterization techniques can, in certain instances, repair a PDA by introducing a coil into the ductus arteriosus, thereby closing the vessel. A small ASD or VSD may be sealed by placing a patch over the defect via a cardiac catheter. (Abadir, Sarquella-Brugada, Mivelaz, Dahdah, & Miró, 2009). Hybrid approaches using catheterization and surgery, or surgery alone, are indicated for repair of more complicated defects.

The primary goals in the medical management of children with left-to-right shunts are (1) to reduce the volume of pulmonary circulation that is overloading the system (i.e., reducing congestive heart failure) and (2) to encourage growth.

Physical therapy intervention may include preoperative and postoperative care, positioning to encourage age-appropriate activities with lowered metabolic costs, monitored exercise programs, and aerobic conditioning. Child and family education concerning the prevention of pulmonary infections, use of supplemental oxygen, and exercise guidelines are also areas for intervention. Children who have undergone repair of defects resulting in left-to-right shunts typically exhibit normal exercise tolerance postoperatively (Bar-Or & Rowland, 2004). Repair of some larger ASDs may result in sinus node injury, resulting in a decreased heart rate response to exercise. Therapists should modify their exercise monitoring in these children. In addition to the immediate cardiovascular impairments, evidence suggests that neurodevelopmental outcomes of children with congenital cardiac defects may be negatively impacted by their cardiac status with changes noted in brain volume and mild motor and language deficits (Limperopoulos et al., 2010; Miatton, De Wolf, François, Thiery, & Vingerhoets, 2007).

Pathophysiology of Right-to-Left Shunts Structural defects that cause too little blood to pass through the lungs cause right-to-left shunts that allow unoxygenated blood to travel to the body. The body subsequently does not receive enough oxygen and will exhibit cyanosis. Cyanotic defects occur in 1,391/million live births and include tricuspid atresia (TA), pulmonary atresia (PA), transposition of the great arteries (TGA), and tetralogy of Fallot (TOF). All cyanotic defects are considered severe, often requiring intervention as neonate or in early infancy (Hoffman & Kaplan, 2002).

TOF occurs in 421/million live births, the most common of all right-to-left shunts (Hoffman & Kaplan, 2002). The four cardiac anomalies that make up the tetralogy include (1) a VSD, (2) an impaired pulmonary outlet (a defect such as a stenotic pulmonic valve, a stricture in the pulmonary artery, or a narrowed infundibulum within the RV), (3) a malpositioned aorta (overriding the VSD), and (4) RV hypertrophy (Fig. 9.5). As an isolated defect, a VSD is considered a left-to-right cardiac shunt, but in TOF, the pulmonary outflow tract defect is usually severe enough to hinder blood flow out of the RV into the pulmonary circulatory system. The blood volume, and therefore pressure within the RV, exceeds the pressure in the LV. Blood will flow from the RV to the LV through the ventricular septal defect, delivering unoxygenated blood to the periphery. The malpositioned aorta only seems to ease the blood flow from RV blood into the aorta. RV hypertrophy is a result of the increased workload of the RV.

Diagnosis A child with a right-to-left shunt will have decreased blood flow through the pulmonary capillaries resulting in normal pulmonary auscultation findings on physical examination. Although systemic blood flow is adequate in volume, it is inadequate in the amount of oxygen transported. SaO_2 values will be low because some blood has bypassed the lungs, bringing down the overall oxygen content of the blood. Cyanosis may be present. The low oxygen content of the blood may cause decreased muscle mass, especially in the extremities; decreased energy for crying or playing; decreased endurance for activity, including feeding; and delayed motor milestones.

Management Right-to-left shunts create concerns related to the degree of systemic cyanosis. In infants with severe structural defects, pharmacological management,

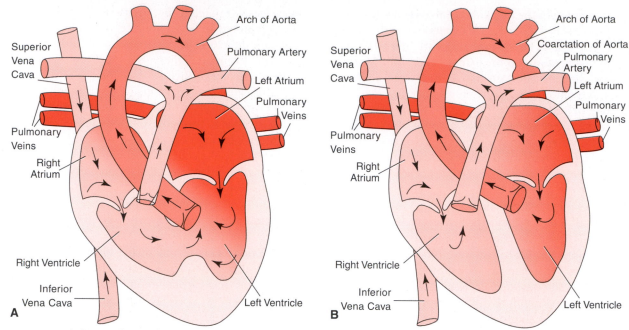

Figure 9.5 (*A*) Tetralogy of Fallot. (*B*) Coarctation of the aorta. (*From Pryor, J., & Prasad, S. [2001]. Physiotherapy for respiratory and cardiac problems [3rd ed., p. 447]. Philadelphia: Churchill Livingstone, with permission.*)

oxygen therapy, and artificial cardiac assistive devices may be used to support the infant until surgical repair is possible. Surgical repair is the definitive treatment for defects resulting in right-to-left shunts. See Table 9.4 for further details of right-to-left shunt abnormalities.

Pathophysiology of Obstructive Cardiac Defects Obstructive cardiac defects result in reduction of blood flow systemically as a result of underdeveloped chambers of the heart or blockages in blood vessels that prevent the proper amount of blood from traveling to the body to meet its needs. Examples include coarctation of the aorta, aortic stenosis, and pulmonary stenosis.

Coarctation of the aorta and valvular stenosis are forms of obstructive cardiac defects. Coarctation of the aorta (a stricture or narrowing of the aortic lumen), and valvular stenosis (a narrowing of the cardiac valves) disrupt normal blood flow through the heart or aorta. Pressure build-up behind the narrowing can cause considerable cardiac and vascular compromise. Decreased blood volume beyond the narrowing can result in decreased growth and development. Table 9.5 provides information about obstructive cardiac defects.

In obstructive defects such as aortic stenosis, the increased circulatory demands of the contracting skeletal muscle create a need for an increase in cardiac output. The obstruction to left ventricular outflow stresses the capability of the circulatory system to meet the demands. In children with significant obstruction, exercise may result in symptoms of angina and fainting and may put the child at increased risk of sudden death (Bar-Or & Rowland, 2004). Guidelines for exercise participation are based on electrocardiogram findings and cardiac pressure gradients using laboratory-based exercise testing. Consensus guidelines are available and should be reviewed by physical therapists (ACSM & AHA, 2007).

Myocardial Disease

Pediatric myocardial disease refers to structural or functional abnormalities of the myocardium that are not secondary to hypertension, pulmonary vascular disease, or valvular or congenital heart disease (Towbin, 1999). This category includes dilated or congestive cardiomyopathies, idiopathic hypertrophic cardiomyopathies, and restrictive cardiomyopathies. The most common cause of acquired heart disease in children is Kawasaki disease, in which vasculitis of the coronary vessels is a predominant feature (Barron et al., 1999). Table 9.6 provides details of cardiomyopathy and Kawasaki disease.

Conditions That Impair Respiration

Respiration refers to the diffusion of gases across the alveolar-capillary membrane (Fig. 9.6). For respiration to occur, oxygen and carbon dioxide must diffuse

(Text continued on page 414)

Table 9.4 Right-to-Left Shunts

Diagnosis	Definition	Etiology	Alterations in Body Functions and Structures	Potential Activity Limitations and Participation Restrictions	Potential Management
Tricuspid atresia	Dysfunctional tricuspid valve in the right atrioventricular septum	Unknown etiology	• Altered structure and function of cardiovascular system (s410/b415–429)* • Blood from right atrium cannot flow through tricuspid valve to the right ventricle; must go through the foramen ovale into left atria • Low oxygen saturation • Poor growth • Poor feeding	• Delay of developmental milestones • Decreased ability to maintain sustained active play (d9200) with peers or family	• Surgical palliation or correction • Physical therapy for pre-/postoperative care, early intervention to encourage development, exercise programs, and parental instruction
Truncus arteriosus	A combined pulmonary artery and aorta, commonly with a ventricular septal defect	Unknown etiology	• Altered structure and function of cardiovascular system (s410/b415–429) • The aorta and pulmonary artery fail to separate, carrying both oxygenated and unoxygenated blood • Poor growth • Poor feeding	• Decreased activity tolerance	• Early (younger than 6 months) surgical repair (Grifka, 1999) • Physical therapy for pre-/postoperative care, early intervention, and parental instruction
Transposition of the great arteries (TGA)	Aorta arises from right ventricle, pulmonary artery from the left ventricle or from the (double outlet) right ventricle	Unknown etiology	• Altered structure and function of cardiovascular system (s410/b415–429) • Unoxygenated blood is pumped from the right ventricle to systemic circulation • Oxygenated blood returns to the lungs	• Defect is not compatible with life, so surgical palliation as neonate is necessary	• Medical management to pharmacologically maintain a patent ductus arteriosus until surgery is possible • Early surgical correction via arterial switch • Physical therapy for pre-/postoperative care, early intervention, and parental instruction

Continued

■ **Table 9.4** Right-to-Left Shunts—cont'd

Diagnosis	Definition	Etiology	Alterations in Body Functions and Structures	Potential Activity Limitations and Participation Restrictions	Potential Management
Total anomalous pulmonary venous return (TAPVR)	Pulmonary venous blood returns to the right atrium or systemic veins rather than to left atrium	Unknown etiology	• Altered structure and function of cardiovascular system (s410/b415–429) • Increased blood return to right atrium with right-sided hypertrophy and increased volume through pulmonary system; an ASD, when present, is the only means for entry to the left atrium • Hypoxemia	• Delay of developmental milestones • Decreased ability to maintain sustained active play (d9200) with peers or family	• Surgical correction in infancy by anastomosis of pulmonary veins to left atrium • Postoperatively may have difficulty with ventilation secondary to stiff, wet lungs from the earlier hyperperfusion caused by defect
Hypoplastic left heart syndrome (HLHS)	Hypoplasia or absence of a left ventricle and hypoplasia of the ascending aorta	Unknown etiology	• Altered structure and function of cardiovascular system (s410/b415–429) • Initially, PDA may allow adequate systemic blood flow • As PDA closes, systemic flow decreases • Hypoxemia • Poor growth • Poor feeding	• Decreased activity tolerance	• Fatal within first month of life if untreated (Fedderly, 1999) • Medical management: supportive care • Multi-stage reconstruction of the heart or cardiac transplantation

*Numbers in parentheses refer to ICF-CY classification.

Table 9.5 Obstructive Cardiac Diseases

Diagnosis	Definition	Etiology	Impairments of Body Functions and Structures	Potential Activity Limitations and Participation Restrictions	Potential Management
Coarctation of the aorta	Stricture, or narrowing, of the aortic lumen, usually at or near site of the ductus arteriosus Increased pressure proximal to the coarctation and decreased distal pressure	Unknown etiology	• Altered structure and function of cardiovascular system (s410/b415–429)* • Significant differences in pulse intensities and blood pressures are found between upper and lower extremities • Increased proximal pressure impedes left ventricular ejection, leading to congestive heart failure and an increased risk for intracranial hemorrhages • Poor growth • Poor feeding • Decreased distal pressure results in lower extremity changes • Decreased skin temperature • Delayed growth and development	• Delay of developmental milestones • Decreased ability to maintain sustained active play (d9200) with peers or family • Increased activity can further increase existing hypertension, necessitating a stress test before participation in an exercise program.	• Surgical repair optimal, between 3 to 10 years of age, reduces the incidence of residual hypertension and associated morbidity and mortality (Fedderly, 1999). • Cardiac stent may be used to enlarge some strictures. • Larger and more complex defects require surgical repair, which may be staged over months or years to accommodate growth-related changes in the cardiac system. • Early surgical correction allows for more normal growth and development but an increased risk of recurrent stenosis (Toro-Salazar et al., 2002).
Aortic or pulmonary stenosis	Aortic or pulmonary valvular stenoses cause obstruction of blood flow from the respective ventricle	Unknown etiology	• Altered structure and function of cardiovascular system (s410/b415–429) • Involved ventricle will hypertrophy in response to resistance provided by the valve's defect • Poor growth • Poor feeding	• Delay of developmental milestones • Decreased ability to maintain sustained active play (d9200) with peers or family • With growth, involved ventricle may fail to meet demands of activity	• Surgical repair or replacement of valve according to severity of symptoms • Physical therapy for pre-/postoperative care, early intervention, and parental instruction

*Numbers in parentheses refer to ICF-CY classification,

Table 9.6 Myocardial Diseases

Diagnosis	Definition	Etiology	Alterations in Body Functions and Structures	Potential Activity Limitations and Participation Restrictions	Potential Management
Dilated cardiomyopathy	Biventricular dilation with loss of systolic contraction, resulting in congestive heart failure Atrioventricular valves may be unable to fully close during systole secondary to ventricular dilation	Unknown etiology	• Altered function of cardiovascular system (b415–429)* • Typically presents with symptoms of congestive heart failure: systolic heart murmur, fatigue, chest pain, syncope, impaired consciousness • Limitations associated with circulatory impairments: tachypnea, diaphoresis, poor peripheral circulation, cyanosis • Failure to thrive • Poor feeding	• Delay of developmental milestones • Decreased ability to maintain sustained active play (d9200) with peers or family	• Medical management is to pharmacologically optimize cardiac function, control associated arrhythmias, and minimize risk of thromboembolism. Antibiotic prophylaxis can be important to prevent bacterial endocarditis. • Surgery may be indicated in children with left ventricular outflow obstruction to relieve the obstruction. • In children for whom medical therapy has failed, heart transplantation may be an option. • Physical therapy to reduce secondary complications associated with progressive congestive heart failure and deconditioning; parental instruction
Hypertrophic cardiomyopathy	Hypertrophy of the myocardium and intraventricular septum Chamber size is lessened, limiting preload and reducing cardiac output.	Unknown etiology	• Altered function of cardiovascular system (b415–429)	• Delay of developmental milestones • Decreased ability to maintain sustained active play (d9200) with peers or family • Typical complications: arrhythmias, hypertrophied septum and ventricular wall obstructs blood flow to aorta • Sudden death	

Table 9.6 Myocardial Diseases—cont'd

Diagnosis	Definition	Etiology	Alterations in Body Functions and Structures	Potential Activity Limitations and Participation Restrictions	Potential Management
Restrictive cardiomyopathy	Restrictive cardiomyopathy results from an abnormal relaxation phase of the ventricle	Unknown etiology	• Altered function of cardiovascular system (b415–429) • Ventricles cannot accept atrial blood volume, resulting in atrial dilation and decreased cardiac output • Complications related to congestive heart failure and formation of thrombus	• Delay of developmental milestones • Decreased ability to maintain sustained active play (d9200) with peers or family	
Kawasaki disease	Vasculitis of coronary vessels in children between ages 6 months and 4 years Resolution within 6 to 8 weeks of onset May result in aneurysms and coronary artery disease	Unknown etiology May be response to infectious exposure	• Altered function of cardiovascular system (b415–429) • Massive myocardial infarction secondary to coronary thrombosis during weeks 3 to 4 of illness (Rowley & Shulman, 1999) • Myocardial infarction symptoms may include shock, vomiting, and unrest rather than chest pain.	• Delay of developmental milestones • Decreased ability to maintain sustained active play (d9200) with peers or family • More specifically activity restriction during acute illness and decreased activity tolerance with significant cardiac involvement	• Pharmacological support including intravenous gamma globulin and aspirin in children with cardiac manifestations • Precautions for competitive contact athletics or endurance training are followed. • Stress tests may be necessary for those with resultant cardiac manifestations before participation in exercise programs.

*Numbers in parentheses refer to ICF-CY classification.

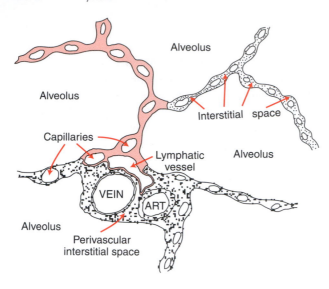

Figure 9.6 Alveolar capillary membrane. *(From Guyton, A. [1996]. Textbook of medical physiology [9th ed., p. 487]. Philadelphia: W.B. Saunders.)*

across the surfactant layer of the alveoli, the alveolar membrane, the interstitial space, the capillary membrane, the plasma, the red blood cell membrane, and finally into the hemoglobin in the red blood cell. Conditions that increase the diffusion distance by widening any of these layers, or otherwise impair gas exchange, will hinder respiration. The most common pediatric conditions that impair respiration are interstitial lung diseases and congestive heart failure. Sickle cell anemia also affects respiration, as well as circulation, by hindering oxygen bonding to hemoglobin and causing vaso-occlusion. Table 9.7 provides details of interstitial lung disease, congestive heart failure, and sickle cell anemia.

Examination and Evaluation

Tests and measurements of the CVP systems are outlined in the *Guide to Physical Therapist Practice* (APTA, 2001). Many of the measurements used with adults who have CVP conditions can, with some modifications in implementation and interpretation, be used when examining infants and children with CVP conditions. Specialized equipment is needed to obtain accurate measurement, such as smaller pediatric stethoscopes, SaO_2 sensors, and blood pressure cuffs. Inherent in all pediatric practice is the effect of age on the ability to communicate, follow commands, and remain attentive to physical therapy examination and intervention. In this section, history, systems review, tests and measures, laboratory tests, and exercise testing are described.

History

Interviewing a child should yield information not only from the child but also from parents, guardians, or other caregivers. When interviewing the parents, the child should be in view, allowing for an initial observation of the child. The information obtained from the child and parent interview includes demographics (age, primary language, race/ethnicity, and gender), social history (family culture, resources, social interactions, and support services), growth and development history (gestational age at birth, labor, delivery, and neonatal events), and details of the living environment (e.g., home, school, daycare). A history of present illness, past medical and surgical history, present medications, and pertinent family history can be obtained with help from a parent or guardian, as described in Chapter 2. Activity level can be determined by watching the child play during the interview and by asking questions concerning the child's participation in physical activities, such as feeding, crying, playing, age at acquisition of motor milestones, and preferred activities. In infants, prolonged feeding times, increased sleeping or napping, or irritability can be symptoms of CVP impairment. Children with CVP compromise may demonstrate age-appropriate fine motor skills but delays in gross motor skills caused by energy constraints. In children with CVP impairments, determining the parents' or caregiver's perception of the child's activities of daily life can also provide important information regarding their comfort with the child's participation in physical activities. The use of standardized parent- or self-reported outcomes of health status focused on physical function, sleep and wake disturbances, and activity and participation can add important information and provides a means to measure the wider impact of specific CVP conditions within the ICF framework. Parents or caregivers may place limits on their

Table 9.7 Conditions That Impair Respiration

Diagnosis	Definition	Etiology	Alterations in Body Functions and Structures	Potential Activity Limitations and Participation Restrictions	Potential Management
Interstitial lung disease	Chronic inflammation of alveolar walls, small airways, arteries, and veins; more peripheral regions of the lungs are generally affected (Bokulic & Hilman, 1994)	Results from infection (e.g., HIV, RSV, CMV), environmental inhalants or toxins (e.g., talcum powder, chlorine, ammonia), treatment induced (e.g., antineoplastic drugs, radiation therapy), neoplastic diseases, metabolic conditions, collagen vascular disease, and neurocutaneous syndromes	• Altered structure and function of respiratory system (s430/b440)* • Disruption of alveolar capillary structures leads to pulmonary fibrosis • Common respiratory signs and symptoms: dyspnea, tachypnea with intercostal and subcostal retractions, nonproductive cough, fatigue, pleuritic chest pain • Decreased growth	• Delay of developmental milestones • Decreased ability to maintain sustained active play (d9200) with peers or family	• Corticosteroids and immunosuppressive agents used to reduce inflammation • Oxygen, nutritional support, and avoidance of environmental exposures • Surgical management is lung transplantation.
Congestive heart failure (CHF)	Inability of the heart to advance blood through cardiac chambers, resulting in congestion of pulmonary and/or systemic circulation	Caused by a congenital left-to-right cardiac defect Obstruction to left ventricular outflow Cardiomyopathy Chronic restrictive lung disease	• Altered function of respiratory system (b440) and cardiovascular system (s410/b410–429) • Clinical signs include tachycardia, tachypnea, arrhythmias, ventricular dilatation, hepatomegaly, peripheral and/or pulmonary edema, poor peripheral perfusion • In infants: poor feeding, lethargy, respiratory tract infections	• Delay of developmental milestones • Decreased ability to maintain sustained active play (d9200) with peers or family	• Surgical correction of causative cardiac defects • Medical treatment includes oxygen and pharmacology to increase myocardial contractility and decrease afterload. • Physical therapy may include maintenance of pulmonary hygiene, developmental stimulation, aerobic exercise training, and parental instruction.

Continued

■ **Table 9.7** Conditions That Impair Respiration—cont'd

Diagnosis	Definition	Etiology	Alterations in Body Functions and Structures	Potential Activity Limitations and Participation Restrictions	Potential Management
Sickle cell anemia	Mutation in hemoglobin that causes a distortion or "sickling" of red blood cell; "sickled cells" reduce life span of the red blood cell as well as cause vaso-occlusion.	Sickle cell anemia is a genetically inherited condition seen primarily in individuals of African descent. Diagnosis can be made through neonatal screening or genetic testing.	• Altered function of hematological system (b430) • Primary presentation is pain • Ischemia • Acute chest syndrome: new pulmonary infiltrate, fever, cough, sputum production, dyspnea, hypoxia, and pain • With repeated acute chest syndrome, restrictive lung disease, pulmonary hypertension, and congestive heart failure (Lane, 1996)	• Delay of developmental milestones • Decreased ability to maintain sustained active play (d9200) with peers or family	• Medical management of acute chest syndrome includes oxygen, pain medication, and intravenous hydration. • Physical therapy directed at improving aeration using airway clearance techniques and breathing exercises during acute episodes

*Numbers in parentheses refer to ICF-CY classification.

child's activity, partly because of their own apprehension rather than physical restrictions related to the actual CVP condition.

Systems Review
General Observation and Palpation

Initial observation of the general appearance, posture, breathing patterns, and comfort during play activities can provide insight into CVP status. The child's preferred posture may have CVP implications. For example, a child whose preferred positioning is supported sitting may have learned to ration his or her limited energy. Less energy expended for maintaining the upright position means more energy for other tasks. Positions may also be chosen that allow muscles to be used primarily for ventilation rather than posture maintenance. Sitting with upper extremities fixed, supporting the shoulder girdle, allows neck and upper extremity muscles to be used as accessory muscles of ventilation (Fig. 9.7). Sleeping in supine position with full shoulder flexion helps elevate the upper chest to assist with breathing. Alterations in speech patterns as a result of breathlessness or changes of position to support speech patterns should be noted.

Skin color can show cyanosis, a sign of acute tissue hypoxia. The bluish-gray skin color of cyanosis is commonly seen about the mouth, eyes, fingertips, and toes. If tissue hypoxia is severe enough, it is also possible to see cyanosis throughout the body. As oxygenation to the tissues improves, the color change reverses, returning the skin to a more normal tone. Cyanosis is more difficult to observe in individuals with naturally darker skin tones. Other integumentary changes may include mottling of the skin, common in infants and children with decreased blood flow to the extremities. Children with cyanotic cardiac disease or congestive heart failure may appear diaphoretic, with cool, moist skin. Clubbing of the fingertips may be noted in individuals with chronic peripheral cyanosis (e.g., right-to-left cardiac shunts, CF) (Fig. 9.8).

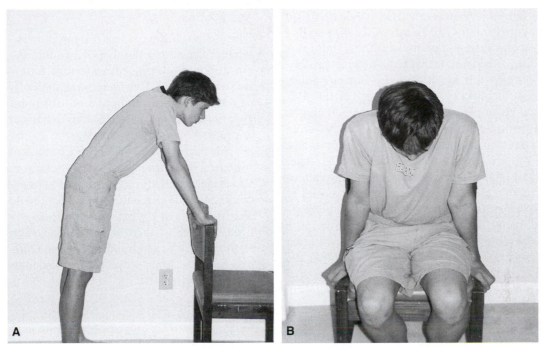

Figure 9.7 Positioning of the upper extremities to assist with ventilation.

Peripheral edema is often associated with heart or liver disease. Because edema is found in gravity-dependent areas of the body, edema in an infant may be found on the skull, the back, or posterior aspects of lower extremities.

General muscular development and amount of adipose tissue in the extremities should also be observed. Children may exhibit poor muscle development and lack of adipose tissue for a number of reasons, including prematurity, poor nutrition from a reduced energy to feed, inadequate oxygenation to the extremities, or decreased absorption of calories.

The observed breathing pattern of a young, healthy infant is not the coordinated, symmetrical pattern one expects in an older child or adult. The RR of the infant is faster, the tidal volume changes from breath to breath, and there is no rhythmic pattern of breathing or a repeating ratio of inspiratory to expiratory time. Overall, the breathing pattern of an infant is typically uncoordinated and unpredictable. Observation of thoracoabdominal movement and the relative timing of inspiration to expiration should be noted.

During periods of respiratory compromise, nostril flaring, head bobbing, and expiratory grunting can be noted. Significant intercostal, substernal, and subclavicular retractions may also be seen in infants, attributable to the compliant ribcage, lack of accessory muscle fixation, and smaller airways.

Tests and Measurements
Vital Signs

Measurement of vital signs in children includes HR, RR, blood pressure (BP), oxygen saturation of arterial blood (SaO_2), and body temperature. Body length and

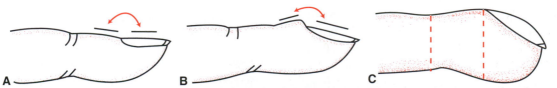

Figure 9.8 Clubbing of the digits. (*A*) Normal. (*B*) Early clubbing with angle present between nail and proximal skin. (*C*) Advanced clubbing. (*Reprinted from R.L. Wilkins & S.J. Drider [1985],* Clinical assessment in respiratory care. *St. Louis: Mosby, with permission from Elsevier.*)

weight and extremity pulses can also provide useful information concerning CVP function. Higher resting HRs are encountered in healthy children, and a rate that would be considered tachycardic in adults may be normal for infants and small children. During periods of high stress, a child's HR can be as high as 180, 190, or even 200 beats per minute. Heart rhythm can be measured through cardiac auscultation, palpation of pulses, or electrocardiography (ECG). Children also have high RR to compensate for the low tidal volumes of the smaller and less compliant thorax. As the pattern of breathing of a child is often variable, RR should be counted for an entire minute to obtain an accurate reporting of breaths per minute. Lower BP in children is partly attributable to the lowered peripheral vascular resistance secondary to shorter blood vessels. As the child grows and develops into adolescence, the vital sign measurements approach the values found in healthy adults. Table 9.8 compares the expected healthy HR, BP, and RR for an infant, child, and adult.

Serial measurements of length and weight of a child are important. Adequate nutritional intake, nutrient absorption by the GI system, and nutrient delivery to the body by the circulatory system are necessary for healthy growth and weight gain. Lung growth is directly related to overall body length. Children with CVP conditions should have their height and weight measured periodically and mapped against the normative height and weight charts. Any change from the expected values can be documented and referrals for appropriate follow-up made.

Palpation of extremity pulses can be helpful in determining alterations in peripheral blood flow patterns in children with cardiac conditions. Decreased extremity pulses may indicate decreased blood flow to the extremities. Differences in upper extremity versus lower extremity pulses may indicate obstruction to blood flow, as occurs in coarctation of the aorta, or a change in pulses with stress may indicate cardiac impairment.

Table 9.8 Comparison of Vital Signs Between Healthy Children and Adults

Vital Signs	Infant	Child	Adult
Heart rate (bpm)	100–140	80–120	60–100
Blood pressure (mm Hg)	80/40	100/60	120/80
Respiratory rate (breaths per minute)	30–40	25–30	12–18

Auscultation

Because the child's cardiac and pulmonary systems are structurally similar to those of an adult, the same general auscultation procedures can be followed. Infants and younger children may have difficulty following commands to breathe in and out for pulmonary auscultation. Asking young children to blow at a tissue or at pretend birthday candles during auscultation may provide deeper breaths and more accurate results. The presence and intensity of pulmonary adventitious sounds (e.g., crackles and wheezes) as well as abnormal cardiac sounds (e.g., murmurs) must be documented. Transmission of abdominal sounds is greater in children because of their smaller size. Warming of the stethoscope's head and allowing the child to hold or play with the stethoscope before auscultation can decrease apprehension.

Range of Motion

ROM of the trunk and upper extremities, focusing on proximal joints and chest wall excursion, should be measured. Because the infant cannot follow the usual commands to measure thoracic excursion, following the infant's respiratory cycle with the therapist's hands in contact with the child's ribcage can be helpful. Exaggerating the exhalation phase of the child's breath with manual pressure will lead to a greater inhalation on the child's next breath, allowing for a more complete evaluation of thoracic mobility. Thoracic symmetry can be assessed at the same time. Observation of any skeletal chest wall abnormalities should be noted.

Laboratory Studies

Children with CVP conditions routinely have multiple laboratory tests to assess cardiac and pulmonary status. The physical therapist must be able to integrate the information from multiple laboratory studies into intervention planning and execution. For example, if lab results indicate relative hypoxemia based on arterial blood gas values, the therapist may need to reassess exercise tolerance and consult with the physician for the need for oxygen during exercise. Another example is the appearance of a new pathogen in the sputum of a child with cystic fibrosis, necessitating a change in medication and pulmonary hygiene program.

Radiology

Radiological laboratory studies are used to define structural and parenchymal abnormalities. Chest radiography, computed tomography (CT) scanning, and magnetic resonance imaging (MRI) can be used to evaluate heart size, amount of pulmonary blood flow, and pulmonary infiltrates or atelectasis. The areas of infiltration identified will direct the physical therapist to the segments of the lung needing intervention. A child's chest radiograph may also demonstrate the alignment of ribs, the amount of ossification of ribs and vertebrae, and the level of the diaphragm.

An echocardiogram uses sound waves to produce a computer-generated picture of the heart. A transthoracic, transesophageal, or even fetal echocardiogram can be performed to look at the structure within the heart. Valvular stenosis or incompetence or congenital defects can be seen and recorded using an echocardiogram. Echocardiography is now considered the standard in diagnoses of congenital cardiac defects.

Right- and left-side heart catheterization can also be used to determine cardiac structural defects in children. A catheter is introduced into the venous system, through which dye is injected to view the right side of the heart, or into the arterial system to evaluate the left side of the heart.

Electrocardiography

ECG is performed and interpreted with results normalized for the differences in body size and cardiovascular maturation. Electrocardiographic differences exist among premature infants, newborns, and older children (Park & Guntheroth, 1992). In the full-term newborn, RV mass exceeds LV mass because of the stresses put on these structures during fetal circulation. At birth, as the pulmonary vascular resistance begins to drop and the systemic resistance rises, there is a shift in the relative size of the RV and LV by about 1 month of age. Not surprisingly, this morphology is reflected in the ECG. The full-term newborn's ECG shows an RV dominance that over a month or so changes to a more adultlike LV dominance. The premature infant may not show an RV dominance because the RV did not have the time to increase its mass before birth. With increasing age, the HR decreases and the duration of intervals (PR interval, QRS duration, QT interval) and voltages all increase.

Arterial Blood Gases

Infants have slightly different baseline values for blood oxygenation (PaO_2), but the interpretation of arterial blood gas values remains the same as in the adult (Table 9.9). Infants with obstructive pulmonary conditions, such as BPD, will demonstrate decreased PaO_2 and increased $PaCO_2$ values. Children with an unrepaired congenital cardiac defect causing a right-to-left

Table 9.9 Comparison of Arterial Blood Gas Values Between Healthy Children and Adults

Value	Infant	Child	Adult
pH	7.35–7.45	7.35–7.45	7.35–7.45
PaO_2	50–70	80–100	95–100
$PaCO_2$	35–45	35–45	35–45
HCO_3^-	22–26	22–26	22–26

shunt will have altered arterial blood gas values, especially a decrease in PaO_2. It is interesting to note that this lower PaO_2 will not readily respond to supplemental oxygen. Because the blood is bypassing the lungs, more supplemental oxygen to the lungs does not necessarily result in higher PaO_2 values.

Pulmonary Function Tests

Pulmonary function tests are effort-dependent and therefore require full cooperation of the child. Children who are able to follow commands and control their breathing patterns, often by 6 to 8 years of age, can perform them. Interpretation of the tests must be normalized for body size. Modifications of testing procedures, or selection of a subset of pulmonary function measures, can make testing possible in younger children. The use of specialized equipment, found predominantly in specialized pediatric pulmonary centers, can make pulmonary function testing possible even in very young children.

Ventilation-Perfusion Scans

Ventilation-perfusion scans are performed to assess the matching of ventilation to perfusion within the lungs, which is helpful in children with cardiac and pulmonary abnormalities. The performance of this test, and interpretation of the results, must take into account the more compliant ribcage, and physical maturation, of the child. The results of this test may be helpful in choosing body positions that optimize ventilation and perfusion matching for a child's daily positioning schedule.

Exercise Testing

Exercise testing in children yields information about the CVP systems (HR, BP, RR, breathing pattern, and oxygen saturation) during different workloads. The results of the exercise test allow a physical therapist to optimally prescribe aerobic exercise. Exercise and activity tolerance can be assessed at all ages, although different modes of exercise may be used. For infants and children under 3 years of age, "formal" exercise tests are not performed. Activity tolerance in infants and very young children can be assessed during crying, feeding, and play activities. Children older than 3 years of age can perform submaximal treadmill and stair exercise tolerance protocols (Bar-Or & Rowland, 2004; Darbee & Cerny, 1995). A more accurate measure of workload can be obtained if the treadmill or stair rails are not used for support, but close supervision is necessary to prevent loss of balance. Children older than 6 years of age can participate in standardized exercise test protocols with the ergometer workload or treadmill speed adjusted for the motor skill level. Exercise test termination criteria are similar to those used in the adult population. Although the body of literature on pediatric exercise testing is growing, children typically serve as their own controls because normative data still need to be developed (Bar-Or & Rowland, 2004; Cerny, 1989). The saturation of oxygen in the arterial blood (Sa_{O_2}) should be monitored in anyone who has a predicted FEV_1 of less than 50%. If there is evidence of exercise hypoxemia during a graded exercise test, a submaximal steady state test, such as a 6- or 12-minute walk test, should be performed. Sustained submaximal exercise can show a greater change in Sa_{O_2} values than a graded test might provide (Nixon, 2003).

In addition to exercise testing, measures of physical fitness that emphasize health-related fitness components are available. The American Alliance for Health, Physical Education, Recreation and Dance (AAHPERD, 1999), 6- and 12-minute walk tests, Presidential Physical Fitness Program, and National Child and Youth Fitness Study are examples of common measures of physical fitness in children. In addition, the NIH Toolbox project (http://www.nihtoolbox.org) also has standardized pediatric physical activity and function measures. The widespread availability of objective monitors of habitual physical activity such as step monitors and accelerometers, as well as heart rate monitors, have allowed these devices to be used in large studies and are often considered the standard for assessing daily energy expenditure.

Physical Therapy Intervention

Physical therapy intervention for the child with impairments of CVP structures and functions, and restrictions in activities and participation, requires a balance between the effects of short-term intervention and long-term outcomes. Children with chronic or progressive CVP conditions may require physical therapy intervention for a lifetime. Teaching family and other caregivers how to

provide long-term maintenance care should be integrated into the initial treatment framework. As the child matures, physical therapy intervention should include methods for more independent physical therapy. The inclusion of mechanical aids and independent exercise programs allows the child with CVP impairments to be more independent in and responsible for his or her own care. Physical therapy intervention includes the child's social, family, and medical well-being, in terms of both the immediate needs of a child during an acute illness and activities to promote long-term function and health. In this section, intervention of airway clearance techniques, breathing exercises, and the prescription of aerobic exercise are discussed.

Airway Clearance Techniques

Airway clearance techniques are indicated for the child with retained secretions that obstruct or limit airflow. Improving secretion clearance can take many forms. A daily regimen of the manual secretion removal techniques of postural drainage, percussion, and shaking is the standard management for retained secretions. Other forms of secretion removal techniques—active cycle of breathing, autogenic drainage, positive expiratory pressure, and chest wall oscillation devices—can be instituted if and when the child is ready to become more independent in his or her care. The following is a brief description of each airway clearance technique. Evidence strongly supporting the use of any form of chest physiotherapy for beneficial long-term outcomes has not emerged within the literature; however, evidence does support short-term positive effects with improved mucus transport noted (van der Schans, Prasad, & Main, 2004).

Manual Secretion Removal Techniques

Postural drainage is a term referring to specific body positions that enlist gravity to drain secretions from a segment of the lung. Manual secretion removal techniques include the use of percussion and shaking in the appropriate postural drainage position to enhance mucociliary clearance of excessive secretions. This combination of techniques requires a caregiver to perform the techniques on the child. It is commonly used with infants, young children, and children who cannot participate in a more independent method of secretion removal.

Optimal body positions used for postural drainage of each lung segment are shown in Figure 9.9. The drainage positions chosen for a treatment session depend on the site of pathology. A child with right middle

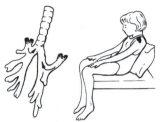

UPPER LOBES Apical Segments

Bed or drainage table flat.

Patient leans back on pillow at 30° angle against therapist.

Therapist claps with markedly cupped hand over area between clavicle and top of scapula on each side.

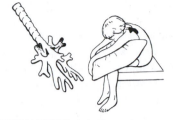

UPPER LOBES Posterior Segments

Bed or drainage table flat.

Patient leans over folded pillow at 30° angle.

Therapist stands behind and claps over upper back on both sides.

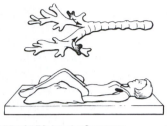

UPPER LOBES Anterior Segments

Bed or drainage table flat.

Patient lies on back with pillow under knees.

Therapist claps between clavicle and nipple on each side.

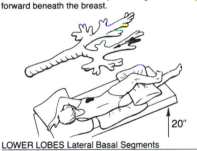

RIGHT MIDDLE LOBE

Foot of table or bed elevated 16 inches.

Patient lies head down on left side and rotates ¼ turn backward. Pillow may be placed behind from shoulder to hip. Knees should be flexed.

Therapist claps over right nipple area. In females with breast development or tenderness, use cupped hand with heel of hand under armpit and fingers extending forward beneath the breast.

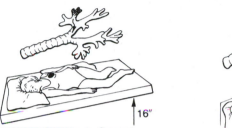

LEFT UPPER LOBE Lingular Segments

Foot of table or bed elevated 16 inches.

Patient lies head down on right side and rotates ¼ turn backward. Pillow may be placed behind from shoulder to hip. Knees should be flexed.

Therapist claps with moderately cupped hand over left nipple area. In females with breast development or tenderness, use cupped hand with heel of hand under armpit and fingers extending forward beneath the breast.

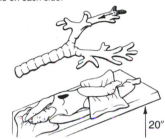

LOWER LOBES Anterior Basal Segments

Foot of table or bed elevated 20 inches.

Patient lies on side, head down, pillow under knees.

Therapist claps with slightly cupped hand over lower ribs. (Position shown is for drainage of left anterior basal segment. To drain the right anterior basal segment, patient should lie on his or her left side in same posture).

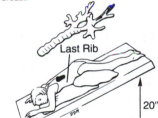

LOWER LOBES Lateral Basal Segments

Foot of table or bed elevated 20 inches.

Patient lies on abdomen, head down, then rotates ¼ turn upward. Upper leg is flexed over a pillow for support.

Therapist claps over uppermost portion of lower ribs. (Position shown is for drainage of right lateral basal segment. To drain the left lateral basal segment, patient should lie on his or her right side in the same posture).

Last Rib

LOWER LOBES Posterior Basal Segments

Foot of table or bed elevated 20 inches.

Patient lies on abdomen, head down, with pillow under hips. Therapist claps over lower ribs close to spine on each side.

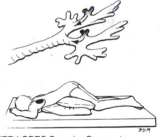

LOWER LOBES Superior Segments

Bed or table flat.

Patient lies on abdomen with two pillows under hips.

Therapist claps over middle of back at tip of scapula on either side of spine.

Figure 9.9 Postural drainage positions for lung segments. The incorporation of head-down positioning should be evaluated on a case-by-case basis in infants and younger children, and in those with medical precautions. *(From J.M. Rothstein, S.H. Roy, & S.L. Wolf [1998],* The rehabilitation specialist's handbook *[2nd ed., pp. 534–534]. Philadelphia: F.A. Davis. Reprinted with permission.)*

lobe syndrome will use the position for the right middle lobe only, whereas a child with CF who has involvement of the entire pulmonary system will use all postural drainage positions during the treatment session. The amount of time each body position is maintained is again dependent on the pathology being treated. From 5 to 20 minutes per position is customary, although gravity drainage positions can be incorporated into a child's positioning schedule and therefore maintained for up to 2 hours.

Postural drainage positions can also be useful in improving ventilation. As this technique places a lung segment in a gravity-independent position, improved ventilation to that lung segment is possible. Continual evaluation of the tolerance to positioning is essential. The prone position has been shown to increase oxygenation levels; however, sleeping in the prone position has been associated with an increased risk of sudden infant death syndrome (SIDS). The Trendelenburg position—head of the bed tipped down with head lower than feet—also requires certain considerations. Children at risk for intraventricular hemorrhage or with acute head injuries may show an increase in their intracranial pressure with the head of the bed flat or in the Trendelenburg position. Acceptable ranges of intracranial pressures should be clear before attempting positioning in this population. Recent studies have demonstrated that tipping (head down) positioning in conjunction with postural drainage positioning increases the potential for microaspiration and increased gastroesophageal reflux (GER), and may actually be relatively harmful in infants and young children. Evidence for the effectiveness of postural drainage in CF is limited (van der Schans et al., 2004). Therapists should actively follow the literature and evidence and utilize head-down positioning with caution in infants and young children. They should balance the positive and negative effects of head-down positioning in older children with chronic lung disease on a case-by-case basis until clear evidence exists to better support decision making. Trendelenburg positioning has, in some instances, been shown to decrease oxygen saturation levels, making it necessary to identify acceptable ranges for Sao_2 before using these positions (Thorensen, Cavan, & Whitelaw, 1988).

Gastroesophageal reflux is not necessarily a contraindication for postural drainage in the Trendelenburg position. Rather, physical therapy interventions should be planned around the child's feeding schedule, so that feeding occurs at least 90 minutes before postural drainage. Estimates of the presence of GER in premature infants are as high as 80% (Newell, Booth, Morgan, Durbin, & McNeish, 1989). Therefore, timing postural drainage treatments around feeding schedules is recommended for all premature infants. Special consideration to the child's positioning can be a simple but effective treatment technique.

Percussion is a force applied to the child's thorax by the caregiver's cupped hand to dislodge secretions within the airways, facilitating airway clearance (Fig. 9.10). Performance of the technique in the neonate may require tenting of the therapist's fingers, as the therapist's whole hand may be too large. With the child in the appropriate postural drainage position, the percussive force is applied to the area of the thorax related to the lung segment being treated. The customary time frame for percussion is between 2 and 5 minutes, although the time frame should be modified to the child's needs and tolerance. Consideration of the use of percussion as a technique for secretion removal must be weighed against possible untoward outcomes. Children who are experiencing pain, such as during the postoperative period or after sustaining a trauma, may need to be adequately medicated before the intervention. Conditions such as hemoptysis, osteoporosis, coagulation disorders, fractured ribs, stress precautions, and fragile hemodynamics may require modification in or negation of the use of this technique.

A bouncing or vibratory force applied to the thorax during exhalation to enhance the normal mucociliary transport of airway secretions toward the glottis for final removal is called **shaking** (Fig. 9.11). The term "shaking" refers to this technique of loosening secretions in the lungs and should not be confused with physically shaking the child. The child is asked to take in a deep breath. As the child exhales, the therapist follows the expiratory movement of the thorax with an intermittent manual force, or "bounce." The high RR

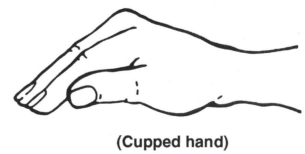

(Cupped hand)

Figure 9.10 Hand position for the technique of percussion. *(From National Cystic Fibrosis Foundation, courtesy of Bettina C. Hilman, MD. From F.J. Brannon, M.W. Foley, J.A. Starr, & L.M. Saul [1998], Cardiopulmonary rehabilitation: Basic therapy and application [p. 427]. Philadelphia: F.A. Davis.)*

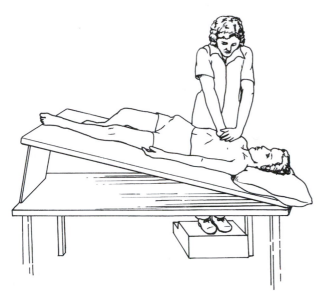

Figure 9.11 Shaking being performed over the involved right middle lobe. *(From the National Cystic Fibrosis Foundation, courtesy of Bettina C. Hilman, MD. From F.J. Brannon, M.W. Foley, J.A. Starr, & L.M. Saul [1998], Cardiopulmonary rehabilitation: Basic therapy and application [p. 427]. Philadelphia: F.A. Davis.)*

of an infant and the inability to follow commands can make shaking difficult to perform. Coordination with the infant's respiratory pattern is essential. The increased compliance of the thorax of an infant makes it difficult to determine how much of the external force from shaking is being translated to the underlying lung. The use of five to seven exhalations for shaking is customary. Precautions for use of the shaking technique are similar to those for percussion.

After secretions are loosened by one of the techniques outlined, clearance of the secretions from the airways is necessary to complete the treatment. Coughing is a natural, often spontaneous, and effective means for clearing secretions from the larger airways. For infants and children who are unable to cough on command because of limitations to cognitive or motor planning abilities, tracheal stimulation delivered manually using a quick, inward thrust on the trachea just above the suprasternal notch will elicit a strong cough reflex (Fig. 9.12).

A child with an obstructive pulmonary disease may have difficulty clearing secretions with coughing because of early closure of the airways. **Huffing** is a technique that may more effectively clear secretions. The child is told to inhale and then forcefully exhale, producing a breathy "ha ha ha" sound. Modifications

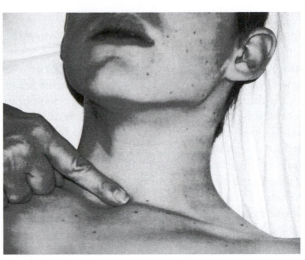

Figure 9.12 Tracheal stimulation for the production of a cough reflex.

of the huff are used in many of the independent secretion removal techniques described in this chapter. This technique may be helpful to clear secretions throughout the day, not just during specified therapy sessions. Children who are able, although somewhat reluctant, to cough on command may become more compliant using coughing or huffing activities. The big bad wolf huffs and puffs, and perhaps can even cough!

For children who are unable to generate the forced expiratory muscle force needed for an effective cough, an assisted cough may improve cough effectiveness. Similar to a coordinated Heimlich maneuver, the therapist's hand is placed just below the xiphoid process (Fig. 9.13). As the child attempts a cough, the therapist pushes inward and under the diaphragm, assisting

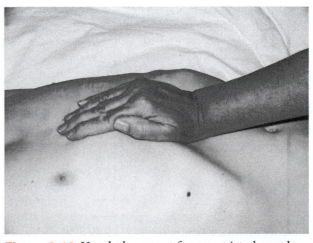

Figure 9.13 Hand placement for an assisted cough.

exhalation. The amount of pressure that the therapist uses on the abdomen is dictated by the child's tolerance. A child with muscular dystrophy will have intact sensation, limiting the amount of pressure that can be used to assist the cough. A child with a spinal cord lesion who lacks abdominal sensation can tolerate more pressure. This coughing technique is usually performed in supine position with the child fully supported on a flat surface. It can be used with the child in other positions, such as upright in a wheelchair or sidelying, but the therapist must ensure that the child's position will be maintained during the assisted cough. For example, the wheelchair brakes must be locked or pillows placed behind the child to maintain sidelying.

Airway suctioning may be necessary to remove airway secretions in children who are on mechanical ventilation or who are unable to generate an effective cough through any other means. Suctioning techniques for children use a small suction catheter. Neonatal suction catheters are 5 to 6 or 8 French gauge. In older children, a size 10 may be used. When suctioning through an artificial airway, take care not to occlude the airway with the suction catheter. The outside diameter of the suction catheter should be only 50% of the internal diameter of the airway (Pryor & Webber, 1998). Suctioning protocols usually encourage preoxygenation. It is recommended that only a 10% increase above the child's present oxygen settings be used. Even short-term hyperoxemia may lead to retinopathy (Roberton, 1996). The negative pressures used in the suction setup should be between 75 and 150 mm Hg (Pryor & Webber, 1998). Finally, take care when choosing suctioning as a method of airway clearance because its use is linked with oxygen desaturation, tachycardia, bradycardia, hypertension, hypotension, pneumothorax, and stridor. Nurses, respiratory therapists, physical therapists, and family members may need to perform suctioning, but proper training is essential.

A combination of postural drainage, percussion, and shaking, followed by airway clearance techniques, may be used to mobilize secretions in infants and young children. Additional evidence is needed to support the use of percussion/vibration in infants requiring ventilatory support (Hough, Flenady, Johnston, & Woodgate, 2008). As the child grows and is able to take on some of the responsibility for his or her pulmonary care, more independent methods of secretion mobilization techniques can be introduced. These often become a primary means of secretion removal when the adolescent or young adult is away from home at college or camp.

Active Cycle-of-Breathing Techniques

Active cycle-of-breathing techniques (ACBT) include a breathing-control phase, thoracic expansion exercises, and the forced expiratory technique to clear secretions from the airways (Fig. 9.14). The breathing-control phase is defined as relaxed diaphragmatic tidal volume breathing. This phase is maintained for a few minutes and is used almost as a physiological and psychological warm-up for what is to come. Thoracic expansion exercises are defined as deep breathing, with a 3-second hold, if possible, at the top of inhalation, followed by a passive exhalation. Three or four thoracic expansion exercises are performed during this phase of ACBT. A return to the breathing-control phase (lasting seconds to minutes depending on the child's level of fatigue) follows thoracic expansion exercises as a rest period and an evaluation time. If the child feels that there are secretions ready to be moved upward, the forced expiratory technique completes the cycle. If secretions are not ready to be moved, the child returns to thoracic expansion exercises, followed by another period of breathing control for rest and evaluation of status. The forced expiratory technique, defined as one or two huffs from tidal volume down to low lung volumes, is used to expel secretions from the airways rather than coughing. The forced expiratory technique is followed by a rest period of breathing control.

Using the active cycle of breathing techniques, secretions are milked from smaller to larger airways. Once the secretions have moved into the larger airways, huffs or coughs from mid- or high-lung volumes remove the secretions. Self-percussion and postural drainage can be added to this technique if warranted. This technique relies on collateral ventilation via the pores of Kohn and channel of Lambert, which develop as the child ages, making this an appropriate technique for older children. Children 8 years of age and older are usually able to participate with this type of independent exercise program. The benefits of this technique have,

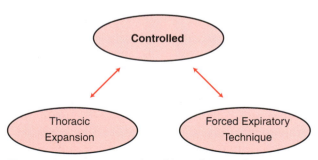

Figure 9.14 Active cycle-of-breathing techniques.

in some instances, been demonstrated to be as effective as postural drainage, percussion, and shaking, with the added benefit of independence from the caregiver (Wilson, Baldwin, & Walshaw, 1995).

Autogenic Drainage

Autogenic drainage uses controlled breathing volumes and velocities in sitting to clear excessive secretions from the airways. There are three phases to autogenic drainage: the unstick phase, the collect phase, and the evacuation phase (Fig. 9.15). Phase 1 uses quiet breathing at low lung volumes (essentially breathing in the expiratory reserve volume) to affect the secretions in the most peripheral airways. Phase 2 uses controlled breathing at low- to mid-lung volumes to mobilize secretions within the middle airways. Phase 3 uses breathing at mid- to high-lung volumes (inspiratory reserve volume) to clear secretions from central airways. Coughing is discouraged during the performance of autogenic drainage. This sequence is repeated until secretions are no longer felt within the thorax. Autogenic drainage requires that the child be able to assess his or her own needs, to locate the position of the secretions within the airways, and to target a segment of the treatment to remove the "felt" secretions. The amount of time spent in each phase is determined by the amount and the location of the pulmonary secretions felt by the child. The entire secretion removal session using autogenic drainage usually takes 30 to 45 minutes to perform. Autogenic drainage has been shown in some instances to be as effective in clearing secretions as postural drainage, percussion, and shaking in children with CF (Davidson, Wong, Pirie, & McIlwaine, 1992). In addition, autogenic drainage offers independence from caregivers and was preferred to manual secretion removal techniques in the referenced study. Autogenic drainage techniques require considerable amounts of time to learn, high concentration, and an ability to "read" the body for adequate performance. It is suggested that a child be at least 8 years old before attempting to use this technique.

Oral Airway and Chest Wall Oscillation Devices

The Flutter device uses an external apparatus to oscillate the airflow throughout the airways. The device itself resembles a pipe with a mouthpiece, a stem, and a covered bowl (Fig. 9.16). Inside this bowl is a steel ball that rests in a plastic seat. The child inhales a breath somewhat greater than tidal volume, approximately three-quarters of vital capacity. A 2- to 3-second hold of the inhaled breath is followed by an active exhalation through the Flutter device. During exhalation through the mouthpiece, the force of the exhaled air begins to raise the steel ball within the pipe bowl. The ball reaches its peak height within the device and then drops back into its plastic seat, causing a backward air pressure that jars the airways. The repeated raising and dropping of the ball throughout the exhalation phase provides an intermittent backward pressure, or oscillation, to the airway. The measurement of expiratory pressure varies from 10 to 25 cm H_2O. The usual procedure is to exhale 5 to 10 breaths that are somewhat greater than tidal volume through the Flutter device, followed by two large exhaled volumes through the Flutter device, and finally a huff or cough to clear mobilized secretions. This routine is repeated until all secretions are cleared from the lungs. The Flutter device has been shown, in some instances, to help in the removal of secretions from airways (Gondor, Nixon, Mutich, Rebovich, & Orenstein, 1999; Konstan, Stern, & Doershuk, 1994). The benefits

Figure 9.15 Phases of autogenic drainage shown on a spirogram of a normal person. Phase 1: Unstick. Phase 2: Collect. Phase 3: Evacuate. (Vt = tidal volume, IRV = inspiratory reserve volume, ERV = expiratory reserve volume, RV = residual volume, FRC = functional residual capacity.) *(From M.H. Schoni. [1989], Autogenic drainage: A modern approach to physiotherapy in cystic fibrosis.* Journal of the Royal Society of Medicine, *82[suppl. 16], 32–37. Reprinted with permission.)*

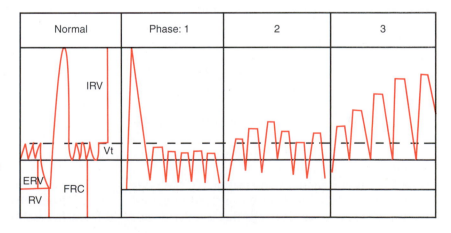

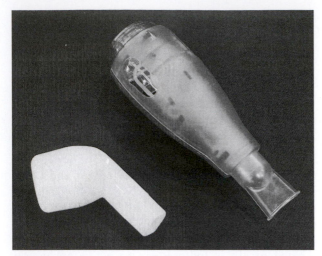

Figure 9.16 Airway oscillation devices: (Left) Flutter device. (Right) Acapella.

of a Flutter device are the relatively quick instruction period, ease of use, and independence from a caregiver. Most children older than 5 or 6 years can use the Flutter device effectively. The Flutter needs to be performed in a position that provides for maximum oscillations of the airways, usually in a seated position, limiting its use in postural drainage positions. Finally, children can keep their Flutter devices with them at school or on overnights for airway clearance when away from home.

Other means of airway oscillations include the Acapella device, which provides positive pressure and vibration to the airway to help mobilize secretions similar to the Flutter device (see Fig. 9.16). The benefit of the Acapella is that it can be used in postural drainage positions.

High-frequency airway oscillations can also be generated through commercially available ventilators. The **intrapulmonary percussive ventilator (IPV)** is a machine that delivers short bursts of air at rates of 150–220 times a minute through a mouthpiece for secretion removal. The use of IPV in children with atelectasis appears to provide more clinically important improvement than in a group using conventional chest physical therapy (positioning, percussion, and vibration) (Deakins & Chatburn, 2002). Research on secretion clearance with high-frequency oscillations versus manual secretion removal techniques has shown similar abilities in clearing secretions (Konstan et al., 1994; Schere, Barandun, Martinez, Wanner, & Rubin, 1998).

High-frequency chest wall oscillation (HFCWO) is another option for achieving the goal of secretion removal. The device is a chest vest that is inflated with

an air-pulsed generator that delivers an external force to the thorax up to 25 times per second. One benefit of HFCWO is that there is no specific position or breathing pattern required on the part of the child. HFCWO has been shown to be comparable to manual secretion removal techniques in clearing secretions and in improving pulmonary function tests during exacerbations of individuals with CF (Arens et al., 1994). Other studies have shown similar results in individuals during exacerbation of their CF (Braggion, Cappelletti, Cornacchia, Zanolla, & Mastella, 1995) and in patients with stable CF (Kluft et al., 1996; Schere et al., 1998).

Noninvasive Ventilation

Noninvasive ventilation (NIV) is based on the cyclical application of a positive pressure (or volume) to the airways using volume or positive-pressure targeted ventilators or respiratory assist devices. While evidence concerning the long-term effectiveness is sparse, NIV may be a useful adjunct to other airway clearance techniques, particularly in children with CF (Moran, Bradley, & Piper, 2009).

Positive Expiratory Pressure

The **positive expiratory pressure (PEP)** technique uses a tight-fitting mask or mouthpiece with a one-way valve to regulate expiratory resistance (Fig. 9.17). The child is seated, breathing at tidal volumes with the mask or mouthpiece securely in place. Inhalation with the mask or mouthpiece in place is unresisted. Because of the PEP provided, exhalation will be an active phase of breathing. Low-pressure PEP uses a resistance of 10 to 20 cm H_2O during mid-exhalation. After approximately 10 breaths, the mask is removed and the child huffs to clear secretions. After a brief rest period, the routine is repeated until all secretions have been cleared from the airways. For children with unstable airways, high-pressure (50 to 120 cm H_2O) PEP can be used. The child breathes up to 10 breaths with the high-pressure PEP mask in place. Huffing is done from high to low lung volumes with the mask in place, helping to stabilize the airways during the huff. High-pressure PEP requires that the resistance be individually set at the point where the child is able to exhale a larger forced vital capacity with the mask or mouthpiece in place than without. In some instances, PEP has been shown to be equally effective as, but not necessarily better than, postural drainage, percussion, and shaking (Elkins, Jones, & van der Schans, 2006; Hofmeyr, Webber, & Hodson, 1986; Oberwaldner, Evans, & Zach, 1986; Steen, Redmond, O'Neill, & Beattie, 1991; Tyrrell, Hiller,

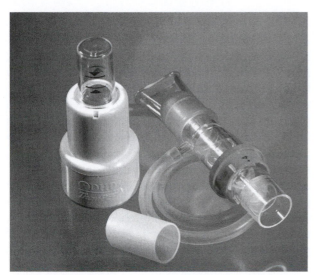

Figure 9.17 Positive expiratory pressure device. *(Photo courtesy of DHD Healthcare Corporation, Wampsville, NY 13163.)*

& Martin, 1986; Van Asperen, Jackson, Hennessy, & Brown, 1987). High-pressure PEP was shown to improve expiratory flow rates, decrease hyperinflation, and improve airway stability when compared with postural drainage, percussion, and shaking in individuals with CF (Oberwaldner, Theiss, Rucker, & Zach, 1991).

The Flutter device, PEP, HFCWO, autogenic drainage, and ACBT have all been compared with manual secretion removal techniques with a range of results. Variations in the performance of each secretion removal technique and differences in measurement make it difficult to conclude efficacy of one treatment over another (Thomas, Cook, & Brooks, 1995). Determination of a treatment plan should consider the availability of care providers, the child's level of responsibility and desire for independence, and the preference of the child (Oermann, Swank, & Sockrider, 2000).

Exercises to Increase Ventilation

Breathing exercises as a means to increase ventilation are the basis for many independent exercise programs for children. In this section, the techniques of diaphragmatic breathing exercises, segmental breathing exercises, ROM exercises, and positioning will be discussed. It is always more enjoyable for the child and the therapist to incorporate a breathing exercise program into age-appropriate play. Blowing bubbles, a toy pinwheel, or tissues can make breathing exercises fun. Blowing a ping-pong ball or a cotton ball across the table into a goal can add a more competitive aspect to a simple set of breathing exercises. The use of pediatric-sized incentive spirometers can also achieve the goal of improved ventilation. Providing written reminders with checklists at the bedside and age-appropriate motivators, such as sticker charts or video game time, may help to increase compliance with breathing exercises.

Diaphragmatic Breathing Exercises

Diaphragmatic breathing can be used to improve ventilation, decrease the work of breathing, and promote relaxation in children. With the child in a semireclining position, place the child's hand just below the xiphoid process. The therapist's hand is now placed over the child's hand. The child is asked to try to feel the therapist's hand rise up during inspiration and fall down during exhalation. Asking the child to forcefully "sniff in" may help the child feel the difference between movement of the diaphragm and abdominal muscle action. The child is asked to take in a slow deep inhalation, using that same movement of the diaphragm. The therapist's hand can provide pressure inward and under the diaphragm during exhalation, making diaphragmatic motion on inhalation more obvious. When the child begins to perform the technique correctly, the tactile cues are slowly taken away. Diaphragmatic breathing is used in breathing control, relaxation, and many independent secretion removal techniques. Diaphragmatic breathing can be encouraged in infants and children by positioning their trunks in flexion while sidelying; prone; on their knees; or supine with the head, neck, hips, and knees supported in flexion. Positioning of upper extremities in a combination of shoulder adduction, extension, and internal rotation will limit upper chest mobility, encouraging diaphragmatic breathing.

Segmental Breathing Exercises

Segmental breathing exercises use a combination of positioning, verbal commands, and tactile cues to enhance ventilation to a particular lung region. Positioning can be used to restrict thoracic motion elsewhere in the chest wall, encouraging the indicated lung segment to expand more fully. For example, a child with right middle lobe collapse can perform segmental breathing exercises while sitting in an armchair. The child places his or her right arm over the back of the chair and leans toward the left armrest. In essence, the left chest has been constrained by the resulting left lateral trunk flexion. The right chest has been opened by the position of the right upper extremity in abduction and by the positioning of the trunk. The child is instructed to inhale slowly and deeply to completely fill his or her chest with air.

The therapist's hands can be placed over the right middle lobe. As the child exhales, a firm pressure, or even the shaking technique, can encourage complete exhalation. Pressure is released, although manual contact is maintained, during the next deep inhalation. Once the child is effective in segmental expansion, the therapist's verbal and tactile cues are slowly withdrawn, leaving the child with an independent breathing exercise program.

Positioning for segmental expansion can use positions other than sitting. Using the appropriate postural drainage position described earlier in this chapter will put the affected lung segment in a gravity-independent position that will enhance ventilation to that segment. Tactile cues from the therapist's hands and appropriate verbal cues can be used to improve ventilation.

Range-of-Motion Exercises

The positions of the upper extremity, trunk, and neck have an effect on thoracic mobility. Shoulder flexion, abduction, and external rotation seem to encourage inhalation. Shoulder extension, horizontal adduction, and internal rotation encourage exhalation. Trunk extension encourages inhalation, and trunk flexion encourages exhalation. Neck extension promotes inhalation, and neck flexion seems to be a natural accompaniment to exhalation. Instructions such as "Stretch to the ceiling and inhale; now touch your toes while you exhale" can be used to coordinate the inhalation motions of upper extremity, trunk, and neck with deep inhalation and the exhalation motions of the body with exhalation. Proprioceptive neuromuscular facilitation patterns for upper-extremity ROM, when coordinated with the breathing cycle, can also be used to enhance ventilation.

Positioning Considerations

Thoughtful positioning can be beneficial to a child's CVP systems as well as to motor development and social interactions. Infant positioning should consider ventilation-perfusion matching, feeding needs, skin integrity, arterial supply and venous return, energy requirements, movement possibilities, and medical precautions. Eventually, children are meant to assume an upright posture. This posture allows them to locomote, to use their upper extremities freely, and to connect with the world face on. It also allows the ribcage to be affected by gravity and angle downward, thus changing the shape of the thorax and the alignment of the ventilatory muscles. Children should be provided the means for upright postures, whether independently or with help from assistive devices such as infant seats, adaptive seating, or adaptive standers.

Exercise and Aerobic Fitness

Aerobic exercise is an integral component of prevention and wellness programs for individuals of all ages. Physical fitness programs in children are beneficial to the establishment of life-long physical fitness. The national initiative *Healthy People 2020* (United States Department of Health and Human Services, 2009) has identified aerobic exercise as a key component of health promotion and wellness. In this section, a brief comparison of child and adult exercise physiological parameters is provided. Issues concerning the development of physical activity and fitness programs for children with CVP conditions, as well as for children of any ability, are also presented. Given the increasing importance of physical activity in all children, physical therapists should utilize resources provided by governmental organizations (National Institutes of Health, Centers for Disease Control and Prevention) and professional organizations (American College of Sports Medicine) to remain current with guidelines for pediatric physical activity and exercise science.

Exercise Response in Children

The exercise response of children demonstrates several important physiological differences when compared with that of adults. Many of the differences are related to relative body size and physical maturation. Therefore, the absolute measurement of an exercise parameter may show a significant difference between an adult and a child, but the relationship of the relative value—that is, when corrected for body size and/or mass—may not.

The cardiac response to exercise in children includes higher resting HR and higher submaximal and maximal HR compared with those of an adult. There is also a lower absolute resting stroke volume, as well as a lower submaximal and maximal stroke volume, attributable to the smaller size of the heart itself. Cardiac output is the product of HR – stroke volume. At rest, there is an absolute decrease in a child's resting cardiac output when compared with that of an adult, because the higher HR is not sufficient to counter the lower stroke volume. However, relative resting cardiac output—that is, a cardiac output corrected for the size and mass of a child—is actually higher than the resting cardiac output of an adult. Relative cardiac outputs at submaximal and maximal exercise are decreased in children compared with those of adults. Resting BP values in children are also typically lower than adult values. During exercise, the pattern of BP response to workload is similar to that in the adult, with systole increasing and diastole remaining essentially stable. However, the slope of the systolic rise is less dramatic in children.

Pulmonary system differences between children and adults are often related to the differences in body size and mass as well. The maturation of the child's pulmonary system also plays a role in exercise ability because the efficiency of the pulmonary system changes over time. Absolute lung volumes, including vital capacity and tidal volume, are directly related to body size and therefore are decreased in children. Higher resting RRs are noted in children. Minute ventilation is the product of RR – tidal volume. At rest, there is an absolute decrease in resting minute ventilation because the higher RR is not sufficient to overcome the lower tidal volume. Absolute minute ventilation is also lower at submaximal and maximal workloads. However, when corrected for size and mass, relative minute ventilation at submaximal and maximal exercise is increased in children compared with that of adults. The work of breathing during exercise is higher in children than in adults because the efficiency of their pulmonary system is not yet optimal. As with adults, ventilation is rarely the limiting system to exercise in healthy children.

Absolute maximal aerobic capacity, or VO_{2max}, is smaller in children than adults. Absolute VO_{2max} increases from childhood through adolescence, mostly caused by an increase in body size. At puberty, males continue to increase their absolute VO_{2max} into adulthood; females tend to plateau (Bar-Or & Rowland, 2004; Cerny & Burton, 2001; Krahenbuhl, Skinner, & Kohrt, 1985). The difference between a child's relative VO_{2max} and that of an adult, although still decreased, is not as dramatic as the difference in absolute VO_{2max} values.

Temperature regulation is also different in children. Although children have a relatively higher skin surface area to body mass ratio, their lower number of sweat glands and lower output from these glands impairs their ability to dissipate heat during exercise at higher environmental temperatures. Children are therefore at a higher risk for heat-related disorders. This high skin surface area also predisposes children to increased heat loss during exercise in cold environmental conditions, making them more susceptible to cold-related disorders. Excellent in-depth overviews of exercise response in children are available in the pediatric rehabilitation literature (Bar-Or & Rowland, 2004; Darbee & Cerny, 1995; Stout, 2000).

Exercise Prescription for Children

Physical fitness programs typically address cardiorespiratory endurance, flexibility, muscular strength, and body composition. Age-appropriate measures of physical fitness can be used to assess general physical fitness levels (Bar-Or & Rowland, 2004; Stout, 2000), and exercise testing can be used to assess more specifically cardiorespiratory endurance. (Refer to the section on laboratory studies for more information on exercise testing.) Current physical activity recommendations for children are for 60 or more minutes a day of physical activity, of which most time should be either moderate- or vigorous-intensity aerobic physical activity and should include vigorous-intensity physical activity at least 3 days a week. Inclusion of both muscle- and bone-strengthening activities should be included on at least 3 days of the week. In addition, limiting periods of inactivity to less than 2 hours and participation in 30 minutes of moderate activity on most days of the week are current physical activity guidelines. The same general exercise prescription parameters of intensity, frequency, duration, and mode that are used to improve CVP endurance in adults also pertain to children.

Intensity The intensity of physical activity should be prescribed at 50% to 85% of the child's maximum capacity, or $V\dot{Y}O_{2max}$. In children with particularly low initial levels of fitness, 40% to 50% of $V\dot{Y}O_{2max}$ may be appropriate. Using the Karvonen formula for prescribing exercise intensity accounts for the child's higher resting HR and the higher maximal exercise HR (Table 9.10). By using 50% to 85% of HR reserve, or 40% to 50% in a child with a low fitness level, one can calculate exercise target HR ranges to ensure exercise training while maintaining a safe exercise session. Rate of perceived exertion (RPE) can also be used with older children to monitor exercise intensity (Table 9.11).

Duration Although the current recommended duration of aerobic activity for health benefits is approximately 60 minutes, it should be adjusted to the child's attention span and kept "fun." The Centers for Disease Control and Prevention (CDC) frequently update recommendations for physical activity (http://www.cdc.gov/physicalactivity/everyone/guidelines/children.html).

■ **Table 9.10** Karvonen's Formula for the Prescription of Exercise Intensity

(HR max – HR rest) × 85% + HR rest = High end of target HR range

(HR max – HR rest) × 50% + HR rest = Low end of target HR range

(HR max – HR rest) × 40% + HR rest = Low end of target HR range with initial low levels of fitness

Table 9.11 Borg Scale of Perceived Exertion

6	
7	Very, very light
8	
9	Very light
10	
11	Fairly light
12	
13	Somewhat hard
14	
15	Hard
16	
17	Very hard
18	
19	Very, very hard

Source: Adapted from G.A. Borg (1982). Psychophysical bases of perceived exertion. *Medicine and science in sports and exercise, 14,* 377–387. Copyright by the American College of Sports Medicine.

Younger children may need a variety of different activities to keep them interested and challenged for 30 minutes at a time. Older children are better able to understand complex rule sets and want to engage in longer games with more complex play.

Frequency   Frequency of exercise is dependent on duration. If the duration of exercise can be 30 minutes, a frequency of 3 to 5 times per week is appropriate. If the duration is less than 30 minutes, the frequency should increase. Shorter, more frequent bouts of physical activity can be used to improve fitness.

Mode   Habitual physical activity (walking to school, free outdoor play, recess) and more structured physical activity (exercise classes, physical education) improve health. Activity modes for children can often be found in age-appropriate forms of play. For infants, encouraging parents and caregivers to place toys slightly out of the infant's reach will require the infant to use larger muscle masses, such as the shoulder, abdominal, and trunk musculature. The additional physical effort required with this activity benefits the CVP systems. Creeping and crawling in safe, interesting, open spaces encourages CVP endurance and promotes motor development as does rolling in children with severe physical limitations. Encouraging the family to take walks together, even if the infant is sitting upright in a stroller, can require greater physical effort than simply sitting or resting at home.

Modes of activities for toddlers and young children are also forms of age-appropriate play. Locomotion in any form—scaling obstacle courses, playing ball, walking, running, chasing soap bubbles, or riding a bike—uses larger muscles and will encourage CVP endurance. Young children enjoy music and dancing. Songs of appropriate tempo and duration can help encourage longer periods of physical activity. School-age children continue to enjoy physical activity with daily periods of typical "playground" activities. Gym class, after-school programs, and simple ball games can promote cardiorespiratory endurance.

As organized sports become more competitive in late elementary school, the distinction between the more athletic and the less athletic child becomes more evident. At this same time, a transformation in body composition related to puberty and changes in interests converge, often resulting in a decline of physical activity. Walking programs, aerobic dance programs, fitness courses, hiking, gardening, or other physical activities that are noncompetitive in nature can provide important alternative aerobic activities to organized sports programs. Technology has both positive and negative impacts on physical activity levels. The increasing reliance on electronic means of communication and entertainment provides more sedentary means of socialization (e.g., texting, computer-based communication, video and computer games) rather than active sports or games with friends. On the other hand, the recent emergence of active video game technology (e.g., Dance Dance Revolution, Nintendo Wii and Wii Fit) may provide more opportunity for "fun" physical activity for older children and adolescents.

Concerns about body composition can be a positive factor in promoting participation in physical fitness for some adolescents, but by high school, adolescents find their "free time" reduced by homework, employment, and other after-school activities. Sports are more competitive than ever, and children may be eliminated from participation or "benched" based on their lack of ability. Less time is allotted to physical education during school, with gym class often held only once or twice a week. If physical fitness habits are not already in place by this age, participation in physical activity will likely be dropped when time is short. Health promotion and wellness programs targeted at the adolescent could be an integral component in promoting physical fitness throughout the life span.

Resistance activities can also be encouraged, provided the proper guidelines and techniques are followed. Strength training that allows for proper breathing, 10 to 15 repetitions with the chosen amount of resistance, and movements that use multiple muscles and span multiple joints can be included into a child's activity program on a twice-weekly basis.

Aerobic Exercise in Children With Impairment of Pulmonary Structures and Function

The potential benefits of aerobic activity in children with chronic CVP disease include (1) an improved sense of well-being, (2) an increase in aerobic capacity and exercise tolerance, (3) an increase in ventilatory muscle strength and endurance, and (4) enhanced secretion clearance (Bar-Or & Rowland, 2004). To ensure safety as well as training, an exercise prescription for children with CVP systems impairments should specify intensity, frequency, duration, and mode. Monitoring and documenting vital signs, including HR, RR, BP, breathing pattern, Sao_2, and RPE during exercise, will help maintain a safe exercise session. Supplemental oxygen should be considered in children with documented hypoxemia during exercise.

The pulmonary system is typically not a limiting factor in aerobic capacity. However, in children with chronic pulmonary disease, exercise tolerance may be limited by pulmonary impairments. To appropriately prescribe exercise intensity for this population, it is helpful to consider pulmonary reserve, the amount of ventilation that is available for exercise, or the difference between resting minute ventilation and maximal minute ventilation. When the pulmonary reserve is very low (i.e., the child has a severe pulmonary limitation), the child will have a higher minute ventilation at rest, will be using a higher percentage of his or her ventilatory ability at lower workloads, and will have a limited ability to perform exercise as a result of pulmonary impairments. In this population, short bursts of high-intensity exercise with interspersed rest periods can be used to produce training. If the pulmonary reserve is larger, a more moderate exercise intensity for a longer duration may be possible. Resumption of a familiar exercise program after a pulmonary exacerbation may require altering the usual exercise intensity until the child can be progressed back to pre-exacerbation levels of exercise. Pediatric physical therapists can encourage children with CVP system impairments to participate in exercise programs that, even at low intensities, can provide aerobic training and encourage long-term participation in physical fitness programs.

Frequency and duration of aerobic exercise are related to the intensity of the activity prescribed. If the duration of exercise can be maintained for 30 minutes, the frequency of that activity should be 3 to 5 times per week. On the other hand, if the activity consists of short bouts of high-intensity exercise, then the exercise needs to be performed on a daily basis. Exercise progression is usually focused on increasing exercise duration until 20 to 30 minutes of continuous exercise is achieved. Exercise intensity can then be progressed to continue aerobic training.

The mode of activity should be judged based on the ability to provide safe and effective conditioning. Activities should be aerobic in nature and have the potential for adjustments in workload. Limitation, or at least modification, of collision sports is necessary in many instances.

The typical environment for the activity mode should be evaluated. Winter sports, including figure skating, ice hockey, and skiing, are performed in an environment that is cold and dry, which may not be optimal for a child with reactive airway disease. Different modes of exercise performed in a warm or more humid environment may allow for longer exercise duration and higher exercise intensity. The timing of pharmacological interventions, particularly the use of bronchodilators, before the exercise session should ensure that the child is optimally medicated during the exercise program. Gentle warm-up activities before the actual exercise session may also help to diminish airway reactivity. The limited thermoregulation ability of children should be considered if the typical environment for an activity is either very hot or very cold. Children with CF need to be concerned with salt depletion in warmer environments, making it more important to replenish both fluids and electrolytes during the exercise session.

Children with secretion retention as part of their pulmonary disease, specifically CF, often find that aerobic exercise aids in secretion clearance. Exercise in conjunction with manual secretion removal techniques has been found to enhance secretion clearance in children with CF. Although exercise alone was not found to be as effective, the combination of exercise and secretion removal techniques seems to be complementary (Bilton, Dodd, Abbot, & Webb, 1992; Sahl, Bilton, Dodd, & Webb, 1989). The benefit of long-term aerobic exercise in children with CF is a slower rate of decline in pulmonary function and an improved sense of well-being (Schneiderman-Walker et al., 2000). A recent review of physical training in children with CF indicates that exercise, aerobic or anaerobic, is not harmful and may be beneficial (Bradley & Moran, 2008).

Inspiratory muscle training has been a treatment technique for adults with chronic lung disease. Inspiratory muscle training, using an inspiratory threshold loading device, may improve the inspiratory muscle endurance, lung function, and quality of life in children with CF, but more research is necessary (Houston, Mills, & Solis-Moya, 2008) The ability to translate this improvement into an improvement in exercise capacity, dyspnea, fatigue, or pulmonary function test scores has had mixed results (Asher, Pardy, Coates, Thomas, & Macklem, 1982; de Jong, van Aalderen, Kraan, Koeter, & van der Schans, 2001; Sawyer & Clanton, 1993). The prescription for exercise using an inspiratory muscle training device varied from study to study, especially in the intensity of exercise prescribed, which may account for the differences in results. Activity training programs targeting the thoracic and shoulder muscles, such as swimming and canoeing, have also been shown to increase ventilatory muscle endurance (Keens et al., 1977).

Children with chronic pulmonary disease have an increased use of the accessory muscles of ventilation. The addition of static stretching of upper extremity, shoulder, back, and neck musculature to a general stretching program can improve flexibility. The American College of Sports Medicine (ACSM, 2008) guidelines for achieving and maintaining flexibility include (1) frequency of 3 times per week, (2) intensity that stretches a muscle group to the point of mild discomfort, and (3) duration of 10- to 30-second hold for each stretch, with 3 to 5 repetitions of each muscle or muscle group.

Aerobic Exercise for Children With Impairments of Cardiac Structures and Functions

Children with cyanotic heart defects will have a decrease in their aerobic capacity. Severe cyanotic cardiac defects may preclude strenuous participation in exercise. However, addressing flexibility or other less cardiac-demanding physical activity, such as modified yoga, can still promote participation in physical activities. After successful cardiac surgical repair, there may be little or no residual restrictions to aerobic capacity, and most children can participate more fully in recreational physical activities. Children with more serious cardiac defects with continued altered hemodynamics postoperatively will need to participate in a modified exercise program using more precise exercise prescription; closer monitoring of vital signs, including arrhythmias; and the ability to supply supplemental oxygen if needed. Children with severe obstructive conditions such as aortic stenosis are at risk for sudden death, fainting, and chest pain and should undergo exercise testing and cardiology evaluation prior to participation in exercise programs. Care should also be taken in children who have undergone Mustard (correction of

transposition of the great arteries) or Fontan (resulting in a single functional ventricle) surgical procedures as they often continue to exhibit decreased exercise tolerance related to decreased VO_{2max}, alterations in peak and resting heart rates, depressed stroke volume with exercise, right ventricular impairment, and oxygen desaturation with exercise (Bar-Or & Rowland, 2004).

Exercise recommendations for children with Kawasaki disease, particularly those with coronary artery involvement or aneurysms, should be made in conjunction with the cardiologist and after exercise testing (Bar-Or & Rowland, 2004).

Children with certain types of impairments of cardiac structures and functions may have pacemakers implanted to ensure an adequate HR response at all times. There are many different types of pacemakers available. A pacemaker is described by (1) where the pacemaker senses the underlying cardiac rhythm (A = atrium, V = ventricle, D = dual [both atrium and ventricle]), (2) where the pacemaker will deliver an electrical impulse (A, V, or D), and (3) what the pacemaker will do when it senses the underlying cardiac rhythm (I = inhibit, T = deliver, or D = either inhibit or deliver an electrical impulse). Therefore, a VVI pacemaker senses the underlying cardiac rhythm within the ventricle, will deliver the impulse to the ventricle, and will inhibit the pacemaker if a timely beat is already sensed within the ventricle. If a child's heart is paced at a constant rate, such as 90 beats per minute, the needed increase in cardiac output during exercise is provided by stroke volume alone. A rate response pacemaker has the ability to consistently readjust its program in response to the child's level of activity. When an increase in the child's activity is sensed, the pacemaker increases its firing rate to account for the increased activity. This increase in HR, along with an increase in stroke volume, will increase cardiac output, similar to what the heart of a healthy child would do.

Children who are candidates for a heart, lung, or heart-lung transplant often participate in a supervised exercise program before and after transplantation. Children who have undergone a heart or a heart-lung transplant have a modified HR response to increased physical activity and exercise. Post–cardiac transplant, there is no direct nervous input to the transplanted heart, and increases in HR are dependent on circulating catecholamines rather than the autonomic nervous system. A longer warm-up is beneficial to prime the heart for increased exercise intensity. HR will stay higher longer after exercise has ceased because the catecholamines remain the system. A longer cool-down period will allow for the slower decline in HR back to resting levels. As

HR lags behind exercise intensity, using an RPE scale is helpful in prescribing exercise intensity. Familiarity with, and acceptance of, an established exercise routine will allow children to improve their activity tolerance and to benefit fully from the transplant procedure.

Physical Fitness for Children of All Abilities

The prevalence of obesity among children and adolescents has been increasing in recent years (Salbe, Weyer, Lindsay, Ravussin, & Tataranni, 2002). Early childhood obesity is the greatest predictor of future obesity, suggesting that early childhood intervention is necessary to prevent and reduce obesity in later childhood and adulthood. The increased incidences of childhood obesity, asthma, and diabetes, coupled with declining physical fitness of our nation's youth, present a serious public-health concern. The prevalence of obesity among children aged 6 to 11 years increased from 6.5% in 1980 to 19.6% in 2008, and among adolescents aged 12 to 19 years increased from 5.0% to 18.1% (Ogden, Carroll, Curtin, Lamb, & Flegal, 2010; National Center for Health Statistics, 2004). Participation in physical fitness and activity programs reduces the risk of chronic illnesses such as coronary artery disease, hypertension, obesity, osteoporosis, and type 2 diabetes. While these chronic diseases are noted in adults, the pathological changes begin in childhood, so improved physical activity and health in childhood will have long-term effects into adulthood.

Children, at both 5 and 10 years of age, who demonstrate a decreased participation in organized sports and an increase in television viewing, are more apt to develop obesity. Surprisingly, only after the child has become obese is a decrease in physical activity noted. Youth-focused fitness programs provide the necessary alternatives to bridge the gap between organized sports and sedentary activities. Family and child activity preferences, and consideration of community resources to support long-term active lifestyles, should be integral concerns in physical fitness program development. To reduce obesity and modify body composition, a physical fitness program should include activities to increase total energy expenditure (Bar-Or, 2000; Bar-Or & Rowland, 2004). Energy expenditure can be increased by selecting activities that involve large muscle groups, such as walking, cycling, rollerblading, skating, swimming, or dancing. The United States Department of Health and Human Services (2008) has developed objectives for physical activity and fitness programs (http://www.cdc.gov/HealthyYouth/physicalactivity/guidelines.htm). The Healthy People 2020 directive should be reviewed by all physical therapists (http://www.healthypeople.gov).

The promotion of physical activity of individuals with physical disabilities is also a public health concern (Heath & Fentem, 1997). Optimal physical fitness should be a goal for children of all abilities. Children with disabilities demonstrate decreased physical work capacity that affects their daily physical activities (Dresen, de Groot, Corstius, Krediet, & Meijer, 1982). Several studies have shown that measures of cardiorespiratory endurance are decreased in children with a variety of neuromuscular conditions, including CP (Lundberg, 1978), spina bifida (Agre et al., 1984), spinal cord injuries (Janssen, van Oers, van der Woude, & Hollander, 1994), muscular dystrophy (Sockolov, Irwin, Dressendorfer, & Bernauer, 1977), and Down syndrome (Dichter, Darbee, Effgen, & Palisano, 1993). Children with neuromuscular impairments may have difficulty participating in traditional fitness programs, but maintaining physical fitness is still critical. The ability of children to complete their activities of daily life without undue fatigue can be enhanced by improving their overall fitness. Weight-loading activities in children with CP can also provide increased bone stores and play a role in osteoporosis prevention (Chad, Bailey, McKay, Zello, & Snyder, 1999).

Equipment

Medical equipment may be helpful in improving, promoting, and maintaining ventilation and mobility. Physical therapists should remain current in their knowledge of equipment types, purpose, indications for use, and proper maintenance of equipment.

Inhalation Devices

Nebulizers and inhalation devices, such as metered-dose inhalers (MDIs), are commonly used to deliver topical medications to the airways of children with airway disease. Educating a child in proper breathing patterns in an appropriate body position can maximize ventilation and optimize deposition of the medication. Physical therapists can assist young children, or children with neuromuscular impairments, in the coordination of breathing with MDI use or suggest the use of adaptive MDIs. Most MDIs now use a spacer device that allows improved particle distribution within the respiratory system.

Vital Sign and Airflow Monitors

Cardiac, apnea, and oxygen saturation monitors are often found within the hospital setting. Premature infants, those at risk for SIDS, or those with sleep apnea are often placed on these monitors at home, although their effectiveness at preventing infant morbidity/mortality has not been proven. Individuals may intermittently use these monitors during rest or sleep. Handheld spirometers are often used to measure expiratory flow rates in individuals with reactive airway diseases to monitor airway function and optimize medical management.

Mechanical Ventilation and Supplemental Oxygen

Equipment to assist with ventilation may include positive and negative pressure ventilators and devices to provide continuous positive airway pressure (CPAP) or bilevel positive airway pressure (BiPAP). Different modes of ventilation are used, depending on the nature of the CVP disease, its severity, and the age and size of the child. Description of these different ventilatory modes is beyond the scope of this text. In children with impaired ventilation, such ventilatory assisting equipment may be used intermittently or all of the time, but most often during sleep or rest times. Children with neuromuscular diseases and associated impairments of respiratory structures and functions with concomitant progressive limitations in activities and participation may maintain adequate mobility by adapting their electric wheelchair for a portable ventilation device.

Supplemental oxygen is used in children as it is in adults. Criteria for the need of supplemental oxygen are an SaO_2 less than 88%, a PaO_2 less than 55 mm Hg, or a significant decrease in oxygenation with activity or during sleep. Supplemental oxygen can be delivered at low pressures via nasal cannula or face mask. In individuals with CF, short-term oxygen therapy improves exercise duration, time to fall asleep, and regular school attendance. However, more research is needed to better define the prescription of chronic oxygen use in individuals with CF (Elphick & Mallory, 2009). Various types of home and portable oxygen tanks and concentrators are available from home-care companies that deliver and maintain the equipment.

Implanted and External Medical Devices

It has become more common for children to have implanted cardiac pacemakers or to receive medications through infusion pumps or in subcutaneous reservoirs for drug delivery. These devices may require additional considerations, particularly with exercise participation. For example, children with insulin pumps need to consider whether the pump is waterproof prior to swimming, and insulin may freeze during participation in winter sports. Contact over implanted medication reservoirs and device, such as from manual percussion, should be done with caution.

Adaptive Supports

Abdominal supports can be used to improve ventilation in children with strength impairments of the abdominal wall. These supports act to increase abdominal pressure and improve the diaphragm's resting position. The more domed the diaphragm resting position, the more effective is the diaphragm contraction as a result of the improved length-tension relationship of that muscle. Children who lack postural control may improve their ability to ventilate with proper thoracic positioning in sitting. In infants and young children, minimization of neck flexion and/or rotation by positioning devices or head restraints adapted to wheelchair, stroller, or car seat can improve ventilation and ensure patent airways.

Service Delivery Models

A variety of service delivery models are found for children with impairments in structure and function of the CVP systems. Direct provision of physical therapy services for individuals with CVP primary impairments is common. In the hospital setting, where children with chronic CVP disease may be periodically admitted, a primary physical therapist is often assigned to provide continuity of care over years of possible hospital admissions. Providing direct physical therapy service over time allows for a close relationship to develop between the therapist and child. However, with changes in health-care coverage, direct services are often provided only during periods of exacerbation, or as respite services for parents and family providing the routine care. The physical therapist who provides intermittent direct care should review the current plan of care and make updates to the program based on the child's age, abilities, tolerance, progression, or current needs of the child and family. Caregiver questions or concerns about the current plan of care within the home setting should be addressed. A review of intervention techniques should be provided, as well as education of new care providers.

Infants and children with complex CVP conditions benefit from collaboration among the many caregivers, including nutritionists, physicians, psychologists, social workers, nurses, physical therapists, occupational therapists, and respiratory therapists. Collaboration among family, medical providers, school, and community can ensure a consistent and supportive environment for the child with CVP conditions. Physical therapists also act as consultants to, or are involved as team members in, a number of areas of pediatric care, including pediatric solid organ transplantation programs, pediatric pulmonary clinics, pediatric neuromuscular clinics, and seating clinics.

Physical therapists play a major role in health promotion and wellness, including promotion of physical fitness in children. The Individuals with Disabilities Education Improvement Act (IDEA) has resulted in greater inclusion of children into regular education programs, including the physical education component. Physical therapists are increasingly involved in after-school recreational programs focused on physical activity or fitness, whether providing direct intervention or consultation in the design of such programs. In particular, the expertise of physical therapists can promote physical fitness for children of all abilities and physical skill levels, including those children with special health-care needs. Physical therapists are also involved in community organizations as consultants for development of appropriate recreational programs for children of all abilities. The design of accessible parks, recreational systems, and sports and fitness programs for children are important health-promotion and wellness roles for the physical therapist. The physical therapist's broad area of expertise provides many avenues to improve the quality of medical care and life for children with CVP conditions.

Summary

Pediatric physical therapy practice considers both the short-term management and enablement of a child and ensuring the best possible outcome across the child's future lifespan. Physical therapy for the child with CVP impairments intervenes at multiple levels of care, from secretion management, thoracic flexibility, breathing exercises, preoperative and postoperative care, to physical activity and fitness training across the lifespan. Physical therapists need to be actively involved in the promotion of physical activity and fitness for children of all abilities. The physical therapy profession is uniquely prepared for this role and can provide continuity in care and management across settings, ages, abilities, and medical status.

DISCUSSION QUESTIONS

1. How does the timing of the embryonic development of the heart relate to structural development of the lungs?

2. Describe the type of shunt (direction of blood flow) created via the ductus arteriosus in utero and the impact of the first few postnatal breaths on the shunt.

3. What are the similarities and differences in impairments and interventions between asthma and exercise-induced bronchospasm?

4. Children with neuromuscular disease may use a wheelchair for locomotion. What effect does seating have on the pulmonary system?

5. Compare the pros and cons of the following interventions for a child with cystic fibrosis: (1) postural drainage positioning, percussion, shaking, and coughing, (2) use of the Flutter device in the seated position, and (3) aerobic exercise program.

6. Explain how a strength and endurance exercise program focused on the trunk and upper extremities can be beneficial to pulmonary system function.

7. What are considerations in the prescription of an aerobic activity program for sedentary, obese adolescents aged 12 to 15 years?

8. A child with an atrial conduction abnormality is treated by a pacemaker. Explain what an AVD pacemaker is, and explain why this device was chosen for this situation. How would this device impact your prescription and monitoring of a program of physical activity or exercise for this child?

Recommended Readings

American College of Sports Medicine (2008). *ACSM's guidelines to exercise testing and prescription* (8th ed.). Baltimore: Williams & Wilkins.

Bar-Or, O., & Rowland, T.W. (2004). *Pediatric exercise science: From physiological principles to health care application.* Champaign, IL: Human Kinetics.

Cerny, F., & Burton, H. (2001). *Exercise physiology for health care professionals.* Champaign, IL: Human Kinetics.

Durstine, J.L., & Moore, G.E. (2003). *ACSM's exercise management for persons with chronic diseases and disabilities.* Champaign, IL: Human Kinetics.

Goodman, C.C., Boissonnault, W.G., & Fuller, K.S. (2003). *Pathology: Implications for the physical therapist.* Philadelphia: W.B. Saunders.

Patrick, K., Spear, B., Holt, K., & Sofka, D. (2001). *Bright futures in practice: Physical activity.* Arlington, VA: National Center for Education in Maternal and Child Health.

Sadowski, S.L. (2009). Congenital cardiac disease in the newborn infant: Past, present, and future. *Critical Care Nursing Clinics of North America, 21*(1), 37–48.

United States Department of Health and Human Services (2009). *Healthy people 2020.* Washington, DC: Author. Available at http://www.healthypeople.gov/HP2020/

References

Abadir, S., Sarquella-Brugada, G., Mivelaz, Y., Dahdah, N., & Miró, J. (2009). Advances in paediatric interventional cardiology since 2000. *Archives of Cardiovascular Diseases, 102*(6–7), 569–82.

Abbott, J., & Gee, L. (2003). Quality of life in children and adolescents with cystic fibrosis. *Pediatric Drugs, 5*(1), 42–56.

Agre, J.C., Findley, T.W., McNally, C., Habeck, R., Leon, A.S., Stradel, L., Birkebak, R., & Schmalz, R. (1984). Physical activity capacity in children with myelomeningocele. *Archives of Physical Medicine and Rehabilitation, 68,* 372–377.

Aitken, M. (1996). Cystic fibrosis, editorial overview. *Current Opinion in Pulmonary Medicine, 2*(6), 435–438.

American Alliance for Health, Physical Education, Recreation, and Dance. *The AAHPERD physical best program.* Reston, VA. (AAHPERD). (1999).

American College of Sports Medicine (ACSM). (2008). *ACSM's guidelines to exercise testing and prescription* (8th ed.). Baltimore: Williams & Wilkins.

American College of Sports Medicine (ACSM) & American Heart Association (AHA). (2007). Exercise and acute cardiovascular events: Placing the risks into perspective: Joint position statement. *Medicine & Science in Sports & Exercise. 39*(5), 886–897.

American Heart Association Council on Cardiovascular Disease in the Young. (2007). Noninherited risk factors and congenital cardiovascular defects: Current knowledge: A scientific statement from the American Heart Association Council on Cardiovascular Disease in the Young. *Circulation, 115,* 2995–3014.

American Physical Therapy Association (APTA) (2001). Guide to physical therapist practice (2nd ed.). *Physical Therapy, 81,* 6–746.

Arens, R., Gozal, D., Omlin, K.J., Vega, J., Boyd, K.P., Keens, T.G., et al. (1994). Comparison of high frequency chest compression and conventional chest physiotherapy in hospitalized patients with cystic fibrosis. *American Journal of Respiratory Critical Care Medicine, 150*(4), 1154–1157.

Asher, M.I., Pardy, R.L., Coates, A.L., Thomas, E., & Macklem, P.T. (1982). The effects of inspiratory muscle training in patients with cystic fibrosis. *American Review of Respiratory Diseases, 126*(5), 855–859.

Baker, J., Olsen, L.W., & Sørense, T.I. (2007). Childhood body-mass index and the risk of coronary heart disease in adulthood. *New England Journal of Medicine, 357*(23), 2329–2337.

Bancalari, E., Abdenour, G.E., Feller, R., & Gannon, J. (1979). Bronchopulmonary dysplasia: Clinical presentation. *Journal of Pediatrics, 95,* 819–823.

Bar-Or, O. (2000). Juvenile obesity, physical activity and lifestyle changes. *The Physician and Sportsmedicine, 28*(11), 51–58.

Bar-Or, O., & Rowland, T.W. (2004). *Pediatric exercise science: From physiological principles to health care application.* Champaign, IL: Human Kinetics.

Barron, K.S., Shulman, S.T., Rowley, A., Taubert, K., Myones, B.L., Meissner, H.C., et al. (1999). Report of the National Institutes of Health Workshop on Kawasaki Disease. *Journal of Rheumatology, 26*(1), 170–190.

Bernstein, S., Heimler, R., & Sasidhara, P. (1998). Approaching the management of the neonatal intensive care graduate through history and physical exam. *Pediatric Clinics of North America, 45*(1), 79–105.

Bilton, D., Dodd, M.E., Abbot, J.V., & Webb, A.K. (1992). The benefits of exercise combined with physiotherapy in the treatment of adults with cystic fibrosis. *Respiratory Medicine, 86*(6), 507–511.

Bokulic, R.E., & Hilman, B.C. (1994). Interstitial lung disease in children. *Pediatric Clinics of North America: Respiratory Medicine II, 41*(3), 543–567.

Borg, G.A. (1982), Psychophysical bases of perceived exertion. *Medicine and Science in Sports and Exercise, 14,* 377–387.

Borowitz, D. (1996). The interrelationship of nutrition and pulmonary function in patients with cystic fibrosis. *Current Opinions in Pulmonary Medicine, 2*(6), 457–461.

Bradley, J.M., & Moran, F. (2008). Physical training for cystic fibrosis. *Cochrane Database of Systematic Reviews*, Issue 1. Art. No.: CD002768. doi: 10.1002/14651858.CD002768.pub2.

Braggion, C., Cappelletti, L.M., Cornacchia, M., Zanolla, L., & Mastella, G. (1995). Short-term effects of three chest physiotherapy regimens in patients hospitalized for pulmonary exacerbations of cystic fibrosis: A cross-over randomized study. *Pediatric Pulmonology, 19*(1), 16–22.

Brannon, F.J., Foley, M.W., Starr, J.A., & Saul, L.M. (1998). *Cardiopulmonary rehabilitation: Basic application.* Philadelphia: F.A. Davis.

Buckingham, M., Meilhac, S., & Zaffran, S. (2005). Building the mammalian heart from two sources of myocardial cells. *Nature Reviews, 6,* 826–835.

Bush, A. (2009). Prenatal presentation and postnatal management of congenital thoracic malformations. *Early Human Development, 85*(11), 679–684.

Cerny, F.J. (1989). Relative effects of bronchial drainage and exercise for in-hospital care of patients with cystic fibrosis. *Physical Therapy, 69*(8), 633–639.

Cerny, F., & Burton, H. (2001). *Exercise physiology for health care professionals.* Champaign, IL: Human Kinetics.

Chad, K.E., Bailey, D.A., McKay, H.A., Zello, G.A., & Snyder, R.E. (1999). The effect of a weight-bearing physical activity program on bone mineral content and estimated volumetric density in children with spastic cerebral palsy. *Journal of Pediatrics, 135*(1), 115–117.

Cordes, K.R., & Srivastava, D. (2009). MicroRNA regulation of cardiovascular development. *Circulation Research, 104*(6), 724–732.

Corey, M., & Farewell, V. (1996). Determinants of mortality from cystic fibrosis in Canada. *American Journal of Epidemiology, 143,* 1007–1017.

Darbee, J., & Cerny, F.J. (1995). Exercise testing and exercise conditioning for children with lung dysfunction. In S. Irwin & J.S. Tecklin (Eds.), *Cardiopulmonary physical therapy* (3rd ed., pp. 563–578). St. Louis: Mosby.

Davidson, A.G.F., Wong, L.T.K., Pirie, G.E., & McIlwaine, P.M. (1992). Long-term comparative trial of conventional percussion and drainage physiotherapy versus autogenic drainage in cystic fibrosis. *Pediatric Pulmonology Supplement 8*, 298.

Deakins, K., & Chatburn, R.L. (2002). A comparison of intrapulmonary percussive ventilation and conventional chest physiotherapy for the treatment of atelectasis in the pediatric patient. *Respiratory Care, 47*(10), 1162–1167.

Decesare, J., Graybill-Tucker, C.A., & Gould, A.L. (1995). Physical therapy for the child with respiratory dysfunction. In S. Irwin & J.S. Tecklin (Eds.), *Cardiopulmonary physical therapy* (3rd ed., pp. 516–562). St. Louis: Mosby.

de Jong, W., van Aalderen, W.M., Kraan, J., Koeter, G.H., & van der Schans, C.P. (2001). Inspiratory muscle training in patients with cystic fibrosis. *Respiratory Medicine, 95*(1), 31–66.

Dichter, C.G., Darbee, J.C., Effgen, S.K., & Palisano, R.J. (1993). Assessment of pulmonary function and physical fitness in children with Down syndrome. *Pediatric Physical Therapy, 5*, 3–8.

Doershuk, C.F., Fischer, B.J., & Matthews, L.W. (1975). Pulmonary physiology of the young child. In E.M. Scarpelli (Ed.), *Pulmonary physiology of the fetus, newborn and child*. Philadelphia: Lea & Febiger.

Dresen, M.H.W., de Groot, G., Corstius, J.J., Krediet, G.H., & Meijer, M.A. (1982). Physical work capacity and daily physical activities of handicapped and non-handicapped children. *European Journal of Applied Physiology, 48*, 241–252.

Elkins, M.R., Jones, A., & van der Schans, C. (2006). Positive expiratory pressure physiotherapy for airway clearance in people with cystic fibrosis. *Cochrane Database of Systematic Reviews*, (2): CD003147. doi: 10.1002/14651858.CD003147. pub3.

Elphick, H.E., & Mallory, G. (2009). Oxygen therapy for cystic fibrosis. *Cochrane Database Systematic Reviews*, (1): CD003884

Eng, P.A., Morton, J., Douglass, J.A., Riedler, J., Wilson, J., & Robertson, C.F. (1996). Short-term efficacy of ultrasonically nebulized hypertonic saline in cystic fibrosis. *Pediatric Pulmonology, 21*(2), 77–83.

Fedderly, R.T. (1999). Left ventricular outflow obstruction. *Pediatric Clinics of North America: Pediatric Cardiology, 46*(2), 369–384.

Fitzgerald, D.A., Hilton, J., Jepson, B., & Smith, L. (2005). A cross-over randomized, controlled trial of dornase alfa before versus after physiotherapy in cystic fibrosis. *Pediatrics, 116*, 4549–554.

Gaultier, C. (1995). Respiratory muscle function in infants. *European Respiratory Journal, 8*(1), 150–153.

Gondor, M., Nixon, P., Mutich, R., Rebovich, P., & Orenstein, D. (1999). Comparison of flutter device and chest physical therapy in the treatment of cystic fibrosis during pulmonary exacerbation. *Pediatric Pulmonology, 28*, 255–260.

Goss, C.H., & Quittner, A. (2007). Patient-reported outcomes in cystic fibrosis. *Proceedings of the American Thoracic Society, 4*, 378–386.

Grifka, R.G. (1999). Cyanotic congenital heart disease with increased pulmonary blood flow. *Pediatric Clinics of North America: Pediatric Cardiology, 46*(2), 405–425.

Gross, S.J., Iannuzzi, D.M., Kveselis, D.A., & Anbar, R.D. (1998). Effect of preterm birth on pulmonary function at school age: A prospective controlled study. *Journal of Pediatrics 133*, 188–192.

Guyton, A. (1996). *Textbook of medical physiology* (9th ed., p. 487). Philadelphia: W.B. Saunders.

Heath, G.W., & Fentem, P.H. (1997). Physical activity among persons with disabilities: A public health perspective. *Exercise and Sport Science Reviews, 25*, 216.

Henderson, A.J. (2008). What have we learned from prospective cohort studies of asthma in children. *Chronic Respiratory Disease, 5*, 225–231.

Herrera-Soto, J.A., Vander Have, K.L., Barry-Lane, P., & Myers, J.L. (2007). Retrospective study on the development of spinal deformities following sternotomy for congenital heart disease. *Spine, 32*(18), 1998–2004.

Hershenson, M.B., Colin, A.A., Wohl, M.E., & Stark, A.R. (1990). Changes in the contribution of the rib cage to tidal breathing during infancy. *American Review of Respiratory Disease, 141*(4 Pt 1), 922–925.

Hintz , S.R., Van Meurs, K.P., Perritt, R., Poole, W.K., Das, A., Stevenson, D.K., Ehrenkranz, R.A., Lemons, J.A., Vohr, B.R., Heyne, R., et al. (2007). Neurodevelopmental outcomes of premature infants with severe respiratory failure enrolled in a randomized controlled trial of inhaled nitric oxide. *Journal of Pediatrics, 151*(1), 16–22, 22.e1–3.

Hoffman, J.I., & Kaplan, S. (2002). The incidence of congenital heart disease. *Journal of American College of Cardiology, 39*, 1890–1900. Review.

Hofmeyr, J.L., Webber, B.A., & Hodson, M.E. (1986). Evaluation of positive expiratory pressure as an adjunct to chest physiotherapy in the treatment of cystic fibrosis. *Thorax, 41*(12), 951–954.

Holloway, E., & Ram, F.S.F. (2002). Breathing exercises for asthma (Cochrane Review). *The Cochrane Library*, Issue 4. Oxford: Update Software.

Hough, J.L, Flenady, V., Johnston, L., & Woodgate, P.G. (2008). Chest physiotherapy for reducing respiratory morbidity in infant's requiring ventilatory support. *Cochrane Database Systematic Reviews, 16*(3): CD006445, DOI: 10.1002/14651858. CD006445.pub.2.

Houston, B.W., Mills, N., & Solis-Moya, A. (2008). Inspiratory muscle training for cystic fibrosis. *Cochrane Database of Systematic Reviews*, (4): CD006112. doi: 10.1002/14651858. CD006112.pub2.

Hulsmann, A.R., & van den Anker, J.N. (1997). Evolution and natural history of chronic lung disease of prematurity. *Monaldi Archives for Chest Disease, 52*, 272–277.

Jacob, S.V., Lands, L.C., Coates, A.L., Davis, G.M., MacNeish, C.F., Hornby, L., Riley, S.P., & Outergridge, E.W. (1997). Exercise ability in survivors of severe bronchopulmonary dysplasia. *American Journal of Respiratory and Critical Care Medicine 155*, 1925–1929.

Janssen, T.W.J., van Oers, C.A.J.M., van der Woude, L.H.V., & Hollander, A.P. (1994). Physical strain in daily life of wheelchair users with spinal cord injuries. *Medicine and Science in Sports and Exercise, 26*, 661–670.

Jongbloed, M.R., Mahtab, E.A., Blom, N.A., Schalij, M.J., & Gittenberger-de Groot, A.C. (2008). Development of the cardiac conduction and the possible relation to predilection sites of arrhythmogenesis. *Scientific World Journal, 3*(8), 239–269.

Keens, T.G., Krastins, J.R., Wannamaker, E.M., Levison, H., Crozier, D.N., & Bryan, A.C. (1977). Ventilatory muscle endurance training in normal subjects and patients with cystic fibrosis. *American Review of Respiratory Disease, 116,* 853–860.

Kirby, M.L., & Waldo, K.L. (1995) Neural crest and cardiovascular patterning. *Circulation Research, 77,* 211.

Klinnert, M.D., Nelson, H.S., Price, M.R., Adinoff, A.D., Leung, D.Y., & Mrazek, D.A. (2001). Onset and persistence of childhood asthma: Predictors from infancy. *Pediatrics, 108*(4).

Kluft, J., Beker, L., Castagnino, M., Gaiser, J., Chaney, H., & Fink, R.J. (1996). A comparison of bronchial drainage treatments in cystic fibrosis. *Pediatric Pulmonology, 22,* 271–274.

Konstan, M.H., Stern, R.C., & Doershuk, C.F. (1994). Efficacy of the Flutter device for airway mucus clearance in patients with cystic fibrosis. *Journal of Pediatrics, 124,* 689–693.

Korhonen, P., Tammela, O., Koivisto, A.M., Laippala, P., & Ikonen, S. (1999). Frequency and risk factors in bronchopulmonary dysplasia in a cohort of very low birth weight infants. *Early Human Development, 54,* 245–258.

Krahenbuhl, G.S., Skinner, J.S., & Kohrt, W.M. (1985). Developmental aspects of maximal aerobic power in children. *Exercise and Sport Sciences Reviews, 13,* 503–538.

Kravitz, R.M. (1994). Congenital malformations of the lung. *Pediatric Clinics of North America: Respiratory Medicine II, 41*(3), 453–472.

Lane, P.A. (1996). Sickle cell disease. *The Pediatric Clinics of North America: Pediatric Hematology, 43*(3), 639–664.

Lara, M., Rosenbaum, S., Rachelefsky, G., Nicholas, W., Morton, S.C., Emont, S., et al. (2002). Improving childhood asthma outcomes in the United States: A blue print for action. *Pediatrics, 109,* 919–930.

Limperopoulos, C., Tworetzky, W., McElhinney, D.B., Newburger, J.W., Brown, D.W., Robertson, R.L., Guizard, N., McGrath, E., Geva, J., Annese, D., et al. (2010). Brain volume and metabolism in fetuses with congenital heart disease: Evaluation with quantitative magnetic resonance imaging and spectroscopy *Circulation, 121*(1), 26–33.

Lundberg, A. (1978). Maximal aerobic capacity of young people with spastic cerebral palsy. *Developmental Medicine and Child Neurology, 20,* 205–210.

Mannino, D.M., Homa, D.M., Oertowski, C.A., Ashizawa, A., Nixon, L.L., Johnson, C.A., et al. (1998). Surveillance for asthma: United States, 1960–1995. *Morbidity and Mortality Weekly Report, 47,* 1–27.

Marshal, B.C., Butler, S.M., Stoddard, M., Moran, A.M., Liou, T.G., & Morgan, W.J. (2005). Epidemiology of cystic-fibrosis related diabetes. *Journal of Pediatrics, 146,* 681–687.

Massery, M. (2006). The patient with multi-system impairments affecting breathing mechanics and motor control. In D. Frownfelter & E. Dean (Eds.), *Cardiovascular and Pulmonary Physical Therapy Evidence and Practice* (4th ed., pp. 695–717). St. Louis: Mosby & Elsevier Health Sciences.

McColley, S. (1998). Bronchopulmonary dysplasia: Impact of surfactant replacement therapy. *Pediatric Clinics of North America, 45,* 573–584.

Miatton, M., De Wolf, D., François, K., Thiery, E., & Vingerhoets, G. (2007). Neuropsychological performance in school-aged children with surgically corrected congenital heart disease. *Journal of Pediatrics, 151*(1), 73–78.

Moran, F., Bradley, J.M., & Piper, A.J, (2009). Non-invasive ventilation for cystic fibrosis. *Cochrane Database Systematic Reviews. 21*(1): CD002769.

Mukhopadhyay, S., Singh, M., Cater, J., Ogston, S., Franklin, M., & Oliver, R. (1995). Nebulised anti-pseudomonal antibiotic therapy in cystic fibrosis: A meta-analysis of benefits and risks. *Thorax, 51,* 364–368.

National Center for Health Statistics. (2004). *Health, United States, 2004 with Chartbook on Trends in the Health of Americans.* Hyattsville, MD: Author.

Newell, S.J., Booth, W., Morgan, M.E., Durbin, G.M., & McNeish, A.S. (1989). Gastroesophageal reflux in preterm infants. *Archives of Disease in Childhood, 64,* 780–786.

Nikolaizik, W., & Schonl, M. (1996). Pilot study to assess the effect of inhaled corticosteroids on lung function in patients with cystic fibrosis. *Journal of Pediatrics, 128,* 271–274.

Nixon, G.M., Glazner, J.A., Martin, J.M. & Sawyer, S.M. (2002). Urinary incontinence in female adolescents with cystic fibrosis. *Pediatrics, 110*(2 Pt. 1), e22.

Nixon, P. (1996). Role of exercise in the evaluation and management of pulmonary disease in children and youth. *Medicine and Science in Sports and Exercise, 28*(4), 414–420.

Nixon, P. (2003). Cystic fibrosis. In J.L. Durstine & G.E. Moore, *ACSM's Exercise management for persons with chronic diseases and disabilities* (pp. 111–116). Champaign, IL: Human Kinetics.

Northway, W., Rosan, R.C., & Porter, D.Y. (1967). Pulmonary disease following respiratory therapy of hyaline membrane disease: Bronchopulmonary dysplasia. *New England Journal of Medicine, 176,* 357–368.

Oberwaldner, B., Evans, J.C., & Zach, M.S. (1986). Forced expirations against a variable resistance: A new chest physiotherapy method in cystic fibrosis. *Pediatric Pulmonology, 2*(6), 358–367.

Oberwaldner, B., Theiss, B., Rucker, A., & Zach, M.S. (1991). Chest physiotherapy in hospitalized patients with cystic fibrosis: A study of lung function effects and sputum production. *European Respiratory Journal, 4,* 152–158.

Oermann, C., Swank, P., & Sockrider, M. (2000). Validation of an instrument measuring patient satisfaction with chest physiotherapy techniques in cystic fibrosis. *Chest, 118,* 92–97.

Ogden, C.L., Carroll, M.D., Curtin, L.R., Lamb, M.M., & Flegal, K.M. (2010). Prevalence of high body mass index in U.S. children and adolescents, 2007–2008. *Journal of the American Medical Association, 303*(3), 242–249.

Park, M.K., & Guntheroth, W.G. (1992). *How to read pediatric ECGs* (3rd ed.). St. Louis: Mosby.

Pierpont, M.E., et al. (2007). Genetic basis for congenital heart defects: Current knowledge: A scientific statement from the American Heart Association Congenital Cardiac Defects Committee, Council on Cardiovascular Disease in the Young. *Circulation, 115,* 3015–3038.

Pilmer, S.L. (1994). Prolonged mechanical ventilation in children. *Pediatric Clinics of North America: Respiratory Medicine II, 41*(3), 473–512.

Pramanik, A.K., (2010). *Respiratory distress syndrome.* http://emedicine.medscape.com/article/976034-overview

Pryor, J., & Prasad, S. (2001). *Physiotherapy for respiratory and cardiac problems* (3rd ed.). Philadelphia: Churchill Livingstone.

Pryor, J., & Webber, B. (1998). *Physiotherapy for respiratory and cardiac problems* (2nd ed., p. 338). Philadelphia: Churchill Livingstone.

Quittner, A.L., Modi, A., & Cruz, I. (2008) Systematic review of health-related quality of life measures for children with respiratory conditions. *Paediatric Respiratory Reviews, 9*, 220–232.

Roberton, N.R. (1996). Intensive care. In A. Greenough, N.R. Roberton, & A. Milner (Eds.), *Neonatal respiratory disorders* (pp. 174–195). London: Arnold.

Rothstein, J.M., Roy, S.H., & Wolf, S.L. (1998). *The rehabilitation specialist's handbook* (2nd ed., pp. 534–535). Philadelphia: F.A. Davis.

Rowley, A.H., Shulman, S.T. (1999). Kawasaki syndrome. *Pediatric Clinics of North America, 46*(2), 313–329.

Sahl, W., Bilton, D., Dodd, M., & Webb, A.K. (1989). Effect of exercise and physiotherapy in aiding sputum expectoration in adults with cystic fibrosis. *Thorax, 44*, 1006–1008.

Salbe, A.D., Weyer, C., Lindsay, R.S., Ravussin, E., & Tataranni, P.A. (2002). Assessing risk factors for obesity in childhood and adolescence: I. Birth weight, childhood adiposity, parental obesity, insulin and leptin. *Pediatrics, 110*, 299–306.

Sawyer, E.H., & Clanton, T.L. (1993). Improved pulmonary function and exercise tolerance with inspiratory muscle conditioning in children with cystic fibrosis. *Chest, 104*(5), 1490–1497.

Schere, T.A., Barandun, J., Martinez, E.R., Wanner, A., & Rubin, E.M. (1998). Effect of high frequency oral airway and chest wall oscillation and conventional chest physical therapy on expectoration in patients with stable cystic fibrosis. *Chest, 113*(4), 1019–1027.

Schneiderman-Walker, J., Pollock, S.L., Corey, M., Wilkes, D.D., Canny, G.J., Pedder, L., et al. (2000). A randomized controlled trial of a 3-year home exercise program in cystic fibrosis. *Journal of Pediatrics, 136*(3), 304–310.

Schoni, M.H. (1989). Autogenic drainage: A modern approach to physiotherapy in cystic fibrosis. *Journal of the Royal Society of Medicine, 82*(suppl. 16), 32–37.

Shah, P.L., Scott, S.F., Knight, R.A., & Hodson, M.E. (1996). The effects of recombinant human DNase on neutrophil elastase activity and interleukin-8 levels in the sputum of patients with cystic fibrosis. *European Respiratory Journal, 9*(3), 531–534.

Smith, J., Travis, S., Greenberg, E., & Welsh, M. (1996). Cystic fibrosis airway epithelia fail to kill bacteria because of abnormal surface fluid. *Cell, 85*, 229–236.

Smyth, A., & Walters, S. (2003). Prophylactic anti-staphylococcal antibiotics for cystic fibrosis (review) *Cochrane Database of Systematic Reviews, 3.*

Sockolov, R., Irwin, B., Dressendorfer, R.H., & Bernauer, E.M. (1977). Exercise performance in 6 to 11 year old boys with muscular dystrophy. *Archives of Physical Medicine and Rehabilitation, 58*, 195–201.

Steen, H.J., Redmond, A.O., O'Neill, D., & Beattie, F. (1991). Evaluation of the PEP mask in cystic fibrosis. *Acta Paediatrica Scandinavica, 80*(1), 51–56.

Stout, J. (2000). Physical fitness during childhood and adolescence. In S.K. Campbell, D.W. Vander Linden, & R.J. Palisano (Eds.), *Physical therapy for children* (2nd ed., pp. 141–169). Philadelphia: W.B. Saunders.

Swartz, M.H. (1994). *Textbook of physical diagnoses: History and examination* (2nd ed.). Philadelphia: W.B. Saunders.

Thomas, J., Cook, D.J., & Brooks, D. (1995). Chest physical therapy management of patients with cystic fibrosis. *American Journal of Respiratory Critical Care Medicine, 151*, 846–850.

Thorensen, M., Cavan, F., & Whitelaw, A. (1988). Effect of tilting on oxygenation in newborn infants. *Archives of Disease in Childhood, 63*, 315–317.

Toro-Salazar, O.H., Steinberger, J., Thomas, W., Rocchini, A.P., Carpenter, B., & Moller, J.H. (2002). Long-term follow-up of patients after coarctation of the aorta repair. *American Journal of Cardiology, 89*(5), 541–547.

Towbin, J.A. (1999). Pediatric myocardial disease. *Pediatric Clinics of North America: Pediatric Cardiology, 46*(2), 289–312.

Treatment Guidelines from the Medical Letter, (2008). *Medical Letter, 6*(76), 83–90.

Tyrrell, J.C., Hiller, E.J., & Martin, J. (1986). Face mask physiotherapy in cystic fibrosis. *Archives of Disease in Childhood, 61*(6), 598–600.

United States Department of Health and Human Services (2009). *Healthy people 2020.* Washington, DC: Author. Available at http://www.healthypeople.gov/HP2020/

Van Asperen, P.P., Jackson, L., Hennessy, P., & Brown, J. (1987). Comparison of a positive expiratory pressure (PEP) mask with postural drainage in patients with cystic fibrosis. *Australian Paediatric Journal, 23*(5), 283–284.

van der Schans, C., Prasad, A., & Main, E. (2004). Chest physiotherapy compared to no chest physiotherapy for cystic fibrosis (Systematic Review). Cochrane Cystic Fibrosis and Genetic Disorders Group. *Cochrane Database of Systematic Reviews, 2.*

Van Essen-Zandvliet, E.E., Hughes, M.D., Waalkens, H.J., Duiverman, E.J., Pocock, S.J., & Kerrebijn, K.F. (1992). Effects of 22 months of treatment with inhaled steroids and/or beta2 agonists on lung function, airway responsiveness and symptoms in children with asthma. *American Review of Respiratory Disease, 146*, 547–554.

Verklan, M.T. (1997). Bronchopulmonary dysplasia: Its effects upon the heart and lungs. *Neonatal Network, 16*(8), 5–12.

Wilkins, R.L., & Drider, S.J. (1985). *Clinical assessment in respiratory care.* St. Louis: Mosby.

Wilson, G.E., Baldwin, A.L., & Walshaw, M.J. (1995). A comparison of traditional chest physiotherapy with the active cycle of breathing in patients with chronic suppurative lung disease. *European Respiratory Journal, 8*(suppl. 19), 171S.

Wilson, C.J., Robbins, L.J., Murphy, J.M., & Chang, A.B. (2007). Is a longer time interval between recombinant human deoxyribonuclease (dornase alfa) and chest physiotherapy better? *Pediatric Pulmonology, 42*, 1110–1116.

World Health Organization (2007). *International Classification of Functioning, Disability and Health—Children and Youth Version.* ICF-CY.

CHAPTER 10

Integumentary System

—Suzanne F. Migliore, PT, DPT, MS, PCS

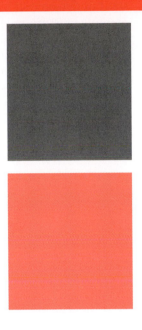

The role of the physical therapist in wound care has evolved over the past several decades. For the physical therapist, the groundwork for learning wound and burn management occurs in the entry-level curriculum. Mechanisms of healing and systems reviews that enhance the knowledge base for caring for a child with open wounds or burns are taught. Physical therapists who desire to be active in wound management need to expand their knowledge through continuing education and, as with any specialty, competency-based training with a mentor. Pediatric clinicians need to be prepared to encounter a wide range of integumentary issues with children. Children are at risk for thermal injuries, pressure ulcers, and traumatic wounds. There are also specific congenital integumentary impairments that will challenge the pediatric clinician's ability to provide timely and age-appropriate interventions. This chapter will serve as an introduction to wound and burn management for the physical therapist as part of an interdisciplinary pediatric wound-management team.

Intervention Settings

Acute-care physical therapists play an integral role on the wound-management team. Therapists work closely with physicians and nurses to achieve wound closure using the various interventions that are discussed in this chapter. In the rehabilitation setting, the physical therapist faces challenges regarding management of chronic wounds and burns after the acute healing process or after grafting. Additionally, the physical therapist must address how the patient will achieve independence with functional skills. For example, in the outpatient setting, therapists are often called on to maximize function and to decrease activity or encourage participation limitations in situations involving open wounds. Therapists also intervene with scar management techniques after wound closure.

School-based therapists need to have background knowledge in the areas of wound and scar management because children with traumatic wounds, pressure ulcers, and burns will eventually return to school after their acute care and rehabilitation. Although school-based therapists may not provide direct wound care, other interventions usually need to be performed throughout the school day. Examples include using static or dynamic splints after a thermal injury, implementing pressure-relieving techniques for a child with a pressure ulcer, and reintegrating a child in school activities after an integumentary injury. Working with teachers and other classmates, the school-based therapist can assist in transitioning a child back to school after prolonged hospitalization. Such children may face issues surrounding cosmesis, body image, and peer acceptance.

Skin Structure and Function

The skin is the largest external organ of the human body, covering a surface area of 2 m². To best understand the etiology of integumentary impairments, physical therapists need to know the anatomy and physiology of the skin. Its primary functions are sensation, metabolism, thermoregulation, and protection from trauma (Rassner, 1994). The skin has two primary layers, the epidermis and the dermis. A schematic drawing of the layers of the epidermis and dermis is shown in Figure 10-1.

Epidermis

The **epidermis,** the outermost layer of the skin, is approximately 0.04 mm thick. There are four layers in the epidermis: the stratum corneum, stratum granulosum, stratum spinosum, and stratum basale. A fifth layer, the stratum lucidum, is found in the soles of the feet and

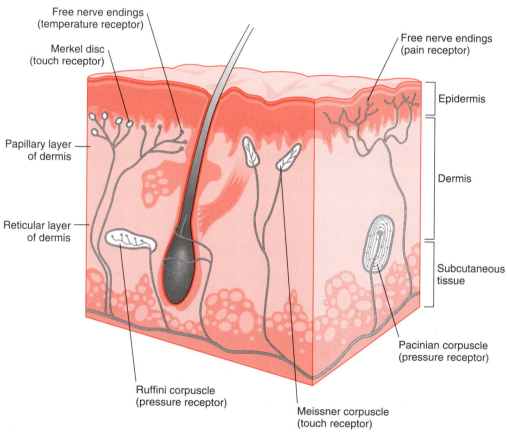

Figure 10.1 Schematic representation of the skin structures.

the palms of the hands (Patterson & Blaylock, 1987). Structures in the epidermis include melanocytes, Langerhans cells, hair follicles, sebaceous and apocrine glands, and eccrine sweat glands. The hair follicle contains primarily epidermal tissue, which plays a key role in reepithelialization of wounds (Falkel, 1994). The epidermis is nonvascular and forms a defensive covering for the dermis. The epidermis varies in thickness throughout the body, with the surfaces of the hands and feet having the deepest thickness. It limits water evaporation from the surface of the skin and molds itself onto the papillary layer of the dermis, forming the epidermal-dermal junction (Gray, 1977).

Dermis

The **dermis** is the "true skin," which is tough, flexible, and highly elastic. Its thickness varies throughout the body. The dermal layer is very thick in the palms of the hands and soles of the feet and very thin in the eyelids and genitalia. The thickness of the skin at the location of an open wound or thermal injury plays a role in the severity of injury. For example, pressure at the sacrum has the potential to cause more damage than pressure at the ischial tuberosity because of the thinness of the skin and the lack of depth of subcutaneous tissues.

The dermis has two layers: the outermost papillary layer and the deeper reticular layer. The reticular layer contains fibroelastic material, mostly collagen. The dermis is highly vascular and contains structures including lymphatic cells, epithelial cells, connective tissue, muscle, fat, and nerve tissue. The vascular supply of the dermal layer supplies nutrition to the epidermis and aids in regulating body temperature (Gray, 1977).

Phases of Wound Healing

The main phases of wound healing are inflammation, proliferation, and maturation. The phases may overlap in the course of wound healing, but each has unique physiological events. Understanding the phases and being able to identify the phase that a wound is in will guide the clinician in choosing appropriate interventions. The ideal outcome of a wound-management program is to influence healing toward wound closure.

Inflammatory Phase

The hallmark signs of the inflammatory process are changes in color, increased skin temperature, swelling, and the presence of pain. The main goal of the inflammatory phase is to rid the wound of debris and prepare the wound for healing by fighting infection. The first part of the inflammatory phase is the vascular response,

with the main goal being to stop the hemorrhage. Catecholamines are then released and produce vasoconstriction; at the same time, collagen and other cells activate platelets and initiate the "clotting cascade" to prevent further bleeding. Increased cell permeability then produces the edema response, which is immediate and continuous for hours (Greenhalgh & Staley, 1994), leading to the second part of the inflammatory phase, the cellular response.

The cellular response is an elaborate and well-orchestrated array of cells migrating toward the area of injury. Neutrophils tend to migrate toward the wound space within the first 24 hours. Their function is to act as phagocytic cells and fight bacteria. The neutrophil helps to keep the wound clean. Wounds with bacterial counts greater than 10^5 are considered infected (Bates-Jensen & Ovington, 2007). Mast cells respond by releasing histamine, which plays a role in cell permeability. During the cellular response, after the body has produced enough platelets for clotting, mast cells change their effect and produce heparin. Heparin then stimulates endothelial cells to migrate toward the wound. Other cells involved in this phase include macrophages, which act to rid the wound of debris. Macrophages have also been linked to the transition to the proliferative phase of wound healing. This transition is accomplished by the macrophage secreting angiogenesis growth factor (AGF). AGF then stimulates endothelial cells and reestablishes the blood flow to the injured area. Through angiogenesis, nutritional supply is reestablished to the wound bed. **Fibroblasts** also appear during the inflammatory phase. Fibroblasts aid in the production of the collagen matrix, which is more clearly defined during the proliferative phase. Late in the inflammatory phase, fibroblasts differentiate into myofibroblasts, which aid in wound contraction. Endothelial and epithelial cells also respond during this phase. From the onset of trauma, the epithelial cells respond from the dermis. These cells begin the resurfacing process known as reepithelialization. The epithelial cells in the inflammatory phase also aid in ridding the wound of necrotic tissue by releasing lytic enzymes (Sussman & Bates-Jensen, 2007).

Proliferative Phase

Two key steps toward wound healing occur during the proliferative phase: fibroplasia and wound contraction. These steps provide the wound bed with needed nutrition and oxygen to allow early progression toward wound closure. Ongoing during this phase are angiogenesis and epithelialization.

Fibroplasia

Fibroplasia is the laying down of the collagen matrix that is known as granulation tissue. The stimulus for fibroplasia, according to Ross (1968), is "an optimal inflammatory response." The angiogenesis that began in the inflammatory phase supplies nutrition and oxygen to this matrix. Cells that respond to the wound during this phase include fibroblasts, myofibroblasts, and endothelial and epidermal cells. The fibroblast is responsible for producing the collagen matrix, which is called procollagen. The procollagen becomes tropocollagen, which eventually forms a collagen fibril. These fibrils are laid down in the wound bed in a disorganized manner. Cross-linkage occurs when the collagen matrix comes together; the better the organization of the matrix, the better the overall improvement in wound tensile strength. When fibroplasia is occurring, the collagen matrix looks like pink or red granules or "buds" piled on top of each other, as seen in Figure 10.2 (Sussman & Bates-Jensen, 2007). During this stage of the proliferative phase, the granulation buds are fragile and cannot sustain any force from an outside trauma. Such trauma can damage the tissue, causing a regression to the inflammatory phase. The potential for regression must be considered when cleansing wounds and applying dressings, which is discussed later in this chapter.

Wound Contraction

During wound contraction, myofibroblasts have the "contractile properties of smooth muscle cells" (Sussman & Bates-Jensen, 2007). The myofibroblast attaches to the wound edges, pulling the epidermal layer toward the center of the wound. The contracting forces appear to come from the cells that are within the granulation tissue (Ross, 1968). The size and shape of the wound will also have an effect on its ability to contract. A linear wound will contract the fastest; circular wounds, such as pressure ulcers, will contract the slowest (Sussman & Bates-Jensen, 2007).

Epithelialization

As described earlier under the inflammatory phase, epithelialization begins immediately after trauma. The ongoing process of reepithelialization or resurfacing of the wound continues during the proliferative phase. The epithelial cells respond to messages from macrophages and neutrophils and advance toward the wound surface in sheets. Epidermal cells in the front of this "sheet" act to rid the wound of debris and allow for resurfacing from the edges of the wound. A moist wound environment is most advantageous for this cell migration. Due to the depth of a full-thickness wound, epidermal cells fail to migrate fully and are unable to resurface the wound. The cells will approach from the wound edges and then appear to roll under the edges, causing epidermal rolling or ridging, as seen with a chronic pressure ulcer. Wounds of this depth and chronic nature will not be able to heal by resurfacing (Sussman, 2007a).

Maturation Phase

During the maturation (or remodeling) phase, three processes occur: collagen lysis, collagen organization, and scar formation. This phase begins a few weeks after trauma and may last for up to 2 to 3 years.

Collagen Lysis/Organization

To regulate fibroplasia during the proliferative phase, the enzyme collagenase is produced. Collagenase has the ability to break the cross-linkages of the tropocollagen; this process is called collagen lysis. During the maturation phase, the balance between collagen synthesis and collagen lysis is a key factor. As a wound matures, collagen lysis takes over and aids in the organization of the collagen bundles. The more organized the bundles, the better the outcome, as seen with a smooth and elastic scar (Sussman & Bates-Jensen, 2007).

Scar Formation

While the organization of the collagen is occurring, the fibronectin that is laid down during fibroplasia is eliminated and large bundles of type I collagen are present.

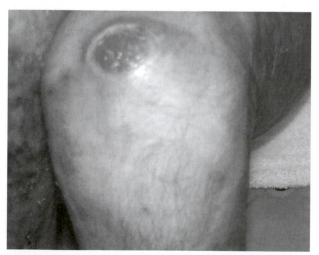

Figure 10.2 Example of granulation buds in a stage II pressure ulcer. See also color plate.

A decrease in the number of small blood vessels occurs, and the new scar, which usually has a bright red appearance, starts to fade. During the maturation phase, an increase in the cross-linkages of collagen fibers will increase the strength of the scar.

While the scar is forming, any diversion from the normal processes might lead to abnormal healing. Wounds that take a longer time to heal may develop hypertrophic (thicker/erythematous) scars. This thickening appears to come from prolonged collagen synthesis and angiogenesis. A **hypertrophic scar** has a raised appearance, as seen in Figure 10.3. A hypertrophic scar that extends above and beyond the original scar site is considered a keloid. The reasons for hypertrophic and keloid type scars are not known. Any event that prolongs the inflammatory phase can lead to excessive scarring. The propensity for raised scars may also be attributed to the location of the wound and to ethnic heritage and age (Ward, 2007).

Recommended readings for a more comprehensive look at wound healing include *Wound healing: Alternatives in management* (Kloth & McCulloch, 2002) and *Wound care: A collaborative practice manual for health professionals* (3rd ed.) (Sussman & Bates-Jensen, 2007).

Integumentary Impairments

To provide appropriate interventions to children with integumentary impairments, the clinician must possess knowledge of the pathophysiology of each body function. The following is a review of some diagnoses with integumentary impairments.

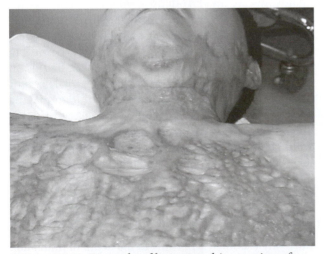

Figure 10.3 Example of hypertrophic scarring after full-thickness burns and skin grafting.

Pressure Ulcers

Despite the usual correlation of pressure ulcers with the geriatric population, the pediatric population is also at risk. Any child who has decreased sensation, inability to communicate pain and discomfort, prolonged bed rest, poor nutrition, or a known integumentary disorder is at risk for pressure ulcers. Children with spina bifida or spinal cord injury have an increased propensity for skin breakdown caused by impaired sensation. Child and caregiver education for skin care and pressure ulcer prevention is imperative.

Pressure occludes blood flow to the local tissues, ultimately causing ischemia and hypoxemia. Four levels of skin breakdown can occur in correlation to the amount of time exposed to pressure. Hyperemia can occur in less than 30 minutes and presents as local redness that dissipates within 1 hour of relief of pressure. Ischemia occurs after 2 to 6 hours of pressure; the erythema that is present takes up to 36 hours to dissipate. Necrosis is the next level of breakdown, and occurs after 6 hours of continuous pressure. Ulceration is the final level of breakdown; it may occur up to 2 weeks after an episode of necrosis.

Factors leading to pressure ulcers include immobility, shear, friction, and moisture. **Shear** is a parallel force that causes ischemia by displacing blood vessels. **Friction** occurs when two surfaces move across each other, abrading and damaging the epidermal and upper dermal layers. Friction and shear occur most commonly during position changes in bed and transfers from bed to other surfaces, including stretchers or wheelchairs. Caution must be taken by all caregivers to avoid friction and shear when moving or transferring children. In children who are incontinent, constant moisture can lead to skin maceration, making the skin more prone to breakdown (Rappl, 2007).

Staging of Pressure Ulcers

Pressure ulcers are described or "staged" according to depth and tissue damage. To provide timely interventions, members of the multidisciplinary team must recognize the stage of the pressure ulcer. In February 2007, the National Pressure Ulcer Advisory Panel (NPUAP) revised the Agency for Health Care Policy and Research (AHCPR) definition of an ulcer as well as the definitions of the various stages, adding two stages to the original four. The NPUAP defines a pressure ulcer as "localized injury to the skin and/or underlying tissue, usually over a bony prominence, as a result of pressure, or pressure in combination with shear and/or friction" (NPUAP, 2007). The stages of pressure ulcers are defined by NPUAP as follows:

- Suspected deep tissue injury: Purple or maroon localized area of discolored, intact skin or a blood-filled blister due to damage of underlying soft tissue from pressure and/or shear. The area may be preceded by tissue that is painful, firm, mushy, boggy, or warm as compared to adjacent tissue. This stage may be difficult to detect in individuals with dark skin tones. Evolution may include a thin blister over a dark wound bed. The wound may further evolve and become covered by thin eschar. Evolution may be rapid, exposing additional layers of tissue even with optimal treatment.
- Stage I: Intact skin with nonblanchable redness of a localized area, usually over a bony prominence. Darkly pigmented skin may not have visible blanching; its color may differ from the surrounding area. The area may be painful, firm, soft, and warmer or cooler than adjacent tissue. This stage may be difficult to detect in patients with dark skin tones.
- Stage II: Partial-thickness skin loss of dermis, presenting as (1) a shiny or dry, shallow open ulcer with a red or pink wound bed without slough or (2) an intact or open/rupture serum-filled blister. This stage should not be used to describe skin tears, tape burns, perineal dermatitis, maceration, or excoriation. Bruising indicates suspected deep tissue injury.
- Stage III: Full-thickness skin loss. Subcutaneous fat may be visible but bone, tendon, or muscle are not exposed. Slough may be present, but does not obscure the depth of tissue loss. Undermining and tunneling may occur. Depth of this stage of pressure ulcer varies by anatomical location. The bridge of the nose, ear, occiput, and malleolus do not have subcutaneous tissue; therefore stage III ulcers in these areas can be shallow. In contrast, areas of significant adiposity can develop extremely deep stage III pressure ulcers.
- Stage IV: Full-thickness tissue loss with exposed bone, tendon, or muscle. Slough or eschar may be present on some parts of the wound bed. Undermining and tunneling are common. Depth varies by anatomical location. Ulcers can extend into muscle and/or supporting structures (e.g., fascia, tendon, or joint capsule), making osteomyelitis possible.
- Unstageable: Full-thickness tissue loss in which the base of the ulcer is covered by slough (yellow, tan, gray, green, or brown) and/or eschar (tan, brown, or black) in the wound bed.

Limitations of these definitions require clinical judgments. For example, stage I ulcers are those with intact skin and may not be assessed accurately in children with darker, pigmented skin. Stage IV pressure ulcers may have associated sinus tracts. If thick, leathery, necrotic, devitalized tissue (**eschar**) is present, the ulcer cannot be correctly staged until it is removed (NPUAP, 2007). Note that as a pressure ulcer heals, it will always be described according to its original stage. Documentation of a "healing stage I, II, III, or IV" ulcer is appropriate; an ulcer should not be downstaged (e.g., from a III to a II) as it heals. (Sussman, 2007a).

The child's participation in life activities is limited according to the stage, size, and location of the pressure ulcer. Pressure ulcers on weight-bearing surfaces will limit mobility, ability to sit, and ambulation. Children may be limited from lying on their backs, sitting up in their wheelchairs, or walking with orthotics. With the most severe pressure ulcers, especially those on the sacrum or ischial tuberosities, the child may be limited to prone positioning while out of bed. For children who are non-ambulatory, being restricted from using their wheelchairs will limit their participation in activities in the home and their ability to participate in school or work.

Thermal Injuries

Thermal injuries are the third most common cause of death in children younger than the age of 1 year, preceded only by nonfirearm homicides and motor vehicle accidents. Between the ages of 1 and 9 years, deaths from thermal injuries are second only to those from motor vehicle accidents. The most common mechanism of burn is scalding, but burns with the highest fatality rate are those from fires, which often involve inhalation injuries. The mechanism of thermal injury may also vary by age. Infants have a higher incidence of scald burns from hot beverages or from being bathed in water that is too hot. Toddlers may pull hot liquids off the stove or sustain electrical injuries from wires or plugs. School-age children are susceptible to playing with matches and have a higher incidence of flame burns than younger children. Adolescents mimic their adult counterparts in the mechanism of injury, which includes flames, chemicals, cooking, smoking materials, or fireworks (Committee on Injury and Poison Prevention, American Academy of Pediatrics, 1997).

Burn Depth Classification

Burns are classified according to the depth of injury and the affected skin structures. The three classifications are superficial, partial thickness, and full thickness.

Superficial Burns **Superficial burns** are caused by ultraviolet exposure, sunburn, or a short flash of heat. Only epidermal layers are affected. The skin is erythematous but does not show any signs of blistering. Healing occurs within 3 to 7 days.

Partial-Thickness Burns **Partial-thickness burns** are split into two categories, superficial and deep, depending on the involved structures. Superficial partial-thickness burns involve damage to the epidermis and some of the papillary dermis. The skin is blistered or weeping, as seen in Figure 10.4. These burns usually heal within 7 to 21 days without surgical intervention. Minimal scarring is expected.

Deep partial-thickness burns involve the epidermis as well as the papillary and reticular layers of the dermis. Additionally, these burns may include fat found in the subcutaneous layer. The skin presents with large blisters or mottled white to cherry-red coloration. These wounds will heal in 21 to 35 days if not infected. Depending on the burn size, deep partial-thickness burns might best be addressed surgically (see the section on surgical interventions). Scarring is likely with a deep partial-thickness burn that is allowed to heal without grafting. With all partial-thickness burns, there is increased pain and sensitivity to temperature.

Full-Thickness Burns **Full-thickness burns** involve all of the epidermis, dermis, and subcutaneous tissue, and may include fascia, muscle, tendon, and bone. The skin appears dry or leathery; no blanching is seen with pressure. With the most severe burns, the skin may appear charred. Hair follicles will pull out easily, and there is little or no pain because of the destruction of pain receptors. These burns are best managed surgically by excision and grafting.

Zones of Burn Wound Classification One difficulty with using the burn depth classification system is that thermal injuries are not traditionally uniform in their presentation. The most severe portion of the burn is typically in the center, with less involved areas surrounding it. Zones of burn wound classification were established to describe the areas involved. The most central zone is the *zone of coagulation,* which is the area of greatest destruction. The center appears white and leathery, and all viable tissue is destroyed. The *zone of stasis* surrounds the zone of coagulation. It is temporarily without blood supply, but vascular response can be restored and the healing process started. If this zone is allowed to dry out, the vascular supply will not reestablish, killing viable tissue and converting the burn to necrotic tissue. This concept is important to remember when topical agents and dressings for burns are reviewed later in this chapter. The outermost zone is the *zone of hyperemia,* which is equal to a superficial burn with intact vascular supply and blanching on pressure (Johnson, 1994).

Burn Size Estimation

In addition to determining the depth of a burn, it is important to determine the total body surface area (TBSA) involved. There are several scales and charts to map out the TBSA; however, they usually underestimate the percentage of involved skin in children (Lund & Browder, 1944). For example, the rule of nines, which is often used in adults with burns, is not as useful with pediatric patients because of the varying sizes of infants, toddlers, and school-age children. Therefore, "[t]he most accurate method of determining surface area burned is by mapping the injured areas on a Lund and Browder-like body chart and then calculating the burned area from body surface area nomograms" (Herndon, Rutan, Alison, & Cox, 1993). The TBSA is determined by age, as seen in Figure 10.5 and Table 10.1. During the initial burn examination, it is important to use the accompanying body chart to identify where the burns are located. This chart can be updated as additional burned areas are identified.

Estimating total body surface area also plays a role in fluid needs, nutritional requirements and overall prognosis. New computer-aided technology is assisting with determining TBSA more accurately. Using a computer-generated full-body diagram decreases the risk of over- or underestimating TBSA (Neuwalder, Sampson, Brueing, & Orgill, 2002).

Burn Severity and Functional Outcomes

The size and location of the burn determines the child's activity restrictions. For example, burns over joints limit range of motion (ROM); loss of muscle

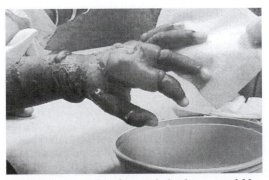

Figure 10.4 Example of partial-thickness scald burn to the hand. Note blistering and weeping of the wound.

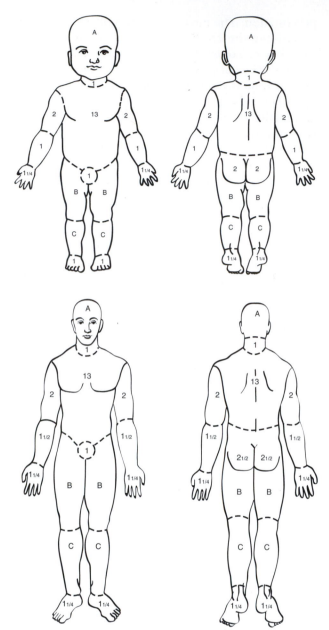

Figure 10.5 Lund and Browder chart for estimation of burn area. Caregivers can mark on the figure where partial- or full-thickness burns are with different colors or hatch marks. *(From C.C. Lund & N.C. Browder [1944]. The estimation of areas of burns.* Surgery, Gynecology, and Obstetrics, *79, 352–358. American College of Surgeons. Reprinted with permission.)*

Table 10.1 Lund and Browder Chart for Estimation of Burn Area

Area	Age (yr)				
	0–1	1–4	5–9	10–15	Adult
Head	9.5	8.5	8.5	5	3.5
Neck	1	1	1	1	1
Anterior trunk	13	13	13	13	13
Posterior trunk	13	13	13	13	13
Right buttock	2.5	2.5	2.5	2.5	2.5
Left buttock	2.5	2.5	2.5	2.5	2.5
Genitalia	1	1	1	1	1
Right upper arm	2	2	2	2	2
Left upper arm	2	2	2	2	2
Right lower arm	1.5	1.5	1.5	1.5	1.5
Left lower arm	1.5	1.5	1.5	1.5	1.5
Right hand	1.25	1.25	1.25	1.25	1.25
Left hand	1.25	1.25	1.25	1.25	1.25
Right thigh	2.25	3.25	4.25	4.25	4.75
Left thigh	2.25	3.25	4.25	4.25	4.75
Right leg	2.5	2.5	2.75	3	3.5
Left leg	2.5	2.5	2.75	3	3.5
Right foot	1.75	1.75	1.75	1.75	1.75
Left foot	1.75	1.75	1.75	1.75	1.75

Source: Lund, C.C., & Browder, N.C. (1944). The estimation of areas of burns. *Surgery, Gynecology, and Obstetrics, 79,* 352–358. American College of Surgeons. Reprinted with permission.

mass or prolonged bed rest may affect strength. Severe burns with high TBSA percentages can cause long-standing contractures and permanent body cosmesis changes. Burns on the hands can limit the child's ability to self-feed, and burns on the plantar surface of the feet will limit the ability to ambulate. A child who sustains facial burns may have limitations with swallowing, talking, and adequate nutritional intake. A referral to speech therapy for oral motor skills may be appropriate. The child's ability to participate in activities of daily living (ADLs), school, play, and sports will be affected until acute burn management and rehabilitation have occurred. The child who is burned may face a lifelong battle with episodes of decreased activities caused by scarring, requiring ongoing scar management. If restrictions are severe enough to limit participation in life activities, consideration is given to surgical interventions.

Surgical Interventions for Thermal Injuries

Partial- and full-thickness burns are typically examined and reexamined throughout their acute healing course to determine whether surgical intervention is necessary. Surgery for thermal injuries may be performed in the acute phase to resume circulation to an area after constriction caused by edema. An **escharotomy** is "a longitudinal incision through the full-thickness burn to the layer of subcutaneous fat of an extremity" (Miller, Staley, & Richard, 1994). This procedure releases the pressure on underlying blood vessels and allows more normal circulation. If the burn is left unaddressed, ischemia may occur and amputation may be necessary.

After acute management, surgical interventions focus on the elimination of devitalized tissue. The burn surgeon must remove or excise the devitalized tissue down to healthy bleeding tissue; this procedure is done with an instrument called a dermatome. Once the eschar has been excised, the surgeon must choose a method to cover the wound. Commonly an autograft, or skin graft, in which the skin is taken from another part of the body and used to cover the burn site, is used. If the TBSA percentage is extensive and limited donor skin is available, cultured skin substitutes or biological or synthetic coverings might be used.

Autografts **Split-thickness skin grafts (STSGs)** are the most common autografts used in surgical management of children with burns. The skin that is harvested from the donor site includes the epidermis and a portion of the dermis. The donor site will heal in 9 to 14 days and is treated like a superficial or partial-thickness burn.

The graft can be applied as a sheet or meshed to cover a greater surface area, as seen in Figure 10.6. The graft must be secured at the burn site, and after approximately 48 hours, blood vessels in the graft connect with vessels in the wound bed, supplying nutrition to the graft. Grafts should adhere or "take" by the fifth to seventh postoperative day. The surgeon will immobilize the grafted area to ensure that the graft takes.

Full-thickness skin grafts (FTSGs) take the entire thickness of the skin, the epidermis and the dermis, stopping short of the subcutaneous fat. They are commonly used for coverage on the palms of the hands or pressure points. The donor site of the FTSG requires primary closure or an STSG to heal.

Cultured Skin Substitutes For children with burns over a large percentage of TBSA, autografts may not be available, or because of frequent reharvesting, the healing process is delayed. With cultured epidermal autografts (CEAs), the child's own epidermal cells are harvested and grown in a laboratory. They are placed on a carrier material that will then be placed on the burn site. These cells take 2 to 3 weeks to grow. Although this is an innovative way to cover burn wounds, these substitutes are often less durable than autografts.

Biological Substitutes For children without adequate donor sites, an allograft (skin from a cadaver) may be used to cover the wound temporarily. Allografts are harvested and stored in a skin bank for use in burn management. The body will eventually reject the allograft, but it can provide wound coverage for 2 to 3 weeks while previous donor sites heal or until cultured skin is available. Heterografts or xenografts are

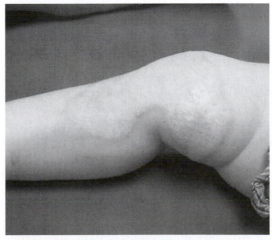

Figure 10.6 Example of meshed split-thickness skin graft.

skin grafts harvested from another species, usually a pig. Heterografts are used as a temporary covering for a wound, protecting it from further external trauma.

Synthetic Substitutes Synthetic dressings are used to aid in the healing of partial-thickness burns or to provide temporary coverage to deeper burns awaiting autografts. One example is Biobrane, "a silastic membrane bonded to a bovine collagen sheet with a nylon backing" (Miller et al., 1994). Blood/sera clot in the product's nylon matrix, which then adheres the dressing to the wound until epithelialization occurs (http://wound.smith-nephew.com/uk/node.asp?NodeId=3562).

Another example is Acticoat. This synthetic dressing is placed over a clean wound bed after débridement. The advantage of this dressing is its ability to be left in place for 3 to 5 days, thereby decreasing the number of painful dressing changes and the potential for disrupting healing tissues.

Aquacel Ag is another type of synthetic dressing that can be used for superficial or deep partial thickness burns. It is an antimicrobial dressing that releases ionic silver as wound exudate is absorbed. It can be left in place as the wound heals, thus avoiding painful dressing changes. (http://www.convatec.com/en/cvtus-aqcagdbpus/cvt-portallev1/0/detail/0/1442/1838/aquacel-ag-dressing.html).

Traumatic Wounds

Motor vehicle accidents account for one of the highest injury rates in children. Many sequelae occur, including traumatic open wounds. These can be in the form of abrasions or road burns, open fractures, and degloving injuries. Degloving injuries are those in which a large portion of the skin is traumatically torn away from the underlying tissue; this commonly happens in pedestrian-versus-car accidents, in which the pedestrian is pulled underneath the car.

Traumatic wounds often require local care and surgical interventions similar to thermal injuries with skin grafts. If the tissue deficit is large enough, a muscle rotational or free flap might be necessary for wound coverage. Rotational muscle flaps are taken from an adjacent muscle group and rotated over the defect, maintaining their vascular supply. A free flap is one in which muscle is taken from another place in the body (e.g., latissimus dorsi or rectus abdominis) and transferred to the defect site. A free flap requires skin grafting (Miller et al., 1994).

As with skin grafts, muscle flaps must avoid external trauma during the initial healing phase. The free flaps typically appear bulky and do not have a smooth, cosmetic appearance. There is also a risk of failure of the flap resulting from poor circulation or reestablishment of the blood supply and nutrition to the flap.

After a muscle flap and graft, the child will be restricted from normal activities until the graft and flap have taken. Often these wounds are associated with fractures, with the status of the healing bone dictating activity and participation levels. Children with degloving injuries have similar restrictions to those with thermal injuries who require skin grafting.

Toxic Epidermal Necrolysis and Stevens-Johnson Syndrome

Toxic epidermal necrolysis (TEN) is a "severe form of erythema multiforme that results in extensive epidermal sloughing" (Sheridan et al., 1999). It is an acute illness involving the epithelial layers of the skin and mucous membrane; the conjunctiva is also involved. TEN involves 30% or more of the TBSA; sloughing involving less than 30% is called borderline TEN (Schulz, Sheridan, Ryan, MacKool, & Tompkins, 2000). Because of the extensive skin involvement and high mortality rate in children who develop TEN, burn units are considered best prepared to deal with the multiple needs of these patients.

If the lesions in the conjunctiva are more extensive than those on the skin, the disease is known as Stevens-Johnson syndrome (SJS). SJS was found to be the most common exfoliating skin disease in children, with an overall majority of patients being male.

The pathophysiologies of TEN and SJS are unknown, but they may be linked to a viral illness or drug interaction. The most common cause of both diseases is the combination of azithromycin and ibuprofen, followed by ibrupofen alone (Dore & Salisbury, 2007). The skin lesions that appear occur at the dermal-epidermal junction. If the disease process affects the oropharyngeal and gastrointestinal systems, there is a high risk of sepsis and death. Children's survival rates improve with intervention strategies that include local wound care, nutritional support, and early detection of sepsis (Sheridan et al., 1999).

If the mucosal involvement is severe, the child will have limited ability to take in adequate calories by mouth. Nutritional supplementation must be considered to allow maximal wound management and increase strength and endurance. Children may encounter the same activity and participation limitations as those with thermal injuries. The severity of the disease and TBSA involved determines the extent of limitations. If medical and wound management is timely and effective, many children will not have long-term sequelae.

Epidermolysis Bullosa

"Inherited epidermolysis bullosa (EB) encompasses 4 major groups of skin diseases" (Fine, Johnson, Weiner & Suchindran, 2008). There are various types of EB, each differing in the way it is inherited, level of separation of the skin, and clinical manifestations. The major subdivisions of EB are determined by the level of skin involvement. The groups are epidermolysis bullosa simplex (EBS), junctional epidermolysis bullosa (JEB), dominant dystrophic epidermolysis bullosa (DDEB) and recessive dystrophic epidermolysis bullosa (RDEB). All of the subtypes are characterized by blister formation, erosion of the skin, and poorly healing ulcers. (Fine et al., 2008).

With JEB, the most severe type is EB letalis, which appears at birth. The skin and mucous membranes are involved. Infants with EB letalis usually do not survive beyond the age of 2 years; many die within the first 3 months of life. In the milder form of JEB, generalized atrophic benign EB, children survive into adulthood. Their appearance at birth is similar to those of the letalis group, but they have less severe skin and mucosal involvement.

DDEB has a wide range of severity, from mild skin eruptions, in which individuals have a normal life span, to severe, in which individuals have many impairments and limitations in normal activities during a painful and shortened life span. One of the most significant complications of DDEB is the propensity to develop squamous cell carcinomas over the bony prominences. This complication is the major cause of death for persons with severe DDEB who survive into adulthood (Atherton, 2000).

Children with EB who survive the neonatal period face a lifetime of skin disruptions, loss of normal joint movement, characteristic loss of fingers and toes, and multiple surgeries and skin grafting procedures. They are usually restricted from normal activities because of concern for skin trauma. With the newborn, special attention must be given to positioning and handling to avoid further trauma. These infants will be limited from participating in normal gross motor activities as a result of their skin disruptions. Throughout their lives, children and adolescents will experience different episodes of activity and participation limitations attributable to new blistering, more extensive skin sloughing, or immobilization after surgery.

In 2008, a longitudinal study of more than 3,000 children with some form of EB was published. Researchers found the risk of death during infancy was greatest in those patients with JEB. Causes of death varied by subtype of EB and included sepsis, pneumonia, respiratory failure, renal failure, and squamous cell carcinoma. "The risk of death among EB infants and children differs markedly by EB subtype in terms of specific cause, magnitude of risk, and timing of onset." Children with EB who survive the first 12 to 24 months of life can live into adulthood with timely and aggressive medical care (Fine et al., 2008).

Prevention

The physical therapist plays a key role in preventing integumentary impairments. Clearly, no one can prevent a congenital skin disorder, but education for families regarding etiology of the disorder and genetic counseling may help parents in family planning. Other injuries, however, are preventable, with child and caregiver education serving as the key. For children with sensory deficits, teaching them how to do daily skin inspections and proper pressure-relieving techniques can decrease the incidence of pressure ulcers. Prescribing pressure-relieving cushions and wheelchairs that provide pressure-relieving positions will also decrease the incidence. Screening tools such as the Norton Risk Assessment, the Gosnell Scale, the Neonatal Skin Risk Assessment, and the Braden Q Scale were developed to identify children at risk for skin breakdown and allow clinicians to choose appropriate interventions to avoid or reduce skin breakdown (Bates-Jensen, 2007).

Prevention education is already in place in the school setting. Children are taught fire prevention and safety, including the dangers of playing with matches, how to "stop, drop, and roll," and how to practice escape routes in their home and school. At home, parents must monitor the temperature of their water heater to decrease the likelihood of scald burns from bath water that is too hot. The physical therapist can play a role in prevention education to patients, families, and the community by reinforcing some of these basic safety suggestions.

Advocating for early referral to physical therapy can aid in preventing skin breakdown in the hospital setting. Even in the intensive care unit, with medically unstable children, positioning programs and devices are appropriate interventions. Often these interventions prevent secondary limitations from prolonged bed rest after a traumatic accident. The incidence of pressure ulcers should decrease with staff education regarding use of proper support mattresses, turning and positioning schedules, and routine skin care and inspections.

Examination and Evaluation

Child History

As with any physical therapy examination, taking a detailed history, including information about age, sex, primary language, social history, developmental history, and general health is important. Knowing the past medical history and related conditions helps the clinician to identify children at risk for skin breakdown or delayed wound healing. More detailed information is needed regarding the current integumentary issue. The child or caregiver should provide an accurate history of the mechanism of injury, but in some cases you may have to rely on information received in the field from emergency medical personnel. The mechanism of injury is important, especially in the case of traumatic or thermal injuries. For example, with a thermal injury, probing what the child was doing and wearing and what was done immediately after the burn are vital to understanding the resulting injury. The timing of medical care and what procedures or interventions were performed before the physical therapist examined the child are all important pieces of information. In the case of suspected child abuse or neglect, matching the pattern of the burn with the history is helpful in making the determination of accident versus abuse (Dressler & Hozid, 2001).

Reviewing the medical chart provides information regarding prior clinical tests and the medical care of the child. The nutritional history and current nutritional status of the child should be documented. Children who are malnourished are at greater risk of skin breakdown. Laboratory findings, especially albumin levels, are important. If serum albumin levels are below 3.5 mg/dL, the child is considered malnourished (Sussman, 2007b). The dietitian should screen all children in the hospital who are at risk for skin breakdown or who have a known integumentary disorder. In the clinic or outpatient setting, a referral to a dietitian might be applicable.

Systems Review

For any child with a potential for integumentary impairments, or with known disorders, a review all of the body systems is necessary. If cardiopulmonary comorbidities exist, they may inhibit mobilization, exercise, or wound healing. In the case of a child with a thermal and inhalation injury, the pulmonary sequelae may outweigh the integumentary disruptions. Children with musculoskeletal impairments, such as contractures, might be at greater risk for skin breakdown, as are children with decreased strength or sensation because of neuromuscular disorders. A detailed examination of the integumentary system is addressed in the next section. It is also necessary to examine the child's cognitive level and ability to communicate. If the child is unable to communicate pain or discomfort at a pressure point, he or she is at risk for skin breakdown. Barriers to learning and preferred learning styles must be identified before choosing child and family education materials.

Tests and Measures

Many tests and measures might be administered during the initial examination of a child with an integumentary disorder. A more in-depth look into the following categories is beneficial to the clinician in performing a comprehensive wound examination and evaluation.

Pain

The ability of the child to detect and determine the amount of pain allows the medical team to address pain management adequately. Therefore, use of pain scales is a must for any physical therapy examination, especially for open wounds or burns. Some scales commonly used in the pediatric population include the CRIES neonatal postoperative pain measurement score (Krechel & Bildner, 1995), the FLACC (Faces/Legs/Activity/Cry/Consolability) behavioral pain assessment tool (Malviya, Voepel-Lewis, Burke, Merkel, & Tait, 2006), the Wong-Baker faces pain rating scale (Wong & Baker, 1988), and the 0-to-10-point verbal rating scale. Each scale is used for specific age ranges or for children who have cognitive or communication disorders that inhibit them from using the appropriate age-related scale. The scales make use of physiological, behavioral, or observational measurements to determine pain (Martin-Herz, Thurber, & Patterson, 2000). Documenting pain scores before, during, and after wound care interventions is vital to identifying the need to change the pain management regimen.

For patients with cognitive impairments, a behavioral scale such as used in the FLACC tool is a reliable and valid measure of pain in children with cognitive impairments. This scale gives clinicians an objective method of pain assessment, which may reduce undertreatment of pain. New descriptors in the revised version of the FLACC tool include verbal outbursts, tremors, increased spasticity, jerking movements, and respiratory pattern changes such as grunting. These new descriptors improve the reliability of the tool among caregivers (Malviya et al., 2006).

Sensory Integrity

A thorough sensory examination including pain, pin-prick, light and deep touch, and temperature provides valuable information to the clinician regarding body structures and functions that may be intact, impaired, or absent. In the case of a thermal injury, the ability to perceive touch and pain may indicate a less severe burn, rather than the painless presentation of a full-thickness burn. For children with pressure ulcers, identifying areas of decreased sensation allows the therapist to choose interventions, such as positioning and pressure-relieving surfaces.

Range of Motion

For children who have sustained a thermal injury, initial examination of available ROM is crucial within the first 24 hours. Immediate interventions should be performed if joints are at risk or show signs of loss of range (see the section on orthotics intervention). Children in the remodeling phase of healing will have scars and scar bands forming. It is a general rule to perform active ROM (AROM) or passive ROM (PROM) for examination purposes within the limits of the scar. "If it's white, it's tight" is a good adage to remember when examining scar tissue. As you are performing PROM, take the scar band/tissue to the point of blanching and then back off by a few degrees; this is the limit of the scar. Pushing the scar past this point may result in skin tears (Humphrey, Richard, & Staley, 1994). Examining the limits of ROM is also important to identify children who are at risk for skin breakdown. A child with significant contractures and decreased ability to move is more prone to skin breakdown.

Gait, Locomotion, and Balance

Identifying the child's ability to mobilize is an important aspect of the initial examination. For children in an intensive care unit setting, mobility may be restricted because of medical stability and technology. For children who are allowed to move, their effectiveness in repositioning themselves and ambulating is important. Documentation should include the amount of assistance needed and the ability of the caregiver to provide assistance. If the child is nonambulatory, it is necessary to assess and document wheelchair mobility skills and pressure-relieving techniques.

Orthotic, Protective, and Supportive Devices

If a child has used orthotics before this episode of care, the physical therapist must assess the age, fit, and effectiveness of each device. If a device is older than 1 year or the child has gone through a recent growth spurt or weight gain, the device may be ill fitting and has the potential to cause skin breakdown. Examine wheelchairs and seat cushions to determine their effectiveness in relieving pressure.

The therapist should also obtain a wearing schedule history; doing so aids in the examination and evaluation of the orthotics. If a child is supposed to wear an orthotic for all mobility and is not wearing the device, there may be a greater risk for skin breakdown. For example, if a child with spina bifida who uses hip-knee-ankle-foot orthoses (HKAFOs) for mobility chooses to crawl around the house and not wear the HKAFOs, he or she runs the risk of creating pressure ulcers or abrasions from friction or shear on the carpet or hard floor on lower extremities that have impaired or absent sensation. On resumption of wearing the HKAFOs, the child and caregiver will need to be diligent in checking the skin and adhering to a wearing schedule. Maintaining a consistent orthotic-wearing schedule helps avoid problems with poor fit of or skin intolerance to the devices.

Integumentary Integrity

Associated Skin

The physical therapist must observe skin integrity of the entire body, especially areas prone to skin breakdown (bony prominences, sacrum, occiput, and trochanters). Identifying any discrepancy with skin coloration, **turgor** (elasticity/tension), nail growth, hair growth, texture, and temperature, is also part of a comprehensive wound examination.

Thermal Injuries

During the initial examination, determining the TBSA percentage is done by mapping the affected areas on the **Lund and Browder chart** (see Fig. 10.5 and Table 10.1). Identifying the structures that have been involved may take several days. Identify the location, joints involved, and depth at each site. For actual burn sites, document the color and texture of the wound, capillary refill, drainage, and odor. Evaluation of these findings allows the clinician to determine burn depth classifications of superficial, partial-thickness, or full-thickness injuries. Presence or absence of blisters, hair follicles, and pain associated with wound care also helps determine burn depth.

For children who are in the remodeling phase of wound healing, identifying the areas of initial thermal injury and those of donor sites is helpful. Check the scars for texture, smoothness, raised appearance, color, and flexibility. Newer scar tissue is bright pink, with more mature scars taking on the coloration of surrounding tissues. Hypertrophic and keloid-type scars have a raised appearance, with keloids presenting out of the boundaries of the original injury site. Check the scar tissue for hyperpigmentation or hypopigmentation. For children with darker pigmented skin, the scars may be hypopigmented (Ward, 2007).

In 1990, Sullivan and colleagues created the Vancouver Scar Scale (VSS)—the first attempt to quantify scars with regards to pliability, vascularity, pigmentation, and height (Sullivan, Smith, Kermode, Mciver, & Courtemanche, 1990). A limitation of the scale, however, is the subjectivity involved in determining scar color, which can result in different scores. Another limitation of the VSS scale is that it was originally developed without considering the variations in skin tones of patients from different racial groups. In 1995, Baryza and Baryza adapted the original VSS by including a plexiglass tool for use with the height and pigmentation subsets. In 2007, Forbes-Duchart and colleagues conducted a clinical trial using a modification of the color scales, which may prove to be useful after more clinical trials are conducted (Forbes-Duchart, Marshall, Strock, & Cooper, 2007).

Pressure Ulcers and Traumatic Wounds

Identifying the location of the wound and its size, depth, and shape are key items in the examination of a pressure ulcer or traumatic wound. Identify any areas of maceration or softening of the skin, which often happens in the periwound area. In intact skin, note the ability to demonstrate capillary refill or blanching. To size the wound, use a tape measure or commercially available plastic measuring tool. There are also commercially available labels with millimeter markings that can be placed on adjacent intact skin to provide a measurement reference in pictures.

Digital photographs are an excellent adjunct to verbal description of the wound. Photographs should be taken on initial examination and at subsequent intervals to demonstrate progression of wound healing or failure of the wound to progress through the phases of healing. The NPUAP encourages clinicians to include the following information in picture documentation of pressure ulcers: (1) patient identification, (2) date and time of picture, and (3) a sample measure such as the millimeter marking labels discussed above (http://www.npuap.org/faq.htm).

To measure wound depth, place a sterile cotton-tipped applicator into the wound until the base is reached. Mark the depth with a pen or break the applicator at the surface opening of the wound; the applicator length can then be measured for the depth of the wound. Be careful that the applicator tip does not become dislodged in the wound during removal. Other options are to use a plastic or rubber feeding tube or suction catheter. The limitation of using these devices is that they may bend when measuring deep wounds, giving inaccurate dimensions.

With stages II through IV wounds, undermining and tunneling must be examined. **Undermining** occurs when the subcutaneous tissue creates a cave under the wound edges. **Tunneling** occurs when sinus tracts form and travel from the apparent wound, deeper into subcutaneous tissues. Measuring the extent of undermining and tunneling gives insight to the status of the tissues below the surface of the skin. To determine the undermining or tunneling, you can use a moist cotton-tipped applicator under the edges of the wound or into a tunnel. Do not force the applicator if resistance is felt; doing so can cause further damage. Once the applicator meets resistance, mark the end of the applicator at the wound edge, remove the applicator, and measure it along a centimeter ruler. The location of the undermining or tunneling can be described according to the hands of a clock. Using 12 o'clock as the top of the wound in relationship to the head, the location can be described according to the hands of the clock at 12, 3, 6, and 9 o'clock (Sussman, 2007c).

Identifying tissue type is the next step in evaluating and examining pressure ulcers and traumatic wounds. This identification can be done using a standard three-color description system: black for devitalized tissue or eschar, yellow for tissue that is possibly infected and in need of débridement, and red for healthy granulation tissue (Cuzzell, 1988). Multiple colors will appear in the wounds during the inflammatory and proliferative phase, but the goal is to achieve all red tissue as the wound heals or is ready for surgical intervention, as seen in Figure 10.7.

Progress in wound healing can be documented by percentages of each color, with the goal of 90% red granulation tissue. With grid photography, the boxes that appear on the photo can be counted and a percentage given to each color. The decrease in the percentages for black and yellow tissue and the increase in the percentages for red tissue can indicate progress in wound healing.

Exudate (drainage) and odor must also be noted during examination. Descriptors for exudate include serous (body fluids), serosanguineous (blood and body fluid), sanguineous (bloody), and purulent (infected

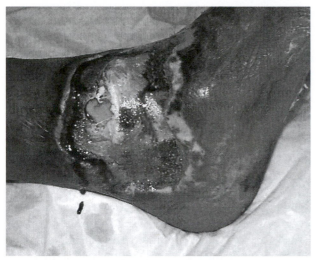

Figure 10.7 Example of red/yellow tissue present in a traumatic wound preoperatively. Black eschar had been surgically removed the day before to reveal underlying tissues.

and malodorous). Normal wound exudate is clear or yellow. Exudate that is yellow, gray, or green and malodorous is usually pus. Color and odor, however, are not always an indication of infection. Document the color and amount of drainage seen on removal of the dressings that cover the wounds (Bates-Jensen & Ovington, 2007).

Identifying any body structure that may be present in an open wound is crucial for determining appropriate interventions. Having a good anatomy text available during the initial examination or for interventions is essential. This will allow the clinician to have a reference available to identify structures that may be present (or absent) in a wound, which will also aid in more accurate documentation of any muscle, tendon, ligament, bone, or vessel that is seen in the wound. Doing so also aids in evaluating the depth of a partial- or full-thickness wound.

Diagnosis, Prognosis, and Plan of Care

After evaluating examination findings, a diagnosis can be formulated. For thermal injuries and open wounds, this diagnosis includes staging of pressure ulcers and determining the depth of a burn or traumatic wound. The prognosis for each wound is specific to the child, depending on the premorbid status, extent of TBSA involved, depth of burn, stage of pressure ulcer, and system impairments.

The plan of care is specific to the type of wound and other activity or participation restrictions the child encounters. Goals for wound management may include keeping the wound site free of infection, ridding the wound of necrotic tissue, preparing the wound bed for surgical intervention, and aiding in wound closure.

Throughout the interventions for wound healing, maintaining a moist wound environment is key. In a moist wound environment, collagen production is greater than in a wound that is exposed to air and allowed to dry out (Alvarez, Rozint, & Meehan, 1997). In a dry environment, epidermal cells are inhibited from migrating and resurfacing the wound. In contrast, in a moist environment, the epithelialization occurs more rapidly because there is no crust or scab formation.

For wounds in the remodeling phase, scar management is the main wound-care goal. Time frames for goals vary according to the type, size, location, nutritional status, and overall medical stability of the child. For example, a healthy child with no other medical history who sustains a 10% TBSA partial-thickness burn usually heals in 10 to 21 days. A child with a stage IV pressure ulcer who is insensate and malnourished and has diabetes could take more than 6 months to heal without surgical interventions. Interventions include those for each identified impairment and for wound care. Frequency of intervention depends on the phase of healing of the wound and on what other impairments are found on examination. For a wound in the acute healing phase (for example, a new burn), the physical therapist in a hospital setting should provide daily interventions. A child in the remodeling phase of healing, without other impairments, may need to be seen only weekly to monthly for child and family education and scar management.

Interventions

According to the American Physical Therapy Association's *Guide to physical therapist practice* (2001), preferred practice patterns for the integumentary system include interventions for primary prevention/risk reduction and interventions for impaired integumentary integrity associated with superficial, partial-thickness, or full-thickness skin loss and scar formation. The following paragraphs describe the interventions.

Coordination, Communication, and Documentation

The complex needs of the pediatric population make coordinating care for the child with integumentary disorders crucial. Often many medical professionals as well as community and family caregivers are involved in the child's care. Sharing of information regarding the plan of care and appropriate interventions is necessary throughout the continuum of care to ensure proper wound management. Throughout the continuum, one key person should make the decisions surrounding the wound-care needs. This individual is typically the primary care physician or surgical specialist (plastic or orthopedic surgeon). Documentation surrounding changes to the plan of care or wound interventions must be shared by the physician and disseminated to all caregivers in a timely fashion. Recognizing when referrals to other professionals are necessary is important throughout the episode of care. The collaboration of hospital-based, school-based, and community therapists is important for integrating one standard of care for the child.

Child-Related Instruction

Child and caregiver instruction is vital to the success of a wound-management program. Often in the care of children, the parent is the primary caregiver in the home and community setting. Identifying any barriers to learning and the learning styles of the child and family is the first step. The family must undergo specific training regarding wound-care techniques, exercises, positioning, orthotic use, and mobility training. Much of the initial instructions is provided in the acute-care setting, but all members of the care team must provide ongoing instruction throughout the episode of care. Teaching the child and his or her family about the integumentary disorder and how to prevent further impairments is important. Children and caregivers who are able to incorporate prevention into their daily routines will avoid recurrent hospitalizations and limitations of ADLs. Children with chronic wounds commonly have multiple medical problems and require increased medical care. Not only is this level of care costly, but it also puts the child at risk for loss of function and social or educational limitations from missing school.

Therapeutic Exercise

ROM and stretching are important interventions for any child with open wounds. For those with pressure ulcers or who are at risk for skin breakdown, maintaining flexibility and avoiding joint contractures is crucial for enhanced quality of life and function for ADLs. For children with thermal injuries, specific attention must be given to ROM. Contraindications to PROM exercises for the child with burns include exposed joints,

tendon exposure over the posterior interphalangeal joint, deep vein thrombosis, compartment syndrome, and a new skin graft.

Passive Range of Motion

PROM may be necessary for children who are in the intensive care unit and unable to participate in active exercises. Scar tissue responds well to a slow, prolonged stretch. Caution must be used when performing PROM for the extensor tendons of the hand because there is risk of rupturing. Children are typically too afraid to allow PROM; therefore, performing PROM while the child is under anesthesia for surgery may be beneficial to examine fully the available range. Precautions must be taken to avoid tearing the skin or causing joint dislocations while the child is under anesthesia. Identifying the true available ROM aids the therapist in daily interventions when the child is awake (Humphrey et al., 1994). For a prolonged stretch, serial casting may be used, as seen in Figure 10.8. Serial casting can be done over closed areas or during wound healing with the surgeon's approval.

Active-Assistive Range-of-Motion Exercises

Active-assistive range of motion (AAROM) exercises are used when children are unable to achieve full ROM independently. AAROM can be used for scar contractures, over escharotomy sites, and in children who have increased physiological demands after an extensive TBSA

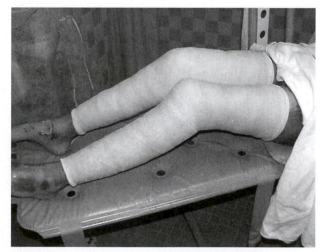

Figure 10.8 Example of serial casting used over healing grafted sites in a child with extensive lower extremity burns. Casts were used for prolonged stretch as well as for wound healing to decrease external trauma to the fragile, healing skin.

percentage burn. As discussed, be aware of the tissue response to stretch during AAROM and PROM. Ideally, ROM should be performed while dressings are off, allowing close monitoring of skin tension and scar blanching and avoiding skin tears (Humphrey et al., 1994). Doing so allows all caregivers to know the available ROM for activities on that specific day and helps ensure that caregivers do not exceed safe ranges for activity.

Active Range-of-Motion Exercises

AROM exercises are the exercises of choice for children with thermal injuries. The child can be in control during these exercises. The muscle-pumping activity that occurs helps reduce edema and increases circulation; it also prevents muscle atrophy. It is also the exercise format chosen immediately after skin grafting to avoid trauma to the newly grafted site. AROM exercises should incorporate the joint involved and combine movements because doing so stretches the scar to the most desired length. For example, for a scar on the anterior shoulder, shoulder flexion and shoulder flexion with elbow extension should be performed to elongate the tissues. Activities such as reaching for a target, shooting baskets, or playing baseball are fun activities that also achieve AROM in various planes of movement. Choosing age-appropriate play activities helps motivate the child to participate in activities that will increase ROM.

Assistive, Adaptive, Orthotic, Protective, and Prosthetic Devices

Before choosing a device for the child, identify limitations in ROM, strength, and mobility. A positioning program may be used in conjunction with devices such as airplane splints, resting hand splints, or ankle contracture boots. For the child with thermal injuries, there are predictable "at-risk" positions that should be avoided. See Figure 10.9 for general positioning guidelines. Listed in Table 10.2 are sites of burns and the preferred position for elongation. These positions are used for positioning programs or for splinting.

For the child at risk for a pressure ulcer or with a known skin disorder, a positioning program is also vital. Children should be repositioned at least every 2 hours to avoid unnecessary pressure. Use the times on a clock as a reminder for which position to choose. For example, at 12 o'clock the child lies supine; at 2 o'clock, right side-lying; at 4 o'clock, left side-lying; and at 6 o'clock, prone. Prone positioning is often overlooked, but it is an effective position for complete pressure relief for the posterior aspect of the body and pulmonary function. Take pictures

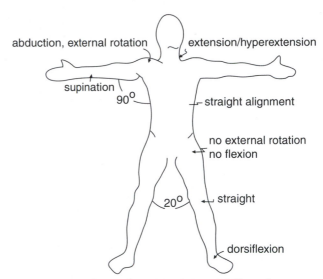

Figure 10.9 General positioning guidelines for the individual with burns. *(From L. Apfel et al. [1994]. Approaches to positioning the burn patient. In R.L. Richard & M.J. Staley [Eds.],* Burn care and rehabilitation *[p. 223]. Copyright F.A. Davis Company. Reprinted with permission.)*

of the child in these positions and post the program at the child's bedside for all caregivers to follow.

Adaptive Devices

In the acute-care setting, the choice of hospital bed/mattress is the first line of defense for maintaining skin integrity. Each institution may have a policy for when a specialty bed is appropriate for a child with integumentary impairment. For example, a specific score on the Braden Q Scale or Norton Scale may qualify the child for a specialty bed. These devices can be as simple as an air mattress overlay, a low air-loss system, gel mattresses, or air-fluidized therapy. In the home-care setting, more generic, commercially available devices include an air mattress or foam mattress. When positioning a child in bed, maintain the head of the bed at the lowest degree possible and limit the time that the head of the bed is elevated because, with this elevation, shearing forces occur at the sacrum and buttocks and can impair blood vessel function (Bergstrom et al., 1994). When the child is medically stable enough to be out of bed, an appropriate seating system must be developed. In the hospital setting, appropriate seating may involve a wheelchair or other type of chair. Any seating system that is used should be an appropriate fit, support the child, and provide pressure relief at the ischium/buttocks. Using a pressure-relieving cushion, rather than a standard pillow, decreases the risk of

Table 10.2 General Positioning Guidelines for the Individual With Burns

Body Area	Contracture Predisposition	Preventive Positioning
Neck	Flexion	Extension Hyperextension
Anterior axilla	Shoulder adduction	Shoulder abduction
Posterior axilla	Shoulder extension	Shoulder flexion
Antecubital space	Elbow flexion	Elbow extension
Forearm	Pronation	Supination
Wrist	Flexion	Extension
Dorsal hand/finger	MCP hyperextension IP flexion Thumb adduction	Metacarpophalangeal flexion Interphalangeal extension Thumb palmar abduction or opposition
Palmar hand/finger	Finger flexion Thumb opposition	Finger extension Thumb radial abduction
Hip	Flexion Adduction External rotation	Extension Abduction Neutral rotation
Knee	Flexion	Extension
Ankle	Plantar flexion	Dorsiflexion
Dorsal toes	Hyperextension	Flexion
Plantar toes	Flexion	Extension

Source: L. Apfel et al. (1994). Approaches to positioning the burn patient. In R.L. Richard & M.J. Staley (Eds.), *Burn care and rehabilitation* (p. 223). Copyright F.A. Davis Company. Reprinted with permission.

developing pressure ulcers. Positioning the child as upright as possible avoids friction and shear at the sacrum.

Assistive Devices

After a thermal injury or during interventions for a pressure ulcer or traumatic wound, the child may require an assistive device for mobilization. For example, a child with a sacral pressure ulcer may be restricted from sitting in a wheelchair and is nonambulatory. Using a prone cart enables the child to get out of bed, avoiding all pressure on the ulcer, and provides a means of independent mobility.

Orthotic Devices

While the child is on prolonged bed rest or medically unstable, use of static splints may be necessary to prevent contractures or to improve ROM. An example of an orthotic device is a posterior ankle resting or foot drop splint. These splints are commercially available in prefabricated sizes; they provide neutral ankle positioning and suspend the heel from the support surface. Often, for the pediatric population, these prefabricated orthotics may not fit well, and fabrication of

an orthoplast-type splint may be required. Prefabricated splints are time saving but often do not fit over bulky dressings. Use of orthoplast-type materials and fabricating custom splints to accommodate dressings and protect grafts or flaps might be necessary (Fig. 10.10).

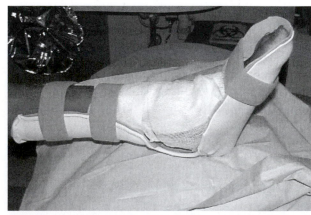

Figure 10.10 Example of orthoplast resting ankle splint fabricated to protect free flap at medial malleolus and maintain ankle range of motion.

For children with thermal injuries, early splinting is the key to preventing further deformities; Table 10.2 lists preventive positions. To maintain or improve ROM, splinting may be necessary, either continuously or during the night to provide a prolonged stretch. Splints may also be used to protect grafted areas after surgery. Splints decrease external trauma or shear to ensure graft adherence (Fig. 10.11). Custom-made orthotics may be prescribed after scar revision surgery to protect the grafted area and to improve ROM (Fig. 10.12).

Protective Devices

Pressure-relieving cushions are effective in protecting the skin from breakdown. For children at risk for a pressure ulcer or with a closed pressure ulcer, an appropriate device must be prescribed. There are many types of pressure-relieving cushions, from high-density foam to gel and Roho cushions. Sitting on a standard pillow should be discouraged because doing so does not relieve pressure. Instructing the child to perform pressure-relieving techniques, such as push-ups or shifting weight, every 15 to 30 minutes is also vital to preventing pressure ulcers.

For children with anterior neck burns, pillows should not be used behind the head because doing so

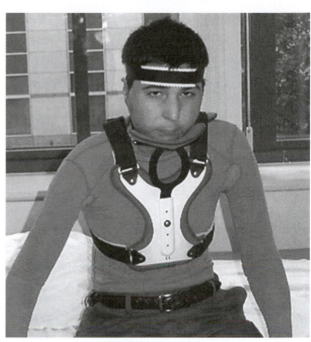

Figure 10.12 Example of a custom head/neck orthosis to protect anterior neck graft site and improve cervical range of motion.

forces the neck into flexion and places the child at risk for neck flexion contractures. A pillow may be used behind the shoulders to extend the neck slightly while the child sleeps.

Avoid using donut-type or ring-style cushions. They may cause circumferential pressure and act as a tourniquet, thus decreasing the blood supply to the area you are trying to protect. Ring-style cushions are known to cause venous congestion and are more likely to cause pressure ulcers than to prevent them. Also avoid positioning a child in the sidelying position with direct pressure over the trochanters. Use of pillows and blanket rolls helps the child to maintain a quarter-turn toward supine and relieve the pressure over the bony prominences. Elevating the affected area (e.g., heels) off the bed is also effective for relieving pressure and healing (Rappl, 2007). Alternatives for areas such as the occiput or bony prominences of the ankle or elbow are gel pillows.

Supportive Devices

After thermal or traumatic injuries, a child may require a skin graft to close the wound. Compression devices aid in vascular support to grafts. When a graft or flap has reached the remodeling phase, scar tissue forms and can continue to form for up to 2 years.

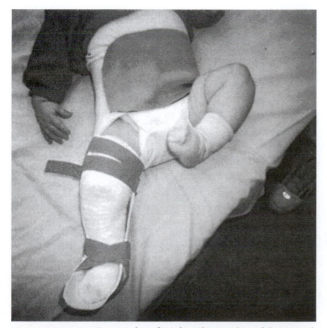

Figure 10.11 Example of orthoplast splint fabricated to restrict right hip and knee flexion to protect skin graft site at the knee.

Compression has been shown to aid in the collagen alignment, thus aiding in scar formation. The main objective of using compression is to balance collagen synthesis and lysis (see the section on Maturation Phase earlier in the chapter). Collagen fibers align parallel to the epidermal surface and have a decreased risk of hypertrophy. Use of compression garments aids in keeping the scars or grafts smoother and less raised and ultimately promotes increased cosmesis. During the remodeling phase, hypertrophic scars begin forming early, so the earlier the pressure or compression is applied, the better the results.

Pressure can be applied as early as 2 weeks after wound closure or graft healing. Pressure can initially be in the form of elastic bandages, cohesive bandages, elastic tubular support bandages, or custom-made pressure garments (Fig. 10.13). These garments should be worn for 23 hours per day, with time out of the garment for hygiene and scar management. Inserts may be needed to obtain even pressure over misshapen or bony prominences. Inserts can be foam, silicone elastomer, gel sheets, or silicone gel pads (Staley & Richard, 1994).

Compression for facial burns can be accomplished with compression garments or plastic face masks. Groce and colleagues (1999) studied the effectiveness of the garment versus the transparent plastic face mask. They found that the compression garment applied lower pressure over the forehead, left cheek, right cheek, and chin than the face mask. They also noted that the full compression garment mask makes

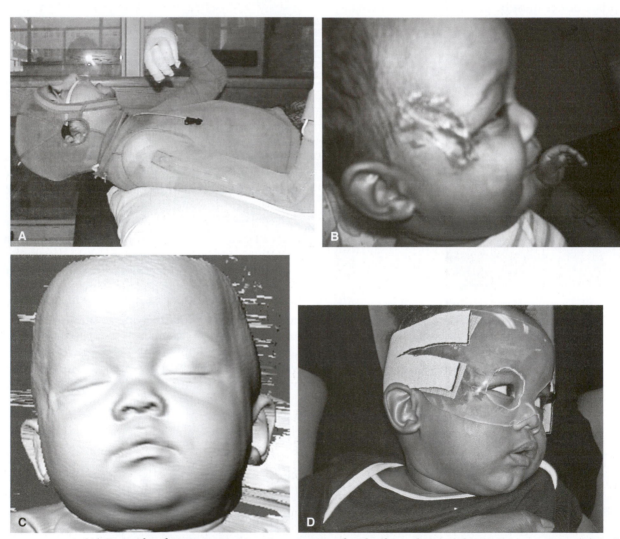

Figure 10.13 (A) Example of custom compression garment for the face, chest, and upper extremities. (B) Patient with facial scar. (C) Digital image from scanner. (D) Patient with custom-made facial mask.

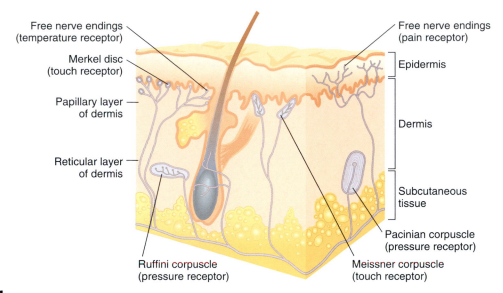

Free nerve endings
(temperature receptor)

Merkel disc
(touch receptor)

Papillary layer
of dermis

Reticular layer
of dermis

Free nerve endings
(pain receptor)

Epidermis

Dermis

Subcutaneous
tissue

Pacinian corpuscle
(pressure receptor)

Ruffini corpuscle
(pressure receptor)

Meissner corpuscle
(touch receptor)

Figure 10.1

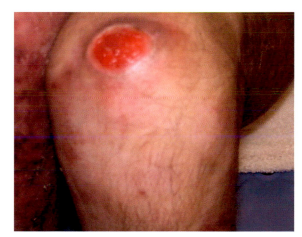

Figure 10.2

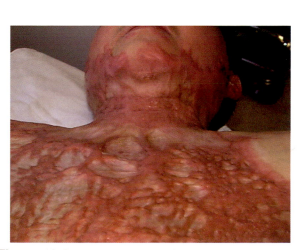

Figure 10.3

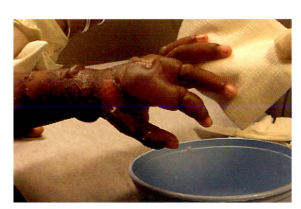

Figure 10.4

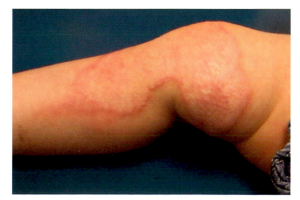

Figure 10.6

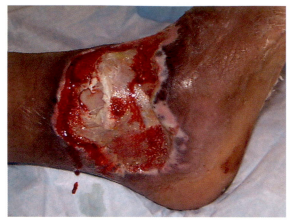

Figure 10.7

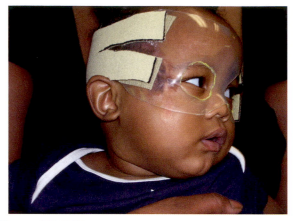

Figure 10.13D

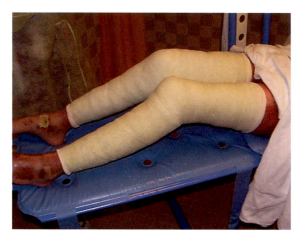

Figure 10.8

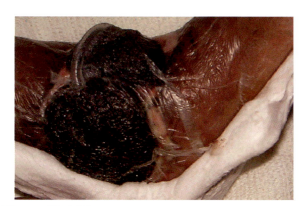

Figure 10.14A

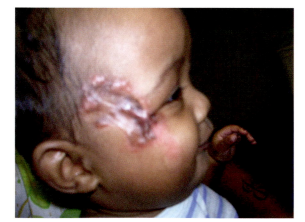

Figure 10.13B

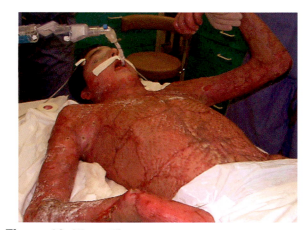

Figure 10.15

the individual appear "sinister," which may cause him or her to withdraw socially. The transparent face mask may give the child a better appearance and improve peer acceptance (Groce, Meyers-Paal, Herndon, and McCauley, 1999).

Custom-made face masks can be made from a plaster mold or using digital imaging. Creating a plaster mold requires sedation or general anesthesia in order for the patient to lie still while the mold is made. This procedure is not cost- or time-effective. However, digital surface scanning allows for quick and accurate scans of the face and neck, without the use of sedation or anesthesia (Fig. 10.13C). These computer-generated models of a patient's face are not only the framework for making the original mask, but they can be used by therapists to adjust the mask as pressure changes are needed. Using the computer-aided models eliminates the need for sedation or anesthesia, increases the turnaround time for mask fabrication and adjustments, and allows for tracking of changes in burn height, volume, and color via the imaging software (Whitestone, Richard, Slemker, Ause-Ellias, & Miller, 1995).

Integumentary Repair and Protection Techniques

Preprocedure Considerations

The role of the parent or caregiver in wound-care techniques has evolved over the past decade. Where once parents and caregivers may have been banned during painful procedures, they are now being encouraged to assist with the child's coping. Doctor's study in 1994 found that parent participation was "mutually beneficial" for the parent and the child. Parental involvement with wound-care procedures took longer, but the parent was able to provide emotional support to the child and also learned how to provide skin care at home (Doctor, 1994). Beckman and colleagues in 2002 reaffirmed these findings. Their study showed that parents want to be present for most pediatric procedures. "They and their children are likely to benefit from the practice." They did recommend education to parents on what to expect during the procedure. Emergency room physicians and nurses believed that parents should be present for some invasive procedures, but as the invasiveness increased, parents should be excluded (e.g., major resuscitation) (Beckman et al., 2002).

A child-life specialist or music therapist with expertise in preparation and distraction techniques can help the child cope with the pain and fear of wound-care procedures. However, activities should be targeted for each age population. For example, an infant can be bundled or held by a parent for comfort. Singing or blowing bubbles can distract a toddler. A school-aged child may want to sing a song or read a book. An adolescent may find relaxation or distraction listening to music through headphones or playing a video game.

Before any painful procedure, whether it is wound care or other interventions, care should be taken to ensure proper premedication for the child. Working with a pain management team in a hospital setting or having the parents administer prescribed pain medicine before an outpatient visit aids in pain relief for the child. Other techniques that may be beneficial during a therapy session are distraction, relaxation or breathing techniques, and guided imagery. The use of a positive reinforcement program may also be beneficial. Such a program may include progress or reward charts using stickers or other rewards when activities or procedures are completed (Martin-Herz et al., 2000).

Débridement

Débridement is "the removal of necrotic and/or infected tissues that interfere with wound healing" (Loehne, 2002). There are two types of débridement: nonselective and selective. When there is necrotic tissue in a wound, débridement must be done for the wound to progress through the healing phases.

Selective débridement can be achieved through enzymatic or autolytic débridement, or by surgical excision. Surgical débridement is the most efficient way to selectively débride necrotic tissue. This sharp débridement can be done in the operating room or may occur in a therapy setting. It should be performed when there is gross necrotic tissue. If an ischemic wound is present, sharp débridement is not indicated unless collateral circulation has been evaluated. Sharp débridement should be done by a trained, skilled clinician and under a doctor's order. Other forms of débridement can include the use of scissors and forceps (in the case of removing blisters from a partial-thickness burn) or gauze to remove sloughing blisters. Individual states' practice acts provide guidelines for the physical therapist regarding débridement. A specially educated and experienced clinician must be able to identify body structures that may be present in the wound bed. This is an advanced skill and should ideally be performed by a clinician who has completed a competency-based training program with a mentor (Bates-Jensen & Apeles, 2007).

The use of topical enzymatic agents is also a form of selective débridement because enzymes digest only necrotic tissue. Proteolytic enzymes are able to débride heavy eschar and denatured proteins. Some wounds contain eschar with undenatured collagen, which can be débrided with the enzyme collagenase. If a thick crust of eschar is present, the eschar may be scored or cross-hatched with a scalpel to allow permeation of the enzymes (Loehne, 2002).

Autolytic débridement is achieved when the body's white blood cells break down necrotic tissue. This form of débridement is accomplished with a moisture-retentive dressing. The moist wound environment promotes rehydration of dry, dead tissue, and the fluid that accumulates has white blood cells in it to break down the necrotic tissue. Dressings that can be used include films, hydrocolloids, and hydrogels (see "Dressings and Topical Agents").

Nonselective débridement removes necrotic and viable tissue from the wound. It can be achieved via wet-to-dry dressings, vigorous agitation in a whirlpool, or pulsed irrigation. This form of débridement is used in wounds that have extensive amounts of necrotic tissue. Caution must be used when using wet-to-dry dressings for nonselective débridement. When the dressing is adherent and then removed, there is a risk of damaging healthy epithelial and granulation tissue along with the necrotic tissue (Loehne, 2002).

Physical Agents and Mechanical Modalities

Hydrotherapy

Whirlpool According to the AHCPR, whirlpool therapy may enhance the removal of necrotic debris from pressure ulcers. Whirlpool therapy should be discontinued, however, when the wound is clean, because of the risk of trauma to healthy granulation tissue (Bergstrom et al., 1994).

Historically, the whirlpool had been used in the management of thermal injuries to cleanse the wounds and remove old topical agents. However, due to the risk of burn wound infections, a change in care led to more use of handheld showering devices and away from immersion in a tank. Mayhall (2003) wrote that the change in epidemiology of burn wound infections over two decades may be due to early excision and closure of burn wounds and replacing immersion hydrotherapy with showering hydrotherapy or local wound care in a patient's room (Mayhall, 2003).

Use of whirlpool therapy involves the risk of cross-contamination from others and the risk of contracting *Pseudomonas aeruginosa*. Despite adequate cleansing between whirlpool users, it is impossible to completely eradicate the risk for contamination of wounds. If whirlpool therapy is used, use of antiseptic agents should be discouraged in the whirlpool because of the cytotoxic effects of most additives. All commonly used antiseptic agents, such as iodine, sodium hypochlorite, and hydrogen peroxide, have cytotoxic effects, even when diluted. (Tap water should be used in whirlpools, as studies showed no increase in the risk for infection in comparison to sterile water or saline (Sussman, 2007d).

Pulsed Lavage Pulsed lavage or irrigation has emerged as an effective method of wound cleansing and nonselective débridement. Pulsed-lavage systems incorporate an irrigation solution (most commonly saline) and an electrically powered device to deliver the agent, in conjunction with wall suction. According to the AHCPR, irrigation pressures should be between 4 psi and 15 psi. At lower ranges, the wound may not be cleansed appropriately; above 15 psi, tissue damage may occur (Bergstrom et al., 1994).

The suction component of pulsed lavage removes debris, bacteria, and the irrigation solution used, and also provides negative pressure, which has been shown to promote granulation tissue formation (Loehne, 2002). Pressure parameters are usually between 60 and 90 mm Hg of continuous suction. The level of suction should be decreased if bleeding occurs or the child complains of pain (Loehne, 2002). Caution must be taken, as with any nonselective débridement device, with body structures that may be present in the wound bed, including tendon, fascia, joint capsule, and blood vessels.

Pulsed lavage is a portable intervention, so it can be done at the bedside and can be localized to the wound site, in contrast to whirlpool therapy, which would partially or fully submerge a body part. Pulsed lavage also has demonstrated an increased rate of granulation tissue formation in comparison to whirlpool treatments (Luedtke-Hoffman & Schafer, 2000).

Svoboda and colleagues performed wound-cleansing trials on animal subjects comparing bulb syringe cleansing with pulsed lavage. Their findings were conclusive for demonstrating that pulsed lavage was more effective than bulb syringe irrigation in reducing the bacterial counts in the wounds. They believed that pulsed lavage was a more effective method of irrigation to remove bacteria in a complex wound (Svoboda et al., 2006).

Dressings and Topical Agents

Dressings are specific to the type of integumentary disorder and vary in their properties. Ideal dressings should be user friendly, protect the surrounding skin from maceration, remove necrotic tissue, maintain a moist wound environment, promote granulation tissue or reepithelialization, relieve pain, stay in place, and be cost effective (Saffle & Schnebly, 1994).

Thermal Injuries Burn wounds should be cleansed once to twice per day. Necrotic tissue and old topical agents that have lost their antimicrobial effects after application should be loosened during this cleansing. Warm water or saline should be used to clean the wound.

Topical antibiotics, such as silver nitrate, mafenide acetate (Sulfamylon), nitrofurazone (Furacin), silver sulfadiazine (Silvadene), and bacitracin, are used to reduce the incidence of infection (Saffle & Schnebly, 1994). Silver sulfadiazine is the most widely used topical agent, although it can cause allergic reactions and transient leukopenia. It has broad-spectrum antimicrobial coverage, softens eschar and aids in its separation, and maintains a moist wound environment.

Topical agents are applied to a contact layer dressing instead of directly to the wound to decrease pain. The contact layer dressing can be gauze or a nonadherent gauze sheet to avoid adherence of the dressing to the wound. These dressings can be secured via a gauze roll, elastic netting, or elastic bandages.

The topical agent used for certain body areas requires special attention. The face is usually dressed with a thin cover of transparent ointment instead of silver sulfadiazine, which can harden and be difficult to remove. Burns on the ear are best treated with mafenide acetate cream because it penetrates more effectively into the tissues and protects ear cartilage from infection. Burns in the perineum are treated with transparent ointments because of the thinness of the dermis and its increased absorptive capacities (Saffle & Schnebly, 1994).

Synthetic Dressings Synthetic dressings that can be used with thermal injuries are Acticoat (discussed earlier) and AQUACEL Ag. AQUACEL Ag is a silver-impregnated hydrocolloid that is absorbent and nontraumatic to burn wound beds. The dressing is placed on the wound and is allowed to become adherent so that it will stay in place for up to 2 weeks, thus decreasing the need for daily dressing changes. (Decreasing the amount of dressing changes can also decrease the pain, fear, and anxiety that typically accompany this procedure.) If the AQUACEL Ag dressing does not adhere, the wound may be full-thickness, thus requiring surgical intervention. With fewer pain management needs and fewer dressing changes, children who had AQUACEL Ag placed have demonstrated shorter hospital stays than children who had other types of dressings placed (Paddock et al., 2007).

Functional Dressings Gauze and other dressings that are applied to burn sites must be placed so that the child may maintain or increase function. For example, fingers and toes should be wrapped individually to avoid sticking together, and gauze should be placed between the fingers to preserve the web space. Dressings should be applied from distal to proximal to reduce edema. As dressings are applied, the therapist should incorporate proper positioning to avoid losing ROM. Using dressings with uniform thickness allows orthotic use over burned areas. Orthotics are fabricated over a dressing, so uniform dressing thickness and technique aids in the appropriate fit of the splint. Burn dressings for an infant or a toddler may need to be more extensively reinforced to prevent the child from pulling or biting on the dressing and disrupting the underlying wound-healing environment. It is often recommended that fingernails be trimmed short to decrease the risk of causing bleeding from scratching.

After a thermal wound has healed, either by reepithelialization or by skin grafting, skin care must continue. Use of a moisturizing lotion is important with skin grafting because of the grafted wound's inability to produce normal body oils. An ideal moisturizer is one that is gentle, hypoallergenic, and alcohol-free, because alcohol has been shown to dry out the skin and may lead to cracking (Saffle & Schnebly, 1994).

In addition to moisturizing the skin, application of lotion can be effective in scar massage. By massaging the skin with lubricating lotion, the scar becomes desensitized via tactile stimulation. The scars should be massaged with hard enough pressure to make them blanch, three to six times per day. Scar massage may make the skin more mobile; however, no permanent decrease in thickness is usually seen (Staley & Richard, 1994).

Pressure Ulcers and Traumatic Wounds As with thermal injuries, pressure ulcers and traumatic wounds require cleansing and application of appropriate dressings. Antiseptic agents, such as povidone-iodine, iodophor, sodium hypochlorite (Dakin's solution), hydrogen peroxide, and acetic acid, are cytotoxic to normal tissue and should be avoided. They have been found to be toxic to fibroblasts, which play a key role in the inflammatory and proliferative phases of healing. Normal saline is the preferred topical agent for cleansing pressure ulcers and traumatic wounds because it is physiological and will not harm tissues (Bergstrom et al., 1994).

Film dressings are moisture and oxygen permeable. They are impermeable to microorganisms and allow easy monitoring of the wound because they are transparent.

They provide a moist wound environment. Film dressings can be used for minor abrasions and lacerations and for stage I ulcers. They can also be used as a secondary dressing to hold a primary dressing over a wound. Film dressings should not be used in a wound with excessive exudates. Examples of film dressings include Opsite, Bioclusive, and Tegaderm.

Foam dressings are produced from polyurethane. They are able to absorb exudates from the wound and maintain a moist environment. Foam dressings can be used for superficial and deep wounds and can be used over skin grafts and minor burns. They can be a secondary dressing to cover an amorphous hydrogel. They can also be used around a tracheostomy tube or gastrointestinal tube. Foam dressings are not effective for use in a dry wound but do not have any true contraindications to use. Examples of foam dressings are Allevyn, Hydrasorb, and Lyofoam.

Hydrogels contain organic polymers with a high water content. There are two types: amorphous and fixed. Amorphous hydrogels are able to absorb water; they are free flowing and easily fit into a cavity space. Fixed hydrogels come in a thin, flexible sheet and swell in size until saturated. They can provide moisture to a dry wound but can also absorb fluid from an exuding wound. Hydrogels can also easily conform to wound or body shape. They are chosen for wounds that are dry to rehydrate eschar and allow autolytic débridement. They should not be used in a wound with a large amount of exudates. Amorphous hydrogels are held in place by a secondary dressing (foam or film) and can stay in place for up to 3 days. Sheet hydrogels are fixed to the skin with tape or cohesive bandage and can also stay in place for 3 to 4 days. Examples of hydrogels are Carrasyn gel, DuoDerm gel, and Intrasite gel.

Hydrocolloids contain gel-forming polymers with adhesives, found on a film or foam. Hydrocolloids can also be in the form of granules, powders, or pastes. The dressing will absorb wound exudates, provide a moist wound environment, and conform to body shape. They can be used for superficial wounds, donor sites, and pressure ulcers. Concern for using this type of dressing in a child with fragile skin is high because of the risk for further skin trauma when removing the dressing. The dressing does not need to be changed for up to 3 to 4 days. Hydrocolloids should not be used in a clinically infected wound or a deep cavity. They will aid in autolytic débridement. An example of a hydrocolloid is Comfeel.

Duoderm and Tegasorb **Alginate dressings** contain calcium, or calcium and sodium salts. When they are applied to a wound, the sodium ions in the wound are exchanged for calcium ions in the dressing, thus acting as a hemostatic agent. They provide a moist wound environment, provide a high absorptive capacity, conform to body shape, and are nonadherent. Alginates are used in exudative wounds, pressure ulcers, and postsurgically at bleeding sites. They come in sheets, rope, or packing alginates. These dressings can stay in place for up to 1 week in clean wounds or changed daily in an infected wound. Examples of alginate dressings are Curosorb, Kaltostat, and Sorbsan (G. Sussman, 2007).

The **vacuum-assisted closure** (V.A.C.) **system** was developed to aid with treatment of traumatic wounds with soft tissue defects and pressure and decrease pain and length of hospitalization. The device itself is a subatmospheric pressure system with a polyurethane foam dressing. Before use of this device, all nonviable tissue had to be removed via surgical débridement (Argenta & Marykwas, 1997).

Mooney and colleagues (2000) conducted a study of the use of the V.A.C. system with children with complex wounds. The children underwent surgical débridement of all nonviable tissue and then application of the system. The V.A.C. system sponge and outflow tube were cut and fit to the appropriate size of the wound and then covered with a transparent film/drape, as seen in Figure 10.14. Continuous negative pressure was used at 125 mm Hg, as close to 24 hours per day as possible. The dressing was changed three times per week. Once a granulating wound bed was achieved, wound coverage was performed through either skin grafting or free flaps. The children required fewer painful dressing changes and less extensive coverage surgeries than children who did not receive treatment with system. The primary goals of the system—stimulating granulation tissue and removing interstitial fluid from the wound—were met. The continuous suction also acted to slowly draw the wound edges together. Mooney et al. (2000) also found that the system was well tolerated by the children and decreased the need for the frequent dressing changes that occur in a more traditional wound management program.

Electrotherapeutic Modalities

Management of wound healing with electrotherapeutic agents has been shown to be safe and effective. These agents include transcutaneous electrical nerve stimulation (TENS) and high-voltage pulsed current (HVPC). These devices can produce physiological responses at the cellular level. TENS causes vasodilation of small blood vessels and increases blood flow to the extremities. HVPC increases tensile strength of the

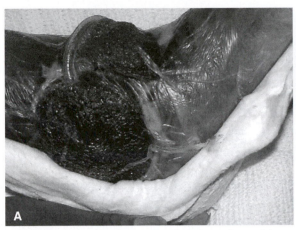
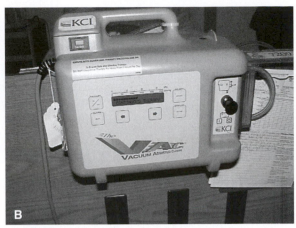

Figure 10.14 *(A)* Vacuum-assisted closure (V.A.C.) system placed on open wound (as seen in Fig. 10.7). Black polyurethane foam dressing in place. *(B)* V.A.C. unit.

scar, increases collagen synthesis and epithelialization, and increases fibroblast production. With HVPC, on days 1 to 5 use 50 pps, 150 V, and negative polarity for 30 to 60 minutes daily. From day 6 until healing, use 80 pps, 90 V, and positive polarity for 30 to 60 minutes daily. If the wound appears to have plateaued, alternate the polarity daily (Unger, 1992).

Electrical Stimulation

"Several in vitro and in vivo studies have reported that ES (electrical stimulation) has either an inhibitory (bacteriostatic) effect or a killing (bactericidal) effect on microorganisms that commonly colonize or infect wounds" (Kloth, 2002a). Other effects reported for ES include increases in the rates of collagen synthesis and epithelialization and improved revascularization and oxygen levels. Kloth (2002a) also reports effects such as acute wound-related pain reduction, augmentation of autolysis, and accelerated wound healing with the use of ES. Precautions for ES include sensation of a light tingling under the electrodes and potential for skin irritation. Contraindications for ES include basal or squamous cell carcinoma in the wound or periwound tissues or melanoma, untreated osteomyelitis, application to the neck or thorax that may send a current through the pericardial area, or when a pacemaker is implanted. For a more in-depth look at ES, see Kloth and McCulloch's (2002a) chapter on electrical stimulation for wound healing in *Wound healing:*

Alternatives in Management
Hyperbaric Oxygen Therapy

Hyperbaric oxygen therapy (HBO) is delivered to an individual by 90% oxygen breathed in a sealed chamber with an atmospheric pressure between 2.0 and 2.5 atmospheres absolute. The use of HBO has been documented for smoke inhalation, enhancement of healing in selected problem wounds, compromised skin grafts and flaps, necrotizing soft tissue infections, and thermal burns (Kloth, 2002b). The improved oxygen delivery has a great effect at the cellular level. Neutrophils, fibroblasts, and macrophages are all dependent on an oxygen-rich environment. Improved oxygenation has also been correlated with decreasing infection and accelerating wound healing. Precautions for using HBO for wound healing include upper respiratory infections, seizures, high fevers, history of spontaneous pneumothorax, history of thoracic surgery, viral infections, and optic neuritis. Contraindications for HBO include antineoplastic medications and untreated pneumothorax.

Outcomes

Because of the wide range of integumentary impairments that have been reviewed, it is not possible to provide one set of guidelines for outcomes. Outcomes for thermal injuries and open wounds include progression of the wound through the stages of wound healing, absence of infection, and an acceptable scar that does not impede functional mobility, ADLs, or community activities and participation. Good wound management is of paramount importance for the child to return to normal activities and participation in ADLs, school, play, and extracurricular activities. Early detection of skin disorders and timely wound care will aid in the child's return to these activities. Care for children with skin disorders should be done at burn centers or trauma centers capable of handling their complex care. Neonatal intensive care units familiar with congenital skin disorders such as EB will also aid in the timely care of newborns with skin disruptions. Children with large TBSA thermal injuries or TEN will have the highest probability for long-term sequelae. Some integumentary disorders and their subsequent impairments will limit the child's quality of life and ability to participate in age-appropriate activities.

Mini-Case Study 10.1
Child History

Ethan is a 14-year-old boy with autism who, at age 13 years, was in his usual state of good health until he was found lying on a burning mattress in his group home. He was transported to a burn center and underwent acute care for approximately 63% TBSA partial- and full-thickness burns to his face, neck, chest, abdomen, back, and extremities. His eyes, forehead, and scalp were spared, along with his perineum and portions of his back, legs, and feet. He required amputations of digits 2, 4, and 5 on his right hand because of the severity of his injuries. He underwent numerous skin grafting procedures and the use of CEA to cover areas when he had no donor sites available. After 3 months in the burn center, he was transferred to a rehabilitation hospital, where he underwent intensive therapy and ongoing wound management. He was discharged to his home 6 months after his original injuries and readmitted to the acute-care setting a month later for neck scar revisions. He had a brief rehabilitation stay and was discharged back home in his parents' care. Barriers to learning for Ethan include expressive language and cognitive deficits, as well as behavioral problems associated with his autism. Barriers to intervention included Ethan's inability to understand why procedures were being done and overall anxiety with any new caregiver.

Impairments in Body Structures and Functions:
Ethan has comorbidities of an extensive TBSA thermal injury and autism. Autism is a syndrome noted in early childhood that can be characterized by abnormal social relationships, language disorders, the presence of rituals, and a compulsive component. In many cases, impaired intellectual development is present (Allison & Smith, 1998).

Integumentary: On arrival at rehabilitation, Ethan had many open wounds and unhealed grafted areas. He was also having intermittent breakdown at the sites that were covered with CEA. He had begun to develop hypertrophic scarring throughout the burned sites.

Goal: To have complete wound closure and to decrease the risk of further skin breakdown as a result of trauma.

Interventions:

1. Daily wound care in a shower room separate from his room

2. Use of a standard procedure for wound care and a scheduled time for the procedure for all caregivers to follow

3. Premedication before interventions for both pain and anxiety

4. Use of a specialty mattress to decrease risk for secondary limitations or pressure sores and to decrease shearing forces on healing tissues

5. Nutrition consultation for adequate intake by mouth with supplemental nasogastric tube feedings at night

6. Use of distraction techniques including favorite DVD movies during dressing changes

7. Use of serial casting not only for prolonged stretching but also to decrease possible trauma to his healing wounds by shearing or scratching

8. Early compression as soon as wounds had healed; initial compression with elastic bandages, then elastic tubular bandages, and eventually custom compression garments

Range of Motion Ethan had deficits in joint ROM at his neck, upper extremities, lower extremities, and trunk caused by scar tissue and tissue shortening that occurred despite therapy in the acute-care setting.

Goal: Ethan will achieve functional use of his neck and extremities for ADLs.

Interventions:

1. PROM/AROM/AAROM exercises geared to his tolerance

2. Positioning program posted at bedside

3. Examination of ROM in the operating room while Ethan is under general anesthesia because of his inability to tolerate PROM to the point of scar blanching; true ROM measurements and restrictions noted and used for ADLs (Fig. 10.15).

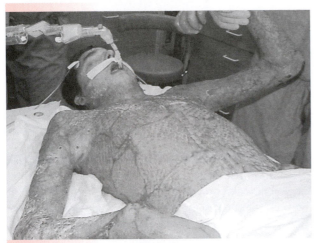

Figure 10.15 Range of motion performed on child while under general anesthesia in the operating room.

4. Orthotic devices such as ankle resting splints, elbow and hand resting splints, knee extension splints, and Watusi rings

5. Serial casting for elbows, hands, and knees to achieve a prolonged stretch and decrease risk of trauma to healing tissues from shearing and scratching by Ethan

6. Use of functional equipment, such as stationary bike or adult-sized tricycle that Ethan appeared to enjoy (Fig. 10.16).

7. Use of distraction techniques including counting and singing a familiar song during PROM

Ethan was referred to the plastic surgery department in July for revision of his neck scar because of significant loss of ROM and cosmesis. Preoperatively, he was unable to extend his head to neutral and had minimal to no rotation to either side. He underwent surgical excision of the scar and skin grafting. He spent 9 days in intensive care, 7 of which were under heavy sedation and on the ventilator to allow proper positioning and ensure that the graft would take postoperatively.

Goal: Ethan will increase neck ROM to at least 50% of normal to aid in ADLs.

Interventions:

1. Postoperative positioning while sedated in neck hyperextension

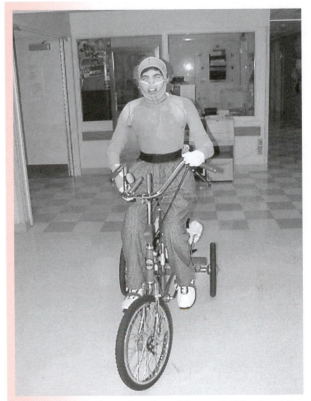

Figure 10.16 Functional and fun activities to gain range of motion and endurance.

2. Use of a head/neck orthosis to maintain neck in neutral to slightly extended position while sitting and mobilizing

3. PROM exercises for neck rotation, side flexion and extension, using singing/counting techniques for distraction and tolerance of intervention (Fig. 10.17)

4. AROM exercises

Mobility Ethan was limited in his ability to ambulate on level surfaces. He required assistance for bed mobility, transfers, and gait.

Goal: Ethan will be independent with all aspects of household and community mobility.

Interventions:

1. Mobilization out of bed to wheelchair

2. Parent education for transfer and guarding techniques

3. Assisted ambulation with handheld assistance because of inability of arms to use assistive device

Continued

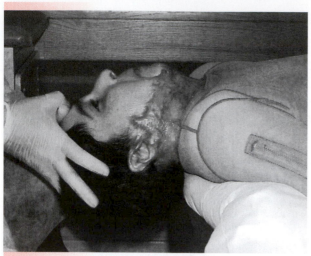

Figure 10.17 Passive range of motion interventions for cervical extension after scar revision.

Endurance Ethan was limited in participating in long therapy sessions, not only because of his attention span but also because of his low endurance and inability to regulate his body temperature as a result of the extensive thermal injury.

Goal: Ethan will be able to participate in ADLs and household mobility without needing frequent rest breaks.

Interventions:

1. Adherence to daily routine and schedule by all staff members

2. Shortened therapy sessions, looking for signs of fatigue that included sitting down, pointing to his wheelchair, or agitation

3. Encouraging Ethan to drink during therapy session, with water bottle always on hand

4. Application of a cool towel to Ethan's face and neck during rest period of therapy session

5. Participation of his parents in therapy sessions to encourage and reassure him

Activity and Participation Restrictions: Ethan was limited from participating in normal ADLs, other community activities, and interactions with his peers because of his prolonged hospitalizations. His parents chose to care for him at home and restrict his participation in school and group home activities because of the nature of the accident.

Outcomes: Ethan continues to have ongoing issues with skin breakdown at sporadic sites throughout his body 9 months after the initial injuries. He wears compression garments for his arms, legs, trunk, and face. His skin is slowly starting to appear smoother, with less apparent hypertrophic scarring present. He continues to have decreased use of his right hand caused by amputations and contractures and has some functional use of his left hand. His neck ROM improved after surgery, but he has already lost range because of scarring. Because of poor tolerance, he uses his neck orthosis only intermittently. Since returning home after surgery, he receives therapy several days per week, and his parents are extremely invested in his care. He is independent ambulating in his house, including up and down stairs. He is able to walk 4 miles daily in a rough terrain setting with supervision. He will require ongoing therapy for an extended period because of his risk for contractures caused by the remodeling process. He will likely need numerous scar revision surgeries and faces a lifetime of episodes of care for wound and scar management, ROM, compression garments, and mobility.

Summary

The physical therapist plays an important role in managing children with open wounds and burns. Knowledge of the structure and function of the integumentary system and related impairments that may occur are essential for delivering quality care. Advanced training in the clinical setting will enhance the intervention skills needed to best serve this population. Competency-based training programs are essential to ensure clinical competence for interventions, especially for débridement and wound-healing techniques.

The physical therapist must also serve as educator for other health-care professionals. Therapists are commonly the most extensively trained health-care professionals in the area of wound, burn, and scar management and must advocate for a wound-management program that enhances moist wound healing and decreases the trauma to the viable tissue. It is vital to keep in mind what phase of healing the wound is in and how best to progress it through all the stages to achieve wound closure, an acceptable-appearing scar, and ultimate function and independence for the child. Continuing education programs that include didactic and laboratory portions for learning new techniques are highly recommended for clinicians of all levels of experience.

DISCUSSION QUESTIONS

1. Describe the key processes in each of the phases of wound healing.

2. How do hypertrophic scars form, and what interventions can be taken to prevent and control them?

3. How can you differentiate the various stages of pressure ulcers?

4. What objective findings would you include in your open wound/thermal injury examination?

5. Discuss the role of proper positioning and ROM for the child with thermal injuries.

6. Describe one modality, other than traditional gauze dressing changes, for achieving wound cleansing and healing.

Recommended Readings

American Burn Association. Retrieved from http://www.Ameriburn.org

Carrougher, G.J. (Ed.) (1998). *Burn care and therapy*. St. Louis: Mosby.

Dystrophic Epidermolysis Bullosa Research Association of America. Retrieved from http://www.DEBRA.org

McCulloch, J.M., & Kloth, L.C. (Eds.) (2010). *Wound healing: Evidence-based management* (4th ed.). Philadelphia: F.A. Davis.

Sussman, C., & Bates-Jensen, B. (Eds.) (2007). *Wound care: A collaborative practice manual for health professionals*. Baltimore, MD: Lippincott Williams & Wilkins.

References

Allison, K.P., & Smith, G. (1998). Burn management in a child with autism. *Burns, 24*, 484–486.

Alvarez, O., Rozint, J., & Meehan, M. (1997). Principles of moist wound healing: Indications for chronic wounds. In D. Krasner (Ed.), *Chronic wound care: A clinical source book for healthcare professionals* (pp. 49–56). King of Prussia, PA: Health Management Publishers.

American Physical Therapy Association (2001). Guide to physical therapist practice (2nd ed.). *Physical Therapy, 81*, 6–746.

Apfel, L., et al. (1994). Approaches to positioning the burn patient. In R.L. Richard & M.J. Staley (Eds.), *Burn care and rehabilitation*. Philadelphia: F.A. Davis Company.

Argenta, L.C., & Marykwas, M.J. (1997). Vacuum-assisted closure: A new method for wound control and treatment: Clinical experience. *Annals of Plastic Surgery, 38*, 563–576.

Atherton, D.J. (2000). Epidermolysis bullosa. In J. Harper, A. Oranje, & N. Prose (Eds.), *Textbook of pediatric dermatology* (Vol. 2, pp. 1075–1095). Malden, MA: Blackwell Science.

Baryza, M.J., & Baryza, G.A. (1995). The Vancouver Scar Scale: An administration tool and its interrater reliability. *Journal of Burn Care and Rehabilitation, 16*(5), 535–538.

Bates-Jensen, B. (2007). Pressure ulcers: Pathophysiology and prevention. In C. Sussman & B. Bates-Jensen (Eds.). *Wound Care: A collaborative practice manual for health professionals* (pp. 336–373). Baltimore: Lippincott Williams & Wilkins.

Bates-Jensen, B., & Apeles, N. (2007). Management of necrotic tissue. In C. Sussman & B. Bates-Jensen (Eds.), *Wound Care: A collaborative practice manual for health professionals* (pp. 197–214). Baltimore: Lippincott Williams & Wilkins.

Bates-Jensen, B., & Ovington, L. (2007). Management of exudate and infection. In C. Sussman & B. Bates-Jensen (Eds.), *Wound care: A collaborative practice manual for health professionals* (pp. 215–233). Baltimore: Lippincott Williams & Wilkins.

Beckman, A., Sloan, B., Moore, G., Cordell, W., Brizendine, E., Boie, E., Knoop, K., Goldman, M., & Geninatti, M. (2002). Should parents be present during emergency department procedures on children and who should make that decision? A survey of emergency physician and nurse attitudes. *Academic Emergency Medicine, 9*(2), 154–158.

Bergstrom, N., Allman, R.M., Alvarez, O.M., Bennett, M.A., Carlson, C.E., Frantz, R.A., et al. (1994). *Treatment of pressure ulcers*. Clinical Practice Guideline, No. 15. Rockville, MD: U.S. Department of Health and Human Services. Public Health Service, Agency for Health Care Policy and Research. AHCPR Publication No. 95-0652.

Committee on Injury and Poison Prevention, American Academy of Pediatrics. Widome, M.D. (Ed.) (1997). *Injury prevention and control for children and youth* (3rd ed., pp. 233–267). Elk Grove Village, IL: Author.

Cuzzell, L.J. (1988). The new RYB color code. *American Journal of Nursing, 88*, 1342–1346.

Doctor, M.E. (1994). Parent participation during painful wound care procedures. *Journal of Burn Care and Rehabilitation, 15*, 288–292.

Dore, J., & Salisbury, R. (2007). Morbidity and mortality of mucocutaneous diseases in the pediatric population at a tertiary care center. *Journal of Burn Care & Research, 28*(6), 865–870.

Dressler, D.P., & Hozid, J.L. (2001). Thermal injury and child abuse: The medical evidence dilemma. *Journal of Burn Care and Rehabilitation, 22*, 180–185.

Falkel, J. (1994). Anatomy and physiology of the skin. In R.L. Richard & M.J. Staley (Eds.), *Burn care and rehabilitation: Principles and practice* (pp. 10–28). Philadelphia: F.A. Davis.

Fine, J., Johnson, L., Weiner, M., & Suchindran, C. (2008). Cause-specific risks of childhood death in inherited epidermolysis bullosa. *The Journal of Pediatrics, 152*(2), 276–280.

Forbes-Duchart, L., Marshall, S., Strock, A., & Cooper, J. (2007). Determination of inter-rater reliability in pediatric burn scar assessment using a modified version of the Vancouver Scar Scale. *Journal of Burn Care & Research, 28*(3), 460–467.

Gray, H. (1977). General anatomy or histology. In T. Pick & R. Howden (Eds.), *Gray's anatomy* (pp. 1135–1143). New York: Bounty Books.

Greenhalgh, D.G., & Staley, M.J. (1994). Burn wound healing. In R.L. Richard & M.J. Staley (Eds.), *Burn care and rehabilitation: Principles and practice* (pp. 70–102). Philadelphia: F.A. Davis.

Groce, A., Meyers-Paal, R., Herndon, D.N., & McCauley, R.L. (1999). Are your thoughts of facial pressure transparent? *Journal of Burn Care and Rehabilitation, 20,* 478–481.

Herndon, D.N., Rutan, R.L., Alison, W.E., Jr., & Cox, C.S., Jr. (1993). Management of burn injuries. In M.R. Eichelberger (Ed.), *Pediatric trauma* (pp. 568–605). St. Louis: Mosby-Year Book.

Huffines, B., & Logsdon, M.C. (1997). The Neonatal Skin Risk Assessment Scale for predicting skin breakdown in neonates. *Issues in Comprehensive Pediatric Nursing, 20*(2), 103–114.

Humphrey, C.N., Richard, R.L., & Staley, M.J. (1994). Soft tissue management and exercise. In R.L. Richard & M.J. Staley (Eds.), *Burn care and rehabilitation: Principles and practice* (pp. 324–360). Philadelphia: F.A. Davis.

Johnson, C. (1994). Pathologic manifestations of burn injury. In R.L. Richard & M.J. Staley (Eds.), *Burn care and rehabilitation: Principles and practice* (pp. 29–48). Philadelphia: F.A. Davis.

Kloth, L.C. (2002a). Electrical stimulation for wound healing. In L.C. Kloth & J.M. McCulloch (Eds.), *Wound healing: Alternatives in management* (3rd ed., pp. 271–315). Philadelphia: F.A. Davis.

Kloth, L.C. (2002b). Adjunctive interventions for wound healing. In L.C. Kloth & J.M. McCulloch (Eds.), *Wound healing: Alternatives in management* (3rd ed., pp. 316–381). Philadelphia: F.A. Davis.

Krechel, S.W., & Bildner, J. (1995). CRIES: A new neonatal postoperative pain measurement score. Initial testing of validity and reliability. *Paediatric Anaesthesia, 5*(1), 53–61.

Loehne, H.B. (2002). Wound débridement and irrigation. In L.C. Kloth & J.M. McCulloch (Eds.), *Wound healing: Alternatives in management* (3rd ed., pp. 203–231). Philadelphia: F.A. Davis.

Luedtke-Hoffman, K.A., & Schafer, D.S. (2000). Pulsed lavage in wound cleansing. *Physical Therapy, 80,* 292–300.

Lund, C.C., & Browder, N.C. (1944). The estimation of areas of burns. *Surgery, Gynecology, and Obstetrics, 79,* 352–358.

Malviya, S., Voepel-Lewis, T., Burke, C., Merkel, S., & Tait, A. (2006). The revised FLACC observational pain tool: improved reliability and validity for pain assessment in children with cognitive impairment. *Pediatric Anesthesia, 16,* 258–265.

Martin-Herz, S.P., Thurber, C.A., & Patterson, D.R. (2000). Psychological principles of burn wound pain in children. II: Treatment applications. *Journal of Burn Care and Rehabilitation, 21,* 458–472.

Mayhall, C.G. (2003). The epidemiology of burn wound infections: Then and now. *Clinical Infectious Diseases, 37,* 543–550.

Miller, S.F., Staley, M.J., & Richard, R.L. (1994). Surgical management of the burned child. In R.L. Richard & M.J. Staley (Eds.), *Burn care and rehabilitation: Principles and practice* (pp. 177–197). Philadelphia: F.A. Davis.

Mooney, J.F., III, Argenta, L.C., Marks, M.W., Marykwas, M.J., & DeFranzo, A.J. (2000). Treatment of soft tissue defects in pediatric patients using the V.A.C. System. *Clinical Orthopedics and Related Research, 376,* 26–31.

National Pressure Ulcer Advisory Panel (NPUAP). (2007). *Pressure ulcer stages revised by NPUAP.* Retrieved from http://www.npuap.org/pr2.htm

Neuwalder, J.M., Sampson, C., Breuing, K., & Orgill, D. (2002). A review of computer-aided body surface area determination: SAGE II and EPRI's 3D burn vision. *Journal of Burn Care & Rehabilitation, 23*(1), 55–59.

Paddock, H., Fabia, R., Giles, S., Hayes, J., Lowell, W., & Besner, G. (2007). A silver impregnated antimicrobial dressing reduces hospital length of stay for pediatric patients with burns. *Journal of Burn Care & Research, 28*(3), 409–411.

Patterson, J.W., & Blaylock, W.K. (1987). *Dermatology* (pp. 1–15). New York: Medical Examination Publishing.

Rappl, L. (2007) Management of pressure by therapeutic positioning. In C. Sussman & B. Bates-Jensen (Eds.), *Wound care: A collaborative practice manual for health professionals* (pp. 374–404). Baltimore: Lippincott, Williams & Wilkins.

Rassner, G. (1994). *Atlas of dermatology* (pp. 7–8). (Walter Burgdorf, trans.). Philadelphia: Lea & Febiger.

Ross, R. (1968). The fibroblast and wound repair. *Biological Review, 43,* 51–91.

Saffle, J.R., & Schnebly, W.A. (1994). Burn wound care. In R.L. Richard & M.J. Staley (Eds.), *Burn care and rehabilitation: Principles and practice* (pp. 119–176). Philadelphia: F.A. Davis.

Schulz, J.T., Sheridan, R.L., Ryan, C.M., MacKool, B., & Tompkins, R.G. (2000). A 10-year experience with toxic epidermal necrolysis. *Journal of Burn Care and Rehabilitation, 21,* 199–204.

Sheridan, R.L., Weber, J.M., Schulz, J.M. Ryan, C.M., Low, H.M., & Tompkins, R.G. (1999). Management of severe toxic epidermal necrolysis in children. *Journal of Burn Care and Rehabilitation, 20,* 497–500.

Staley, M.J., & Richard, R.L. (1994). Scar management. In R.L. Richard & M.J. Staley (Eds.), *Burn care and rehabilitation: Principles and practice* (pp. 380–418). Philadelphia: F.A. Davis.

Sullivan, T., Smith, J., Kermode, J., Mciver, E., & Courtemanche, D.J. (1990). Rating the burn scar. *Journal of Burn Care and Rehabilitation, 11,* 256–260.

Sussman, C. (2007a). Assessment of the skin and wound. In C. Sussman & B. Bates-Jensen (Eds.), *Wound care: A collaborative practice manual for health professionals* (pp. 85–122). Baltimore: Lippincott Williams & Wilkins.

Sussman, C. (2007b). The diagnostic process. In C. Sussman & B. Bates-Jensen (Eds.), *Wound care: A collaborative practice manual for health professionals* (pp. 2–20). Baltimore: Lippincott Williams & Wilkins.

Sussman, C. (2007c). Wound measurements and prediction of healing. In C. Sussman & B. Bates-Jensen (Eds.), *Wound care: A collaborative practice manual for health professionals* (pp. 123–143). Baltimore: Lippincott Williams & Wilkins.

Sussman, C. (2007d). Whirlpool. In C. Sussman & B. Bates-Jensen (Eds.), *Wound care: A collaborative practice manual for health professionals* (pp. 644–664). Baltimore: Lippincott Williams & Wilkins.

Sussman, C. & Bates-Jensen, B. (2007) Wound healing physiology: Acute and chronic. In C. Sussman & B. Bates-Jensen (Eds.), *Wound care: A collaborative practice manual for health professionals* (pp. 21–51). Baltimore: Lippincott Williams & Wilkins.

Sussman, G. (2007) Management of the wound environment with dressings and topical agents. In C. Sussman & B. Bates-Jensen (Eds.), *Wound care: A collaborative practice manual for health professionals* (pp. 250–267). Baltimore: Lippincott Williams & Wilkins.

Svoboda, S., Bice, T., Gooden, H., Brooks, D., Thomas, D., & Wenke, J. (2006). Comparison of bulb syringe and pulsed lavage irrigation with use of a bioluminescent musculoskeletal wound model. *The Journal of Bone & Joint Surgery, 88*, 2167–2174.

Unger, P.G. (1992). Electrical enhancement of wound repair. *Physical Therapy Practice, 80*, 41–49.

Ward, R.S. (2007). Management of scar. In C. Sussman & B. Bates-Jensen (Eds.), *Wound care: A collaborative practice*

manual for health professionals (pp. 309–318). Baltimore: Lippincott Williams & Wilkins.

Whitestone, J., Richard, R., Slemker, T., Ause-Ellias, K., & Miller, S. (1995). Fabrication of total-contact burn masks by use of human body topography and computer-aided design manufacturing. *Journal of Burn Care & Rehabilitation, 16*(5), 543–547.

Wong, D., & Baker, C. (1988). Pain in children: Comparison of assessment scales. *Pediatric Nursing, 14*(1), 9–17.

Service Delivery Settings

SECTION
3

—Susan K. Effgen, PT, PhD, Section Editor

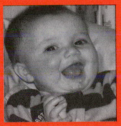
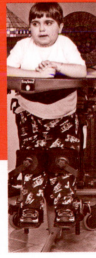
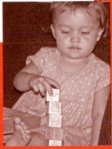
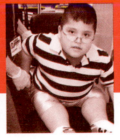
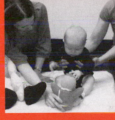
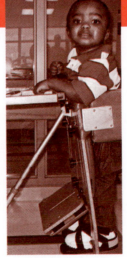
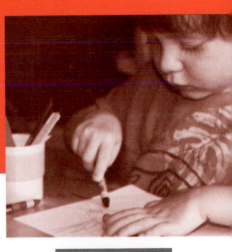

CHAPTER 11

Early Intervention

—Jane O'Regan Kleinert, PhD, CCC-SLP

—Susan K. Effgen, PT, PhD, FAPTA

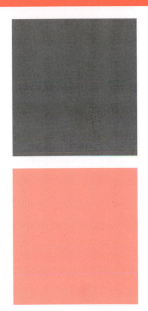

This chapter will discuss early identification, examination, evaluation, and intervention services for children from birth to 3 years of age with disabilities. The federal legislation that guides these services and current evidenced-based practice in early intervention will be discussed. Guiding principles for this chapter include family-centered services, support-based (contextual) models, interdisciplinary and trans-disciplinary team models, evidence-based practice, providing services in natural environments, and using activity-based instruction whenever possible.

What Do We Mean by "Early Intervention"?

The term *early intervention* (EI) is used in a variety of ways in a variety of disciplines. Conventional wisdom tells us it is best to intervene quickly when problems are suspected, before major problems occur. In medicine, competent physicians practice EI when they strive to provide intervention for illness as soon as symptoms are detected. The kindergarten teacher practices EI when he or she screens the class at the beginning of the school year to determine which children may need extra help learning to read. Even the wary homeowner who watches for signs of a leaky roof or basement is practicing early identification and intervention in an effort to ward off major and expensive household repairs. In other words, EI involves early detection and intervention of problems to minimize negative effects and reduce future potential problems as cost-effectively as possible.

When physical therapists engage in EI with infants and young children with delays, disabilities, or potential disabilities, they are doing essentially the same things as the individuals previously described. Pediatric therapists work with families, physicians, and others interested in the well-being of young children to *identify* potential or emerging problems or established developmental physical and cognitive problems as early as possible and to *intervene* quickly and efficiently to correct or minimize the problem/delay and to *maximize* the child's developmental potential, whatever that may be.

Definitions of Early Intervention

Federal legislation (PL 99-457), adopted in 1986, provided federal funding to the states for provision of early identification and intervention services to infants and young children aged 0 to 36 months who have, or are at risk of having, disabilities, and their families. This legislation was part of the Individuals with Disabilities Education Improvement Act (IDEA) and is discussed in this and the following chapter.

"The term 'early intervention services' means developmental services that:

[A] are provided under public supervision;

[B] are provided at no cost except where Federal or State law provides for a system of payments by families, including a schedule of sliding fees;

[C] are designed to meet the developmental needs of an infant or toddler with a disability, as identified by the individualized family service plan team, in any 1 or more of the following areas: (i) physical development, (ii) cognitive development, (iii) communication development, (iv) social or emotional development, or (v) adaptive development" (IDEA, 2004, 20 U.S.C.1432 § 632).

Although this legislation provides the "legal" definition of EI programs, experts in the field provide additional information regarding EI services and programs. Rune Simeonsson, a renowned educator and researcher in the area of EI, notes that the overall goal of EI "is to prevent disabilities in infants and young children by reducing or removing physical and social barriers and by promoting their growth, development, and well-being through stimulation and provision of support" (Simeonsson, 2000, p. 6). Simeonsson believes that EI providers must see each child as an individual, be comprehensive, address the child and his or her family as a unit, and take the individual family's social and cultural context into account.

Guralnick (2000) sees the provision of early, comprehensive assessment from many disciplines all working in harmony with the family as a vital element of EI and lists four guiding principles of EI: (a) family-centered services, (b) use of natural environments, (c) inclusion of children with disabilities in activities and settings with typically developing children, and (d) integration and coordination at all levels of EI (Guralnick, 2005). Bailey (1997) has stressed the importance of addressing the "at-risk" child when we speak of EI. As specified in IDEA 2004, "[t]he term 'at-risk infant or toddler' means an individual under 3 years of age who would be at risk of experiencing a substantial developmental delay if early intervention services were not provided to the individual" (IDEA, 2004, 20 U.S.C. 1431 § 631).

In addition, the EI pioneer Carl Dunst (Dunst, Trivette, & Jodry, 1997) reminds us that a child's and family's social support systems influence EI programs. He recommends a support-based service delivery model in which the interventionist provides or makes available the supports that would enable a family to optimize their child's development (Dunst, 2002). Specialized hands-on services provided by professionals is downplayed, while use of family routines as opportunities for practice is encouraged.

Authorities in EI come from many fields of research and study. They have come together as a workgroup for the National Early Childhood Technical Assistance Center to develop principles for providing early intervention (Workgroup, 2008) outlined in Table 11.1. These principles are elaborated throughout this chapter.

Purposes of Early Intervention

IDEA 2004 Part C lists the following primary purposes of EI services and needs that EI services are designed to meet:

"[1] to enhance the development of infants and toddlers with disabilities, to minimize their potential for developmental delay, and to recognize the significant brain development that occurs during a child's first 3 years of life;

[2] to reduce the educational costs to our society, including our Nation's schools, by minimizing the need for special education and related services after infants and toddlers with disabilities reach school age;

[3] to maximize the potential for individuals with disabilities to live independently in society;

[4] to enhance the capacity of families to meet the special needs of their infants and toddlers with disabilities; and

[5] to enhance the capacity of State and local agencies and service providers to identify, evaluate, and meet the needs of all children, particularly minority, low-income, inner city, and rural children, and infants and toddlers in foster care." (IDEA, 2004, 20 U.S.C.1431 § 631).

Table 11.1 Key Principles for Providing Early Intervention Services

1. Infants and toddlers learn best through everyday experiences and interactions with familiar people in familiar contexts.
2. All families, with the necessary supports and resources, can enhance their children's learning and development.
3. The primary role of the service provider in early intervention is to work with and support the family members and caregivers in a child's life.
4. The early intervention process, from initial contacts through transition, must be dynamic and individualized to reflect the child's and family members' preferences, learning styles and cultural beliefs.
5. IFSP outcomes must be functional and based on children's and families' needs and priorities.
6. The family's priorities needs and interests are addressed most appropriately by a primary provider who represents and receives team and community support.
7. Interventions with young children and family members must be based on explicit principles, validated practices, best available research and relevant laws and regulations.

Source: Workgroup on Principles and Practices in Natural Environments (February 2008). *Seven key principles: Looks like/doesn't look like.* OSEP TA Community of Practice—Part C Settings. Retrieved from http://www.nectac.org/topics/families/families.asp

You need to know that IDEA is updated or "reauthorized" by the federal government on a regular basis. The last reauthorization was in 2004, but the regulations for Part C were not published until 2011. Each time the law is reauthorized, EI therapists must be aware of the changes in the law. The American Physical Therapy Association, Section on Pediatrics and other national organizations such as the Council for Exceptional Children (CEC), will offer regular updates and easy to read summaries of changes in the law. One especially nice example is the document from the CEC-Division for Early Childhood entitled: Final Regulations Side-by-Side Comparison (2011). You can find the full reference under "Recommended Readings" at the end of this chapter.

Who Receives Early Intervention Services?

States are allowed to develop their own specific eligibility guidelines, but the federal legislation on EI includes the following description of children who may receive EI services. "The term 'infant or toddler with a disability'—

[A] means an individual under 3 years of age who needs early intervention services because the individual—
(i) is experiencing developmental delays, as measured by appropriate diagnostic instruments and procedures in 1 or more of the areas of cognitive development, physical development, communication development, social or emotional development, and adaptive development; or

(ii) has a diagnosed physical or mental condition that has a high probability of resulting in developmental delay; and

[B] maybe also include, at a State's discretion—
(i) at-risk infants and toddlers (IDEA, 2004, 20 U.S.C. 1431 § 631).

Some states include children who are at risk for having a developmental delay if EI is not provided. Children may receive EI services until the age of 36 months, or their third birthday.

What Services May Be Available to Children in Early Intervention?

Again, IDEA helps answer this question. Services include assessment and intervention in a large variety of areas and disciplines, including primary service coordination; audiology (hearing) and vision services; some health, medical, and nursing services; nutrition; occupational therapy; physical therapy; psychological services; social work services; speech/language pathology services; and some transportation services. Specialized instruction provided by specially trained educators, assistive technology services, and family support and respite services are also included in EI programs.

Physical therapy examination, evaluation, and intervention are important services needed by many children who participate in EI. It is important to note that physical therapy is considered a primary service in EI rather than a related service. This means that in EI, unlike services to school-aged children in which the physical therapy program must relate to the educational program, physical therapy services stand alone regardless of a child's educational/cognitive needs. Therefore, an infant with cystic fibrosis or a toddler with juvenile idiopathic arthritis might receive physical therapy services even though there may not be an educational need for services.

One further, very important point regarding EI services should be mentioned here. In the reauthorization of IDEA 2004, the federal government placed special emphasis on the increasing diversity of the population in the United States and emphasized the need for teachers and specialists who are able to represent and work with families and children with "limited English proficiency." Physical therapists working in EI must be aware of and honor the wide diversity represented by the families and children in their caseloads.

What Are the Components of Early Intervention?

The components of EI are determined by the federal regulations of Part C of IDEA, best practice, and evidence-based practice. Best practices are those goals, strategies, interventions, and principles that have been agreed on as reflecting the highest level of quality by certain professions, disciplines, and practitioners in those various fields.

In the following sections, the term **assessment** is used frequently because it is the word for the examination and evaluation of the child. In addition, many providers in early childhood special education and

speech-language pathology use the term "assessment" to refer to the initial and, especially, the ongoing examination and evaluation of a child's status. This is not meant to conflict with the physical therapist's use of the words "examination" and "evaluation," which have specific meaning within physical therapy. Rather, the term "assessment" is used to familiarize you with the terms most commonly used in the field of EI and within IDEA.

Individualized Planning for Each Child and Family

The federal regulations of Part C in IDEA define for us the what, who, where, when, how, and why of EI; however, states have a great deal of latitude in how these regulations are implemented. There is tremendous variability in state implementation of EI, so the focus of this chapter is the federal rules and accepted best practices.

Family-centered services should be flexible, individualized programs based on the family needs, emphasizing the strengths of the child with goals created by shared decision making by family members and professionals as equal partners (Dunst, 2002). Each child and family must have an **Individualized Family Service Plan (IFSP)**. The IFSP has several main components outlined by the federal law, which are presented in Table 11.2. Each state has an IFSP form to describe the proposed EI program for a specific child and family. Although

---

Table 11.2 Content of an Individualized Family Service Plan (IDEA, 2004, 20 U.S.C.1436 § 636(d))

1. A statement of the infant's or toddler's present levels of physical development, cognitive development, communication development, social or emotional development, and adaptive development, based on objective criteria
2. A statement of the family's resources, priorities, and concerns relating to enhancing the development of the family's infant or toddler with a disability
3. A statement of measurable results or outcomes expected to be achieved for the infant or toddler and the family, including preliteracy and language skills, as developmentally appropriate for the child, and the criteria, procedures, and timelines used to determine the degree to which progress toward achieving the results or outcomes is being made and whether modifications or revisions of the results or outcomes or services are necessary
4. A statement of specific early intervention services based on peer-reviewed research, to the extent practicable, necessary to meet the unique needs of the infant or toddler and the family, including the frequency, intensity, and method of delivering services
5. A statement of the natural environments in which early intervention services will appropriately be provided, including a justification of the extent, if any, to which the services will not be provided in a natural environment
6. The projected dates for initiation of services and the anticipated length, duration, and frequency of the services
7. The identification of the service coordinator from the profession most immediately relevant to the infant's or toddler's or family's needs (or who is otherwise qualified to carry out all applicable responsibilities) who will be responsible for the implementation of the plan and coordination with other agencies and persons, including transportation services
8. The steps to be taken to support the transition of the toddler with a disability to preschool or other appropriate services

Source: Individuals with Disabilities Education Improvement Act of 2004, 20 U.S.C. 1436 § 636(d).

forms may vary in appearance, they usually include the following elements.

Demographics

These are simply the basic identifying information for the child, family, service providers, and agencies to be involved in the plan.

History

Included in this section might be the child's past medical, prenatal, birth, and developmental histories, family history, and any past intervention the child may have received. See Figure 1.2 for content areas important to physical therapists.

Child's Current Level of Functioning

This section includes a summary of the child's current strengths and needs. This information comes from recent assessments by a team of interventionists and the family and includes the child's abilities in the major developmental areas of cognition, communication, physical, social/emotional, and adaptive skills. It is vitally important that all members of the EI team focus on the child's strengths as well as needs. For too long parents have had to endure long recitals of their child's deficits when they attended the planning meetings, with no attention being given to the positive, typical aspects of their child. Parents who have had such past experiences often comment after attending an IFSP meeting in which their child's strengths are recognized, "This is the first time anyone has had positive things to say about my child." This is a chilling commentary on the medical, educational, and therapeutic fields, and an occurrence that should no longer be tolerated.

Family's Concerns, Priorities, and Resources

This is the section of the IFSP in which the family members identify their primary concerns regarding their child, and their own needs in fostering their child's optimal development. They then list the priority *outcomes* they envision from the EI program. We may be more familiar with seeing the word "goals" used rather than "outcomes." Using the word *outcomes,* however, implies a more active program that focuses on the whole team working toward the same result. IDEA 2004 directs that outcomes should be measurable and developmentally appropriate. Fortunately, parents are more likely to express outcomes in terms of activity or participation such as wanting their child to walk around the house and sit independently at a local restaurant.

They rarely express goals in terms of impairments in body structure or function (Randall & McEwen, 2000).

Finally, the family reflects on the resources that are available to them to assist in achieving the outcomes they have selected. These resources include not only the agencies and providers at the IFSP meeting but also any community resource, family, or friends who may help support the family's and child's optimal development.

Early Intervention Services

Next, the team, including the family as a full participating equal member, designs the intervention program that is to help achieve the selected outcomes. This section includes the intervention strategies each provider will use and where, when, how often, and for how long the intervention services will be implemented. Interventions should occur in the child's natural environment and strategies should be evidence-based. This element of the IFSP are discussed in the sections on assessment and intervention.

Service Coordinator

Each family is provided with a **service coordinator** (also referred to as a *primary service coordinator*), who serves as a case manager for the family and child's EI program. The service coordinator should be "from the profession most immediately relevant to the infant's or toddler's or family's needs" (IDEA, 2004, 20 U.S.C. 1436 § 636(d)). The service coordinator is involved with the family from initial referral and will be available to the family to help facilitate all areas of the EI process. The service coordinator coordinates other team members, evaluations, IFSP development, interventions, and finally, the smooth transition from EI to public preschool programs when the child reaches 3 years of age.

Transition Plan

EI programs seek to provide "seamless" transition of services from EI to the early childhood program offered by the local public school system for the child. Long before the child approaches age 3 years, when he or she must transition out of EI, the local school system should have been advised of the child's needs and become a member of the IFSP team. In this way, the child and family are not left alone when EI services stop at age 3 years. Unfortunately, physical therapists have not been as engaged in the transition process as they should be. They rarely attend transition team meetings, but do report working with families on the transition process

(Myers & Effgen, 2006). Physical therapists who have strong communication and collaboration in their programs have greater involvement in the transition planning process (Myers et al., 2011). (See Chapter 12 on preschool and school-age services.)

Family-Centered Services and Intervention

The components of family-centered services and intervention are covered in Chapter 3. However, there cannot be a discussion of EI without including this overriding concept: **Family-centered services** and intervention imply the full involvement of the family in *all* aspects of the EI program. This involvement includes active participation of the family in assessment, planning, and intervention. It is easy to see that, as professionals, physical therapists cannot address the needs of an infant or toddler without the full participation of the most vital individuals in that child's life. What possible impact can physical therapists have on a child by visiting him or her only 1 or 2 hours per week? What of the remaining 166 hours of the week? Unless family members select the outcomes that are important to them and their child, agree with the intervention program, and help develop and implement that program within their individual abilities, how can therapists be expected to really affect a child's development? Family-centered services and intervention also imply that the family serves as an advocate for the child. In this position, family members may not always agree with what the professional believes is "best" for the child. The therapist must be ready to listen and work with the family until the EI program is acceptable to all concerned, if possible. This is vital since opportunities for the child to engage in high volumes of task-specific practice of an activity in a meaningful context is critical to achieve of the desired outcomes (Hickman, Westcott, McCoy, Long, & Rauh, 2011).

As in all aspects of the EI program, communication with the family must be in the family's primary language, and interpreters should be available when needed. This consideration includes not only those who speak a language other than English but also those individuals who are deaf or hard of hearing. In addition, we must be sensitive to the cognitive abilities of some parents and be sure that they fully understand what is being developed and decided in any EI program. The 2004 reauthorization of IDEA stresses the importance of our awareness of the increasing numbers of families and children who may have limited English proficiency.

Implementation of Early Intervention Within Natural Environments

Natural environments are "settings that are natural or typical for a same-aged infant or toddler without a disability, may include the home or community settings" (*Federal Register*, 2011). Researchers and specialists in a variety of disciplines note that children act and react differently in familiar, secure locations, such as the home, than when in an unfamiliar setting (Dunst, Hamby, Trivette, Raab, & Bruder, 2000; Woods, 2008). Physical therapists are more likely to achieve the most reliable examination information and the most typical behaviors in intervention if they work with the child and his or her family within their natural environment.

In addition, it is usually much easier for the family if the interventionist can come to the child's home or daycare setting. This approach causes less disruption of the family's daily life. Seeing a child for intervention in a hospital or office is using an artificial environment. What if the family does not have the equipment used in the office? What if prescribed activities never occur in the family's daily life or in the daycare setting? How are family members going to implement intervention strategies the other 166 hours per week if the intervention strategies and materials are not readily part of their lives? For these reasons, IDEA directs that assessment and intervention occur in the family's natural environments, not that of the therapist or interventionist.

Natural environments can include the child's home, daycare setting, local playground, or perhaps a playgroup site. Natural environments encourage and stimulate the easy carryover of intervention objectives into the family's everyday life. The family can see how everyday materials found in the home can be used to aid in the child's development. Seeing the child in his or her daycare setting helps caregivers to become active in his or her EI program and to use their time with the child to help optimize his or her development. The therapist must be flexible in finding and adapting therapeutic strategies to the equipment, toys, and activities available to the child on a daily basis. In addition, the therapist must be a model and teacher to the child's caretakers so they can carry out therapeutic activities with the child when the therapist is not present. Specific strategies for this are discussed later in this chapter in the intervention section.

Activity-Based Instruction

Conducting EI activities in the child and family's natural environment leads directly to the concept of **activity-based instruction.** This concept has also been referred as "routines-based instruction" or, when used in reference to curriculum planning and implementation, as "activity-based intervention." "Activity-based intervention is a child-directed, transactional approach where multiple learning opportunities are embedded into authentic activities and logically occurring antecedents, and timely feedback are provided to ensure functional and generative skills are acquired and used by the children" (Pretti-Frontczak, & Bricker, 2004, p.11). Activity-based instruction is similar to the concept of activity-focused intervention (Valvano, 2004; Valvano & Rapport, 2006) applied to the principles of motor development and learning discussed in Chapter 8.

Activity-based instruction is a concept that was developed in the field of special education in which teachers and interventionists strive to make intervention strategies as functional and integrated into the child's daily routine as possible. Working in the natural environment facilitates the ability to develop functional objectives and strategies that fit the family's lifestyle and the desired outcomes they have for their child (Bricker & Waddell, 2002). In years past, when therapists developed goals and interventions without the family's input, they often selected strategies or goals that could be implemented only by a therapist. Or they showed the family intervention strategies that required them to set aside specific, lengthy time periods of the day in which they did "therapy" with their child. Unfortunately, families have more to do than carry out "homework" assignments that the therapist assigns to them, with no regard to the time, or energy, that must be available to the family for them to complete the assignment each week. In the authors' experience, all too often, a parent would quickly fill in the "homework" data sheets that she or he had been given to complete throughout the week while sitting waiting for the therapist! Therapists need to learn that unless the suggestions given to families for daily activities with their children fit easily into the family's routines, are functional, and are easy to complete while the parents care for the other children, go to work, clean the house, and care for grandmother, those "home programs" may as well be pitched in the trash. The use of activity-based instruction or activity-focused intervention will be discussed in more detail in the intervention section of this chapter.

Teaming

Teaming is a vital part of the EI process. In Chapter 1, you learned about the various models of teaming and how the members interact; therefore, we will only briefly review these models as they relate to EI. Part C of IDEA requires team input during examination, evaluation, and intervention with the young child and family. Regular interaction and planning among all team members is necessary in EI. Team collaboration does not stop after the evaluation, but continues as long as the IFSP is in place.

There are several types of teams seen in EI. As described in Chapter 1, the **multidisciplinary team** is the oldest form of teaming and has the least active interaction among team members. There are no set channels of interaction and consultation. A multidisciplinary team could individually assess and report their findings without ever seeing each other. This type of team is clearly not sufficient to meet the requirements of Part C, which *requires* that each assessment conducted in EI include *multiple sources* of input and involve *interaction of the family and other evaluators*; however, IDEA Part C uses the term multidisciplinary to really describe an interdisciplinary or transdisciplinary team process. The interdisciplinary or transdisciplinary team is the preferred mode of EI team interaction (Mellin & Winton, 2003).

The **interdisciplinary team** offers more interaction among the team members than the multidisciplinary team, and there are typically formal channels of communication established among the professionals. Often, the team may submit one combined assessment report that includes information from all the professionals. Although this is an improved model of teaming, it still does not guarantee well-integrated development of intervention programming.

The **transdisciplinary team** is a frequently used model of team assessment and program development in EI (Hickman et al., 2011; Orelove, Sobsey, & Silberman, 2004). In this model, the team members are encouraged to share information, skills, and programming *across* disciplines and with the family. Some of this sharing involves *role release* and will be discussed under intervention. Team members may assess the child together, and even treat together at times, to ensure themselves and the family that *all team members are sharing goals and strategies for the child's optimal development*. When assessment and programming are developed with all the team members and the family together, and strategies are shared across disciplines, the child receives constant reinforcement of all the important outcomes strategies, rather than receiving input only when the physical therapist, speech-language pathologist, or occupational therapist happens to be in the home or with the child.

Keeping best practice and Part C regulations in mind, physical therapists should no longer examine a child and independently develop and implement an intervention program. They must serve as part of a larger team, including a variety of disciplines and the child's family. Somewhat counter to this important concept of team assessment, program planning, and intervention is an unfortunate trend in some locations to have one group of professionals perform the assessment and another group provide the intervention. This is done under the misguided assumption that too many children are being recommended for services by assessment teams that will provide the services. Perhaps this has occurred; however, the use of two teams creates additional work, expense, and duplication of assessment services. In this model, once the assessment team determines that intervention is required, the child is referred for services, and another team provides the intervention. Under most circumstances the second team, based on professional codes of conduct and state practice acts, must reassess the child before intervention can be provided. A physical therapist should always examine and evaluate a client before developing a plan of care and providing intervention (American Physical Therapy Association, 2001).

The composition of the individual child's IFSP team should be individualized, with different team members constituting teams for different children. The primary IFSP team may include smaller teams. For example, a child with cerebral palsy may be seen by a team that includes an occupational therapist, a physical therapist, a developmental interventionist, and a speech-language pathologist, whereas a child with a language delay might have a team consisting of only a developmental interventionist and a speech-language pathologist.

The child may also see teams of professionals at a center that specializes in a specific disability. Often children who have been diagnosed with autism travel to a center that specializes in that disability for assessment and consultation. There the child may see another set of occupational therapists, physical therapists, speech-language pathologists, psychologists, social workers, physicians, and so on. Again, this specialized team must be careful to include the input of the EI team that sees the child on a regular basis. Unfortunately, this is not always the case, and early interventionists, whether part of the home-based team or the specialized consultation team, must work diligently to be sure that interaction between the two teams occurs so that the child and family are not given conflicting information or confusing input.

How Are These "Best Practice" Components of Early Intervention Integrated Into Assessment/Evaluation and Intervention Strategies?

The primary components of a quality EI program were just discussed. These components included the IFSP, family-centered services and intervention, assessment/intervention within the child's natural environment, activity-based instruction, and teaming. How these components play out in the two major parts of the EI process, assessment/evaluation and intervention, can now be seen.

Assessment/Evaluation

Individualized Family Service Plan and Family-Centered Services

IDEA provides specific timelines regarding how many days may pass between the referral of a child to the EI system and when the first contact with the family must occur. In addition, each state has specific guidelines regarding how many days may pass before an assessment is completed after the child is referred to a provider and how soon the assessment report must be completed. Typically, a state requires that the results of the assessment must be given to and discussed with the family *before* the IFSP meeting. Therapists must be aware of the guidelines of the state in which they practice and adhere closely to those guidelines. Each state has specific formats for reporting assessment/evaluation results.

As noted by Bagnato, Neisworth, and Pretti-Frontczak (2010), assessment or "measurement is not merely an administrative exercise. It must be practical, sensible, and representative and must benefit the child and family in tangible ways." They note that conventional testing is flawed and that many measures just highlight the child's limitations and do not demonstrate the child's everyday skills and uniqueness. However, most states still recommend a particular instrument to use to determine "eligibility" for EI. This instrument may be (but is not necessarily) a standardized instrument that establishes functioning levels in the five developmental areas outlined by Part C of IDEA. Although this instrument may be sufficient to determine that a child is eligible for the state's EI program, it may not be sufficient to program for a child's individual needs in any particular area. After a child qualifies for EI and the developmental areas of need are determined, a more complete assessment/evaluation is usually conducted by professionals in each appropriate discipline that address the child's specific areas of need. The family's concerns must also be a driving force in determining which assessments are to be completed.

Part C also requires that assessments include *multiple sources of information.* This means not only that *more than one* evaluator gives input *as well as the family,* but *that this input must come from more than one type of measure.* Simply giving the child a commercially available instrument is not sufficient for assessment under Part C. The child should be observed in natural activities and natural environments that allow numerous opportunities for the child to display true functioning levels and strengths.

Part C states some very clear requirements for the conducting and reporting of the EI assessments. Under Part C, the assessment should include the family's input. Before any interaction with the child, the therapist contacts the family to determine their primary concerns regarding the child's development—a top-down approach to assessment.

The family must give written consent for assessment. The family should be present throughout the assessment, whether it is conducted only by the physical therapist or in a team setting involving other disciplines. It can be especially helpful to give the family some form of a family-friendly checklist or home assessment to record their own impression of their child's developmental levels.

This information is then integrated into the written report as the parental input, information that is required under Part C. Such an activity also allows *parents to give their own assessment input,* if they desire, during the IFSP meeting. The assessment must be in the family's primary language and should be culturally sensitive. If the therapist does not speak the family's primary language, an interpreter should be present. This requirement includes obtaining an interpreter for the deaf or hearing impaired.

If any standardized instruments are used in the evaluation, every effort should be made to use only instruments that have been standardized on a population similar to the family's cultural and socioeconomic background. Because this may not always be possible, care must be taken in interpreting and reporting the results of instruments that do not fit these requirements.

Natural Environments

Assessments should be conducted within the child's natural environment. As stated earlier in this chapter, that setting may be the child's home, daycare setting, the playground, a family friend's home, or any other setting where typically developing children are found. The therapist's office, a hospital, or a developmental center designed specifically for children with special needs usually does not qualify as a "natural environment." The use of the natural environment allows naturalistic observation of play and other daily routines that are required under Part C. The natural environment helps to ensure that therapists are being culturally sensitive and family centered and provides a much more realistic picture of the child's real, functional abilities. Although a child may be hesitant to climb stairs in the office building, he or she may be quite adept at this skill at home or on the playground.

Activity-Based Assessment

In the field of EI, authorities have long been concerned that standardized assessment/evaluation instruments are not functional or realistic, do not give a "real-life" or an "authentic" picture of a child and his or her daily routines, and frequently are not sensitive to the family's culture (Neisworth & Bagnato, 2004). Rich information about the child and his or her skills can be drawn from observation and interactions with the child in everyday play and activities.

Activity-based or authentic assessment can be conducted by using a commercially available, criterion-referenced instrument, or from trained observations. Some of the more popular commercial instruments are listed in Appendix 3.A. These instruments are usually conducted in the child's home or daycare setting and involve a team of early interventionists as well as the family. The child is observed with his or her siblings or peers during a variety of activities. Professionals record information that applies to their discipline and expertise, and the team discusses and scores the assessment as a group.

A commercial instrument is not necessary to complete an activity-based assessment. The physical therapist may choose to observe and "play" with the child in his or her natural environment and allow the child to select favorite, natural, functional activities through which he or she demonstrates strengths and areas of need. This approach allows the child to demonstrate his or her true functional abilities while enjoying natural activities.

Using specific instruments, which allow only certain materials and activities, may severely limit the functionality of the assessment as well as its accuracy. Therapists should try to come to the home at a time when the child is usually going to be involved in activities that will best demonstrate his or her skills in a certain area. If a therapist needs to observe a child's self-feeding skills, it makes sense to try to come during the child's typical mealtime. This reduces the disruption of the family's schedule and increases the likelihood of seeing the child's real skill level.

Teaming

The types of teams that are seen in EI have already been discussed. The type of team you participate in may well influence how your assessments are conducted. The assessment should be at least of an interdisciplinary nature. This means that the individuals involved with the assessment of a particular child have (1) discussed concerns with the family, (2) discussed what areas of assessment and what tools are to be used with the other team members, (3) determined, with the family, what are the best times and locations for the assessment, and have coordinated this with other team members so that the family's schedule is not unduly disrupted, (4) discussed the results of assessments with the family and with other team members before the IFSP meeting, and (5) worked to coordinate and integrate assessment information in the reporting process. Each individual interdisciplinary team member then conducts the actual assessment of the child usually on a one-to-one basis as appropriate.

Best practice indicates that *transdisciplinary assessments* may be an especially efficient and effective form of assessment in a child's EI years. The initial aspects of the assessment process might be similar to the interdisciplinary approach. Each team member talks to the family before the assessment to secure the family's concerns about their child. The team also decides together which instruments are to be used and, with the family, when and where the assessment will be conducted. How the actual assessment is conducted, however, can be quite different from the way it is conducted in the interdisciplinary team approach.

Transdisciplinary teams frequently use **arena assessment,** as discussed in Chapter 1, when the resources for proper service delivery are available. In this style of assessment, team members are all together for the assessment along with the family and child (Fig. 11.1). Which team members will be included in the assessment process for a particular child will be determined by the family's areas of concern for their child's development. A team might include a physical therapist, a speech-language pathologist, an occupational therapist, an early childhood educator (developmental interventionist), possibly a social worker or psychologist and, of course, the service coordinator as well as the family.

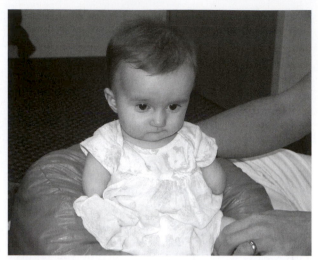

Figure 11.1 Infant with limb deficiencies participating in an arena assessment.

In an arena assessment, the team selects one or more assessment instruments that include sections for each of the five developmental areas (cognition, communication, physical, adaptive, and social/emotional skills) typically addressed in EI. Some commonly used assessments in EI include the Bayley Scales of Infant Development II, Hawaii Early Learning Profile, Carolina Curriculum, and the Assessment, Education, and Programming System for Infants and Children (AEPS).

In an arena assessment, all members are present for the assessment, but only one or two may actually interact directly with the child. This approach reduces the number of adults to whom the child must become accustomed. The team usually selects the members who will be working directly with the child based on the family's primary concern about the child's development. For instance, if the parent is very concerned about the child's ability to move and walk, the physical therapist may be the primary evaluator. If the child is not yet talking and has a feeding disorder, the speech-language pathologist and occupational therapist may lead the assessment. The other team members observe and prompt the primary evaluator(s) to complete various tasks with the child that they need to observe.

In the arena assessment, the parent will answer developmental and history questions with all team members present. This approach decreases the repetitious nature of multiple individual assessments. Usually, one or more team members can talk with the family quietly during the assessment and secure their opinion of their child's performance during the assessment, when adjustments and adaptations can readily be made to enhance the child's performance. One of the team members can quietly suggest to the primary evaluator(s) that they try some alternative activity or input to facilitate the child's participation or interaction that the parent has suggested. Parents are often frustrated when they know that their child could perform a task if the evaluator merely stated a direction differently or allowed the child to use the assessment material in a different manner. Remember, unless administering a standardized instrument, the goal is to see if there is any way a child can complete a task by accessing his or her *strengths,* rather than simply noting the weaknesses and what cannot be done. This approach to assessment allows the parent to have a more active role and reinforces to the family how much their input is valued. When the primary instrument has been completed, various members of the team may need to complete more specific examinations with the child while the rest of the team observes or interacts with the family. The physical therapist might need to examine body structures and functions that might impair the child's performance of activities.

Materials and activities should be familiar to the child and be appropriate for his or her age and cultural background. As noted above, the team should make the assessment as functional and activity based as possible. Remember, the assessment should be reflective of the child's actual functional abilities and should be as enjoyable as possible for the child and family.

Assessment Report

When the written report is developed, each team member contributes within his or her area of expertise, and a single, well-integrated report and recommendations are developed from the assessment based on the priorities of the family. Use of activity-related goals and objectives should increase independence and participation of the infant in daily routines (Valvano & Rapport, 2006). Early intervention assessment reports, as in all EI reports, must use **family-friendly language**. The assessment report should be easily understandable to the child's parents or caregiver. Families vary in their education, cognitive levels, cultural background, and reading skills. If a technical term or professional jargon is necessary in a report, a simple explanation should accompany that term immediately after it is used. For example, if the physical therapy notes that a child appears to be "hypertonic," the therapist might report this as follows: "Muscle tone examination revealed hypertonicity in the legs. This means that Billy's legs are

stiff and difficult to bend." The report must be understandable to family members regardless of their educational or language background.

Intervention

Individualized Family Service Plan

The IFSP includes the outcomes decided on by the family and team, and it guides the child's intervention program. These outcomes are written in the family's words. The team then develops strategies that are aimed at accomplishing the outcomes the family desires for their child. These outcomes are similar to intervention goals but they are recorded in the family's words. For example, an outcome may read: "Bob and Nancy want Billy to walk across the kitchen." The therapist then works with the family toward designing programming to fulfill this outcome. The child might need to begin working toward the outcome of "walking" at a much earlier developmental level. The therapist does not try to dash the family's dream of their child walking, even if he or she is not ready for this stage. The IFSP is developed around the family's outcome statements and is being written before the child is even 3 years of age. Remember that few can predict what any particular child may achieve at so early an age. On the other hand, honesty with families about the child's current developmental levels and prognosis is critical. For some diagnoses, such as cerebral palsy, evidence-based guidelines regarding motor prognosis are becoming available (Rosenbaum et al., 2002). Therapists may discuss with the family the stages a baby passes through on the way to walking and decide with them where to begin therapy. Perhaps they will begin with the child bearing weight and rocking on all fours. The plan for the child's intervention for the next 6 months becomes the strategies used to achieve the "walking" outcome the family has selected. This plan, along with the **functional, activity-based techniques** used when working with the child and family, fits well under the "strategies" section of the IFSP. Just remember that the important elements of the planned strategies must include how to embed the intervention plan into the family's daily routines, natural environment, and activities.

Family-Centered Intervention

As in all stages of the EI program, intervention must fully include the family, be designed around the family's routines and activities, and be easily completed within the family's busy schedule. Strategies for these requirements will be discussed toward the end of this chapter.

In addition, intervention is scheduled as closely as possible to the family's requests so as to not disrupt their daily routine. The therapist works with the family and service coordinator to find times for home visits that are optimal for the child's performance and the family's full participation.

The family is a full member of the intervention team. Therapists do not enter a child's home, provide therapy alone with the child, make a few written suggestions, and leave. It is very important that the family or caregiver be present throughout the intervention visit and have active participation in the session. Materials, toys, and equipment used should be those found in the home, if possible, so that the family can easily follow through on the activities and strategies. Any interventions that can be taught to the family should be practiced while the therapist is present. When family members cannot be present for a session, consider videotaping the session and leaving it for the family to watch later. This allows them to actively involve themselves in the intervention and learn what activities may be helpful for their child.

Natural Environments

Intervention should be conducted in natural environments (Bruder, 2001; Workgroup, 2008). In fact, IDEA 2004 requires a justification if services to a specific family or child are not provided in the natural environment (IDEA, 2004, 20 U.S.C. 1435 § 635(a)(16)(B)). Natural environments are where typical children would be found and include the home, daycare setting, playground, a playgroup with typical peers, or even at Grandma's house. Children are much more interactive and perform better in familiar environments. It's also been found that including the siblings in the intervention session gives the child wonderful models. The child is often much more likely to imitate his or her brother or sister than the less-than-appealing adult therapist! By working in the child's natural environment, therapists increase the likelihood that the primary caregiver can be available to participate in the sessions. This is especially true when visiting the daycare setting. These caregivers are usually eager to carry over a child's EI goals if they are included in the sessions and taught what they can do to contribute to the child's EI program.

Activity-Based Instruction

As already described, the concept of activity-based instruction originated in the area of special education and has been contributed to by many individuals (Pretti-Frontczak & Bricker, 2004; Pretti-Frontczak,

Barr, Macy, & Carter, 2003; Valvano & Rapport, 2006). In the past, educators found that children with disabilities were often being taught and receiving therapy services in rigid, nonfunctional ways. There was no intrinsic reinforcement for the child in the activity in which he or she was participating. The goals were selected from developmental profiles, without regard to a particular child's interest or functional needs.

Activity-based instruction and activity-focused intervention, on the other hand, looks at what the child enjoys doing, how target skills can be embedded into interesting activities or daily routines, and the functionality of an activity and goal. Why must a child stack blocks if there is no interest in block stacking? Therapists should analyze the skills block stacking involves (e.g., grasping, alternating use of hands, visual perception, and coordination) and then find ways to stimulate these skills in activities that are interesting to the child. Maybe the child prefers to construct a fort with blocks or to stack cookies. Why not stimulate the same motor skills and make use of the intrinsic reinforcement that fun activities offer the child? Children who have been mistakenly labeled "uncooperative" may merely be indicating that they do not like the activity selected for them. Remember, EI is largely child directed, not adult directed. It requires creativity and perseverance at times to fit the goals into the child's daily activities or favorite games, but it can be done, and the payoff is a happily engaged child and a positive caregiver or parent.

Activity-based instruction also means that therapeutic strategies fit into the child's and family's daily routine. This practice is in line with task-specific practice but requires that the tasks be carefully planned within the daily routines. For example, it certainly makes more sense to schedule a session on sensory or tactile input and reaching during bath time than to come at some other time of day that will disrupt the busy schedule of the family. This scenario also allows the parents or caregivers to be fully involved with the session because they would be bathing the child at the time anyway. Helpful strategies for implementing activity-based instruction will be discussed toward the end of the chapter.

Teaming in Intervention

As already noted, the preferred models of EI team intervention are the interdisciplinary model and the transdisciplinary model (Hickman et al., 2011; Mellin & Winton, 2003). As discussed before in the interdisciplinary model, the intervention team and the family may talk regularly and meet periodically in IFSP meetings (at least every 6 months) to develop outcomes together. The actual implementation of those outcomes and the strategies that support them, however, are typically completed separately, with each team member visiting the family and child on an individual basis. Ideally, the team members talk or correspond on a regular basis, sharing their strategies and concerns. Often, written copies of each therapist's programs and suggestions are circulated among the team. The parents or caregivers are present, if possible, at all therapy sessions and are given demonstrations and written suggestions for home carryover of therapeutic goals. Intervention in any team model should incorporate the principles of activity-based, functional instructions and curriculum, and occur in the child's and family's natural environment.

As already noted, the transdisciplinary team has constant communication among team members. Team members and the family work together to consolidate programming so that each session, regardless of what discipline is involved, reinforces all outcomes and strategies that have been developed for a child's intervention program.

Another version of this approach is termed "**coaching**," which utilizes conversation and self-observation to support families and other team members in gaining skills to facilitate the child's development in natural situations and then to self-evaluate the result. "Coaching . . . provides a structure for developing and nurturing partnerships with both families and colleagues and reconceptualizes the role of an early childhood practitioner as a collaborative partner working alongside family members and other caregivers," (Hanft, Rush, & Shelden, 2004).

Special educators endorse this collaborative/consultative intervention model, which holds that "all intervention occurs between specialists' visits" (McWilliam, 2003). This means that the interventionist partners with the family during home visits to share strategies to support the child's development so that the family can continuously foster their child's development when the specialist is not present.

However, the use of the words "consultative model" can be confusing to therapists who, because of their training, typically think of "consultation" as infrequent or remote interactions with the child and family. It is easy to see how misconceptions can occur among the various disciplines that work in EI. Physical therapists who work in EI must maintain ongoing discussion and communication with colleagues in other fields to avoid confusion involving discipline-specific vocabulary.

Regardless of the vocabulary used, all EI specialists know the importance of empowering and supporting families during home visits so that family members can learn to support and foster their child's development in each area of need and become comfortable with this process—whether or not a therapist or teacher is present at any one time (Workgroup, 2008). Physical therapists were involved in family-focused and ecological approaches to EI long before suggested by federal law (Effgen & Berger, 1978).

Therapists need to partner with the family and other team members for the child's optimal success. For example, if a child's IFSP lists the outcomes of sitting up, eating from a spoon, drinking from a cup, and talking (as prioritized by the child's parents), all of the therapists must work toward these desired outcomes. The physical therapist should have very specific strategies to facilitate the child's ability to sit and must provide the other team members with training and demonstrations to allow them to reinforce the strategies for the sitting outcome, which will allow the child to sit with stability when working on feeding skills.

At the same time, the physical therapist has much to offer the speech-language pathologist in terms of working with the child's respiration to facilitate the oral/vocal output that leads to oral speech. Also facilitating such outcomes is the family, who will be with the child all week when no professional is present. The family will want to encourage the child's progress as much as, or more than, any of the therapists.

As part of the transdisciplinary team, how does one fulfill all of these responsibilities in, perhaps, only an hour per week? Are therapists not just there to see that the child learns to sit and later walk if possible? How can therapists also be responsible for reinforcing the goals of other professionals? How can therapists "allow" others (family and colleagues) to carry out activities with the child for which the physical therapist has trained for years? Three very important elements of the transdisciplinary intervention approach help answer these weighty questions: *integrated programming, cotreatment,* and *role release.*

Integrated programming specifically involves the development of strategies for the parent-selected outcomes that are developed *as a team.* When the team develops the strategies for "talking," the speech-language pathologist and family will, of course, take the lead. However, the speech-language pathologist will ask the physical therapist to include specific strategies that the full team can be taught, which will improve the child's respiration so that vocalization is more likely.

If the child is not yet an oral speaker, the speech-language pathologist will develop an augmentative communication system. This could include the use of manual signs, a simple picture board, or an electronic device. In this situation, the speech-language pathologist teaches the other team members to use this system of communication, and it becomes as much the responsibility of the physical therapist, occupational therapist, and special educator to utilize this system when communicating with the child as it is for the speech-language pathologist and family.

The strategies section of the IFSP is then developed as a *unit* by the team and family, with all disciplines offering input to *each outcome,* not only the one or two that seem to fall solely within one's own discipline. Everyone must help find opportunities for the child to engage in high-volume, task-specific practice of target behaviors (Hickman et al., 2011).

Cotreatment is a situation in which two or more of the professionals are involved in the child's intervention in a single session. There are situations in which this is a necessity. If a child has severe cerebral palsy (CP) and has great difficulty sitting or moving, or even achieving a stable position for oral feeding, it may be almost impossible for a speech-language pathologist to set up a feeding program with the family without the hands-on input and *demonstration and instruction* from the physical therapist, with both the speech-language pathologist and family present and actively involved.

Likewise, the physical therapist may be at a loss in communicating with a child with a severe communication disorder. This may occur if a child is nonverbal, has a severe physical handicap, or perhaps has been diagnosed with autism. In this situation, the physical therapist will want the speech-language pathologist to be present to *demonstrate and instruct* during a physical therapy session to help the physical therapist learn to interact with the child.

If communication is poor, the physical therapist may mistake a child's frustration at not understanding or being understood as a behavioral problem. When such a problem is left unchecked, therapy sessions may become unfruitful. Parents become frustrated with the therapist as well, thinking that the child does not like the physical therapy sessions, when, in fact, there is only a communication problem. Cotreatment, in which the speech-language pathologist helps analyze the problem and offers training and demonstration for improved means of communication, may markedly improve the sessions.

Cotreatment is not done on a weekly basis. In fact, some payors mistakenly think that a cotreatment session is not a full session of treatment by each of the professionals present, although this is not true. In the cotreatment session, both therapists are actively involved at all times, and the sessions may well be much more productive than an individual 1-hour session by individual therapists. Nevertheless, the reality is that some payors do not support this mode of intervention, and it may be difficult to schedule such sessions with the family's and therapists' busy schedules. However, intermittent, regularly scheduled cotreatment sessions, or cotreatment sessions on an "as needed" basis, are still highly beneficial to the child, family, and therapists and are usually possible in most situations.

The last strategy, that of **role release,** grows directly out of cotreatment sessions, integrated planning strategies, and transdisciplinary services. In role release, the primary therapist for a specific outcome—say, the physical therapist for an independent sitting outcome—decides what are the most important strategies that must be completed with the child on a regular basis to learn the task of sitting. Such strategies or therapeutic techniques might include encouraging head control, sitting with support, and then reducing the degree of support and reduction of the limitations of body structure and function, such as increasing range of motion and trunk strength. Although the physical therapist is highly adept at these strategies, intervention occurring once a week for 1 hour cannot accomplish much progress with the child's development unless some strategies or techniques can be repeated regularly throughout the week.

Many intervention strategies can be safely demonstrated, practiced, and then carried out by the family and other interventionists. Videotaped demonstrations, photographs, written instructions, hands-on instructions, and regular monitoring by the physical therapist will allow the child to benefit from "intervention" all week long. For example, parents have been taught successfully somewhat complex interventions, such as providing treadmill training for infants with Down syndrome (Ulrich, Lloyd, Tiernan, Looper, & Angulo-Barroso, 2008).

The "coaching" model would also fit into this paradigm (Hanft et al., 2004; Rush & Sheldon, 2011). All professionals will have certain strategies that they can safely share with their colleagues and the child's family. They will also have strategies that only they are trained or licensed to complete, and these are not part of role release.

However, unless an effort is made to share some of the therapist's expertise with the team, when feasible and safe, the child will not get the consistent input needed to make rapid and consistent progress. Some therapists like to keep a written log of the strategies they have taught to the family and to the other therapists, and then periodically monitor the use of these strategies.

All of the strategies discussed so far are considered best or preferred practice in the area of EI. How can therapists implement these excellent ideas when they are bound by a heavy caseload and busy schedule? In addition, how can parents be asked to add more responsibilities to their already full days? The next section of this chapter will try to answer some of these concerns.

Strategies to Encourage Intervention: Cataloging and Matrix Development

Families who have children with disabilities are especially busy and may have difficulty fitting in everything they are recommended to do with their child each day. Suggestions may be made about home carryover of the therapy activities that are shared with families, but they may not have the time, person power, or energy to follow all of the suggestions. When this occurs, many parents or caregivers begin to feel guilty. If therapists are not sensitive to the many stressors and demands each family has, they may inadvertently contribute to parents' or caregivers' feelings of "not doing enough" for their child with a disability.

Suppose you are working with a family that has three children. They have a set of 3-year-old twins and an 8-month-old infant who has just been diagnosed with CP. The father works for a trucking firm and drives several days at a time. Therefore, his wife must care for their three children alone, several days per week. There are no grandparents or close relatives nearby.

You are the physical therapist seeing the baby who has CP. The baby has poor head control, is not sitting yet, and has difficulty grasping her toys. She "stiffens" when her diaper is changed or when placed on her tummy. You believe that she needs a variety of developmental activities completed throughout the day, and you suggest these to the mother. The mother calmly but clearly tells you that there is no way she can possibly add anything else to her busy schedule. She is distressed that she cannot complete all the activities the therapists are recommending for her child. What will you do?

Two excellent strategies have been developed in the disciplines of special education and early childhood special education that are well suited for this situation. They are called **cataloging** and **matrix development** (Browder & Martin, 1986; Wilcox & Belamy, 1987) and have been used in the areas of education and EI for

some time. The following paragraphs illustrate how they can be applied to this situation.

Cataloging

Cataloging involves making a simple log of all of the baby's daily activities from morning to night. The therapist, or any other member of the team, meets with the parents at a convenient time and asks them to outline the baby's day. Activities usually include a sequence such as getting up, changing diapers, eating breakfast (or nursing), taking a bath, and swinging in the baby seat while Mom gets the other children up, fed, and dressed. The baby may then ride in the car while her siblings are taken to preschool, go with mom to the grocery store, then pick up the siblings, come home, eat, and take a nap. All of this is probably done before noon! You can see right away how useful cataloging is for the therapist who often has no idea what a family deals with daily.

When the catalog is completed, the family is assured that no one wants to add any more stress to their daily lives. Rather, the purpose is to see if the therapeutic activities can be embedded into the family's existing schedule. For example, the baby may have her diaper changed up to eight times per day. That is an activity that occurs regularly and cannot be omitted. Why not just show the parents how they can perform some trunk rotation activities each time the baby's diaper is changed?

Mom will place the baby on the changing table, and before taking off the diaper and raising the baby's legs to clean her and place the new diaper on, she bends the hips and knees, gently rocking the legs and trunk from side to side. Remember, the baby stiffens every time her diaper is changed, and this makes diapering unpleasant for her and Mom. By embedding some relaxation activities into the diapering routine, diapering can be made more enjoyable for everyone. Later, active leg abduction activities may be added to maintain ROM. Most of the objectives can be accomplished by embedding them into the baby's daily routine.

Matrix Development

Once the catalog of the baby's day is completed and the parents have been shown how they can embed specific activities into their daily routine, the baby's catalog entries are placed in the first column of a "**matrix**" (Table 11.3).

The matrix is a chart that lists the baby's daily activities in the first column and the main outcome areas or specific outcomes across the top row. In the

Table 11.3 Completed Matrix With Several Embedded Strategies

Information	Communication Outcomes	Physical Outcomes	Cognitive Outcomes	Adaptive Outcomes	Social/Emotional Outcomes
7 a.m. Wake up	Call baby's name				
Change diaper		Do relaxation activity			
Nurse/eat				Assist with lip closure	
Bath		Sensory input			
Dress			Show each item of clothing and name it		
8 a.m. Twins get up, eat, dress		Sitting upright while assisting in dressing			Twins talk to baby, baby responds with smile
9 a.m. Take twins to preschool	Sing in the car				
Go to grocery store			Have baby look at each item as it goes into the cart		
Run errands					
11:30 a.m. Pick up twins	Twins call baby's name as they get in the car, baby looks				
Change diaper		Relaxation activity and sensory input			
Mom fixes lunch					
Eat		Properly positioned for eating		Lip closure	
Change diaper		Relaxation activity and sensory input			
1 p.m. Take nap		Position for sleeping			

boxes by each of the baby's main activities, embed a therapeutic activity that is easily completed within the daily routine.

In the transdisciplinary model, all of the therapists contribute to one matrix, so as not to overload the family. If the baby has feeding goals, they can be easily inserted into snack times or mealtimes. Occupational therapy sensory programs can fit nicely into bath time. The speech-language pathologist might suggest that the parents call the baby's name each time they intend to pick her up to help her learn to recognize and respond to voice and then words.

Do not overload the family. Begin with only one outcome for each therapy at first. When the family becomes familiar with the matrix concept and the activities, they will decide for themselves what to do throughout the day. A completed matrix is presented in Table 11.3. Using the strategies of cataloging and matrix development assists the early interventionist in making maximum use of the child's natural environments, and will incorporate activity-based instruction into the family's daily routines.

Occasionally, the team will determine that the child requires more intervention than can be provided by the EI team. The intensity and frequency of services generally vary across, and even within, states. This variability is often not based on the child's needs but on the resources available in each individual state. The therapist must discuss with the entire team the extent of required additional services.

In some states, the team can request and receive permission to provide additional services. If these needed services are not available through the EI system, the therapist has the ethical obligation to work with the team to seek appropriate services in the community. Children who might require more extensive physical therapy services than the EI system can provide include those with complex medical needs, those who are at critical transition periods, and those whose parents or care providers are clearly unable to carry out the recommended activities. Children should not be punished because of the limitations of the EI system or their caregivers, and efforts should be made to obtain necessary services.

What Do Other Disciplines Expect of the Physical Therapist in the Team Setting?

If you are lucky enough to have the opportunity to work in a strong interdisciplinary or transdisciplinary setting, your colleagues in occupational therapy, speech-language pathology, special education, and so on will ask you for consultation, inservicing, demonstrations, cotreatment, team assessment, and planning. They will also expect that you will come to them for the same type of input. Each member of the team is responsible for these activities within their area of expertise. Only in this way can a strong team be built.

Some of the most common areas of consultation and demonstration that the physical therapist offers to colleagues in EI include positioning and seating for daily activities, feeding, play, and transportation; providing information on age-appropriate movement activities; assisting in improving respiratory development, which will facilitate louder and easier speech sounds and babbling; helping to determine which body part should be used to activate an augmentative communication device or adapted toy play; and identifying proper body mechanics for care providers. Indeed there is evidence that increases in motor skills facilitate speech and language development. According to Iverson (2010), there is evidence "that the emergence and continued development of new motor abilities during the first eighteen months has far-reaching consequences that extend to other developing systems, including language" (p. 258).

The physical therapist will also be expected to carry over and reinforce the therapeutic strategies of other disciplines. The speech-language pathologist may give input regarding how to help the child learn and understand language, and how to use the child's augmentative communication system. The speech-language pathologist may also ask the physical therapist to model certain vocalizations when the baby's movement typically elicits vocalizations. The special educator will have suggestions about what toys are best for play during therapy or what directions the baby needs to learn to follow.

The behavioral specialist may ask that all members of the team respond to the child's disruptive behavior in a certain manner, because consistency of responses is of critical importance. The occupational therapist may provide suggestions for each team member to follow as he or she introduces activities that include sensory stimulation and functional hand use. Research stresses the interplay among development as well. There is evidence that social and cognitive development mediate what motor activities the infant attempts (Adolf, Tamis-Lemonda, & Karasik, 2010). Physical therapists will want to take into account cultural, experiential, social and cognitive differences when designing interventions.

Clearly, the physical therapist has much to offer the EI team and will have many opportunities to learn from colleagues. Inexperienced physical therapists will learn a great deal from all members of the team; however, they should also seek an experienced physical therapist as a mentor so that they can develop skills and knowledge within their own discipline.

Summary

EI is an exciting and challenging area of practice. It provides the opportunity to work closely with numerous different professionals focused on a single goal of meeting the needs of the young child and family, but rarely at the same time. Service delivery in natural environments as required in EI can be a challenge for some professionals, but as the benefits unfold, the obstacles are overcome. EI can offer the physical therapist constant learning opportunities and many rewards. It also provides an employment situation where part-time work is usually available, so the therapist can stay in practice while raising a family or while working in a variety of service delivery settings.

DISCUSSION QUESTIONS

1. What are the benefits of observation and evaluation in the natural environment?

2. Are there any problems or limitations with intervention in the natural environment, and if so, how might they be overcome?

3. What is the role of the physical therapist in activity-based instruction?

4. In family-centered care, why is it important to understand the family's daily routine? How does cataloging assist the therapist and family?

Recommended Readings

Adolf, K.E., Tamis-Lemonda, C., & Karasik, L.B. (2010). Cinderella indeed- A commentary on Iverson's: 'Developing language in a developing body: The relationship between motor development and language development.' *Journal of Child Language, 37,* 269–273.

Council for Exceptional Children-Division of Early Childhood-Infant Toddler Coordination Association (2011). IDEA Part C: Early Intervention Program for Infants and Toddlers With Disabilities: Final Regulations Side-by Side Comparison. Retrieved from http://www.directionservice.org/cadre/finalregscompare.cfm

Guralnick, M. (2005). *The developmental systems approach to early intervention.* Baltimore: Paul H. Brookes.

Hickman, R., Westcott McCoy, S., Long, T.M., & Rauh, M.J. (2011). Applying contemporary developmental and movement science theories and evidence to early intervention practice. *Infants & Young Children, 24*(1), 29–41.

Individuals with Disabilities Education Improvement Act of 2004, 20 U.S.C. (2004). Retrieved from http://www.copyright.gov/legislation/pl108-446.pdf

Iverson, J. (2010). Developing language in a developing body: The relation between motor development and language development. *Journal of Child Language, 37,* 229–261.

McEwen, I. (Ed.) (2009). *Providing physical therapy services under Parts B & C of the Individuals with Disabilities Education Act (IDEA)* (2nd ed.). Alexandria, VA: Section on Pediatrics, American Physical Therapy Association.

Valvano, J., & Rapport, M.J. (2006). Activity-focused interventions for infants and children with neurological conditions. *Infants and Young Children, 19*(4), 292–307.

References

Adolf, K.E., Tamis-Lemonda, C., & Karasik, L.B. (2010). Cinderella indeed- A commentary on Iversons: 'Developing language in a developing body: The relationship between motor development and language development.' *Journal of Child Language, 37,* 269–273.

American Physical Therapy Association (2001). Guide to physical therapist practice (2nd ed.). *Physical Therapy, 81,* 6–746.

Bagnato, S.T., Neisworth, J.T., & Pretti-Frontczak, K. (2010). *Linking authentic assessment and early childhood intervention: Best measures for best practices* (2nd ed.). Baltimore: Paul H. Brookes.

Bailey, D. (1997). Evaluating the effectiveness of curriculum alternatives for infants and preschoolers at high risk. In M. Guralnick (Ed.), *The effectiveness of early intervention.* Baltimore: Paul H. Brookes.

Bricker, D., & Waddell, M. (2002). *Curriculum for birth to three years: AEPS assessment, evaluation, and programming system for infants and children* (2nd ed.). Baltimore: Paul H. Brookes.

Browder, D., & Martin, D.K. (1986). A new curriculum for Tommy. *Teaching Exceptional Children, 18*(4), 261–265.

Bruder, M.B. (2001). Infants and toddlers: Outcomes and ecology. In M. Guralnick (Ed.), *Early childhood inclusion: Focus on change.* Baltimore: Paul H. Brookes.

Council for Exceptional Children-Division of Early Childhood-Infant Toddler Coordination Association (2011). IDEA Part C: Early Intervention Program for Infants and Toddlers With Disabilities: Final Regulations Side-by Side Comparison. Retrieved from http://www.directionservice.org/cadre/finalregscompare.cfm

Dunst, C.J. (2002). Family-centered practices: Birth through high school. *Journal of Special Education, 36*(3), 139–147.

Dunst, C.J., Hamby, D., Trivette, C.M., Raab, N., & Bruder, M.B. (2000). Everyday family and community life and children's naturally occurring learning opportunities. *Journal of Early Intervention, 23,* 151–164.

Dunst, C., Trivette, C.M., & Jodry, W. (1997). Influences of social support on children with disabilities and their families. In M. Guralnick (Ed.), *The effectiveness of early intervention.* Baltimore: Paul H. Brookes.

Effgen, S.K., & Berger, M. (1978, June 19). Physical therapy in family-focused intervention. American Physical Therapy Association National Conference, Las Vegas, NV.

Federal Register. (2011). Part 303—Early intervention program for infants and toddlers with disabilities. §303.26 Natural environments. Vol. 76, No. 188, p. 60250.

Guralnick, M. (2000). *Interdisciplinary clinical assessment of young children with developmental disabilities.* Baltimore: Paul H. Brookes.

Guralnick, M. (2005). *The developmental systems approach to early intervention.* Baltimore: Paul H. Brookes.

Hanft, B.E., Rush, D.D., & Shelden, M. (2004). *Coaching families and colleagues in early childhood.* Baltimore: Paul H. Brookes.

Hickman, R., Westcott McCoy, S., Long, T.M., & Rauh, M.J. (2011). Applying contemporary developmental and movement science theories and evidence to early intervention practice. *Infants & Young Children, 24*(1), 29–41.

Individuals with Disabilities Education Improvement Act of 2004 (2004). Retrieved from http://www.copyright.gov/legislation/pl108-446.pdf

Iverson, J. (2010). Developing language in a developing body: The relation between motor development and language development. *Journal of Child Language, 37,* 229–261.

McWilliam, R.A. (2003, May). *The McWilliam model for providing services in natural environments: Key practices in a consultative model.* Retrieved from http://www.vanderbiltchildrens.com/uploads/documents/Consultative_Model—1_Day.ppt

Mellin, A.E., & Winton, P. (2003). Interdisciplinary collaboration among intervention faculty members. *Journal of Early Intervention, 25,* 173–188.

Myers, C.T., & Effgen, S.K. (2006). Physical therapists' participation in early childhood transition. *Pediatric Physical Therapy, 18*(3), 182–189.

Myers, C.T., Effgen, S.K., Blanchard, E., Southall, A., Wells, S., & Wilford, E. (2011). Factors predicting physical therapists' involvement and facilitation of involvement in early childhood transitions. *Physical Therapy, 91*(5), 656–664.

Neisworth, J.T., & Bagnato, S.J. (2004). The mismeasure of young children: The authentic assessment alternative. *Infants and Young Children, 17,* 198–212.

Orelove, F., Sobsey, D., & Silberman, R. (2004). *Educating children with multiple disabilities: A collaborative approach* (4th ed.). Baltimore: Paul H. Brookes.

Pretti-Frontczak, K.L., Barr, D.M., Macy, M., & Carter, A. (2003). Research and resources related to activity-based intervention, embedded learning opportunities, and routines-based instruction. *Topics in Early Childhood Special Education, 23,* 29–39.

Pretti-Frontczak, K., & Bricker, D. (2004). *An activity-based approach to early intervention* (3rd ed.). Baltimore: Paul H. Brookes.

Randall, K. E., & McEwen, I. R. (2000). Writing patient-centered functional goals. *Physical Therapy, 80*(12), 1197–1203.

Rosenbaum, P.L., Walter, S.D., Hanna, S.E., Palisano, R.J., Russell, D.J., Raina, P., & Galuppi, B.E. (2002). Prognosis for gross motor function in cerebral palsy: Creation of motor development curves. *Journal of the American Medical Association, 288*(11), 1357–1363.

Rush, D., & Sheldon, M. (2011). *The early childhood coaching handbook.* Baltimore: Paul H. Brookes.

Simeonsson, R. (2000). Early childhood intervention: Toward a universal manifesto. *Infants and Young Children, 12*(3), 4–9.

Ulrich, D.A., Lloyd, M.C., Tiernan, C.W., Looper, J.E., & Angulo-Barroso, R.M. (2008). Effects of intensity of treadmill training on developmental outcomes and stepping in infants with Down syndrome: A randomized trial. *Physical Therapy, 88,* 114–122.

Valvano, J. (2004). Activity-focused motor interventions for children with neurological conditions. *Physical and Occupational Therapy in Pediatrics, 24,* 79–107.

Valvano, J., & Rapport, M.J. (2006). Activity-focused interventions for infants and children with neurological conditions. *Infants and Young Children, 19*(4), 292–307.

Wilcox, J., & Belamy, T. (1987). *A comprehensive guide to the activities catalog: An alternate curriculum for youth and adults with severe disabilities.* Baltimore: Paul H. Brookes.

Woods, J. (2008). Providing early intervention in natural environments. *The ASHA Leader, 14,* 15–17.

Workgroup on Principles and Practices in Natural Environments (February 2008). *Seven key principles: Looks like/doesn't look like.* OSEP TA Community of Practice—Part C Settings. Retrieved from: http://www.nectac.org/topics/families/families.asp

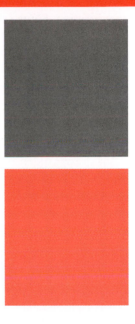

CHAPTER 12

Schools

—Susan K. Effgen, PT, PhD, FAPTA

P hysical therapists have worked in school settings from almost the beginning of the profession. Work in these school settings requires collaboration with teams of individuals, including numerous professionals, paraprofessionals, and, of course, the child and parents. School systems are major employers of pediatric physical therapists and are interesting, fun places to work. In this chapter, the unique aspects of school-based physical therapy will be discussed. Local, state, and federal laws regulate all school services and are discussed in some detail. The most significant law is the Individuals with Disabilities Education Act (IDEA). You have probably gone to school with children with disabilities because of this important United States federal law, first enacted in 1975. This law has a major impact on the education and delivery of related services for preschoolers and school-aged children with disabilities, and is the focus of this chapter.

History of Physical Therapy in Schools

Physical therapists have a long, rich history of serving children with special needs, in special schools set aside for those with physical disabilities. Those schools, many of which were residential, were started in the late 1800s and became common in the early 20th century. Most major cities had special schools for "crippled children" where physical therapists worked. In fact, in the 1930s, a master's thesis was written on physical therapy in the Chicago city schools (Vacha, 1933). Since that time, services to children with disabilities have expanded from serving just those with physical disabilities to including children with a wide range of disabilities, including intellectual impairment and mental illness, children who were not adequately served until the late 20th century. The role of physical therapists in schools continued to expand slowly, until the exponential increase in responsibility and need resulting from major federal legislation in 1975, when the United States Congress passed PL 94-142, the Education of All Handicapped Children Act. This landmark legislation provided that all children aged 6 to 21 years were entitled to a free appropriate public education that included "related services" such as physical therapy, occupational therapy, speech-language pathology, and transportation. Until that time, each local school system had the privilege of determining which children would receive an education. Some systems, especially in large cities, provided extensive services to many children with special needs. Other systems had requirements, such as that the child must to able to walk, independently use the bathroom, or not have mental retardation, to be eligible to receive an education. This national inequity in the availability of a public education, which forced families to move to areas that would serve their children with special needs, ended with PL 94-142.

Since 1975, the Education of All Handicapped Children Act has been amended seven times. In 1986, the reauthorization included the provision of early intervention (EI) services for infants and toddlers with disabilities, as discussed in Chapter 11. In 1990, the act's name was changed to the Individuals with Disabilities Education Act. IDEA and Section 504 of the Rehabilitation Act of 1973 guide physical therapy services in school settings, and a thorough knowledge of these federal laws is critical for the provision of school-based services for children and young adults aged 3 to 21 years.

Individuals With Disabilities Education Act

IDEA 2004, PL 108-446, notes, "Improving educational results for children with disabilities is an essential element of our national policy of ensuring equality of opportunity, full participation, independent living, and economic self-sufficiency for individuals with disabilities" [20 USC 1400, § 601(c)(1)]. The purpose of IDEA was "to ensure that all children with disabilities have available to them a free appropriate public education that emphasizes special education and related services designed to meet their unique needs and prepare them for further education, employment and independent living" [20 USC 1400, § 601(d)(1)(A)].

The phrase "prepare them for employment and independent living" was new in IDEA 97 and was a critical addition for helping to meet the needs of children with more severe disabilities. It was probably added to

expand the very strict interpretation of education as meaning only traditional academic areas, used by some systems. Many school systems have had a difficult time understanding the importance of a life skills curriculum in which children with significant disabilities learn to function in society even though they may never be able to read or write. Congress and advocacy groups believed that being prepared for independent living and, perhaps, employment, was for some children more important and functional than learning to read.

The original Education of All Handicapped Children Act, enacted in 1975, included seven major provisions that were very new, if not radical, regarding the education of children with special needs at that time. These provisions included:

- *Zero Reject.* "All children" meant all children. There was to be **zero reject** of children in schools; even children with the most severe physical and mental disabilities were to be provided with an education.
- *Least Restrictive Environment.* Children were also to receive their education in what was termed the **least restrictive environment (LRE)**. "To the maximum extent appropriate, children with disabilities . . . are educated with children who are not disabled" [PL108-446, 20 USC 1412, § 612(a)(5)(A)]. Thus, the concept of mainstreaming and, later, integration, natural environments, and inclusion began to influence provision of all educational and related services as discussed later in this chapter.
- *Right to Due Process.* Parents were now to become active partners in their child's education. They had the **right to due process,** which included impartial hearings, the right to be represented by counsel, and the right to a transcript of meetings. Later legislation provided for reimbursement of legal fees to parents if they prevailed in a court case. Interpreters were to be provided as necessary at meetings.
- *Parent Participation.* **Parent participation** was now welcomed, and parents were to be major decision makers in determining their child's educational program.
- *Nondiscriminatory Evaluation.* **Nondiscriminatory evaluation** was required, and every child receiving special education was to have an Individualized Education Program (IEP).
- *Individualized Education Program (IEP).* The **IEP** is the foundation of service delivery and will be discussed in detail. The IEP team meeting might determine that the child needs related services.
- *Related Services.* **Related services** "as may be required to assist a child with a disability to benefit

from special education" [PL108-446, 20 USC 1401, § 602(26)(A)]. Related services assist children in meeting their educational needs in a variety of ways and include physical therapy, occupational therapy, speech-language pathology, transportation, audiology, psychological services, recreation, rehabilitation counseling, orientation and mobility services, and medical services for diagnostic or evaluation purposes only.

Since the passage of PL 94-142 in 1975, many of the original provisions of the law that were once thought unusual or controversial are well-accepted, routine practice. The components of IDEA that still require some refinement, include the *IEP, LRE, School Climate and Discipline*, and *State and District-Wide Assessment*. The management of discipline is a major issue in schools. Advocates fear that, all too often, children with behavior disorders are not being provided with appropriate services and are being expelled from school so that the local education agency (LEA) or school system can avoid dealing with the problem. In IDEA 97, requirements were made that appropriate positive behavioral interventions and strategies be determined for each child. State and district-wide assessment is related to the push for outcomes data that are so critical in *No Child Left Behind*. How to test children with disabilities and whether to include them in state- or district-wide assessment are ongoing areas of concern and debate. These two issues, although very important, are not within the province of physical therapy. The IEP and LRE are important to physical therapists and require discussion.

Individualized Education Program

The IEP is developed after a multidisciplinary team has evaluated the child. The term *multidisciplinary* is used in educational circles to reflect interdisciplinary services. *Multidisciplinary* is defined by IDEA as "involvement of two or more disciplines or professions in the provision of integrated and coordinated services" (*Federal Register*, 1989). As you can see, that definition of practice is more in keeping with the definition of *interdisciplinary*. The evaluation process varies from LEA to LEA and state to state. The multidisciplinary team might first screen the child to determine what professionals would be most appropriate to participate in the evaluation. If the child has serious reading problems but no other noticeable problem, the physical therapist would not be involved in the evaluation. On the other hand, if after the evaluation by an educator and psychologist, subtle gross motor and coordination problems are noted, a physical therapist might be asked to

perform a more in-depth examination of coordination, perceptual motor development, and gross motor skills to determine whether these problems affect educational performance.

Examination and Evaluation

In the educational environment, evaluation refers to the procedures used "to determine whether a child is a child with a disability . . . and to determine the educational needs of such child" [20 USC 1412 § 614(a)(1)(C)(i)(I)]. "In conducting the evaluation, the local educational agency shall . . . use a variety of assessment tools and strategies to gather relevant functional, developmental, and academic information, including information provided by the parent" [20 USC 1414, § 614(b)(2)(A)]. The evaluation procedures should include instruments that are technically sound, nondiscriminatory regarding race and culture, and administered in the child's native language [20 USC 1414, § 614(b)(2)]. A child should be evaluated in all areas of suspected disability, which would include physical and developmental factors [20 USC 1414, § 614(b)(2)]. The functional and developmental assessments are part of the federal mandates.

The initial evaluation of the child will assist in determining if the child has a disability. "The term 'child with a disability' means a child—(i) with mental retardation, hearing impairments (including deafness), speech or language impairments, visual impairments (including blindness), serious emotional disturbance (referred to in this title as 'emotional disturbance'), orthopedic impairments, autism, traumatic brain injury, other health impairments, or specific learning disabilities; and (ii) who, by reason thereof, needs special education and related services" [20 USC 1401, § 602(3)]. The diagnostic categories for special education are listed in Table 12.1.

Based on the evaluation, the child's eligibility for special education and related services is determined by the multidisciplinary team. If the child qualifies for special education, within 30 calendar days, the IEP team, sometimes called the Admissions and Release Committee (ARC) or Multidisciplinary Team (MDT), must meet to develop a written IEP. Only after it is decided that the child qualifies for special education does the team determine the extent of need for various related services that will assist the child to benefit from special education.

The purpose of therapy in a school setting is to meet the educational needs of the child and to assist in helping them prepare for further education, employment, and independent living. To determine how to best meet those

■ Table 12.1 Federal Definitions of Child With a Disability

Autism "means a developmental disability significantly affecting verbal and nonverbal communication and social interaction, generally evident before age 3, that adversely affects a child's educational performance. Other characteristics often associated with autism are engagement in repetitive activities and stereotyped movements, resistance to environmental change, change in daily routines, and unusual responses to sensory experiences. The term does not apply if a child's educational performance is adversely affected primarily because the child has an emotional disturbance."

Deaf-blindness "means a concomitant hearing and visual impairments, the combination of which causes such severe communication and other developmental and educational needs that they cannot be accommodated in special education programs solely for children with deafness or children with blindness."

Deafness "means a hearing impairment that is so severe that the child is impaired in processing linguistic information through hearing, with or without amplification, that adversely affects a child's educational performance."

Developmental delay: "The term child with a disability for children aged 3 through 9 may, at the discretion of the State and LEA . . . include a child (1) Who is experiencing developmental delays, as defined by the State and as measured by appropriate diagnostic instruments and procedures, in one or more of the following areas: physical development, cognitive development, communication development, social or emotional development, or adaptive development, and (2) Who, by reason there of, needs special education and related services."

Emotional disturbance "means a condition exhibiting one or more of the following characteristics over a long period of time and to a marked degree that adversely affects a child's educational performance: (A) An inability to learn that cannot be explained by intellectual, sensory, or health factors. (B) An inability to build or maintain satisfactory interpersonal relationships with peers and teachers. (C) Inappropriate types of behavior or feelings under normal circumstances. (D) A general pervasive mood of unhappiness or depression. (E) A tendency to develop physical symptoms or fears associated with personal or school problems. The term includes schizophrenia. The term does not apply to children who are socially maladjusted, unless it is determined that they have an emotional disturbance."

Hearing impairment "means an impairment in hearing, whether permanent or fluctuating, that adversely affects a child's educational performance but that is not included under the definition of deafness."

Mental retardation "means significantly subaverage general intellectual functioning existing concurrently with deficits in adaptive behavior and manifested during the developmental period that adversely affects a child's educational performance."

Multiple disabilities "means concomitant impairments (e.g., mental retardation-blindness, mental retardation-orthopedic impairment, etc), the combination of which causes such severe educational needs that they cannot be accommodated in special education programs solely for one of the impairments. The term does not include deaf-blindness."

Orthopedic impairment "means a severe orthopedic impairment that adversely affects a child's educational performance. The term includes impairments caused by congenital anomaly (e.g., clubfoot, absence of some member), impairments caused by disease (e.g., poliomyelitis, bone tuberculosis, etc.), and impairments from other causes (e.g., cerebral palsy, amputations, and fractures or burns that cause contractures)."

Other health impairment "means having limited strength, vitality, or alertness, including a heightened alertness to environmental stimuli, that results in limited alertness with respect to the educational environment, that (i) Is due to chronic or acute health problems such as asthma, attention deficit disorder or attention deficit hyperactivity disorder, diabetes, epilepsy, a heart condition, hemophilia, lead poisoning, leukemia, nephritis, rheumatic fever, and sickle cell anemia; and (ii) Adversely affects a child's educational performance."

Specific learning disability is "a disorder in one or more of the basic psychologic processes involved in understanding or in using language, spoken or written, that may manifest as an imperfect ability to listen, think, speak, read, write, spell, or do mathematical calculations, including such conditions as perceptual disabilities, brain injury, minimal brain dysfunction, dyslexia, and developmental aphasia. . . . The term does not include learning problems that are primarily the result of visual, hearing, or motor disabilities, of mental retardation, of emotional disturbance, or of environmental, cultural, or economic disadvantage."

Speech and language impairment "means a communication disorder such as stuttering, impaired articulation, a language impairment, or a voice impairment that adversely affects a child's educational performance."

Traumatic brain injury "means an acquired injury to the brain caused by an external physical force, resulting in total or partial functional disability or psychosocial impairment, or both, that adversely affects a child's educational performance. The term applies to open or closed head injuries resulting in impairments in one or more areas, such as cognition; language; memory; attention; reasoning; abstract thinking; judgment; problem-solving; sensory, perceptual, and motor abilities; psychosocial behavior; physical functions; information processing; and speech. The term does not apply to brain injuries that are congenital or degenerative or brain injuries induced by birth trauma."

Visual impairment including blindness "means an impairment in vision including blindness means an impairment in vision that, even with correction, adversely affects a child's educational performance. The term includes both partial sight and blindness."

Source: [20 U.S.C. 1401(3)(A) and (B); 1401(26). *Code of Federal Regulations*, 34 CFR §300.7(b), (c). Available at http://cfr.vlex.com/vid/300-7-child-with-disability-19761359]

needs, a comprehensive physical therapy examination is required to determine the most appropriate recommendations for the intervention plan. All of the areas of physical therapy examination discussed throughout this text must be considered for each individual child, although an examination and evaluation of each system might not be indicated. As outlined in Table 1.2 (see Chapter 1), the *Pediatric Physical Therapy Evaluation and Plan of Care* might be followed. What is included in any specific examination will depend on the child's age, diagnosis, and level of cognitive functioning, as well as the specific purpose of the examination and evaluation. Screening or eligibility evaluations are different from the initial examination for services or reevaluation for continued physical therapy services.

Frequently, the therapist will want to administer a standardized test of motor performance to document present level of performance and to monitor progress. Unlike the tests in EI, this evaluation of physical performance is not required to determine eligibility. Commonly used tests include the Peabody Developmental Motor Scales (Folio & Fewell, 2000) for younger children and older children with significant motor skill restrictions; and the Bruininks Oseretsky Test of Motor Proficiency II (Bruininks & Bruininks, 2005) for children who are ambulatory but have some movement limitations or restrictions in activities. For children with cerebral palsy (CP) or Down syndrome, the Gross Motor Function Measure (GMFM) (Russell, Rosenbaum, Avery, & Lane, 2002) is a very useful tool. In addition to standardized tests of motor performance, tests of functional ability are frequently indicated; these include the Pediatric Evaluation of Disability Inventory (PEDI) (Haley, Coster, Ludlow, Haltiwanger, & Andrellos, 1992) and the School Function Assessment (SFA) (Coster, Deeney, Haltiwanger, & Haley, 1998). The SFA is used to determine the student's current level of participation in the school setting and performance of functional activities, as well as the supports needed to perform those functional tasks at school. The SFA is a judgment-based questionnaire that is completed by one or more school professionals who have observed the student performing typical school tasks. The items are written in measurable, behavioral terms that can easily be used in the later writing of the child's IEP. This assessment helps to highlight problems the child might be having in performing common functional tasks at school that are frequently overlooked in measurements of standard motor performance. The sections of the SFA, outlined in Table 12.2, indicate its suitability for assessing common school tasks. This assessment is especially helpful to therapists who are new to educational settings because it highlights the areas of importance to school functioning and assists the therapist in planning appropriate school-based programs. The School Outcomes Measure that is in development involves collecting a minimal data set to measure groups of students' performance in school-based therapy (McEwen, Arnold, Hansen, & Johnson, 2003).

Table 12.2 Sections of the School Function Assessment

Part I Participation
Playground/Recess
Transportation
Bathroom/Toileting
Transitions
Mealtime/Snack Time

Part II Task Supports: Physical Tasks
Travel
Maintaining and Changing Positions
Recreational Movement
Manipulation With Movement
Using Materials
Set-up and Clean-up
Eating and Drinking
Hygiene
Clothing Management

Part II Task Supports: Behavioral Tasks
Functional Communication
Memory and Understanding
Following Social Conventions
Compliance With Adult Directives and School Rules
Task Behavior/Completion
Positive Interaction
Behavior Regulation
Personal Care Awareness
Safety

Part III Activity Performance: Physical Tasks
Travel
Maintaining and Changing Positions
Recreational Movement
Manipulation With Movement
Using Materials
Set-up and Clean-up
Eating and Drinking
Hygiene
Clothing Management
Up/Down Stairs
Written Work
Computer and Equipment Use

Continued

■ **Table 12.2** Sections of the School Function
■ Assessment—cont'd

**Part III Activity Performance: Cognitive/
Behavioral Tasks**
Functional Communication
Memory and Understanding
Following Social Conventions
Compliance With Adult Directives and School Rules
Task Behavior/Completion
Positive Interaction
Behavior Regulation
Personal Care Awareness
Safety
**Adaptations Checklist: Adaptations Routinely
Used**
Activities of Daily Living
Architectural
Behavioral
Classroom Work
Cognitive
Communication
Computer
Seating/Mobility/Transportation
Other Adaptations

Source: Coster, W., Deeney, T., Haltiwanger, J., & Haley, S.
(1998). *School function assessment.* San Antonio, TX: The Psychological Corporation

Classroom observation should be part of the assessment of all children being considered for services. This naturalistic observation is critical to understanding the child's true abilities in a natural setting. Although a physical therapist is not required by law to conduct a classroom observation, this observation can be critical in determining the limitations in the child's activities and also assist in clarifying any questions the therapist might have regarding the scoring of the SFA by other school personnel. For example, knowing the type of stairs in the school, how many children are generally in the hallway, and how far away the school buses park is important in determining realistic goals for stair climbing and getting through the school to the bus.

The examination of a preschooler might take place in the classroom, whereas the examination of a school-aged child might be better in a private setting where other children cannot observe and the class would not be disrupted. The examination might also be done as an arena assessment with other professionals, as discussed in Chapters 1 and 11. An arena assessment decreases the amount of handling of the child and allows the professionals to problem-solve together and easily share information.

The actual write-up of the evaluation might be done as suggested in Table 1.2 or will follow the conventions of the LEA. The report is written in **lay language** so that the family and other team members can understand the report. Any "medical terms" that the therapist believes must be used should be explained carefully. Using lay language is no excuse for an incomplete report. Proper documentation of the child's status is critical in determining change in status over time and the outcomes of intervention. The school-based evaluation report does *not* include specific goals and objectives for the child. Goals and objectives are determined with the entire IEP team at the IEP meeting.

IEP Meeting

Once all of the necessary examinations and evaluations are performed and the child's eligibility for special education is determined, the IEP team meets. The team includes:

- parents
- a regular education teacher
- a special education teacher
- a representative from the public agency who is knowledgeable and qualified to provide specially designed instruction
- an individual who can interpret the instructional implications of the evaluation results
- at the discretion of the parent or agency, other knowledgeable individuals, including related service personnel
- if appropriate, the child [20 USC 1414, § 614 (d)(1)((B)]

This is a very important meeting in planning the child's program, and physical therapists should participate to the fullest extent possible. Some LEAs welcome and expect therapist participation, whereas others consider the participation of therapists to be an added expense and attempt to restrict participation to a limited number of people. If the child requires physical therapy to succeed in school, the therapist must be there to advocate for the child and to explain to the team how the therapist might assist the child and teachers in helping the child achieve his or her individual educational goals. The role of the therapist as a consultant is critical during the IEP process, and if therapists are not there, they cannot assist.

The content of the IEP is dictated by IDEA and must include the following:

(I) a statement of the child's present levels of academic achievement and functional performance, including—

(a) how the child's disability affects the child's involvement and progress in the general curriculum;

(b) for preschool children, as appropriate, how the disability affects the child's participation in appropriate activities; and

(c) for children with disabilities who take alternate assessments aligned to alternate achievement standards, a description of benchmarks or short-term objectives;

(II) A statement of measurable annual goals, including academic and functional goals, designed to—

(a) meet the child's needs that result from the child's disability to enable the child to be involved in and progress in the general curriculum; and

(b) meet each of the child's other educational needs that result from the child's disability;

(III) a description of how the child's progress toward meeting the annual goals . . . will be measured and when periodic reports on the progress the child is making toward meeting the annual goals . . . will be provided;

(IV) a statement of the special education and related services and supplementary aids and services, based on peer-reviewed research to the extent practicable, to be provided to the child, or on behalf of the child, and a statement of the program modifications or supports for school personnel that will be provided for the child—

(a) to advance appropriately toward attaining the annual goals;

(b) to be involved in and make progress in the general curriculum . . . and to participate in extracurricular and other nonacademic activities; and

(c) to be educated and participate with other children with disabilities and nondisabled children in the activities described in this subparagraph;

(V) an explanation of the extent, if any, to which the child will not participate with nondisabled children in the regular class and in the activities. . . .

(VI) (a) a statement of any individual appropriate accommodations that are necessary to measure the academic achievement and functional performance of the child on State and districtwide assessments. . . .

(VII) the projected date for the beginning of services and modifications . . . and the anticipated frequency, location, and duration of those services and modifications; and

(VIII) beginning not later than the first IEP to be in effect when the child is 16, and updated annually thereafter—

(a) appropriate measurable postsecondary goals based upon age appropriate transition assessments related to training, education, employment, and, where appropriate, independent living skills;

(b) the transition services (including courses of study) needed to assist the child in reaching those goals; and

(c) beginning not later than 1 year before the child reaches the age of majority under State law, a statement that the child has been informed of the child's rights under this title, if any, that will transfer to the child on reaching the age of majority. [20 USC 1414, § 614 (d)(1)]

How all of the preceding information is developed and written up varies from LEA to LEA. The physical therapist must be involved in the IEP meeting to determine the child's measurable annual goals and benchmarks or short-term objectives for those taking alternate assessments. These goals are *not* discipline specific and relate to the overall academic and functional needs of the child. They are child goals and, as appropriate, should include goals involving functional performance and the motor domain. Consensus among experts in pediatric occupational and physical therapy indicates that objectives should:

- relate to functional skills and activities
- enhance the child's performance in school
- be understood easily by all individuals
- be free of professional jargon
- be realistic and achievable within the typical IEP time frame (Dole, Arvidson, Byrne, Robbins, & Schasberger, 2003)

These experts suggest that if a skill or an activity cannot be observed or measured during the child's normal school day, then it might not be relevant to the child's educational needs. They also note, although there is no consensus, that generalization of skills across settings is important. In addition to the IEP goals, the physical therapist in the majority of states will also have to write specific physical therapy goals for the child for the plan of care. The goals in the plan of care should be based on the IEP goals. See Table 12.3 for an example of an integrated IEP goal and the physical therapy goals in the plan of care.

The IEP team then decides the frequency and intensity of participation by various related service personnel as well as the location of services. These decisions should be based on what is best for the child and not what is convenient for the LEA or service providers. In the past, all too often, children were sent to a special school away from the local school they would have otherwise attended because therapy services were offered only at that special school. Services should be available in all educational environments. Some children might be best served

Table 12.3 Sample IEP Goal and Physical Therapy Plan of Care

IEP Goal (APTA, 2009)

In one year, Juan will follow the morning routines independently without verbal guidance for 3 days in a row. Morning routines includes getting off the bus, walking to the correct door, going up the steps and through the door, finding and opening his locker, hanging up his coat, entering the classroom, and sitting at his desk ready to start the academic portion of the day.

Responsible parties: classroom teacher, PT, and OT

Physical Therapy Plan of Care Goals

1. Within 6 months Juan will require stand-by assistance to get off the bus.

2. In one year, Juan will independently get off the bus.

3. Within 6 months Juan will require stand-by assistance to go up the two school stairs and open the door.

4. In one year, Juan will independently go up the two school stairs and open the door.

Juan does not require the intervention of a physical therapist to walk to the correct door, find and open his locker, hang up his coat, enter the classroom, and sit at his desk. The therapist will be available for consultation related to those issues as required.

---

in a somewhat restrictive environment for certain aspects of their education, whereas other children can function in the general education environment with supports provided from special education and related service personnel. The decision about location of services is a critical component of the IEP meeting. Therapists should always strive for services in the least restrictive and least intrusive environment; however, they must also be aware that "it is important to consider the student's privacy, dignity, and the perceptions of peers when selecting both where services will be provided and what strategies will be used" (Giangreco, 1995, p. 62). Some interventions are best provided in a private area, although there should be frequent reevaluation to determine the continued need for an isolated environment.

While the IEP meeting is progressing, the decisions are written down and the team and parents agree in writing to the recommendations. If the parents do not agree, they have the right to appeal the decisions and to have mediation or a due process hearing. The rights of the parents and child are well defined in IDEA. Related services have been the focal point of many disputes between parents and school districts. These disputes usually involve (1) adequacy of physical therapy services, (2) qualifications of the service providers, (3) the need for physical therapy during the extended school year (summer), (4) compensatory physical therapy, and (5) type of intervention provided (Jones & Rapport, 2009).

During the due process procedures, the child will continue his or her current educational services and placement, unless everyone agrees otherwise. This is termed "stay put." For a child new to the special education system, this might mean no services. On the other hand, for a child already in the system where perhaps there is a recommendation for fewer services or a change of environment that the parent does not desire, the ability to "stay put" while the plan is appealed might be attractive to the child and family.

Once the IEP is accepted, the services should be provided as stated. This is a time when physical therapy, if indicated, is most important. The therapist needs to consult with the child's teachers regarding their needs; check for accommodations the child might need to participate fully in the classroom; have equipment needs determined, ordered, or constructed; and, if indicated, instruct all personnel working with the child in proper positioning and lifting techniques. In addition, safe positioning while traveling on the school bus and management of architectural barriers need to be addressed, as does a safe evacuation from the building if there is a fire or other emergency.

Intervention

As already noted, school-based intervention must focus on the educational needs of the child as determined by the IEP team. Some LEAs are very liberal in that they consider educational benefit and openly accept that the purpose of an education is to prepare individuals for employment and independent living. Other systems take a very strict view of educational relevance and attempt to limit education to traditional academic skills and severely restrict intervention focused on life skills and achieving independent living. A child might be eligible for physical therapy in one LEA and ineligible in another LEA just several miles away. There is even greater variation in service provision from state to state.

Some children might clearly require physical therapy intervention but might not be eligible for that intervention because it is not needed for them to benefit from education. For services to be provided under IDEA, a student must be eligible for special education, and then related services can be provided. In situations where the child requires physical therapy but is not eligible for special education, the therapist must explain to the parents why physical therapy is not indicated in the school setting and perhaps assist the parents in obtaining physical therapy services through another setting. There is a professional obligation to inform the parents of the need for physical therapy; however, the physical therapist does not have an obligation to provide that therapy through the school system if it is not required for the child to benefit from education. An example of this situation is a child with mild CP who is fully ambulatory and functions well with classroom supports. Physical therapy intervention might help the child achieve a more efficient, attractive gait pattern. Some might say that a more efficient gait pattern will assist the child in navigating the school environment and therefore might improve his or her educational performance and employment outlook. Physical therapy might be provided in that LEA but not in another LEA. The therapist must be careful about providing therapy that is not clearly educationally relevant and not absolutely required by the child. Remember that time used for physical therapy means time away from other academic tasks. This can be a critical loss of academic time, especially for that child with mild CP, who might be preparing for college and for whom time out of physics class can be very detrimental to educational performance. On the other hand, for a preschooler, increased intervention now might be very appropriate to perhaps lessen the amount of intervention required later. Unfortunately, there is a lack of research on the most sensitive and effective times and ages for intervention, although there is agreement that in general, the earlier the intervention, the better (Harris, 1997).

Coordination, Communication, and Documentation The *Guide for physical therapist practice* (APTA, 2001) indicates that major areas of intervention are coordination, communication, and documentation. These are very critical areas for school-based practice. As part of a team, the physical therapist must coordinate intervention with the other professionals in the school system and professionals serving the child in the community. This includes coordination and consultation with physical education teachers regarding fitness, gross motor skill development (Cohn 2007), and recreational activities.

Many children also receive therapy outside of the school setting, and the therapists must work together and coordinate their intervention efforts. This, of course, includes communication, both verbal and written.

The LEA, in response to state and federal rules and regulations, generally determines the format of the documentation in school-based settings; however, the therapist still must comply with the state physical therapy practice acts, which might have more extensive requirements for documentation than required by the LEA. The documentation template suggested in the *Guide* (APTA, 2001) has limited applicability in pediatric practice. Use of more traditional methods of pediatric physical therapy documentation has now been reinstated in many LEAs because of the increasing trend of seeking reimbursement from Medicaid. As therapists work on the goals and objectives written in the child's IEP, they must break down those generic educational goals and objectives into the specific components that will be addressed during intervention. For example, the goal for the child in school might be to select and get his or her lunch independently in the cafeteria. One of many related physical therapy goals might be that the child be able to carry the lunch tray from the food service line to a table without dropping it. To achieve this goal, the therapist might have specific objectives related to improving the child's balance while walking, increasing upper extremity strength to hold a full tray, and improving coordination. These goals and objectives are not part of the IEP; however, they are clearly related to the IEP goal and might be necessary as documentation of physical therapy intervention for reimbursement.

Child-Related Instruction A priority area of intervention in school settings is child, family, and team instruction. Some therapists might rarely actually touch a child, yet they are providing appropriate intervention if they are serving the child through instruction and consultation in the school setting. A consultative service delivery model (see Chapter 1) might be the most appropriate model, whereas other children might require consultation plus direct service and a collaborative model.

The potential areas of child-related instructions are extensive. For example, if a child is using a power wheelchair, not only must the child be instructed in how to use the device, but so must the parents, teachers, teachers' aides, bus drivers, and others responsible for the child's safety and mobility throughout the school day. Perhaps new ramps must be installed to meet the size and weight requirements of the wheelchair; perhaps there is a need to modify the bathroom and rearrange the classroom seating arrangement to accommodate the radius required to maneuver the wheelchair.

Instruction is a team effort. The physical therapist not only provides instruction but also receives instruction from the other disciplines serving the child. In one setting, the physical therapist might provide expert education in power wheelchairs, but in another setting, it might be the occupational therapist who provides the instruction to the team. In school settings there is rarely a strict line of professional demarcation, and therapists must be prepared for role release as required under a transdisciplinary model of service delivery (Rainforth, 1997).

Procedural Interventions As noted in the *Guide* (APTA, 2001), the physical therapist selects, applies, or modifies the procedural interventions that will be provided to a child in a school setting. The therapist applies therapeutic exercise that includes conditioning, self-care, and functional training for home, school, and play. These would not be referred to as "procedural interventions" in an educational setting; "strategies," or perhaps "interventions," would be more appropriate terminology.

Physical therapy interventions available to the child in special education are diverse. Each IEP team determines the extent and type of services based on the evaluation findings and the team's recommendations. The physical therapist does not independently determine the extent, type, and frequency of physical therapy services in a school setting. There is a trend away from one-to-one service delivery, yet the importance of more than just consultation cannot be overstated. The use of flexible service delivery models that may combine different frequency and intensity options are probably best suited for achieving specific goals and objectives (Hanft & Place, 1996; Swinth & Hanft, 2002; Trahan & Malouin, 2002). The traditional model of one-to-one service for a certain number of minutes per week should be reconsidered. Perhaps, for a certain child, daily intervention for the first few weeks of school can best meet his or her needs, followed by only monitoring for the remainder of the school year. For other children, group intervention can

be the most effective, or at least as effective as one-to-one intervention (LaForme Fiss, Effgen, Page, & Shasby, 2009). The IEP goals, objectives, and frequency of services cannot be changed without another IEP meeting; however, as long as there is no change in the objectives and overall amount of time, adjustments in scheduling of services are possible without another IEP meeting (*Federal Register*, 1992, p. 44839). This decision should be based on professional judgment.

There are school systems in the United States that are willing and able to provide all recommended physical therapy services, including aquatics and therapeutic riding for their children with special needs. On the other hand, some school systems rebel at the thought of putting in ramps for wheelchairs and see no need for the physical therapist to teach a child stair climbing. Therapists must educate administrators regarding the services a physical therapist can offer and the most appropriate degree of service delivery in their community. Mature therapists who are members of the APTA, Section on Pediatrics, do not appear to have problems with overinvolvement or influence from administration (Effgen, 2000), although many therapists, perhaps not as experienced and professionally involved, have noted that their school administrations often interfere with professional decision making.

The specific interventions to be used by the physical therapist might be discussed at the IEP meeting, but they, along with educational strategies to be used, are not part of the IEP. The physical therapists' major intervention in school settings was found to be teaching/learning techniques, followed by handling/physical interventions (McDougall et al., 1999). The interventions a therapist uses will vary according to the needs of the individual child, the age of the child, placement of the child, the policies of the LEA regarding degree of intervention, parental input, team opinion, therapist experience, and numerous other factors. The service delivery model used will also vary according to the preceding factors. Initially, the therapist should consult with the classroom teachers to see what their needs are regarding the child. Frequently the therapist will need to provide coordination, communication, documentation, and child-related instruction first, then classroom modifications and transportation considerations, followed by specific procedural interventions if indicated. For example a child might walk most safely with a walker (Fig. 12.1), but the child has only crutches. The therapist might have to obtain a walker through the school system and then make certain that the child is

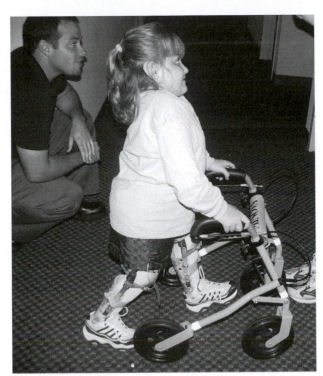

Figure 12.1 Child walking safely with walker at school.

safe with the walker by providing some intervention and establishing the parameters of safe use of the walker within the school. The therapist would then consult with and instruct classroom teachers, aides, and physical therapist assistants (PTAs) in how the child may safely walk with the walker throughout the building. In the meantime, the therapist or PTA might still be providing direct interventions on the use of crutches in the school building, meeting the IEP objective of being able to safely walk with crutches to the cafeteria when other children are in the halls.

The physical therapist, along with other team members, will decide on the assistive technology, adaptive equipment, and augmentative and alternative communication needs of the child, as discussed in Chapters 17 and 18. IDEA makes it very clear that the assistive technology needs of the child will be met to allow the child to benefit from a free and appropriate public education. How supportive an LEA is in meeting these needs varies greatly and is a reflection of the financial resources of that LEA.

Reexamination

The frequency of reexamination should be based on the individual needs of the child, the child's response to intervention, and the requirements of individual state practice acts. Unfortunately, additional time for a complete reexamination is rarely provided in an educational setting. IEP meetings are held at least annually (the option of triannual IEP meetings is recommended in the IDEA 2004 reauthorization), and the therapist should perform a reexamination at least that often to assist in determining the program for the following year. An official, complete reexamination is required only every 3 years (the triannual evaluation), although even that evaluation can be waived if considered unnecessary by the entire IEP team, including the family. More frequent physical therapy reexamination of every 30 to 90 days is usually required by individual state physical therapy practice acts.

Discharge

The termination or "graduation" from physical therapy services is not a unilateral decision made by the physical therapist in an educational setting. The team, during the IEP meeting, decides on the services that will or will not be provided for the child during the next school year. In one study (Effgen, 2000), the most important factor in terminating services was the child's attainment of the functional goals. This is in keeping with accepted professional practice. The severity of the child's disability also influenced continuation of services, as did the input of parents and caretakers. As already noted in this study, the mature, professionally active respondents were not unduly influenced by administration in their decisions regarding termination of service delivery.

Least Restrictive Environment

As already mentioned, the location of the child's education and all service delivery should be in schools with children who are not disabled. "Each public agency shall ensure that to the maximum extent appropriate, children with disabilities, including children in public or private institutions or other care facilities, are educated with children who are nondisabled; and that special classes, separate schooling or other removal of children with disabilities from the regular education environment occurs only if the nature or severity of the disability is such that education in regular classes with the use of supplementary aids and services cannot be achieved satisfactorily" (*Federal Register* [1997], 34 CFR § 300.550). It is believed that the majority of children who are eligible for special education and related services are able to participate in the general education curriculum with some adaptations and modifications. This provision of IDEA is intended to "ensure that children's special education and related services are in addition to and are affected by the general education curriculum, not separate from it."

The concept of LRE involves much more than mere physical location of services. There are four key elements to inclusion (Turnbull, Turnbull, Shank, & Smith, 2004):

- Students receive their education in the school they would have attended if they did not have a disability.
- Students are placed in classrooms according to the natural proportion of the exceptionality to the general population. This suggests that because about 10% of the general school population has disabilities, no more than 10% of the children in a classroom should have a disability.
- Teaching and learning for all students should be restructured so that special education and related services can support the general education classroom. Curriculum, instruction, and evaluation should be universally designed.
- School and general education placements should be age and grade appropriate.

Meeting the mandate for inclusive education has not been easy. Initially, when PL 94-142 was enacted in 1975, the concept of a continuum of placement options was encouraged. Taylor (1988), however, eloquently noted that children with disabilities were "caught in the continuum" and had to earn their way out. The inclusion movement has now tried to limit the use of more restrictive settings by creating partnerships between special education and general education (Turnbull et al., 2004). Many schools now have separate spaces for all children to use for different purposes as a way to facilitate learning for everyone. Major decreases in the restrictive environments of special schools and residential facilities have been replaced with 96% of students with disabilities now being educated in regular school buildings (U.S. Department of Education, 2010, p. 72). The amount of time they spend in regular classrooms is varied as indicated in Figure 12.2.

Physical therapists must determine how they can best meet the physical therapy needs of the child to allow the child's full participation in the general education curriculum. Therapists' involvement in LRE occurs on at least three levels. First, there are the *architectural considerations*. Perhaps merely adding a ramp or railing to the front stairs of the school would allow the child direct access to the school. Perhaps push doors or enlarged knobs would allow all children to open doors more easily. Lockers in middle and high schools can be difficult or inconvenient for any child, and care should be taken

Percentage of students ages 6 through 21 with disabilities receiving special education and related services by educational environment

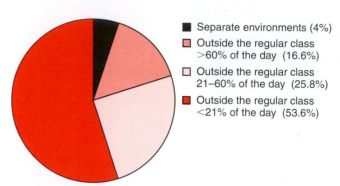

- ■ Separate environments (4%)
- ▨ Outside the regular class >60% of the day (16.6%)
- □ Outside the regular class 21–60% of the day (25.8%)
- ■ Outside the regular class <21% of the day (53.6%)

Figure 12.2 Percentage of students ages 6 through 21 with disabilities receiving special education and related services by educational environment. *(U.S. Department of Education. (2010). Office of Special Education and Rehabilitative Services, Office of Special Education Programs, 29th Annual Report to Congress on the Implementation of the Individuals with Disabilities Education Act, 2007, vol. 1, p. 72, Washington, DC: Author.)*

to make certain that the child's locker is in an accessible location and can easily be locked and unlocked.

Consultation with all teachers is another critical component, as discussed under the intervention process. Physical therapists have always worked closely with special education teachers; however, to truly assist in optimizing an inclusive educational environment, we must anticipate the needs of general education teachers. The general education teacher might never have had a child with a disability or with this particular disability in the classroom. The therapist might be the only health-care professional available to provide information regarding the child's diagnosis and specific needs. Nurses can provide this information, but not all states or LEAs have school nurses. Will the teachers need to be instructed in proper positioning for the child? Will they need to learn proper body mechanics to avoid injury to themselves and the child? Who will check for pressure sores? How does the adaptive equipment work? Who gets called if equipment breaks? What are the physical limitations and expectations for the child? What can and should the child do? How can learned helplessness be prevented? How can obesity be prevented in all children in the classroom? Is the child safely positioned on the school bus? These are just a few of the questions the general education teacher might have for the therapist.

The final area that the therapist must address regarding LRE and full inclusion is the *specific needs of the individual child.* Besides consultation with the special education and general education teachers, does the child require direct services (procedural interventions)? If direct services are indicated, where and when will those services be provided to be the least obtrusive to the child's daily educational routine? There is a growing body of evidence that functional physical therapy (Ketelaar, Vermeer, Hart, van Petegem-van Beek, & Helders, 2001) and therapy provided in natural education settings might result in superior skill acquisition (Karnish, Bruder, & Rainforth, 1995). The location of direct services is significantly influenced by the child's age, classroom placement, cooperation of the teachers, and degree of disability. Providing direct services in a preschool classroom is generally accomplished quite easily, even for a child with significant disabilities (Guralnick, 2001). However, for a high-school child, even a simple activity, such as adjusting a wheelchair seat or desk height, cannot be accomplished easily during the regular classroom routine without calling attention to the child and disrupting the class. The child's dignity must be maintained (Giangreco, 1995). Different service delivery models are discussed in Chapter 1. No one service delivery model should be considered "best practice," and it is unlikely that any one model is adequate to meet the complex needs of all children (Massey Sekerak, Kirkpatrick, Nelson, & Propes, 2003). The LRE for service delivery will depend on each individual child and is likely to change during the years of the child's education.

Working in the general education environment does place some burdens on therapists, which can be overcome with planning and administrative support. Therapists need to travel to schools. This takes time and requires increased staff. The therapist must also bring equipment to the schools or have duplicate equipment available at each location. Again, this can be costly if the equipment is used for only one child. If there is only one related service provided in a school setting at any one time, there is professional isolation. Therapists are not able to speak with other therapists within and outside their discipline while they are seeing a child, and this isolation means that there is little peer review of the performance of therapists in school settings. School administrations must be sensitive to this isolation and allow therapists to meet frequently to discuss the children they serve and coordinate intervention. In addition, therapists should set up journal clubs and special-interest groups where they can meet with colleagues to seek advanced knowledge and skills.

Transition Services

Transitions, whether they are from EI to preschool, from preschool to elementary school, from elementary school to middle and high school, or from school to the adult community, are critical periods in the life of any child and family. These periods of transition are especially complex and frequently quite difficult for a child with a disability. The child must leave a familiar setting where he or she knows everyone and is familiar with the physical environment. The child must now go to a new setting where the people, the environment, and even the adaptive equipment might be new. In some small LEAs, the therapist will transition with the child, but in larger systems, the child will have an entirely new team of professionals to work with in the new setting. The degree of adjustment will, of course, depend on the child and the setting, and in no small part on appropriate transition planning by all team members.

The transition from EI, which is covered under Part C of IDEA, to preschool, which is Part B of IDEA, can be particularly difficult for parents. Families must adjust to the different rules and regulations; different levels of service delivery, specifically the shift in focus from development of all developmental skills to only those that are educationally relevant; new service delivery models; new personnel and philosophies; and usually different lead agencies (Hanson et al., 2000). The child goes from receiving home-based services to preschool classrooms with new caregivers and new equipment. A transition plan should have been started between 90 days and 6 months before the child's third birthday to make the transition as "seamless" as possible. The transitions from preschool to kindergarten and then to primary school, middle school, and high school are equally important and complex, but specific planning for these transitions is not required or outlined in IDEA.

When transitioning during the school years, just the change in equipment can be devastating for a child who, for example, uses a power wheelchair and an augmentative communication system. The physical and occupational therapists must plan ahead to make certain the child has the same type of access to the power drive on the wheelchair and the same access to the computer, and the teachers need to make certain the computer programs are the same. If they are to be different, exposure to the new equipment or systems should have occurred long before the transition to the new school. It can take months to receive new equipment in a school setting, and the planning for transition must be started long before the actual event.

One of the most significant transitions in the life of a child and the family is when he or she leaves school. This is especially complicated for a child with significant disabilities who has limited options. Therefore, transition planning and services are required leading to postschool activities. Under IDEA 04, **transition services** are a coordinated set of activities for a child with a disability that,

(A) is designed to be within a results-oriented process, that is focused on improving the academic and functional achievement of the child with a disability to facilitate the child's movement from school to post-school activities, including post-secondary education, vocational education, integrated employment (including supported employment), continuing and adult education, adult services, independent living, or community participation;
(B) is based on the individual child's needs, taking into account the child's strengths, preferences, and interests; and
(C) includes instruction, related services, community experiences, the development of employment and other post-school adult living objectives, and, when appropriate, acquisition of daily living skills and functional vocational evaluation. [20 USC 1401, § 602(34)]

Transition planning must begin at age 16 years (earlier if the IEP team determines it is appropriate). The Tri-Alliance of the American Occupational Therapy Association, the American Speech-Hearing-Language Association, and APTA worked together to have related services included in the IEP team for transition planning for children with disabilities. In addition to the usual members of the IEP team, transition service participants should also include representatives of agencies likely to be responsible for providing transition services or paying for those services and related service providers as appropriate.

Transition services should focus on personal/social skills, daily living skills, and occupational/vocational skills so that the young adult may have a meaningful postsecondary school career and positive life outcomes. Consideration must be given to the child's long-term goals and needs. Therapists must help in determining what physical skills the child must have in multiple environments to achieve his or her goals and be successful in the community.

Common themes in promising practices in transition, according to Flexer and Baer (2008, pp. 15–26), include the following:

- Student self-determination (social skills training and self-advocacy)
- Ecological approaches (use of formal and informal supports, career education)
- Individualized backward planning (person-centered planning that starts with the student's future goals and works backward to the present situation)
- Service coordination (interagency and interdisciplinary collaboration)
- Community experiences (paid work experiences, career education, and exposure to social situations)
- Access and accommodation technologies (assistive technology)
- Supports for postsecondary education
- Systems change strategies (secondary curricular reform and inclusion)
- Family involvement (parent involvement)

The issues involving transitions at each stage are complex and require the full participation of a dedicated team of professionals along with the child and the parents. Physical therapists have the skills and background to assist in making transitions go more smoothly for children with physical disabilities.

Who Receives School-Based Physical Therapy?

IDEA

The vast majority of children who receive school-based physical therapy services do so under IDEA, based on the deliberations of the IEP team. Ideally, the physical therapist would have performed an examination, written up an evaluation, and attended the IEP meeting to assist in determining goals, objectives, and services. The physical therapist may attend the IEP meeting at the recommendation of the LEA or at the request of the parents. Therapists are not required to attend all IEP meetings, nor are they barred from attending meetings. During the meeting, they should indicate in what areas physical therapy services might help the child to benefit from his or her education. Then the team decides whether physical therapy services are needed and, if so, the frequency, duration, and location of services.

Although any child eligible for special education might also be eligible for physical therapy as a related service, therapists tend to serve children with restrictions in motor activities: those with the federal classifications (see Table 12.1) of developmental delay, mental retardation, multiple disabilities, orthopedic impairment, other health impairment, and traumatic brain injury. Children who have problems in locomotion, walking, climbing stairs, or using wheelchairs and who have restrictions in activities of daily living will make up the majority of the therapist's caseload. The diagnoses of the children commonly served include CP, myelomeningocele, Down syndrome (especially in preschool and high school), Duchenne muscular dystrophy, osteogenesis imperfecta, arthrogryposis, intellectual impairment, and general developmental delay (in children up to age 9 years of age). Therapists might also assist in meeting the needs of children with autism, pervasive developmental disorder (PDD), and developmental coordination disorder (DCD). An example of the team approach to meeting the complex needs of a child with autism is given in Mini-Case Study 12.1. Autism is a developmental disability that affects the child's verbal and nonverbal communication and social interaction. Children with autism are likely to have restricted, repetitive, and stereotyped patterns of behavior, interests, and activities. Their sensory issues have been well described in the literature (Tomchek & Case-Smith, 2009). Less well known are the problems children with autism have in fine and gross motor development. A common misconception that is not supported by the literature is that children with autism have relative strengths in their gross motor skills (Provost, Heimeri, & Lopez, 2007).

Section 504 of the Rehabilitation Act

Children with diagnoses such as cystic fibrosis (CF) or juvenile idiopathic arthritis (JIA) might also be served by a physical therapist in a school if they qualify for special education. If they do *not* qualify for special education under the rules and regulations of IDEA, they cannot receive related services, including physical therapy, under IDEA. They might, however, qualify for services under Section 504 of the Rehabilitation Act of 1973 (PL 93-112). Section 504 is an antidiscrimination statute designed to ensure that federal funding recipients, such as public schools, treat individuals with disabilities fairly. School systems that receive federal funds are not allowed to exclude qualified individuals with a disability from participation in programs offered by the school. The definition of "qualified handicapped person" under Section 504 is broader than under IDEA and includes any individual who "has a physical or mental impairment which substantially limits one or more major life activities" (*Federal Register*, 1988). Life activities "means functions such as

caring for one's self, performing manual tasks, walking, seeing, hearing, speaking, breathing, learning and working." Therefore, a child with a diagnosis such as CF or JIA, who does not require special education but who has physical impairments that substantially limit life activities, such as breathing or walking, could qualify for physical therapy services in the school setting. A recent U.S. Department of Education, Office of Civil Rights Guidance Letter expanded the definition of and services to students with disabilities. This change should allow more students to receive needed services under Section 504 (Ali, 2012). Also, these services do not follow the strict rules and regulations of IDEA, and there is great variability of services under Section 504 across the nation.

Athletics in Schools

Adaptive physical education for children with disabilities is required under IDEA. Some very large or affluent school systems have athletic trainers and physical therapists on their staffs to meet the needs of school athletes, but there is generally no mandate for such services. This is a specialized area of practice and is discussed in Chapter 13.

What Do Other Disciplines Expect of the Physical Therapist in the Team Setting?

As in EI, team involvement is critical for successful service delivery in school settings. Therapists are expected to share their expertise, as will other members of the team. Time should be set aside for team meetings and communication. All too often, the only team member who is in the child's school consistently is the teacher. Other team members usually have to serve several schools, especially when children are in general education classrooms. Unfortunately, telephone communication is difficult in school settings, and therapists must consistently strive to determine the best ways of communicating with other team members and parents. The traditional small spiral notebook that went home with the child every day and was where teachers, therapists, and parents wrote might still be the best means of communication in many situations. However, therapists should make use of all available technology to help improve communication during the school day.

Unlike EI, in which any discipline might have primary responsibility for the child and might serve as case manager, once the child reaches school age (3 years of age), the teacher(s) become(s) the primary service provider and coordinator of services. All team members must work closely with teachers to help meet their needs and to see that they are interested and able to assist in carrying out the activities the therapist recommends for the child. If the child needs to practice stair climbing and the teacher has arthritis and cannot climb stairs, alternative arrangements must be made to assist the child in practicing stair climbing. Always taking the elevator to the second floor art class does not allow the child practice time in stair climbing or time transitioning from class to class with peers on the stairwell.

Speech-language pathologists and others need input for children with multiple disabilities or severe physical disabilities on positioning for feeding, functional activities, and access to communication systems. Therapists also assist teachers and others in determining alternative positions to decrease the child's pain, maintain range of motion, and prevent skin breakdown.

Professional Development

As in all areas of practice, the therapist must have a plan for professional development. The educational environment is unique, and advanced competencies should be obtained (Chiarello, Effgen, Milbourne, & Campbell, 2003; Rapport & Effgen, 2004). A few states require special certification to work in school settings. This certification has not been difficult to obtain, but as practice becomes more specialized and the legal requirements more complex, additional states might start to require certification and additional competencies. Another way of providing evidence of clinical competence is certification as a pediatric clinical specialist (PCS) by the American Board of Physical Therapy Specialties. This general pediatric certification provides evidence of a broad base of knowledge in pediatrics, including school-based therapy. Because there are fewer postprofessional academic specialty programs in pediatrics as a result of the Doctor of Physical Therapy becoming the entry-level degree, the PCS will become the primary way to document competence in pediatric physical therapy.

An unfortunate problem in school-based settings is professional isolation, in which the therapist is not challenged, does not observe state-of-the-art practice, and has no role models from whom to learn or receive evaluation. School systems offer continuing education/inservice programs, but rarely do these programs address issues specific to the professional development needs of the therapists. School-based therapists need to determine their own professional development plan, either with the support and assistance of the school system or independently, to guarantee their continued professional competence.

Mini-Case Study 12.1
Preschool Child With Autism

Developed by Deborah Widelo, MSPT, PCS

Parents' Concerns

Chris's parents want him to socialize with peers, be more cooperative, and perform on an age-appropriate level.

Child's History

Chris is 4 years 4 months old and attends preschool in the public school system. He was evaluated last year as he turned 3 years old and transitioned from the home-based Early Intervention (EI) Program to a school-based preschool program. At that time, Chris did not have a specific medical diagnosis, but qualified for EI based on developmental delay. He had a past medical history significant for ear infections. Areas of concern based on the initial preschool screening include language, behavior, vision, hearing, articulation, self-help, and social skills. Chris did not and does not take medication.

Examination and Evaluation

The physical therapy examination and evaluation included parent interview, one-on-one examination of the neuromusculoskeletal system at the preschool, and administration of the Peabody Developmental Motor Scales (PDMS), Second Edition, for standardized assessment of gross motor skills.

Chris was 41 months old at the time of the examination and was well developed physically. He communicated with sounds, imitating some words. He used facial expressions and body language to effectively make his wants and needs known. Vision and hearing were within normal limits. Chris did not make eye contact with other children or adults. He was tactilely defensive and responded with an emotional outburst when he spilled a drink on his clothing. When presented with an unfamiliar task, Chris began to line objects up on the tabletop and required 30 minutes of redirection and sensory activities to disrupt that pattern of behavior. ROM and strength were within normal limits; Chris was able to move his extremities and trunk through full joint exertions and against gravity in all planes of motion. Muscle tone was normal. Chris demonstrated symmetrical head, trunk, and hip alignment in sitting and standing.

Chris demonstrated protective extension responses in all planes of movement and had quick protective (parachute) reactions. Equilibrium reactions were present in hands/knees position, tall kneeling, and standing. Static and dynamic sitting and standing balance were normal. He was able to stand on either foot for 2 to 3 seconds as he kicked his opposite foot to hip level. His father studies martial arts, and Chris was able to mimic many of his postures, positions, and activities but was not able to motor plan to perform these tasks upon request.

Chris was independent and safe walking on level surfaces and on uneven surfaces. He used a handrail to walk up and down steps with a reciprocal gait pattern. He was independent in transferring between level surfaces and uneven surfaces.

Chris demonstrated the following gross motor skills: hop with two feet 17 consecutive times, jump forward 12 inches and down from an object 12 inches high, jump over a hurdle 2 inches high, stand on either leg for 2 to 3 seconds, walk tandem on a visual line for 6 feet, walk on tiptoes with arms overhead with motivation, somersault, throw a large ball 6 feet with directionality, throw a tennis ball 5 feet with two hands, catch a large ball from a distance of 5 feet clasping it to his chest, and catch a tennis ball from 4 feet clasping it to his chest.

On the PDMS, Chris demonstrated an age equivalent of 35 months (25th percentile, Z-score of −0.67) for stationary skills; an age equivalent of 32 months (16th percentile, Z-score of −1.00) for locomotion; and an age equivalent of 36 months (37th percentile, Z-score of −0.33) for object manipulation. His gross motor quotient was 87 (19th percentile, Z-score of −0.87).

Summary of Findings
Strengths included independent mobility, good ball-throwing skills, and some advanced gross motor skills (such as the somersault). Areas of concern included behavioral breakdown with structured tasks, transitions between activities, and difficulty following directions for task completion. No physical impairment of body structure or function that would affect Chris in the preschool environment was identified, although his behavior affected numerous activities.

IEP/Admissions and Release Committee Meeting
The IEP Team/Admissions and Release Committee (ARC) met to discuss the evaluation results. The data from the Physical Therapy Evaluation were combined with information gathered from the occupational therapist, speech-language pathologist, and psychologist. (The physical therapist and occupational therapist performed their evaluation jointly, as did the speech-language pathologist and psychologist.)

Chris's present level of educational performance indicated a need for physical therapy in his initial preschool years to address following directions and attention to tasks during gross motor activities, per IEP/ARC consensus. An IEP was developed and physical therapy was recommended for the following academic objectives:

1. Chris will be able to transition from one activity to another when given a visual/verbal directive with no disruptive behavior.
2. Chris will participate in a small-group activity with emphasis on interactive play for 1 minute without leaving the group area.

Based on the recommendations of the team, which included his parents, Chris was placed in special education, with related services, for developmental delay and speech and language impairment. He was scheduled for ten 20-minute sessions of physical therapy for his first year of preschool. Modifications in the school environment, recommended by the physical therapist and occupational therapist, included adaptive seating on a disc seat for visual and tactile cues during sitting activities. He was to use a rocker board during circle time for vestibular stimulation within his personal space. Physical therapy was integrated in the regular classroom program with demonstration of sensory diet activities before structured task activities individually and with his peers, to provide models of successful interaction for the preschool staff. The occupational therapist provided a visual schedule, visual timers, and behavior modification strategies.

Reexamination
During his first 6 months of preschool, Chris made 10% progress on his first objective and 20% progress on his second objective. This means that he still required maximal physical assistance to transition between activities while he demonstrated tantrum behavior. He would stand with his peers at the water table or art table for 10 to 20 seconds but with no interactive play.

Further Testing
Chris's mother pursued further medical and psychological testing, and Chris was diagnosed with autism by the end of his first year of preschool.

Autism is identified when a child exhibits a cluster of the following characteristics, across a range of severity from mild to profound, and collected across multiple settings:

- Deficits in developing and using verbal or nonverbal communication for receptive or expressive language
- Deficits in social interactions, including social cues, emotion expression, personal relationships, and reciprocal interaction
- Repetitive ritualistic behaviors, including insistence on following routines and persistent preoccupation and attachment to objects
- Abnormal response to environmental stimuli

Follow-up

Chris received occupational therapy over the summer through an outpatient agency. When he returned for his second year of preschool, his previous educational objectives remained in place because he did not master those objectives during the last school year. Modifications and strategies within the classroom included use of a minitrampoline for proprioceptive input, a sit and spin, and a rocking chair for vestibular input. The occupational therapist instituted a bear hug vest for deep pressure during transitions, a visual schedule, visual time lines, and a visual timer to help him self-organize.

At this time, 2 months into his second year of preschool, Chris is able to transition between activities and play areas with verbal and tactile cues 80% of the time. Tantrums and verbal outbursts occur with disruptions in the "normal" preschool routine and requirements for task completion. Chris continues to play independently, with no peer interaction. Physical therapy continues for only eight 20-minute sessions for this school year, and he will be followed as he transitions into kindergarten next year. At that time, he will be due for reevaluation and might be discharged from physical therapy because other professionals might better be able to meet his needs. Occupational therapy will continue to work with the regular education teachers and resource room special educators to facilitate meeting his sensory needs, especially during transitions, in addition to visual cues/prompts to assist him with on-task activities and following directions.

Physical Therapy for Children With Autism

For students with the diagnosis of autism in the school system, physical therapy is indicated on an individual basis to reinforce attention to task, following directions during gross motor activities and gross motor skill development. As the student progresses through the educational levels, the need for physical therapy might decrease as students with autism have adequate mobility skills and other needs take priority for intervention. Occupational therapy has been effective in providing input for tailoring activities to meet the student's sensory needs for self-organization and time management for long-term success.

Summary

School-based practice offers many rewards for the physical therapist. Unlike many other settings, the school gives the therapist the opportunity to follow the child for many years, sometimes throughout the child's entire education. The therapist gets to observe the natural progression of a disability, the immediate and long-term impact of interventions, the effectiveness or lack of effectiveness of interventions, and the implications of their work on the child's quality of life and functioning in real life situations. The therapist also gets to work with and learn from members of other disciplines. For many therapists, the opportunity to work in their own local school system and to support their community is an added advantage to school-based employment. School-based therapists must, however, make certain that they continuously update their professional knowledge and skills because working in isolation can restrict their professional development and might impede the progress of the children they serve.

DISCUSSION QUESTIONS

1. Discuss how determining goals differs in a school setting compared with other settings in which physical therapists practice.
2. Why is eligibility for special education so important for provision of physical therapy in school settings?
3. What is the difference in eligibility requirements under IDEA versus Section 504 of the Rehabilitation Act?
4. Discuss ways of making intervention in a general education classroom successful.

Recommended Readings

Hanft, B., & Shepherd, J. (Eds.) (2008). *Collaborating for student success: A guide for school-based occupational therapy.* Bethesda, MD: American Occupational Therapy Association.

McEwen, I. (Ed.) (2009). *Providing physical therapy services under Parts B & C of the Individuals with*

Disabilities Education Act (IDEA). Alexandria, VA: Section on Pediatrics, American Physical Therapy Association.

McEwen, I.R., & Sheldon, M.L. (1995). Pediatric therapy in the 1990s: The demise of the educational versus medical dichotomy. *Physical and Occupational Therapy in Pediatrics, 15*(2), 33–45.

PL 108-446, Individuals with Disabilities Education Improvement Act of 2004. Retrieved from http://www.copyright.gov/legislation/pl108-446.pdf

Resources on IDEA and School Practice

Consortium for Citizens with Disabilities (CCD)
http://www.c-c-d.org
CCD addresses a broad range of federal legislative and legal issues.

Council for Exceptional Children (CEC)
http://www.cec.sped.org
CEC is a professional organization dedicated to improving the educational success of individuals with disabilities. They have numerous resources available.

National Early Childhood Technical Assistance Center (NECTAC).
http://www.nectac.org/idea/idea.asp
NECTAC provides numerous resources, including links to the IDEA law and rules and regulations.

Wrightslaw
http://www.wrightslaw.com
Wrightslaw provides information about special education law and advocacy for children with disabilities.

References

Ali, R. (2012). Dear colleague letter. Office of the Assistant Secretary. U.S. Department of Education, Office for Civil Rights. Retrieved from http://www2.ed.gov/about/offices/list/ocr/letters/colleague-201109.html

American Physical Therapy Association (APTA). (2001). *Guide to physical therapist practice* (2nd ed.). *Physical Therapy, 81*, 6–746.

American Physical Therapy Association (APTA), Section on Pediatrics, IDEA Conference Faculty. (2009). *Examples of team based goals.* Retrieved from http://www.pediatricapta.org/members/school.cfm

Bruininks, R.H., & Bruininks, B.D. (2005). *Bruininks-Oseretsky test of motor proficiency* (2nd ed.). Circle Pines, MN: AGS Publishing.

Chiarello, L., Effgen, S., Milbourne, S., & Campbell, P. (2003). Specialty certification program in early intervention and school-based therapy. *Pediatric Physical Therapy, 15*, 52–53.

Cohn, S.L. (2007). School-based practice: Physical therapists collaborating with physical education teachers. Give it a try! *Physical and Occupational Therapy in Pediatrics, 27*(3), 1–4.

Coster, W., Deeney, T., Haltiwanger, J., & Haley, S. (1998). *School function assessment materials.* San Antonio, TX: The Psychological Corporation.

Dole, R.L., Arvidson, K., Byrne, E., Robbins, J., & Schasberger, B. (2003). Consensus among experts in pediatric occupational and physical therapy on elements of Individualized Education Programs. *Pediatric Physical Therapy, 15*(3), 159–166.

Effgen, S.K. (2000). Factors affecting the termination of physical therapy services for children in school settings. *Pediatric Physical Therapy, 12*(3), 121–126.

Federal Register (1989). Section 104, 3(j), June 22, p. 26313.

Federal Register (1992). September 29, Part II, Department of Education, 34 CFR Parts §300 and §301, Assistance to States for the Education of Children with Disabilities Program and Preschool Grants for Children with Disabilities, Final Rule, Vol. 57, No. 189, p. 44839.

Federal Register (1997). 34 CFR 111, Parts §300 and §301, 7-1-02 Edition. Part II, Department of Education, Assistance to States for the Education of Children with Disabilities Program and Preschool Grants for Children with Disabilities (IDEA 97). In print and available at http://www.access.gpo.gov/nara/cfr/waisidx_02/34cfrv2_02.html

Fischer, J.L. (1994). Physical therapy in educational environments: Moving through time with reflections and visions. *Pediatric Physical Therapy, 6*(3), 144–147.

Flexer, R.W., & Baer, R. M. (2008). Transition planning and promising practices. In R.W. Flexer, T.J. Simmons, P. Luft, & R.M. Baer (Eds.), *Transition planning for secondary students with disabilities* (3rd ed., pp. 3–28). Upper Saddle River, NJ: Pearson Prentice Hall.

Folio, M.R., & Fewell, R.R. (2000). *Peabody developmental motor scales* (2nd ed.). Austin, TX: Pro-ed.

Giangreco, M.F. (1995). Related services decision-making: A foundational component of effective education for students with disabilities. *Occupational and Physical Therapy in Educational Environments, 15*, 47–67.

Guralnick, M.J. (Ed.) (2001). *Early inclusion: Focus on change.* Baltimore: Paul H. Brookes.

Haley, S.M., Coster, W.J., Ludlow, L.H., Haltiwanger, J.T., & Andrellos, P.J. (1992). *Pediatric evaluation of disability inventory.* San Antonio, TX: The Psychological Corporation.

Hanft, B.E., & Place, P.A. (1996). *The consulting therapist: A guide for OTs and PTs in schools.* St. Louis: Elsevier Science & Technology Books.

Hanson, M.J., Beckman, P.J., Horn, E., Marquart, J., Sandall, S.R., Greig, D., & Brennan, E. (2000). Entering preschool: Family and professional experiences in this transition process. *Journal of Early Intervention, 23,* 279–293.

Harris, S.R. (1997). The effectiveness of early intervention for children with cerebral palsy and related motor disabilities. In M.J. Guralnick (Ed.), *The effectiveness of early intervention* (pp. 327–347). Baltimore: Paul H. Brookes.

Jones, M., & Rapport, M.J.K. (2009). Court decisions, State Education Agency hearings, letters of inquiry, policy interpretation, and investigations by Federal agencies related to school-based physical therapy. In I. McEwen (Ed.), *Providing physical therapy services under Parts B & C of the Individuals with Disabilities Education Act (IDEA)*. Alexandria, VA: Section on Pediatrics, American Physical Therapy Association.

Karnish, K., Bruder, M.B., & Rainforth, B. (1995). A comparison of physical therapy in two school based treatment contexts. *Physical and Occupational Therapy in Pediatrics, 15*(4), 1–25.

Ketelaar, M., Vermeer, A., Hart, H., van Petegem-van Beek, E., & Helders, P.J.M. (2001). Effects of a functional therapy program on motor abilities of children with cerebral palsy. *Physical Therapy, 81*(9), 1534–1545.

LaForme Fiss, A., Effgen, S.K., Page, J.L. & Shasby, S. (2009). Effect of sensorimotor groups on gross motor acquisition for young children with Down syndrome. *Pediatric Physical Therapy, 21*(2), 158–166.

Massey Sekerak, D., Kirkpatrick, D.B., Nelson, K.C., & Propes, J.H. (2003). Physical therapy in preschool classrooms: Successful integration of therapy into classroom routines. *Pediatric Physical Therapy, 15*(2), 93–103.

McDougall, J., King, G.A., Malloy-Miller, T., Gritzan, J., Tucker, M., & Evans, J. (1999). A checklist to determine the methods of intervention used in school-based therapy: Development and pilot testing. *Physical and Occupational Therapy in Pediatrics, 19*(2), 53–77.

McEwen, I.R., Arnold, S.H., Hansen, L.H., & Johnson, D. (2003). Interrater reliability and content validity of a minimal data set to measure outcomes of students receiving school-based occupational therapy and physical therapy. *Physical and Occupational Therapy in Pediatrics, 23*(2), 77–95.

PL 108-446, Individuals with Disabilities Education Improvement Act of 2004 Retrieved from http://www.copyright.gov/legislation/pl108-446.pdf

Provost, B., Heimeri, S., & Lopez, B.R. (2007). Levels of gross and fine motor development in young children with autism spectrum disorder. *Physical and Occupational Therapy in Pediatrics, 27*(3), 21–36.

Rainforth, B. (1997). Analysis of physical therapy practice acts: Implications for role release in educational environments. *Pediatric Physical Therapy, 9*, 54–61.

Rapport, M.J.K., & Effgen, S.K. (2004). Personnel issues in school-based physical therapy. *Journal of Special Education Leadership, 17*(1), 7–15.

Russell, D., Rosenbaum, P., Avery, L. & Lane, M. (2002). Gross Motor Function Measure (GMFM-66 & GMFM-88) user's manual. *Clinics in Developmental Medicine, No. 159,* London, England: Mac Keith Press

Swinth, Y., & Hanft, B. (2002). School-based practice: Moving beyond 1:1 service delivery. *OT Practice,* September 16.

Taylor, S. (1988). Caught in the continuum: A critical analysis of the principle of least restrictive environment. *Journal of the Association for Persons with Severe Handicaps, 13*(1), 41–53.

Tomchek, S.D., & Case-Smith, J. (2009). *Occupational therapy practice guidelines for children and adolescents with autism.* Bethesda, MD: American Occupational Therapy Association.

Trahan, J., & Malouin, F. (2002). Intermittent intensive physiotherapy in children with cerebral palsy: A pilot study. *Developmental Medicine and Child Neurology, 44,* 233–239.

Turnbull, R., Turnbull, A., Shank, M., & Smith, S.J. (2004). *Exceptional lives: Special education in today's schools* (4th ed., pp. 61–76). Upper Saddle River, NJ: Pearson Prentice Hall.

U.S. Department of Education. (2010). Office of Special Education and Rehabilitative Services, Office of Special Education Programs, *29th Annual Report to Congress on the Implementation of the Individuals with Disabilities Education Act, 2007,* vol. 1, Washington, DC: Author.

Vacha, V.B. (1933). History of the development of special schools and classes for crippled children in Chicago. *Physical Therapy Review, 13,* 21–26.

CHAPTER 13

Sports Settings for the School-Aged Child

—Donna Bernhardt Bainbridge, PT, EdD, ATC

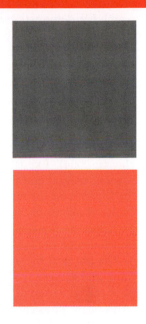

National health initiatives have become focused on the promotion of healthy living as a best practices method to reduce risk factors for disease. These efforts have emphasized an increase in **physical activity** (PA) and **fitness** as key methods to reduce risk, especially for overweight and obesity (Centers for Disease Control and Prevention [CDC], 2008, 2010a; Department of Health and Human Services, 2007; Floriani & Kennedy, 2007; Fox, 2004; Goran & Treuth, 2001; Hills, King, & Armstrong, 2007; Nowicki & Flodmark, 2007; Sothern, 2004; Steinbeck, 2001). As a result, children are encouraged to become involved in PA or recreational and sport activities at a much younger age.

PA levels of children and adolescents are still below the levels established in *Healthy People 2010* (2001). According to the 1990 Youth Risk Behavior Survey (YRBS), Heath and colleagues (1994) reported that approximately 37% of all students in grades 9 through 12 engaged in vigorous physical activity for at least 20 minutes three or more times per week. By the 1997 survey, the percentage of participation had increased to 63.8% (Pratt, Macera, & Blanton, 1999). Participation was higher for males than females (72.3% versus 53.5%) and demonstrated differences in ethnic and racial groups. Changes in PA reported in 9th through 12th grades in the YRBS from 1991–2009 indicated no changes in percentages meeting the recommended levels of PA (34.7%), or attendance at physical education classes at least one day per week (56.4%). Computer use more than 3 hours daily did increase between 2003 and 2009 (22.1 to 24.9 %), while television watching more than three hours daily decreased from 1999 to 2009 (42.8 to 32.8%) (CDC, 2010a).

Current estimates suggest that between 20 and 30 million youth aged 5 to 17 years participate in community-sponsored athletic programs (Adirim & Cheng, 2003; Patel & Nelson, 2000); however, Damore (2002) suggests that suburban preschool and school-aged children are more active than urban children in the same age groups. These rates did not include the elementary ages or community programs. A Fact Sheet from the World Health Organization suggests that PA is low in all children, but declines from age 11 to age 15 years due to the increasingly sedentary nature of many forms of recreation, modes of transportation, and increasing urbanization (World Health Organization, 2007).

Early participation in exercise and sports extends a physically active and athletic life over many decades. Research has demonstrated that more PA in adolescence increases a sense of psychological well-being in adults, and may improve self-rating of physical health in adulthood (Sacker & Cable, 2006). Additionally, higher levels of PA from youth to adulthood are associated with lower risk of abdominal obesity in women (Yang, Telama, Viikari, & Raitakari, 2006), while decreasing levels of PA are related to overall obesity in both genders and severe abdominal obesity in females (Tammelin, Laitinen, & Nayha, 2004). Exposure to sports during significant years of mental and physical development establishes the foundation for future exercise beliefs and training habits. However, the increase in years of PA and athletic participation can also increase total time exposure and thus the potential for injury.

The physical therapist is uniquely qualified to promote and restore wellness, fitness, and health in the physically active child/adolescent in a variety of settings (American Physical Therapy Association [APTA], 2010). Physical therapists and physical therapist assistants have positive roles to play in promotion of healthy lifestyles, wellness, and injury prevention (APTA, 2009).

The purposes of this chapter are to outline the unique risks of participation in recreational and sport activities by physically active youth with and without disability, and to discuss the role of the physical therapist in fitness and sports. Two currently established models—the in-school athletic wellness model and the community-based Special Olympics model—will detail the role and involvement of the physical therapist in sports programs for both the able child and the school-aged child/adolescent with a disability.

Risk of Injury

Children and Adolescents With No Disabilities

More than 1 million serious sports-related injuries occur each year to adolescents aged 10–17 years (Bijur

et al., 1995). Taylor and Attia (2000) reviewed all sports-related (SR) injuries in children between 5 and 18 years seen in the Emergency Department (ED) over a 2-year period. They noted 677 injuries, with 71% occurring in males. Sports that were most commonly implicated were basketball (19.5%), football (17.1%), baseball/softball (14.9%), soccer (14.2%), inline skating (5.7%), and hockey (4.6%). Sprains/strains were most frequent, accounting for 90% of all injuries, followed by fractures, contusions, and lacerations. Conn, Annest, and Gilchrist (2003) evaluated SR injury events in the national health interview survey for 1997–1999. They reported that the estimates for SR injuries were about 42% higher for 5- to 24-year-olds than shown in ED data. The highest average annual rates were for children aged 5 to 14 years (59.3 per 1000) and 15 to 24 years (56.4 per 1000). Injury rates were twice as high in males.

Injury patterns of children 5 to 21 years of age (mean age 12.2 years) presenting to four EDs found a total of 1,421 injuries in 1,275 patients (Damore, Metzl, Ramundo, Pan, & Van Amerongen, 2003). They noted that sports injuries accounted for 41% of all musculoskeletal injuries, and 8% of all ED visits. Injuries to head, forearms, and wrists were most common in cycling, while hand injuries were common in football and basketball. Soccer accounted for most of the knee injuries, while basketball caused most foot and ankle injuries. Conn and colleagues (2006) used the National Electronic Surveillance System to examine injuries related to violent sports behavior. An estimated 0.25% of all sports and recreational injuries were related to violence (65.6% pushing or hitting), with the highest incidence in those age 10–14 years. The majority were head and neck injuries (52%), 24% of which were traumatic brain injuries. Playground-related injuries were most common in children under 9 years, cycling in those 10–14 years, and basketball for 15–19 year olds.

A study by Radelet and colleagues (2002) observed 1,659 children aged 7 to 13 years during two seasons of community baseball, softball, indoor and outdoor soccer, and football. Their definition of injury, broader than the accepted definition, included any injury that the coach examined on field, any injury requiring first aid, as well as any injury preventing participation. They noted injury rates of 1.7 for baseball, 1.0 for softball, 2.1 for soccer, and 1.5 for football per 100 athlete exposures. Rates were significantly higher for games versus practice for all sports except softball. However, the frequency of injury per team per season was 4 to 7 times higher in football, with more severe injuries. The types of injuries were consistent with other studies. Contact was a leading cause for severe injury in baseball (contact with ball) and football (contact with player). Interestingly, children between the ages of 8 and 10 years were more frequently injured than were younger or older children, perhaps because of their transition to more advanced levels of play. Brown and colleagues (2001) noted that 27% of cervical injuries seen in a trauma center were related to sports, and football accounted for 29% of those injuries.

An estimated 1.6–3.8 million sports- and recreation-related concussions occur in the United States each year (Langlois, Rutland-Brown, & Wald, 2006). During 2001–2005, children and youth ages 5–18 years accounted for 2.4 million sports-related ED visits annually, of which 6% (135,000) involved a concussion (CDC, 2007). Yang and colleagues (2008) have documented a total of 755 nonfatric pediatric (ages 5–18 years) hospitalizations for sports-related concussions. Browne and Lam (2006) noted 592 sports-related concussions at one ED during 2000–2003. Of these, 72% were males, with 51% over the age of 10 years. Only 25% were related to sports; the remainder were recreational injuries, mostly falls (55%) or collision. Nearly 25% were admitted for further observation and evaluation. A survey of ED visits for sports-related concussions in pre–high school and high school athletes demonstrated that 35% of all visits were for 8- to 13-year-olds, who accounted for 40% of all concussions reported. The authors further stated that from 1997 to 2007, visits for concussion in the 8- to 13-year-old group has doubled, while the visits for the 14- to 19-year-old group increased by >200% even though participation had declined (Bakhos, Lockhart, Myers, & Linakis, 2010).

Data suggests that athletes who have had one concussion are more likely to have another. Children and teens are more likely to get a concussion and take longer than adults to recover (CDC, 2007). More conservative guidelines for management of concussion have been promoted by many organizations (Guskiewcz et al., 2004).

Children and adolescents are becoming more involved in **extreme variations of sports**, as well as in increased risk taking with everyday sports. Various authors note significant injury rates during cycling (Gerstenbluth, Spirnak, & Elder, 2002; Ortega, Shields & Smith, 2004; Winston et al., 2002); exercycling (Benson, Waters, Meier, Visotsky, & Williams, 2000); cheerleading (Shields & Smith, 2006); equestrian (Jagodzinski & DeMuri, 2005; McCrory & Turner, 2005); gymnastics (Singh, Smith, Fields, & McKenzie, 2008); trampoline use (Shankar, Williams, & Ryan, 2006); all-terrain vehicle use (Brown, Koepplinger, Mehlman, Gittelman, & Garcia

2002; Levine, 2006); snowboarding and skiing (Drkulec & Letts, 2001; Skokan, Junkins, & Kadish, 2003); soccer (Adams & Schiff, 2006; Powell, Tanz, & Robert, 2004); and inline skate, skateboard, and scooter use (Kubiak & Slongo, 2003; Mankovsky, Mendoza-Sagaon, Cardinaux, Hohlfeld, & Reinberg, 2002; Nguyen & Letts, 2001; Powell & Tanz, 2000a, 2000b). Although many of these injuries are contusions, fractures, and sprains/strains, these authors noted significant numbers of renal injuries, head and neck injuries, and hand trauma.

Children and Adolescents With Disabilities

Several studies have investigated whether children and youth with disabilities are at greater risk for injury. Sinclair and Xiang (2008) used the National Health Interview Survey data from 1997–2005 to compare medically attended injuries in children ages 0–17 years with and without disability. While characteristics of the injury episodes were not significantly different, children with a single disability had a significantly higher prevalence of injury (3.8% versus 2.5%). However, if sociodemographic variables were controlled, only children with emotional or behavioral problems had a higher injury risk.

Xiang and colleagues (2005) reported a higher percentage of nonfatal injuries in children with disabilities (4.2% vision disability, 3.2% mental retardation, 4.5% attention deficit/hyperactivity disorder, 5.7% asthma) versus 2.5% for typically developing children. Likewise, Canadian children who reported a disability had a 30% increased risk for a medically attended injury, multiple injuries, or serious injury (Raman, Boyce, & Pickett, 2007).

Students with disabilities had an injury rate of 4.7/100 students per year (Ramirez, Peek-Asa, & Kraus, 2004). Children with multiple disabilities had a 70% increased odds of injury compared with those with intellectual (odds ratio [OR] 1.7) or physical disability (OR 1.4).

Minimal data have been collected on the **incidence and type of sports injuries** that occur in persons with disabilities. A 1995 study by Taylor and Williams in the United Kingdom reports the same overall rate of injury. A survey of the 1990 Junior National Wheelchair Games demonstrated injury rates of 97% in track, 22% in field events, and 91% in swimming among 83 athletes (Wilson & Washington, 1993). Among the 20 medical problems noted in 19 athletes in the International Flower Marathon, 13 were injuries: 8 soft tissue injuries and 5 abrasions/ulcers (Hoeberigs, Deberts-Eggen, & Deberts, 1990).

A study of 210 athletes in 8 special education high schools noted 38 injuries among 512 athletes (a rate of 2 per 1,000 athlete exposures) (Ramirez et al., 2009). The sample included children with learning, intellectual, or emotional disability; multiple disability including traumatic brain injury; and autism. The highest injury rate (3.7 per 1,000) occurred in soccer. Although few in number, youth with autism had the highest risk for injury (five times greater). Those with a seizure history had injury rates >2.5 times those with no seizures. The athletes with disabilities, when compared to typically developing peers, had less severe injuries, fewer strains and sprains, no fractures or concussions. They also required less time away from sport and fewer absences from school.

Injury Types Specific to Children and Adolescents

Although children and adolescents can sustain many of the same injuries as adults, they are more susceptible to **unique injuries** related to psychological, developmental, and physiological components. Lack of psychological and developmental maturity for an activity can predispose a child to injury. Tanner scales and psychological attributes, such as attention and ability to follow directions, are often used to assess developmental and psychological readiness.

Evidence from clinical and biomechanical studies suggests that growing articular cartilage has a lower resistance to repetitive loading that may result in microtrauma to the cartilage or to the underlying growth plate. This tissue damage can lead to early onset of osteoarthritis or to asymmetry in growth (Chen, Diaz, Loebenberg, & Rosen, 2005; Hogan & Gross, 2003; Hutchinson & Ireland, 2003; Oeppen & Jaramillo, 2003). The repetitive loading of distance running or jumping might lead to knee osteoarthritis or growth plate disturbance with subsequent permanent alteration of growth (Caine, Difiori, & Maffulli, 2006).

Another weakness of growing articular cartilage is **shear stress**, especially at the elbow, knee, and ankle (Adirim & Cheng, 2003; Malanga & Ramirez-Del Toro, 2008). Research suggests that a segment of the subchondral bone becomes avascular, separates from the articular cartilage, and becomes a loose body known as osteochondritis dissecans. This repetitive shear is implicated in osteochondritis dissecans of the talus in runners, of the capitellum in "Little League elbow," and in epiphyseal displacement (Cassas & Cassettari-Wayhs, 2006)

The third area of weakness in growing cartilage is the **apophysis**. Evidence suggests that overuse stresses the apophyseal growth center, especially if it is an insertion point for the musculotendinous unit, and causes microavulsion fractures. This process is implicated in Osgood-Schlatter disease, Sever disease, and ischial or anterior-superior iliac spine apophysitis (Cassas & Cassettari-Wayhs, 2006; Patel & Nelson, 2000; Vandervliet et al., 2007).

The biomechanical properties of bone also alter with growth. As bone becomes less cartilaginous and stiffer, the resistance to impact decreases. Sudden overload may cause the bone to bow or buckle. The **epiphysis**, the area of growth in the long bones, is more susceptible and may shear or fracture. Examples of this process include avulsion-fracture of the anterior cruciate ligament, avulsion-fracture of the ankle ligament, or growth plate fractures. Because of the difficulty of radiographic analysis, any injury to the epiphyseal area is considered a fracture and treated as such to avoid potential growth disturbance (Caine et al., 2006; Siow, Cameron, & Ganley, 2008; Vandervliet et al., 2007).

A final issue of concern is the longitudinal growth of bones, which often occurs in spurts, with slower secondary elongation of soft tissue. This process causes periods of loss of relative musculotendinous flexibility during periods of rapid bone growth. A coincident occurrence of bone growth and **overuse injury** has been noted (Oeppen & Jaramillo, 2003; Soprano, 2005). Physical therapy prevention focuses on reducing the occurrence, severity, and duration of overuse injuries. These roles are defined more thoroughly in the following models of prevention and management.

Many **physiological differences** distinguish children from adults and affect performance. Children have smaller hearts and lower blood volume; this results in a lower stroke volume with compensatory higher heart rate. Children also have a lower glycolytic capacity, limiting anaerobic performance, and a slowly maturing nervous system. Improvements in balance, agility, coordination, and speed parallels maturation of this system. This neural maturation also affects gains in muscle strength and neuromuscular control (Fawkner & Armstrong, 2004).

Setting-Based Service Delivery Models

The physical therapist is involved in prevention and wellness activities, screening, and the promotion of fitness and positive health behaviors, such as avoidance of smoking, drugs, and alcohol. These goals are directed toward the prevention or reduction of risk for injury. **Primary prevention** is focused toward prevention of disease or injury in a potentially susceptible population. **Secondary prevention** focuses on decreasing the duration, severity, or sequelae of injury/illness through early diagnosis and prompt intervention. **Tertiary prevention** limits the degree of disability and promotes restoration of function in those with chronic or irreversible diseases. These roles can be defined in the following multidisciplinary models of service delivery.

School-Based Model

The school-based model, one that is funded in whole or part by the school district, has been instituted successfully in many high schools (Bernhardt-Bainbridge, 2006). School personnel may include coaches, school nurses, health educators, and nutritionists. Personnel usually retained on contract are a physician and physical therapist, both preferably with expertise in sports medicine, and possibly a certified athletic trainer (ATC). These programs are designed to provide education in positive health behaviors, promote wellness, reduce the risk of injury, and provide early management of injuries.

The components of the prevention model include a **preparticipation examination**, development of an appropriate training and conditioning program, proper supervision, and protection during practice and events. The physical therapist can play an integral part in most of these components.

Preparticipation Screening Examination

The purposes of the preparticipation screening are to determine general health, detect any conditions that might limit participation or predispose to injury, assess maturity and fitness levels, identify sports that may be played safely, and educate the athlete and his or her family (Bernhardt-Bainbridge, 2006). The usefulness of these screenings has been demonstrated in several studies (Drezner, 2000; Fuller et al., 2000; Kurowski & Chandran, 2000; Lyznicki, Nielsen, & Schneider, 2000; Maron, 2002; Maron et al., 2007; Pigozzi et al., 2005; Tanaka et al., 2006). Most states require a preparticipation screening to meet legal and insurance requirements. Although an individual examination is most commonly performed, the multistation examination that objectively screens not only the general health but also aerobic conditioning, strength, flexibility, balance, and power is more cost and time efficient. A complete entry-level examination and evaluation and an annual reevaluation that includes a brief physical examination, a physical maturity assessment, and an examination of all new problems are recommended (Saglimbeni, 2010).

The **components** of the preparticipation examination are a medical history; a physical examination, including cardiovascular and eye examinations; a musculoskeletal examination; body composition assessment; physical maturity evaluation; and sports-specific functional tests (American College of Sports Medicine, 2011; Bernhardt-Bainbridge, 2006). A standard preparticipation medical questionnaire and examination has been created by several medical professional organizations, and can be obtained from the American Academy of Family Physicians (2010). This new fourth edition also has an expanded medical history for special needs athletes.

The physician must perform and sign off on the physical examination and systems testing. The physician or nurse should assess physical maturity. As a specialist in the neuromusculoskeletal system, the physical therapist can perform the history and musculoskeletal examination. Several personnel, including the physical therapist, ATC, or coach, can perform the standardized functional testing.

The physical therapist, ATC, or nurse can assess body composition with one of several field tests: body mass index (BMI) (use the BMI calculator for children and teens ages 2–19 years found in Tables 13.1 and 13.2), skinfold assessment using age- and population-specific equations, or anthropometric measures such as waist circumference. Lower to upper acceptable levels of body fat are 5% to 31% for males aged 6 to 17 years, and 12% to 36% for females of similar age (Lohman, Houtkooper, & Going, 1997).

The preparticipation examination guides the team physician in determining the **level of athletic clearance** (Table 13.3 and Appendix 13.A). The examination also defines each athlete's strengths and limitations. These levels are the foundation for an individualized training and conditioning program with the following elements: energy training, strength and endurance training, speed work, and nutritional counseling (Birrer & Brecher, 1987).

The preparticipation examination can also be used to **screen** youth and adolescents for involvement in risky health behaviors, such as tobacco and alcohol use, use of recreational drugs or substances to enhance performance—both legal and illegal (Armsey & Hosey, 2004), and unsafe sexual practices (Nsuami et al., 2003). In addition to actual questions, the examiner can be alert for reported changes in behavior, poor grades, loss of attention, irritability, and weight changes.

The importance of screening for performance-enhancing drugs is supported by the fact that more and

Table 13.1 Body Mass Index Conversion Table

How do you find your BMI risk level?*

1. Use a weight scale on a hard, flat, uncarpeted surface. Wear very little clothing and no shoes.
2. Weigh yourself to the nearest pound.
3. With your eyes facing forward and your heels together, stand very straight against a wall. Your buttocks, shoulders, and the back of your head should be touching the wall.
4. Mark your height at the highest point of your head. Then measure your height in feet and inches to the nearest 1/4 inch and convert the measurement to inches only.
5. Find your height in feet and inches in the first column of the Body Mass Index Risk Levels table. The ranges of weight that correspond to minimal risk, moderate risk (overweight), and high risk (obese) are shown in the three columns for each height.

Height	Minimal Risk (BMI <25)	Moderate Risk (BMI 25–29.9):Overweight	High Risk (BMI ≥30): Obese
4'10"	118 lb. or less	119–142 lb.	143 lb. or more
4'11"	123 lb. or less	124–147 lb.	148 lb. or more
5'0	127 lb. or less	128–152 lb.	153 lb. or more
5'1"	131 lb. or less	132–157 lb.	158 lb. or more
5_2"	135 lb. or less	136–163 lb.	164 lb. or more
5'3"	140 lb. or less	141–168 lb.	169 lb. or more
5'4"	144 lb. or less	145–173 lb.	174 lb. or more
5'5"	149 lb. or less	150–179 lb.	180 lb. or more
5'6"	154 lb. or less	155–185 lb.	186 lb. or more
5'7"	158 lb. or less	159–190 lb.	191 lb. or more
5'8"	163 lb. or less	164–196 lb.	197 lb. or more
5'9"	168 lb. or less	169–202 lb.	203 lb. or more
5'10"	173 lb. or less	174–208 lb.	209 lb. or more
5'11"	178 lb. or less	179–214 lb.	215 lb. or more
6'0"	183 lb. or less	184–220 lb.	221 lb. or more
6'1"	188 lb. or less	189–226 lb.	227 lb. or more
6'2"	193 lb. or less	194–232 lb.	233 lb. or more
6'3"	199 lb. or less	200–239 lb.	240 lb. or more
6'4"	204 lb. or less	205–245 lb.	246 lb. or more

*To calculate your exact BMI value, multiply your weight in pounds by 705, divide by your height in inches, then divide again by your height in inches. BMI calculator for children and teens ages 2–19 years also available from the CDC (2011) at http://apps.nccd.cdc.gov/dnpabmi/Calculator.aspx
Source: Adapted from National Institutes of Health, National Heart, Lung, and Blood Institute (1998). Obesity Education Initiative: Clinical guidelines on the identification, evaluation, and treatment of overweight and obesity in adults. *Obesity Research 6* (suppl. 2), 51S–209S; American Heart Association (2003). Body composition tests. Available from http://www.heart.org/HEARTORG/GettingHealthy/NutritionCenter/Body-Composition-Tests_UCM_305883_Article.jsp

more young athletes are using these drugs (Gregory & Fitch, 2007; Laos & Metzl, 2006), with a 3% to 5% overall doping prevalence among children. Higher incidence is noted in boys, older adolescents, and competitive athletes. Use of anabolic steroids, as early as 8 years of age, has increased since 1990, especially in girls (Laure, 2000). Research reported that 3% to 12% of adolescent boys and 1% to 2% of girls reported use of steroids (Bahrke, Yesalis, & Brower, 1998; Yesalis & Bahrke, 2000). The 2002 "Monitoring the Future"

Table 13.2 Body Mass Index Percentiles for Underweight, at Risk for Overweight, and Overweight* in Children and Adolescents (Ages 2–20 Years)

Underweight	BMI-for-age <5th percentile
Healthy weight	BMI-for-age = 5th percentile to <85th percentile
Overweight	BMI-for-age = 85th percentile to <95th percentile
Obese	BMI-for-age ≤95th percentile

*Growth Charts for boys and girls can be found in Figure 2.3.

Source: Centers for Disease Control and Prevention, National Center for Chronic Disease Prevention and Health Promotion (2003, April). *Nutrition & physical activity*. Retrieved from http://www.cdc.gov/growthcharts/

study, supported by the National Institute on Drug Abuse and conducted by the Institute for Social Research at the University of Michigan, indicated a significant increase of steroid use by school-age children. Eighth-grade students had increased usage from 1.9% in 1991 to 2.5% in 2002, while tenth-grade students showed an increase from 1.8 to 2.5%. By twelfth grade, usage was 4%, up from 2.1% in 1991.

The Youth Risk Behavior Surveillance Study in 2009 noted that 6.4% of all high school students had used cocaine, while 4.1% had used methamphetamines (CDC, 2010a). Over 3.3% of all high school students reported lifetime use of steroid tablets/injections without a doctor's prescription.

Steroids are used to increase strength, weight, power, speed, and aggressiveness (Casavant, Blake, Griffith,

Table 13.3 Athletic Fitness Scorecards

Athletic Fitness Scorecard for Boys

Test	0: Below average	1: Above average	2: Good	3: Very good	4: Excellent
Strength: Pull-ups (no)	Fewer than 7	7 to 9	10 to 12	13 to 14	15 or more
Power: Long jump (in)	Fewer than 85	85 to 88	89 to 91	92 to 94	95 or more
Speed: 50-yd dash (sec)	Slower than 6.7	6.7 to 6.4	6.3 to 6.0	5.9 to 5.6	5.5 or less
Agility: 6-c agility (c)	Fewer than 5–5	5–5 to 6–3	6–4 to 7–2	7–3 to 8–1	8–2 or more
Flexibility: Forward flexion (in)	Not reach ruler	1 to 2	3 to 5	6 to 8	9 or more
Muscular endurance: Sit-ups (no)	Fewer than 38	38 to 45	46 to 52	53 to 59	60 or more
Cardiorespiratory endurance: 12-min run (mi)	Fewer than $1\frac{1}{2}$	$1\frac{1}{2}$	$1\frac{3}{4}$	2	$2\frac{1}{4}$ or more

Athletic Fitness Scorecard for Girls

Test	0: Below Average	1: Above Average	2: Good	3: Very Good	4: Excellent
Strength: Pull-ups (no)	Fewer than 2	2 to 3	4 to 5	6 to 7	8 or more
Power: Long jump (in)	Fewer than 63	63 to 65	66 to 68	69 to 71	72 or more
Speed: 50-yd dash (sec)	Slower than 8.2	8.2 to 7.9	7.8 to 7.1	6.9 to 6.0	5.9 or less
Agility: 6-c agility (c)	Fewer than 3–5	3–5 to 4–3	4–4 to 5–2	5–3 to 6–2	6–3 or more
Flexibility: Forward flexion (in)	Fewer than 3	3 to 5	6 to 8	9 to 11	12 or more
Muscular endurance: Sit-ups (no)	Fewer than 26	26 to 31	32 to 38	39 to 45	46 or more
Cardiorespiratory endurance: 12-min run (mi)	Fewer than $1\frac{1}{4}$	$1\frac{1}{4}$	$1\frac{1}{2}$	$1\frac{3}{4}$	2 or more

Your Score

Strength	Power	Speed	Agility	Flexibility	Muscular endurance	Cardiorespiratory endurance
Your Score						
Rating (0–4)						

Source: Athletic fitness scorecards (1988). *Patient Care*, October 30, Montvale, NJ: Medical Economics Publishing.

Yates, & Copley, 2007). Other substances used to increase muscle performance include DHEA, branched chain and essential amino acids, caffeine, cannabis, creatine, EPO and its derivatives, growth hormone, and dietary supplements containing nandrolone and testosterone (Armsey & Green, 1997; Bramstedt, 2007; Calfee & Fadale, 2006; Kreider, Miriel, & Bertun, 1998; Laure, Lecerf, Friser, & Binsinger, 2004; Lorente, Peretti-Watel, & Grelot, 2005). Dietary substances including ephedra and carnitine have been used to increase energy and endurance, suppress appetite, and promote weight loss (Bell, McLellan, & Sabiston, 2002; Haller & Benowitz, 2000).

With the exception of studies of the effect of creatine on muscle during resistance training, research has not supported the efficacy of these substances for performance enhancement. Little research has examined these substances in adults; no research yet exists on the population under the age of 21 years. Research has reported potential risk and harm with ingestion of substantial amounts of several substances, including steroids, nandrolone, and ephedra (Calfee & Fadale, 2006; Kerr & Congeni, 2007; Matich, 2007; van den Berg, Neumark-Sztainer, Cafri, & Wall, 2007), while the effects of branched amino acids are mixed (Hoffman et al., 2008; Negro, Giardina, Marzani, & Marzatico, 2008; Nicholas, 2008). The use of ephedrine-containing compounds has been banned by most professional and collegiate sports organizations, as well as the National Federation of State High School Associations (2003).

Risk factors for substance abuse include poor or single parent family situation, poor health perception, other drug consumption, antisocial behavior, depression, and clumsiness. Good communication with a parent, academic achievement, regular sports participation, serious and organized personality, and mother at home were cited as protective factors (Challier, Chau, Predine, Choquet, & Legras, 2000; Stronski, Ireland, Michaud, Narring, & Resnick, 2000).

Dietary supplements are not approved by the Food and Drug Administration, so actual ingredients are not listed on the bottle, nor are safety and effectiveness validated (Congeni & Miller, 2002). The few protections offered to the consumer include a USP label, a nationally known manufacturer, and appropriate and accurate claims supported by research. Herbal substances are being used by adolescents in increasing numbers to feel or perform better (Yussman, Wilson, & Klein, 2006).

Training and Conditioning

Fitness should be a year-round endeavor for the child and youth. The athletic child can develop a fitness program that also trains him or her for improved performance in the activity of choice. Because the body does not respond in a linear manner across all physiological systems, and to maintain interest in the program, a training program is organized into components: off-season, preseason, in-season, and after season. For the child and youth, these programs should emphasize fun, cooperation, team play, and learning.

The focus of **off-season** energy training is development of an aerobic-based, long-duration activity with low- to moderate-intensity work, such as running or swimming. A general base of muscular endurance and strength is also developed to balance the body and to reduce risk of activity-related injuries to the musculoskeletal system.

The goals of **preseason** training are more focused preparation for activity related to strength, balance, and the cardiovascular demands of the activity. Anaerobic efficiency (higher intensity for shorter duration) may be developed in the preseason period, as well as focused strength and speed (Fig. 13.1) (Bernhardt-Bainbridge, 2006).

The **in-season** period is the time for maintenance of condition. The program focuses on specific areas that might be more at risk for injury or limitation. The postseason is a short period designed to allow the body to rest and recuperate. Child athletes should perform activities that they enjoy but that are not their usual choices. For example, the soccer player might choose to swim or cycle.

Strength training for prepubescent and pubescent athletes has been demonstrated to increase strength without alteration of muscle mass (Bernhardt et al., 2001; Faigenbaum, Loud, O'Connell, Glover, & Westcott, 2001; Faigenbaum, Milliken, & Westcott, 2003; Falk & Eliakim, 2003; Gabbett, Johns, & Reimann, 2008; Ingle, Sleap, & Tolfrey, 2006; Malina, 2006; Stratton et al., 2004). Training has several parameters that make it safe for the youth. Instruction in proper technique with constant supervision is necessary. Activities should be nonballistic and performed through full range of motion with no, or very light, weight. An emphasis on negative or eccentric work should be avoided. Apparatus should be scaled to the size of the youth (Kraemer & Fleck, 2005). Many examples of sports-specific strength programs exist in the literature (Faigenbaum et al., 2001). A program can be designed for either the individual athlete or the team. All programs should be coordinated with the coach and performed under direct supervision of an adult. In many cases, such as in children with cerebral palsy or Down syndrome, the

TRAINING CONTINUUM

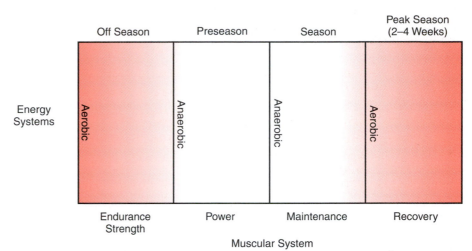

Figure 13.1 Strength-endurance training continuum.

training program should be reviewed with a physical therapist to ensure safety and appropriateness.

Proper training requires **good nutrition** as the fuel for energy production. Nutritional requirements for the younger athlete have been documented (American Heart Association et al., 2011; Gonzalez-Gross, Gomez-Lorente, Valtuena, Ortiz, & Melendez, 2008; Hoch, Goossen, & Kretschmer, 2008; Maughan, 2002; Unnithan & Goulopoulou, 2004) (see Appendix 13.B1 and 13.B2). Attention should also be directed to adequate caloric intake, as active children burn more calories and can have a balanced diet that has too few calories (U.S. Department of Health and Human Services and U.S. Department of Agriculture, 2010). Education of youth and families should be a part of any training program and can be used as an opportunity to encourage young athletes to choose healthy methods for achieving their performance goals without the use of steroids, dietary aids, or performance enhancing substances. This education should be reinforced by both the family and the coach. Some children may have problems with either excess weight and/or excess body fat. If a youth has excess body fat, exercise may convert some fat weight to lean mass. Difficulties with excess leanness and eating disorders are being identified more frequently in the preadolescent population. If a special nutrition program and counseling for weight loss or gain is indicated, it should be supervised by a nutritionist and/or nurse.

Hydration is an important issue with children because they require more liquid per proportional weight than adults. Children also have more difficulty dealing with thermal stress than do adults. Their greater surface area-to-body mass ratio facilitates greater heat gain on

hot days and greater heat loss on colder days. Children produce less sweat, and less total evaporative heat loss, and more metabolic heat per pound of body weight during exercises such as walking and running. Finally, although children can acclimatize, they do so at a slower rate than adults (Naughton & Carlson, 2008).

Thus, the physical therapist or ATC must closely monitor **environmental temperature and humidity**. Field precautions and practice recommendations are noted in Table 13.4. Recommendations for hydration include prehydration of 3 to 12 ounces (3 to 6 ounces for less than 90 pounds body weight; 6 to 12 ounces for more than 90 pounds) 1 hour before activity and 3 to 6 ounces just before activity. During activity, 3 to 9 ounces (3 to 5 ounces for less than 90 pounds and 6 to 9 ounces for more than 90 pounds) should be ingested every 10 to 20 minutes relative to the temperature and humidity. Then 8 to 12 ounces should be consumed for each 1/2 pound of weight lost in 2 to 4 hours after activity (Casa et al., 2000).

Significant research has evaluated the **type of fluid** to be ingested by children. Children will not ingest enough water to remain hydrated or to rehydrate after activity (Bergeron, Laird, Marinik, Brenner, & Waller, 2009; Casa, Clarkson, & Roberts, 2005; Decher et al., 2008). However, if flavor is added to the water, the volume of intake is improved substantially (Passe, Horn, & Murray, 2000). Sports drinks have been shown to improve energy in both intensive and endurance exercise (Davis, Welsh, & Alerson, 2000; Galloway & Maughan, 2000; Meadows-Oliver & Ryan-Krause, 2007). In addition to flavor, well-constituted sports drinks have a simple low-carbohydrate content that

Table 13.4 Restraints on Activities at Different Levels of Heat Stress

WBGT*		Restraints on Activities
°C	°F	All activities allowed, but be alert for prodromes (symptoms) of heat-related illness in prolonged events
<24	<75	
24.0–25.9	75.0–78.6	Longer rest periods in the shade; enforce drinking every 15 minutes
26–29	79–84	Stop activity of unacclimatized persons and other persons with high risk; limit activities of all others (disallow long-distance races, cut down further duration of other activities)
<29	>85	Cancel all athletic activities

*WBGT is *not* air temperature. It indicates wet bulb globe temperature, an index of climatic heat stress that can be measured on the field by the use of a psychrometer. This apparatus, available commercially, is composed of 3 thermometers. One (wet bulb [WB]) has a wet wick around it to monitor humidity. Another is inside a hollow black ball (globe [G]) to monitor radiation. The third is a simple thermometer (temperature [T]) to measure air temperature. The heat stress index is calculated as WBGT = 0.7 WB temp + 0.2 G temp + 0.1 T temp. It is noteworthy that 70% of the stress is due to humidity, 20% to radiation, and only 10% to air temperature.
Source: American Academy of Pediatrics. Committee on Sports Medicine and Fitness (2000). Climatic heat stress and the exercising child and adolescent. *Pediatrics, 106,* 158–159, with permission.

provides energy and speeds fluid absorption and sodium to stimulate the thirst mechanism (Passe et al., 2000; Rivera-Brown, Ramirez-Marrero, Wilk, & Bar-Or, 2008; Wilk, Rivera-Brown, & Bar-Or, 2007).

Successful hydration programs involve not only fluid intake but also fluid availability. Cool fluids infuse into the system more readily, so accessible liquids should be chilled, or ice should be provided (Greydanus & Patel, 2002). Education of everyone involved with the activity is of paramount importance to ensure continued compliance. Knowledge of the common signs of dehydration—irritability, headache, nausea, dizziness, weakness, cramps, abdominal distress, and decreased performance—assist those involved with early recognition and intervention (Bytomski & Squire, 2003; Casa et al., 2000).

Supervision and Protection

The **coach** is the primary supervisor of the athlete. The American Academy of Pediatrics (2007) recommends that all coaching staff members complete a certification course. Coverage of practices and competitions by qualified medical personnel (physician, physical therapist, or ATC) is a second level of supervision. These individuals provide immediate containment and correct management of injury or illness.

Providing the young athlete with high-quality **equipment** that is correctly fitted should be mandatory for safe participation (Ceroni, De Rosa, De Coulon, & Kaelin, 2007; Geary & Kinirons, 2008; Kroncke,

Niedfeldt & Young, 2008; Roccia, Diaspro, Nasi, & Berrone, 2008). This equipment includes footwear, head and eye protection, padding, and mouth guards. Although the coaching staff is responsible for provision of appropriate equipment, it is often the physical therapist or athletic trainer who fits or modifies the equipment to the size or physical needs of the athlete. Physical therapists may also fabricate specialized equipment such as orthotics, soft casts or splints, and braces for athletes who are injured.

Playing areas should be well lit and free from obstacles and possess shock-absorbing qualities. Equipment modifications known to decrease injury (e.g., breakaway bases) should be used (Ceroni et al., 2007; Janda, 2003), and equipment and playing areas should be scaled to the size of the athletes (Hogan & Gross, 2003). The knowledge of the physical therapist can be vital to correct choice or alteration of surface and equipment for safety of the athletes (i.e., wooden floors for dance activities).

Infectious disease transmission has always been a concern, but in recent years the occurrence of human immunodeficiency virus (HIV) and methicillin-resistant *Staphylococcus aureus* (MRSA) have made this a significant issue. HIV is spread by sexual contact with an infected person, through the contact with blood or bodily fluids of an infected person with open area of a noninfected person, by sharing needles or syringes with someone who is infected, or less commonly through transfusions of infected blood or blood clotting factors.

Currently, there are no documented cases of HIV being transmitted during participation in sports. The very low risk of transmission during sports participation would involve direct body contact in which bleeding might be expected to occur. If someone is bleeding, his or her participation in the sport should be interrupted until bleeding stops, and the wound is antiseptically cleaned and securely bandaged. There is no risk of HIV transmission through sports activities where bleeding does not occur (CDC, 2010b).

Several factors increase the risk for development of MRSA, including male-to-male sexual contact, history of intravenous drug usage, and known contact with individuals with this bacterium. Other risk factors include contact sports, i.e. football, wrestling, rugby and soccer, and a history of recurrent boils (CDC, 2003; Cohen & Grossman, 2004; Cohen & Kurzrock, 2004; Nguyen, Mascola, & Bancroft, 2005).

Recommendations from the National Federation of State High School Associations (NFHS) Sports Medicine Advisory Committee (2007) include the following suggestions for infectious disease reduction:

- All clothing for practice and competition needs to be cleaned daily.
- Participants in equipment-intense sports, i.e. football, hockey, need to properly clean equipment on a routine basis with an approved disinfectant.
- Wrestling mats and gymnastic equipment need to be disinfected (1:100 solution of bleach and water) before practice and several times daily in a tournament.
- Personal sporting equipment, i.e., gloves, knee pads, should not be shared.
- A whirlpool or cold tub should not be used if there are open wounds, or scratches.
- Athletes should shower immediately after practice and competition and consider showering multiple times during tournaments using soap from liquid dispensers and personal towels.
- If a child has a skin infection, treat the child and remove him from competition and practice; if he has an active infection, he should be treated with an appropriate antibiotic. All players should be screened for similar infections on a daily basis. If multiple outbreaks develop on a team, contact the Public Health Department for assistance. Multiple outbreaks could indicate there are carriers for the bacteria on the team; consider nasal cultures on all team members, including coaches, to determine the carriers. Consider treating all infected and carrier individuals with antibiotics with a contact sport.

Mini-Case Study 13.1
A School Model

J.B. is a 14-year-old boy attending his preparticipation screening for high school junior varsity football. The physical therapist documents a right knee injury in middle-school football last year. J.B. reports that he had pain on the inside of his knee with minimal swelling. His knee was not examined by any medical personnel and the injury caused him to lose 2 weeks of play.

Examination by the physical therapist reveals no tenderness over the knee joint line. However, J.B. has tenderness at the origin of the infrapatellar tendon. Stability testing reveals no laxity of the anterior or posterior cruciate or lateral collateral ligaments. Slight laxity of the medial collateral ligament is noted. The physical therapist further documents that girth of the right thigh is decreased by 1 inch. Hip and knee range of motion is normal, but right hamstring flexibility is 15° less than the left side. Single-leg standing balance with eyes open is reduced by 15 seconds on the right lower extremity compared to the left. Functional reach is 4 inches less on the right side than the left.

The coach notes that timed single leg squats on the right leg are 50% of the left. Controlled lateral step-ups can be performed on a 12-inch step with the left leg but only a 6-inch step with the right. Cutting to the right is more cautious.

J.B. is referred to the physical therapist for development of a preseason training program to increase strength, balance, and power of the right lower extremity.

The preseason training program will have four components. First, J.B. is placed on a strengthening program for both lower extremities, with emphasis on the right. He is instructed in several weight machine exercises (leg press, short arc quads, seated hamstring curls, and unilateral toe lifts with knees straight and bent). These exercises are done with single leg so he can focus on development of strength in his right leg. He is also instructed in a series of closed chain exercises including half squats, alternate leg lunging, and squat to toes.

The second component is balance training. J.B. is taught a number of simple to more complex balance exercises that train both static and dynamic balance on both and single legs. These drills can gradually progress in cutting, running, and diagonal activities as related to football.

The third component is stretching exercises to equalize flexibility on the right leg. Stretching is done at the end of each exercise session. Focus is placed on the hamstrings, quads, calf muscles, anterior hip, iliotibial band, and hip rotators.

The final component is power. This portion of the program is delayed until both balance and strength have improved. Once those criteria are met, the development of power using plyometrics, quick strength movements, and single repetition exercises with higher weight can be employed.

J.B.'s coach and parents are informed of the situation. The coach will supervise his program at school. He will be reexamined by the physical therapist every 2 weeks. When the strength and balance of the right side are 85% of the left, the physical therapist will release J.B. for play.

Community-Based Model

Many community-based models of sports participation exist for normally abled children and children with disabilities. Peewee Football and Little League are two well-known examples of programs for children with no disabilities. Special Olympics is one of the best-developed integrative models for children and adults with intellectual and/or developmental disabilities and will be used as an example of a community-based model.

The Kennedy Foundation spearheaded years of research and development of models and materials for sport skill assessment and programming, which has culminated in an adaptation of the President's Physical Fitness Test for skill evaluation of persons with intellectual disability. The merger of testing and need for sports opportunity resulted in the first Special Olympics Games in 1968. The success of these games led to the establishment of Special Olympics, Inc. in 1968, and the subsequent development of over 200 accredited National and International Special Olympics Programs in 180 countries. The mission of the Special Olympics is similar to that of the school model: "to provide year-round sports training and athletic competition in a variety of Olympic-type sports for children and adults with intellectual disabilities, giving them continuing opportunities to develop physical fitness, demonstrate courage, experience joy, and participate in a sharing of gifts, skills, and friendship with their families, other Special Olympics athletes, and the community" (Special Olympics International, 2003).

The Special Olympics, recognizing the disparity in health care for their members and the need to address routine health care, developed the *Healthy Athlete* program.

This program is a series of health services and education that address the most significant areas of disparity. Current venues include Opening Eyes—a visual examination with eyeglass and protective eyeware fabrication; Healthy Hearing—an auditory examination, referral, and limited fabrication of hearing aides; Special Smiles—a dental examination, education, and mouth guard fabrication; Fit Feet—a podiatric evaluation and education in foot and shoe care; Health Promotion—an assessment of BMI and bone mineral density, education in nutrition, skin protection, substance avoidance, and bone health; MedFest—a medical examination and introduction to Special Olympics; and FUNfitness—a fitness screening with education about how to improve overall fitness.

Developed by APTA, **FUNfitness** is a fitness screening program in which physical therapists screen athletes for selected flexibility, functional strength, balance, and aerobic conditioning (APTA, 2003; Special Olympics, 2011a). Based on the results of the screening, physical therapists educate athletes, parents, and coaches about correct and safe methods for improvement. Data collected at state, regional, and world games are being entered into an international database on the athletes.

The components of this model are similar to those of the school model. Physical therapists have participated in the primary care of these individuals to prepare them for participation and to manage their ongoing physical needs. In the fitness and wellness model, the physical therapist has an integral role in prevention through the screening of flexibility, functional strength, balance, and aerobic conditioning in FUNfitness. Physical therapists are the ideal professionals to develop year-round fitness and health promotion programs for these individuals to promote wellness and reduce the occurrence and impact of secondary conditions, such as overweight and obesity, poor nutrition, and poor physical condition.

Preparticipation Screening Examination

The Special Olympics **preparticipation screening** is an individual physician examination. Persons must have an intellectual disability; a cognitive delay as determined by standardized measures such as intelligence quotient or other generally accepted measures; or a closely related development disability, i.e., functional limitations in both general learning and adaptive behavior to be eligible. The athlete must be at least 8 years of age to compete; no upper age limit for competition exists. An athlete must complete an Athlete Registration Packet, which contains a medical examination signed by a physician who is familiar with the athlete. A new medical application must be submitted every 3 years unless a significant change in health occurs, necessitating a more current medical examination. Any athlete with a diagnosis of Down syndrome must obtain a full radiological examination for atlantoaxial instability and be examined for cardiac anomalies. Jacob and Hutzler (1998) have reported successful use of the Sports-Medicine Assessment Protocol in athletes with neurological disorders as an additional tool to assess neurological function.

A new Special Olympics preparticipation examination, modeled after the examination adopted by the American Academy of Family Physicians, was piloted in 2007, and has been modified for utilization (Appendix 13.C). Children with intellectual disability (ages 2–7 years) can participate in the Young Athletes program.

Training and Conditioning

After athletes have been cleared to participate, they may choose any of 30 summer or winter sports. Each sport has a specific **Sports Skills Assessment** designed to determine the athlete's present level of function and to monitor training progress. Once a level of function (Level I or Level II) is determined, the athlete follows a specific training and conditioning program that is outlined in the Sports Skills Program (Special Olympics International, 2001).

These sports-specific program booklets contain sections on coaching techniques, warm-up, clothing, equipment, sportsmanship, and rules, as well as specific pathways for developing strength, flexibility, fitness, and power. The final sections address the development of specific skills for the sport. Each skill is broken down into sequential task progression with a complete task performance analysis and coaching suggestions. The specific training is designed for an 8- to 12-week session before the competition.

Longer training and **year-round conditioning** are encouraged so that fitness becomes a lifestyle behavior. This expanded training can be performed in community organizations, in special adapted physical education programs, or with special coaches individually or in groups. Physical therapists can utilize the results of the FUNfitness screening as a basis for development of these programs in either the schools or the community. The physical therapist can educate and oversee fitness mentors who will conduct weekly programs, monitor progress, and advance the physical activity programs as indicated. Research is beginning to document the efficacy of training programs for children with disabilities (Edouard, Gautheron, D'Anjou, Pupier, & Devillard, 2007), including cerebral palsy (Fragala-Pinkham, Haley, Rabin, & Kharasch, 2005; Unger, Faure, & Frieg, 2006; Verschuren, Ketelaar,

Takken, Helders, & Gorter, 2008) and intellectual disability (Lotan, Henderson, & Merrick, 2006; Ordonez, Rosety, & Rosety-Rodriguez, 2006; Shields, Taylor, & Dodd, 2008; Smith, Kubo, Black, Holt, & Ulrich, 2007).

Supervision and Participant Safety

Special Olympics recommends that all **coaches** participate in the Coaches Training Program. Three levels of coaching education are available: the Volunteer Coach Certification Course, the Principles of Coaching Course, and the Advanced Coach Certification Course (Special Olympics International, 1994a). Those wishing to become officials must participate in an orientation and must learn specific Special Olympics sport rules (Special Olympics, 2011b).

Physicians, physician assistants, physical therapists, athletic trainers, and emergency medical services personnel provide medical coverage at game events. They maintain adequate hydration for the environmental conditions and manage injury and illness related to participation. They also monitor the use and need for special equipment or orthotics secondary to physical disability or injury.

Several levels of competition and participation have been designed for athletes based on age, gender, and ability to ensure safe participation. Competitive divisions are established so that each participant has an equal chance of winning based on performance scores, not chronological age. Divisions are structured so that the difference between the best and the worst scores is only 10% to ensure fair play.

The **Motor Activities Training Program** (MATP) was designed to provide comprehensive motor activity and recreation training for people with severe intellectual disability or multiple disabilities. The emphasis of MATP is on training in motor skill and dexterity and on participation rather than competition. After an 8-week training program, participants may take part in a Training Day to demonstrate a "personal best" (Special Olympics International, 1994b).

The **Unified Sports Program**, launched in 1989, is also an option. This pioneering program brings together equal numbers of athletes with and without intellectual disability, of similar age and ability, on competitive teams. Each state holds at least one annual competition for qualifying athletes from each area. The states then send representative athletes to the World Games, which are held every other year in the same manner as the Olympic Games. World Games, previously only held in the United States, have been held internationally since 2003.

Mini-Case Study 13.2
Community Model

K.T. is a 10-year-old girl who has mild intellectual disability and myelomeningocele at T12/L1. She is wheelchair independent. Her physical therapist introduces K.T. and her family to the local Special Olympics coordinator. A physical examination is arranged with a local pediatrician, who clears her to participate without restrictions. A physical therapist performs an examination and evaluation of her strength, balance, mobility, and endurance. Her strength is 4–/5 in her upper extremity muscles, 3+/5 in her scapular and core muscles. Balance is good in static sitting, but only fair + in dynamic seated activities. Mobility in her upper extremities is within functional limits, but she has tightness in her anterior hip (–10 degrees modified Thomas Test), hamstrings (–40 degrees passive knee extension, and calf muscles (–10 degrees neutral position). Her endurance to use of her wheelchair is only 15 minutes before fatigue (HR elevated to 130 bpm, and respiratory rate 35).

K.T. decides to participate in wheelchair running and is introduced to the local coach, who places her in the appropriate competition level for her age and skill. The coach and physical therapist modify the Special Olympics training program. K.T. begins training twice weekly, once with her coach and once with her parents.

Her physical therapist designs a general fitness program that will prepare K.T. for her sport. Based on the examination and evaluation, the physical therapist outlines a program that consists of:

- First daily aerobic activity to improve her conditioning and endurance. She works with K.T. to choose several aerobic activities related to wheelchair running so K.T. can cross train and avoid injuries; these activities include swimming and upper body cycling. The length of the activity and the intensity are alternately increased as tolerated.

- The second component of her fitness program is strength training three times weekly. K.T. enjoys using the weight machines at the YWCA, so her physical therapist designs a program to strength her upper extremity and core muscles. She works initially on muscle endurance (2 sets × 15 reps), then changes to strength training (2 sets × 6 reps).

- The third component of her fitness program is balance training. The physical therapist develops several balance exercises that K.T. can perform both in her wheelchair, and seated on a regular chair.

- Finally, K.T. is given a series of stretches for her upper and lower body and trunk that she performs at the completion of each fitness session. She holds each stretch for 15 seconds, and performs each exercise 5 times.

K.T. is reexamined by her physical therapist every 2 weeks for reevaluation and progression of her program. The physical therapist also modifies her wheelchair and her seating for more efficient and safe function during sport. K.T. trains for 12 weeks before she is ready to compete in a state Special Olympics Games. In discussion with her coach and physical therapist, K.T. decides that at the age of 14 years, she will enter a Unified Sports Wheelchair Running Team for racing and relay.

Summary

Participation in sports and recreation is a vital part of the life of both children and young adults. The elements of safe and successful participation are similar for children with or without a disability. The two models described differ primarily in location, cost, and base of support. Both can apply to all athletes regardless of ability.

The physical therapist has an important role in each model, both in prevention and wellness and in primary care for the management of the athlete. The prevention role encompasses musculoskeletal screening with tests and measurements, formulation of intervention to increase sports function and overall fitness, and education in injury risk prevention. The primary care management might consist of intervention to manage an injury, modification of equipment, or fabrication of special orthotics, prosthetics, or other devices. The broad scientific and medical knowledge of physical therapists makes them integral and vital members of the prevention and management team.

Acknowledgment: Special thanks to David Evangelista, Director, Healthy Athletes, for his insightful comments on this chapter.

DISCUSSION QUESTIONS

1. Describe the evidence-based knowledge of types and incidence of injuries in children and youth during sports and recreation.

2. Discuss the unique developmental and physiological characteristics of children that distinguish them from adults.

3. Outline several of the unique injuries incurred by children.

4. Discuss the primary components of any sports model for children and youth.

5. Outline the similarities and differences in models for normally abled children and children with disabilities.

Recommended Readings

ACSM's Guidelines for exercise testing and prescription (8th ed.). (2009). Hagerstown, MD: Lippincott Williams & Wilkins.

Alter, M. (2004). *Science of flexibility* (3rd ed.). Champaign, IL: Human Kinetics.

Bar-Or, A. & Rowland, T. (2004). *Pediatric exercise medicine*. Champaign, IL: Human Kinetics.

Centers for Disease Control and Prevention. (2011). *BMI Calculator for Child and Teen for ages 2–19 years.* Retrieved from http://apps.nccd.cdc.gov/dnpabmi/Calculator.aspx

Durstine, J.L., & Moore, G. (2009). *ACSM's Exercise management for persons with chronic disease and disabilities* (3rd ed.). Champaign, IL: Human Kinetics.

Faigenbaum, A., & Westcott, W. (2009). *Youth strength training: Programs for health, fitness and sport*. Champaign, IL: Human Kinetics.

Heyward, V. (2010). *Advanced fitness assessment and exercise prescription* (6th ed.). Champaign, IL: Human Kinetics.

Hopper, C., Fisher, b., Munoz, K. (2008). *Physical activity and nutrition for health*. Champaign, IL: Human Kinetics.

Horowicz, S., Kerker, B., Ownes, P., & Zigler, E. (2001). *The health status and needs of individuals with mental retardation*. Washington, DC: Special Olympics, Inc.

Kraemer, W., & Fleck, S. (2004). *Strength training for young athletes*. Champaign, IL: Human Kinetics.

Maffulli, N., & Bruns, W. (2000). Injuries in young athletes. *European Journal of Pediatrics, 159*, 59–63.

Nicole, N., Barry, M., Dillingham, J., & McGuire, M. (2002*). Nonsurgical sports medicine: Preparticipation exam through rehabilitation*. Baltimore: Johns Hopkins University Press.

President's Council on Physical Fitness, Sport & Nutrition. Presidential Active Lifestyle Award. Retrieved from https://www.presidentschallenge.org/challenge/active/index.shtml

Rowland, T. (2005). *Children's exercise physiology*. Champaign, IL: Human Kinetics.

United States Department of Health and Human Services. (2001). *Surgeon General's call to action to prevent and decrease overweight and obesity*. Washington, DC: Author.

Recommended Websites

American College of Sports Medicine
http://www.acsm.org
ACSM is the largest sports medicine and exercise science organization in the world. It is dedicated to advancing and integrating scientific research to provide educational and practical applications of exercise science and sports medicine.

American Physical Therapy Association
http://www.apta.org
The APTA seeks to improve the health and quality of life of individuals in society by advancing physical therapist practice, education, and research, and by increasing the awareness and understanding of physical therapy's role in the nation's health-care system. Information is available for both comsumers and professionals at this web site.

National Athletic Training Association
http://www.nata.org
The National Athletic Trainers' Association (NATA) mission is to enhance the quality of health care provided by certified athletic trainers and to advance the profession.

National Center on Physical Activity and Disability
http://www.ncpad.org
The National Center on Physical Activity and Disability (NCPAD) is an information center concerned with physical activity and disability. The mission of NCPAD is to promote the substantial health benefits that can be gained from participating in regular physical activity. Their slogan is Exercise is for EVERY body. This site provides information and resources that can enable people with disabilities to become as physically active as they choose to be.

National Youth Sports Safety Foundation
http://www.nyssf.org/
The National Youth Sports Safety Foundation, Inc. (NYSSF) is an educational organization established to promote the safety and well-being of youth participating in sports. The Foundation is dedicated to reducing the number and severity of injuries youth sustain in sports and fitness activities through the education of health professionals, program administrators, coaches, parents, and athletes.

Special Olympics, Inc.
http://www.specialolympics.org
The mission of Special Olympics is to provide sports training and athletic competition in a variety of Olympic-type sports for children and adults with intellectual disabilities, giving them continuing opportunities to develop physical fitness, demonstrate courage, experience joy and participate in a sharing of

gifts, skills and friendship with their families, other Special Olympics athletes and the community. Special Olympics reaches out through a wide range of trainings, competitions, health screenings, and fund-raising events with information available on their web site.

References

Adams, A.L., & Schiff, M.A. (2006). Childhood soccer injuries treated in U.S. emergency departments. *Academic Emergency Medicine, 13*(5), 571–574.

Adirim, T.A., & Cheng, T.L. (2003). Overview of injuries in the young athlete. *Sports Medicine, 33,* 75–81.

American Academy of Family Physicians & American Academy of Pediatrics, Committee on Sports Medicine and Fitness. (2007). Recommendations for participation in competitive sports. *Pediatrics, 81,* 737.

American Academy of Family Physicians, American Academy of Pediatrics, American College of Sports Medicine, American Medical Society for Sports Medicine, American Orthopedic Society for Sports Medicine, & American Osteopathic Academy of Sports Medicine. (2010). *Preparticipation physical examination.* Retrieved from http://www.aafp.org/online/en/home/clinical/publichealth/sportsmed/preparticipation-evaluation-forms0.html

American Academy of Pediatrics. (2007). Organized athletics for children and preadolescents. *Pediatrics, 107*(6), 1459–1462. Retrieved from http://aappolicy.aappublications.org/cgi/content/full/pediatrics;107/6/1459

American Academy of Pediatrics, Committee on Sports Medicine and Fitness. (2000). Climatic heat stress and the exercising child and adolescent. *Pediatrics, 106,* 158–159.

American Academy of Pediatrics, Committee on Sports Medicine and Fitness. (2001). Medical conditions affecting sports participation. *Pediatrics, 107,* 1205–1209.

American College of Sports Medicine, 2011. Pre-Participation Physical Examinations. Brochure of ACSM's Consumer Information Committee. Retrieved at http://www.acsm.org/docs/brochures/pre-participation-physical-examinations.pdf

American Heart Association. (2003). Body composition tests. Adapted from Obesity Education Initiative: Clinical Guidelines on the Identification, Evaluation, and Treatment of Overweight and Obesity in Adults, National Institutes of Health, National Heart, Lung, and Blood Institute, *Obesity Research 1998, 6*(Suppl. 2), 51S–209S. Retrieved from http://www.heart.org/HEARTORG/GettingHealthy/NutritionCenter/Body-Composition-Tests_UCM_305883_Article.jsp

American Heart Association. (2011). Dietary recommendations for children. Retrieved from http://www.heart.org/HEARTORG/GettingHealthy/NutritionCenter/Dietary-Recommendations-for-Healthy-Children_UCM_303886_Article.jsp

American Physical Therapy Association (APTA). (2009). *Health promotion and wellness by physical therapists and physical therapist assistants,* HOD P06-93-25-50. Retrieved from http://www.apta.org/uploadedFiles/APTAorg/About_Us/Policies/HOD/Health/HealthPromotion.pdf.pdf#search=%22hod policies on promotion of health%22

American Physical Therapy Association (APTA). (2010). *Physical education, physical conditioning, and wellness advocacy,* HOD P06-04-22-18. Retrieved from http://www.apta.org/uploadedFiles/APTAorg/About_Us/Policies/HOD/Practice/PhysicalEducation.pdf#search=%22Physical Education Physical Conditioning Wellness Advocacy%22

Armsey, T.D., & Green, G.A. (1997). Nutritional Supplements: Science vs Hype. *Physician and Sportsmedicine, 25*(6), 77–92.

Armsey, T.D., & Hosey, R.G. (2004). Medical aspects of sports: Epidemiology of injuries, preparticipation physical examination, and drugs in sports. *Clinics in Sports Medicine, 23*(2), 255–279.

Athletic fitness scorecards (1988). *Patient Care,* October 30, Montvale, NJ: Medical Economics Publishing.

Bahrke, M.S., Yesalis, C.E., & Brower, K.J. (1998). Anabolic-androgenic steroid abuse and performance-enhancing drugs among adolescents. *Child and Adolescent Psychiatric Clinics of North America, 7*(4), 821–838.

Bakhos, L.L., Lockhart, G.R., Myers, R., and Linakis, J.G. (2010). Emergency department visits for concussion in young child athletes. *Pediatrics, 126*(3), e550–556.

Bell, D.G., McLellan, T.M., & Sabiston, C.M. (2002). Effect of ingesting caffeine and ephedrine on performance. *Medicine and Science in Sports and Exercise, 34,* 344–349.

Benson, L.S., Waters, P.M., Meier, S.W., Visotsky, J.L., & Williams, C.S. (2000). Pediatric hand injuries due to home exercycles. *Journal of Pediatric Orthopedics, 20,* 34–39.

Bergeron, M.F., Laird, M.D., Marinik, E.L., Brenner, J.S., Waller, J.L. (2009). Repeated-bout exercise in the heat in young athletes: Physiological strain and perceptual responses. *Journal of Applied Physiology, 106*(2), 476–485.

Bernhardt, D.T., Gomez, J., Johnson, M.D., Martin, T.J., Rowland, T.W., Small, E., et al. (2001). Strength training by children and adolescents. *Pediatrics, 107,* 1470–1472.

Bernhardt-Bainbridge, D. (2006). Sports injuries in children. In S.K. Campbell, D.W. VanderLinden, & R.J. Palisano (Eds.), *Physical therapy for children* (3rd ed., pp. 517–556). Philadelphia: W.B. Saunders.

Birrer, R.B., & Brecher, D.B. (1987). *Common sports injuries in youngsters.* Oradell, NJ: Medical Economics Books.

Bijur, P.E., Trumble, A., Harel, Y., Overpeck, M.D., Jones, D., & Scheidt, P.C. (1995). Sports and recreation injuries in US children and adolescents. *Archives of Pediatric Adolescent Medicine, 149,* 1009–1016.

Bramstedt, K.A. (2007). Caffeine use by children: The quest for enhancement. *Substance Use Misuse, 42*(8), 1237–1251.

Brown, R.L., Brunn, M.A., & Garcia, V.F. (2001). Cervical spine injuries in children: A review of 103 patients treated consecutively at a level 1 pediatric trauma center. *Journal of Pediatric Surgery, 36,* 1107–1114.

Brown, R.L., Koepplinger, M.E., Mehlman, C.T., Gittelman, M., & Garcia, V.F. (2002). All-terrain vehicle and bicycle crashes in children: Epidemiology and comparison of injury severity. *Journal of Pediatric Surgery, 37,* 375–380.

Browne, G.J., & Lam, L.T. (2006). Concussive head injury in children and adolescents related to sports and other leisure physical activities. *British Journal of Sports Medicine, 40*(2), 163–168.

Bytomski, J.R., & Squire, D.L. (2003). Heat illness in children. *Current Sports Medicine Reports, 2*(6), 320–324.

Caine, D., DiFiori, J., & Maffulli, N. (2006). Physeal injuries in children's and youth sports: Reasons for concern? *British Journal of Sports Medicine, 40*(9), 749–760.

Calfee, R., & Fadale, P. (2006). Popular ergogenic drugs and supplements in young athletes. *Pediatrics, 117*(3), e577–589.

Casa, D.J., Armstrong, L.E., Hillman, S.K., Montain, S.J., Reiff, R.V., Rich, B.S.E., Roberts, W.O., & Stone, J.A. (2000). National Athletic Trainers' Association position: Fluid replacement for athletes. *Journal of Athletic Training, 35*, 212–224.

Casa, D.J., Clarkson, P.M., & Roberts, W.O. (2005). American College of Sports Medicine roundtable on hydration and physical activity: Consensus statements. *Current Sports Medicine Reports, 4*(3), 115–127.

Casavant, M.J., Blake, K., Griffith, J., Yates, A., & Copley, L.M. (2007). Consequences of use of anabolic androgenic steroids. *Pediatric Clinics of North America, 54*(4), 677–690.

Cassas, K.J., & Cassettari-Wayhs, A. (2006). Childhood and adolescent sports-related overuse injuries. *American Family Physicians, 73*(6), 1014–1022.

Centers for Disease Control and Prevention (CDC). (2003a). Methicillin-resistant *Staphylococcal aureus* infections among competitive sports participants: Colorado, Indiana, Pennsylvania, and Los Angeles County, California, 2000–2003. *Morbid Mortal Weekly Report, 52*, 793–795.

Centers for Disease Control and Prevention (CDC), National Center for Chronic Disease Prevention and Health Promotion (2003b). *Nutrition & physical activity.* Retrieved from http://www.cdc.gov/growthcharts/

Centers for Disease Control and Prevention (CDC). (July 27, 2007). Nonfatal traumatic brain injuries from sports and recreation activities: United States, 2001–2005. *Morbid Mortal Weekly Report, 56*(29), 733–737. Retrieved from http://www.cdc.gov/mmwr/preview/mmwrhtml/mm5629a2.htm

Centers for Disease Control and Prevention (CDC). (2008). *Physical activity and the health of young people.* Retrieved from http://www.cdc.gov/healthyyouth/physicalactivity/pdf/facts.pdf

Centers for Disease Control and Prevention (CDC). (2010a). Youth risk behavior surveillance-United States, 2009. *Morbid Mortal Weekly Report, 59*(SS-5), 1–36. Retrieved from http://www.cdc.gov/mmwr/pdf/ss/ss5905.pdf

Centers for Disease Control and Prevention (CDC). (2010b). *HIV transmission.* Retrieved from http://www.cdc.gov/hiv/resources/qa/transmission.htm

Ceroni, D., De Rosa, V., De Coulon, G., & Kaelin, A. (2007). The importance of proper shoe gear and safety stirrups in the prevention of equestrian foot injuries. *Journal of Foot and Ankle Surgery, 46*(1), 32–39.

Challier, B., Chau, N., Predine, R., Choquet, M., & Legras, B. (2000). Associations of family environment and individual factors with tobacco, alcohol, and illicit drug use in adolescents. *European Journal of Epidemiology, 16*, 33–42.

Chen, F.S., Diaz, V.A., Loebenberg, M., & Rosen, J.E. (2005). Shoulder and elbow injuries in the skeletally immature athlete. *Journal of American Academy of Orthopedic Surgery, 13*(3), 172–185.

Cohen, P.R., & Grossman, M.E. (2004). Management of cutaneous lesions associated with an emerging epidemic: community acquired methicillin-resistance *Staphylococcal aureus* skin infections. *Journal of American Academy of Dermatology, 51*, 132–135.

Cohen, P.R., & Kurzrock, R. (2004). Community-acquired methicillin-resistant *Staphylococcal aureus* skin infection: An emerging clinical problem. *Journal of American Academy of Dermatology, 50*, 277–280.

Congeni, J., & Miller, S. (2002). Supplements and drugs used to enhance athletic performance. *Pediatric Clinics of North America, 49*(2), 435–461.

Conn, J.M., Annest, J.L., Bossarte, R.M., & Gilchrist, J. (2006). Non-fatal sports and recreational violent injuries among children and teenagers, United States, 2001–2003. *Journal of Science and Medicine in Sport, 9*(6), 479–489.

Conn, J.M., Annest, J.L., & Gilchrist, J. (2003). Sports and recreation related injury episodes in the U.S. populations, 1997–99. *Injury Prevention, 9*, 117–123.

Damore, D.T. (2002). Preschool and school age activities: Comparison of urban and suburban populations. *Journal of Community Health, 27*, 203–211.

Damore, D.T., Metzl, J.D., Ramundo, R., Pan, S., & Van Amerongen, R. (2003). Patterns in childhood sports injury. *Pediatric Emergency Care, 19*(2), 65–67.

Davis, J.M., Welsh, R.S., & Alerson, N.A. (2000). Effects of carbohydrate and chromium ingestion during intermittent high-intensity exercise to fatigue. *International Journal of Sport Nutrition and Exercise Metabolism, 10*, 476–485.

Decher, N.R., Casa, D.J., Yeargin, S.W., Ganjo, M.S., Levreault, M.L., Dann, C.L., James, C.T., McCaffrey, M.A., Oconnor, C.B., & Brown, S.W. (2008). Hydration status, knowledge, and behavior in youths at summer sports camps. *International Journal of Sports Physiology and Performance 3*(3), 262–278.

Department of Health and Human Services, Office of the Surgeon General (2007). *Overweight and Obesity: What You Can Do.* Retrieved from http://www.surgeongeneral.gov/topics/obesity/calltoaction/fact_whatcanyoudo.htm

Drezner, J.A. (2000). Sudden cardiac death in young athletes. Causes, athlete's heart, and screening guidelines. *Postgrad Medicine, 108*, 37–44, 47–50.

Drkulec, J.A., & Letts, M. (2001). Snowboarding injuries in children. *Canadian Journal of Surgery, 44*, 435–439.

Edouard, P., Gautheron, V., D'Anjou, M.C., Pupier, L., & Devillard, X. (2007). Training programs for children: Literature review. *Annuals of Physical Medicine and Rehabilitation, 50*(6), 499–509.

Faigenbaum, A.D., Loud, R.L., O'Connell, J., Glover, S., & Westcott, W.L. (2001). Effects of different resistance training protocols on upper-body strength and endurance development in children. *Journal of Strength and Conditioning Research, 15*, 459–465.

Faigenbaum, A.D., Milliken, L.A., & Westcott, W.L. (2003). Maximal strength testing in healthy children. *Journal of Strength and Conditioning Research, 17*(1), 162–166.

Falk, B., & Eliakim, A. (2003). Resistance training, skeletal muscle, and growth. *Pediatric Endocrinology Review, 1*(2), 120–127.

Fawkner, S.G., & Armstrong, N. (2004). Longitudinal changes in the kinetic response to heavy-intensity exercise in children. *Journal of Applied Physiology, 97*(2), 460–466.

Floriani, V., & Kennedy, C. (2007). Promotion of physical activity in primary care for obesity treatment/prevention in children. *Current Opinions Pediatrics, 19*(1), 99–103.

Fox, K.R. (2004). Childhood obesity and the role of physical activity. *Journal of Royal Society of Health, 124*(1), 34–39.

Fragala-Pinkham, M.A., Haley, S.M., Rabin, J., & Kharasch, V.S. (2005). A fitness program for children with disabilities. *Physical Therapy, 85*(11), 1182–1200.

Fuller, C.M., McNulty, C.M., Spring, D.A., Arger, K.M., Bruce, S.S., Chryssos, B.E., Drummer, E.M., Kelley, F.P., Newmark, M.J., & Whipple, G.H. (2000). Prospective screening of 5,615 high school athletes for risk of sudden cardiac death. *Medicine and Science in Sports and Exercise, 32*, 1809–1811.

Gabbett, T.J., Johns, J., & Reimann, M. (2008). Performance changes following training in junior rugby league players. *Journal of Strength Conditioning Research, 22*(3), 910–917.

Galloway, S.D., & Maughan, R.J. (2000). The effects of substrate and fluid provision on thermoregulatory and metabolic responses to prolonged exercise in a hot environment. *Journal of Sports Science, 18*, 339–351.

Geary, J.L., & Kinirons, M.J. (2008). Post thermoforming dimensional changes of ethylene vinyl acetate used in custom-made mouthguards for trauma prevention: A pilot study. *Dental Traumatology, 24*(3), 350–355.

Gerstenbluth, R.E., Spirnak, J.P., & Elder, J.S. (2002). Sports participation and high grade renal injuries in children. *Journal of Urology, 168*, 2575–2578.

Gonzalez-Gross, M., Gomez-Lorente, J.J., Valtuena, J., Ortiz, J.C., & Melendez, A. (2008). The "healthy lifestyle guide pyramid" for children and adolescents. *Nutrition Hospital (Sp.), 23*(2), 159–168.

Goran, M.I., & Treuth, M.S. (2001). Energy expenditure, physical activity, and obesity in children. *Pediatrics Clinics of North America, 48*(4), 931–953.

Gregory, A.J., & Fitch, R.W. (2007). Sports medicine: Performance-enhancing drugs. *Pediatrics Clinics of North America, 54*(4), 797–806.

Greydanus, D.E., & Patel, D.R. (2002). Sports doping in the adolescent athlete: The hope, hype and hyperbole. *Pediatric Clinics of North America, 49*, 829–855.

Guskiewcz, K.M., Bruce, S.L., Cantu, R.C., Ferrara, M.S., Kelly, J.P., McCrea, M., Putukian, M., & Valovich McLeod, R.C. (2004). National Athletic Trainers' Association position statement: management of sport-related concussion. *Journal of Athletic Training, 39*, 280–297. Retrieved from http://www.nata.org/sites/default/files/MgmtOfSportRelated Concussion.pdf

Haller, C.A., & Benowitz, N.L. (2000). Adverse cardiovascular and central nervous system events associated with dietary supplements containing ephedra alkaloids. *New England Journal of Medicine, 343*, 1833–1838.

Healthy People 2010. (2001). *Physical Activity and Fitness: Progress toward Healthy People 2010 Targets.* Retrieved from http://www.healthypeople.gov/Data/midcourse/html/focusareas/FA22ProgressHP.htm

Heath, G.W., Pratt, M., Warren, C.W., & Kann, L. (1994). Physical activity patterns in American high school students: Results from the 1990 Youth Risk Behavior Survey. *Archives of Pediatric and Adolescent Medicine, 148*, 1131–1136.

Hills, A.P., King, N.A., & Armstrong, T.P. (2007). The contribution of physical activity and sedentary behaviours to the growth and development of children and adolescents: implications for overweight and obesity. *Sports Medicine, 37*(6), 533–545.

Hoch, A.Z., Goossen, K., & Kretschmer, T. (2008). Nutritional requirements of the child and teenage athlete. *Physical Medicine Rehabilitation Clinics of North America, 19*(2), 373–398.

Hoeberigs, J.H., Deberts-Eggen, H.B., & Deberts, P.M. (1990). Sports medicine experience from the International Flower Marathon for disabled wheelers. *American Journal of Sports Medicine, 18*, 418–421.

Hoffman, J.R., Ratamass, N.A., Ross, R., Shanklin, M., Kang, J., & Faigenbaum, A.D. (2008). Effect of a pre-exercise energy supplement on the acute hormonal response to resistance exercise. *Journal of Strength and Conditioning Research, 22*(3), 874–882.

Hogan, K.A., & Gross, R.H. (2003). Overuse injuries in pediatric athletes. *Orthopedic Clinics of North America, 34*(3), 405–415.

Hutchinson, M.R., & Ireland, M.L. (2003). Overuse and throwing injuries in the skeletally immature athlete. *Instructional Course Lectures, 52*, 25–36.

Ingle, L., Sleap, M., & Tolfrey, K. (2006). The effect of a complex training and detraining programme on selected strength and power variables in early pubertal boys. *Journal of Sports Science, 24*(9), 987–997.

Jacob, T., & Hutzler, Y. (1998). Sports-medical assessment for athletes with a disability. *Disability Rehabilitation, 20*, 116–119.

Jagodzinski, T., & DeMuri, G.P. (2005). Horse-related injuries in children: A review. *Wisconsin Medical Journal, 104*(2), 50–54.

Janda, D.H. (2003). The prevention of baseball and softball injuries. *Clinical Orthopedics& Related Research, 409*, 20–28.

Kerr, J.M., & Congeni, J.A. (2007). Anabolic-androgenic steroids: Use and abuse in pediatric patients. *Pediatric Clinics of North America, 54*(4), 771–785.

Kraemer, W.J., & Fleck, S. (2005). *Strength training for young athletes* (2nd ed.). Champaign, IL: Human Kinetics.

Kreider, R.B., Miriel, V., & Bertun, E. (1998). Amino acid supplementation and exercise performance: Analysis of the proposed ergogenic value. *Sports Medicine, 16*, 190–209.

Kroncke, E.L., Niedfeldt, M.W., &.Young, C.C. (2008). Use of protective equipment by adolescents in inline skating, skateboarding, and snowboarding. *Clinical Journal of Sports Medicine, 18*(1), 38–43.

Kubiak, R., & Slongo, T. (2003). Unpowered scooter injuries in children. *Acta Paediatrica, 92*, 50–54.

Kurowski, K., & Chandran, S. (2000). The preparticipation athletic evaluation. *American Family Physician, 61*, 2683–2690, 2696–2698.

Langlois, J.A., Rutland-Brown, W., & Wald, M.M. (2006). The epidemiology and impact of traumatic brain injury: A brief overview. *Journal of Head Trauma Rehabilitation, 21*(5), 375–378.

Laos, C., & Metzl, J.D. (2006). Performance-enhancing drug use in young athletes. *Adolescent Medicine Clinics, 17*(3), 719–731.

Laure, P. (2000). Doping: Epidemiological studies. La *Presse Medical (Fr.), 29*(24), 1365–1372.

Laure, P., Lecerf, T., Friser, A., & Binsinger, C. (2004). Drugs, recreational drug use and attitudes towards doping of high school athletes. *International Journal of Sports Medicine, 25*(2), 133–138.

Levine, D. (2006). All terrain vehicle, trampoline and scooter injuries and their prevention in children. *Current Opinions Pediatrics, 18*(3), 260–265.

Lohman, T.G., Houtkooper, L., &.Going, S. (1997). Body fat measurement goes high tech: Not all are created equal. *ACSM's Health & Fitness Journal, 7*, 30–35.

Lorente, F.O., Peretti-Watel, P., & Grelot, L. (2005). Cannabis use to enhance sportive and non-sportive performances among French sport students. *Addictive Behaviors, 30*(7), 1382–1391.

Lotan, M., Henderson, C.M., & Merrick, J. (2006). Physical activity for adolescents with intellectual disability. *Minerva Pediatrica, 58*(3), 219–226.

Lyznicki, J.M., Nielsen, N.H., & Schneider, J.F. (2000). Cardiovascular screening of student athletes. *American Family Physician, 15*, 2332.

Malanga, G.A., & Ramirez-Del Toro, J.A. (2008). Common injuries of the foot and ankle in the child and adolescent athlete. *Physical Medicine and Rehabilitation Clinics of North America, 19*(2), 347–371.

Malina, R.M. (2006). Weight training in youth-growth, maturation, and safety: An evidence-based review. *Clinical Journal of Sports Medicine, 16*(6), 478–487.

Mankovsky, A.B., Mendoza-Sagaon, M., Cardinaux, C., Hohlfeld, J., & Reinberg, O. (2002). Evaluation of scooter-related injuries in children. *Journal of Pediatric Surgery, 37*, 755–759.

Maron, B.J. (2002). The young competitive athlete with cardiovascular abnormalities: Causes of sudden death, detection by preparticipation screening, and standards for disqualification. *Cardiac Electrophysiology Review, 6*, 100–103.

Maron, B.J., Thompson, P.D., Ackerman, M.J., Balady, G., Berger, S., Cohen, D., Dimeff, R., Douglas, P.S., Glover, D.W., Hutter, A.M., Krauss, M.D., Maron, M.S., Mitten, M.J., Roberts, W.O., Puffer, J.C., & American Heart Association Council on Nutrition, Physical Activity, and Metabolism. (2007). Recommendations and considerations related to preparticipation screening for cardiovascular abnormalities in competitive athletes: 2007 update: A scientific statement from the American Heart Association Council on Nutrition, Physical Activity, and Metabolism: endorsed by the American College of Cardiology Foundation. *Circulation, 115*(12), 1643–1645.

Matich, A.J. (2007). Performance-enhancing drugs and supplements in women and girls. *Current Sports Medicine Reports, 6*(6), 387–391.

Maughan, R. (2002). The athlete's diet: Nutritional goals and dietary strategies. *Proceedings of the Nutrition Society, 61*, 87–96.

McCrory, P., & Turner, M. (2005). Equestrian injuries. *Medicine and Sport Science, 48*, 8–17.

Meadows-Oliver, M., & Ryan-Krause, P. (2007). Powering up with sports and energy drinks. *Pediatric Health Care, 21*(6), 413–416.

National Federation of State High School Associations. (2003). *Heat stress and athletic participation*. Position paper. Indianapolis, IN: Author.

National Federation of State High School Associations. (2007). *MRSA in sports participation*. Position Statement and Guidelines. Indianapolis, IN: Author.

National Institutes of Health, National Heart, Lung, and Blood Institute (1998). Obesity Education Initiative: Clinical guidelines on the identification, evaluation, and treatment of overweight and obesity in adults. *Obesity Research 6*(suppl. 2), 51S–209S.

Naughton, G.A., & Carlson, J.S. (2008). Reducing the risk of heat-related decrements to physical activity in young people. *Journal of Science and Medicine in Sport, 11*(1), 58–65.

Negro, M., Giardina, S., Marzani, B., & Marzatico, F. (2008). Branched-chain amino acid supplementation does not enhance athletic performance but affects muscle recovery and the immune system. *Journal of Sports Medicine and Physical Fitness, 48*(3), 347–351.

Nguyen, D., & Letts, M. (2001). In-line skating injuries in children: A 10-year review. *Journal of Pediatric Orthopedics, 21*, 612–618.

Nguyen, D.M., Mascola, L., & Bancroft, E. (2005). Recurring methicillin-resistant *Staphylococcal aureus* infections in a football team. *Emerging Infectious Disease, 11*(4), 526–532.

Nicholas, C. (2008). Legal nutritional supplements during a sporting event. *Essays Biochemistry, 44*, 45–61.

Nowicki, P., & Flodmark, C.E. (2007). Physical activity-key issues in treatment of childhood obesity. *Acta Paediatrica Supplement, 96*(454), 39–45.

Nsuami, M., Elie, M., Brooks, B.N., Sanders, L.S., Nash, T.D., Makonnen, F., Taylor, S.N., & Cohen, D.A. (2003). Screening for sexually transmitted diseases during preparticipation sports examination of high school adolescents. *Journal of Adolescent Health, 32*, 336–339.

Oeppen, R.S., & Jaramillo, D. (2003). Sports injuries in the young athlete. *Top Magnetic Resonance Imaging, 14*(2), 199–208.

Ordonez, F.J., Rosety, M., & Rosety-Rodriguez, M. (2006). Influence of 12-week exercise training on fat mass percentage in adolescents with Down syndrome. *Medicine Science Monitor, 12*(10), CR416–419.

Ortega, H.W., Shields, B.J., & Smith, G.A. (2004). Bicycle-related injuries to children and parental attitudes toward bicycle safety. *Clinics in Pediatrics, 43*(3), 251–259.

Passe, D., Horn, M., & Murray, R. (2000). Impact of beverage acceptability on fluid intake during exercise. *Appetite, 35*, 219–225.

Patel, D.R., & Nelson, T.L. (2000). Sports injuries in children. *Medical Clinics of North America, 844*, 983–1007.

Pigozzi, F., Spataro, A., Alabiso, A., Parisi, A., Rizzo, M., Fagnani, F. Di Salvo, V., Massazza, G., & Maffulli, N. (2005). Role of exercise stress test in master athletes. *British Journal of Sports Medicine, 39*(8), 527–531.

Powell, E.C., & Tanz, R.R. (2000a). Cycling injuries treated in emergency departments: Need for bicycle helmets among preschoolers. *Archives of Pediatric and Adolescent Medicine, 154*, 1096–1100.

Powell, E.C., & Tanz, R.R. (2000b). Tykes and bikes: Injuries associated with bicycle-towed child trailers and bicycle-mounted child seats. *Archives of Pediatric and Adolescent Medicine, 154*, 352–353.

Powell, E.C., Tanz, R.R., & Robert, R. (2004). Incidence and description of scooter-related injuries among children. *Ambulatory Pediatrics, 4*(6), 495–499.

Pratt, M., Macera, C.A., & Blanton, C. (1999). Levels of physical activity and inactivity in children and adults in the United States: Current evidence and research issues. *Medicine and Science in Sports & Exercise, 31*, S526–S533.

Radelet, M.A., Lephart, S.M., Rubenstein, E.N., & Mayers, J.B. (2002). Survey of the injury rate for children in community sports. *Pediatrics, 110*, e28.

Raman, S.R., Boyce, W., & Pickett, W. (2007). Injury among 1107 Canadian students with self-identified disabilities. *Disability Rehabilitation, 29*(22), 1727–1735.

Ramirez, M., Peek-Asa, C., & Kraus, J.F. (2004). Disability and risk of school-related injury. *Injury Prevention, 10*(1), 21–26.

Ramirez, M., Yang, J., Bourque, L., Javien, J., Kashani, S., Limbos, M.A., Peek-Asa, C. (2009). Sports injuries to high school athletes with disabilities. *Pediatrics, 123*(2), 690–696.

Rivera-Brown, A.M., Ramirez-Marrero, F.A., Wilk, B., & Bar-Or, O. (2008). Voluntary drinking and hydration in trained, heat-acclimatized girls exercising in a hot and humid climate. *European Journal of Applied Physiology, 103*(1), 109–116.

Roccia, F., Diaspro, A., Nasi, A., & Berrone, S. (2008). Management of sport-related maxillofacial injuries. *Journal of Craniofacial Surgery, 19*(2), 377–382.

Sacker, A., & Cable, N. (2006). Do adolescent leisure-time activities foster health and well-being in adulthood? Evidence from two British cohort studies. *European Journal of Public Health, 16*(3), 332–336.

Saglimbeni, A. (2010). Sports physicals. Retrieved from http://emedicine.medscape.com/article/88972-overview

Shankar, A., Williams, K., & Ryan, M. (2006). Trampoline-related injury in children. *Pediatric Emergency Care, 22*(9), 644–646.

Shields, B.J., & Smith, G.A. (2006). Cheerleading-related injuries to children 5 to 18 years of age: United States, 1990–2002. *Pediatrics, 117*(1), 122–129.

Shields, N., Taylor, N.F., & Dodd, K.J. (2008). Effects of a community-based progressive resistance training program on muscle performance and physical function in adults with Down syndrome: A randomized controlled trial. *Archives of Physical Medicine & Rehabilitation, 89*(7), 1215–1220.

Sinclair, S.A., & Xiang, H. (2008). Injuries among U.S. children with different types of disabilities. *American Journal of Public Health, 98*(8), 1510–1516.

Singh, S., Smith, G.A., Fields, S.K., & McKenzie, L.B. (2008). Gymnastics-related injuries to children treated in emergency departments in the United States, 1990–2005. *Pediatrics, 121*(4), e954–960.

Siow, H.M., Cameron, D.B., & Ganley, T.J. (2008). Acute knee injuries in skeletally immature athletes. *Physical Medicine and Rehabilitation Clinics of North America, 19*(2), 319–345.

Skokan, E.G., Junkins, E.P., & Kadish, H. (2003). Serious winter sport injuries in children and adolescents requiring hospitalization. *American Journal of Emergency Medicine, 21,* 95–99.

Smith, B.A., Kubo, M., Black, D.P., Holt, K.G., & Ulrich, B.D. (2007). Effect of practice on a novel task—walking on a treadmill: Preadolescents with and without Down syndrome. *Physical Therapy, 87*(6), 766–777.

Soprano, J.V. (2005). Musculoskeletal injuries in the pediatric and adolescent athlete. *Current Sports Medicine Reports, 4*(6), 329–334.

Sothern, M.S. (2004). Obesity prevention in children: physical activity and nutrition. *Nutrition, 20*(7–8), 704–708.

Special Olympics. (2011a). *Healthy athletes resources.* Retrieved from http://resources.specialolympics.org/Topics/Healthy_Athletes/Healthy_Athletes_Resources.aspx

Special Olympics. (2011b). *Sports info, rules and coaching guides.* Retrieved from http://resources.specialolympics.org/sports.aspx

Special Olympics International (1994a). *Special Olympics general session information pamphlet.* Washington, DC: Author.

Special Olympics International (1994b). *Special Olympics fact sheet.* Washington, DC: Author.

Special Olympics International (2001). *Special Olympics Winter World Games medical data.* Washington, DC: Author.

Special Olympics International (2003). *The mission of the Special Olympics.* Retrieved from http://www.specialolympics.org

Steinbeck, K.S. (2001). The importance of physical activity in the prevention of overweight and obesity in childhood: A review and an opinion. *Obesity Review, 2*(2), 117–130.

Stratton, G., Jones, M., Fox, K.R., Tolfrey, K., Harris, J., Maffulli, N., Lee, M., Frostick, S.P., & REACH Group. (2004). BASES position statement on guidelines for resistance training in young people. *Journal of Sports Science, 22*(4), 383–390.

Stronski, S.M., Ireland, M., Michaud, P., Narring, F., & Resnick, M.D. (2000). Protective correlates of stages in adolescent substance use: A Swiss national study. *Journal of Adolescent Health, 26,* 420–427.

Tammelin, R., Laitinen, J., & Nayha, S. (2004). Change in the level of physical activity from adolescence into adulthood and obesity at the age of 31 years, *International Journal of Obesity Related Metabolic Disorders, 28*(6), 775–782.

Tanaka, Y., Yoshinaga, M., Aran, R., Tanaka, Y., Nomura, Y., Oku, S., Nishi, S., Kawano, Y., Tei, C., & Armina, K. (2006). Usefulness and cost effectiveness of cardiovascular screening of young adolescents. *Medicine and Science in Sports & Exercise, 38*(1), 2–6.

Taylor, B.L., & Attia, M.W. (2000). Sports-related injuries in children. *Academy of Emergency Medicine, 7,* 1376–1382.

Taylor, D., & Williams, T. (1995). Sports injuries in athletes with disabilities: Wheelchair racing. *Paraplegia, 33,* 296–299.

Unger, M., Faure, M., & Frieg, A. (2006). Strength training in adolescent learners with cerebral palsy: A randomized controlled trial. *Clinical Rehabilitation, 20*(6), 469–477.

Unnithan, V.B., & Goulopoulou, S. (2004). Nutrition for the pediatric athlete. *Current Sports Medicine Reports, 3*(4), 206–211.

U.S. Department of Health and Human Services and U.S. Department of Agriculture. (2010). *Dietary guidelines for Americans.* Washington, DC: Author

van den Berg, P., Neumark-Sztainer, D., Cafri, G., & Wall, M. (2007). Steroid use among adolescents: Longitudinal findings from Project EAT. *Pediatrics, 119*(3), 476–486.

Vandervliet, E.J., Vanhoenacker, F.M., Snoeckx, A., Gielen, J.L., Van Dyck, P., & Parizel, P.M. (2007). Sports-related acute and chronic avulsion injuries in children and adolescents with special emphasis on tennis. *British Journal of Sports Medicine, 41*(11), 827–831.

Verschuren, O., Ketelaar, M., Takken, T., Helders, P.J., & Gorter, J.W. (2008). Exercise programs for children with cerebral palsy: A systematic review of the literature. *American Journal of Physical Medicine & Rehabilitation, 87*(5), 404–417.

Wilk, B., Rivera-Brown, A.M., & Bar-Or, O. (2007) Voluntary drinking and hydration in non-acclimatized girls exercising in the heat. *European Journal of Applied Physiology, 101*(6), 727–734.

Wilson, P.E., & Washington, R.L. (1993). Pediatric wheelchair athletes: Sports injuries and prevention. *Paraplegia, 31,* 330–337.

Winston, F.K., Weiss, H.B., Nance, M.L., Vivarelli-O'Neill, C., Strotmeyer, S., Lawrence, B.A., & Miller, T.R. (2002). Estimates of the incidence and costs associated with handlebar-related injuries in children. *Archives of Pediatric and Adolescent Medicine, 156,* 922–928.

World Health Organization (2007). Percentage of physically active children and adolescents. WHO—Europe Fact Sheet.

Xiang, H., Stallones, L., Chen, G., Hostetler, S.G., & Kelleher, K. (2005). Nonfatal injuries among U.S. children with disabling conditions. *American Journal of Public Health, 95*(11), 1970–1975.

Yang, X., Phillips, G., Xiang, H., Allareddy, V., Heiden, E., & Peek-Asa, C. (2008). Hospitalisations for sport-related concussions in U.S. children aged 5 to 18 years during 2000–2004. *British Journal of Sports Medicine, 42*(8), 664–669.

Yang, X., Telama, R., Viikari, J., & Raitakari, O.T. (2006). Risk of obesity in relation to physical activity tracking from youth to adulthood. *Medicine and Science in Sports & Exercise, 38*(5), 919–925.

Yesalis, C.E., & Bahrke, M.S. (2000). Doping among adolescent athletes. *Baillières Best Practices and Research in Clinical Endocrinology and Metabolism, 14,* 25–35.

Yussman, S.M., Wilson, K.M., & Klein, J.D. (2006). Herbal products and their association with substance use in adolescents. *Journal of Adolescent Health, 38*(4), 395–400.

◼ Appendix 13.A Medical Conditions and Sports Participation

Condition	May Participate*
Atlantoaxial instability (instability of the joint between cervical vertebrae 1 and 2)	Qualified yes
Bleeding disorder	Qualified yes
Carditis (inflammation of the heart)	No
Hypertension	Qualified yes
Congenital heart disease (structural heart defects present at birth)	Qualified yes
Dysrhythmia or heart murmur	Qualified yes
Cerebral palsy	Qualified yes
Diarrhea	No
Anorexia nervosa or bulimia nervosa	Qualified yes
Functionally one-eyed athlete, loss of an eye, detached retina, previous eye surgery, or serious eye injury	Qualified yes
Fever	No
Heat illness, history of	Qualified yes
Hepatitis	Yes
Human immunodeficiency virus infection	Yes
Kidney, absence of one	Qualified yes
Liver, enlarged	Qualified yes
Malignant neoplasm	Qualified yes
Musculoskeletal disorders	Qualified yes
Neurologic disorders	Qualified yes
Seizure disorder, well controlled	Yes
Seizure disorder, poorly controlled	Qualified yes
Obesity	Qualified yes
Organ transplant recipient	Qualified yes
Ovary, absence of one	Yes
Pulmonary compromise, including cystic fibrosis	Qualified yes
Asthma	Yes
Sickle cell disease	Qualified yes
Sickle cell trait	Yes
Skin disorders (boils, herpes simplex, impetigo, scabies, molluscum contagiosum)	Qualified yes
Spleen, enlarged	Qualified yes
Testicle, undescended or absence of one	Qualified yes

*Determination of participation and the need for evaluation should be done by a physician with appropriate knowledge and experience who can assess the safety of a given sport for an athlete with the condition.
Source: American Academy of Pediatrics, Committee on Sports Medicine and Fitness (2001). Policy Statement: Medical conditions affecting sports participation. *Pediatrics, 107*(5), 1205–1209. Retrieved from http://aappolicy.aappublications.org/cgi/content/full/pediatrics;107/5/1205#T2

Life Stage Group	Vitamin A (µg/d)a	Vitamin C (mg/d)	Vitamin D (µg/d)b,c	Vitamin E (mg/d)d	Vitamin K (µg/d)	Thiamin (mg/d)	Riboflavin (mg/d)	Niacin (mg/d)e	Vitamin B6 (mg/d)	Folate (µg/d)f	Vitamin B12 (µg/d)	Pantothenic Acid (mg/d)	Biotin (µg/d)	Choline (mg/d)g
Infants 0 to 6 mo	400*	40*	10	4*	2.0*	0.2*	0.3*	2*	0.1*	65*	0.4*	1.7*	5*	125*
6 to 12 mo	500*	50*	10	5*	2.5*	0.3*	0.4*	4*	0.3*	80*	0.5*	1.8*	6*	150*
Children 1–3 y	**300**	**15**	**15**	**6**	30*	**0.5**	**0.5**	**6**	**0.5**	**150**	**0.9**	2*	8*	200*
4–8 y	**400**	**25**	**15**	**7**	55*	**0.6**	**0.6**	**8**	**0.6**	**200**	**1.2**	3*	12*	250*
Males 9–13 y	**600**	**45**	**15**	**11**	60*	**0.9**	**0.9**	**12**	**1.0**	**300**	**1.8**	4*	20*	375*
14–18 y	**900**	**75**	**15**	**15**	75*	**1.2**	**1.3**	**16**	**1.3**	**400**	**2.4**	5*	25*	550*
Females 9–13 y	**600**	**45**	**15**	**11**	60*	**0.9**	**0.9**	**12**	**1.0**	**300**	**1.8**	4*	20*	375*
14–18 y	**700**	**65**	**15**	**15**	75*	**1.0**	**1.0**	**14**	**1.2**	**400**i	**2.4**	5*	25*	400*

NOTE: This table (taken from the DRI reports, see www.nap.edu) presents Recommended Dietary Allowances (RDAs) in **bold type** and Adequate Intakes (AIs) in ordinary type followed by an asterisk (*). An RDA is the average daily dietary intake level, sufficient to meet the nutrient requirements of nearly all (97%–98%) healthy individuals in a group. It is calculated from an Estimated Average Requirement (EAR). If sufficient scientific evidence is not available to establish an EAR, and thus calculate an RDA, an AI is usually developed. For healthy breastfed infants, an AI is the mean intake. The AI for other life stage and gender groups is believed to cover the needs of all healthy individuals in the groups, but lack of data or uncertainty in the data prevent being able to specify with confidence the percentage of individuals covered by this intake.

a As retinol activity equivalents (RAEs). 1 RAE = 1 µg retinol, 12 µg β-carotene, 24 µg α-carotene, or 24 µg β-cryptoxanthin. The RAE for dietary provitamin A carotenoids is two-fold greater than retinol equivalents (RE), whereas the RAE for preformed vitamin A is the same as RE.
b As cholecalciferol. 1 µg cholecalciferol = 40 IU vitamin D.
c Under the assumption of minimal sunlight.
d As α-tocopherol. α-Tocopherol includes *RRR*-α-tocopherol, the only form of α-tocopherol that occurs naturally in foods, and the 2*R*-stereoisomeric forms of α-tocopherol (*RRR*-, *RSR*-, *RRS*-, and *RSS*-α-tocopherol) that occur in fortified foods and supplements. It does not include the 2S-stereoisomeric forms of α-tocopherol (*SRR*-, *SSR*-, *SRS*-, and *SSS*-α-tocopherol), also found in fortified foods and supplements.
e As niacin equivalents (NE). 1 mg of niacin = 60 mg of tryptophan; 0–6 months = preformed niacin (not NE).
f As dietary folate equivalents (DFE). 1 DFE = 1 µg food folate = 0.6 µg of folic acid from fortified food or as a supplement consumed with food = 0.5 µg of a supplement taken on an empty stomach.
g Although AIs have been set for choline, there are few data to assess whether a dietary supply of choline is needed at all stages of the life cycle, and it may be that the choline requirement can be met by endogenous synthesis at some of these stages.

Appendix 13.B2 Dietary Reference Intakes (DRIs): Recommended Dietary Allowances and Adequate Intakes, Elements

Life Stage Group	Calcium (mg/d)	Chromium (µg/d)	Copper (µg/d)	Fluoride (mg/d)	Iodine (µg/d)	Iron (mg/d)	Magnesium (mg/d)	Manganese (mg/d)	Molybdenum (µg/d)	Phosphorus (mg/d)	Selenium (µg/d)	Zinc (mg/d)	Potassium (g/d)	Sodium (g/d)	Chloride (g/d)
Infants															
0 to 6 mo	200*	0.2*	200*	0.01*	110*	0.27*	30*	0.003*	2*	100*	15*	2*	0.4*	0.12*	0.18*
6 to 12 mo	260*	5.5*	220*	0.5*	130*	11	75*	0.6*	3*	275*	20*	3	0.7*	0.37*	0.57*
Children															
1–3y	700	11*	340	0.7*	90	7	80	1.2*	17	460	20	3	3.0*	1.0*	1.5*
4–8y	1,000	15*	440	1*	90	10	130	1.5*	22	500	30	5	3.8*	1.2*	1.9*
Males															
9–13y	1,300	25*	700	2*	120	8	240	1.9*	34	1,250	40	8	4.5*	1.5*	2.3*
14–18y	1,300	35*	890	3*	150	11	410	2.2*	43	1,250	55	11	4.7*	1.5*	2.3*
Females															
9–13y	1,300	21*	700	2*	120	8	240	1.6*	34	1,250	40	8	4.5*	1.5*	2.3*
14–18y	1,300	24*	890	3*	150	15	360	1.6*	43	1,250	55	9	4.7*	1.5*	2.3*

NOTE: This table (taken from the DRI reports, see www.nap.edu) presents Recommended Dietary Allowances (RDAs) in bold type and Adequate Intakes (AIs) in ordinary type followed by an asterisk (*). An RDA is the average daily dietary intake level; sufficient to meet the nutrient requirements of nearly all (97-98 percent) healthy individuals in a group. It is calculated from an Estimated Average Requirement (EAR). If sufficient scientific evidence is not available to establish an EAR, and thus calculate an RDA, an AI is usually developed. For healthy breastfed infants, an AI is the mean intake. The AI for other life stage and gender groups is believed to cover the needs of all healthy individuals in the groups, but lack of data or uncertainty in the data prevent being able to specify with confidence the percentage of individuals covered by this intake.

Appendix 13.C Special Olympics Health History, Physical Examination, and Recommendations for Participation

SPECIAL OLYMPICS	HEALTH HISTORY	MEDFEST

Athlete Name: Date of Birth: ☐ Male   ☐ Female

☐ African   ☐ American Indian/Eskimo   ☐ Middle Eastern   ☐ Asian/Pacific Islander   ☐ Australian Aboriginal

☐ Caucasian   ☐ Hispanic/Latin American   ☐ Mix (check all that apply)   ☐ Other:

Social Security # (if US citizen):   Day Phone #:   Night Phone #:

Health Insurance Company: Policy #:

Athlete's Address: City: State:

Parent/Guardian Name: Day Phone #:   Night Phone #:

Parent/Guardian Address: City: State:

Primary Care Physician's Name: Day Phone #:

Primary Care Physician's Address: City: State:

Emergency Contact Name: Day Phone #:   Night Phone #:

Do you have any religious objections to medical treatment?   ☐ No   ☐ Yes, Please Describe:

Where do you live?   ☐ With Parents or Other Family Members   ☐ Independently   ☐ Group Home   ☐ Institution/Facility

Please list any medications, vitamins or dietary supplements below (include birth control or hormone therapy, if applicable).

Medication, Vitamin or Supplement	Dosage	Times per Day	Medication, Vitamin or Supplement	Dosage	Times per Day

Please check which of the following vaccines the athlete has had.

☐ Anthrax   ☐ Influenza (flu)   ☐ Pertussis (DTP)   ☐ Small Pox
☐ Chickenpox (VZV)   ☐ Japanese Encephalitis   ☐ Pneumococcus   ☐ Tetanus (DTP)
☐ Diphtheria (DTP)   ☐ Lyme Disease   ☐ Polio   Year of last dose: _____
☐ Hepatitis A   ☐ Measles (MMR)   ☐ Rabies   ☐ Tuberculosis
☐ Hepatitis B   ☐ Meningococcus   ☐ Rotavirus   ☐ Typhoid Fever
☐ Hemophilus Influenza B   ☐ Mumps (MMR)   ☐ Rubella (MMR)   ☐ Yellow Fever

List any allergies	List any special diet needs

List all past or ongoing medical conditions	List all past surgeries

List any medical conditions which run in your family	Which sports are you interested in playing?

Please answer the following questions (circle questions you do not know the answer to).

How long has it been since you visited an emergency room?			How long has it been since you visited a physician?	☐ Yes ☐ No
How many times did you visit an emergency room last year?			How many times did you visit a physician last year?	☐ Yes ☐ No
Have you ever had a seizure in your lifetime?	☐ Yes	☐ No	Do you take birth control or another hormone therapy? ☐ Yes ☐ No	
Have you had a seizure in the last 12 months?	☐ Yes	☐ No	Have you taken antibiotics in the past month?	
Has any family member or relative died while exercising?	☐ Yes	☐ No	Do you have burning or discomfort when urinating?	
Has any relative died of a heart problem before age 40?	☐ Yes	☐ No	Do you currently have any symptoms of a cold or flu?	
Do you currently have any chronic or acute infection?	☐ No	☐ Yes, please describe?		
Have you ever had an abnormal Electrocardiogram (EKG)?	☐ No	☐ Yes, why?		
Have you ever had an abnormal Echocardiogram (Echo)?	☐ No	☐ Yes, why?		
Has a doctor ever limited your participation in sports?	☐ No	☐ Yes, why?		

■ **Appendix 13.C** Special Olympics Health History, Physical Examination, and Recommendations
■ for Participation—cont'd

What is the medical cause of the athlete's intellectual disability?	List any additional conditions or syndromes (see list below)

Adams-Oliver Syndrome	Ehler-Danlos Syndrome	Kearns-Sayre Syndrome	Townes-Brocks Syndrome
Allagile Syndrome	Eisenmenger Syndrome	Laurence-Moon-Biedle Syndrome	Treacher Collins Syndrome
Apert Syndrome	Ellis Van Crevald Syndrome	Leopard Syndrome	Tuberous Sclerosis
Cantrell Syndrome	Emery-Dreifuss Dystrophy	Marfan Syndrome	Turner Syndrome
Carpenter Syndrome	Fanconi Anemia	Mucopolysaccharidosis	VACTERL Syndrome
Cayler Syndrome	Farber Syndrome	Muscular Dystrophy	VATER Syndrome
CHARGE Syndrome	Fetal Alcohol Syndrome	Osler-Weber-Rendu Syndrome	Velo-Cardio-Facial Syndrome
Congenital Rubella Syndrome	Fragile X Syndrome	Progeria	Von Hippel Lindau Syndrome
De Lange Syndrome	Friedreich Ataxia	Scimitar Syndrome	William-Beuren Syndrome
Dejerin-Soltas Syndrome	Hemorrhagic Telangiectasia	Shones Syndrome	Williams Syndrome
DiGeorge Syndrome	Heterotaxy Syndrome	Shprintzen Syndrome	Wolff-Parkinson-White Syndrome
Down Syndrome	Holt-Oram Syndrome	Smith Magenis Syndrome	Zellweger Syndrome
Dubowitz Syndrome	Ivemark Syndrome	Smith-Lemli-Opitz Syndrome	
Edwards Syndrome	Kartagener Syndrome	TAR Syndrome	

Please indicate if you have ever had any of the following conditions (circle questions you do not know the answer to).

SECTION 1 (CR)	SECTION 2 (TR)	SECTION 3 (ER)
Chest Pain During or After Exercise ☐ Yes ☐ No	Atlanto-Axial Instability ☐ Yes ☐ No	Asthma ☐ Yes ☐ No
Dizziness During or After Exercise ☐ Yes ☐ No	Broken Bones (More Than One) ☐ Yes ☐ No	Diabetes (Type I) ☐ Yes ☐ No
Fainting During or After Exercise ☐ Yes ☐ No	Concussions (More Than One) ☐ Yes ☐ No	Diabetes (Type II) ☐ Yes ☐ No
Headache During or After Exercise ☐ Yes ☐ No	Dislocated Joints (More Than One) ☐ Yes ☐ No	Ectodermal Dysplasia ☐ Yes ☐ No
Irregular Heart Rate ☐ Yes ☐ No	Easy Bleeding ☐ Yes ☐ No	Heat Exhaustion ☐ Yes ☐ No
Loss of Consciousness ☐ Yes ☐ No	Enlarged Spleen ☐ Yes ☐ No	Heat Stroke ☐ Yes ☐ No
Shortness of Breath ☐ Yes ☐ No	Hepatitis ☐ Yes ☐ No	Sickle Cell Disease ☐ Yes ☐ No
Skipped Heart Beats ☐ Yes ☐ No	Osteogenesis Imperfecta ☐ Yes ☐ No	Sickle Cell Trait ☐ Yes ☐ No
	Osteopenia or Osteoporosis ☐ Yes ☐ No	Single Kidney ☐ Yes ☐ No
	Spina Bifida ☐ Yes ☐ No	Thyroid Disease ☐ Yes ☐ No
Arrhythmogenic Right Ventricular Hypertrophy ☐ Yes ☐ No		SECTION 4 (PR)
Dilated Cardiomyopathy ☐ Yes ☐ No	Burner, stinger or pinched nerve in neck, arms, shoulders/hands ☐ Yes ☐ No	Aggressive Behavior (AB) ☐ Yes ☐ No
Endocarditis ☐ Yes ☐ No		AB during the past year? ☐ Yes ☐ No
Heart Defect ☐ Yes ☐ No	Difficulty controlling bowels ☐ Yes ☐ No	Self-Injurous Behavior (SIB) ☐ Yes ☐ No
Heart Disease ☐ Yes ☐ No	Difficulty controlling bladder ☐ Yes ☐ No	SIB during the past year? ☐ Yes ☐ No
Heart Infection ☐ Yes ☐ No	Numbness in arms or hands ☐ Yes ☐ No	Autism ☐ Yes ☐ No
Heart Murmur ☐ Yes ☐ No	Numbness in legs or feet ☐ Yes ☐ No	Attention Deficit/ Hyperactivity ☐ Yes ☐ No
High Blood Pressure ☐ Yes ☐ No	Tingling in arms or hands ☐ Yes ☐ No	
High Cholesterol ☐ Yes ☐ No	Tingling in legs or feet ☐ Yes ☐ No	Bipolar Mood Disorder ☐ Yes ☐ No
Hypertrophic Cardiomyopathy ☐ Yes ☐ No	Weakness in arms or hands ☐ Yes ☐ No	Depression ☐ Yes ☐ No
Left Ventricular Hypertrophy ☐ Yes ☐ No	Weakness in legs or feet ☐ Yes ☐ No	Psychosis ☐ Yes ☐ No
Long QT Syndrome ☐ Yes ☐ No	Recent change in coordination ☐ Yes ☐ No	Schizophrenia ☐ Yes ☐ No
Pericarditis ☐ Yes ☐ No	Recent change in ability to walk ☐ Yes ☐ No	
Racing Heart Beat ☐ Yes ☐ No		

Athletes with Down Syndrome, please answer the following questions.

If the athlete has Down Syndrome, Special Olympics requires a full radiological examination establishing the absence of Atlanto-Axial Instability before he/she may participate in sports or events which, by their nature, may result in hyperextension, radical flexion or direct pressure on the neck or upper spine. The sports and events for which such a radiological examination is required are: judo, equestrian sports, gymnastics, diving, pentathlon, diving starts in swimming, butterfly stroke, high jump, alpine skiing, snowboarding, squat lift, and football (soccer) competition.

Has an x-ray evaluation for Atlanto-Axial instability been done? ☐ Yes ☐ No | If yes, was it positive for Atlanto-Axial instability? ☐ Yes ☐ No

Please sign and date.

Athlete Signature	Date	Legal Guardian Signature	Date
Print Name		Print Name	

Continued

Appendix 13.C Special Olympics Health History, Physical Examination, and Recommendations for Participation—cont'd

VITAL MEASURES

Height:		Weight:		BMI:		Temp:		Medication Risks:		☐ bmi ☐ bmd ☐ lqt ☐ sun ☐ csp
BP Right:		BP Left:		Pulse:		O2 Sat.:		R. T-Score:		L. T-Score:

	Near Vision		Can't	Far Vision					Can't	Hearing	1000 Hz		2000 Hz		4000 Hz		Can't
	Pass	Fail	Evaluate		20/20	20/30	20/40	>20/40	Evaluate		Pass	Fail	Pass	Fail	Pass	Fail	Evaluate
Right	☐	☐	☐	Right	☐	☐	☐	☐	☐	Right	☐	☐	☐	☐	☐	☐	☐
Left	☐	☐	☐	Left	☐	☐	☐	☐	☐	Left	☐	☐	☐	☐	☐	☐	☐

PHYSICAL EXAM

HEAD AND NECK

Oral Hygiene	☐ Good	☐ Needs Improvement	
Right Ear Canal	☐ Clear	☐ Cerumen Impaction	☐ Foreign Body
Left Ear Canal	☐ Clear	☐ Cerumen Impaction	☐ Foreign Body
Right Tympanic Membrane	☐ Clear	☐ Infection	☐ Perforation
Left Tympanic Membrane	☐ Clear	☐ Infection	☐ Perforation
Thyroid Enlargement	☐ No	☐ Yes, describe:	
Lymph Node Enlargement	☐ No	☐ Yes, describe:	

CARDIAC EXAMINATION

Heart Murmur (supine)	☐ No	☐ 1/6 ☐ 2/6	☐ 3/6	☐ 4/6	☐ 5/6	☐ 6/6
Heart Murmur (upright)	☐ No	☐ 1/6 ☐ 2/6	☐ 3/6	☐ 4/6	☐ 5/6	☐ 6/6
Heart Rhythm	☐ Regular ☐ Irregular					

CHEST EXAMINATION

Lung (right)	☐ Clear	☐ Not Clear, describe:
Lung (left)	☐ Clear	☐ Not Clear, describe:

EXTREMITIES

Right Leg Edema	☐ No	☐ 1/4	☐ 2/4	☐ 3/4 ☐ 4/4
Left Leg Edema	☐ No	☐ 1/4	☐ 2/4	☐ 3/4 ☐ 4/4
Radial Pulse Symmetry	☐ Yes	☐ R>L	☐ L>R	
Dorsalis Pulse Symmetry	☐ Yes	☐ R>L	☐ L>R	
Cyanosis	☐ No	☐ Yes, describe:		
Clubbing	☐ No	☐ Yes, describe:		

ABDOMINAL EXAMINATION

Abdominal Tenderness	☐ No	☐ RUQ	☐ RLQ	☐ LUQ	☐ LLQ
Hepatomegaly	☐ No	☐ Yes			
Splenomegaly	☐ No	☐ Yes			
Bowel Sounds	☐ Yes	☐ No			
Kidney Tenderness	☐ No	☐ Right			

NEUROLOGICAL EXAMINATION

Right Triceps Reflex	☐ 2/4	☐ 0/4	☐ 1/4	☐ 3/4	☐ 4/4
Left Triceps Reflex	☐ 2/4	☐ 0/4	☐ 1/4	☐ 3/4	☐ 4/4
Right Patellar Reflex	☐ 2/4	☐ 0/4	☐ 1/4	☐ 3/4	☐ 4/4
Left Patellar Reflex	☐ 2/4	☐ 0/4	☐ 1/4	☐ 3/4	☐ 4/4
Abnormal Gait	☐ No	☐ Yes, please describe:	☐ Non-ambulatory		
Tremor	☐ No	☐ Yes, please describe:			
Spasticity	☐ No	☐ Yes, please describe:			

NOTES

RANGE OF MOTION

Mobility =	hyper	full	partial	little	none
Neck	☐	☐	☐	☐	☐
Right Shoulder	☐	☐	☐	☐	☐
Left Shoulder	☐	☐	☐	☐	☐
Right Elbow	☐	☐	☐	☐	☐
Left Elbow	☐	☐	☐	☐	☐
Right Wrist	☐	☐	☐	☐	☐
Left Wrist	☐	☐	☐	☐	☐
Right Hand	☐	☐	☐	☐	☐
Left Hand	☐	☐	☐	☐	☐
Spine	☐	☐	☐	☐	☐
Right Hip	☐	☐	☐	☐	☐
Left Hip	☐	☐	☐	☐	☐
Right Knee	☐	☐	☐	☐	☐
Left Knee	☐	☐	☐	☐	☐
Right Ankle	☐	☐	☐	☐	☐
Left Ankle	☐	☐	☐	☐	☐

STRENGTH

Strength =	full	partial	little	none
Neck	☐	☐	☐	☐
Right Shoulder	☐	☐	☐	☐
Left Shoulder	☐	☐	☐	☐
Right Elbow	☐	☐	☐	☐
Left Elbow	☐	☐	☐	☐
Right Wrist	☐	☐	☐	☐
Left Wrist	☐	☐	☐	☐
Right Hand	☐	☐	☐	☐
Left Hand	☐	☐	☐	☐
Spine	☐	☐	☐	☐
Right Hip	☐	☐	☐	☐
Left Hip	☐	☐	☐	☐
Right Knee	☐	☐	☐	☐
Left Knee	☐	☐	☐	☐
Right Ankle	☐	☐	☐	☐
Left Ankle	☐	☐	☐	☐

RECOMMENDATIONS

☐ Athlete has been cleared for participation in all sports

☐ Athlete has been cleared for participation in the following sports only, pending further medical evaluation and clearance:

☐ Alpine Skiing	☐ Bocce	☐ Figure Skating	☐ Judo	☐ Snowshoeing	☐ Tennis
☐ Aquatics	☐ Bowling	☐ Floor Hockey	☐ Power Lifting	☐ Softball	☐ Volleyball
☐ Athletics	☐ Cross County Ski	☐ Football (Soccer)	☐ Roller Skating	☐ Speed Skating	
☐ Badminton	☐ Cycling	☐ Golf	☐ Sailing	☐ Table Tennis	
☐ Basketball	☐ Equestrian	☐ Gymnastics	☐ Snowboarding	☐ Team Handball	

☐ Athlete is restricted from participation in all sports pending further medical evaluation and clearance.

SCREENER SIGNATURE AND DATE:

Appendix 13.C Special Olympics Health History, Physical Examination, and Recommendations for Participation—cont'd

Referrals Based on Health History
☐ High-risk medication for Long-QT syndrome. EKG and further medical evaluation is strongly advised.
☐ Possible at-risk medication for Long-QT syndrome. EKG and further medical evaluation is advised.
☐ Possible at-risk medication for osteoporosis. Bone density testing and medical evaluation is advised.
☐ Possible at-risk medication for sun sensitivity. Sun protection and further medical evaluation is advised.
☐ Possible at-risk medication for weight gain, if overweight, further medical evaluation is advised.
☐ Possible at-risk medication for constipation, further medical evaluation is advised.
☐ No medical cause of intellectual disability is noted, further medical evaluation is advised.
☐ Seizure activity within the past 12 months, partial restriction (see below) pending further medical evaluation and clearance.

Referrals Based on Vital Measures
☐ BMI indicates obesity, nutritional counseling is strongly advised.
☐ BMI indicates overweight, nutritional counseling is advised.
☐ BMI indicates underweight, nutritional counseling is advised.
☐ Blood Pressure is greater than 160/100, participation restricted pending further medical evaluation.
☐ Blood Pressure is greater than 140/90, further medical attention is advised.
☐ Blood Pressure is less than 90/50, participation restricted pending further medical evaluation.
☐ Blood Pressure difference between right and left is greater than 20mm/hg, further medical attention is strongly advised.
☐ Pulse is greater than 100 beats per minute, further medical evaluation is advised.
☐ Pulse is less than 60 beats per minute, further medical evaluation is advised.
☐ Pulse is irregular, participation restricted pending further medical evaluation.
☐ Oxygen Saturation is less than 90%, further medical evaluation is advised.
☐ T-score is less than −1, indicating low bone density, further medical evaluation is advised, nutritional counseling is advised.
☐ Oral temperature greater than 37.5°C (99°F), participation restricted pending further medical evaluation.
☐ Screening indicates possible vision deficit, further vision evaluation is advised (or Opening Eyes)
☐ Screening indicates possible hearing deficit, further hearing evaluation is advised (or Healthy Hearing)

Additional Referrals
☐ Dental evaluation is suggested (or Special Smiles)
☐ Podiatric evaluation is suggested (or Fit Feet)
☐ Nutrition/lifestyle evaluation is suggested (or Health Promotion)
☐ Physical Therapy evaluation is suggested (or FUN Fitness)
☐ Medical attention is needed for the following:

Medical Clearance
☐ Athlete has been cleared for participation in all sports.
☐ Athlete has been cleared for participation in the following sports only, pending further medical evaluation and clearance:

☐ Alpine skiing	☐ Bowling	☐ Football (Soccer)	☐ Sailing	☐ Team Handball
☐ Aquatics	☐ Cross Country Ski	☐ Golf	☐ Snowboarding	☐ Tennis
☐ Athletics	☐ Cycling	☐ Gymnastics	☐ Snowshoeing	☐ Volleyball
☐ Badminton	☐ Equestrian	☐ Judo	☐ Softball	
☐ Basketball	☐ Figure Skating	☐ Power Lifting	☐ Speed Skating	
☐ Bocce	☐ Floor Hockey	☐ Roller Skating	☐ Table Tennis	

☐ Athlete is restricted from participation in all sports pending further medical evaluation and clearance.

Additional Notes

(This athlete assessment is taken from the Special Olympics MedFest Manual, pages 46-49 which can be located at http://media.specialolympics.org/soi/files/healthy-athletes/MedFest%20Manual%202010.pdf.)

CHAPTER 14

Pediatric Acute-Care Hospital

—Stacey Caviston, PT, DPT, PCS

—Suzanne F. Migliore PT, DPT, MS, PCS

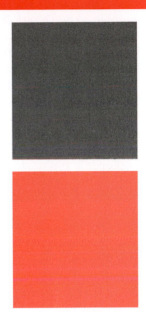

According to the National Association of Children's Hospitals and Related Institutions (NACHRI) (2009), "Children's hospitals are the most specialized and regionalized centers of care for children in the United States. They provide the majority of highly specialized inpatient care for children with complex and rare conditions." The majority of children's hospitals are nonprofit organizations that help train one-third of all pediatricians and over 50% of all pediatric specialists. They are premiere institutions focused on quality patient care and innovative research, and advocate health promotion and injury prevention.

In 2006, there were over 250 children's hospitals across the United States, with 44% of these children's hospitals within larger adult-based institutions. Another 36% are specialty children's hospitals for orthopedic, rehabilitation, or psychiatric diagnoses. Only 20% of the hospitals were considered free-standing. Each year

3 million children require hospitalization for illness or injury, and one-third of these admissions will be at a children's hospital. The leading reasons for admission to children's hospitals include respiratory (16.8%), gastrointestinal (11.9%), neonatal (11.9%), neurological (9.8%), and orthopedic (6.7%) issues. If the children's hospital is also a trauma center, those figures may change to reflect diagnoses such as multitrauma and burns.

Within the pediatric acute-care hospital, there are many specialized areas of practice for the physical therapist, including the neonatal intensive care unit, pediatric intensive care unit, cardiac intensive care unit, and medical and surgical units with subspecialties such as pulmonary, oncology, orthopedics, and general pediatrics. The physical therapist plays a vital role on the interdisciplinary health-care team within the acute-care setting. This fast-paced environment will challenge the physical therapist to stay current with age-specific competencies and diagnostic processes, as well as being psychologically prepared to work with children and their families, often following a devastating diagnosis, illness, or injury. This chapter will take a look at the complex role of the acute-care physical therapist.

Interdisciplinary Team

The **interdisciplinary team** in the acute-care setting consists of a large group of individuals, each with their own area of specialty, working together to best serve the child's and family's needs. The primary physician team guiding a child's care in the hospital setting can be as small as just the attending physician or can include a nurse practitioner and/or a physician's assistant. In a teaching hospital, the team also includes a fellow and/or a resident who are training under the attending physician. Other physician specialists may also be consulted to work on the interdisciplinary team based on the child's diagnosis. For example, a child admitted to the hospital for a femur fracture is usually under the orthopedic physician service and does not typically require the consultation of other physician specialists. However, a child admitted after a car accident who has a femur fracture in addition to a head injury would require the orthopedic team, but also possibly the critical care, neurosurgical, and even neurology teams. The child's primary medical team in the acute setting is determined by the child's greatest medical need. Other teams then act in the consultative role.

A child's nursing team consists of the bedside nurse, who is intimately involved in the child's daily care, as well as a certified nursing assistant who works with the nurse. A nurse specialist can also be brought in to assist the primary nursing team. An example of this need is a child who has decreased skin integrity. A nurse with advanced training in treating wounds or burns may be consulted to assist with care.

Social workers, the hospital or family's community chaplain, and staff of the child life department work closely with nursing to address a child's psychosocial needs. The child life department in a pediatric hospital consists of child life specialists and assistants, art therapists, and/or music therapists. These services work with children and families to normalize the hospital environment and allow children an outlet for their emotions during a hospital admission. Education is also a part of the child life department. Teachers work bedside or in small groups with children admitted to the hospital for extended periods of time to address their school needs. The goal of most children and families is to keep up with their education so that when they are healthy enough to be discharged to home they can return to school in their grade level with their peers.

When a language barrier prevents appropriate communication, interpreters or the language line can be used. Some hospitals staff interpreters for languages that are frequently encountered in their surrounding community, where others use consultants for all their interpreter needs. The language line can be used to communicate with families when an interpreter is not available. This system consists of a phone with a dual headset. The medical professional holds one receiver and speaks. The interpreter on the call then relays the information to the child or family member who is holding the other receiver.

Physical therapists, occupational therapists, and speech and language pathologists are individually consulted in the acute-care setting of a hospital. These professions work closely together to address a child's needs. In pediatrics the needs tend to overlap more than those of an adult, however, each service works within their scope of practice to meet the needs of the children and their families.

Dietitians and nutritionists are also important members of the interdisciplinary team. These professionals work closely with the medical team to meet the nutrition needs of the pediatric population. They are involved with children who are able to eat by mouth to ensure healthy choices are available to all, especially those who have been prescribed specific diets, such as those with diabetes. The nutrition department also works closely with the medical team to make recommendations for children who are not able to eat by mouth. These populations include those on formulas being fed by tube or those children who require total parenteral nutrition (TPN).

The child's discharge planning needs are coordinated by a representative from case management, who seeks input from the entire interdisciplinary team. This individual coordinates with caregivers and insurance companies to ensure the timely acquisition of the needed services, medications, and equipment to make discharge as smooth and successful as possible.

Laboratory Values

A physical therapist working in the acute environment must be able to access and interpret a child's laboratory values to make appropriate clinical decisions. While specific guidelines for laboratory values can be setting or facility specific, physical therapists must be aware of both the ranges of normal for their specific patient population as well as the implications for making decisions surrounding whether to treat and/or whether treatment plans should be adjusted based on laboratory values. Examples of laboratory values that directly impact physical therapy care in the acute environment are hemoglobin and platelet levels. Hemoglobin norms vary by age and gender. The norm for a child is 11–13 g/100 mm, whereas the norms for adult males are 13–18 g/100 mm and for adult females 12–16 g/100 mm. In the pediatric acute-care setting, for children whose baseline falls within the normal ranges, intervention is typically deferred when their hemoglobin level falls below 8 g/100 mm. For those children whose baseline ranges are typically already below 8 g/100 mm, clinical discussions should occur among the medical team on whether interventions are indicated. While this laboratory value is a guideline, patient symptoms should be closely monitored. Please refer to Table 22.2 for exercise guidelines and activity level in accordance with platelet count.

Diagnostic Imaging

Multiple modes of diagnostic imaging are utilized in the acute setting to both diagnose and guide medical care. A physical therapist in the acute setting should be aware of the different types of imaging techniques and their general purpose, and should be able to adapt their treatment interventions in a timely manner based on results of diagnostic imaging.

X-ray

Plain film x-rays are used quite frequently in the acute setting. This mode of imaging is fast and relatively inexpensive. It is most commonly used to detect fractures of bones but is also used frequently in the intensive care unit (ICU) to ensure proper placement of endotracheal tubes and to diagnose or monitor lung function. While an x-ray is typically a poor indicator of soft tissue integrity, the presence of effusion or calcification within soft tissue can been seen on an x-ray.

Computerized Tomography

Computed tomography (CT) is a noninvasive x-ray technique. A CT reading consists of multiple images taken at predetermined intervals of the body structure selected for examination. The CT scanner then accumulates the images taken to re-create the structure into a two- or three-dimensional image. CT imaging is used to diagnose bone and soft tissue disorders, tumors, abdominal trauma, and head trauma. A CT scan can be completed relatively quickly, in about 15 minutes; however, the child must lie still for accurate images to be obtained, which can be a problem with infants and children. When a good scan is obtained, CT imaging can be up to 100 times more sensitive than a plain film x-ray. CT imaging is completed with or without contrast, depending on the structure being examined (Erkonen, 1998).

Magnetic Resonance Imaging

Magnetic resonance imaging (MRI) uses external magnetic fields and radiofrequency waves to evaluate soft tissues of the spine, extremities, joints, central nervous system, and other body viscera. While MRI is not a good tool for evaluating for fracture of bones, it has become the method of choice for examining joint pathologies (Erkonen, 1998). MRI takes longer to complete than CT scans, approximately an hour, and children must lie still for adequate images to be obtained. For this reason, a large number of children must be sedated for an MRI to be completed.

Diagnostic Ultrasound

Diagnostic ultrasound (US) is a noninvasive procedure that uses sound waves to obtain images of body structures. US is used in the acute setting to detect the location of tumors and cysts within areas such as the abdomen, breasts, and thyroid, to evaluate cardiac function (echocardiogram), and to examine blood vessels for possible clots. It is also used in the neonatal ICU to determine intraventricular bleeding. It is not a good tool for examining bones or the lungs. US imaging can be completed quickly and is relatively inexpensive compared to CT and MRI.

Lines, Tubes, and Drains

A physical therapist practicing in the acute environment should have knowledge of the purpose and clinical considerations surrounding the many types of lines and tubes that are utilized in the acute-care setting. The following lines and tubes are used with children for purposes such as monitoring a child's hemodynamic status, draining fluids after a medical procedure, and/or administering medications.

Lines

Peripheral IV

A **peripheral IV (PIV)** (Fig. 14.1) is inserted through the skin of an extremity into a peripheral vein. It is typically less than 3 inches in length. It is used to administer fluids or medication when the anticipated need is less than 6 days. A PIV is not typically used for blood

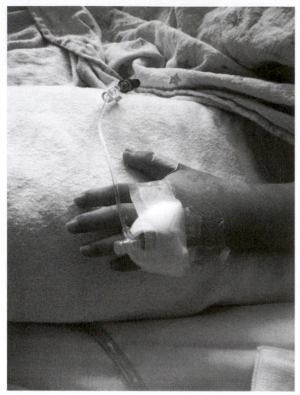

Figure 14.1 A child with a peripheral IV (intravenous) catheter in the left hand.

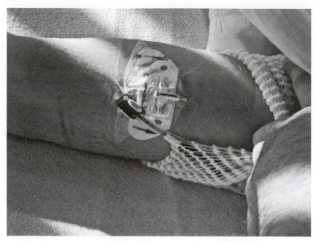

Figure 14.2 An adolescent with a peripherally inserted central venous catheter (PICC line) in the right upper extremity.

draws, but blood can be drawn at the initial insertion of the line. While a therapist should be aware of the location of a PIV and cautious to not displace it, there aren't any contraindications for movement of an extremity with a PIV.

Peripherally Inserted Central Venous Catheters

A **peripherally inserted central venous catheter (PICC)** line (Fig. 14.2) is a line inserted into a peripheral vein and then threaded to a larger vessel such as the vena cava (Marino, 1998). A PICC line is typically placed in an upper extremity, but can be inserted in a lower extremity. This type of line is utilized for children who require administration of IV medication for longer than a week, such as long-term antibiotic treatment or for children with a history of poor peripheral venous access (Children's Hospital of Philadelphia [CHOP], 2009a).

Arterial Line

An arterial line or arterial catheter (Fig. 14.3) is inserted into a child's artery, most commonly in the upper extremity, as a means to continually monitor blood

pressure and pulse. Since blood pressure readings from the arterial line are dependent upon position, it is imperative that a physical therapist take note of the position of the extremity housing an arterial line. Any movement of this extremity such as range of motion (ROM) or position changes will affect the blood pressure reading on the bedside monitor. Joints surrounding arterial line placement in children are frequently

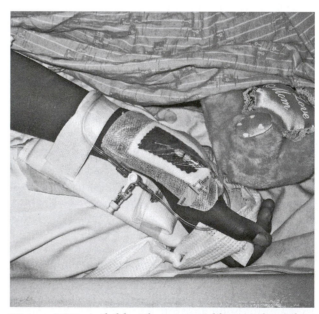

Figure 14.3 A child with an arterial line in the right upper extremity. The white padded board secured to the child's wrist immobilizes the joint to protect the line.

stabilized using an IV board to maintain accurate reading and interpretation of results as well as the integrity of the line. An arterial line is also used for blood draws to assess a blood gas levels. Since arteries carry oxygen rich blood from the heart and lungs throughout the body, a measure of the body's levels of oxygen and carbon dioxide from an arterial line can provide information on the functioning of a person's heart and lungs.

Nontunneled Central Venous Catheter

A nontunneled **central venous catheter (CVC)** (Figure 14.4) is a temporary catheter, utilized when the anticipated need is less than one month. It is inserted percutaneously into a central vein. The uses of this type of line include medication administration, monitoring of vital signs, and temporarily for dialysis or apheresis procedures. Examples of nontunneled CVCs are femoral lines, subclavian lines, internal jugular lines, or umbilical lines. The most common site in children for this type of line is femoral due to ease of location. Precautions for treating children with nontunneled CVCs include avoiding extreme motions, which could disturb the integrity of the line, for example, hip flexion greater than 90° in children with a femoral line (Children's Hospital of Philadelphia, 2009b).

Tunneled, Cuffed Central Venous Catheter

A tunneled central venous catheter (Fig. 14.5) is indicated for children with long-term medication administration, parenteral therapy needs, and/or frequent blood draws. Tunneled CVCs can be used for months or even years. This type of line is inserted into the superior

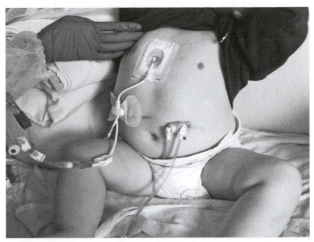

Figure 14.5 A toddler with a broviac line and stat lock on the chest as well as a gastric tube in the abdomen.

or inferior vena cava by way of a larger peripheral vessel. An example of a tunneled CVC is a broviac line. A **broviac** line is used frequently in children who require long-term chemotherapy and/or parenteral means of nutrition. While a tunneled CVC does have a cuff to assist with both decreasing infection risk and keeping the line in place, children often also have a stat lock externally to secure the line.

Implanted Central Venous Catheter or Port

A **port** is very similar to a tunneled, cuffed CVC in its purpose and internal location, but it is different in external appearance. Children with a tunneled CVC have external infusion lines, whereas a port is completely internal. The port itself is composed of a metal or plastic reservoirlike device with a thin diaphragm top. It is surgically placed within subcutaneous tissue and the line is threaded into a central vein. A port is indicated for children with long-term, intermittent need for chemotherapy, long-term antibiotics, and/or blood draws. A port is accessed with a needle that is inserted through the skin above the port site. While the risk of infection and precautions for life activities are lower with a port than with a tunneled CVC, a child does have to undergo a needle stick for each use. For this reason, ports are used less commonly with children.

Feeding Tubes

Nasogastric Tube

A **nasogastric (NG) tube** (Fig. 14.6) is a small tube that is inserted through a child's nose, down the esophagus, and into the stomach. The tube is externally secured to

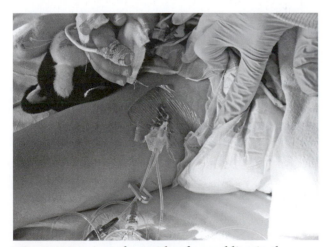

Figure 14.4 An infant with a femoral line in the right leg.

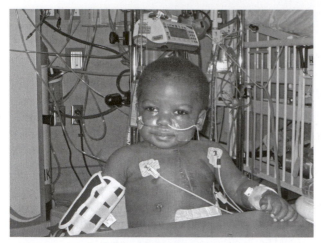

Figure 14.6 A child with both a nasogastric tube (tube in left nare) and a nasal cannula (clear tubing in center of upper lip area). This child also has a peripheral IV in his left wrist and a scar on his chest from previous open-heart surgery.

the child's face with adhesive. This type of tube is used to administer medications or nutrition to a child who is unable to ingest these products by mouth. An NG tube can also be used to remove stomach acids. It is temporary and can easily be dislodged or pulled out.

Orogastric Tube

An **orogastric (OG)** tube runs from a child's mouth down into the stomach. Its means of insertion, purpose, and ability to be removed easily are the same as those of the NG tube.

Gastric Tube

A **gastric tube (G-tube)** (Fig. 14.5) is a tube inserted through a surgical opening from the abdomen into the stomach. It is also used to deliver medications and nutrition into a child's stomach when the child is unable to ingest these products by mouth. A G-tube is a more long-term solution and therefore is placed only when a child will have a long-term need for nutrition or medication administration. A G-tube can, however, be removed and the site of insertion closed if a child no longer requires this means of administration.

Jejunal Tube

A **jejunal tube (J-tube)** is also inserted through a surgical opening from the abdomen and is placed into a child's jejunum. A J-tube is necessary when a child is both unable to ingest nutrition and/or medication by mouth and is unable to initiate and tolerate digestion

in the stomach. A J-tube can be removed if it is no longer medically necessary.

Gastric-Jejunal Tube

A **gastric-jejunal tube (G-J tube)** is, as the name implies, a combination of the types of tubes previously discussed. With this type of tube system the J-tube is housed within the G-tube as it passes from the abdomen, through the stomach. The J-tube portion of this system then is pushed through the stomach and into the jejunal portion of the small intestine. A G-J tube is used when a child can tolerate some medications or nutrition in the stomach, but also needs a portion to be administered into the jejunum.

Respiratory Tubes

Nasal Cannula

A **nasal cannula** (Fig. 14.6) is a thin flexible tube running from an oxygen source to a child's nostrils. Nasal cannulas are used to administer oxygen to support oxygenation.

Noninvasive Ventilatory Support

Continuous positive airway pressure (CPAP) (Fig. 14.7) is a noninvasive means of assisting ventilation. CPAP is administered via an interface, typically a mask, which creates a seal around the child's mouth and nose. A bedside CPAP machine delivers continuous positive pressure through tubes connecting to the mask. This pressure, which is individually prescribed by a physician, works to keep the child's airways open and thus allow for improved ventilation. CPAP was developed

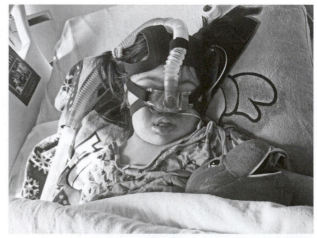

Figure 14.7 A child on continuous positive airway pressure (CPAP) via mask interface. The slender tube on the left side of her face is a nasogastric tube.

initially to treat sleep apnea but is also utilized in the acute-care setting to assist ventilation in the hopes of preventing the need for intubation as well as supporting a child in the short term after extubation.

Biphasic or **bilevel positive airway pressure (BiPAP)**, like CPAP, is delivered via mask, tubes, and a respiratory machine bedside. The difference between BiPAP and CPAP is that with BiPAP there are two levels of pressure provided: inspiratory positive airway pressure and expiratory positive airway pressure. The expiratory pressure in this mode is slightly lower than the inspiratory pressure to allow for easier exhalation. When working with children who are on CPAP or BiPAP during a treatment session, care must be taken to ensure that the interface or mask remains in place. Disrupting the seal that is created between the interface and the child's face will immediately result in a decrease in the airway pressure a child is receiving and could quickly impact ventilation. For this reason, children on CPAP and BiPAP are typically on continuous heart rate and pulse oximeter monitoring.

Endotracheal Tubes

An **endotracheal (ET) tube** (Fig. 14.8) can be inserted through a child's mouth or nose and extends down the airway. It maintains an open airway and is used in conjunction with a ventilator to assist with mechanical ventilation. Oral intubation is the most common means for this process in children with lower levels of arousal (Marino, 1998). However, one concern with this type of intubation is the possibility that a child can bite down and occlude the tube and prevent air from passing through the tubing into the lungs. A bite block can be

used to prevent this type of tube clamping. Therapists working in the intensive care environment should monitor this behavior and response, as biting the endotracheal tube can be a sign of stress in a noncommunicative child.

If a child consistently bites down on the tube, the medical team may determine it necessary to switch to nasal intubation. When a child is intubated nasally (Fig. 14.9), the ET tube passes through one nostril and down into the child's airway. The tube is secured to the child and connected to the ventilator in the same way as with oral intubation, but the child's mouth is free to move. This allows those who are more alert to mouth words as a means of communication with both family and healthcare providers.

Tracheostomy

A **tracheostomy** is a surgical procedure in which a tube is inserted through the skin in a child's anterior neck and directly into the trachea. The tube is first sutured in place, and then held in place with tracheal ties to maintain its placement. While all adult tracheostomy tubes have cuffs surrounding the tube within the airway securing it in place, children do not always need this cuff due to the size of the trachea and tracheal tubes used with children. This tracheal tube is then hooked via flexible tubing to a ventilator, which, depending on the acuity of the child, either completes or supports ventilation. This means of ventilation surpasses the child's entire upper airway, including the mouth and nose.

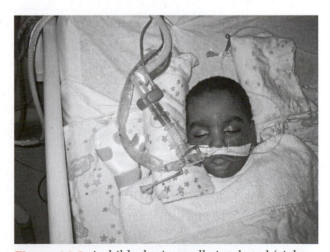

Figure 14.9 A child who is nasally intubated (right nare) and has a nasogastric tube in the left nostril. The blanket roll on the right side of the child's head is both promoting neutral alignment of the neck as well as supporting the ventilator tubing.

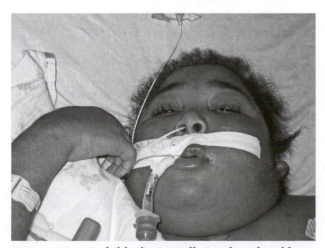

Figure 14.8 A child who is orally intubated and has a nasogastric tube in the right nare.

A tracheostomy (Fig. 14.10) is performed when a child requires prolonged mechanical ventilation. The benefits of tracheostomy over endotracheal intubation are increased comfort, improved effectiveness of clearing secretions, and increased stability of the airway. This increased comfort and airway stability allow the child increased freedom of movement and therefore decreased secondary complications that occur with prolonged bedrest (Marino, 1998). These complications include, but are not limited to, deep vein thrombosis, decreased strength, decreased endurance, and decreased independence with functional mobility and activities of daily living.

Chest Tubes

Chest tubes (Fig. 14.11) are surgically inserted through a child's chest wall and into the space between the ribs and lungs. In this location, chest tubes allow either air or fluid (i.e., **pneumothorax** or **hemothorax**) to drain from this space, thus decreasing pressure on the lungs and allowing the lungs to more fully inflate. Depending on the child's diagnosis, there could be one or multiple chest tubes. Chest tubes either drain into a sealed collection container bedside or can be hooked to wall suction from this container to assist with fluid drainage. Clinical considerations when working with a child with a chest tube include monitoring complaints of and/or symptoms of pain at the insertion site, maintaining integrity of the seal around the insertion site, and assisting with maintaining accurate measurement of drainage from the tube. It is imperative to maintain accurate measurements

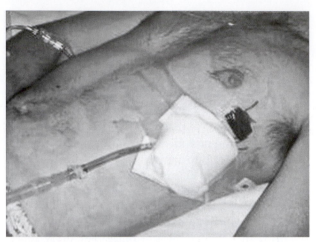

Figure 14.11 An adolescent in supine with a chest tube on the left side of his chest. The thick dressing over the insertion site both helps to secure the tube in place and creates a seal over the area.

of rates and amount of drainage from a chest tube as these values are integral pieces of information the surgical team uses to determine when to remove a chest tube.

Drains

Jackson Pratt Drain

A Jackson-Pratt (JP) drain (Fig. 14.12) is used postsurgically to allow fluid to drain from the body. It consists of tubing running from the body near the operative site, through a surgical incision site, to a bulb that has been compressed prior to being attached to the tubing. This compression initiates a small amount of suction to assist with drainage of fluid from the area.

Ventriculostomy

A **ventriculostomy** or external ventricular drain (EVD) is an acute means of draining excessive cerebrospinal fluid from a child's ventricular system. In children, excessive cerebrospinal fluid is especially dangerous due to the anatomical boundaries of the skull. Because the skull encloses the brain in a bony covering, there is little margin for excessive fluid or swelling. As fluid builds either within or surrounding the brain within the skull, pressure is applied to the brain itself and can quickly cause damage to critical areas of the brain. Examples of acute needs for a ventriculostomy include increased intracranial pressure as a result of a traumatic head injury or after a tumor resection or shunt malfunction.

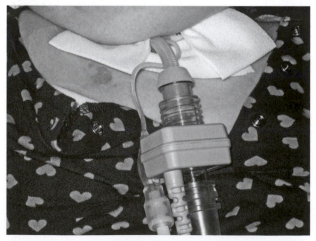

Figure 14.10 This photo shows a tracheostomy. The white padding is used to protect the child's skin where the tracheostomy ties are secured.

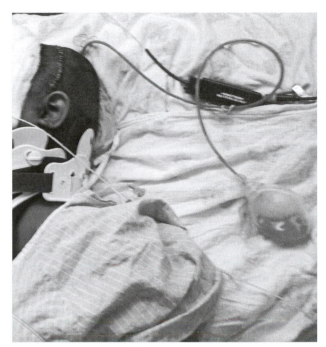

Figure 14.12 An adolescent status post neurosurgery for evacuation of head bleed with a Jackson-Pratt (JP) drain from the head. A cervical collar is in place while c-spine evaluation is pending and a nasogastric tube is in her nose.

The ventriculostomy setup consists of a tube inserted by a neurosurgeon running from a ventricle (Fig. 14.13A) to an external collection device. The external collection device is hung at a specific height (Fig. 14.13B) in relation to the child's head to allow gravity to facilitate the desired output. For example, a collection device hung below the level of a child's head would allow gravity to assist with drainage of fluid from the head to the device, whereas a collection device hung above the head would require increased pressure within the ventricular system to overcome gravity and allow fluid to drain out of the brain into the collection device. Implications for physical therapists working with children who have ventriculostomies include close monitoring of the child's position in relation to the collection device as well as signs and symptoms of increased and decreased intracranial pressure.

As indicated previously, ventriculostomies are used acutely to treat children with a new need for assistance managing flow of cerebrospinal fluid. If a chronic need is diagnosed, a child is often evaluated by a neurosurgeon for a shunt, most commonly a ventriculoperitoneal (VP) shunt.

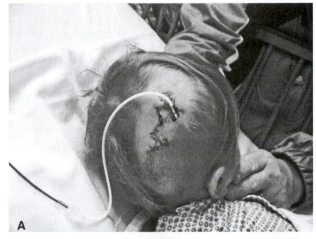

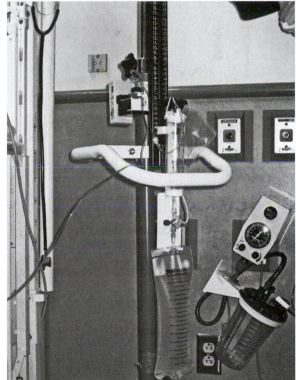

Figure 14.13 (*A*) A ventriculostomy tube in a toddler's head. Notice the dark colored sutures securing the tube in place, as well as the healing incision from previous neurosurgery. (*B*) A ventriculostomy apparatus at bedside. The box attached to the IV pole is a laser level used for accurately aligning the apparatus with the patient. The upright graduated cylinder and bag are used to collect and monitor cerebrospinal fluid output.

Dialysis

Dialysis is a means of supporting a child in acute or chronic renal failure by assisting with the clearance of electrolytes, metabolites, and toxins. Dialysis in children is as successful as in adults; however, it is usually temporary in children. Children who receive long-term dialysis fit into two categories: those recovering from acute renal failure who are anticipated to recover and those who are awaiting kidney transplant. There are two means of delivering dialysis: **hemodialysis** or peritoneal dialysis. Hemodialysis is performed via access to the circulatory system, either via external cannulas or internal arteriovenous fistulas. In this procedure, the blood is filtered by a medical device external to the body and then warmed and returned to the body via the cannulas or fistula. When necessary, hemodialysis is completed three times per week and lasts approximately 4 hours each visit. This procedure is more efficient and precise than peritoneal dialysis but requires more specialized care, including anticoagulant therapy (MedlinePlus, 2009).

Peritoneal dialysis must be completed between one and four times a day. It is performed by administering dialysis fluid through a catheter in the child's abdomen. Peritoneal dialysis utilizes the peritoneal cavity as a membrane for exchange of waste products between the administered dialysis fluid and the child's underlying blood vessels. This fluid is exchanged every 4 to 6 hours through the indwelling abdominal catheter. While it is less efficient than hemodialysis, peritoneal dialysis is the treatment of choice for children with poor cardiovascular function, vascular access, or tolerance to anticoagulation. In addition, peritoneal dialysis can be completed in the home setting versus hemodialysis, which must be completed in a medical setting (MedlinePlus, 2009).

Extracorporeal Membrane Oxygenation

Extracorporeal membrane oxygenation (ECMO) is a cardiopulmonary bypass technique utilized for treating infants and children who have reversible cardiac and/or respiratory conditions. This technique provides long-term pulmonary and/or cardiac support for those whose lungs and/or hearts are so severely damaged or diseased that they are unable to function on their own to support life. There are two common types of ECMO, venovenous (VV) ECMO and venoarterial (VA) ECMO. In both types, blood is drained from the venous system through a large cannula, oxygenated via the ECMO circuit, and returned to the body. In VV ECMO, blood is returned to the child's venous system and no cardiac support is provided to the child. In VA ECMO, blood is returned to the arterial system bypassing the child's heart (Emedicine, 2006). While ECMO has been proven effective in saving lives, it is often used as a last-resort modality because of the risks that go along with its use. These risks include but are not limited to severe infection, blood clotting resulting in emboli or deep vein thrombosis, or severe bleeding due to the anticoagulant requirement to maintain the circuit (Ravishankar et al., 2006).

Pain Management

Working with children in the acute-care environment can be challenging, especially when the child is experiencing pain. Whether from injury or illness, or pain experienced from procedures, managing a child's pain can be difficult. As physical therapists, we must recognize and evaluate a child's response to our interventions and work with the interdisciplinary team to ensure proper pain management during our sessions.

Pain Scales

The **Joint Commission (JC)**, formerly the Joint Commission for Accreditation of Hospital Organization (JCAHO), has established guidelines to measure pain in acute-care hospitals. Their current standard is that pain is assessed and documented on every individual, on every encounter. Physical therapists are also accountable to this standard, and must select an appropriate pain scale and perform a thorough evaluation of a child's pain including where the pain is, the intensity, the duration of the pain, and any aggravating or alleviating factors. For children, there are several reliable and valid pain scales to quantify and track a child's pain, as discussed in Chapter 3. Reliable and valid pain scales appropriate for neonates include the CRIES (cry, requires O_2, increased vital signs, expression, sleeplessness), the CHIPPS (children's and infants' postoperative pain scale), and the NIPS (neonatal infant pain scale) (Suraseranivongse et al., 2006).

For a child who is nonverbal, or not of an age to participate in a self-reporting scale, a behavioral pain scale is needed. Two such scales are the Face, Legs, Activity, Cry and Consolability (FLACC) behavioral pain scale (Merkel et al., 1997; and Nilsson et al., 2008) and the Children's Hospital of Eastern Ontario Pain Scale (CHEOPS) (McGrath et al., 1985), both for children up to 7 years of age. For children who are cognitively intact and able to participate in reporting their pain, there are also several scales to choose from. The Wong-Baker Faces scale (Wong & Baker, 1988) asks children, ages 3 to 7 years, to pick from 5 different faces according to their pain level.

Pharmacological Interventions
Patient-Controlled Analgesia

There are many modes of administering pharmacological agents to help in controlling pain in children. While this chapter will not explore specific mediations, modes of delivery are important to recognize when working with a child in the acute setting. One such mode is **patient-controlled analgesia (PCA)**. PCA is used to treat pain related to surgery, burns, sickle cell disease, and mucositis. Because PCA allows the children themselves to titrate the amount needed to achieve a comfortable level, it decreases the risk of peaks and troughs with traditionally given opioids by a nurse on an as-needed basis. The ability to self-manage pain makes the PCA an appropriate method for addressing fluctuating pain situations. Schiessl and colleagues studied the use of PCA for pain control in dying children and found that PCA proved to be an ideal, dependable, and feasible mode of analgesia administration (Schiessl, Gravou, Zernikow, Sittl, & Griessinger, 2008).

Children who are too young or developmentally delayed are often not able to verbalize pain or advocate for pain medicine due to cognitive, motor, or verbal limitations. They may often be undermedicated and in distress during medical interventions. Since they are unable to use PCA, family- or nurse-controlled PCA may be another option to IV or intramuscular injections. Czarnecki and colleagues (2008) studied the effectiveness of parent- or nurse-controlled analgesia in children with developmental delay. Their data supported parent- or nurse-controlled analgesia in this population based on the participants' pain scores, mean opioid requirements, and frequency of side effects. The authors do note the safety concerns regarding this practice, with the potential of unauthorized persons activating the PCA. Each institution should have very specific policies and procedures and parent/caregiver education in place prior to implementing this mode of analgesia. They believe that with proper education, medication management, and monitoring parent- or nurse-controlled analgesia is an effective modality.

Peripheral Nerve Blockade

Children undergoing surgery or procedures in a day surgery program may be discharged to home the same day. Pain management with a PCA or epidural catheter would be impossible in the home setting. A newer mode for pain control is **continuous peripheral nerve blockade (CPNB)**. The CPNB is a reliable alternative for providing adequate pain control with fewer side effects, which has more recently been used in adult surgical cases. Ludot and colleagues (2008) studied the feasibility of using CPNB in children postoperatively at home. The main finding from this observational study was that CPNB with an infusion pump was effective and feasible and allowed for an ambulatory (one-day) stay or shortened hospitalization in children. The authors did conclude that child and family selection and compliance was a key factor to success, as families were responsible for looking for signs and symptoms of infection or malfunction of the device and bringing the child back to the hospital for catheter removal.

Precautions/Contraindications for Physical Therapy

In the acute-care hospital, there are numerous precautions and contraindications for physical therapy. Some specific precautions surround orthopedic or neurosurgical procedures and are written as orders from the physicians. Some may be procedural precautions such as bedrest following a lumbar puncture or cardiac catheterization. On the oncology unit, blood count levels may dictate what types of interventions are warranted (see Chapter 22). One event that usually sparks debate on whether therapy is indicated is following a **deep vein thrombosis (DVT)**.

Deep Vein Thrombosis

Venous thromboembolism is a result of venous stasis, vein injury, and increased coagulation (Virchow's triad). Stasis occurs when children are immobile and blood pools in the extremities, usually the legs. Children who are hospitalized are at risk for DVT due to immobility, medical illness, and devices such as central venous catheters. Signs and symptoms of a DVT include pain, swelling, and increased temperature of a limb. Children who develop DVT may then also be at risk for the serious complication of pulmonary embolism and even death (Kehl-Pruett, 2006).

In children, vein injury is most common when a central venous catheter is placed. The disruption of blood flow and subsequent DVT are associated with significant morbidity (>90% of DVTs in neonates and 60% of DVTs in children are associated with central lines) (Andrew, Monagle, & Brooker, 2000). Vu and colleagues (2008) published a cross-sectional study looking at the prevalence of DVT in pediatric inpatients. They found the prevalence of lower-extremity DVT in hospitalized children had increased significantly since

1997. They also found that comorbidities such as irritable bowel syndrome, surgical procedures, and obesity increased the risk of DVT. Their results showed that children with DVT had a twofold increase in risk for death compared to those without DVT (Vu, Nobuhara, Lee, & Farmer, 2008).

Prevention

Mechanical prophylactic measures for preventing DVT include exercises, ROM, graded compression stockings, and pneumatic compression devices. Each of these can improve venous return and reduce venous stasis in leg veins. These interventions may be initiated by nurses or physical therapists, especially in an intensive care unit setting. Active ROM exercises, especially at the ankle, are easy for children to participate in. However, if they are not cognitively aware or able, passive ROM may substitute for actively moving the muscle and decreasing venous pooling. Often, parents are instructed in these techniques, as they desire to help with their child's care.

Graded compression stockings may be used in conjunction with active ROM exercises to assist with preventing DVT in those at low risk. Proper fit is important to provide appropriate compression, but garments too tight may cause a tourniquet effect. Off-the-shelf stockings may fit adolescents, but younger children may be more difficult to fit. Other graded compression materials may be considered, including elastic bandage wrapping, or elastic stockinette.

Intermittent pneumatic compression devices can also assist in decreasing venous stasis by creating pressure on leg muscles. This pressure assists in venous blood return and decreasing blood pooling. Again, the size of the devices may make it difficult for use in very small children.

In patients with a great risk of bleeding, mechanical compression devices such as compression stockings or pneumatic compression devices can be a suitable alternative in thromboprophylaxis. These devices are often issued to patients at risk for DVT, or post operatively, and are in place until the patient is up and walking independently (Lippi, Favaloro, & Cervellin, 2011).

Pharmacological Measures

Anticoagulants are used as preventive and post-DVT interventions. These anticoagulants may include aspirin, Coumadin, and low molecular weight heparin (Kehl-Pruett, 2006). Enoxaparin (Lovenox) is a low molecular weight heparin used in children. Children with known DVT are started on Lovenox and monitored via blood counts for coagulation levels. Once at a therapeutic medication level, further intervention can be initiated by a physical therapist.

Implications for Physical Therapy

Physical therapists play a key role in detection of DVT in children. As a therapist may be working closely with a child on a daily basis, providing evaluation and interventions, he or she may be able to recognize the signs and symptoms of DVT and alert the medical staff. During diagnosis, providing therapy to the unaffected limbs should be continued. Ambulation or out-of-bed activities should be suspended until the child is determined to be anticoagulated to decrease the risk of pulmonary embolus. With the use of Lovenox, the time that a patient is on "bedrest" awaiting anti-coagulation levels may be quick, even as quick as the same day of the initial doses. Once medically cleared, it is important to resume mobility as soon as possible, as bedrest has been shown to increase the risk of DVT occurrence or reoccurrence. Early ambulation has not been associated with an increased risk for embolism in anticoagulated patients with acute DVT. Following the acute phase, steps should be taken to prevent postthrombotic syndrome (PTS). PTS begins with the blood flow obstruction of the thrombus and incompetent venous valves that were damaged by the clot or the medical interventions used to break up the clot. Interventions used to reduce the severity of PTS include early ambulation and gradient compression stockings (Blumenstein, 2007).

Regulatory Agencies

In addition to organizational and departmental policies and procedures, the physical therapist working in the acute-care hospital will need to be knowledgeable about regulations from agencies such as the state **Department of Health** and **the Joint Commission**. Each state has its own Department of Health, with its own policies and procedures. The Department of Health has the responsibility for licensing and oversight of hospital organizations in each state. They conduct licensure and safety surveys and handle complaint and incident investigations. Refer to your state government website for your local department of health and hospital regulations.

The Joint Commission

The Joint Commission (JC) is a not-for-profit organization that accredits and certifies health-care organizations in the United States. The JC's mission is "to continuously improve health care for the public, in collaboration with other stakeholders, by evaluating health care organizations and inspiring them to excel in providing safe and effective care of the highest quality and value" (JC, 2011a).

National Patient Safety Goals

Each year, the JC publishes new national patient safety goals (NPSGs), which must be met by any hospital seeking accreditation. The purpose of the NPSGs is to improve overall patient safety. These goals focus on problems that can occur and how to safely and effectively solve them. For 2011–2012, goals include proper identification of patients, improving staff communication, using medications safely, preventing infection, identifying patients at risk for suicide, and preventing surgical mistakes (JC, 2011b).

Infection Prevention and Control

Both the DOH and JC have standards written to assist with the decrease of hospital-acquired infections. Standards regarding hand hygiene and disinfecting and sanitizing equipment have been implemented due to the increased morbidity and mortality associated with infections. The advent of drug-resistant organisms has also increased the importance of protecting the children and health-care workers from these infections. Both agencies have provided guidance for such programs such as universal precautions, influenza immunizations for health-care workers, and guidelines for preventing surgical site and blood stream infections. Therapists working in the acute-care hospital must follow the guidelines put forth by these agencies and their organizations.

Common Infections in the Hospital Setting

Children in the acute-care setting are exposed to and at risk for contracting many different infections. Whether from an injury or illness, these infections can prolong their hospital stay, increase the severity of their illness, or even lead to death. Therapists need to be aware of these commonly seen infections and appropriate steps to take to prevent spreading the organisms to other children.

Methicillin-Resistant Staphylococcus Aureus

According to the Centers for Disease Control and Prevention (CDC) (2009a), **methicillin-resistant *Staphylococcus aureus* (MRSA)** is a dangerous type of bacteria that is resistant to certain antibiotic medications and can cause skin or other infections. MRSA is contracted via direct contact with an infected person or by sharing personal items that have come in contact with an infected person. Signs and symptoms of MRSA skin infections include a bump or infected area that is red, swollen, painful, and warm to the touch, accompanied by a fever. MRSA has become the most frequent cause of skin and soft tissue infections, with outbreaks seen in sports teams and child-care attendees. In the hospital setting, in addition to skin infections, bloodstream infections from MRSA have been seen, leading to greater lengths of stay and higher mortality. In 2007, the *Journal of the American Medical Association* published findings from a study of 9 U.S. communities and the incidence of MRSA. Most of the cases they report were health-care associated, with over 90,000 infections overall in the study, an increase of almost 20% from 3 years prior. Overall their findings concluded that MRSA is a major public health problem that is no longer just limited to acute-care sites (Klevens et al., 2007). Children in the acute hospital setting will be either on isolation or cohorted with others with the same infection. Staff working with them will utilize universal precautions during treatment. Close attention to cleaning, sanitizing, and disinfecting everything they come in contact with is key to preventing spread of the infection, as well as proper hand hygiene by health-care workers.

Vancomycin-Resistant Enterococci

According to the CDC (2009b), enterococci are bacteria that are normally present in the human intestines and in the female genital tract, but they are also found in the environment. These bacteria can sometimes cause infections. Vancomycin is an antibiotic that is commonly used to treat infections caused by enterococci. In some children, enterococci have become resistant to Vancomycin, thus being called **VRE**. The approach from the health-care team is the same as with MRSA to decrease spreading of the infection within the hospital setting.

Clostridium Difficile

***Clostridium difficile* (C-diff.)** is a bacterium that causes diarrhea and more serious intestinal conditions such as colitis. It is common to see this infection in children in the acute-care setting. The CDC reported increased rates and increased severity of C-diff. in 2005. The recent changes to the infection may be due to changes in antibiotic use, a new more virulent strain, or antimicrobial resistance. The new strain is capable of producing greater quantities of toxins A and B and more resistant to traditional antibiotic therapy. C-diff.

is detected by a laboratory study of a stool sample. Once a child is known to have this infection, he or she is put on isolation precautions. Staff working with these children will use universal precautions, good hand hygiene, preferably with soap and water to prevent contamination with spore-forming bacteria, and good cleaning and disinfecting of equipment.

Respiratory Syncytial Virus

Respiratory syncytial virus (RSV) is a viral organism that can cause upper and lower respiratory tract infections. It is most common in children under the age of 1 and causes bronchiolitis and pneumonia. In the United States, RSV is most prevalent during the winter months. For most children, RSV can be managed on an outpatient basis, but approximately 2% of children developing RSV will be admitted to the hospital for management of their symptoms. Children at higher risk for developing RSV are those between 6 weeks and 6 months of age, premature infants, infants and children with breathing or heart problems, and those with weakened immune systems.

RSV is highly contagious and is transmitted via contact with infectious material from another individual or inanimate object. Secretions from the eye, mouth, or nose can contain the virus. The virus may also survive for many hours on inanimate objects such as doorknobs, bedrails, and toys.

Signs and symptoms include lethargy, irritability, poor feeding, apnea, nasal discharge, fever, wheezing, rapid breathing, cough, and nasal flaring. RSV is diagnosed via a culture of the child's nasal discharge in conjunction with a chest x-ray. Treatment is supportive for the symptoms, including keeping the infant or child hydrated, bronchodilators, and supplemental oxygen. Severe cases of RSV in immune-compromised children may result in an ICU stay and mechanical ventilation until respiratory symptoms subside. In the hospital setting, prevention is still the main focus so as not to pass on RSV to anyone else. As with the other infections discussed, these infants/children are on isolation, and staff must follow universal precautions (CHOP, 2009c).

Burkholderia Cepacia Complex and Pseudomonas Aeruginosa

One other infection unique to the pediatric acute-care setting is Burkholderia cepacia complex (Bcc), which is seen in those having **cystic fibrosis (CF)**. Bcc is a known virulent pathogen that can cause an accelerated clinical deterioration of a child with CF. Bcc is spread by passing the infection from person to person. For children with CF and Bcc, they have more problems with their respiratory status and can become very ill, very quickly. Children with CF are also at great risk for developing *Pseudomonas aeruginosa*, with most acquiring their first infection by age 3 years. With over 90% of children with CF dying due to respiratory failure, the majority of cases are from one of these two infections. Infection occurs from coming in close contact with infected children or their personal items, such as a toothbrush or eating utensils. Patient-to-patient transmittal in a nosocomial setting has been documented, thus leading to calls for strict segregation of this population in the hospital setting. Conway (2008) found overwhelming evidence to support such strict segregation and isolation in the CF population to decrease the risk of cross-contamination in the hospital. In one acute-care hospital, children with CF are on isolation, must wear masks when leaving their rooms for testing, receive physical therapy in their room, and are segregated and isolated upon arrival for clinic appointments.

Interventions

Therapists in the acute-care setting will need to be prepared to provide interventions under stressful circumstances, for children of all ages and diagnoses. The interventions listed here are based on impairment and limitations in activity, rather than diagnosis. Many interventions are already discussed in the systems chapters in this book.

Positioning

Children in the hospital or in bed for a prolonged period of time are at risk for many different impairments, which can be addressed by good positioning. These include pressure ulcers, decreased ventilation, loss of flexibility, muscular weakness, and loss of function. Therapists can intervene for children in the acute-care setting by providing adequate supportive positioning depending on the impairment. Utilizing pressure-relieving surfaces such as low air loss mattresses, wheelchair cushions, supportive devices to keep heels off the bed, and bony prominences protected are often the first type of interventions a therapist may provide in an ICU setting. In addition, providing support to promote midline positioning for the head/neck to avoid a secondary **torticollis** may be appropriate for a child who is intubated for an extended period of time. Utilizing towel rolls and positioning devices to keep lower extremities in neutral will prevent the "frog leg" position and loss of flexibility at the hips while in bed. Positioning programs posted at the bedside are also forms of written handoff communication to all caregivers, including the parents, so therapeutic positioning and programs can be followed daily. Teaching parents and caregivers the premises of the positioning program and how to help the child will go a long way toward trying to ensure the appropriate carryover and compliance with therapy programs.

Splinting and Serial Casting

Children demonstrating an injury or loss of functional ROM may be appropriate for splinting or serial casting in the acute-care setting. Splints may be fabricated to protect joints following an injury such as a burn, tendon disruption, or fracture. Children suffering from a traumatic brain injury who may be demonstrating increased tone in their lower legs might be appropriate for serial casting to regain flexibility. The difficulty with serial casting in the acute-care setting is often intravenous access in an emergency situation. For example, a child who has suffered a traumatic injury may have several central and peripheral IV access lines. In an emergency, the foot or lower leg may be used as a peripheral access site. If there are casts on both lower legs, then in an emergency physicians would have less access to veins. Casting in the acute-care setting is an interdisciplinary decision, with the child's acuity and need for peripheral IV access two of the main factors to consider.

Mobility

Depending on the reason for hospitalization, a child may or may not be allowed out of bed. Clearance to mobilize a child is made by the attending physician or designee and is made with respect for the child's level of medical or surgical stability. For instance, a child who was involved in a motor vehicle accident may have a C-spine collar in place until a C-spine injury can be ruled in or out. This may take several days to clear if the child is in critical condition and unable to participate in an examination. Removal of the collar, or **"C-spine clearance,"** must be done by either orthopedics or trauma surgeons in most hospital settings and must be a written order. This will decrease the chance of mobilizing a child prior to ruling out a spinal cord injury.

Once a child is cleared to get out of bed, physical therapy plays an important role in providing the teaching and training to the child, staff, and family members, especially when the child has a new mobility restriction or loss of previous function. Children who are intubated may not be allowed out of bed but may be allowed to sit upright in bed or over the edge of the bed. In this situation, it is helpful to have nursing or respiratory therapy present in the case of any issues with the endotracheal tube. Children who require a tracheostomy due to prolonged ventilation are allowed to move around in bed and get out of bed. Out-of-bed orders are usually written once the first tracheostomy tube change has been done, which is between 5 and 7 days following placement.

In the ICU setting especially, preparing the environment surrounding the bedside is often the most important step for a therapist prior to getting the child out of bed. For a child who has multiple tubes or lines and who may be medically fragile, working with the nursing staff to determine the medical status prior to the start of therapy is imperative. Having the nurse participate in the transfer out of bed will also give the therapist another set of eyes to monitor the child's autonomic status (inclusive of HR/RR/BP), while the therapist focuses on physically helping the child out of bed. Checking that lines and tubes are not tangled and have enough slack to move easily with the child from the edge of the bed to the wheelchair or bedside chair is also an imperative safety step prior to moving a child out of bed. Children who are disoriented or confused should not be left alone in a wheelchair or bedside chair and should have at least a seatbelt and adult supervision. If during the transfer, monitor leads needed to be disconnected, make sure the child is reconnected to the monitor prior to leaving the room.

Child and Family-Centered Care

Within the pediatric acute-care hospital setting, physical therapists must be prepared to treat not only the child, but their family or caregivers as well. Keeping the focus on what is best for the child and family is the meaning of family-centered care. The American Academy of Pediatrics described **family-centered care** as principles including "respecting the child and family, honoring racial, ethnic, cultural and socioeconomic diversity and its effect on the families' perception of care, supporting and facilitating choices for the child and family, ensuring flexibility with facility policies/procedures to be tailored for beliefs and cultural values of each child and family, sharing information, providing support for children and families and collaborating amongst all caregivers and children/families" (American Academy of Pediatrics Committee on Hospital Care, 2003).

The Institute of Family-Centered Care defines patient- and family-centered care as "an approach to the planning, delivery, and evaluation of health care that is grounded in mutually beneficial partnerships among health care providers, patients, and families" (Carmen, Teal, & Guzzetta, 2008). Carmen and colleagues describe four core concepts of patient- and family-centered care. These core concepts include dignity and respect, information sharing, participation, and collaboration. Healthcare professionals working under these concepts are expected to listen to children and their families and respect their perspectives and choices, communicate effectively, allow the children and families to participate in decisions and include families and caregivers in many aspects of the development of hospital policies and procedures. Including children and families on hospital-wide committees and assisting with amenity selection and design of patient rooms are just some ways pediatric hospitals can incorporate the ideas, desires, and opinions of children and families with administrative decisions.

Planning for and providing patient- and family-centered care in an emergency department setting can be quite challenging in the acute-care hospital setting. Factors such as overcrowding and addressing the most acute cases first may not allow health-care professionals the ability to provide patient- and family-centered care. There are many areas in the emergency department where patient- and family-centered care practice could be reflected. Working toward keeping the parent or caregiver and child together during triage and registration; allowing the family to choose to stay present for a potentially painful or uncomfortable procedure; establishing interpreter services (not other family members) to allow for effective communication and to decrease misunderstood medical terminology; identifying the child's needs for comfort measures, both pharmacological and nonpharmacological, and physical space needs; and allowing for children and their families to participate in the establishment of policies and procedures for the emergency department are all examples of patient- and family-centered care (O'Malley, Brown, & Krug, 2008).

Another challenging area to practice the vision of patient- and family-centered care is in the postanesthesia care unit (PACU). Hospitals should focus on the entire continuum of elective or emergent operative procedures. For elective procedures, allowing children and families to have all questions answered and time to prepare for the process with child life therapists is essential. During the procedure, keeping the parents informed of the status of the procedure, how the procedure is going, and when to expect their child to be in the PACU affords parents some peace of mind during a potentially

stressful period of separation from their child. Once the child's surgery or procedure is finished and they have been brought to the PACU, opinions differ as to whether to let families into the PACU early on in the postanesthesia phase.

Potential benefits for allowing families to visit their children in the PACU include providing reassurance for the child, assisting with the child becoming oriented upon awakening, decreasing the need for physical and pharmacological restraints, decreasing analgesic requirements, increasing child and parent satisfaction, and decreasing recovery time. Barriers and or myths to allowing parents to visit the PACU are safety concerns, staff resistance to change in practice, privacy concerns, parent as a potential patient, and delays in PACU discharges. One hospital has adopted patient- and family-centered care in this environment from preprocedure education and support, to intraoperative communication updates from a family services nurse coordinator who physically goes to each operating room suite for an update, to allowing families into the PACU as soon as their child is medically stable (Kamerling, Lawler, Lynch, & Schwartz, 2008). For physical therapists providing care in the operating room suite or PACU, keeping the principles of patient- and family-centered care in mind while in this intense environment is key to successful child and parent interactions.

Suspected Child Abuse or Neglect

In 2007, the CDC (2009c) reported that state and local child protective services investigated 3.2 million reported cases of child abuse or neglect. Of these cases, 794,000, or 10.6 per 1,000 children, were found to be victims of abuse or neglect. Over 1,700 of these cases resulted in the death of a child. More women than men were found to be the perpetrators (56% to 42%) and girls were slightly more at risk than boys to be victims.

According to each state's practice act, a physical therapist as a health-care provider is often a mandatory reporter of **suspected child abuse and neglect**. The website, Child Welfare Information Gateway, provides information on child welfare laws/statues and mandatory reporting (http://www.childwelfare.gov/systemwide/laws_policies/state/).

The American Academy of Pediatrics published several articles in their 2008 journal, *Pediatrics*, dedicated to child abuse and neglect. Goad reported on the failure of health-care providers to report situations. He reported the provider's previous experience with child protective services, poor communication, and fear that reporting would cause families to withdraw from medical care were among the reasons. Goad proposed several steps to improve the collaboration of health-care professionals evaluating and investigating suspected abuse: expanded training on the roles of other professionals involved, requiring medical consultation, reducing the child protective services workload to allow sufficient time for investigation, clarifying confidentiality requirements, and establishing local teams of medical staff, child protective service staff, and law enforcement professionals (Goad, 2008).

A study (Jones et al., 2008) of 434 primary care physicians revealed four major themes of reporting child abuse. They included familiarity with the family, elements of the case history, use of available resources, and perception of the expected outcome (would child protective services actually intervene). Factors that facilitated reporting cases included inconsistent history, lack of explanation for the injury, injury pattern, previous injuries, exclusion of other medical diagnoses, and delay on the caregiver's part for seeking medical attention.

In the acute-care setting, therapists work with help from physicians and social workers to pull together information surrounding an injury or accident when a child is involved and to help determine whether there is a reportable case of neglect or abuse. The same items found in the Jones et al. study are prudent for therapists to remember when working with a suspected child abuse or neglect case. Seeking to gain relevant information from interviewing family members, matching the injury to the developmental age and abilities of the child, ruling out other factors such as a metabolic or genetic issues, and matching the pattern of injury to the history will help therapists and the team decide whether there has been abuse. Once established, law enforcement agencies are called in as well as child protective services to apprehend the perpetrator and establish a safe plan for discharging the child home. Therapists play a role on the acute-care team to recognize the signs and symptoms of abuse or injuries that occurred due to neglect. Working with the interdisciplinary team and providing diagnoses and evaluation findings are important for children with traumatic injuries or burns that have occurred from an intentional act. Therapists should also be involved in prevention programs such as hospital-based neonatal programs that promote mother-infant bonding, parent education programs, and home visits (Gocha, Murphy, Dholakia, Hess, & Effgen, 1999).

Types of Physical Abuse

Children who have been abused may present with a single injury or a pattern of injuries. Common injuries seen that are intentionally inflicted include rib fractures, bruises, retinal hemorrhages, burns consistent with immersion or dunking, spiral fractures, fractures of long bones in nonambulatory children, solid organ trauma from a blow to the abdomen, head trauma, and skull fractures. (Legano, McHugh, & Palusci, 2009). Full body radiographs, head CT, MRI, and ophthalmologic examinations are all crucial in determining the presence and extent of the injuries. Sexual abuse is also common. A comprehensive medical evaluation of the child, inclusive of the genitals, and an understanding of normal anatomy and atypical normal variants must be taken into consideration when examining the child. Findings that might indicate sexual abuse include laceration or bruising of the labia, penis, scrotum, or perineum as well as laboratory findings of sexually transmitted infection.

Types of Neglect

Physical Neglect

Children who have improper access to food may present with inadequate growth or failure to thrive. Families will be screened for medical conditions that might affect growth as well as mental health issues, depression, substance abuse, and overall knowledge of normal growth and development. Inadequate or ill-fitting clothes may also be a sign of neglect. Children who present without basic hygiene might be dirty or foul smelling and have poor dental hygiene, and may be suffering from neglect. Interventions may include education on appropriate hygiene and referrals to community-based agencies for support and resources.

Medical Neglect

Medical neglect often includes parents or caregivers who are noncompliant or nonadherent with a treatment program or recommendations that might result in harm to the child. First, barriers to following a treatment plan must be assessed (e.g., financial, transportation, language) with accommodations put in place to give families every opportunity to comply. Delaying or failing to get medical attention is also a form of neglect. Determining the reason for the delay must be established to prevent further occurrences or harm to the child. A written contract with the family may be necessary to keep the family in compliance with the medical plan of care.

Emotional Neglect

Children who do not receive adequate affection and nurturing from parents or caregivers may be at risk for emotional neglect. Parental mental health issues, substance abuse issues, or poor parental supervision may all play a role. Emotional neglect may also occur in the case of an unwanted pregnancy or if the child has a disability (Legano et al., 2009).

Educational Neglect

Children of school age who are not enrolled in school or miss an excessive amount of school are considered to be having educational neglect. Working with both the family and school to ensure attendance and/or any special support that is required is essential.

Effects of Neglect on Children

Any form of neglect can have a negative bearing on a child's psychological or physical well-being. In younger children, neglect may be associated with cognitive and language delays, poor coping abilities, and less positive social interactions. In school-aged children, neglect is often associated with severe cognitive problems. MRIs done on maltreated children have shown brain changes, such as a smaller area of the corpus callosum and decreased cranial and cerebral volumes (Legano et al., 2009).

Physical therapists must understand and recognize the signs and manifestations of abuse and neglect and work with the interdisciplinary team in the acute-care setting to provide a safe environment at discharge as well as a comprehensive plan of care that can be followed by the caregiver who will have custody of the child at discharge.

Intervention Frequency

While many settings such as schools, rehabilitative hospitals, and outpatient services may have written guidelines for **frequency and intensity of intervention** according to funding sources, there is little evidence to support or guide selecting an intervention frequency in the acute-care hospital. Families, physicians, and therapists may all have differing opinions of how frequently a child may be seen while they are in the hospital. Clinical decision making for therapists should encompass the reason for hospitalization, the acuity of the illness or injury, the loss of previous level of function, and, for those children with chronic medical conditions, the frequency of readmission. Along with these criteria, the child's ability to participate in therapy

as well as documented progress may help when determining initial or change in frequency.

Intervention frequency guidelines for an acute-care pediatric hospital have been developed by Bailes, Reder, and Burch (2008). They developed four frequency modes, taking into consideration factors such as potential to participate, benefit from the therapy process, critical period for skill acquisition or potential regression, level of support present to assist the child in attaining goals, and amount of clinical decision making needed from a therapist. Their modes included an intensive mode, with 3–11 visits per week, which was appropriate for a child who had a condition that was changing rapidly or who required a high frequency to achieve a new skill or recover function lost due to surgery, illness, or trauma. Their next mode was the weekly or bimonthly mode, which included sessions 1–2 times per week to once every other week. Children receiving these frequencies did not have a condition that was changing rapidly—for example, those on their ventilator unit who have complex medical needs and discharge planning is extended. Their periodic frequency mode incorporated monthly visits and was utilized mostly on an outpatient or clinic basis. The therapist in this mode was primarily updating and monitoring a home program. The last role they discuss is a consultative frequency mode. Consultative services might be required if a child improves or regresses, or if there is a change in development or technology. For example, a child receiving community-based therapy services may need a consultation for a piece of durable medical equipment in the hospital setting following surgery. Overall, the authors believed that their guidelines had been well received and that complaints from physicians and parents regarding decreasing services were less when they were included in the discussion of the guideline (Bailes et al., 2008).

At one large, urban, level I trauma center and children's hospital, therapists are also met with the debate over treatment frequency. Therapists too have a **level of service model**, with an algorithm to assist therapists in making the judgment of how frequently to see a child in the acute care setting.

Those children whose discharge is pending are seen daily by a physical therapist, or in the case of training may need to be seen twice daily on the day before or of discharge to ensure a safe discharge home with appropriate caregiver training. Those children who have sustained an illness or injury or are postoperative and have suffered loss of functional abilities are seen daily. A majority of children following neurosurgery (e.g., brain tumor resection), multitrauma, burns, or traumatic brain injury are seen daily in preparation for transitioning to the rehabilitation unit, where their frequency changes to two times per day. Children in the acute-care setting who are not pending transition to a rehabilitation setting and are making progress with therapy and toward their goals are seen five times per week. Those children not making daily progress in their therapy goals, and whose families are able to assist them with their programs, are seen 1–3 times per week. Those children admitted for medical (non–physical therapy related) reasons who receive therapy services in the community may not receive therapy services while in the hospital due to their inability to participate, or anticipated short length of stay. Children who are receiving therapy services in the community, and may be admitted for an extensive length of time for a medical procedure, may be followed 1–2 times per week in accordance to their community-based service frequency. Children admitted to the hospital whose family or caregiver may have specific questions or concerns regarding therapy, orthotics, or durable medical equipment may receive a consultation from a therapist, but if they do not meet the above criteria for services, they may be seen only for the consultation and referred to an appropriate specialty clinic.

The most difficult part in addressing frequencies with parents and physicians is their expectations for the amount of services their child should get. Parents may assume that since they are in the hospital, their child with a chronic medical condition and developmental delay will get services daily, when in reality they may fall in the 1–2 times per week category unless they have suffered a loss of skills. The other difficult discussion is with the family of a child who has suffered a traumatic injury. You may see a child daily initially to address ROM, positioning, tone management, and skin protection. If the child does not improve and in fact may not survive the injuries, and his or her ability to participate or make progress toward goals is in question, the frequency might be decreased. Open communication with the interdisciplinary team as well as the parents is crucial. Parents must feel empowered to help their child, yet also not feel like the team is "giving up." Parents are usually reassured that the therapist will continually reevaluate the child, and if their status improves, the frequency can be adjusted again.

End of Life Care

In many acute-care hospitals, working with children and families enduring end of life decisions often causes much stress and anxiety for all involved. In the pediatric setting, dealing with a dying child and grieving family can often be overwhelming for the interdisciplinary team. Many children's hospitals have established Pediatric Advance Care Teams (PACT) to work with children, families, and the medical team to establish treatment plans for children at the end of life. The goal of the PACT is to help children live as well as possible and as long as possible. The World Health Organization in 2006 established criteria for pediatric palliative care and these include caring for the child's body, mind, and spirit; continuity of care from diagnosis and continuing whether curative interventions are pursued; expertise and involvement of an interdisciplinary team along with the family and community resources (Duncan, Spengler, & Wolf, 2007). Goals of involving the PACT team in a child's care may include opening up discussions with the family to look at their goals, providing assistance with quality of life decisions, managing symptoms, serving as a liaison with homecare or hospice, and meeting the wishes of the child and family for end of life care at home or in the hospital. The team will also provide support not only for the child and family but also for the interdisciplinary team during the time leading up to and following the child's death (Duncan et al., 2007). Supporting the family after the time of death either via phone calls, sympathy cards, or a hospital-based memorial may be ways to assist the family during their grieving and recovery process. Therapists must be sensitive to the needs of the child and family during this time, but also aware of their therapeutic relationship with the family in order to not become too emotionally attached to the situation. Bearing the emotional burden of a dying patient is difficult for any clinician, and even more so when a child is involved. Working with team counselors and social workers may be a way for the therapist to express grief over the loss of a child, and decrease the risk of emotional stress or burnout.

Transition From the Acute-Care Setting

When a child is discharged from the acute setting, the physical therapist works with the interdisciplinary team as well as the family to both make recommendations for services and assist with locating the recommended services in the child's community. The interdisciplinary team collaborates to determine the child's needs after discharge. For example, a child who has limitations in functional mobility, completing their activities of daily living, and communicating with others would benefit from an inpatient rehabilitation admission to address all areas of impairment, whereas a child who presents with limitations in only one of these areas and whose caregivers are able to care for them in the home setting could best be served with an episode of outpatient services in the discipline where they are demonstrating limitations. Based on all the variables impacting a child's function, it is important for the entire interdisciplinary team to work together to make an individualized discharge plan for each child.

Options for physical therapy services in the community vary from inpatient rehabilitation admissions to outpatient services. Children who demonstrate a significant difference in their functional mobility from baseline and who are unable to negotiate their home environment safely would benefit from an inpatient rehabilitation admission. Those children who present with a large decline in their functional status from baseline but are able to negotiate their home environment safely with the assistance of a caregiver, are able to be transported to and from a medical center, and who would benefit from intensive therapy services may qualify for a day hospital admission. In this setting, children receive 3–6 hours of therapy (PT, OT, and/or speech) during the day in a medical setting, then return home in the evening with their family. This level of service is not offered in all communities and is not covered by all insurance providers.

An episode of outpatient physical therapy is recommended for children who present with impairments and activity limitations that will improve with direct physical therapy provided at a frequency of 2–3 times per week. Examples of children referred to outpatient physical therapy include those postoperative from orthopedic surgeries for an episode of strengthening and conditioning, children with a newly diagnosed developmental delay or those with a new onset of loss of gross motor skills, and those children and parents who would benefit from education and prescription of a home program to progress independence in the community.

Children under school age who present with gross motor delays or disabilities often qualify for early intervention services. State-run early intervention programs serve children in the community who have a developmental delay or disabilities, as discussed in Chapter 11. A caregiver or health-care professional can make a referral for early intervention services. Therapists who provide early intervention services work with children and their caregivers in their home or daycare facility to provide intervention and education for caregivers to progress a child's developmental skills.

Children with long-standing physical therapy needs are often followed in a clinic setting based on their underlying diagnosis. An example of such a clinic is Cerebral Palsy Clinic. Children are followed every 6 months or more frequently as need and at each visit are evaluated by an interdisciplinary team. When changes occur based on growth, acquisition or loss of functional skills, or limitations in activities and participation, or when equipment needs arise, children are referred for an episode of outpatient physical therapy to address the current needs.

Summary

The pediatric physical therapist in an acute-care setting must be well prepared to provide examinations, interventions, and consultations for a wide age range of children with various diagnoses. Working within an interdisciplinary team, the acute-care therapist must be prepared to demonstrate excellent communication skills, flexibility with scheduling, and the ability to provide child- and family-focused care. Therapists need to be prepared to make sound clinical decisions in accordance to their institution's policies as well as abide by any regulatory agencies they may encounter.

Acute-care pediatric physical therapists should have a broad clinical background encompassing pediatric diagnoses, medical and surgical interventions, hematological studies, and diagnostic imaging results and interpretations and be comfortable with the complex technology often encountered in the acute-care setting. Mentorship from experienced staff will aid in gaining confidence and competency for providing care especially in the intensive care unit. Therapists who practice in this setting are often those who enjoy a challenge, can think quickly on their feet, can adapt to an ever-changing environment, have great time management and communication skills, and are truly learning something new every day.

DISCUSSION QUESTIONS

1. Discuss your role as a physical therapist in providing patient-family centered care.
2. Name 3–5 common contraindications or precautions for providing care in the acute-care setting.
3. Describe the differences between invasive and noninvasive mechanical ventilation.
4. List the warning signs of abuse or neglect that you may identify upon initial examination.

5. Discuss the differences between the adult and pediatric populations when considering recommendations for discharge from the acute-care setting.

Recommended Readings

Custer, J., Rau, R., & Lee, C. (Eds.) (2008). *The Harriet Lane handbook.* Philadelphia: Elsevier Health Sciences.

Frank, G., Shah, S., Zaoutis, L., & Catallozzi, M. (Eds.). (2005). *The Philadelphia guide: Inpatient pediatrics.* Philadelphia: Lippincott Williams & Wilkins.

Nichols, D., & Helfaer, M. (Eds.) (2008). *Rogers' handbook of pediatric intensive care.* Philadelphia: Lippincott Williams & Wilkins.

Zaoutis, L., & Chang, V. (Eds.) (2007). *Comprehensive pediatric hospital medicine.* Philadelphia: Elsevier Health Sciences.

References

American Academy of Pediatrics Committee on Hospital Care (2003). Family-centered care and the pediatrician's role. *Pediatrics, 112,* 691–696.

Andrew, M., Monagle, P.T., & Brooker, L. (2000). *Thromboembolic complications during infancy and childhood.* Hamilton, ON: B.C. Decker.

Bailes, A.F., Reder, R., & Burch, C. (2008). Development of guidelines for determining frequency of therapy services in a pediatric medical setting. *Pediatric Physical Therapy, 20,* 194–198.

Blumenstein, M.S. (2007). Early ambulation after deep vein thrombosis: Is it safe? *Journal of Pediatric Oncology Nursing, 24*(6), 309–313.

Carmen, S., Teal, S., & Guzzetta, C.A. (2008). Development, testing and national evaluation of a pediatric patient-family-centered care benchmarking survey. *Holistic Nursing Practice, 22*(2), 61–74.

Centers for Disease Control and Prevention (CDC). (2009a). *Methicillin-resistant staphylococcus aureus.* Retrieved from http://www.cdc.gov/mrsa/

Centers for Disease Control and Prevention (CDC). (2009b). *Vancomycin-resistant enterococci.* Retrieved from http://www.cdc.gov/

Centers for Disease Control and Prevention (CDC). (2009c). *Violence prevention.* Retrieved from http://www.cdc.gov/ViolencePrevention/childmaltreatment/

Children's Hospital of Philadelphia (CHOP). (2009a). *Peripherally inserted central venous catheter.* Retrieved from http://www.chop.edu/service/radiology/interventional-radiology/peripherally-inserted-central-catheter-picc.html

Children's Hospital of Philadelphia (CHOP). (2009b). *Nontunneled central venous catheter.* Retrieved from http://www.chop.edu/service/radiology/interventional-radiology

Children's Hospital of Philadelphia (CHOP). (2009c). *Respiratory syncytial virus.* Retrieved from http://www.chop.edu/healthinfo/respiratory-syncytial-virus-rsv.html

Child Welfare Information Gateway. (2009). *Child abuse reporting number.* Retrieved from http://www.childwelfare.gov/systemwide/laws_policies/state/

Conway, S. (2008). Segregation is good for patients with cystic fibrosis. *Journal of the Royal Society of Medicine, 101,* S31–35.

Czarnecki, M.L., Ferrise, A.S., Jastrowski-Mano, K.E., Garwood, M.M., Sharp, M., Davies, H., & Weisman, S.J. (2008). Parent/nurse-controlled analgesia for children with developmental delay. *The Clinical Journal of Pain, 24*(9), 817–824.

Duncan, J., Spengler, E., & Wolfe, J. (2007). Providing pediatric palliative care, PACT in action. *American Journal of Maternal Child Nursing, 32*(5), 279–287.

Emedicine. (2006). *Extracorporeal Membrane Oxygenation.* Retrieved from http://www.emedicine.com/PED/topic2895.htm

Erkonen, W. (Ed.) (1998). *Radiology 101: The basics and fundamentals of imaging.* Philadelphia: Lippincott Williams & Wilkins.

Goad, J. (2008). Understanding roles and improving reporting and response relationships across professional boundaries. *Pediatrics, 122,* S6–9.

Gocha, V.A., Murphy, D.M., Dholakia, K.H., Hess, A.A., & Effgen, S.K. (1999). Child maltreatment: Our responsibility as health care professionals. *Pediatric Physical Therapy, 11*(3), 133–139.

Joint Commission (JC). (2011a). *About us.* Retrieved from http://www.jointcommission.org/about_us/about_the_joint_commission_main.aspx

Joint Commission (JC). (2011b). *Standards information.* Retrieved from http://www.jointcommission.org/standards_information/npsgs.aspx

Jones, R.J., Flaherty, E.G., Binns, H.J., Price, L.L., Slora, E., Abney, D., Harris, D.L., Christoffel, K.K., & Sege, R.D. (2008). Clinicians' description of factors influencing their reporting of suspected child abuse: Report of the child abuse reporting experience study research group. *Pediatrics, 122,* 259–266.

Kamerling, S.N., Lawler, L.C., Lynch, M., & Schwartz, A.J. (2008). Family-centered care in the pediatric post anesthesia care unit: Changing practice to promote parental visitation. *Journal of Perianesthesia Nursing, 23*(1), 5–16.

Kehl-Pruett, W. (2006). Deep vein thrombosis in hospitalized patients: A review of evidence-based guidelines for prevention. *Dimens Critical Care Nursing, 25*(2), 53–59.

Klevens, R.M., Morrison, M.A., Nadle, J., Petit, S., Gershman, K., Ray, S., Harrison, L.H., Lynfield, R., Dumyati, G., Townes, J.M., Craig, A.S., Zell, E.R., Fosheim, G.E., McDougal, L.K., Carey, R.B., & Fridkin, S.K. (2007). Active Bacterial Core surveillance (ABCs) MRSA Investigators. *JAMA, 298*(15), 1763–1771.

Legano, L., McHugh, M.T., & Palusci, V.J. (2009). Child abuse and neglect. *Current Problems in Pediatric Adolescent Health Care, 39*(31), e1–e26.

Lippi, G., Favaloro, E., & Cervellin, G. (2011). Prevention of venous thromboembolism: Focus on mechanical prophylaxis. *Seminars in Thrombosis and Hemostasis, 37*(3), 237–251.

Ludot, H., Berger, J., Pichenot, V., Belouadah, M., Madi, K., & Malinovsky, J.M. (2008). Continuous peripheral nerve block for postoperative pain control at home: A prospective feasibility study in children. *Regional Anesthesia and Pain Medicine, 33*(1), 52–56.

Marino, P. (1998). *The ICU book* (2nd ed.). Baltimore: Williams & Wilkins.

McGrath, P.J., Johnston, G., Goodman, J.T., Schillinger, J., Dunn, J., & Chapman, J. (1985). CHEOPS: A behavioral scale for rating postoperative pain in children. In H.L. Fields (Ed.), *Advances in pain research and therapy* (pp. 395–402). New York: Raven Press.

MedlinePlus. (2009). *Dialysis.* Retrieved from http://vsearch.nlm.nih.gov/vivisimo/cgi-bin/query-meta?v%3Aproject=medlineplus&query=dialysis

Merkel, S.I., Voepel-Lewis, T., Shayevitz, J.R., & Malviya, S. (1997). The FLACC: a behavioral scale for scoring postoperative pain in young children. *Pediatric Nursing, 23,* 293–297.

National Association of Children's Hospitals and Related Institutions (NACHRI). (2009). *All Children Need Children's Hospitals.* Retrieved from http://www.childrenshospitals.net

Nilsson, S., Finnstorm, B., & Kokinsky, E. (2008). The FLACC behavioral scale for procedural pain assessment in children age 5–16 years. *Pediatric Anesthesia, 18,* 767–774.

O'Malley, P.J., Brown, K., & Krug, S.E. (2008). Patient and family-centered care of children in the emergency department. *Pediatrics, 122,* e511–521.

Ravishankar, C., Dominguez, T., Kreutzer, J., Wernovsky, G., Marino, B., Godinez, R., Priestley, M., Gruber, P., Gaynor, W., Nicolson, S., Spray, T., & Tabbutt, S. (2006). Extracorporeal membrane oxygenation after Stage I reconstruction for hypoplastic left heart syndrome. *Pediatric Critical Care Medicine, 7*(4), 319–323.

Schiessl, C., Gravou, C., Zernikow, B., Sittl, R., & Griessinger, N. (2008). Use of patient-controlled analgesia for pain control in dying children. *Support Care Cancer, 16,* 531–536.

Suraseranivongse, S., Kaosaard, R., Intakong, P., Pornsiriprasert, S., Karnchana, Y., Koapinpruck, J., & Sangjeen, K. (2006). A comparison of postoperative pain scales in neonates. *British Journal of Anesthesia, 97*(4), 540–544.

Vu, L.T., Nobuhara, K.K., Lee, H., & Farmer, D.L. (2008). Determination of risk factors for deep venous thrombosis in hospitalized children. *Journal of Pediatric Surgery, 43,* 1095–1099.

Wong, D., & Baker, C. (1998). Pain in children: Comparison of assessment scales. *Pediatric Nursing, 14*(1), 9–17.

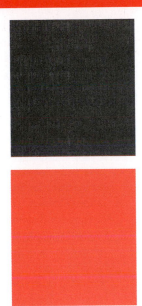

CHAPTER 15

Neonatal Intensive Care Unit

—RACHEL UNANUE ROSE, PT, PhD, PCS

T he **neonatal intensive care unit (NICU)** is a technologically advanced setting that provides services to infants who require highly specialized services. Infants who are served in the NICU are at high risk both medically and developmentally, requiring a team approach to their complex care. Physical therapists who work in the NICU provide examination, evaluation, and intervention to these high-risk infants. NICU care is a specialized area within pediatric physical therapy, involving a different approach than that used in other types of pediatric settings. Due to the physiological, medical, and developmental issues facing infants in the NICU, physical therapists working in the NICU require pediatric experience and advanced training (Sweeney, Heriza, & Blanchard, 2009). Advanced training is necessary to safely provide services to these fragile infants and their families. This chapter provides a basic overview of service delivery in the NICU.

Further study is required for physical therapists wishing to work in a NICU, especially the most intensive level III nursery.

Infants Served

The NICU serves infants with a variety of diagnoses. Infants admitted to the NICU are born both preterm and full-term. Infants who show signs of central nervous system (CNS) impairment, specific neuromuscular or orthopedic problems, multiple medical or genetic problems, abnormal feeding behaviors, and other symptoms that put infants at risk for developmental problems are often referred to physical therapy in the NICU (McCarton, Wallace, Divon, & Vaughn, 1996; Taylor, Klein, Schatschneider, & Hack, 1998) (Table 15.1).

Full-term infants are those infants born between 37 and 42 weeks gestation. Infants who are born less than 37 weeks gestation are considered premature (Darcy,

Table 15.1 Common Diagnoses of Infants in the Neonatal Intensive Care Unit

Premature birth: Less than 38 weeks' gestation

Low birth weight: Less than 2,500 grams

Very low birth weight: Less than 1,500 grams

Small for gestational age (SGA): Less than the 10th percentile

Large for gestational age (LGA): Greater than the 90th percentile

Microcephaly: Occipital frontal head circumference of less than the third percentile for the infant's gestational age at birth

Hypoxic ischemic encephalopathy: Full-term infant who has had a significant episode of intrapartum asphyxia

Genetic syndromes and diseases: Chromosomal abnormalities, gene disorders, unusual patterns of inheritance

Compromised respiration: Infant requires medical or mechanical assistance to achieve functional respiration

Persistent feeding problems: Infant is unable to take in adequate calories orally without special assistance

Seizure disorder: Neonatal seizures identified at or shortly following birth

Amniotic band syndrome: Intrauterine development of amniochorionic strands leading to limb and digital amputations or constrictions and other deformities

Myelomeningocele: Malformation of the spinal cord resulting from defective closure of the neural tube

2009; Engle, Tomashek, Wallman, & Committee on Fetus and Newborn, 2007; Vergara & Bigsby, 2004). Infants are also classified according to weight. Infants who are born weighing less than 2,500 grams are considered **low birth weight (LBW)** (Vergara & Bigsby, 2004). Infants weighing less than 1,500 grams are **very low birth weight (VLBW),** and those weighing less than 1,000 grams are considered **extremely low birth weight (ELBW)**. Gestational age and birth weight should be assessed and interpreted independently of one another. Infants born preterm and weighing less than 1,000 grams at birth are at the greatest risk for cerebral palsy (CP) and other motor, cognitive, and behavioral disorders (Foulder-Hughes & Cooke, 2003; Laptook, O'Shea, Shankaran, Bhaskar, & NICHD Neonatal Network, 2005; Walden et al., 2007). Of the infants born at or less than 1,500 grams, 5% to 15% exhibited major motor deficits, while another 25% to 50% exhibited less severe developmental disabilities (Volpe, 1997).

Infants are further classified based on size for gestational age. If their weight falls in less than the

10th percentile, they are considered **small for gestational age (SGA)**. If their weight in greater than the 90th percentile, they are considered **large for gestational age (LGA)**. SGA does not imply that an infant is very small and LGA does not imply that an infant is very heavy. A preterm infant who weighs more than what is typical for his or her gestational age at birth would be classified as LGA. An infant who is heavier, but whose weight is lower than what is expected for gestational age, would be classified as SGA (Vergara & Bigsby, 2004).

Infants born prematurely are at risk for CNS complications. Premature birth may lead to visual and hearing impairments, learning disabilities, behavioral disorders, neurological disorders, and developmental disorders (Kilbride & Daily, 1998; McGrath, Sullivan, Lester, & Oh, 2000). CP is the most prevalent developmental disorder related to premature birth. Approximately 40% of children with CP were born prematurely (Bennett, 1999).

One common complication associated with premature birth is **intraventricular hemorrhage (IVH)** (Bayram, Kayserili, Agin, Bayram, & Unalp, 2008; Linder et al., 2003; Vergani et al., 2004). The premature brain is at risk for IVH due to the lack of supporting elements in the brain around the ventricles resulting from neuronal migration, a lack of cerebrovascular autoregulation causing changes in arterial pressure to be passively transmitted to the cerebral vessels, and asphyxia in the preterm infant (Aicardi, 1992). IVHs are graded I to IV, with I being the least severe and IV being the most severe (Mantovani & Powers, 1991). Approximately 35% to 50% of infants born before 32 weeks' gestation or with birth weights less than 1,500 grams are diagnosed with an IVH (Duncan & Ment, 1993; Volpe, 1998). ELBW infants with grade I and II IVH have poorer neurodevelopmental outcomes than ELBW infants with normal head ultrasounds and no IVH (Patra, Wilson-Costello, Taylor, Mercuri-Minich, & Hack, 2006). Another complication of preterm birth is **periventricular leukomalacia (PVL).** PVL is the primary ischemic lesion of infants born prematurely and is located in the white matter around the lateral ventricles (Aicardi, 1992; Candy & Hoon, 1996; Hamrick et al., 2004; Rivkin, 1997; Volpe, 1995, 1997). Spastic diplegia, a form of CP, is the most common long-term outcome of PVL (Candy & Hoon, 1996; Rivkin, 1997; Volpe, 1995).

Infants born prematurely are also at risk for other medical complications, such as chronic respiratory disease, cardiovascular disorders, hearing loss, anemia, retinopathy of prematurity, and feeding difficulties (Vergara & Bigsby, 2004; Weisglas-Kuperus, Baerts, Smrkovsky, & Sauer, 1993).

Late preterm infants are infants born between 34 and 37 weeks' gestation (Darcy, 2009; Engle et al., 2007). Often, these infants are the size and weight of some term infants and are often treated by parents and health care professionals as developmentally mature and at low risk of morbidity. However, the late preterm infant is physiologically and metabolically immature and should not be treated like a full-term infant. Late preterm infants are at an increased risk for developing medical complications resulting in higher rates of morbidity and mortality. Late preterm infants also have an increased rate of readmission to the hospital compared to full-term infants. Limitations associated with late preterm birth include respiratory difficulties, difficulty with body temperature regulation, elevated bilirubin, feeding difficulty, hypoglycemia, sepsis, and possible neurodevelopmental disabilities (Darcy, 2009; Engle et al., 2007).

Neonatal Intensive Care Unit

Levels of Care

NICUs have improved the morbidity and mortality of high-risk infants and are designed to meet a wide range of special needs (Fig. 15.1). The American Academy of Pediatrics (AAP) Committee on Fetus and Newborn (2004) describes the three levels of care provided by NICUs as Level I: Basic Neonatal Care, Level II: Specialty Neonatal Care, and Level III: Subspecialty Neonatal Care. Level I, or Basic Care, NICUs are well-newborn nurseries that evaluate and provide routine care for healthy newborns and that are also capable of providing resuscitation. A Level II, or Specialty Care, NICU is a special care nursery that provides care to infants who are more than 32 weeks gestational age and weigh more than 1,500 grams. These units also resuscitate and stabilize infants prior to transfer to a Level III nursery. Level III, or Subspecialty Care, NICUs provide comprehensive care to extremely high-risk newborn infants and infants with complex and critical illnesses.

Level III units can be further divided into units that provide extracorporeal membrane oxygenation (ECMO) and those that do not (AAP, 2004). ECMO is a heart-lung bypass machine used to support critically ill neonates whose heart and lungs need to rest or heal. Infants who are placed on ECMO have blood oxygenated externally and then returned to the body. ECMO is most commonly used for infants with congenital diaphragmatic hernia, persistent pulmonary hypertension of the newborn, and sepsis (Ford, 2006; Tulenko, 2004).

Physical therapists rarely see infants in Level I nurseries; however, they may be consulted for an infant with a specific neuromuscular issue. Physical therapists in Level II nurseries provide handling and development for the specific needs of infants in the unit. In Level III nurseries, physical therapists are working with fragile and critically ill infants and their families. Physical therapists must have specific skills in observation, handling, and development to provide recommendations for infants and their families (Fig. 15.2).

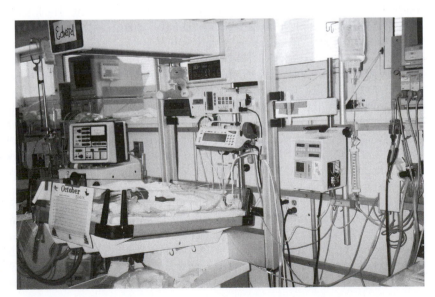

Figure 15.1 Infant in typical technologically rich NICU.

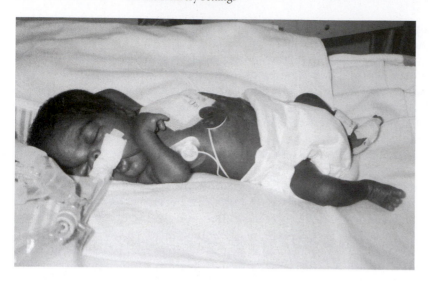

Figure 15.2 Closer view of the infant, who is intubated and connected to cardiac, respiratory, and temperature monitors.

Lighting and Noise

The NICU is an unfamiliar setting for many families. Not only is the high-tech environment overwhelming to families, but to infants as well. Technology brings with it an increase in sensory stimulation for infants in the NICU. Environmental noise is a major source of stress for infants in the NICU. The AAP (1997) recommends noise levels in the NICU should be monitored by caregivers and maintained at or below 45 dB (AAP, 1997). One study found that noise levels in the NICU were substantially lower in 2005 compared to a previous study performed in the same NICU in 1989 (Thomas & Uran, 2007). However, inside the isolette, sound levels were the same or higher in 2005. Sound levels related to caregiving equipment (59–68 dB), motor operations (60 dB), and opening or closing portholes and porthole plastic sleeves (58–72 dB) were a major contributor to overall sound levels within the isolette. This study suggests that sound continues to be a challenge in the NICU, particularly inside the isolette. Although this study did not test the effect of nursing and caregiving practice on sound level, staff largely determines the reduction in room sound.

Lighting is another source of sensory stimulation for infants in the NICU. Guidelines developed by the Consensus Committee to Establish Recommended Standards for Newborn ICU Design (2002) include adjustable ambient lighting from 10 to 600 lux, controls to darken artificial and natural lighting, framed lighting to reduce illumination onto adjacent bedsides, and at least one source of natural lighting visible from patient care areas, but no closer than 2 feet from an infant's bedside (Vergara & Bigsby, 2004). The AAP recommends that lighting levels in the NICU should be less than 646 lux (Lasky & Williams, 2009). Light levels tend to be within guidelines more often than sound levels, with higher light levels found in open beds compared to isolettes (Lasky & Williams, 2009).

Developmentally Supportive Care

Individualized developmental care is a model of care in the NICU developed by Als and colleagues (1986). Developmental care is based on the synactive theory of development and the knowledge that infants discharged home from the NICU are at risk for developmental delays (Als et al., 1986, 1994; Brown & Heermann, 1997). The synactive theory proposed by Als and colleagues (1986) examines the infant's ability to respond to external stimuli. The infant is evaluated in five systems: the autonomic, motor, state organizational, attention and interaction, and self-regulatory systems. Behavioral cues are identified through observations centered on caregiving activities. Based on these behavioral observations, an individualized plan of care is developed for each infant to encourage and support development and optimal recovery and rest (Als et al., 1986). The individual plan may have recommendations regarding lighting, sound levels, and facilitation of self-regulatory behaviors. Developmentally supportive care is a best practice and is the standard of care for Level III NICUs.

The **Newborn Individualized Developmental Care and Assessment Program (NIDCAP)** provides the framework for developmentally supportive care (Lawhon & Hedlund, 2008). NIDCAP is a model for clinical observation of infants in the NICU. The infant communicates to the observer through behavioral responses how his or her autonomic, motor, and state subsystems are functioning. Behavioral cues are interpreted and care is provided through individualized developmentally supportive care to promote self-regulation, behavioral organization, and overall development. The implementation of NIDCAP observations and developmentally supportive care have improved patient outcomes and decreased the cost of hospitalizations. These improved outcomes include decreased incidence of IVH, improved weight gain, shorter duration of ventilatory support, and decreased length of stay (Als et al., 1986, 1994; Brown & Heermann, 1997; Lawhon & Hedlund, 2008). In addition, infants who are treated after implementation of NIDCAP care have higher levels of motor development in the arms and trunk compared to infants prior to NIDCAP care (Ullenhag, Persson, & Nyqvist, 2009).

Pain Management

The NICU environment frequently exposes the infant to painful or stressful stimuli. Pain has been studied extensively in preterm infants. They respond to noxious stimuli with a clear flexor withdrawal as early as 26 weeks postconceptional age (Andrews & Fitzgerald, 1994) and display physiological changes associated with a heelstick (Stevens & Johnston, 1994; Walden et al., 2001). Caregiver interventions, such as tucking and swaddling, provide infants with comfort during painful procedures (Prince, Horns, Latta, & Gerstmann, 2004). In addition, sucrose is helpful in reducing physiological and behavioral responses to pain (Abad, Diaz, Domenech, Robayna, & Rico, 1996; Johnston, Stremler, Horton, & Friedman, 1999; Maone, Mattes, Bernbaum, & Beauchamp, 1990; Stevens, Taddio, Ohlsson, & Einarson, 1997). Therapists in the NICU should identify and make recommendations for strategies to reduce an infant's response to painful procedures.

Family-Centered Care

Family-centered care, as noted throughout the text, is a model of service delivery to infants and their families that recognizes the family as a constant in the infant's life (Rosenbaum, King, Law, King, & Evans, 1998). Family-centered care is based upon a partnership between health-care professionals and families of infants in the NICU (Griffin, 2006; Sweeney, Heriza, Blanchard, & Dusing, 2010). Families in the NICU participate in caregiving and decision making and are provided with complete, accurate information about their infant. Each family's individual strengths and needs are identified, as well as their cultural beliefs and values. Family-centered care promotes collaboration between the physical therapist and the parents (Dunst, Johanson, Trivette, & Hamby, 1991; Griffin, 2006; Harrison, 1993; Johnson, 1990; Rosenbaum et al., 1998; Shelton & Stepanek, 1995). Physical therapists working in the NICU should involve parents in their interventions to provide the best care to the infant and their families.

Role of Physical Therapy

The physical therapist is a member of a team of caregivers and professionals providing medical and developmental care to infants in the NICU. The team in the NICU may include physicians, nurses, respiratory therapists, nutritionists, physical therapists, occupational therapists, and speech therapists. Physical therapists are actively involved in the examination, evaluation, and intervention of high-risk infants.

Examination and Evaluation

Physical therapists receive referrals from the neonatologist or nurse practitioner to initiate services to high-risk infants in the NICU. Referrals may be made at varying times throughout the infant's stay, depending on the facility. Infants in the NICU may be referred at a specific time during their stay based on a timeline developed in that unit with the neonatologists, nurses, and therapists. The majority of infants will be referred at this time, with a few referred earlier or later depending on their medical status. In other facilities, infants may be referred to therapy based on their medical or birth history and once stable.

Sweeney and colleagues (2009) developed an algorithm for clinical decision making in the NICU. The pathways are outlined for examination, intervention, and reexamination. During the examination process, the NICU team and family determine the strengths and needs of the infant, from which appropriate goals are developed. The initial examination begins with a chart review; observation of the infant and caregivers; discussions with the neonatologist, nursing staff, and the family; and handling or additional diagnostic procedures, if appropriate (Sweeney et al., 2009). Based on the information obtained through the history and observation of the infant, the physical therapist formulates a strategy for the physical therapy examination (Fig. 15.3).

History

Prenatal, birth, and medical history are reviewed and documented in the initial examination, as well as the infant's current medical status. Important information from the history includes Apgar scores, which indicate physiological function (Table 15.2). Apgar scores

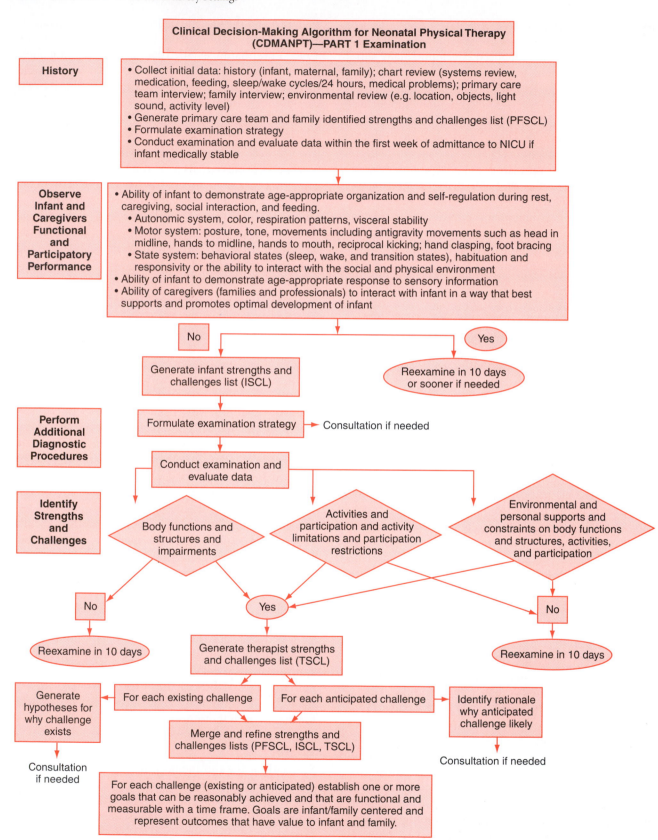

Figure 15.3 Clinical decision-making algorithm for neonatal physical therapy practice: Part 1: Examination. *(Reprinted from Sweeney, J.K, Heriza, C.B., & Blanchard Y. (2009). Neonatal physical therapy, Part I: Clinical competencies and neonatal intensive care unit clinical training models.* Pediatric Physical Therapy, 21, 304, *with permission.)*

Table 15.2 Apgar Scores*

Apgar Score			
Sign	0	1	2
Heart Rate	Absent	Below 100 bpm	Over 100 bpm
Respiration	Absent	Slow, irregular	Good, crying
Muscle tone	Limp	Some flexion	Active movement
Grimace (reflex irritability)	No Response	Grimace	Cough or sneeze
Color (appearance)	Blue, pale	Body pink, extremities blue	Completely pink

* 0, 1, or 2 points are given for each sign based on observation of the infant at 1, 5, and sometimes 10 minutes after birth.

are assigned at 1 and 5 minutes after birth. When low scores are assigned at 1 and 5 minutes, an additional score at 10 minutes may be assigned. Scores of 8 to 10 at 1 minute after birth are normal. If Apgar scores at both 1 and 5 minutes are 0 to 3, the infant requires resuscitation and there is a risk of neonatal death. The possibility of the infant developing a neurological complication is also associated with extremely low Apgar scores, and particularly with a low score assigned at 10 minutes (Moster, Lie, Irgens, Bjerkedal, & Markestad, 2001).

The infant's gestational age at birth should be noted, as well as the number of weeks since birth and their postconceptional age. Infants will respond differently based on their gestational age at birth and their postconceptional age at the time of the examination. Medical history, including time ventilated, presence of IVH, and genetic anomalies, are important information that provide a picture of how the infant is functioning. Medical complications and ongoing medical issues will give insight into how well an infant will tolerate handling. In addition, sleep/wake patterns, type of feeding and frequency, and medications are also important to note in the history. These may also influence caregiving and therapeutic interventions. At this time, both the family and medical team will identify a list of strengths and challenges.

Observation

Prior to the therapist placing hands on the infant, information can be obtained through observation alone. Appearance includes the type of bed the infant is in—isolette, open bed, or crib. What is attached to the infant at the time of the initial examination? This may include a ventilator, oxygen via a nasal cannula, peripheral or central intravenous (IV) lines, feeding tubes, ostomies, and physiological monitors (heart rate, respiration, and oxygen saturation). This information gives the therapist a picture of the infant in his resting state. The therapist is also able to see how organized the infant is at rest in terms of autonomic, motor, and state systems.

In addition to the infant's appearance at rest, the therapist observes the infant during caregiving by family or nursing. Through this observation, the therapist learns how organized the infant is with stimulation and his ability to self-regulate. The therapist also learns how the family or nursing staff responds to the infant's behavioral cues and supports or promotes optimal development for the infant during routine caregiving (Sweeney et al., 2009).

Tolerance to Handling

Although the physical therapist has observed how well the infant tolerates caregiving activities, handling and position changes during physical therapy examinations have been shown to cause physiological and behavioral signs of stress in infants born preterm (Sweeny, 1986, 1989). Throughout the physical therapy examination, the infant should be monitored for tolerance to handling. All infants are attached to monitors that allow physiological signs of stress to be monitored (Table 15.3). **Physiological signs** of stress may include changes in oxygen saturation, respiratory rate, and

Table 15.3 Neonatal Methods of Coping With Stimulation

Self-Calming
- Hand to face or mouth
- Sucking on hand, fingers, thumb, pacifier
- Maintaining flexed posture
- Hands or feet to midline
- Closing eyes, gaze aversion
- Drowsy state to control stimulation

Assisted Calming
- Nesting, positioning in flexion
- Holding in flexion
- Slow rocking
- Swaddling
- Quiet voice

heart rate. However, physical therapists should also observe the infant's tolerance to handling through behavioral signs of stress. **Behavioral signs** of stress include changes in color, hiccoughs, finger splay, stiffening extremities into extension, frowning, and turning away from or averting gaze away from a noise or the therapist's face. The examination may be modified or stopped based on the infant's tolerance to handling either physiologically or behaviorally (Table 15.4). A conservative approach to handling and positioning should be followed based on the potential for harm.

The infant's tolerance to handling and position changes is evaluated during the initial examination. The position of the infant and any positioning devices needed to maintain a position are noted. Often, infants have a head preference to one side, which should be noted. Recommendations on positioning should be given to family and nursing staff to help properly position infants, especially those infants who are difficult to position and those with a head preference to one side.

Behavioral State and Alertness

All infants have various states of alertness, drowsiness, and sleep. CNS maturity is indicated by an infant's ability to move through a variety of behavioral states and to maintain a state of alertness. The infant's state has the ability to affect examination findings. Drowsy infants may appear to have low tone because they are unable to maintain a level of alertness in response to handling and position changes. Infants may move quickly between different states of sleep, alertness, and crying (Table 15.5) (Brazelton, 1984). Infants born prematurely may move erratically from one state to

■ Table 15.4 Neonatal Signs of Stress

Physiological	Behavioral
Increased heart rate	Gaze aversion
Decreased heart rate	Finger splays
Decreased respiratory rate	Trunk extension
Increased blood pressure	Facial grimace
Decreased oxygen saturation	Leg extension
Apnea	Tuning out/drowsiness
Bradycardia	Hyperalertness
Skin color changes	Arm salute

Source: Kahn-D'Angelo, L. (1995). The special care nursery. In S.K. Campbell (Ed.), *Physical therapy for children* (pp. 787–822). Philadelphia: W.B. Saunders, with permission.

■ Table 15.5 Behavioral States of Sleep and Arousal

Deep sleep	No movement of body or eyes. Optimal for growth and recovery.
Light sleep	Body jerks and eye movements seen. Heart and respiratory rate responses to noise and lights noted on bedside monitors.
Drowsiness	Transitional state between sleep and wakefulness. Eyes may open briefly. Little spontaneous movement. Behavioral signs of stress often present.
Quiet alertness	Eyes open and eye contact made. Relaxed face and facial expressions. Movements smooth. Ready for interaction.
Active alertness	Eyes open or closed. Facial grimace or hyperalert appearance common. Large-ranged, constant movements of extremities seen. Trunk extension often seen. Behavioral signs of stress present. Increased heart and respiratory rates.
Crying	Eyes closed. Crying. Stressed facial expression. Extremity and trunk movements seen. Increased heart and respiratory rates.

Source: Brazelton, T.B. (1984). Neonatal Behavioral Assessment Scale (2nd ed.). *Clinics in Developmental Medicine, No. 88.* Philadelphia: J.B. Lippincott, with permission.

another and spend little time in the quiet alert state (Kahn-D'Angelo & Rose, 2006). Responding to behavioral signs of stress and assisting with self-regulatory behaviors may facilitate a more alert state. When the infant is awake, visual and auditory reactions can be observed and documented.

Active Movement and Strength

Movement and strength can both be examined initially through general observations. The type of movements seen should be documented. Movements may initially be global and jerky, but with time should become smooth and more purposeful. Active movements may include hands to midline, hands to mouth, and lower extremity movements into extension. Any asymmetries in movement should be noted. Strength is observed through antigravity movements of the head, neck, trunk, and extremities. Generally, lower extremity movements are into extension, but gradually movement into flexion should be seen. Although a preterm infant is not expected to have head control, attempts at head control in all positions should be seen.

Muscle Tone and Reflexes

Muscle tone is evaluated through the assessment of resistance to passive movement, observation of movement, and reflex testing. Recoil of arms and legs gives the physical therapist information about the infant's muscle tone. Generally, muscle tone may be decreased in infants born prematurely and infants born at term who are ill. Infants with decreased tone may fall into the surface they are on. They will often be in extension and have a difficult time overcoming the effects of gravity. The development of reflexes and the symmetry of responses to reflex testing can provide information about an infant's neuromotor system. The optimal state for reflex testing is the quiet alert state.

Feeding

Feeding by mouth is a landmark skill for infants in the NICU. Learning to suck, swallow, and breathe can be a difficult and long process for an infant and his family. Depending on the facility and the involvement of other therapies (occupational therapy or speech-language pathology), physical therapists may be involved in the evaluation of feeding skills. Infants may have problems with discoordination or disorganization of sucking, swallowing, and breathing, difficulty maintaining an alert state for feedings, and abnormalities in oral motor skills.

Intervention

Once the examination and evaluation are completed, the physical therapist makes recommendations for further follow-up and intervention if indicated. The physical therapist will identify strengths and challenges in body function and structures, activity, and participation levels of the ICF (Sweeney et al., 2009). This may include ongoing physical therapy intervention while the infant is in the hospital or reexamination by the physical therapist in another week or two.

Physical therapy intervention in the NICU may vary depending on the disciplines of the other team members in the NICU. Physical therapy interventions might include range of motion (ROM), positioning, facilitation of behavioral organization, handling to promote sensory and motor development, feeding, parent education, and screening of infants at risk for disability (Kahn-D'Angelo & Rose, 2006; Rapport, 1992). Field and colleagues (2010) performed a review of massage therapy studies in the NICU. Infants who received massage in the NICU had better weight gain than those who did not. In addition, infants who received passive movement of their limbs had better weight gain and also an increase in bone density. Weight gain was also associated with shorter hospital stays (Field, Diego, & Hernandez-Reif, 2010).

Based on the infant's individual needs, therapists may be involved through consultation to the family and nurses or by providing direct physical therapy intervention. The physical therapy plan of care is individualized based on the infant's needs, as well as the needs of the family. The physical therapy plan changes as the infant grows, develops, and stabilizes.

Using the clinical decision-making algorithm for intervention in the NICU, the physical therapist develops a plan based on goals developed from the examination and evaluation (Sweeney et al., 2009). Interventions are implemented based on the systems: autonomic, motor, behavioral state, and attention-interaction. Interventions include education and consultation and procedural interventions provided by the physical therapist, family, and nurses. The physical therapist can provide direct handling to the infant to address impairments in body structures and function, limitations in activity, and restrictions in participation (Sweeney et al., 2009) (Fig. 15.4).

Controversy exists over the effects of stimulation in the NICU (Field et al., 1986; Gorski, Hole, Leonard, & Martin, 1983; Leib, Benfield, & Guidubaldi, 1980; Long, Lucey, & Philip, 1980; Long, Philip, & Lucey, 1980; Scarr-Salapatek & Williams, 1973). Research from the 1980s identified harmful effects associated with stimulation and the need for careful monitoring of infants in the NICU (Gorski et al., 1983; Long, Lucey, & Philip, 1980; Long, Philip, & Lucey, 1980). Long, Philip, and Lucey (1980) reported a correlation between hypoxemia and excessive handling of LBW infants. Drops in $TcPO_2$ were reduced with careful monitoring. They also found that sudden noises caused agitation and crying, which lead to hypoxemia and increases in intracranial pressure, heart rate, and respiratory rate. Within 5 minutes of chest physical therapy and close social interaction, Gorski and colleagues (1983) reported significant increases in subtle and gross behavioral and physiological distress in stable neonates.

In contrast to these studies reporting the negative physiological changes associated with sensory stimulation,

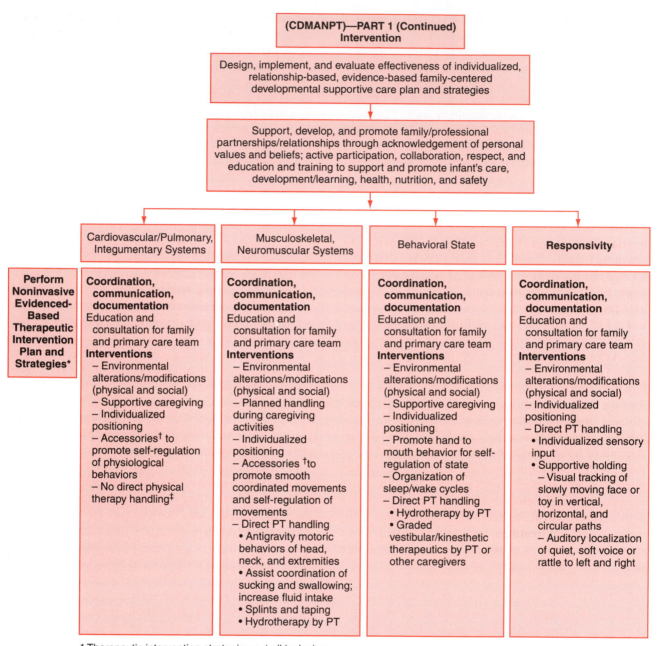

Figure 15.4 Clinical decision-making algorithm for neonatal physical therapy practice: Part 1: Intervention. *(Reprinted from Sweeney, J.K., Heriza, C.B., & Blanchard Y. (2009). Neonatal physical therapy, Part I: Clinical competencies and neonatal intensive care unit clinical training models. Pediatric Physical Therapy, 21, 304, with permission.)*

other studies exist to support sensory programs for infants in the NICU (Field et al., 1986; Fucile & Gisel, 2010; Leib et al., 1980; Scarr-Salapatek & Williams, 1973). Infants receiving sensory programs, including a combination of visual, tactile, kinesthetic, and auditory stimulation, had greater weight gain, increased motor activity, increased levels of alertness, greater developmental advantage, and shorter hospital stays (Field et al., 1986; Leib et al., 1980; Scarr-Salapatek & Williams, 1973). Infants who received an oral or tactile-kinesthetic intervention, or a combination of the two, had greater weight gain or motor function than a control group of infants (Fucile & Gisel, 2010).

There is evidence to support physical therapy intervention in the form of developmental activities and positioning (Bjornson et al., 1992; Girolami & Campbell, 1994; Kelly, Palisano, & Wolfson, 1989; Lekskulchai & Cole, 2001). Two studies support the use of positioning and developmental interventions (Bjornson et al., 1992; Kelly, Palisano, & Wolfson, 1989). Kelly and colleagues (1989) showed that healthy preterm infants responded to developmental activities with increasing heart rate and no changes in oxygen saturation (SaO_2). Bjornson and colleagues (1992) studied the effects of body position on the SaO_2 of preterm infants with respiratory distress syndrome who were ventilated. Results of the study showed that SaO_2 remained within clinically acceptable levels in supine, sidelying, and prone positions, with prone producing a greater SaO_2. A study by Girolami and Campbell (1994) supports a specific type of physical therapy intervention and its effect on motor and postural control. Results of this study support neurodevelopmental treatment as an effective method for improving motor and postural control in infants born preterm, without harmful effects on physiological variables and poor weight gain. The positive effects of an intervention program designed specifically to facilitate motor development with parent participation on the motor and postural control of preterm infants has been demonstrated (Lekskulchai & Cole, 2001).

Studies also support involving parents in their infant's care (Melnyk et al., 2006; Parker, Zahr, Cole, & Brecht, 1992; Rice, 1977). Parker and colleagues (1992) used a program of education and training individualized around the infant's behavioral and developmental functioning. Positive benefits of parent education were shown for mothers of low socioeconomic status (Parker et al., 1992). Rice (1977) used a structured program of tactile-kinesthetic stimulation involving parent participation and showed significant progress in terms of weight gain, neurological development, and mental

development. Melnyk and colleagues (2006) provided parents with information on the appearance and behavioral characteristics of preterm infants and how best to implement this information in their parenting. Parents who received this information reported less stress and depression compared to the control group. In addition, infants whose parents received the information were discharged home earlier than the control group infants.

Positioning

Proper positioning is one intervention that is provided to the infant and through education to caregivers. Proper positioning encourages flexion, midline orientation, and symmetry, enhances self-calming behaviors, and promotes ease of breathing (Fig. 15.5). Proper positioning can facilitate visual and auditory development and the development of head control. Physical therapists work with the nursing staff and parents to provide proper positioning to infants. In supine, the goal of positioning is to promote hip and knee flexion, promote midline orientation, and prevent scapular retraction. Positioning devices may be used to help position an infant. Evidence supports the use of positioning devices to encourage flexion and midline positioning of the head (Vaivre-Douret & Golse, 2007). These may include blanket rolls, specialized snuggles or buntings, and special beanbags. Arms may be positioned with rolls along the sides of the trunk to prevent scapular retraction and promote elbow flexion with hands together or at midline. Rolls may also be used to provide hip and knee flexion and prevent hip abduction and external rotation. Prone positioning provides maximal support to the chest wall and anchors the respiratory muscles and rib cage, which helps ease breathing (Bjornson et al., 1992). Prone positioning also facilitates

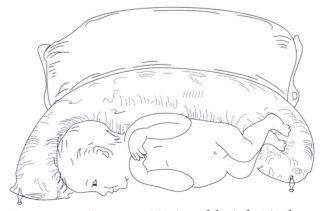

Figure 15.5 Proper positioning of the infant in the NICU.

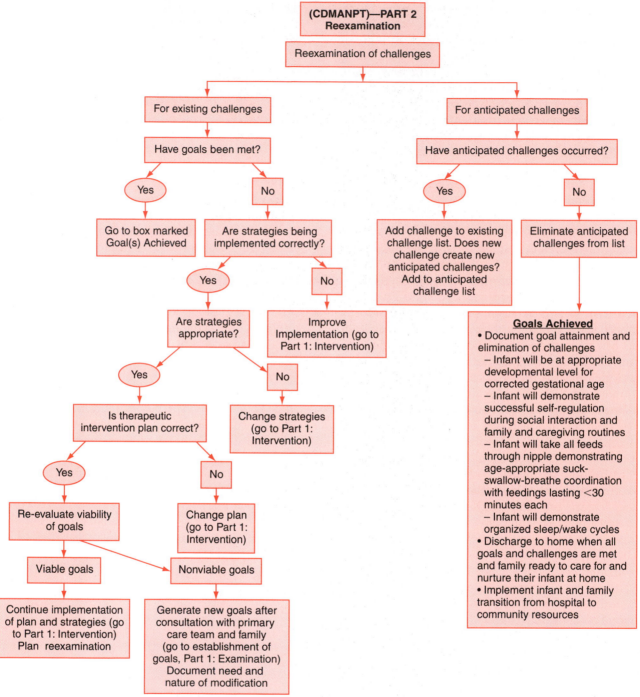

Figure 15.6 Clinical decision-making algorithm for neonatal physical therapy practice: reexamination.

flexion and aids in the development of postural muscles as infants lift and clear their face.

Sidelying facilitates flexion and is a nice position for infants to bring hands together and hands to mouth. Often infants develop a head preference to one side while in the NICU. Problem solving and educating best positioning with family and nursing is important to encourage the infant to turn to the opposite side. Frequently, this is done by turning the bed around to have the head of the bed at the opposite side.

Educating families in proper sleep positions at home is also important. The AAP recommends that infants sleep in the supine position (Gibson, Cullen, Spinner, Rankin, & Spitzer, 1995). The prone position is not recommended due to correlations between prone sleeping and sudden infant death syndrome (SIDS). Sidelying is also not recommended because infants are more likely to roll from their side onto their stomachs, placing them at risk for SIDS (Li et al., 2003; Moreno, Furtner, & Rivara, 2009). Since the Back to Sleep campaign began in 1994, supine sleeping has increased and prone sleeping has decreased for all infants (Colson et al., 2009). Although the trend has shown a decrease in prone sleeping, fewer African American infants are placed in supine to sleep. Since 2001, supine sleeping has reached a plateau, with concern that the trend may be heading in the opposite direction (Colson et al., 2009). Infants born prematurely have a higher incidence of SIDS when sleeping in prone than infants born full-term (Saiki et al., 2009). Infants in the NICU are placed in a variety of positions to sleep, including prone with consistent monitoring. It is recommended that infants begin sleeping supine in the NICU before discharge. Parents must be instructed to follow the Back to Sleep guidelines when their infant is discharged home and be instructed in the benefits of *tummy time* when the infant is awake and being watched.

Range of Motion/Active Movement

Some infants need a program for ROM to maintain or increase passive ROM. A ROM program can be initiated by the physical therapist and the nursing staff that families can then implement on a daily basis. Infants with osteopenia may benefit from ROM performed by therapists, nursing, and family multiple times a day. Some infants may need a program to improve or encourage active movement of the extremities. This may be achieved through facilitation of self-calming behaviors such as hand to mouth or hand to midline. Tactile stimulation to facilitate active movement may also be used. Proper positioning to promote antigravity movement is another method to increase active movement.

Reexamination and Discharge Planning

Physical therapists are continuously reevaluating infants during their interventions. The plan of care for infants in the NICU is dynamic, changing as the infant grows and changes. Sweeney and colleagues (2009) developed an algorithm for clinical decision making for reexamination in the NICU (Fig. 15.6; see facing page). Physical therapists use reexamination to determine whether there are changes in the infant's status, whether goals and outcomes were achieved, and whether modification in the intervention plan is needed to achieve the goals. Recommendations should be made for follow-up at discharge. This may be a referral to an early intervention program or outpatient/home health physical therapy.

Summary

This chapter provides only a very general, brief overview of the NICU setting. The NICU provides highly specialized medical care to fragile infants. The physical therapist is an active member of the NICU team, providing examination, evaluation, and interventions to infants and their families. As a subspecialty of pediatric physical therapy, physical therapists working in the NICU must have specialized knowledge and training to provide safe and effective care. Neonatal physical therapy is one area where there is a potential to do harm. Physical therapists must keep up with current literature on interventions and development to provide the best services to infants and their families. Sweeney and colleagues (2009) developed clinical training models and proficiencies for therapists in the NICU. In addition, a decision-making algorithm was developed to provide a flow chart for clinical reasoning.

Mini-Case Study 15.1
Infant in the NICU

History: James was born at 26 weeks weighing 960 grams. James's mother is a 24-year-old whose pregnancy was uncomplicated until she presented to the hospital in labor. An emergency cesarean section was performed due to fetal distress. James was limp at birth with no respiratory effort. Apgar scores were 3 at 1 minute, 5 at 5 minutes, and 8 at 10 minutes. James was intubated in the delivery room and remained on the ventilator for 6 weeks. Multiple attempts were made to wean him from the ventilator. James remained on supplemental oxygen for 5 weeks after he was extubated. His head ultrasound revealed a bilateral grade II IVH.

Examination: James was referred to physical therapy at 21 days of life (29 weeks' postconceptional age). The physical therapy examination included a chart review to obtain prenatal, birth, and medical history, a systems review, and tests and measures. At the time of the examination, James was asleep in the prone position in an isolette and was orally intubated. His heart rate at rest was 147 beats per

Continued

minute, respiratory rate of 42 breaths per minute, and oxygen saturation of 93%. James was pink and appeared comfortable. There was no visible edema or scars. He had a central line in his right forearm and a nasogastric tube for feedings. James's nurse reported that he did not tolerate a lot of handling and preferred to be positioned in prone. While the therapist was in the room, James's nurse changed his diaper. When hands were placed on him, he displayed some stress signs, but maintained his vitals within acceptable ranges. His nurse repositioned him in supine for the diaper change. With the change in position, James's oxygen decreased to the low 70s and he displayed multiple stress signs. James's nurse responded to his stress signs by bringing his hands and legs in close to his body. James slowly increased his oxygen saturation, but continued to remain in the 70s. His nurse increased his oxygen to help him return to more acceptable levels. His nurse identified position changes and routine caregiving as a challenge for James in his ability to maintain his vitals within acceptable limits and maintain a calm state. She said he was also a little stiff when she moved him around.

After observing his nurse during the diaper change and discussing James with her, the physical therapist decided to continue with the hands-on portion of the examination. When the therapist placed her hands on James, he displayed an increase in stress signs such as straightening extremities with tension, finger splay, tremors, arching, and a decrease in oxygen saturation to the low 70s again. The therapist brought his arms and legs in close to his body and used gentle deep pressure to help him calm, and slowly James's oxygen saturation returned to acceptable levels. The therapist waited until James was calm and had maintained his oxygen saturation at an acceptable level of greater than 85% for several minutes before proceeding. ROM, tone, and primitive reflexes were assessed. James had full ROM in his extremities with tightness at end range of shoulder flexion and hip flexion bilaterally. His tone was increased in his extremities. Many of the primitive reflexes were absent at this time. James did have a palmar grasp bilaterally.

Through observation both during caregiving and during the physical therapy examination, the physical therapist noted any active movements and stress signs. James showed an increase in stress signs with handling, which included finger splay, stop signs, straightening extremities with tension, and arching. James did not display self-calming behaviors. With facilitation from the therapist, James was able to bring hands to midline and hands to mouth for calming. He also calmed with containment of his extremities into a flexed position and gentle deep pressure at his head and bottom. Sucking on a pacifier also helped James to self-calm. James required frequent rest breaks to maintain a calm state during the examination.

James displayed minimal active movements. The movements observed by the physical therapist were global and jerky, and lower extremity movement was primarily into extension. Without positioning devices, James's upper extremities were in a position of scapular retraction with shoulder abduction and external rotation. In this position, James displayed limited antigravity movement in his upper extremities.

James briefly opened his eyes during the examination but did not transition to an awake, alert state. When presented with an auditory or visual stimulus, James displayed an increase in stress signs. James received all feedings through his nasogastric tube. He would suck on a pacifier during his feedings.

No family was present during the examination. James's parents do not visit very often. They are married, have 2 other young children at home, and live 2 hours away. His mother does not have a lot of help with her other children and does not have a car to drive to the hospital. Dad cannot take off from work as a mechanic because of financial reasons. They do have all the necessary baby equipment for James. When James is ready, he will be discharged home. Since James's parents were not present during the examination, the physical therapist called his mother at home. The role of physical therapy was explained to her. She was asked if there were any strengths or challenges that she has identified on any of her visits to the hospital. Her biggest concern was that he did not like to be touched. Her goal was to hold him without James's oxygen levels dropping.

Physical therapy reexamination occurs on an ongoing basis. As James grows and develops, the plan of care will change according to his needs and the needs of his family. After each reexamination, the therapist will call James's mother and update her on how he is doing in terms of his physical therapy goals.

Summary of Examination and Evaluation

Limitations in body structure: Tightness at end range of hip flexion and shoulder flexion. Increased tone in all extremities.

Limitations to activities: Poor tolerance to handling and stimulation with signs of stress. Unable to self-calm without facilitation.

Strengths: Full ROM in all extremities. Brief transition to awake state.

Physical Therapy Diagnosis

Practice Pattern 5C: Impaired Motor Function and Sensory Integrity Associated with Nonprogressive Disorders of the Central Nervous System—Congenital Origin or Acquired in Infancy or Childhood (American Physical Therapy Association, 2001).

Physical Therapy Plan of Care

The physical therapy plan of care will change with James's changing needs. As James grows and develops, the plan of care will be modified. Initially, the physical therapist will provide less direct intervention, but as James grows, the physical therapist will increase the frequency of intervention.

Parent Education: Instruct parents on how to perform gentle ROM, how to read their infant's behavioral cues, gentle handling techniques, and positioning. As James gets older and closer to discharge home, developmental activities can be provided to parents to incorporate into play at home. Since James's parents are not able to visit often, the therapist will set up a time to meet with them when they are planning to visit.

Positioning: Instruct nursing and family when available on proper positioning to encourage midline position and flexion in supine and prone, and proper positioning in sidelying to encourage flexion and hands together. Proper positioning can also help to promote self-calming.

Gentle ROM and Handling: ROM should be performed to decrease the tightness noted at the end range of shoulder flexion and hip flexion. ROM can be carried out daily by nursing and family once instructed.

State Transitions: Facilitate state transitions from sleep state to awake state. As James transitions to an awake state, the therapist can help to promote transitions to an awake alert state during treatment. When James is able to transition to and maintain an awake alert state, activities can be performed to promote visual tracking.

Developmental Activities: As James gets older, the physical therapist will begin working on increasing head and trunk control in all positions.

Discharge Plan

At discharge, James will be referred to an early intervention program. The early intervention program services infants from birth to 3 years of age and will provide these services in the home. The therapists in the early intervention program will evaluate his development and provide follow-up services. James will also be referred to the Newborn Follow-Up Clinic. This clinic has a physical therapist who will reexamine James after discharge home. The therapist will be able to follow up on the early intervention services James is to receive.

DISCUSSION QUESTIONS

1. Why is correcting for gestational age important? Until what age should you continue to correct for gestational age?

2. What is the recommended position for the infant while sleeping at home? How might this position for sleeping affect the infant's motor development?

3. Explain the importance of flexor muscle tone in the neonate. Why is positioning the infant in flexion important for development of movement?

4. What are some behavioral and physiological signs of stress used by the infant? Why is it important for the physical therapist and other caregivers to adapt the infant's care plan to minimize stress?

5. What is developmentally supportive care in the NICU? How does developmentally supportive care promote neonatal recovery?

6. What is periventricular leukomalacia? Discuss the correlation between the incidence of premature birth and periventricular leukomalacia with the outcome of cerebral palsy.

Recommended Readings

Als, H., & Gilkerson, L. (1997). The role of relationship-based developmentally supportive newborn intensive care in strengthening outcome of preterm infants. *Seminars in Perinatology, 21*(3), 178–189.

Kahn-D'Angelo, L., Blanchard, Y., McManus, B. (2012). The special care nursery. In S.K. Campbell, R.J. Palisano, & M.N. Orlin (Eds.). *Physical therapy for children* (4th ed., pp. 903–943). St. Louis: Elsevier Saunders.

Neonatology on the Web. Available from http://www.neonatology.org/index.html

Sweeney, J.K., Heriza, C.B., & Blanchard, Y. (2009). Neonatal physical therapy. Part I: Clinical competencies and neonatal intensive care unit clinical training models. *Pediatric Physical Therapy, 21*, 296–307.

Sweeney, J.K., Heriza, C.B., Blanchard, Y., & Dusing, S.C. (2010). Neonatal physical therapy. Part II: Practice frameworks and evidence-based practice guidelines. *Pediatric Physical Therapy, 22*, 2–16.

Sweeny, J.K., & Swanson, M.W. (2007). Low birth weight infants: Neonatal care and follow-up. In D.A. Umphred (Ed.). *Neurological rehabilitation* (5th ed.). St. Louis, MO: Mosby.

Vergara, E.R., & Bigsby, R. (2004). *Developmental & therapeutic interventions in the NICU.* Baltimore: Paul H. Brookes.

Wolf, L.S., & Glass, R.P. (1992). *Feeding and swallowing disorders in infancy: Assessment and management.* San Antonio, TX: Therapy Skill Builders.

References

Abad, F., Diaz, N.M, Domenech, E., Robayna, M., & Rico, J. (1996). Oral sweet solution reduces pain-related behaviour in preterm infants. *Acta Paediatrica, 85*, 854–858.

Aicardi, J. (1992). Neurological diseases in the perinatal period. In J. Aicardi (Ed.), *Clinics in developmental medicine* (pp. 47–105). New York: Cambridge University Press.

Als, H., Lawhon, G., Brown, E., Gibes, R., Duffy, F.H., McAnulty, G., & Blickman, J.G. (1986). Individualized behavioral and environmental care for the very low birth-weight preterm infant at high risk for bronchopulmonary dysplasia: Neonatal intensive care unit and developmental outcome. *Pediatrics, 78*, 1123–1132.

Als, H., Lawhon, G., Duffy, F.H., McAnulty, G.B., Gibes-Grossman, R., & Blickman, J. (1994). Individualized developmental care for the very low birth-weight preterm infant: Medical and neurofunctional effects. *JAMA, 272*, 853–858.

American Academy of Pediatrics (AAP) Committee on Environmental Health. (1997). Noise: A hazard for the fetus and newborn. *Pediatrics, 100*, 724–727.

American Academy of Pediatrics (AAP) Committee on Fetus and Newborn. (2004). Levels of neonatal care. *Pediatrics, 114*, 1341–1347.

American Physical Therapy Association (APTA). (2001). Guide to Physical Therapist Practice (2nd ed.). *Physical Therapy, 81*(1), 347–364.

Andrews, K.A., & Fitzgerald, M. (1994). The cutaneous withdrawal reflex in human neonates: Sensitization, receptive fields, and the effects of contralateral stimulation. *Pain, 56*, 95–101.

Bayram, M., Kayserili, E., Agin, H., Bayram, E., & Unalp, A. (2008). Evaluation of short-term neurodevelopmental outcomes in the premature patients with periventricular-intraventricular hemorrhage. *Journal of Pediatric Neurology, 6*, 351–356.

Bennett, F.C. (1999). Developmental outcome. In G.B. Avery, M. Fletcher, & M.G. MacDonald (Eds.), *Neonatology: Pathophysiology and management of the newborn* (pp. 1479–1497). Philadelphia: Lippincott Williams & Wilkins.

Bjornson, K.F., Deitz, J.C., Blackburn, S.T., Billingsley, F., Garcia, J., & Hays, R. (1992). The effect of body position on the oxygen saturation of ventilated preterm infants. *Pediatric Physical Therapy, 4*, 109–115.

Brazelton, T.B. (1984). Neonatal Behavioral Assessment Scale (2nd ed.). *Clinics in Developmental Medicine, No. 88.* Philadelphia: J.B. Lippincott.

Brown, L.D., & Heermann, J.A. (1997). The effect of developmental care on preterm infant outcome. *Applied Nursing Research, 10*(4), 190–197.

Candy, E.J., & Hoon, A.H. (1996). Neuroradiology. In A.J. Capute & P.J. Accardo (Eds.), *Developmental disabilities in infancy and childhood: Vol. I. Neurodevelopmental diagnosis and treatment* (2nd ed., pp. 393–422). Baltimore: Paul H. Brookes.

Colson, E.R., Rybin, D., Smith, L.A., Colton, T., Lister, G., & Corwin, M.J. (2009). Trends and factors associated with infant sleeping position: The national infant sleep position study, 1993–2007. *Archives of Pediatrics & Adolescent Medicine, 163*(12), 1122–1128.

Darcy, A.E. (2009). Complications of the late preterm infant. *Journal of Perinatal & Neonatal Nursing, 23*(1), 78–86.

Duncan, C.C., & Ment, L.R. (1993). Intraventricular hemorrhage and prematurity. *Neurosurgical Clinics of North America, 4*, 727–734.

Dunst, C.J., Johanson, C., Trivette, S.M., & Hamby, D. (1991). Family-oriented early intervention policies and practices: Family-centered or not? *Exceptional Parent, 58*, 115–126.

Engle, W.A., Tomashek, K.M., Wallman, C., & the Committee on Fetus and Newborn. (2007). "Late-preterm" infants: A population at risk. *Pediatrics, 120*, 1390–1401.

Field, T., Diego, M., & Hernandez-Reif, M. (2010). Preterm infant massage therapy research: A review. *Infant Behavior and Development, 33*, 115–124.

Field, T.M., Schanberg, S.M., Scafidi, F., Bauer, C.R., Vega-Lahr, N., Garcia, R., Nystrom, J., & Kuhn, C.M. (1986). Tactile/kinesthetic stimulation effects on preterm neonates. *Pediatrics, 77*, 654–658.

Ford, J.W. (2006). Neonatal ECMO: Current controversies and trends. *Neonatal Network, 25*(4), 229–238.

Foulder-Hughes, L.A., & Cooke, R.W.I. (2003). Motor, cognitive and behavioral disorders in children born very preterm. *Developmental Medicine and Child Neurology, 45*, 97–103.

Fucile, S. & Gisel, E.G. (2010). Sensorimotor interventions improve growth and motor function in preterm infants. *Neonatal Network, 29*(6), 359–366.

Gibson, E., Cullen, J.A., Spinner, S., Rankin, K., & Spitzer, A.R. (1995). Infant sleep position following new AAP guidelines. *Pediatrics, 96*(1), 69–72.

Girolami, G.L., & Campbell, S.K. (1994). Efficacy of a neuro-developmental treatment program to improve motor control in infants born prematurely. *Pediatric Physical Therapy, 6*, 175–184.

Gorski, P.A., Hole, W.T., Leonard, C.H., & Martin, J.A. (1983). Direct computer recordings of premature infants and nursery care: Distress following two interventions. *Pediatrics, 72,* 198–202.

Griffin, T. (2006). Family-centered care in the NICU. *Journal of Perinatal and Neonatal Nursing, 20*(1), 98–102.

Hamrick, S.E.G., Miller, S.P., Leonard, C., Glidden, D.V., Goldstein, R., Ramaswamy, V., Piecuch, R., & Ferriero, D.M. (2004). Trends in severe brain injury and neurodevelopmental outcome in premature newborn infants: The role of cystic periventricular leukomalacia. *Journal of Pediatrics, 145,* 593–599.

Harrison, H. (1993). The principles of family-centered neonatal care. *Pediatrics, 92,* 643–650.

Johnson, B.H. (1990). The changing role of families in health care. *Children's Health Care, 19,* 234–241.

Johnston, C.C., Stremler, R., Horton, L., & Friedman, A. (1999). Effect of repeated doses of sucrose during heel stick procedure in preterm neonates. *Biology of the Neonate, 75*(3), 160–166.

Kahn-D'Angelo, L. (1995). The special care nursery. In S.K. Campbell (Ed.), *Physical therapy for children* (pp. 787–822). Philadelphia: W.B. Saunders.

Kahn-D'Angelo, L., & Rose, R.A.U. (2006). The special care nursery. In S.K. Campbell, D.W. Vander Linden, & R.J. Palisano (Eds.), *Physical therapy for children* (3rd ed., pp. 1053–1097). St. Louis: Saunders Elsevier.

Kelly, M.K., Palisano, R.J., & Wolfson, M.R. (1989). Effects of a developmental physical therapy program on oxygen saturation and heart rate in preterm infants. *Physical Therapy, 69,* 467–474.

Kilbride, H.W., & Daily, D.K. (1998). Survival and subsequent outcome to five years of age for infants with birth weights less than 801 grams born from 1983 to 1989. *Journal of Perinatology, 18*(2), 102–106.

Laptook, A.R., O'Shea, T.M., Shankaran, S., Bhaskar, B., & NICHD Neonatal Network. (2005). Adverse neurodevelopmental outcomes among extremely low birth weight infants with a normal head ultrasound: Prevalence and antecedents. *Pediatrics, 115,* 673–680.

Lasky, R.E., & Williams, A.L. (2009). Noise and light exposures for extremely low birth weight newborns during their stay in the neonatal intensive care unit. *Pediatrics, 123,* 540–546.

Lawhon, G., & Hedlund, R.E. (2008). Newborn individualized developmental care and assessment program training and education. *Journal of Perinatal & Neonatal Nursing, 22*(2), 133–144.

Leib, S.A., Benfield, D.G., & Guidubaldi, J. (1980). Effects of early intervention and stimulation on the preterm infant. *Pediatrics, 66,* 83–90.

Lekskulchai, R., & Cole, J. (2001). Effect of a developmental program on motor performance in infants born preterm. *Australian Journal of Physiotherapy, 47,* 169–176.

Li, D.K., Petitti, D.B., Willinger, J., McMahon, R., Odouli, R., Vu, H., & Hoffman, H.J. (2003). Infant sleeping position and the risk of sudden infant death syndrome in California, 1997–2000. *American Journal of Epidemiology, 157*(5), 446–455.

Linder, N., Haskin, O., Levit, O., Klinger, G., Prince, T., Naor, N., Turner, P., Karmazyn, B., & Sirota, L. (2003). Risk factors for intraventricular hemorrhage in very low birth weight premature infants: A retrospective case-control study. *Pediatrics, 111*(5), e590–e595.

Long, J.G., Lucey, J.F., & Philip, A.G.S. (1980). Noise and hypoxemia in the intensive care nursery. *Pediatrics, 65,* 143–145.

Long, J.G., Philip, A.G.S., & Lucey, J.F. (1980). Excessive handling as a cause of hypoxemia. *Pediatrics, 65,* 203–207.

Mantovani, J.F., & Powers, J. (1991). Brain injury in preterm infants: Patterns on cranial ultrasound, their relationship to outcome, and the role of developmental intervention in the NICU. *Infants and Young Children, 4*(2), 20–32.

Maone, T.R., Mattes, R.D., Bernbaum, J.C., & Beauchamp, G.K. (1990). A new method for delivering a taste without fluids to preterm and term infants. *Developmental Psychobiology, 23,* 179–191.

McCarton, C.M., Wallace, I.F., Divon, M., & Vaughan, H.G. (1996). Cognitive and neurologic development of the premature, small for gestational age infant through age 6: Comparison by birth weight and gestational age. *Pediatrics, 98*(6), 1167–1178.

McGrath, M.M., Sullivan, M.C., Lester, B.M., & Oh, W. (2000). Longitudinal neurologic follow-up in neonatal intensive care unit survivors with various neonatal morbidities. *Pediatrics, 106*(6), 1397–1405.

Melnyk, B.M., Feinstein, N.F., Alpert-Gillis, L., Fairbanks, E., Crean, H.F., Sinkin, R.A., Stone, P.W., Small, L., Tu, X., & Gross, S.J. (2006). Reducing premature infants' length of stay and improving parents' mental health outcomes with the creating opportunities for parent empowerment (COPE) neonatal intensive care unit program: A randomized, controlled trial. *Pediatrics, 118,* e1414–e1427.

Moreno, M.A., Furtner, F., & Rivara, F.P. (2009). Infant sleep position: Back to sleep. *Archives of Pediatrics & Adolescent Medicine, 163*(2), 1168.

Moster, D., Lie, R.T., Irgens, L.M., Bjerkedal, T., & Markestad, T. (2001). The association of Apgar score with subsequent death and cerebral palsy: A population-based study in term infants. *Journal of Pediatrics, 138*(6), 798–803.

Parker, S.J., Zahr, L.K., Cole, J.G., & Brecht, M.L. (1992). Outcome after developmental intervention in the neonatal intensive care unit for mothers of preterm infants with low socioeconomic status. *Journal of Pediatrics, 120*(5), 780–785.

Patra, K.P., Wilson-Costello, D., Taylor, H.G., Mercuri-Minich, N., & Hack, M. (2006). Grades I–II intraventricular hemorrhage in extremely low birth weight infants: Effects on neurodevelopment. *Journal of Pediatrics, 149,* 169–173.

Prince, W.L., Horns, K.M., Latta, T., & Gerstmann, D.R. (2004). Treatment of neonatal pain without a gold standard: The case for caregiving interventions and sucrose administration. *Neonatal Network, 23*(4), 33–45.

Rapport, M.J.K. (1992). A descriptive analysis of the role of physical and occupational therapists in the neonatal intensive care unit. *Pediatric Physical Therapy, 4,* 172–178.

Rice, R.D. (1977). Neurophysiological development in premature infants following stimulation. *Developmental Psychology, 13,* 69–76.

Rivkin, M.J. (1997). Hypoxic-ischemic brain injury in the term newborn: Neuropathology, clinical aspects, and neuroimaging. *Clinics in Perinatology, 24,* 607–625.

Rosenbaum, P., King, S., Law, M., King, G., & Evans, J. (1998). Family-centered service: A conceptual framework and research review. In M. Law (Ed.), *Family-centered assessment and intervention in pediatric rehabilitation* (pp. 1–20). New York: Haworth Press.

Saiki, T., Rao, H., Landolfo, F., Smith, A.P.R., Hannam, S., Rafferty, G.F., & Greenough, A. (2009). Sleeping position, oxygenation and lung function in prematurely born infants studied post term. *Archives of Disease in Childhood: Fetal and Neonatal Edition, 94,* F133–F137.

Scarr-Salapatek, S. & Williams, M.L. (1973). The effects of early stimulation on low-birth weight infants. *Child Development, 44,* 94–101.

Shelton, T.L., & Stepanek, J.S. (1995). Excerpts from family-centered care for children needing specialized health and developmental services. *Pediatric Nursing, 21,* 362–364.

Stevens, B.J., & Johnston, C.C. (1994). Physiological responses of premature infants to painful stimulus. *Nursing Research, 43*(4), 226–231.

Stevens, B., Taddio, A., Ohlsson, A., & Einarson, T. (1997). The efficacy of sucrose for relieving procedural pain in neonates: A systematic review and meta-analysis. *Acta Paediatrica, 86,* 837–842

Sweeney, J.K. (1986). Physiologic adaptation of neonates to neurological assessment. *Physical and Occupational Therapy in Pediatrics, 6*(3/4), 155–169.

Sweeney, J.K. (1989). Physiological and behavioral effects of neurological assessment in preterm and full-term neonates (abstract). *Physical and Occupational Therapy in Pediatrics, 9*(3), 144–146.

Sweeney, J.K., Heriza, C.B., & Blanchard, Y. (2009). Neonatal physical therapy. Part I: Clinical competencies and neonatal intensive care unit clinical training models. *Pediatric Physical Therapy, 21,* 296–307.

Sweeney, J.K., Heriza, C.B., Blanchard, Y., & Dusing, S.C. (2010). Neonatal physical therapy. Part II: Practice frameworks and evidence-based practice guidelines. *Pediatric Physical Therapy, 22,* 2–16.

Taylor, H.G., Klein, N., Schatschneider, C., & Hack, M. (1998). Predictors of early school age outcomes in very low birth weight children. *Developmental and Behavioral Pediatrics, 19*(4), 235–243.

Thomas, K.A., & Uran, A. (2007). How the NICU environment sounds to a preterm infant: Update. *American Journal of Maternal Child Nursing, 32*(4), 250–253.

Tulenko, D.R. (2004). An update on ECMO. *Neonatal Network, 23*(4), 11–18.

Ullenhag, A., Persson, K., & Nyqvist, K.H. (2009). Motor performance in very preterm infants before and after implementation of the newborn individualized developmental care and assessment programme in a neonatal intensive care unit. *Acta Paediatrica, 98,* 947–952.

Vaivre-Douret, L., & Golse, B. (2007). Comparative effects of 2 positional supports on neurobehavioral and postural development in preterm neonates. *Journal of Perinatal & Neonatal Nursing, 21*(4), 323–330.

Vergani, P., Locatelli, A., Doria, V., Assi, F., Paterlini, G., Pezzullo, J.C., & Ghidini, A. (2004). *Obstetrics and Gynecology, 104,* 225–231.

Vergara, E.R., & Bigsby, R. (2004). *Developmental & therapeutic interventions in the NICU* (pp. 59–75, 97–113). Baltimore: Paul H. Brookes.

Volpe, J.J. (1995). *Neurology of the newborn* (3rd ed.). Philadelphia: W.B. Saunders Company.

Volpe, J.J. (1997). Brain injury in the premature infant: Neuropathology, clinical aspects, pathogenesis, and prevention. *Clinics in Perinatology, 24,* 567–587.

Volpe, J.J. (1998). Neurologic outcome of prematurity. *Archives of Neurology, 55,* 297–300.

Walden, M., Penticuff, J.H., Stevens, B., Lotas, M.J., Kozinetz, C.A., Clark, A, & Avant, K.C. (2001). Responses of preterm neonates to pain. *Advances in Neonatal Care, 1*(2), 94–106.

Walden, R.V., Taylor, S.C., Hansen, N.I., Poole, W.K., Stoll, B.J., Abuelo, D., Vohr, B.R. (2007). Major congenital anomalies place extremely low birth weight infants at higher risk for poor growth and developmental outcomes. *Pediatrics, 120,* e1512–e1519.

Weisglas-Kuperus, N., Baerts, W., Smrkovsky, M., & Sauer, P.J.J. (1993). Effects of biological and social factors on the cognitive development of very low birth weight children. *Pediatrics, 92,* 658–665.

CHAPTER 16

Rehabilitation Settings

—Heather Atkinson, PT, DPT, NCS

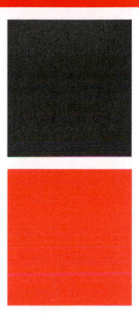

Pediatric rehabilitation is a unique and important facet of the health-care system, and physical therapy plays a significant role. As a member of the interdisciplinary team, the physical therapist provides comprehensive care to both children and families with the ultimate goal of maximal recovery and function in life. To be successful with this extraordinary opportunity, physical therapists must possess not only the skill to deliver family-centered, culturally competent, and age-appropriate care, but also the fundamental knowledge and ability to make evidence-based clinical decisions that drive best practice and advance the field of pediatric health care and rehabilitation.

Core values central to rehabilitation have historically included the promotion of overall happiness with the ultimate goal of increased patient freedom or maximized independence. In more recent years, with the propensity of managed health care, fairness and equitable access to treatment has also become a central core value, sparking many ongoing ethical debates about frequency and duration of treatment (Dougherty, 1991; Reder, 2009). These ethical considerations arise as the philosophy in the rehabilitation field is shifting from compensation to recovery of function. While teaching compensatory techniques to a child with a new neurological injury may expedite the discharge process, taking the necessary time to focus on recovery of function could result in neuroplastic changes, with consequential improved long-term outcomes (Taub, 2002). As rehabilitation teams and payors struggle to determine the most cost-effective plans that will yield the best outcomes, physical therapists play a crucial role in advocating for their patients with the support of evidence-based plans of care and measurable outcomes.

Once a child has become medically stabilized, he or she will begin the journey of recovery. These journeys can take many forms, and may include admission to an acute rehabilitation setting, day hospital, or outpatient rehabilitation. Some children may receive outpatient services at a facility typically geared toward adults. While the principles of physical therapy remain the same despite age, specific and important nuances exist in the pediatric population that are important for all clinicians to consider when working with a pediatric client.

Pediatric Rehabilitation Settings

Pediatric rehabilitation may occur within the same hospital where the acute care was provided, but may also occur in a freestanding rehabilitation hospital. In a study of pediatric trauma facilities, Osberg and colleagues explored variables that triggered discharge to inpatient rehabilitation versus home (Osberg, DiScala, & Gans, 1990). Severity of injury and degree of impairment were major influencing factors in the decision to refer a child to inpatient rehabilitation; however, these authors also found that children were more likely to be admitted to inpatient rehabilitation if an onsite rehabilitation facility existed at the acute trauma center. While this is not always available, the authors suggest that the presence of an onsite rehabilitation facility should be external to the decision as to whether a child is appropriate for rehabilitation, and admission should be decided based on the child's individual needs and goals (Osberg et al., 1990). Physical therapists in acute-care centers may also advocate for the most appropriate placement based on their evaluation, prognosis, and established goals.

Once a child is admitted to inpatient rehabilitation, a diverse team of professionals will be dedicated to providing an intense level of care to the child and family. While the main focus in a critical care setting is achieving medical stability, the goal of rehabilitation is to restore function. Pediatric rehabilitation differs from that for adults in several ways.

Staff All staff are specially trained in the treatment of children. Many disciplines offer and encourage board certifications and ongoing professional development for this specialized population. A thorough understanding of all domains of development (motor, cognitive, language, social, and emotional) is necessary in order to effectively care for a child (see Table 16.1).

Delivery of Service While adult settings may have one therapist serving multiple patients at one time, pediatric settings demand 1:1 ratios due to the nature of the client. While individual therapy is typically 1:1, interdisciplinary

Table 16.1 Professional Development

Development of Expertise in Pediatric Rehabilitation

In a study of the development of expertise in pediatric rehabilitation therapists, King and colleagues examined the clinical decision-making abilities of novice, intermediate, and expert clinicians from the fields of physical, occupational, and speech therapy. The authors found three important characteristics unique to expert providers.

- First, expert clinicians possess a great deal of content knowledge. This includes a strong ability to approach the child and family holistically and see the big picture. Expert clinicians possess a broader sense of role and are driven to support, educate, and empower patients and families. Content knowledge unique to expert clinicians also includes the ability to prioritize what is most important to the family, and to refrain from personal judgments.

- A second characteristic defining expertise was a broad sense of self-awareness. The authors found that as expertise develops, both self-confidence and humility increase. Expert clinicians are also better able to define realistic expectations for themselves and their clients.

- Third, therapists considered to be expert clinicians were able to manufacture maximal client change. When probed in more detail, expert clinicians commonly employ the strategies of patient and family engagement, the selection of meaningful activities, and manageable treatment regimes to optimize patient outcome.

These three major distinctions between novice and expert clinicians suggest a multifaceted outline for professional development. Vehicles to facilitate the journey from novice to expert clinician must also be multifaceted and include more than training in clinical or technical skills. Professional development should also include the practice of self-reflection, seeking feedback, and requesting mentorship. As clinicians adopt a philosophy of deliberate practice and lifelong learning, improved long-term outcomes can be realized for children and families.

Source: King et al. (2007). The development of expertise in pediatric rehabilitation therapists: changes in approach, self-knowledge, and use of enabling and customizing strategies. *Developmental Neurorehabilitation*, *10*(3), 223–240.

groups are sometimes utilized as an adjunct to help meet other needs such as peer interaction. Groups may be arranged by age, such as teen or preschool recreation groups, or by function, such as a school or cognitive group, community group, and dining group.

Benefits Most insurance plans for children will provide inpatient rehabilitative care for as long as medically necessary. Outpatient benefits vary, and can range from full coverage to none at all. Several HMOs allow only 30 consecutive days of therapy per condition, per lifetime. This restriction can be devastating for a child with a new chronic disability, as a child's needs can change dramatically over the course of a lifetime. Therapists, social workers, and child advocates often work with the family to explore other options for coverage and alternative sources of funding. When impossible, the therapist is forced to choose the best time and manner to provide service.

Goals for Discharge The overall goal of any rehabilitation setting is to return the child to the least restrictive and fullest life possible. For children, this means returning to school and play activities. Typically, mobility and daily living goals for discharge from an inpatient rehabilitation setting are set at the level of contact guard to minimal assistance rather than independence, as children generally have a caregiver available to provide assistance at home. Occasionally, adolescents are admitted who were independent prior to admission and need to be independent upon discharge due to lack of family support. In these cases, the team will work with the insurance company to negotiate a longer admission.

Caregivers Typically, caregivers are encouraged to stay with their child throughout the admission, and many facilities offer the option of overnight stays. Therapists must recognize the supreme importance of family education and begin planning for transition to home and discharge from therapy from day one.

Environment Pediatric rehabilitation settings often have developmentally friendly decor and surroundings. Playrooms are often available, as well as electronic gaming stations to help pass the time while at rest.

Ethical Issues A therapist may encounter various ethical issues specific to caring for children and their families. Examples include the question of parental control versus the right of a child to make choices about his or her care, eligibility criteria for therapy and discharge, how to handle waiting lists, how to manage education regarding sexuality, and how to honestly convey negative information to families (Flett & Stoffell, 2003; Matthews, Meier, & Bartholome, 1990). The American Physical Therapy Association (APTA) offers a framework for ethical decision making that clinicians can use as a resource to discuss with a trusted mentor.

Similar to those for adults, several organizations exist to provide support, oversight, and education to rehabilitation facilities to ensure standardized and optimal care for children. The Joint Commission and the Commission on Accreditation of Rehabilitation Facilities (CARF) are accrediting bodies that demand ongoing excellence in patient safety and quality of care. Specific to children, the National Association of Children's Hospitals and Related Institutions (NACHRI) is a group dedicated to advocacy, education, research, and health promotion and also has an arm devoted to advancing public policy for children's health. Many other pediatric-focused groups exist to provide education and support for both professionals and families of children with disabilities. It is of great importance for physical therapists to use these organizations as a guide and resource so they can have a clear understanding of current trends and standards of practice in rehabilitation in order to most effectively and safely care for their patients.

Continuum of Care

Pediatric and adult health systems have a similar range in continuum of care; however, pediatric settings have some specific nuances that are important to consider.

Acute-Care Hospital Physical therapy begins in the acute-care setting, and therapists often work with both the acute-care team and the rehabilitation team to determine whether the child is a candidate for an inpatient rehabilitation admission. If the team believes the child would benefit from intensive therapy, acute-care physical therapists work with the family and other team members to generate goals for the rehabilitation admission. They also coordinate closely with therapists in the rehabilitation setting to facilitate a smooth transition of care. Please see Chapter 14 for details.

Inpatient Rehabilitation The inpatient rehabilitation unit serves children who are still dealing with major physical, sensory, language, and/or cognitive effects of a new injury or condition. These children need intensive therapy services and are not yet safe to go home. Children receive approximately 3 combined hours of occupational, speech, and physical therapy per day, 7 days per week. Children also go to other programs such as school, art therapy, music therapy, and psychological support. Caregivers and children receive comprehensive education on diagnosis, rehabilitation, coping, recovery, and future needs. Therapy is focused on recovery of lost function as well as compensatory techniques to allow safe and successful return to home and school (see Table 16.2).

Day Hospital Rehabilitation If the child is safe to return home but still requires intense therapy services, the child may be entered into a day hospital rehabilitation program. This program provides full-day therapy services 5 days per week but allows the child to be home at night

Table 16.2 Continuum of Rehabilitative Care

Setting	Acute Inpatient Rehabilitation	Day Hospital Rehabilitation	Outpatient Rehabilitation	Long-Term Care	Home Care
Therapy Need	Intense Daily 7x/week Child unsafe to go home	Intense Daily 5x/week Child safe to be home evenings and weekends, still requires high level of therapy	Moderate Nondaily 1–3x/week Episodes of care typically last 6–12 weeks	Low Nondaily 1x/week Services extremely limited	Low Nondaily 1x/week Services extremely limited
Admission Criteria	Must have at least 2 services (PT, OT, speech) Must tolerate intensive therapy	Must have at least 2 services (PT, OT, speech) Must tolerate intensive therapy	Typically has defined need for discipline specific service	Family unable to manage care at home; child unlikely to regain more function	Child typically must be bed bound
Goals for Discharge	Functioning at the level of contact guard to minimal assistance If dependent, family independent and safe with all needs	Functioning at the level of supervision to independence	Return to independence, sports, or community activities	Cessation of progress toward goals	Cessation of progress toward goals
Considerations	Most desirable during acute recovery phase	Not widely available; plans are sometimes limited	Coverage may be limited; plan to optimize benefit	Not widely available; limited therapy involvement	Not widely available for pediatrics; limited community resources

and on weekends. Children and family are able to practice new skills in real environments but also receive daily guidance, support, and progression from the rehabilitation team.

Outpatient Rehabilitation When the child is ready to return to school and home, he or she may still require outpatient therapy to improve skills and abilities. Typically outpatient services are provided at a frequency of 1 to 3 times per week for a defined period of time (Bailes, Reder, & Burch, 2008). Once goals are achieved, the child is discharged from outpatient rehabilitation. Sometimes children return several months later for another episode of outpatient rehabilitation if new goals arise due to a change in medical or functional status.

Long-Term Care Pediatric nursing homes or adult nursing homes with pediatric beds exist to care for children unable to be placed in a setting with their caregivers. Therapy services are often available on a very limited basis.

Home Care Home physical therapy in the adult population offers the opportunity to practice important functional skills in real environments; however, pediatric home physical therapy is a very limited resource. Typically children must be completely bed bound to qualify for services. Occasionally home therapy services can be justified for a child who is severely immunocompromised, but services are often very limited due to the lack of resources.

School Therapy (see Chapter 12) The rehabilitation team and the child's school may determine that the child requires PT, OT, and/or speech services in school. The goal of school physical therapy is to provide the child with access to education so he or she can have full participation, independent living, and economic self-sufficiency. School therapists can work only on the goals that the individualized education team determines are important for the child. Therefore, there might be some goals or skills for which therapy is also provided by the medical-based outpatient rehabilitation team.

Early Intervention (see Chapter 11) If the child is not yet in school (under 3 years of age), he or she may qualify for early intervention services. Early intervention is provided in the child's natural environment (home, daycare). Early intervention addresses overall development in all areas (gross motor, fine motor, language, cognitive, social, and emotional).

In today's managed care environment, children are receiving shorter lengths of stays in all environments, including the acute-care setting. Consequently, inpatient rehabilitation is admitting children with increased acuity and complexity of care. For a child who has suffered a severe brain injury, this may entail several weeks or months in a minimally conscious state, with decreased participation of the child and limited ability of the team to progress goals. If the child emerges into a more conscious state and is cognitively and behaviorally ready to engage in intensive rehabilitation, benefits may be exhausted or the family may no longer wish to commit to hospitalization. In these cases, transition to a day hospital is ideal to continue to allow an intense level of service. Alternatively, some children may be sent home from rehabilitation after caregivers are independent with the basics of dependent care, and then readmitted if the child begins to show change and readiness for intensive therapy.

Some children may not have day hospital coverage, and clinicians must be creative with their overall plan of care to optimize benefits. If a child is continuing to make rapid progress and requires daily skilled reassessment, the team and family may opt to maintain inpatient status until progress begins to slow.

Pediatric health care is a dynamic system. Children may enter the system at any point if new goals arise. Because children are constantly growing and developing, many benefit from a long-term follow-up plan. Many pediatric hospitals and rehabilitation settings have multidisciplinary clinics that reevaluate the child on a regular basis. Intervals may be every 3 to 6 months or annually, depending on the needs of the child. Typically a clinic visit will entail a reevaluation by a team of specialized professionals and may include a physician, nurse, physical, occupational, and speech therapist, social worker, and neuropsychologist. Each member of the team performs a screening evaluation and discusses what recommendations they may have for the family. Recommendations may include various medical interventions, another episode of therapy services, additional equipment, a change in the home regimen, or consultation with the school team. Long-term follow-up plans, whether performed by a team of professionals or a single clinician, is vital to adequately follow a child's growing needs.

The Team and Family-Centered Care

The team caring for a child in a rehabilitation setting is typically diverse and specialized, as noted in Table 16.3. There are a variety of individuals outside the hospital that also participate with the rehabilitation team including the community team, school team, and family. Teams can function together in a variety of ways and the relationship depends on the culture of the organization and the experience of the various members.

As discussed in Chapter 1, the *multidisciplinary* team consists of a variety of disciplines that work together to provide care. Expertise of each discipline is recognized and respected as the team works toward an overall goal for the child, but there is little collaboration between disciplines. The disciplines on an *interdisciplinary* team respect the expertise of each member but collaborate closely in evaluation, treatment, and the development of goals. There is close coordination and carryover of interventions among team members. For instance, the physical therapist will intimately know the goals of the occupational therapist and speech-language pathologist and will try to incorporate those strategies into physical therapy. There may be scheduled cotreats between disciplines, which provides a higher level of care to the child and also educates the different team members on activities that can be carried out in later treatment sessions. All aspects of care are closely coordinated and there are frequent meetings to ensure good continuity of care. On a *transdisciplinary* team, members educate each other on providing therapeutic interventions from each discipline and may choose a primary interventionist(s) to deliver care. Team members have a great deal of trust and allow role release. This model requires ongoing communication and teamwork.

In addition to the rehabilitation team, the community team, and the school team, the family also functions

Table 16.3 Potential Team Members for Each Child

The Rehab Team	The Community Team	The School Team	The Family
Attending physician	Insurance company	School district	Immediate caregivers
Consultant physician	Equipment vendors	Child study team	Extended family
Nursing staff	Primary care physician	Principal	Friends
Physical therapist	Community providers	Teacher	Neighbors
Occupational therapist	Community resources	School psychologist	Religious organizations
Speech-language	Charities	School nurse	
pathologist	Athletic coach	Education aide	
Psychologist	Orthotist	Physical therapist	
Neuropsychologist	Prosthetist	Occupational therapist	
Music therapist		Speech-language pathologist	
Art therapist			
Child life specialist			
Teacher			
Social worker			
Case manager			

as a team. Each family unit can be viewed as its own team, with different members taking on various roles. These roles can be significantly altered with a catastrophic injury, and the family will need much support from all involved to regain a new sense of the family unit's functioning after such an injury occurs. Ongoing support will be required as the child recovers, grows older, and family dynamics continue to change. It is important for all team members to recognize the supreme importance of the family as the key member of the child's life. The family is the only team unit that transcends every other team, and cares for the child over the lifetime (see Fig. 16.1). While medical and school teams may attempt to support lifespan needs, the family is the only true constant and should be revered as such. Outside team members should be cautious not to judge the function of the family and should rather aim to work with it, and collaborate with the family on how they can best achieve a lifestyle that will meet the needs of every member of the family.

It is critical for the various teams in a child's life—the rehabilitation team, the community team, the school team, and the family—to communicate and collaborate with one another to meet common goals. In a review of the rehabilitation literature, Nijhuis and colleagues described five key elements of team collaboration: communication, decision making, organization, goal setting, and team process (Nijhuis et al., 2007). In addition, the importance of family was recognized to

be integral to the various teams in a child's life (Nijhuis et al., 2007). Because of this, the investigators propose family involvement as the sixth key element of team collaboration for pediatric rehabilitation (Nijhuis et al.,

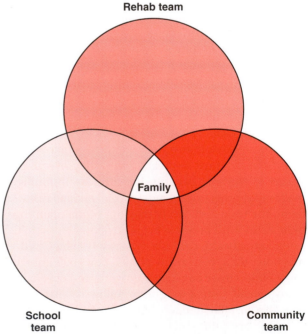

Figure 16.1 The family transcends every team involved in the child's life and is the only team to care for the child over a lifetime.

2007). More research would be helpful in understanding the relationship between these components and how to facilitate more effective collaboration in individual settings (Nijhuis et al., 2007).

Coordination of Care

Because of the large number of individuals involved with a child's care at any one time during rehabilitation, strategies must be employed to allow effective coordination. One common strategy is the traditional meeting. Meetings can have many different purposes and outcomes. In pediatric rehabilitation, typical meetings may include the following:

Team meetings: Discuss overall progress and discharge planning
Family meetings: Review care to date and address questions and discharge needs
School meetings: Plan for transition back to the school setting
Behavior meetings: Bring the team to consensus on the best strategy to use with new behaviors, assuring consistency and success for the child
Responsiveness meetings: Review the plan for each team member in caring for a child in a minimally conscious state

In addition to formal meetings, team members communicate constantly throughout the day either verbally or through various technologies. Documentation, whether written or electronic, should reflect the efforts of the team to communicate and coordinate care. As technology continues to advance, it will be possible to hold virtual meetings that include every member of the child's team. As information becomes more accessible, team members must be constantly vigilant in ensuring patient privacy.

The Role of Physical Therapy

The role of the physical therapist in the pediatric setting is similar to that in the adult setting. The principles of examination, evaluation, diagnosis, prognosis, plan of care, intervention, and outcomes set forth in the *Guide to Physical Therapist Practice* (APTA, 2001) still hold true; however, there are some important considerations when dealing with a pediatric client.

Examination Depending on the setting, physical therapists may perform their examination with other team members present. Typically the family is requested to participate to serve as developmental historians, decrease possible stranger anxiety, motivate the child, and begin the partnership to achieve goals. Age-appropriate

tests and measures are selected and administered to collect data.

Evaluation While synthesizing the data from the examination, the therapist also considers many factors that could have an influence on the overall diagnoses, prognosis, and plan of care. These include developmental skill in all domains, behavior and motivation, family needs, goals, ability to participate, and anticipated discharge setting. In addition, age of onset and nature of progress thus far are important considerations in formulating the plan of care and could indicate capacity for neuroplasticity and motor learning as well as overall potential for recovery.

Plan of Care In formulating the plan of care, the pediatric therapist should expect the need to constantly reassess and progress goals. The family is instrumental in establishing objective, measurable, and realistic goals. This is the ideal time to begin anticipating discharge and lifelong needs.

Intervention Various physical therapy approaches exist for treating the pediatric population. The past 20 years of rehabilitation have seen a major shift in focus from improving focal movement to increasing function in a meaningful activity that results in social reintegration, independence, and community participation (Anderson & Catroppa, 2006; Ylvisaker et al., 2005). As mentioned previously, new insights into potential neuroplasticity and cortical reorganization also play a major factor in a clinician's decision making when choosing intervention strategies. Physical therapists have an obligation to utilize interventions demonstrating the strongest evidence (Jewell, 2008; Kaplan, 2007). In addition to being based on evidence, interventions should be age-appropriate and motivating to the child. Activities may need to be adapted to the developmental level of the child. Creativity and flexibility is key; clinicians may need to frequently change the activity to keep the child engaged and motivated. Therapists should also be wary of the tendency to be self-limiting; children can frequently tolerate challenges well and respond positively to rewards (see Figs. 16.2–16.7)

Outcomes Therapists should select age-appropriate outcome measures to monitor effectiveness of their plan of care. Several developmental standardized tests exist that assess a child's motor skills. Selecting appropriate outcome measures pre- and posttreatment not only will help guide treatment for that specific child but also can potentially be used in sharing information to the professional community through a case study, single subject design, or more sophisticated research design involving multiple subjects. In addition to physical

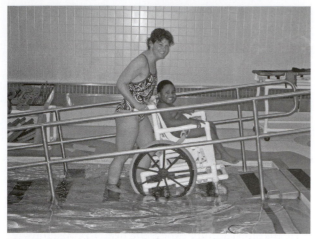

Figure 16.2 Some rehabilitation facilities may include a therapeutic pool. Ramps and aquatic wheelchairs may be available for children who are nonambulatory.

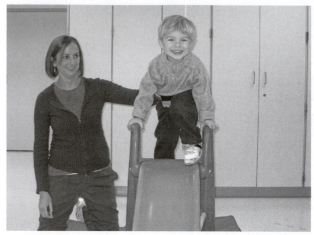

Figure 16.4 Using a therapeutic reward such as a sliding board can also help work on goals such as stair climbing and motor planning.

therapy–focused measures, there are also interdisciplinary outcome measures that the entire rehabilitation team may utilize. These measures include the Functional Independence Measure for Children (WeeFIM) and the Pediatric Evaluation of Disability Inventory (PEDI). These can be useful tools in evaluating the effectiveness of a rehabilitation program and determining what measures may need to be employed for quality improvement (Chen, Heinemann, Bode, Granger, & Mallinson, 2004; Dumas, Haley, Ludlow, & Rabin, 2002;

Iye, Haley, Watkins, & Dumas, 2003). When used systematically for a large number of patients, outcome measures can track trends in progress and help provide insight to potential needed changes in programming or allocation of resources (Majnemer & Limperopoulos, 2002). In addition, the ability to share vast amounts of valid and reliable outcome data through a national database has the potential to generate creative discussion among leaders in rehabilitation and to improve the overall effectiveness of rehabilitative care.

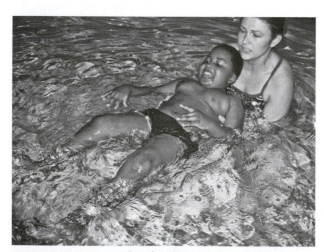

Figure 16.3 Example of a physical therapy session in the pool. The water can be very motivating and can be a useful adjunct to land-based goals of improving strength, flexibility, and mobility.

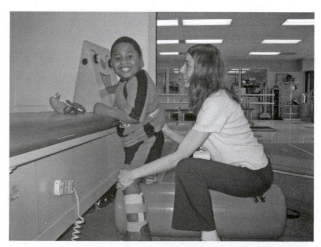

Figure 16.5 Strengthening exercises such as squats and sit to stands can be accomplished by incorporating a developmentally appropriate game.

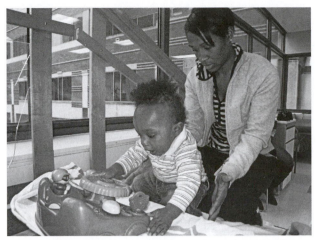

Figure 16.6 Manipulating the environment and placing toys just out of reach can be a useful tool to engage even the youngest client in practicing a challenging movement.

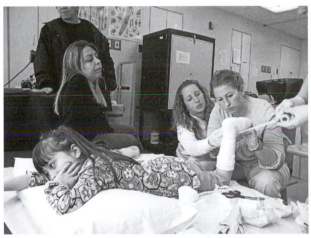

Figure 16.7 In some rehabilitation facilities, physical therapists may perform serial casting to gain passive range of motion around a joint. Physical therapists may also fabricate temporary orthoses until a custom device is warranted.

Discharge Planning

No matter how long the estimated length of stay, discharge planning should begin at admission. The following should be considered when formulating the overall plan.

Goals Because a child is continually growing and developing, it is always possible to write another goal for therapy. Clinicians must discern the difference between skilled therapy needs and typical development. It is helpful to determine specific goals and estimated length of stay with the family upon admission.

Home Evaluation Important questions include where the child will go after discharge, whether modifications will be required, and whether an alternative living situation may need to be considered. It is often difficult for the family to conceptualize life at home with their child in the early days of rehabilitation, especially if the child requires a wheelchair and the ultimate goal is for the child to walk. Despite continuing to work on ambulation goals, it is usually beneficial to plan early and to anticipate more modifications than what may truly be needed at the time of discharge, as modifications can take a long time and may require searching for community resources and funding. Even if a child is able to regain ambulation skills, a wheelchair may be needed on a temporary basis, and the home and family may need recommendations for safety. Being inside the family's home can give therapists a truer picture of the life and activity the family is striving to return to and can help suggest activities the child still needs to work on in the hospital setting. Occasionally the child may be able to attend the home evaluation with the caregivers, which can present a unique opportunity to assess the child in the natural environment, provide hands-on caregiver training, and determine what other activities may need to be simulated and practiced back at the rehabilitation setting (see Fig. 16.8).

School Reentry The process for planning the transition back to school begins on day one. As overall length of stay has significantly shortened over the past several

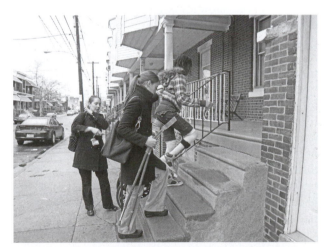

Figure 16.8 A physical and occupational therapist may perform a home evaluation with the child present. This is an excellent opportunity for the child and family to practice skills in their own environment and to reveal what skills may still need to be practiced before discharge.

years, rehabilitation therapists have been prompted to bridge even more closely with school and community supports (Rice et al., 2004). An education coordinator from the hospital may request permission from the parents to retrieve records from the school to shed light on the child's past performance and determine whether an Individualized Education Plan (IEP) or 504 Plan already existed. Ideally, frequent and ongoing communication between the school, rehabilitation team, and family will occur throughout the admission. As the child nears discharge, a meeting with the school team, rehabilitation team, and family is typically held to discuss the child's current functioning, educational needs, and recommendations for any accommodations or modifications. The school may request additional tests such as a neuropsychological examination or standardized tests from therapies. School personnel may observe the child during rehabilitation. The district determines the most appropriate setting and learning environment for the child as well as whether the child will require an IEP or 504 Plan. Support services such as physical therapy, occupational therapy, and speech-language pathology may be put into place to help the child achieve the educational objectives. The child may return to the same classroom in the same school or he or she may be enrolled in an entirely different school. If the child is in a day hospital rehabilitation program, the team may advocate for a gradual return to school so the child may continue to participate in rehabilitation but also begin the process of the ultimate goal of returning to school. This option can allow for ongoing monitoring, support, and practice of skills during this complex experience. Alternatively, if a child is discharged home, he or she may receive homebound instruction until all educational and supportive planning is put into place.

Once the school setting is determined, it may be helpful for members of the rehabilitation team to visit the school to evaluate the need for any modifications specific to the child's needs. It can also be helpful for members of the rehabilitation team to meet with the teachers and the class to educate the students on a returning student's new diagnosis. Understanding why a classmate may look or sound different can help prepare the class and potentially improve acceptance and peer reintegration.

Community Reentry During the hospital admission, it is very helpful to practice skills learned in the physical therapy gym in the outside community. Negotiating uneven terrain, crossing the street, interacting with the public, shopping, and taking public transportation are important skills the child will need for discharge (see Figs. 16.9–16.11).

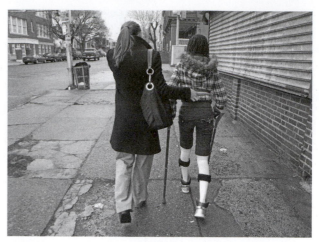

Figure 16.9 It is important for children to practice negotiating crossing the street and ambulating over uneven terrain in preparation for discharge home.

Family Education Family education takes on a different dynamic in the pediatric setting. Therapists need to assess the family's learning style to provide effective education, but they must also deliver age-appropriate education to children of all ages and developmental abilities. Education needs in the rehabilitation setting can at times seem overwhelming to the family. A comprehensive family support program, inclusive of both family education and social supports, has the potential to decrease caregiver burden and improve caregiving ability, which may consequentially increase health-related quality of life (Aitken et al., 2005). It can be very

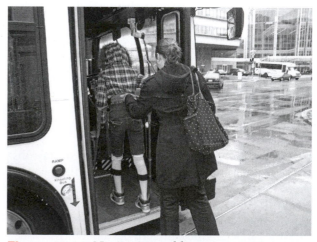

Figure 16.10 Navigating public transportation or other common community activities can put rehabilitation skills to a real-world test.

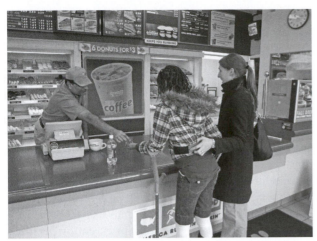

Figure 16.11 Practicing making a small purchase in a local establishment can challenge mobility, balance, fine-motor, problem-solving, language, cognitive, and social skills.

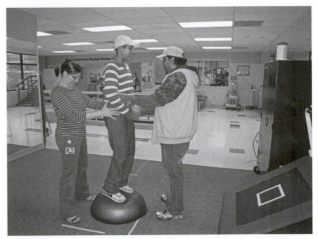

Figure 16.12 Having a parent participate in therapy can be extremely motivating for the child and rewarding for the parent.

helpful to generate a calendar or list of all needed education from all disciplines. This can assure that every need is met and facilitate collaboration between all team members to help with carryover and generalization of newly learned skills. Incorporating the family into therapy whenever possible can accomplish many things for the child, caregiver, and therapist. For the child, family involvement can be a great source of comfort and safety and could facilitate a strengthening of the caregiver-child bond. For the caregiver, it can provide the building blocks for family education required for a safe discharge. Sometimes in the early phases even the smallest bit of participation such as catching or tossing a ball can help caregivers feel empowered in this new and strange situation. Caregiver participation also provides the knowledge necessary to form the foundation for advocacy for the child. For the therapist, observing and truly listening to the child and parent during therapy can provide tremendous enlightenment on the best ways to motivate the child and provide the most effective care (see Figs. 16.12–16.13).

Equipment (see Chapters 17 and 18) The child may need temporary or custom equipment such as a walker, stander, wheelchair, or orthotic devices. A car seat or booster seat for safe transport may be required. Typically, therapists coordinate equipment evaluations with outside vendors and the family. It is important for clinicians to develop relationships with vendors who possess expertise in pediatric equipment as technology is constantly evolving. Occasionally, loaner equipment

may need to be arranged for discharge as custom equipment may take months to arrive (see Figs. 16.14–16.15).

Health-Care Followup This includes recommendations for any outpatient services, home therapy, home nursing or home health aides, and school-based or early intervention services. Because resources for home health care are scarce, it is helpful to start looking for these services as early in the rehabilitation stay as possible.

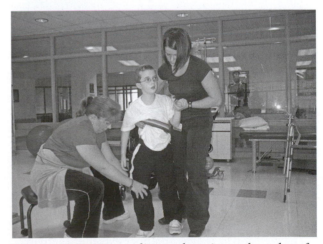

Figure 16.13 Depending on learning style and preference, some parents may choose to become intimately involved early on in the rehabilitation process. The caregiver shown has been educated on how to properly assist with limb advancement and how to help the child avoid knee hyperextension.

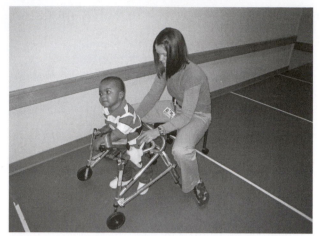

Figure 16.14 During the rehabilitation process, children may trial a variety of assistive devices during their recovery. The example pictured is a posterior rolling walker, which promotes upright posture in children with the tendency to flex forward. For a small child, the therapist may choose to sit on a rolling stool while guarding to help preserve proper body mechanics.

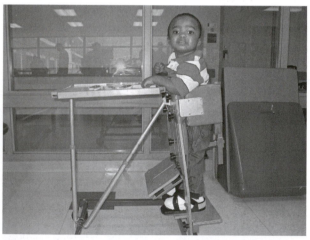

Figure 16.15 A physical therapist may institute a standing program during inpatient rehabilitation to help work on upright tolerance and pre-walking goals. Devices for standing may include a traditional tilt table, supine stander, or prone stander (pictured). In a prone stander, a child can work on head and neck extension as well as an upper extremity activity. Typically, nursing staff and families may help complete the standing program outside of the physical therapy session.

Future Directions

As we move forward into the decades to come, one can anticipate that drivers such as technology, evidence-based practice, and advanced education will be influential factors in shaping the future of pediatric rehabilitation.

As technology continues to advance, so too will the delivery of health care and pediatric rehabilitation. With the advent of the electronic medical record, less time can be spent on asking redundant questions and more time can be spent in direct contact with the child and family. Ultimately, improved communication and documentation among professionals will allow for better safety and outcomes. From an intervention perspective, both virtual reality and telemedicine are rapidly expanding fields with many direct applications to physical therapy. In a virtual reality environment, children can practice negotiating household and community environments as well as sports and leisure activities. For children, virtual rehabilitation is frequently very motivating, and new frontiers are beginning to be explored for orthopedic, neurological, and burn populations (Erren-Wolters, van Dijk, de Kort, Ijzerman, & Jannink, 2007; Fitzgerald et al., 2007; Grealy & Heffernan, 2000; Koenig et al., 2008). Telemedicine is a developing field that allows medical professionals to treat patients and families from a distance using communication technology, thereby delivering state-of-the-art care for people who are otherwise unable to access it due to their living circumstances (Theodoros & Russell, 2008). Parents who are not able to be at the hospital due to work or distance may be able to participate in their child's physical therapy session or care conference via webcam. Technology will also have a major influence on evidence-based practice. Search engines are becoming more user-friendly, which empowers clinicians to actively utilize evidence within busy clinic settings to improve overall care. In addition, strategically designed databases can allow for the analysis of large amounts of information and recommendations to the professional community. Advances in technology may also facilitate an improvement in available outcome measures as well as increased usage and standardization in practice (Jette, Halbert, Iverson, Miceli, & Shah, 2009).

While evidence-based practice is not a new concept, it is becoming more embedded into the fabric of clinical decisions for all members of the interdisciplinary team. Throughout this text, evidence-based practice is described for each of the body systems that would be appropriate to use in a rehabilitation setting. As the body of literature accumulates and therapists continue to integrate evidence into everyday practice, better outcomes will be realized for children and families.

Finally, education and advanced degrees also have the power to influence the future of rehabilitation. In the field of physical therapy, greater emphasis is being placed on postprofessional education programs such as residencies and fellowships. These intense training programs work to develop clinicians who possess advanced skills in clinical decision making and critical inquiry with the ultimate goal of achieving board-certified specialization in pediatrics by APTA. Pediatric specialists exemplify clinical excellence, professionalism, and leadership and serve as a resource for the pediatric community. By engaging in a career dedicated to lifelong learning, physical therapists have an excellent opportunity to lead and shape the future of rehabilitation.

Mini-Case Study 16.1
One Child's Journey Through Rehabilitation

History: Bobby is a 12-year old boy who underwent a liver transplant due to cholecystosis, a disease of the gallbladder. After the procedure he suffered a rapid and severe electrolyte imbalance resulting in central pontine myelinolysis. Consequently, he became paralyzed from the neck down and required ventilatory support through a tracheostomy. Prior to the hospitalization, he was independent with all age-appropriate mobility and gross motor skills.

Social History: Bobby lived with his parents and three brothers. He previously attended the sixth grade in a parochial school. He enjoyed swimming, playing with his brothers, and feeding his fish.

Physical Therapy Course: Physical therapy began in the intensive care unit of the hospital and focused on maintaining range of motion (ROM) and skin integrity. The family learned how to perform passive exercises. At this time, Bobby was unresponsive to commands. Over the course of 8 weeks, Bobby began to open his eyes and track people in his room. At the same time, he developed severe spasticity in his arms and legs, necessitating serial casting. Therapists and the family began to realize that Bobby could communicate yes and no answers by blinking. He was fully dependent for all mobility and head control and could tolerate sitting out of bed in a wheelchair for 30 minutes. As Bobby's body began to heal, he no longer required pressure assistance from the ventilator and was transitioned to room air through his tracheostomy. After 4 months in acute care, Bobby was medically stabilized and ready for transition from the acute-care setting. The team and family determined that Bobby would benefit from inpatient rehabilitation to work on maximizing any potential functional skills that would ease the burden of care on his family.

Upon admission to inpatient rehabilitation, physical therapy focused on eliciting any active movement possible, through facilitation and electric stimulation. Bobby began to gradually show trace to poor movements in a few muscle groups (digits, elbows, hamstrings). He continued to require maximal assistance for all mobility but was beginning to hold his head up for 60 seconds. His brothers were trained in how to help Bobby actively move through gravity-eliminated planes. Therapy utilized a tilt table to work on pre-standing activities. Bobby's mother positioned Bobby with nightly splints and knee immobilizers to help maintain ROM.

Bobby then received Botox injections to some of his spastic muscles, which allowed his weaker muscles to move through a greater ROM. He was decannulated and started to mouth and eventually speak words with very low volume. Therapy worked on increasing sitting balance, bed mobility, transfers, and standing with full support in the parallel bars.

As Bobby developed more head and trunk control he became very motivated for walking. Physical therapy included body weight support locomotor training, as well as ambulation in the parallel bars with bilateral ankle foot orthoses, knee immobilizers, and maximal assistance. Gradually, Bobby developed more strength and was able to walk with a rolling walker for 50 feet with moderate assistance.

During the course of his rehabilitation, Bobby worked with a large team of professionals. This included occupational therapy for his activities of daily living, speech-language pathology for his feeding and language skills, and psychology and child life for coping with his illness and hospitalization. He had a case manager who worked with the rehabilitation team and the insurance company to negotiate more time in rehabilitation based on his progress and goals yet to achieve. Bobby also worked on school readiness by participating in a school group with a teacher who assessed what his back-to-school needs would be.

Continued

Discharge Planning: Because of Bobby's dramatic progress and continued potential for more recovery, the rehabilitation team desired to maintain Bobby's inpatient status and high level of intensive service. The family, however, had been in the hospital for 7 months and needed to return home to rebuild a sense of normalcy. Bobby then transitioned to a day hospital, where he attended a full day of rehabilitation 5 times per week and was able to practice skills learned in his home environment with his family. Prior to this, a home evaluation was performed and recommendations were made for safety and how to help integrate Bobby back into typical family life. Several meetings were made with his parochial school to determine whether Bobby could continue to meet his educational needs in that environment. The rehabilitation team visited the school and assessed the stairwells, classrooms, cafeteria, and other places Bobby would need to visit and made recommendations to the school on the type of support he would need. Eventually, Bobby returned to school on a part-time basis. He attended school 3 times per week in the morning and then went for day hospital rehabilitation in the afternoon. The rehabilitation team was invited to visit the classroom with Bobby present to explain to the class what Bobby had been through over the past year and why he may look different now. The physical therapist brought a variety of splints that Bobby had used while an inpatient, which Bobby's classmates were eager to try on. The children asked many questions and fears were alleviated. Many classmates volunteered to help Bobby with different tasks for which he still required assistance. Bobby was then transitioned from a day hospital rehabilitation setting to outpatient rehabilitation, where he continues to receive outpatient physical therapy 2 times per week. Bobby's current goals are community ambulation with crutches and household ambulation without an assistive device.

Summary

Pediatric rehabilitation is an exciting place to work, where physical therapists are part of a diverse team providing service to children with a wide range of ages and diagnoses. Witnessing a child who is rapidly recovering from a neurological insult can be rewarding yet challenging as the therapist contemplates the influence of physical therapy on neuroplastic potential. For a child with a poor prognosis for functional recovery, therapists play an important role in helping a child and family adjust to a life-changing diagnosis as they educate caregivers in optimizing their child's abilities. In all cases, physical therapists have the unique opportunity to be not only a teacher, a guide, and an advocate, but also a coach who can empower children to maximize their fullest potential. Despite this awesome and humbling opportunity, it is often said that "patients are the best teachers." The nature of pediatric rehabilitation allows for a large amount of time spent with each child, and that time is often spent actively listening to the deepest concerns or greatest joys they are experiencing during this significant life event. Meaningful therapeutic relationships can evolve, which can have a profound and lasting effect for not only the child and family, but also the physical therapist. A career in pediatric rehabilitation can be challenging and rewarding, and provide the backdrop for professional development and lifelong learning.

DISCUSSION QUESTIONS

1. Compare and contrast pediatric and adult rehabilitation settings.

2. Following the patient management model in the *Guide to Physical Therapist Practice*, describe aspects of physical therapy management unique to pediatric rehabilitation.

3. Using examples, illustrate how physical therapy goals may vary according to setting along the rehabilitation continuum of care.

4. Discuss the role of the family in the pediatric rehabilitation setting.

5. Describe elements of discharge planning necessary for pediatric rehabilitation.

Recommended Readings

Bailes, A.F., Reder, R., & Burch, C. (2008). Development of guidelines for determining frequency of therapy services in a pediatric medical setting. *Pediatric Physical Therapy, 20*(2), 194–198.

King, G., Currie, M., Bartlett, D.J., Gilpin, M., Willoughby, C., Tucker, M.A., et al. (2007). The development of expertise in pediatric rehabilitation therapists: changes in approach, self-knowledge, and use of enabling and customizing strategies. *Developmental Neurorehabilitation, 10*, 223–240.

Web-Based Resources

American Physical Therapy Association: Ethics and Professionalism
   http://www.apta.org/ethics
Commission on Accreditation of Rehabilitation Facilities
   http://www.carf.org
The Joint Commission
   http://www.jointcommission.org

References

Aitken, M. E., Korehbandi, P., Parnell, D., Parker, J. G., Stefans, V., Tompkins, E., et al. (2005). Experiences from the development of a comprehensive family support program for pediatric trauma and rehabilitation patients. *Archives of Physical Medicine & Rehabilitation, 86,* 175–179.

American Physical Therapy Association (APTA). (2001). Guide to physical therapist practice (2nd ed.). *Physical Therapy, 8,* 9–746.

Anderson, V., & Catroppa, C. (2006). Advances in postacute rehabilitation after childhood-acquired brain injury; a focus on cognitive, behavioral and social domains. *American Journal of Physical Medicine and Rehabilitation, 85,* 767–778.

Bailes, A.F., Reder, R., & Burch, C. (2008). Development of guidelines for determining frequency of therapy services in a pediatric medical setting. *Pediatric Physical Therapy, 20*(2), 194–198.

Chen, C.C., Heinemann, A.W., Bode, R.K., Granger, C.V., & Mallinson, T. (2004). Impact of pediatric rehabilitation services on children's functional outcomes. *American Journal of Occupational Therapy, 58,* 44–53.

Dougherty, C.J. (1991). Values in rehabilitation: Happiness, freedom and fairness. *Journal of Rehabilitation, 57*(1), 7–12.

Dumas, H.M., Haley, S.M., Ludlow, L.H., & Rabin, J.P. (2002). Functional recovery in pediatric traumatic brain injury during inpatient rehabilitation. *American Journal of Physical Medicine & Rehabilitation, 81,* 661–669.

Erren-Wolters, C.V., van Dijk, H., de Kort, A.C., Ijzerman, M.J., & Jannink, M.J. (2007). Virtual reality for mobility devices: Training applications and clinical results: A review. *International Journal of Rehabilitation Research, 30,* 91–96.

Fitzgerald, D., Foody, J., Kelly, D., Ward, T., Markham, C., McDonald, J., et al. (2007). Development of a wearable motion capture suit and virtual reality biofeedback system for the instruction and analysis of sports rehabilitation exercises. Conference Proceedings: Annual International Conference of the IEEE Engineering in Medicine & Biology Society. 2007:4870–4874, Lyon, France. doi: 10.1109/IEMBS.2007.4353431

Flett, P.J., & Stoffell, B.F. (2003). Ethical issues in paediatric rehabilitation. *Journal of Paediatrics & Child Health, 39,* 219–223.

Grealy, M.A., & Heffernan, D. (2000). The rehabilitation of brain injured children: The case for including physical exercise and virtual reality. *Pediatric Rehabilitation, 4,* 41–49.

Iye, L.V., Haley, S.M., Watkins, M.P., & Dumas, H.M. (2003). Establishing minimal clinically important differences for scores on the pediatric evaluation of disability inventory for inpatient rehabilitation. *Physical Therapy, 83,* 888–898.

Jette, D.U., Halbert, J., Iverson, C., Miceli, E., & Shah, P. (2009). Use of standardized outcome measures in physical therapist practice: Perceptions and applications. *Physical Therapy, 89,* 125–135.

Jewell, D.V. (2008). *Guide to evidence-based physical therapy practice.* Boston: Jones & Bartlett.

Kaplan, S.L. (2007). *Outcome measurement & management: First steps for the practicing clinician.* Philadelphia: F.A. Davis.

King, G., Currie, M., Bartlett, D.J., Gilpin, M., Willoughby, C., Tucker, M.A., et al. (2007). The development of expertise in pediatric rehabilitation therapists: Changes in approach, self-knowledge, and use of enabling and customizing strategies. *Developmental Neurorehabilitation, 10,* 223–240.

Koenig, A., Wellner, M., Koneke, S., Meyer-Heim, A., Lunenburger, L., & Riener, R. (2008). Virtual gait training for children with cerebral palsy using the Lokomat gait orthosis. *Studies in Health Technology & Informatics, 132,* 204–209.

Majnemer, A., & Limperopoulos, C. (2002). Importance of outcome determination in pediatric rehabilitation. *Developmental Medicine & Child Neurology, 44,* 773–777.

Matthews D.J., Meier, R.H., & Bartholome, W. (1990). Ethical issues encountered in pediatric rehabilitation. *Pediatrician, 17,* 108–114.

Nijhuis, B.I.G., Reinders-Messelink, H.A., Blécourt, A.C.E., Olijve, W.G., Groothoff, J.W., Nakken, H., & Postema, K. (2007). A review of salient elements defining team collaboration in paediatric rehabilitation. *Clinical Rehabilitation, 21,* 195–211.

Osberg, J.S., DiScala, C., & Gans, B.M. (1990). Utilization of inpatient rehabilitation services among traumatically injured children discharged from pediatric trauma centers. *American Journal of Physical Medicine & Rehabilitation, 69*(2), 67–72.

Reder, R. (2009). Proceedings from Combined Sections Meeting, American Physical Therapy Association, '09: Clinical and Operational Best Practice: Identifying Meaningful Outcomes and Appropriate Service Delivery in Pediatric Settings. Las Vegas, NV.

Rice, S.A., Allaire, J., Elgin, K., Farrell, W., Conaway, M., & Blackman, J.A. (2004). Effect of shortened length of stay on functional and educational outcome after pediatric rehabilitation. *American Journal of Physical Medicine & Rehabilitation, 83,* 27–32.

Taub, E. (2002). New treatments in neurorehabilitation founded on basic research. *Nature Reviews Neuroscience, 3,* 228–236.

Theodoros, D., & Russell, T. (2008). Telerehabilitation: Current perspectives. *Studies in Health Technology & Informatics, 131,* 191–209.

Ylvisaker, M., Adelson, P.D., Braga, L.W., Burnett, S.M., Glang, A., Feeney, T., et al. (2005). Rehabilitation and ongoing support after pediatric TBI: Twenty years of progress. *Journal of Head Trauma Rehabilitation, 20,* 95–109.

CHAPTER 17

Assistive Technology: Positioning and Mobility

—Maria Jones, PT, PhD

—Trina Puddefoot, PT, MS PCS, ATP

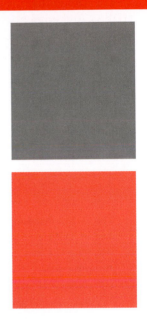

Assistive technology (**AT**) includes devices and services used to enhance abilities and participation of children with disabilities, while reducing limitations that may arise as a result of impairments of body functions and structures. These children have limitations that prevent them from performing activities in the same manner as their peers. The limitations are attributable to neuromotor or musculoskeletal impairments, including muscle contractures, skeletal deformities, and inadequate balance and control of muscle groups that affect children's ability to produce the movement necessary to perform specific skills and activities. Physical therapists, as members of an intervention team, may recommend AT in the areas of positioning, mobility, and communication for children with disabilities to prevent or decrease the influence of neuromotor or musculoskeletal impairments (Henderson, Skelton, & Rosenbaum, 2008; McEwen &

Lloyd, 1990; Minkel, 2000; Washington, Deitz, White, & Schwartz, 2002). Historically, professionals in rehabilitation and educational environments have used AT to support therapeutic intervention.

With continued advancement of technology and legislation in the United States addressing the provision of AT during the past 25 years, options for devices are more readily available. Although therapists and families may still use handmade devices fabricated from low-cost materials, other options are now commercially available. Physical therapists, along with parents and other service providers, can evaluate a child's need for AT devices and services and make appropriate recommendations to meet those needs (Carlson & Ramsey, 2000; Galvin & Scherer, 1996; Gillen, 2002). This chapter describes the laws and processes used to meet the AT needs of children, as well as the role physical therapists play in the selection, acquisition, and implementation of AT, with a focus on positioning and mobility. Chapter 18 provides information for the physical therapist using augmentative communication and other technologies.

Assistive Technology Legislation

Many laws in the United States address AT and provide a legislative framework designed to ensure that children with disabilities receive the AT they need. These laws are summarized in Table 17.1 and in Chapter 1.

The Individuals with Disabilities Education Act (IDEA) Amendments of 2004 continue to identify six AT services that a child may need to acquire or use AT: (1) evaluation, (2) funding, (3) modification, repair, and replacement of devices, (4) coordination of services, (5) training of children and their families, and (6) training of others who will support children's use of AT. AT evaluation is necessary to determine whether a child requires AT and to identify appropriate device(s) or service(s). Funding for the device(s) and/or service(s) occurs after the assessment, when the Individualized Education Plan (IEP) team has decided upon an appropriate device and service. Once obtained, devices may require modification to ensure that they meet the child's unique needs and abilities. Examples include customizing a keyboard or building up a handle on a spoon. In addition, devices must be repaired and sometimes replaced to ensure that they remain in working order. The IEP team should identify all necessary AT services and include them in the IEP. IDEA also addresses the need for coordinated services. If a school pursues other funding sources to obtain devices and/or services, the process must be coordinated, as it can be time consuming. The team will benefit from designating

Table 17.1 Federal Laws Related to Assistive Technology (AT)

The Rehabilitation Act of 1973 (PL 93-112) and Amendments	Individuals With Disabilities Education Improvement Act and Amendments of 2004 (IDEA) (PL 108-446) and Its Precursors	Technology-Related Assistance for Individuals With Disabilities Act of 1988 (PL 100-407) and Amendments	The Americans With Disabilities Act of 1990 (ADA) (PL 101-336)
• Protects civil rights of people with disabilities from discrimination in programs or activities that receive federal financial assistance. • Definitions of disability are broader than those defined by IDEA. • Some children qualify for services under this definition, although not meeting eligibility criteria of IDEA. • AT devices and/or services may be considered reasonable accommodation when needed by children to access and participate in their public education.	• Defines AT device and service. • Schools must provide AT at no cost to the parent when determined by the Individualized Education Program (IEP) team to be needed and addressed in the IEP. • The need for AT must be considered as part of IEP development for each child who qualifies for special education and related services and also when reviewing or revising the IEP. • For children birth to 36 months, Part C ensures that the need for AT is addressed in the Individualized Family Service Plan (IFSP).	• First legislation to provide the definition of AT device and service. • Provides federal funding for states to establish training and service delivery systems for AT. • Supports the creation of systems change to eliminate barriers to the acquisition of AT. • Services vary from state to state, but may include information and referral, demonstration, loan libraries of devices, and training.	• Protects civil rights of people with disabilities. • Prevents discrimination in employment, public services, accommodations, transportation, and telecommunications. • Includes definitions of AT devices and services. • Provides for reasonable accommodations, such as AT, to make employment or public services accessible.

someone to be responsible for completing the paperwork and ensuring that the process is moving forward. In the event that the school district cannot identify another funding source or that another agency denies a request for funding the device or service, the school is still responsible for providing AT identified in the IEP.

The IEP team also addresses services (5) and (6)—training the child, family, school personnel and other people who are responsible for providing care in the child's life and will support the use of AT in the school, home, vocational, and community environments. All of the identified services are essential to ensure the child becomes proficient in using the device(s) in a variety of contexts. Although previous amendments to IDEA added AT as one of the special factors that teams had to consider for all children when developing IEPs, IDEA 2004 extended the consideration of special factors to include the IEP review and revision process. Not only do teams have to consider whether a child requires AT in order to have a free and appropriate public education as defined by IDEA, but now they also must reconsider whether the child requires AT when reviewing or revising the IEP.

The Process for Providing Assistive Technology Services

Although legislation mandates the provision of AT devices and services when appropriate and necessary, few defined processes exist for therapists to use when making AT decisions. Physical therapists, however, must consider critical elements when evaluating, recommending, and implementing AT for children (Angelo, 2000).

Gathering Background Information

The use of a referral form, the review of educational records, and interviews with children, parents, caregivers, or school staff are methods for obtaining background information about children with disabilities. Referral forms often include personal information, such as age, medical diagnosis, health information, and potential funding sources. A review of education records yields information about educational performance and the results of educational evaluations, including academic performance, cognitive abilities, strengths, and weaknesses. Interviews with children, parents or caregivers, and important team members, such as teachers, related service providers, and friends, provide not only information regarding abilities and needs but also different perspectives (Reed & Lahm, 2004).

The AT evaluation team gathers background information regarding the child's abilities. What are the child's motor, sensory, cognitive, language, and social strengths? What are the child's current abilities that allow him or her to use AT today? What improvements can be made to the child's abilities that will result in increased performance? The needs of the child are also important when assessing for AT. What does the child need to do that he or she currently cannot do? Are there activities in which the child cannot participate, but could perform part of a task with AT? The child's history of technology use also is important. Has the child tried or used technology before? If so, what was tried, and were the results successful or unsuccessful? Information should be gathered regarding not only present environments but also future environments. For example, if a child who maneuvers a power wheelchair independently is currently in elementary school but will be transitioning to middle school during the following school year, the physical therapist should evaluate the middle-school environment to ensure that no architectural barriers exist that will prevent the student from continued independent mobility.

Gathering Objective Data for Decision Making

Observation is one way to gather data. Physical therapists and other team members must observe children in the context of natural environments and during daily routines to evaluate how children function in different environments and to help identify barriers, which could interfere with the use of AT (Henderson et al., 2008; Reed & Lahm, 2004). Identifying barriers is a critical part of the evaluation process. Observing children in the context of familiar activities can provide information about their cognitive, physical, visual, and communication skills. The use of an environmental evaluation tool, such as the Activity/Standards Inventory (Beukelman & Mirenda, 2005), can assist in identifying discrepancies of participation. Beukelman and Mirenda (2005) identify the following opportunity barriers that may be present in the environment and may interfere with the success or use of AT: policy, practice, attitude, knowledge, and skill. When opportunity barriers are present, the team must propose solutions to address them.

Formal and informal testing is another means for gathering objective data for decision making. The team should identify what information is lacking and then select the appropriate tests to gather the needed information. Professionals from the various disciplines should be knowledgeable regarding formal tests related to their areas of expertise.

Assistive Technology Evaluation

To identify and obtain AT for children, service providers, including physical therapists, need to provide an AT evaluation. A systematic evaluation process ensures that AT device selection decisions are based on information regarding the child's abilities, needs, and environments. The AT evaluation is characterized by a team approach, focuses on functional evaluation techniques provided in the natural environment, and is ongoing in nature (Reed & Lahm, 2004). Although most AT evaluations are not standardized, the evaluation process should be systematic and use a framework for effective decision making.

A team approach is critical in the AT evaluation process. No single professional possesses knowledge and expertise about all areas of AT. The child's positioning needs, vision, cognitive/linguistic abilities, and computer hardware and software needs are some of the child-oriented areas that the team considers. Children and their parents are essential team members. Other team members may come from a wide range of professions, including physical therapy, occupational therapy, speech-language pathology, education, psychology or psychometry, optometry/ophthalmology, audiology, adaptive physical education, recreation therapy, music therapy, and rehabilitation engineering. Professionals with a special interest in AT may become certified as an assistive technology professional (ATP) through the Rehabilitation Engineering and Assistive Technology Society of North America (RESNA). The ATP certification identifies professionals who have demonstrated competency in the broad field of assistive technology, meeting the eligibility criteria and passing the ATP examination (RESNA, 2010). It is important that all team members contribute information regarding the child's abilities, needs, environments, and tasks that must be considered in the evaluation and that they actively work together to identify possible AT solutions (Reed & Lahm, 2004).

AT evaluations should occur in the child's home and other natural environments. For very young children, this may include settings outside the home where the child receives care (e.g., Grandma's house, child care center). If the child is in school, the evaluation should occur in the classroom and other environments (cafeteria, playground, restroom, gym, and so on) where the child participates during the school day. For older children and young adults, the evaluation might include

school and work environments. Because the evaluation procedures are not standardized, information may be gathered by observing a child during typical daily routines, such as playing with siblings, sitting at the desk, eating in the cafeteria, and playing at centers with other children. The evaluation and recommendations are functional because they remain focused on the child's abilities and needs for specific activities that occur as part of daily routines. For example, even though the child may have limited use of his or her hands to access a communication system, his or her functional abilities could include the use of eye gaze for communication purposes. Identifying and focusing on specific tasks that are relevant in present and future environments ensure that the evaluation is functional.

Feature Match With Child's Abilities

Scherer and Craddock (2002) describe a process of AT selection in which the needs of the child are assessed, documented, and then matched to the device that most closely offers the required features. First, the evaluation team identifies the child's needs and abilities. This information is then matched with specific features of AT to develop a list of potential systems for trial purposes. For example, if environmental needs for the child indicate that the system should be portable and easy to support, the team should not consider devices that are not portable or that require extensive support. Using a feature match approach helps narrow the options to those most relevant for a specific child.

Trial

After the AT team has proposed a system or systems, a field test is essential in determining the effectiveness of the proposed system(s). Field tests are useful if more than one system meets the need, or to document a child's use of the system to secure funding. Trials of the system in the natural environment and for identified tasks help determine whether the system will accomplish the identified need. A field test helps children and their families determine whether they prefer one device over another, because they have the opportunity to manage the device in the context of their daily routines. A systematic procedure of data collection should be used to assess the effect of the device on the desired outcomes.

Recommendations

Team members should complete a report that summarizes and synthesizes the information gathered during the evaluation process and provides recommendations for AT devices and services that can be submitted to an appropriate funding source to secure payment for the recommended AT. Funding of AT is discussed in Chapter 18. All team members review the report and reach an agreement regarding implementation of the recommendations. The report includes recommendations for the specific system, including requirements and components, and for AT services needed to support the system (Reed & Lahm, 2004). If a child, teacher, or caregiver needs training, recommendations should address how much training is required, and who will provide the training.

Training and Implementation

Acquiring AT devices is usually just the preliminary step in the AT process. Team members may believe that a device is the "answer" or "cure" for problems identified in the evaluation process, but significant training in the use of a device is necessary for successful generalization across settings (Campbell, Milbourne, Dugan, & Wilcox, 2006; McNevin, Wulf, & Carlson, 2000).

When training children to use AT devices, all team members should incorporate motor learning principles. *Motor learning* is defined as processes that lead to relatively permanent changes in a person's ability to produce a skilled action as a result of practice or experience (Schmidt & Lee, 2005). As discussed here and in Chapter 8, physical therapists should incorporate concepts such as transfer of behavior or generalization, practice, and feedback when training a child to use AT.

Transfer of Behavior

Children with disabilities often have difficulty transferring behaviors or generalizing skills into new environments or situations (Brown, Effgen, & Palisano, 1998). When training a child to use AT, physical therapists must design practice and provide feedback to ensure that the skills performed transfer and generalize across all device use environments (Campbell et al., 2006; Jones, McEwen, & Hansen, 2003; McNevin et al., 2000; Reichle & Sigafoos, 1991).

Practice

For children to become proficient in the use of AT, they must practice using the AT in one or more environments. For example, if a child is learning to use a powered wheelchair for mobility, practice must include using the wheelchair in places such as the hallways of the child's school, on sidewalks going to the bus, and in the grocery store. Practicing powered mobility in a wide-open space, such as a gym, or setting up an obstacle course is less likely to be effective in helping the child to gain independence.

Organization of practice opportunities is another important consideration when designing training in the use of AT. Children with disabilities require more practice opportunities to develop a motor skill than do children without disabilities. All team members must provide an increased number of well-designed practice opportunities within daily activities to assist children in becoming proficient and competent users of AT (Campbell et al., 2006; Jones et al., 2003; Sommerville, Hildebrand, & Crane, 2008).

Feedback

Feedback (i.e., knowledge of results or consequences) refers to use of intrinsic and extrinsic factors to facilitate development of a motor skill. Intrinsic factors include proprioception and kinesthesia. Extrinsic factors include visual, auditory, or tactile cues that children receive from people and objects within their environment. Although feedback is important and may be provided continuously during initial acquisition of a skill, it must be faded out quickly for actual learning and refinement of the skill to occur. Fading out ensures that the child does not become dependent on the feedback to perform the skill (Larin, 2000; Maslovat, Brunke, Chua, & Franks, 2009; Reichle & Sigafoos, 1991). (For a more detailed discussion of motor learning, see Chapter 8.)

Categories of Assistive Technology

In 1992, RESNA identified 10 categories of AT for children in educational environments:

- Positioning
- Mobility
- Augmentative communication
- Access
- Computer-based instruction
- Environmental control
- Activities of daily living
- Recreation/leisure/play
- Vision technology
- Assistive listening

These categories are the basis of AT intervention and serve as the framework for the following sections and Chapter 18.

Positioning

Positioning children with disabilities plays an important role in their ability to function and participate within the environment. Optimal positioning improves head position and control (McEwen & Lloyd, 1990), permits greater control of the arms and head (Myhr & von Wendt, 1991; Stavness, 2006), improves ability to eat, digest, and breathe (Miedaner & Finuf, 1993; Nwaobi & Smith, 1986), improves postural alignment (Washington et al., 2002), facilitates adult-child interaction (McEwen, 1992), and improves ability to listen, speak and communicate (Bay, 1991; Hulme, Bain, Hardin, McKinnon, & Waldron, 1989).

Positioning refers to the alignment of body parts in relation to one another and to the surrounding environment. For example, children without disabilities may sit while working at the computer, stand while washing dishes, and lie on their stomachs while playing Nintendo Wii. They use various positions throughout the day, depending on the activity they are performing. For children with disabilities, therapists recommend positioning systems that provide proper alignment to promote improved function, movement, and participation in activities.

Positioning Systems

Two basic categories of positioning systems exist: recumbent and upright systems. Recumbent systems provide support in supine, prone, or sidelying positions and are frequently used by children with severe physical disabilities as a means of alternative positioning throughout the day. Recumbent positioning systems (Fig. 17.1) include wedges, bolsters, mats, and sidelyers. In general, recumbent positioning systems should not be used during the day because they may have the potential to exclude children from participating in activities along with their peers. Physical therapists must consider the effect recumbent positions have on

adult and peer interaction with the child and the movement demands of the tasks required in that position (Bergen, Presperin, & Tallman, 1990; Carlson & Ramsey, 2000; McEwen, 1992).

In contrast to recumbent positioning systems, **upright positioning** systems support the child in either a seated or standing position. Physical therapists recommend seating systems for children who use wheelchairs as their primary means of mobility, but they may also recommend them for children with less obvious physical disabilities, such as developmental coordination disorders (DCD). Children with DCD may need seating supports to improve sitting posture in class, especially when doing written work. Although limited research is available to describe the effect of adaptive positioning for children with disabilities (Chung et al., 2008; Harris & Roxborough, 2005), a positive impact of adaptive seating on health, function, participation and family life has been reported (Hulme, Gallacher, Walsh, Niesen, & Waldron, 1987; McNamara & Casey, 2007; Rigby, Ryan, & Campbell, 2009; Ryan et al., 2009). Careful assessment of the needs of the child and the features of the seating system is needed, as recommendations for adaptive seating cannot be generalized across populations and outcomes (McNamara & Casey, 2007; Chung et al., 2008). Physical therapists recommend standing systems to provide alternative positioning throughout the day, allow access to normal work surfaces, such as cabinets and sinks, and provide weight-bearing opportunities for children who are unable to stand independently.

Types of Seating Systems

Seating systems can be divided into four categories: sling, planar, generically contoured, and custom contoured. Each type of support surface has different effects on a child's position. **Sling systems** are the industry standard for mobility bases. Sling systems are usually vinyl or cloth material, which allows for folding during transportation. However, they provide little support because the material gives way to the weight and movement of the child, causing a "hammock" effect. Postural deviations commonly caused by sling seating systems include pelvic asymmetries and adducted and internally rotated hips.

In contrast to sling seating systems, **planar seating systems** provide a firm base of support for children, preventing the development of common postural deviations. Planar systems are flat seat and back supports, often constructed of a plywood or plastic base with 1 to 2 inches of foam and covered with upholstery. Some pediatric mobility bases, such as the one shown in

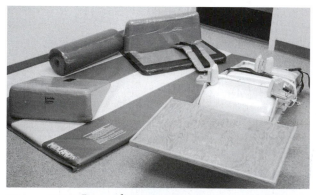

Figure 17.1 Recumbent positioning systems (left to right): Tumble Forms wedge, bolster, and sidelyer and Rifton prone support scooter.

Figure 17.2, come standard with a planar seating system. Modular components, such as lateral trunk supports, lateral thigh supports, hip guides, and medial thigh supports, are often used in conjunction with planar seating systems to provide the level of support to meet a child's needs. Planar seating systems provide adequate support for children with mild postural problems, symmetrical posture, and no structural deformities.

If planar seating systems do not provide the level of support a child needs to sit upright, cushions that are **contoured** can be considered. Generally, commercially available or off-the-shelf cushions are contoured and approximate the shape of the body in their design and construction (Fig. 17.3). Contoured seats provide adequate support for children with moderate postural problems, flexible postural asymmetries, and few, if any, structural deformities (Washington et al., 2002).

For children with the most severe physical disabilities, seating systems in the first three categories often do not provide the level of support needed to enhance function. **Custom-contoured** seating systems are specifically molded to a child's body and are designed to match that child's body contours. Because the seating systems are specifically molded to a child's body, they can accommodate for leg length discrepancies, pelvic asymmetries, and trunk asymmetries. Custom-contoured

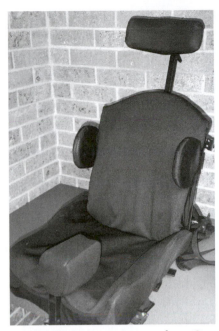

Figure 17.3 Jay Fit Seating System from Sunrise Medical.

systems are often used to accommodate fixed structural deformities. With the continued advancement of technology, custom-contoured seating systems, such as those shown in Figure 17.4, are comparable in price with other seating systems and are readily available.

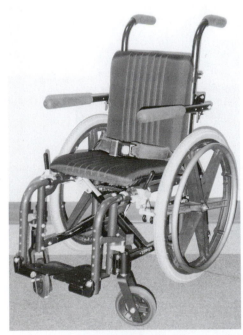

Figure 17.2 Zippie 2 manual wheelchair with planar seating system.

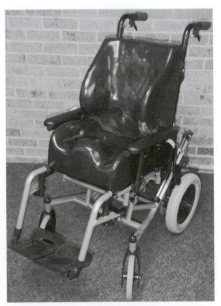

Figure 17.4 Custom-contoured seating system fabricated at the Oklahoma Assistive Technology Center.

Standing Systems

Therapists recommend standing systems to provide an alternative position for children who remain in a seated position throughout most of their day. **Standing systems** are also used as a means of weight bearing for children who otherwise could not stand. Common standing systems include prone, supine, and upright standers (Fig. 17.5). Most standers have table or tray attachments that allow the child to play or perform other activities while standing. The benefits of standing include elongation of the hamstrings (Gibson, Sprod, & Maher, 2009), knee and hip flexor and ankle plantarflexor musculature, maintenance or improvement in bone mineral density (Caulton et al., 2004), and facilitation of optimal musculoskeletal development of the hip, knee, and ankle joints (Stuberg, 1992). A child who requires the use of a stander will often have a wheelchair and seating system and a separate standing system. Wheelchairs with standing capabilities are available and allow the same system to serve both functions.

Benefits of Proper Positioning

When a child is in an optimal position, the therapist can begin to assess the impact of positioning on the child's performance of daily activities. Bergen and colleagues (1990) identified nine benefits of optimal positioning:

1. Normalize or decrease abnormal neurological influence on the body.

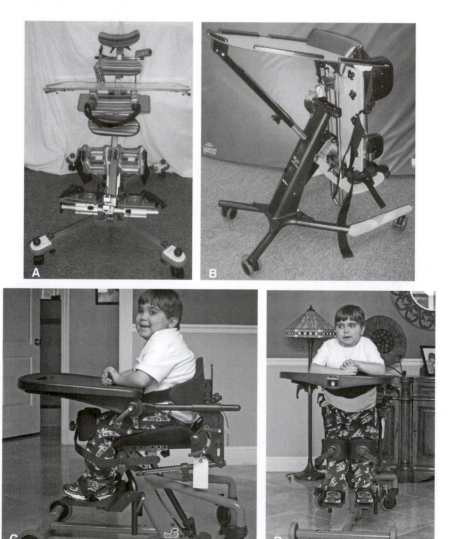

Figure 17.5 (*A*) Snug Seat Giraffe stander. (*B*) Rifton prone stander, (*C*) Easy Stand Bantam seated position, and (*D*) Easy Stand Bantam standing position.

2. Increase range of motion, maintain neutral skeletal alignment and control, and prevent skeletal deformities and muscle contractures.
3. Manage pressure and prevent or decrease the potential for decubitus ulcers.
4. Upgrade stability to increase function.
5. Promote increased tolerance of desired position (comfort).
6. Enhance function of autonomic nervous system.
7. Decrease fatigue.
8. Facilitate components of normal movement.
9. Facilitate maximum function with minimal pathology.

Physical Examination for Seating Systems

The goal of positioning intervention is to determine the position in which the child has the most control with the least amount of support or restriction. The physical examination should take place in both supine and sitting positions. The supine examination eliminates the effect of gravity on the spine and allows examination of passive movement of the pelvis, hips, and knees. The sitting examination provides information about the child's ability to maintain the head and trunk in a neutral and functional position against gravity.

The physical examination provides information used to determine the level of support a child needs in a seating system. The primary focus of the physical examination is to determine whether a child's postural changes are flexible or fixed. Flexible deformities can be eliminated or corrected with manual support. Fixed deformities cannot be eliminated or corrected with manual support. When designing a seating system, flexible deformities must be corrected, providing the supports necessary to position a child in neutral alignment. The seating system must accommodate fixed or structural deformities and not apply corrective forces, preventing progression of those deformities, while providing a comfortable and functional position for the child (Carlson & Ramsey, 2000; McDonald, Surtees, & Wirz, 2003). As part of the physical examination, physical therapists determine the impact of hip and knee movement on the position of the pelvis. With the child in supine, physical therapists measure hip and knee range of motion, ensuring that the child can flex the hip to at least 90° with the knee positioned at 90° (Fig. 17.6). If a child has limited hip or knee movement, adjustments must be made to the seat-to-back angle or knee flexion angle of the wheelchair. In addition, when examining the child's hip flexion, physical therapists must ensure that the lumbar curve

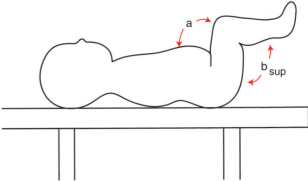

Figure 17.6 In supine, physical therapists measure (*a*) hip and (*b*) knee angles to determine whether the child can achieve at least 90° of hip flexion with the knee at 90°. This will determine the seat-to-back angle and footrest angle of the wheelchair. *(From Bergen, A.F., Presperin, J., & Tallman, T. [1990]. Positioning for function: Wheelchairs and other assistive technologies [p. 15]. Valhalla, NY: Valhalla Rehabilitation Publications. Adapted with permission.)*

does not flatten when bringing the hip to 90° and straightening the knee as seen when the child has tight hamstring musculature (Fig. 17.7). Additional measurements taken during the physical examination are summarized in Figure 17.8. The examination continues to include the hips, thighs, knees, trunk, head, and arms, but the pelvis provides the foundation for postural support.

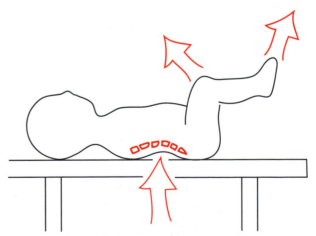

Figure 17.7 While measuring the hip flexion and knee flexion angle, physical therapists must ensure that the lumbar curve does not flatten as a result of hamstring tightness. *(From Bergen, A.F., Presperin, J., & Tallman, T. [1990]. Positioning for function: Wheelchairs and other assistive technologies [p. 14]. Valhalla, NY: Valhalla Rehabilitation Publications. Adapted with permission.)*

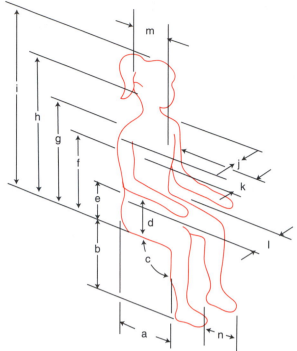

Figure 17.8 Physical therapists take the following measurements in sitting: (*a*) behind hips to popliteal fossa (right and left), (*b*) popliteal fossa to heel (right and left), (*c*) knee flexion angle, (*d*) seat surface to hanging elbow, (*e*) seat surface to pelvic crest, (*f*) seat surface to axilla, (*f*) seat surface to top of shoulder, (*h*) seat surface to occiput, (*i*) seat surface to top of head, (*j*) shoulder width, (*k*) chest width, (*l*) hip width, (*m*) trunk depth, and (*n*) foot length. *(From Bergen, A.F., Presperin, J., & Tallman, T. [1990]. Positioning for function: Wheelchairs and other assistive technologies [p. 17]. Valhalla, NY: Valhalla Rehabilitation Publications. Adapted with permission.)*

Pelvis

The physical examination in sitting begins by palpating the anterior superior iliac spines (ASISs) with your thumbs to determine whether the child's pelvis is level. If the thumbs are level, the child's pelvis is level. If the thumbs are not level, a pelvic obliquity is present. If one thumb tip is more forward than the other, this indicates the presence of pelvic rotation (Fig. 17.9). Initially, if thumbs are not level or if one is more forward than the other, the physical therapist should try to reposition the child to see whether repositioning will result in neutral alignment. If repositioning does not resolve the identified deviation, the pelvic deformity should be accommodated in the seating system. The position of the ASISs in relation to each other is critical in describing pelvic deformities.

Some children cannot maintain their pelvis in a neutral position without support, so therapists add pelvic supports for stability. A pelvic positioning belt (e.g., seat belt or lap belt) is the most common support used to stabilize the pelvis. Physical therapists should closely evaluate the angle at which the pelvic belt is secured to a wheelchair and ensure that the belt can be easily removed by the child and caregiver. A general rule is to position the belt at a 45° angle, bisecting the pelvic/femoral angle to maintain a neutral pelvis (Fig. 17.10a). Some children may require additional stability but may also need to shift the pelvis forward to reach. If this is the case, a pelvic belt angle closer to 90° may prove beneficial (Fig. 17.10b). Pelvic belts that are positioned too high can cause the child to move into a posterior pelvic tilt (Fig. 17.10c) (Bergen et al., 1990). Other pelvic supports include sub-ASIS bars and anterior knee blocks (Rigby, Reid, Schoger, & Ryan, 2001).

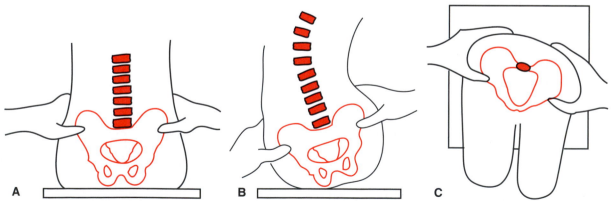

Figure 17.9 Common pelvic positions: (*A*) neutral pelvis, (*B*) pelvic obliquity, and (*C*) pelvic rotation. *(Courtesy of Corinne Vance.)*

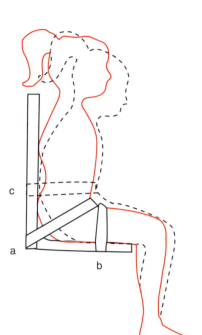

Figure 17.10 Three common seat belt configurations: (*a*) belt at 45° angle to maintain a neutral pelvis, (*b*) belt at 90° angle for increased stability, allowing forward shift, (*c*) belt positioned too high causing posterior pelvic tilt. (*Courtesy of Corinne Vance.*)

Hips

Hip range of motion is critical in determining the seat-to-back angle of a wheelchair. When examining a child's pelvic position in supine, therapists must pay close attention to the effect of hip flexion and knee extension on the position of the pelvis. These factors are used to determine the seat-to-back and knee angle within a mobility base and seating system. A child whose pelvic mobility is not affected by hip flexion or knee extension requires much less support than one who has significant movement limitations. Because children with physical disabilities often present with tight hip flexors/extensors and hamstrings, the pelvis may be fixed in an anterior or a posterior tilt, requiring more support to accommodate the deformities. When examining hip movement, physical therapists should determine whether a child can achieve 90° of hip flexion while maintaining neutral pelvic alignment. If a child does not have 90° of hip flexion, then the angle of the back in relationship to the seat (the seat-to-back angle) must be reclined to accommodate the lack of hip flexion.

Thighs

For most children, sitting with the thighs in slight abduction is optimal. When examining a child's thigh position, therapists should observe whether the child's thighs are too close together or too far apart. Thighs that are too close together indicate a postural deviation commonly caused by muscle imbalance and/or stiffness that pulls the knees together. When a child's thighs are too far apart, it is often indicative of muscle weakness or low muscle tone. Lateral and medial thigh supports (adductor and abductor supports) are designed to control postural deviations of the thighs. Lateral thigh supports bring a child's legs into adduction, and medial thigh supports separate the legs into a neutral or slightly abducted position. Medial thigh supports are not intended and should not be used to stretch tight adductors or to prevent the child from sliding forward in the chair. Hip guides provide lateral control across the greater trochanter to keep the hips from moving laterally in the seating system.

Knee and Foot Supports

When examining a child's knee movement, therapists must consider the impact of tight hamstring musculature on hip movement and pelvic position. Because the hamstring muscles cross both the hip and knee joints, tightness in the hamstrings can cause the hip to extend as the knee is extended, pulling the pelvis into a posterior tilt. The footrest angle should be determined based on a child's available knee movement with the hip flexed and while maintaining the pelvis in a neutral position. Footrests that are too far in front of the seating system cause children with tight hamstrings to lose the neutral alignment of their hips and pelvis. In addition, the footrest height should support the entire foot while maintaining thigh contact with the seating system.

Most mobility bases include leg and foot support options. Footrest options on wheelchairs include the footrest hanger, footplate, and accessories. The angle of the footrest hanger is critical to proper positioning. Physical therapists should use the child's knee angle to determine the angle of the footrest hanger. The standard footrest hanger is generally angled at 60° or 70°, which is often too far in front of the chair to benefit children with tight hamstring musculature. Most chairs now have other options available, including 80°, 90°, elevating, and contracture platforms. The tighter a child's hamstrings, the closer the footrests need to be to the front edge of the chair. In extreme cases, the footrests must angle under the seat to accommodate tight hamstring musculature (Fig. 17.11). Several

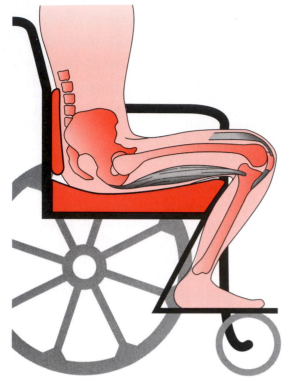

Figure 17.11 When a child has tight hamstring muscles, the footrests must angle under the seat to accommodate for the tightness and allow the pelvis to stay in neutral alignment.

footplate options are available and can be attached to the footrest hanger. Options include individual, solid, flip-up, angle adjustable, and dynamic (Fig. 17.12). If a child has a leg length discrepancy, the therapist should order individual footplates, which allow for independent adjustment of each side to accommodate for the differences in length. If a child transfers independently

in and out of the wheelchair, flip-up footplates will not interfere with transfers. If a child has structural foot deformities either in plantarflexion or dorsiflexion, angle-adjustable footplates allow therapists to angle the footplate to support the entire length of the child's foot. Other leg/foot support accessories include calf pads, calf straps, heel loops, foot straps, and shoe holders. Most of the leg/foot accessories serve one of two functions: (1) preventing the feet from sliding off the back of the footplates or (2) stabilizing the feet on the footrests.

Trunk

When the pelvis and lower body are supported, physical therapists further examine the position of the trunk, head, and arms. When positioning the trunk, physical therapists begin by providing support along the posterior aspect of the child's body, then the lateral aspect, and finally the anterior aspect. Posterior support (seat and back cushions) should provide a stable base of support for the pelvis, trunk, and lower body. Lateral trunk supports (scoliosis pads) and anterior trunk supports (chest straps, shoulder harnesses, H-straps) are commonly used supports for the trunk. Lateral trunk supports center the body over the pelvis and correct flexible trunk deformities. Anterior trunk supports are designed to facilitate thoracic extension of the spine, allowing the child to rest against the back support.

Head

Frequently, after a child's hips, pelvis, and trunk are supported in a seating system, the child's head will often be in a neutral, upright position. However, children may require specialized head supports, even after the rest of the body is supported in a neutral position. Head positioning is crucial for children with severe neuromotor

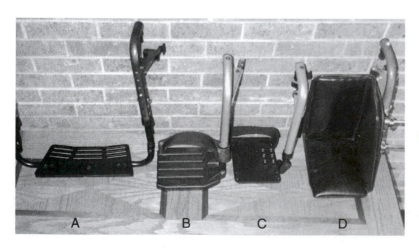

Figure 17.12 Footrest options: (*A*) 90° hanger with one-piece footplate, (*B*) 60° hanger with individual composite footplate, (*C*) 90° hanger with individual angle adjustable footplate, and (*D*) 70° hanger with Miller solid footbucket.

impairments because it affects their ability to visually attend to their environment. Specialized head supports are available and should be used much in the same manner as trunk supports (posterior first, followed by lateral, and last anterior). Most headrests provide a combination of posterior head and neck support. The neck support incorporated into many headrests fits below the occiput and supports the cervical spine. Posterior head supports range in size depending on the amount of surface area with which the child needs contact. Children with more significant needs may require the use of lateral and anterior head and neck supports (Fig. 17.13). These should be incorporated into a system only when posterior supports do not meet the child's needs, because they tend to interfere with peripheral vision. Headrests also can serve as a control mechanism for a power wheelchair, communication device, and computer controls for children with severe physical disabilities.

Arms

The final consideration in the design of a seating system is the position of a child's arms. Physical therapists should ensure that the child's arms are supported in a forward position. The height and angle of armrests and trays influence a child's arm position, so they need to be appropriately adjusted. Armrests and trays are the most commonly used arm supports for children. Armrest options on most wheelchairs include desk length, full length, fixed height, height adjustable, fixed, removable, and swing-away; they come in a variety of shapes and styles. Some children who propel their wheelchairs may not require arm supports, and armrests can be omitted from their systems. Armrests are often necessary if the child uses a tray because the tray is generally secured to the armrests. Trays are commonly recommended for children with limited shoulder movement and upper trunk strength. Trays also provide children a surface from which they can eat, play, and work when they encounter an environment that is not accessible.

Simulation

Based on the findings in the record review, interview with the child and family, and physical examination, the physical therapist can now simulate different seating systems. Seating simulators (Fig. 17.14) are commercially available and allow easy adjustment of linear components, seating angles, and contouring. Simulators also allow physical therapists to evaluate the effect of recline and tilt-in-space on a child's trunk and head position. They are especially useful for examining children with severe physical disabilities.

Simulation may include a process as simple as trying two or three off-the-shelf seating systems. In other situations, it may involve intimate molding around a child's body and adjusting various seating angles, including seat-to-back angle and tilt-in-space, to determine the optimal position. When simulating a seating system, physical therapists should provide as little support as is required for the child to sit upright and participate in activities across environments.

Mobility

Children with disabilities often cannot move freely about their environment. The ultimate goal for mobility is to get from one place to another in a defined period of time and still have the energy necessary to function in the new environment. When considering mobility options for children, team members must consider whether the child can move independently from place to place. Team members must also consider the child's future environments and potential for independence. Mobility aids such as walkers, crutches, canes, and manual and powered wheelchairs can promote independence for children (see Figs. 17.2, 17.15 to 17.18). Physical therapists play a significant role in determining the type of mobility aids children need to be as independent and functional as possible. Table 17.2 summarizes factors that physical therapists must consider when selecting walking aids for children.

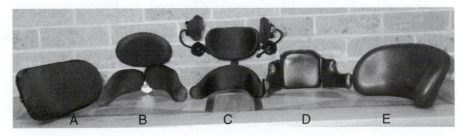

Figure 17.13 Headrest options. (*A*) Whitmyer Plush 1, (*B*) Whitmyer SOFT-1, (*C*) Stealth, (*D*) AEL Tri-Pad Headrest, and (*E*) OttoBock Combination Head/Neckrest.

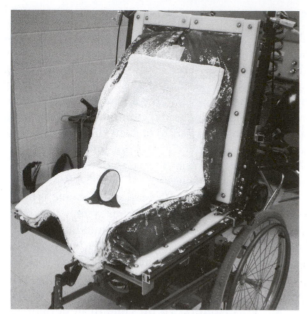

Figure 17.14 The Flamingo Seating Simulator from Tallahassee Therapeutic.

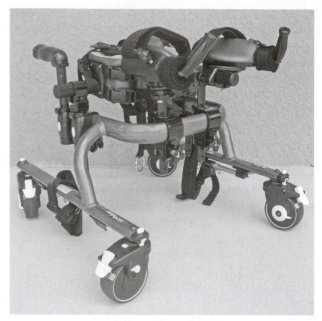

Figure 17.16 Mobility aids. Rifton Pacer gait trainer.

Children with disabilities use a variety of mobility aids. For example, the use of mobility aids for children with spinal cord injuries and myelodysplasia varies widely depending on the level of lesion and age. Children with injuries from T11 to L2 may use knee-ankle-foot orthoses or reciprocating gait orthoses in combination with forearm crutches for indoor mobility only, whereas children whose level of injury is L3 to S2 may require only ankle-foot orthoses in combination with forearm crutches or a cane. Lofstrand crutches or wheeled walkers may be used in a small percentage of children with juvenile rheumatoid arthritis who experience pain, contracture, or weakness in their lower extremities that prevents efficient weight bearing. Children with arthrogryposis multiplex congenita often require the use of a power wheelchair for efficient community mobility. Children with cerebral palsy (CP) often require manual or power wheelchairs for independent and efficient mobility. Children with CP or myelomeningocele who walk independently often

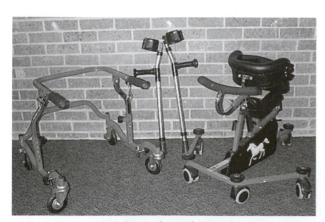

Figure 17.15 Mobility aids. Left to right: Wenzelite reverse walker, Lumex forearm crutches, and Pony prone support walker.

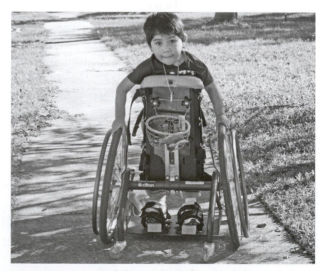

Figure 17.17 Mobility aids. Rifton mobile prone stander.

need an alternative form of mobility, such as a power wheelchair, as they grow and have to travel greater distances at a faster pace to keep up with their peers (David & Sullivan, 2005; Franks, Palisano, & Darbee, 1991).

As previously described, children may use a combination of mobility aids depending on environmental demands. For example, a child may use a walker in home and school environments to walk short distances within rooms but may use a power wheelchair for community and outside mobility where longer distances of greater duration are required.

Effects of Mobility on Other Aspects of Development

Children with limited mobility experiences often fall behind in other areas of development because they must rely on others to move them about their environment. Therapists cannot allow years to pass while waiting for a child to walk, because motor skills develop rapidly during the first 3 years of life and become the bridge to more advanced learning, socialization, and psychological development (Jones et al., 2003; Lynch, Ryu, Agrawal, & Galloway, 2009; Ragonesi, Chen, Agrawal, & Galloway, 2010).

Therapists must augment a child's mobility to prevent or minimize the detrimental effects caused by immobility.

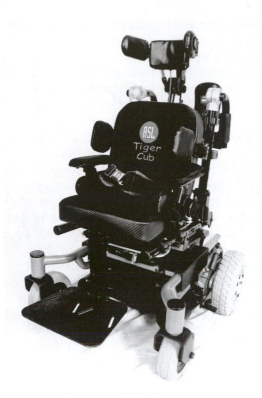

Figure 17.18 Power mobility devices. Invacare/ASL Tiger Cub.

Table 17.2 Choosing Walking Aids for Children

Device	Advantages	Disadvantages
Cane	Small Require use of only one hand Can use quad base to increase stability Good for decreasing pain with weight bearing	Small base of support Safe for weight bearing as tolerated only Requires sequencing and coordination
Crutches	Allow fast movement Able to go up and down stairs Allow non–weight bearing (NWB) and partial weight bearing (PWB) Inexpensive Very maneuverable	Small base of support Require sequencing and coordination Require use of both hands Require good balance Require good strength in arms and uninvolved leg Require at least fair strength in involved leg
Walker	Increased stability Minimal sequencing needed Will work for young child Allows NWB and PWB Can add wheels for easier maneuverability	Cannot maneuver on stairs Larger and more cumbersome than crutches
Gait trainer	Increased stability Can work for children who do not have good postural stability Can work for children who cannot maintain consistent weight bearing Good for long distances	Cumbersome Hard to transport in car or public transportation Hard to maneuver in home Cannot maneuver up and down stairs Costly to purchase

Equipment used to augment mobility includes walkers, canes, crutches, ladder frames, walking frames, splints, orthotics, tricycles, bicycles, and manual and powered wheelchairs. Augmented mobility must be viewed as a tool that promotes independence and continued development rather than a stumbling block that prevents the development of ambulation (Butler, 1997; Jones et al., 2003; Lynch et al., 2009; Ragonesi et al., 2010).

Types of Mobility Bases

Children who cannot walk without the assistance of mobility aids frequently rely on a wheelchair to move about in their environments. Children's needs change over time because of growth and development; therefore, children need adaptable systems and/or multiple systems throughout their lives to ensure that AT promotes and supports their development. Physical therapists work with families to determine when children need their "first chair." During typical development, most children begin moving independently (in an upright position) between 12 and 15 months of age. If children with disabilities do not have a means of independent, self-produced locomotion by this age, physical therapists assist families in determining the type of mobility base that provides the most independence and function to augment the child's mobility (Jones et al., 2003). Features of a wheelchair that are critical to consider when ordering include method of propulsion (manual or power), frame style (folding or rigid), size, and model. Physical therapists should carefully review all of the features of a mobility base with the family before ordering a specific chair (McDonald et al., 2003). They match features of a mobility base with information obtained during their interview with the child and/or family, record review, and physical examination. Team members also ensure that, when delivered, the mobility base and seating system are adjusted to meet the child's needs. Mobility bases can be divided into two basic categories according to the method of propulsion: manual and power. Manual wheelchairs can be further divided into chairs for independent mobility and dependent transport chairs. Children who rely on others to move them within and between environments use dependent transport chairs.

Manual Wheelchairs for Independent Mobility Wheelchairs for independent mobility encompass a wide array of frame styles, sizes, and models. Most fold, allowing the chair to become more compact for transportation. Weight of the wheelchair is an important factor because it affects the ease of propulsion, especially for young children. Chairs are generally classified by their weight and include standard, lightweight, and ultra-lightweight frames.

Standard wheelchairs weigh in excess of 45 pounds and are often difficult for children with disabilities to propel. They generally fold for transportation but have limited adjustability for efficient wheelchair propulsion and growth. **Lightweight chairs** weigh between 30 and 36 pounds and have options available that improve their adjustability for wheelchair propulsion and growth. Lightweight chairs usually allow adjustment of the rear wheel position to allow a child to reach the wheels for propulsion. In general, they also allow for adjustment of seat width, seat depth, and back height. The frame adjustability is especially important for children, allowing accommodation of their current size but having versatility to adjust for future growth. **Ultra-lightweight chairs** weigh less than 30 pounds. Chairs in this category can be folding or rigid. Folding frames are beneficial when families must fold the chair for transportation. The folding frame is achieved either with a cross-brace (x-frame) or a folding back (Fig. 17.19). *Folding frames*, because of the "flex" in the frame, require more energy to propel than do rigid frames. *Rigid frames* are more responsive and energy efficient for children to propel independently but often require that families have vans or alternate chairs to use for transportation outside of the school or home.

Manual Wheelchairs for Dependent Mobility Manual chairs for dependent mobility are most often used for children who cannot propel their wheelchairs independently. Family members push the wheelchair, moving the children from place to place. Therefore, when choosing a chair for dependent mobility, the family must also be considered a "user" of the chair. As with manual wheelchairs for independent mobility, various frame styles are available. Manual wheelchairs for dependent mobility can generally be divided into tilt-in-space wheelchairs and strollers (Fig. 17.20).

Manual **tilt-in-space wheelchairs** allow adjustment of the frame in relationship to the surrounding environment. Children may require tilt-in-space for position changes throughout the day to prevent the development of pressure ulcers. Children with poor head and trunk control, significant musculoskeletal impairments, and poor endurance may also require tilt-in-space. Team members should consider the child's visual orientation when using tilt-in-space to avoid decreasing a child's visual interaction with people. Adjustments should be made to the seating system or other parts of the frame to limit the degree of tilt-in-space needed as much as possible to facilitate a horizontal eye gaze.

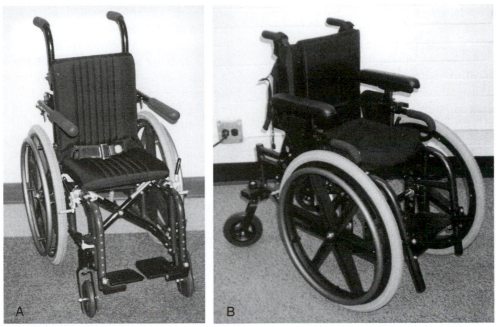

Figure 17.19 (*A*) Zippie 2 manual wheelchair with x-frame and (*B*) Zippie GS manual wheelchair with a folding back.

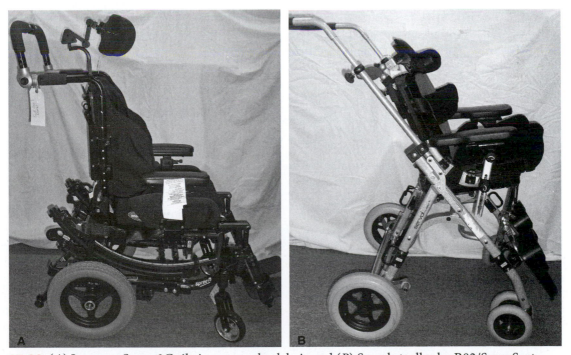

Figure 17.20 (*A*) Invacare Spree 3G tilt-in-space wheelchair and (*B*) Serval stroller by R82/Snug Seat.

Tilt-in-space wheelchairs are often designed with an adjustable seat-to-back angle. An adjustable seat-to-back angle is important when obtaining a wheelchair for a child who has limited hip mobility (less than 90° of hip flexion), shortened hamstring musculature, or structural kyphosis, or who cannot sit in an upright position because of fatigue or the effects of gravity. Manual chairs with an adjustable seat-to-back angle can generally be adjusted from 90° of hip flexion to a recline angle ranging from 90° to 120° to accommodate a child's structural deformities.

Strollers are designed for very young children. Parents of young children who are receiving their first mobility base may be more receptive to a stroller that looks the least like a wheelchair; however, therapists should offer the full range of mobility base options available. Strollers often are easier to fold for transport, making them a preferred option for many parents. Strollers that are easy to fold, however, are not generally designed to provide extensive positioning support, so they may not be beneficial for children with severe physical disabilities. Many of today's commercially available strollers are designed with firm seats and backs and offer the option to add various positioning components. They also can be adapted with custom-contoured seating systems. Strollers are not intended for permanent use by older children, and their use should be limited to young children or as a backup method of transportation for older children.

Powered Mobility Bases

For children who cannot maneuver a manual wheelchair independently, but for whom independent mobility is a goal, powered mobility bases should be considered. Children who will never ambulate, whose ambulation is inefficient, or whose abilities have declined as a result of trauma or progressive neuromuscular disorders should be assessed for power mobility. Hays (1987) believes that power mobility should be provided for children who have a mismatch between cognitive and motor skills. Typical 8- to 9-month-olds are mobile by crawling and typical 12-month-olds can walk; however, children who have the cognitive skills of a 12-month-old, but are immobile, have a mismatch between their cognitive and motor skills. These children should be assessed for power mobility, especially when considering the potential developmental consequences that they may experience due to their immobility (Campos et al., 2000). The decision to introduce power mobility should be based on the team's assessment of many factors such as motivation, understanding of cause

and effect, attention, problem solving, and the identification of a consistent access method (RESNA, 2008). Too often, young children are denied the use of power mobility based on age alone. However, children as young as 7–12 months of age have successfully used power mobility (Lynch et al., 2009; Zazula & Foulds, 1983).

Continued advancements in the field of powered mobility have made independence a reality for many children with disabilities. Most power wheelchairs for children are direct-drive chairs, which provide a direct connection between the motors and wheels. Direct-drive chairs offer the greatest range of control options. Some powered mobility bases also offer seat height adjustment and standing options. Power tilt and recline systems can be added to these chairs, allowing for position changes throughout the day to prevent the development of ulcers, pain, or fatigue, as well as to improve function.

Scooters and add-on battery packs are options available for children, but are less commonly used. Scooters are equipped with either three or four wheels and are controlled with a tiller on which the controls are positioned. Control and positioning/seating options are often limited with scooters, requiring good upper extremity movement and independent sitting balance. Scooters are better suited for indoor than outdoor use.

Add-on battery packs can be attached over the rear wheels of a manual wheelchair to convert it to a powered mobility base. Power packs perform better on level surfaces and are not designed for rigorous outdoor use.

Controls for powered wheelchairs are either *proportional* or *microswitch*. Typical power wheelchairs are controlled through a joystick mechanism, although other electronic control systems also are available. Typically, the joystick is mounted on the armrest and controls the speed and direction of the chair in a 360° arc of movement. Alternative mounting options and joystick sizes are available. For children who cannot use a proportional control, other electronic controls or microswitches are available. Electronic controls include sip-and-puff options, chin controls, head controls, and foot controls. Microswitch controls consists of four separate switches that control a single direction of the chair (forward, backward, right, left). Figure 17.21 illustrates some popular wheelchair controls.

Physical therapists, in collaboration with other team members, play a critical role in researching, presenting,

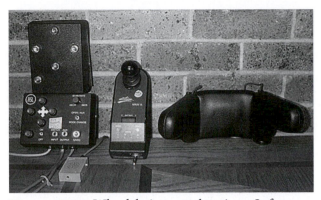

Figure 17.21 Wheelchair control options. Left to right: ASL single switch direction scan, standard joystick and ASL head array.

trying, and possibly developing appropriate control systems to provide children with a means of independent mobility. The physical therapist's contributions are as follows:

1. identifying potential voluntary movement patterns that the child can reliably control
2. identifying the potential body part that the child will use to operate the control mechanism
3. determining the type of control mechanism that best interfaces with the child's movement pattern
4. evaluating a child's ability to activate, control direction, and release the wheelchair control mechanism
5. determining how to secure the control mechanism to the mobility base
6. assessing the effectiveness of potential options during trials

Physical therapists, whether recommending a manual or powered wheelchair, work with durable medical equipment suppliers to review the finer details of the chair. The wheelchair's overall size, ability to accommodate a child's current size and future growth, and adjustability of component parts, such as seating angles, footrests, armrests, and turning radius, as well as ease of maneuvering, disassembly, and transport, are details that physical therapists and durable medical equipment suppliers discuss with the child and family. Such details are crucial in making an appropriate, informed recommendation.

Summary

AT devices and services allow children with disabilities to participate in activities alongside their peers. Devices are designed to promote independence, improve activities and participation, and enhance the lives of children with disabilities. AT allows children to overcome neuromotor, musculoskeletal, and sensory impairments and to eliminate secondary limitations in activities and participation that arise as a result of such impairments. Physical therapists play a key role in the selection, acquisition, modification/customization, and implementation of AT devices, ensuring that children receive—and can effectively use—the AT they need across all environments. AT is an integral part of a child's therapeutic program and cannot be viewed as a separate task for which therapists have no responsibility. Physical therapists work with families and other team members to provide AT evaluations, complete paperwork necessary to apply for funding, design and provide practice opportunities when training children to use AT, and provide ongoing support and follow-up to ensure that the AT provided continues to meet a child's changing needs. AT devices change rapidly, as do the needs of children. Therefore, physical therapists must stay current on AT devices available to meet children's needs. As with other areas of practice, continued research evaluating the impact and use of AT is critical.

DISCUSSION QUESTIONS

1. What are the critical elements that provide information as part of the assistive technology decision-making process?
2. What factors should you consider when training children to use assistive technology?
3. What factors should you consider when determining the type of seating system to recommend for a child?
4. What factors should you consider when determining the type of wheelchair to recommend for a child?

Recommended Readings

Angelo, J. (1997). *Assistive technology for rehabilitation therapists.* Philadelphia: F.A. Davis.

Furumasu, J. (Ed.). (1997). *Pediatric powered mobility: Developmental perspectives, technical issues, clinical approaches.* Arlington, VA: Rehabilitation Engineering and Assistive Technology Society of North America.

Reed, P., & Lahm, E. (Eds.). (2004). *Assessing students' needs for assistive technology: A resource manual for school district teams.* Oshkosh, WI: Wisconsin Assistive Technology Initiative.

References

Angelo, J. (2000). Factors affecting the use of a single switch with assistive technology devices. *Journal of Rehabilitation Research and Development, 37*(5), 591–598.

Bay, J.L. (1991). Positioning for head control to access an augmentative communication machine. *The American Journal of Occupational Therapy, 45*, 544–549.

Bergen, A.F., Presperin, J., & Tallman, T. (1990). *Positioning for function: Wheelchairs and other assistive technologies.* Valhalla, NY: Valhalla Rehabilitation Publications.

Beukelman, D., & Mirenda, P. (2005). *Augmentative and alternative communication: Supporting children and adults with complex communication needs* (3rd ed.). Baltimore: Paul H. Brookes.

Brown, D.A., Effgen, S.K., & Palisano, R.J. (1998). Performance following ability-focused physical therapy intervention in individuals with severely limited physical and cognitive abilities. *Physical Therapy, 78*(9), 934–947.

Butler, C. (1997). Wheelchair toddlers. In J. Furumasu (Ed.), *Pediatric powered mobility: Developmental perspectives, technical issues, clinical approaches* (pp. 1–5). Arlington, VA: Rehabilitation Engineering and Assistive Technology Society of North America.

Campbell, P.H., Milbourne, S., Dugan, L.M. & Wilcox, M.J. (2006). A review of evidence on practices for teaching young children to use assistive technology devices. *Topics in Early Childhood Special Education, 26*, 3–13.

Campos, J.J., Anderson, D.I., Barbu-Roth, M.A., Hubbard, E.M., Hertenstein, M.J., & Witherington D. (2000). Travel broadens the mind. *Infancy, 1*(2), 149–219.

Carlson, S.J., & Ramsey, C. (2000). Assistive technology. In S.K. Campbell, D.W. Vander Linden, & R.J. Palisano (Eds.), *Physical therapy for children* (2nd ed., pp. 671–708). Philadelphia: W.B. Saunders.

Caulton, J.M., Ward, K.A., Alsop, C.W., Dunn, G., Adams, J.E. & Mughal, M.Z. (2004). A randomized controlled trial of standing programme on bone mineral density in nonambulant children with cerebral palsy. *Archives of Disease in Childhood, 89*, 131–135.

Chung, J., Evans, J., Lee, C., Lee, J., Rabbani, Y., Roxborough, L. & Harris, S.R. (2008). Effectiveness of adaptive seating on sitting posture and postural control in children with cerebral palsy. *Pediatric Physical Therapy, 20*, 303–317.

David, K.S., & Sullivan, M. (2005). Expectations for walking speeds: Standards for students in elementary schools. *Pediatric Physical Therapy, 17*(2), 120–127.

Franks, C.A., Palisano, R.J., & Darbee, J.C. (1991). The effect of walking with an assistive device and using a wheelchair on school performance in students with myelomeningocele. *Physical Therapy, 71*(8), 570–577.

Galvin, J.C., & Scherer, M.J. (1996). *Evaluating, selecting, and using appropriate assistive technology.* Gaithersburg, MD: Aspen Publishers.

Gibson, S.K., Sprod, J.A., & Maher, C.A. (2009). The use of standing frames for contracture management for nonmobile children with cerebral palsy. *International Journal of Rehabilitation Research, 32*, 316–323.

Gillen, G. (2002). Improving mobility and community access in an adult with ataxia. *American Journal of Occupational Therapy, 56*(4), 462–466.

Harris, S.R., & Roxborough, L. (2005). Efficacy and effectiveness of physical therapy in enhancing postural control in children with cerebral palsy. *Neural Plasticity, 12*, 229–243.

Hays, R.M. (1987). Childhood motor impairments: Clinical overview and scope of the problem. In K.M. Jaffe (Ed.), *Childhood powered mobility: Developmental technical and clinical perspectives: Proceedings of the RESNA first Northwest Regional Conference* (pp. 1–10). Washington, DC: RESNA.

Henderson, S., Skelton, H., & Rosenbaum, P. (2008). Assistive devices for children with functional impairments: Impact on child and caregiver function. *Developmental Medicine and Child Neurology, 50*, 89–98.

Hulme, J.B., Bain, B., Hardin, M., McKinnon, A., & Waldron, D. (1989). The influence of adaptive seating devices on vocalization. *Journal of Communication Disorders, 22*, 137–145.

Hulme, J.B., Gallacher, K., Walsh, J., Niesen, S., & Waldron, D. (1987). Behavioral and postural changes observed with use of adaptive seating by clients with multiple handicaps. *Physical Therapy, 67*(7), 1060–1067.

Jones, M.A., McEwen, I.R., & Hansen, L. (2003). Use of power mobility for a young child with spinal muscular atrophy. *Physical Therapy, 83*, 253–262.

Larin, H.M. (2000). Motor learning: Theories and strategies for the practitioner. In S.K. Campbell, D.W. Vander Linden, & R.J. Palisano (Eds.), *Physical therapy for children* (2nd ed., pp. 170–197). Philadelphia: W.B. Saunders.

Lynch, A., Ryu, J.C., Agrawal, S., & Galloway, J.C. (2009). Power mobility training for a 7-month-old infant with spina bifida. *Pediatric Physical Therapy, 21*, 362–368.

Individuals with Disabilities Education Act Amendments of 1997, PL 105-17, 20 U.S.C. §§1400 et seq.

Maslovat, D., Brunke, K.M., Chua, R., & Franks, I. (2009). Feedback effects on learning a novel bimanual coordination pattern: Support for the guidance hypothesis. *Journal of Motor Behavior, 41*(1), 45–54.

McDonald, R., Surtees, R., & Wirz, S. (2003). A comparison between parents' and therapists' views of their child's individual seating systems. *International Journal of Rehabilitation Research, 26*(3), 235–243.

McEwen, I.R. (1992). Assistive positioning as a control parameter of social-communicative interactions between students with profound multiple disabilities and classroom staff. *Physical Therapy, 72*(9), 634–646.

McEwen, I.R., & Lloyd, L.L. (1990). Positioning students with cerebral palsy to use augmentative and alternative communication. *Language, Speech, and Hearing Services in Schools, 21*, 15–21.

McNamara, L., & Casey, J. (2007). Seat inclinations affect the function of children with cerebral palsy: A review of the effect of different seat inclines. *Disability and Rehabilitation: Assistive Technology, 2*(6), 309–318.

McNevin, N.H., Wulf, G., & Carlson, C. (2000). Effects of attentional focus, self-control, and dyad training on motor learning: Implications for physical rehabilitation. *Physical Therapy, 80*(4), 373–385.

Miedaner, J., & Finuf, L. (1993). Effects of adaptive positioning on psychological test scores for preschool children with cerebral palsy. *Pediatric Physical Therapy, 5*, 177–182.

Minkel, J.L. (2000). Seating and mobility considerations for people with spinal cord injury. *Physical Therapy, 80*(7), 701–709.

Myhr, U., & von Wendt, L. (1991). Improvement of functional sitting position for children with cerebral palsy. *Developmental Medicine and Child Neurology, 33*(3), 246–256.

Nwaobi, O.M., & Smith, P.D. (1986). Effect of adaptive seating on pulmonary function of children enhance psychosocial and cognitive development. *Developmental Medicine and Child Neurology, 28,* 351–354.

Ragonesi, C., Chen, X., Agrawal, S., & Galloway, J.C. (2010). Power mobility and socialization in preschool: A case report on a child with cerebral palsy. *Pediatric Physical Therapy, 22*(3), 322–329.

Reed, P., & Lahm, E. (Ed.). (2004). *Assessing students' needs for assistive technology: A resource manual for school district teams.* Oshkosh, WI: Wisconsin Assistive Technology Initiative.

Reichle, J., & Sigafoos, J. (1991). Establishing spontaneity and generalization. In J. Reichle, J. York, & J. Sigafoos (Eds.), *Implementing augmentative and alternative communication: Strategies for learners with severe disabilities* (pp. 157–171). Baltimore: Paul H. Brookes.

Rehabilitation Engineering and Assistive Technology Society of North America (RESNA). (2008). *RESNA position on the application of power wheelchairs for pediatric users.* Rehabilitation and Engineering Society of North America, Arlington, VA: RESNA Press.

RESNA. (2012). *Becoming certified.* Retrieved March 3, 2012 from http://www.resna.org/certification/becoming-certified.dot

RESNA Technical Assistance Project (1992). *Assistive technology and the individualized education program* (updated). Washington, DC: RESNA Press.

Rigby, P., Reid, D., Schoger, S., & Ryan, S. (2001). Effects of wheelchair-mounted rigid pelvic stabilizer on caregiver assistance for children with cerebral palsy. *Assistive Technology, 13*(1), 2–11.

Rigby, P.J., Ryan, S.E., & Campbell, K.A. (2009). Effect of adaptive seating devices on the activity performance of children with cerebral palsy. *Archives of Physical Medicine and Rehabilitation, 90,* 1389–1395.

Ryan, S.E., Campbell, K.A., Rigby, P.J., Fishbein-Germon, B., Hubley, D., & Chan, B. (2009). The impact of adaptive seating devices on the lives of young children with cerebral palsy and their families. *Archives of Physical Medicine and Rehabilitation, 90,* 27–33.

Scherer M.J., & Craddock, G. (2002). Matching person and technology (MPT) assessment process. *Technology & Disability, 14*(3), 125–131.

Schmidt, R.A., & Lee, T.D. (2005). *Motor control and learning: A behavioral emphasis.* Champaign, IL: Human Kinetics.

Sommerville, J.A., Hildebrand, E.A., & Crane, C.C. (2008). Experience matters: The impact of doing versus watching on infants' subsequent perception of tool-use events. *Developmental Psychology, 44*(5), 1249–1256.

Stavness, C. (2006). The effect of positioning for children with cerebral palsy on upper-extremity function: A review of the evidence. *Physical & Occupational Therapy in Pediatrics, 26*(3), 39–53.

Stuberg, W.A. (1992). Considerations related to weight-bearing programs in children with developmental disabilities. *Physical Therapy, 72,* 35–40.

Washington, K., Deitz, J.C., White, O.R., & Schwartz, I.S. (2002). The effects of a contoured foam seat on postural alignment and upper extremity function in infants with neuromotor impairments. *Physical Therapy, 82*(11), 1064–1076.

Zazula, J.L., & Foulds, R.A. (1983). Mobility device for a child with phocomelia. *Archives of Physical Medicine and Rehabilitation, 64,* 137–139.

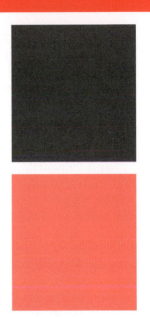

CHAPTER 18

Assistive Technology: Augmentative Communication and Other Technologies

—Maria Jones, PT, PhD

—Trina Puddefoot, PT, MS, PCS, ATP

Children with disabilities often require multiple assistive technology (AT) devices to meet their needs across environments. Physical therapists, in collaboration with other team members, will assess for other technologies after addressing the child's positioning. As discussed in Chapter 17, proper positioning promotes improved function, movement, and participation in activities. When a child is well positioned and can move about his or her environment independently, the need for communication and other technologies increases. This chapter provides information pertinent to physical therapists working as members of AT teams when addressing the remaining categories of AT.

Augmentative Communication

Augmentative and alternative communication (AAC) is the use of means other than speech to assist children in communication. The term "augmentative" includes the use of systems that support existing speech to assist children in communicating a message. In essence, all speakers use augmentative techniques from time to time. Speakers often augment their messages with facial expressions and gestures, or by pointing to visual supports in the environment in an effort to make sure the message is understood. "Alternative" communication describes systems that are intended to be the primary communication systems for children who are nonspeaking. AAC systems consist of a wide variety of techniques, systems, and intervention strategies to assist children in becoming proficient communicators.

For any given AAC user, a core group of people, including the child, family, and professionals from two or three disciplines, typically assume the role of AAC team (Reed & Lahm, 2004). Each person provides essential information. For example, the child identifies his or her abilities, limitations, needs, and desires. Family members provide information about any pertinent medical and educational history; day-to-day communication needs; family dynamics, strengths, and needs; family resources; and environmental considerations. Educators discuss current and projected educational abilities, learning needs and potential, and use of materials in the classroom. Speech-language pathologists discuss current receptive and expressive communication abilities, current and future communication abilities, needs, opportunities, and barriers and provide communication intervention. When children who use AAC or may potentially use AAC also have physical disabilities that limit their motor control, a physical therapist can make a contribution by (1) assessing motor control, (2) identifying body part(s) and movement(s) that the child may use to control AAC devices, (3) assessing positioning and ensuring that positioning systems promote optimal motor control and use of devices, (4) designing a system that best matches the motor abilities of the child, and (5) designing intervention strategies to promote functional use of the AAC system (McEwen, 1997). AAC systems are broadly categorized as unaided or aided.

Unaided Systems

Unaided systems are naturally available to us and do not require the addition of something external. Examples of unaided systems are gestures, body language, vocalizations or speech, facial expressions, signals, and manual signs. For some children, behaviors, such as crying, smiling, or tensed or relaxed body tone, may serve as communication systems. Gestures may be conventional or idiosyncratic in nature. Conventional gestures are behavioral postures or movements that are generally interpreted by society as having a specific meaning (e.g., head nod for yes, head shake for no, hand wave for hello/good-bye). Idiosyncratic gestures are unique to a child, and familiar communication partners have assigned their meaning, limiting their use to unfamiliar or novel communication partners. The use of body language also assists in the expression of a communication message. Moving closer to a person usually indicates interest, whereas moving away generally indicates lack of interest or a desire to terminate a conversation.

Although a child may have limited capabilities for producing speech, vocalizations and word approximations can still be effectively used to augment communication. For example, vocalizations combined with facial expressions can effectively communicate messages, such

as accept and protest, or yes and no. Vocalizations may also effectively provide a means of gaining someone's attention. Word approximations are often recognized by parents, friends, and caretakers, thus enhancing communication in certain situations.

Manual signs and sign languages are formal systems in which conventionalized gestures are assigned relatively abstract meanings and communication with these gestures is based on specific rules (Blischak, Lloyd, & Fuller, 1997). Just as with spoken language, there are many sign languages. For example, the sign that represents the word "doctor" may not be produced the same way across languages. American Sign Language (ASL) is the language most often used by the deaf community in the United States.

Aided Systems

Aided communication systems add something to a person to assist with communication. Aided systems may consist of manual communication systems (e.g., communication boards, communication notebooks, or communication wallets) or electronic systems such as voice output communication devices. Walser and Reed (2004) categorize aided augmentative communication systems as follows: simple communication boards, simple voice output devices, leveling or layering devices, devices using icon sequencing, dynamic display devices, and devices that spell with a speech synthesizer/written text (Fig. 18.1).

Communication boards are designed using objects, photographs, graphic symbols (line drawings), or letters/words to represent messages for communication. Decisions about the type of representation to use depend on many factors, such as the child's visual, cognitive-linguistic, and academic abilities. Communication boards can have any number of accessible symbols to create messages. Communication boards are also designed based on how the child will access or send the message to another person, such as eye gaze or pointing.

Simple voice output devices have single-symbol/single-message capabilities. A message is stored in a single location using digitized or recorded speech. The message is easily programmed or recorded by another person. Programming consists of pushing a button and recording the message into the microphone. Children retrieve or deliver messages by activating the device by touch or through a switch. Simple voice output devices have a vocabulary capacity from 1 message to more than 100 messages.

Leveling or layering devices operate by storing vocabulary in levels, which are like pages in a book.

Figure 18.1 Different types of AAC devices: (*a*) Fabricated communication board (low-tech), (*b*) Dynavox Mayer-Johnson, VMax with EyeMax accessory (dynamic display device with eye gaze input system), (*c*) PRC, Vantage™Lite (dynamic display device), (*d*) Enabling Devices, four-level communication builder (level-based system), (*e*) Ablenet iTalk2 (dual-message communicator), (*f*) AMDI, Tech/Speak (recorded speech), (*g*) Attainment company, Go Talk 20+, (*h*) Ablenet BIGmack, (*i*) Ablenet FL4SH, and (*j*) Apple, iPod Touch (commercial device with communication app.).

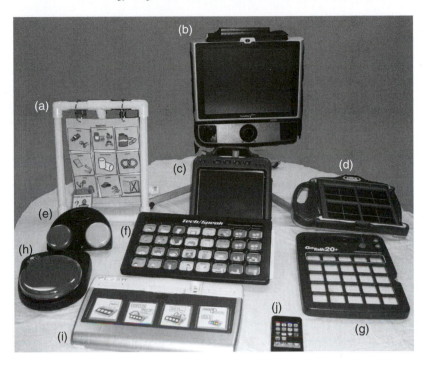

Level-based systems increase the amount of stored vocabulary or messages without the need for reprogramming and also provide a system for organizing the vocabulary. The vocabulary or message storage capacity depends on the number of levels available on the device, as well as the memory capacity. Some level-based systems use digitized speech and others use synthesized or computer-generated speech. Synthesized requires less memory than digitized, but programming is more complicated. Level systems allow vocabulary storage based on activities or environments. For example, if a system has the capacity for four levels, vocabulary may be stored as follows:

Level 1: Circle time vocabulary
Level 2: Snack time vocabulary
Level 3: Story time vocabulary
Level 4: Getting ready for bed vocabulary

Touching a button or turning a dial changes the levels. The display for the vocabulary is usually a paper overlay and has to be physically changed to match the voice messages.

Dynamic display devices automatically change the visual display on the screen of the device based on user input. This feature makes the display or message choices "dynamic" as opposed to "fixed" or "static." Pages or levels of vocabulary are linked when programming the device. Making a choice on one screen links the user to another screen with more vocabulary options. These systems can use picture symbols, letters for spelling, or word prediction, depending on a child's abilities. To access a message such as "I would like a glass of milk," the child might first select the picture on a screen representing foods. This selection causes a display of food categories to appear, such as drinks, vegetables, fruits, desserts, and so on. The child then chooses "drinks." A display with the following choices might appear: water, milk, juice, and so on. The child now selects "milk" from the array of choices to indicate the desire for milk. Most dynamic display systems have touchscreen capabilities but also have other methods of access for children who cannot use a touchscreen.

Another group of devices use icon sequencing or Unity to store and retrieve messages. When using Unity, a message is stored and recalled using a two- or three-picture symbol sequence. Unity relies on a child's ability to make multiple associations with a picture and sequence two or three symbols to create a message. With Unity, a two-symbol sequence can be used to store the name of a color, such as the rainbow icon that represents "colors" and the sun icon to represent "yellow." The message "What color is it?" might be stored under the question mark icon (?) and the rainbow icon.

For children who have functional literacy skills (at least third-grade level), teams may consider devices that have "text-to-speech" capabilities. Such devices operate like a talking keyboard—the user types in a message and the device speaks the typed message. Some of these devices have rate enhancement strategies to increase the speed of message generation for children who have difficulty with motor control. Rate enhancement strategies may include letter prediction, word prediction, or abbreviation expansion. The letter prediction feature assists by predicting the next letter to be typed. Word prediction assists by predicting the word a person is typing. After that word is selected, it may predict the next word. Abbreviation expansion allows a child to store a word, phrase, or sentence message by assigning the message a string of letters. When the child types the letter string, the message expands to include the full text stored, decreasing the number of keystrokes necessary to retrieve messages. The child must have the ability to assign letter codes to specific messages and remember the letter codes to retrieve the message. For example, NMJ might represent "My name is Maria Jones."

Access for Communication Systems or Computers

Access refers to how children will use or provide input to a communication device or computer. Most children turn on a portable device by pushing the play button. For children with disabilities this may not be possible; therefore, they need some other means of accessing devices or tools within their environment. Two basic forms of access include direct selection or indirect selection (scanning).

Direct Selection

Direct selection involves the child directly interacting with the device or system. One example of direct selection is using both hands to access a computer keyboard. Children may also use direct selection with a head pointer, chin pointer, mouthstick, or hand splint. When using these options, children make physical contact with the device or system. They can, however, make a direct selection without making physical contact. For example, children can use their eyes, a light pointer, or their voices to select activities or make choices. New technology continues to develop, making it easier to find a method of direct selection for accessing a system. Whenever possible, identifying a method for direct selection is preferred because it is usually faster and less cognitively demanding than indirect selection.

Indirect Selection

Children who cannot use direct selection must rely on indirect selection to access devices. **Indirect selection** involves the use of a switch in combination with an encoding system, such as scanning or Morse code. Switches provide an interface between the child and the device or system he or she is controlling (Angelo, 2000). Scanning provides a child with access to a group of items, such as the alphabet, pictures, or icons on a computer. The system scans through the group of items, making only one item available at a time. For example, if a student wants to type his name, "Chris," he must activate the switch to begin scanning, wait for the cursor to pass over the "A" and "B," and be ready to activate the switch again when the cursor highlights "C." This process is then repeated for each letter in his name. Scanning is slower than direct selection but requires reliable motor control of only one movement. Figure 18.2 illustrates movement options available for switch control for AAC or computer access.

A wide variety of switches is commercially available (Fig. 18.3). Categories of switches include pressure, pneumatic, motion, photosensitive, physioelectric, and sound activated. Applying *pressure* causes activation of pressure switches. *Pneumatic* switches are activated by air, such as sip and puff switches and air cushion switches. The release of air into the switch results in activation. Examples of *motion* switches are mercury or infrared switches. Examples of *photosensitive* switches include blink switches. *Physioelectric* switches detect muscle movements such as tension and relaxation for activation. *Sound* switches are activated when sound is detected. With the wide variety of switches available, teams can identify a means of indirect selection for children with varying degrees of physical abilities.

The evaluation process for selecting a method of indirect selection involves identifying (1) movement patterns that the child can reliably and voluntarily control, (2) the joint or body part that the child will use to access the switch, (3) the type of switch that best interfaces with the child's movement pattern, and (4) how the switch will be secured. The physical therapist should be an integral part of the evaluation process. The physical therapist's contributions are to (1) determine whether a child has the motor control necessary for unaided AAC, (2) identify body part(s) and movement(s) to control AAC devices, (3) assess positioning and ensure that positioning systems promote optimal motor control and use of devices, (4) design a system that best matches the motor abilities of the child, (5) design intervention strategies to promote development of motor control for functional use of the AAC system, and (6) determine methods to assess the effect of the device on the desired outcomes.

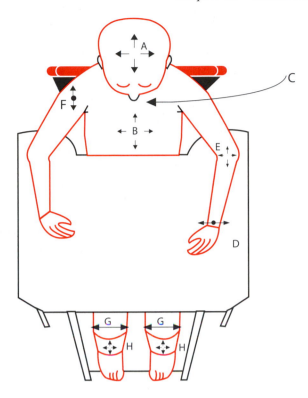

A. Head Control - forward/backward and left/right movement of the head

B. Chin Control - forward/backward and left/right movement of the chin, as with a chin-controlled joystick

C. Mouth/Tongue/Lip or Puff/Sip Control

D. Hand Control - up/down and left/right hand movement

E. Arm/Elbow Control - movement of the elbow outward or sliding the arm forward and backward

F. Shoulder Control - elevation/depression or protraction/retraction of the shoulder

G. Leg/Knee Control - inward/outward movement of the knee

H. Foot Control - left/right and up/down movement of the foot

Figure 18.2 Potential movement and control sites. *(From D.M. Bayer (1984), DU-IT. Control Systems Group, Inc. 8755 TR 513, Shreve, OH. Adapted with permission.)*

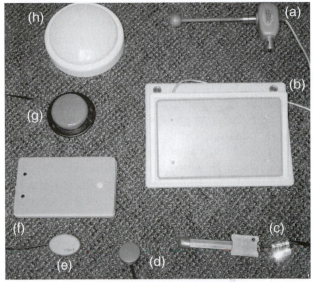

Figure 18.3 Different types of switches: (*a*) Enabling Devices, Ultimate switch, (*b*) Enabling Devices, Plate switch, (*c*) Zygo, Leaf switch, (*d*) AbleNet, Spec switch, (*e*) Ellipse switch, (*f*) Don Johnson Bass switch, (*g*) AbleNet, Jellybean switch, (*h*)WATI Light switch.

The next phase of the evaluation includes observing how the child accesses the switch. A child's ability to activate and release the switch can be categorized in three ways: (1) the child has timed or controlled initiation and release, (2) the child has untimed initiation and timed release, or (3) the child has untimed initiation and release. The way the child activates and releases the switch determines the type of scanning that is appropriate. Factors considered include scan technique and scan pattern.

Scan techniques include automatic, inverse, and step. *Automatic* means that the child activates the switch and the indicator automatically moves through the scan pattern. When the desired target is lighted, the child again hits the switch to indicate the desired selection. Children need controlled initiation and release activation of the switch for this method. In *inverse* (i.e., directed) scan technique, the child initiates and maintains contact with the switch. As long as the child maintains contact with the switch, the indicator light moves through the scan pattern. When the indicator is on the desired target, the child releases the switch to make the selection. Children with good ability to maintain contact and perform controlled releases are often matched with this type of scan technique. In *step* scan, one-to-one correspondence exists between switch activation or release and movement through the scan pattern. Children who have difficulty with timed or controlled movements may be matched with this type of scan technique.

Scan pattern refers to how the indicator moves through the array of choices presented on the communication or computer display. Scan patterns include circular, linear, and group-item. *Circular* scans move item by item through a circular pattern, like a second hand on a clock. A dial scan or clock communicator are examples of devices that use a circular scan pattern. A child who can activate and hold a switch and has timed release to stop the "scan" on the appropriate choice may use a circular pattern. *Linear* scans move item by item and line by line from left to right, as in the Tech/ Scan 8. *Group-item* scans move through the array of choices first by highlighted groups of choices (i.e., row or quadrant) and then item by item through the options available in that particular group. Row-column, column-row, and quadrant scanning are options of group-item scan patterns. When using row-column scanning, an entire row is highlighted at once. When the row containing the desired choice is lit, the child activates the switch, indicating the item is in that row. The scanning continues to highlight each individual item in that row. The child then activates the switch a second time when the cursor reaches the desired choice. The child must have quick, controlled activation and release of a switch to use linear or group-item scanning.

Computer-Based Instruction

Children who have physical, sensory, or other disabilities may not be able to access a computer with a standard keyboard or mouse. However, computers can be adapted in many ways to enable children with disabilities to use them (Lahm, Walser, & Reed, 2004; Walser & Reed, 2004). Currently, both Mac and Windows operating systems provide features in the control panel to make a computer more accessible. Sometimes the use of these features alone may provide sufficient adaptation to make the computer accessible; however, these features are typically used in combination with other

access methods. Physical therapists should become familiar with the built-in accessibility features when assessing children's needs for adapted computer access. With the constant changes in technology, updating knowledge of available products is important.

In addition to features built into computer operating systems, options for assisting direct access to computers are available. These include keyguards, keycaps, and arm supports. **Keyguards** fit over the keyboard and are attached using Velcro. They are made of metal or Plexiglas and have holes drilled through them to match the layout of the keyboard. They are helpful for children who have difficulty isolating or targeting keys on the keyboard or communication device because they more definitively separate the keys and prevent accidental keystrokes. When selecting a keyguard, make sure the keyguard matches the keyboard or communication device. Keycaps are labels or stickers that are secured to the keyboard. They provide greater visual contrast and larger print. Keycaps may be helpful for children who have low vision or visual perceptual difficulties. **Arm supports** provide forearm stability and assist with movement for children with limited strength.

Children who cannot access a computer when provided with adaptations to a standard keyboard may have to rely on an alternative keyboard for access. Alternative keyboards include those that provide a larger keyboard area for access (expanded keyboards) and those that provide a smaller keyboard area for access (mini-keyboards) (Fig. 18.4). Children who have

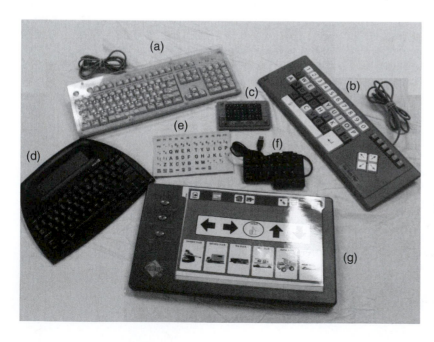

Figure 18.4 Alternative keyboards: (*a*) ORCCA Technology, Keyguard, (*b*) Greystone Digital, Big Keys plus, (*c*) Frog Pad (one-handed keyboard), (*d*) Neodirect, Neo2, (*e*) Viziflex Seels, Large Print Keyboard labels, (*f*) Matias Corporation, half-keyboard, and (*g*) Intellitools, Intellikeys.

limited range of motion may use mini-keyboards. Children who need larger areas to target may use expanded keyboards. Most alternative keyboards are designed to plug directly into the computer.

If children cannot access a computer using standard, modified, or alternative keyboards, voice recognition software may be an option. Voice recognition software is installed on the computer and the child uses voice commands to input information into the computer. Children must have fairly good articulation skills and consistent speech patterns to benefit from voice recognition. Voice recognition is often not useful for children with cerebral palsy or traumatic brain injuries who may have problems with articulation and difficulty coordinating phonation with respiration.

Students who need adaptation to a keyboard may also require alternative mouse access. A wide variety of alternatives are available, including Touch Windows, touchpads, trackballs, different mouse styles, keypad mouse, joysticks, and pointing systems such as those illustrated in Figure 18.5.

Pointing systems allow a child to control the cursor and provide input through head and/or eye movements. In pointing systems, a sensor attached to the computer translates head or eye movements. When the cursor is in the desired location, the child can perform mouse clicks either by "dwelling" on the location for a predetermined length of time or by activating a separate switch. To provide total "hands-free" computer access, these systems are used in combination with on-screen keyboards. An on-screen keyboard is a software program that, when installed and activated, places a visual keyboard on the computer screen. The child uses the pointing device such as a mouse, touchscreen, or head pointing system to have total keyboard control.

Environmental Control

Environmental control units (ECUs) promote a child's interaction, independence, and control of appliances or devices in the environment. Benefits related to the use of environmental control include improved personal satisfaction, increased participation in daily activities, and possible reduction in cost for personal care attendants (Jutai, Rigby, Ryan, & Stickel, 2000). ECUs can allow children to participate in activities that they would otherwise be unable to do. For example, a child can help prepare a snack by turning a blender on and off to make milkshakes.

ECUs consist of three main components: the input device, the control unit, and the appliance. The input

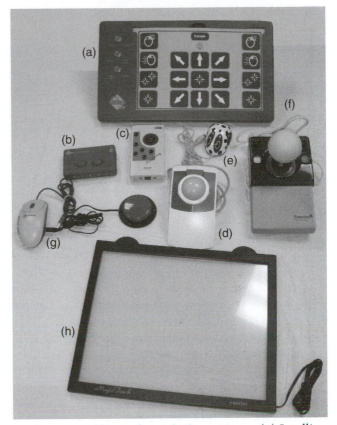

Figure 18.5 Alternative pointing systems: (*a*) Intellitools, Intellikeys with mouse overlay, (*b*) Intellitools, Intelliswitch, (*c*) Penny & Giles, Headway (optical mouse emulator), (*d*) Ergoguys LLC, Kidtrac trackball, (*e*) Infogrip, Kiddymouse, (*f*) Traxsys Input Products, Roller II Joystick, (*g*) Infogrip switch-adapted mouse with AbleNet Jelly Bean switch, and (*h*) KeyTech, Magic Touch.

device controls the ECU by either direct selection or scanning using switches. The control unit is the "brain" of the appliance, translating the input signal into an output action, giving the appliance a direction. Last, the appliance or a piece of electronic equipment responds to the child's input. Table 18.1 provides a summary of control strategies for ECUs.

Activities of Daily Living

AT is often used to promote independence in activities of daily living (ADLs). Team members must consider whether a child can manage daily care activities and must evaluate how AT can assist the child's performance. Children with disabilities often require AT in the areas of toileting, grooming/hygiene, and eating. Toileting devices include a footstool to increase sitting

■ Table 18.1 Advantages and Disadvantages of Various Control Strategies for Environmental Control
■ Units (ECUs)

Type of ECU Control	Advantages	Disadvantages
Ultrasound (uses high-frequency sound waves).	Child does not have to point the control directly at the control box. Systems are wireless, portable, and small.	The transmitter must be in the same room as the control box.
Infrared (activated from a remote control).	Systems are portable.	Child must point the remote directly at the control box with nothing obstructing the signal.
Radio control (translate control codes to appliances).	Transmission cannot be blocked by objects, making it possible to signal an appliance in one room while in another room.	Radio frequencies are limited in the distance they can travel, ranging between 50 and 200 feet. Interference from another control unit is possible.
AC power uses existing electrical wiring to send input to activate appliances. The input device can be remote or be part of the control unit that is plugged into the wall. The appliances are plugged into a module that is plugged into an electrical outlet.	AC power does not require additional wiring, but modules must be programmed.	Systems require several electrical outlets and older electrical wiring can pose problems.

stability, grab bars, raised toilet seats, and supportive potty chairs. Grooming/hygiene equipment often used by children and their families includes bath or shower chairs and can range from adapted toothbrushes to architectural modifications to a home. Many products are commercially available depending on the needs and age of the child (Fig. 18.6). Adaptive eating utensils, such as spoons with built-up handles, cut-out cups, and scoop plates (Fig. 18.7), can assist a child in becoming independent during mealtime routines. Physical therapists, along with other team members, especially the

family and occupational therapist, can improve a child's level of independence by using AT for ADLs.

Recreation/Leisure/Play

The ability to play is an important part of childhood. Play is a child's work. A child who cannot participate in play activities is missing an opportunity to experience normal development. Children with physical disabilities may not be able to manipulate toys independently or move around the environment to explore. Children with sensory impairments may also have reduced opportunities

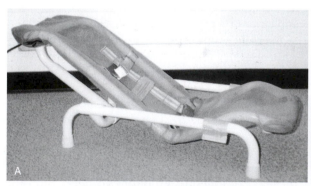
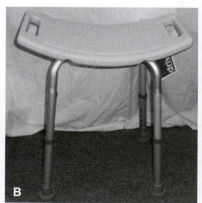
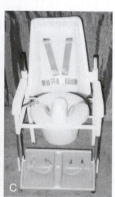

Figure 18.6 (*a*) Columbia reclining bath chair. (*b*) Drive Medical bath bench. (*c*) High-back potty chair.

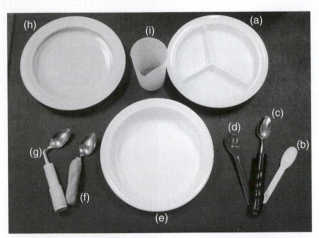

Figure 18.7 Eating/drinking utensils: (*a*) partitioned scoop plate, (*b*) child's feeding spoon, (*c*) weighted handle spoon, (*d*) the maroon spoon, (*e*) melamine scoop dish, (*f*) spoon with modeling clay, (*g*) Homecraft angled spoon, (*h*) plate with inside edge. (*i*) Nosey cut-out cup.

for independent exploration and have a need for adapted toys and play materials. As a result, the play experiences for children with disabilities may be qualitatively and quantitatively different from play experiences for children who are developing typically. As children become older, the need for recreation/leisure activities becomes important. The area of recreation/leisure should be considered and addressed as part of the intervention program for all children with disabilities (King, Petrenchik, Law, & Hurley, 2009; Shikako-Thomas, Majnemer, Law, & Lach, 2008).

Therapists should consider the need for AT to facilitate recreation/leisure/play activities whenever children with disabilities cannot play independently or interact with others during play or other recreation/leisure activities (Besio, 2002; Lane & Mistrett, 1996, 2002). Given the options available today, no child should sit on the sidelines and just "watch" other children play. For some children, toys or materials may need to be stabilized to make them more accessible. Therapists can use materials such as Velcro, Dycem, or other nonslip material, play boards, and C-clamps to stabilize play materials and toys and promote independent play opportunities. Velcro placed on toys or puzzle pieces can make them easier to handle. When hook Velcro is placed on the play materials, they attach to any Velcro-sensitive surface such as indoor/outdoor carpet, tempo loop fabric, or loop Velcro. Building up handles or adding materials to increase the diameter of toys and objects can make them

easier to grasp and hold. Attaching beads, blocks, or shower curtain rings to play items can make them easier to manipulate. For children who are unable to interact directly with toys and other recreational devices, the use of simple technology components such as switches, battery adapters, ECUs, and latch timers may provide options for play. With the wealth of computer programs, children of all ages and abilities are enjoying video and computer games. Switches provide an alternative means for children with disabilities to access computers, tape recorders, battery-operated toys, or even electrical appliances, as previously discussed. Switches can be purchased commercially or home made. Switches are used in combination with switch interfaces to provide computer access. Likewise, battery adapters are used with battery-operated devices and ECUs are used with electrical appliances.

For a detailed description of switches, refer to the previous section on AAC. Battery adapters or interrupters can be made simply and inexpensively or can be purchased commercially. The battery adapter is placed between the battery(ies) and a contact terminal to "interrupt" the power to the motor. The switch is then plugged into the battery adapter; when the device is turned on, it will run when the child activates the switch.

A computer may provide a recreation/leisure activity. Software exists to cover a wide range of personal interests such as music, drawing, and games. Access to the Internet can provide a source of recreation/leisure to those who have an interest in "surfing" the Internet or telecommunicating with others online. As the technology field evolves, computers may change the world of opportunities for children with disabilities more than anything else in the 21st century.

Children in school environments may require specialized equipment to facilitate their access to and participation in playground and recess activities. Several companies market adaptive playground equipment. In addition to specialized equipment, therapists can modify games to allow all children to participate in these activities. Physical therapists should be active participants in their communities' ADA and playground committees so that community "play" environments are accessible to all children.

Visual Technology

Visual impairments can significantly affect functioning in major areas of life. Depending on the nature and severity of the impairment, a child's ability to independently access the environment, to use materials and tools of daily activities, and to access a computer may be affected. The use of AT can help children with visual impairments be as successful and independent as possible.

Visual impairments significantly affect children's independent mobility skills. A lack of awareness of the environment may contribute to reduced exploration, which affects the developmental process for young children and safety in travel at any age. Orientation and mobility specialists and AT devices can assist children with visual impairments to be more independent. An orientation and mobility specialist can teach children to navigate environments by using canes, guide dogs, and electronic travel aids.

Visual impairments also significantly affect children's use of tools and appliances needed in daily life. Many devices designed to allow children with visual impairments to be more independent are commercially available and include devices that talk or provide audible feedback (e.g., talking thermometers, talking clocks, talking calculators, books on tape), Braille devices (e.g., clock faces with Braille, Braille instruction manuals, and Braille label makers), and large-print items.

Visual impairments also affect reading and writing abilities. For children with low vision, the use of low-vision aids such as magnifiers, large-print books, closed-circuit television systems, larger computer monitors, and computer-based programs that combine optical character recognition, large font, screen magnification, color contrasts, and speech capabilities can make print accessible. For children who are blind, a Braille system or computer-based system that reads the text and graphic information on screen makes print accessible.

To facilitate writing, children with visual impairments may require the use of raised line paper, writing guides, or broad tip felt markers. Children who use Braille as their writing system may rely on a slate and stylus, devices such as the Braille N Speak or Type N Speak, or computer-based systems with Braille translation software and a Braille printer.

When working with children with visual impairments, physical therapists need to alter their intervention. For example, physical therapists need to have a variety of toys that provide auditory or tactile feedback, not just visual. They also need to talk with the child throughout activities, explaining what they are doing and providing verbal feedback to the child regarding changes in the environment.

Assistive Listening

The terms "hard of hearing" and "deaf" are used to describe children with hearing losses. Hearing loss is often described as mild, moderate, severe, or profound. The terms "mild" and "moderate" indicate that a child has difficulty understanding speech that is not amplified. The term "severe" indicates that amplification is required to hear speech. "Profound" loss indicates the inability to understand speech that is amplified. Hard of hearing usually describes a child who can understand speech with the ear with difficulty. **Deaf** usually describes a child who cannot hear or understand speech with amplification.

For children with hearing impairments, the use of AT is needed for communication, environmental control, ADLs, recreation and leisure, and reception of auditory information. Devices are available to send a visual signal such as a strobe light, flash of light, or vibrating signal on alarm clocks, doorbells, smoke detectors, or telephones to alert children via a visual instead of auditory signal. Assistive listening devices can aid in the reception of auditory information. Most children with a hearing loss have a personal amplification device, such as a hearing aid, that an audiologist individually prescribes. However, the use of other assistive devices in combination with personal devices may be needed in environments that are very noisy. If a child uses an assistive listening device, physical therapists need to make sure that they use the transmitter during intervention so that the child can hear auditory cues provided by the therapist. Although assistive listening systems aid in the reception of auditory information, some children require or may prefer to use sign language to receive information. In most instances, the use of oral interpreters is required.

Captioning is another method for enhancing reception of auditory information. In captioning, text appears at the bottom of a screen and provides a transcription of the aural information. Open captioning does not require the use of a special decoder to access the captioning. Closed captioning requires a special decoder to access the captioned information.

People who are deaf require AT to use the telephone. Since the implementation of the ADA, this technology is more readily available. A device called the telecommunications device for the deaf (TDD) or TTY (TeleType) makes telephones accessible. To use a TDD, both parties must have access to a device. The receiver of the telephone is placed in the coupler of the TDD, and the conversation is typed on it and transmitted over the telephone lines to the other TDD. When both parties do not have access to TDDs, a relay system is needed. Relay services are available in all states to ensure accessibility. A person at the relay service has a TDD and acts as an interpreter/transcriptionist between the party who has access to the TDD and the party who does not.

The expressive communication of a child may be affected, depending on the onset and severity of the hearing loss. ASL is considered the native language of the people who are deaf, but not all people with a hearing loss rely on sign language for communication. Children who have combined physical and hearing impairments may have difficulty using sign language for communication. Physical therapists play a critical role in determining whether a child has the motor control necessary to use sign language as a functional means of expressive communication. Cochlear implants may benefit children who are deaf or severely hard of hearing. Cochlear implants are different from hearing aids because they are surgically implanted to stimulate the auditory nerve and bypass the damaged portion of the ear. Children who receive cochlear implants also often receive intensive therapy to enhance speech and language development.

Funding

Funding has long been a barrier to the acquisition of AT devices. As awareness of the benefits of AT has increased, service providers have led the way in accessing funding sources. As members of the AT team, physical therapists must be familiar with funding options for AT. They must understand the basic differences between funding agencies to ensure that technology is paid for by the most appropriate funding source.

Differences Between Funding Sources

Public or private sources of funding may be available to pay for AT devices and services for children. Private sources are not under government control and can be divided into national, statewide, and regional/local programs. Federal or state governments, laws, or acts control public sources of funding. The U.S. government classifies sources under their control as either discretionary or entitlement programs.

Discretionary programs are not required to provide all services to every eligible child under the program. Authorizing personnel within the agency, usually a case manager or counselor, determines whether the agency will provide the service or equipment. Discretionary programs have a limit on the money available to serve children under the program within a given year. Vocational rehabilitation is an example of a discretionary program.

Entitlement programs provide all services to every eligible child under the program. In an entitlement program, once children meet eligibility criteria, they are guaranteed all the benefits of the program. Medicaid is an example of an entitlement program. Governments control entitlement programs by either limiting eligibility criteria or narrowing the cost, duration, and scope of services provided under the program.

Some of the more common funding sources of payment for AT devices for children are (1) Medicaid (Title XIX of the Social Security Act), including Early, Periodic, Screening, Diagnosis, and Treatment (EPSDT); and state waiver programs; (2) early intervention (birth to 3 years) programs and local school districts, as part of Individuals with Disabilities Education Act (IDEA); (3) private insurance; and (4) service clubs and organizations (Golinker & Mistrett, 1997; Judge, 2000). Medicaid is a federal/state medical assistance program for selected people with low incomes or children who come from families with low incomes. Medicaid coverage varies from state to state, and therapists should become familiar with Medicaid procedures in their state. Early intervention programs, which serve children from birth to age 3 under IDEA, can pay for AT that is required by children to achieve Individualized Family Service Plan (IFSP) outcomes. Local school districts, as part of IDEA, pay for AT that is required by children to benefit from their educational program. A child's Individualized Education Program (IEP) team determines the AT needs. Private insurance is a contract between the company (or individual) and the insurance provider or carrier. Companies or employers determine the coverage. Private insurance coverage varies widely between and within companies. Two families who may be covered by the same insurance company will not necessarily have the same insurance benefits unless their employer is also the same. Many private insurance companies have nurse case managers on staff who can provide assistance when trying to determine what coverage is available. In general, they can also provide information about the medical review process, which is used to determine whether AT is covered by a family's policy.

Physical therapists must be proficient at completing the paperwork necessary to apply for AT funding and services, such as certificates of medical necessity for private insurance and Medicaid or letters of justification for private funding sources. Although no "magic words" exist to ensure that a funding agency will approve recommended AT, physical therapists can use terms that are specific or familiar to the agency. If therapists apply to Medicaid, their justification must be written in terms of "medical necessity." If a child's educational team determines that a local school district should purchase the equipment, the justification must demonstrate the impact of the AT on the child's educational performance. If therapists approach vocational rehabilitation, documentation must show how the technology supports the vocational goals or employment opportunities.

In addition to using specific or familiar terms when completing funding requests, therapists must also include necessary components. Necessary components for a certificate of medical necessity or justification letter include (1) the child's diagnosis and/or general physical condition as it applies to AT recommendations, (2) a description of limitations in the child's abilities as they relate to the need for AT, (3) a description of current AT, (4) a prognosis relating to how the recommended AT serves to "resolve" the limitations described previously, (5) a description of AT critical features, including the purpose of each feature and how it relates to increased function for the child, and (6) the list of all team members involved in the selection of the AT. It is also beneficial and sometimes necessary to include pictures and/or videotapes of the child during simulation or while using trial AT (Taylor & Kreutz, 1997).

Continued Assessment and Intervention

After a child receives AT, physical therapists along with the family and other team members provide follow-up assessment and intervention to support the child's successful use of AT (Long, Huang, Woodbridge, Woolverton & Minkel, 2003). Team members follow the progress of the child and continue to ask questions such as "Is this device helping the family achieve the desired outcomes?" If not, team members should reassess to determine what needs to be changed so that the child can achieve the targeted outcomes. Particular attention should to be given to factors associated with the successful long-term use of AT. These include child and family satisfaction, involvement of the child and family in the AT process, adequate training, knowledge level of parents, and continued maintenance of the device (Copley & Ziviani, 2004; Huang, Sugden, & Beveridge, 2009; Benedict, Lee, Marujo, & Farel, 1999; Lesaur, 1998; Long et al., 2003). The physical therapist and other team members may also fit, modify, or adapt the device; train the child, family, caregivers, and other professionals; and provide continued assessment, with the goal of assisting the child to achieve desired outcomes.

Physical therapists can use many different tools to assess the child and factors related to achievement of identified outcomes, such as the level of satisfaction with the device; the child's level of independence with functional activities; participation within the home, school, and community setting; and changes in the child's and family's quality of life. A tool previously designed for adults that authors modified for use with children is the Quebec User Evaluation of Satisfaction with assistive Technology (QUEST) (Routhier, Vincent, Morisette, & DeSaulnier, 2001). Other tools are designed specifically for children and can give information about the impact of an intervention on a child's level of independence, such as the Pediatric Evaluation of Disability Inventory (PEDI) (Haley et al., 2010).

Despite a systematic approach to evaluation, device selection, and ongoing assessment, modifications to the intervention plan are sometimes needed. The child and team members may require additional training or the device may require adaptation to ensure that it functions as intended, to assist the child and family in achieving targeted outcomes. Physical therapists and other team members must have knowledge about the latest technological advances and translate research findings into practice to assist in meeting the unique and constantly changing needs of children and their families.

Summary

This chapter describes augmentative communication and other technologies that may benefit children with disabilities. Assessment for augmentative communication and other technologies takes place after addressing a child's positioning needs. The AT described in this chapter allows children with disabilities to accomplish tasks that they would otherwise be unable to do (Hammell, Lai, & Heller, 2002). Whether saying "I love you" to a friend or relative, or simply turning the television on or off, AT provides for independence and a sense of control over the environment. Children with AT needs require ongoing support and intervention from physical therapists and other service providers to ensure that they are successful in obtaining and using technology.

Difficulties in obtaining AT for children can often be a barrier to the use of technology. Funding is a crucial part of the process. Without funding, AT can never be put into action and the possibilities remain hidden. The information presented in this chapter provides therapists with the basic information needed to approach various funding agencies, access AT for children, and evaluate the effectiveness of AT, once implemented.

DISCUSSION QUESTIONS

1. What contributions can a physical therapist make when assessing a child with physical disabilities for augmentative communication?

2. What is the difference between direct selection and indirect selection? Give an example of each.

3. Describe different modifications that can be made for a child who needs to use a computer but has limited motor skills.

4. What are the different components of an environmental control unit?

5. Describe the differences between a discretionary program and an entitlement program.

6. How would you justify equipment differently if you were approaching a school system for funding versus an insurance company?

References

Angelo, J. (2000). Factors affecting the use of a single switch with assistive technology devices. *Journal of Rehabilitation Research and Development, 37*(5), 591–598.

Benedict, R.E., Lee, J.P., Marrujo, S.K., & Farel, A.M. (1999). Assistive devices as an early childhood intervention: Evaluating outcomes. *Technology and Disability, 11*, 79–90.

Besio, S. (2002). An Italian research project to study the play of children with motor disabilities: The first year of activity. *Disability and Rehabilitation, 24*, 72–79.

Blischak, D.M., Lloyd, L.L., & Fuller, D.R. (1997). Terminology issues. In L.L. Lloyd, D.R. Fuller, & H.H. Arvidson (Eds.), *Augmentative and alternative communication: A handbook of principles and practices*. Boston: Allyn & Bacon.

Copley, J., & Ziviani, J. (2004). Barriers to the use of assistive technology for children with multiple disabilities. *Occupational Therapy International, 11*(4), 229–243.

Golinker, L., & Mistrett, S.G. (1997). Funding. In J. Angelo & S. Lane (Eds.). *Assistive technology for rehabilitation therapists* (pp. 211–234). Philadelphia: F.A. Davis.

Haley, S.M., Costa, W.I., Kao, Y.C., Dumas, H.M., Fragala-Pinkham, M.A., Kramer, J.M., Ludlow, L.H., & Moed, R. (2010). Lessons from the use of pediatric evaluation of disability inventory: Where do we go from here? *Pediatric Physical Therapy, 22*, 69–75.

Hammell, J., Lai, J.S., & Heller, T. (2002). The impact of assistive technology and environmental interventions on function and living situation status with people who are aging with developmental disabilities. *Disability and Rehabilitation, 24*, 93–105.

Huang, I.C., Sugden, D., & Beveridge, S. (2009). Assistive devices and cerebral palsy: Factors influencing the use of assistive devices at home by children with cerebral palsy. *Child: Care, Health and Development, 35*(1), 130–139.

Judge, S.L. (2000). Accessing and funding assistive technology for young children with disabilities. *Early Childhood Education Journal, 28*(2), 125–131.

Jutai, J., Rigby, P., Ryan, S., & Stickel, S. (2000). Psychosocial impact of electronic aids to daily living. *Assistive Technology, 12*(2), 123–131.

King, G., Petrenchik, T., Law, M., & Hurley, P. (2009). The enjoyment of formal and informal recreation and leisure activities: A comparison of school-aged children with and without physical disabilities. *International Journal of Disability, Development and Education, 56*(2), 109–130.

Lahm, E.A., Walser, P., & Reed, P. (2004). Computer access. In P. Reed & E. Lahm (Eds.), *Assessing students' need for assistive technology: A resource manual for school district teams* (pp. 64–74). Oshkosh, WI: Wisconsin Assistive Technology Initiative.

Lane, S.J., & Mistrett, S. (1996). Play and assistive technology issues for infants and young children with disabilities: A preliminary examination. *Focus on Autism and Other Developmental Disabilities, 11*(2), 96–104.

Lane, S.J., & Mistrett, S. (2002). Let's play! Assistive technology interventions for play. *Young Exceptional Children, 5*(2), 19–27.

Lesaur, S. (1998). Use of assistive technology with young children with disabilities: Current status and training needs. *Journal of Early Intervention, 21*(2), 146–159.

Long, T., Huang, L., Woodbridge, M., Woolverton, M., & Minkel, J. (2003). Integrating assistive technology into an outcome-driven model of service delivery. *Infants and Young Children, 16*(4), 272–283.

McEwen, I.R. (1997). Seating, other positioning, and motor control. In L.L. Lloyd, D.R. Fuller, & H.H. Arvidson (Eds.), *Augmentative and alternative communication: A handbook of principles and practices*. Boston: Allyn & Bacon.

Reed, P., & Lahm, E. (Eds.). (2004). *Assessing students' needs for assistive technology: A resource manual for school district teams*. Oshkosh, WI: Wisconsin Assistive Technology Initiative.

Routhier, F., Vincent, C., Morisette, M.J., & DeSaulnier, L. (2001). Clinical results of an investigation of paediatric upper limb myoelectric prosthesis fitting at the Quebec Rehab Institute. *Prosthetics and Orthotics International, 25*, 119–131.

Shikako-Thomas, K., Majnemer, A., Law, M., & Lach, L. (2008). Determinants of participation in leisure activities in children and youth with cerebral palsy: Systematic review. *Physical & Occupational Therapy in Pediatrics, 28*(2), 155–169.

Taylor, S.J., & Kreutz, D. (1997). Powered and manual wheelchair mobility. In J. Angelo & S. Lane (Eds.), *Assistive technology for rehabilitation therapists* (pp. 117–158). Philadelphia: F.A. Davis.

Walser, P., & Reed, P. (2004). Augmentative and alternative communication. In P. Reed & E. Lahm (Eds.), *Assessing students' need for assistive technology: A resource manual for school district teams* (pp. 95–106). Oshkosh, WI: Wisconsin Assistive Technology Initiative.

Case Studies

—Donna J. Cech, PT, DHS, PCS

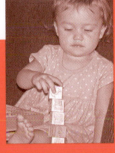
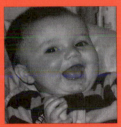
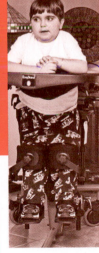
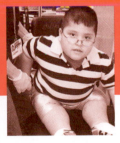
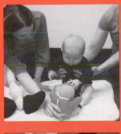
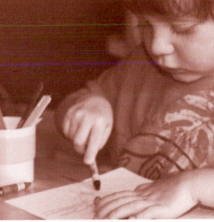
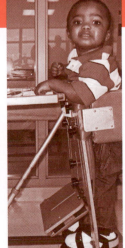

CHAPTER 19

Case Study

Cerebral Palsy

—Donna Cech, PT, DHS, PCS

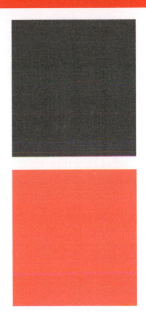

This case study focuses on the physical therapy management of Kayla, a young woman with spastic, diplegic cerebral palsy (CP). Kayla is now 20 years old and a sophomore in college. She was born prematurely and has received physical therapy services in a variety of settings since infancy. She has been followed for early intervention, early childhood, school-based, outpatient, and home health physical therapy services. At this time she does not regularly see a physical therapist, but does continue with occasional sessions to monitor adaptive equipment and to address episodes of foot pain or back pain. Kayla walks in her home/dormitory settings and on campus using bilateral forearm crutches. For longer distances, she uses a motorized cart.

Children and young adults with CP are reportedly less socially and physically active than their peers without a physical disability (Shikako-Thomas, Majnemer, Law, & Lach, 2008; Engel-Yeger, Jarus, Anaby, & Law, 2009; Maher, Williams, Olds, & Lane, 2007). Individuals with CP frequently present with impairments of range of motion (ROM), soft tissue mobility, strength, coordination, and balance, resulting in motor control difficulties. CP implies damage to the immature cortex, involving the sensorimotor system. Associated problems with vision, seizures, perception, and cognition may be seen if areas of the cortex associated with these functions are also damaged. Although the cortical lesion is nonprogressive, as the infant grows and strives to become more independent, functional limitations become more apparent, as do restrictions in activities and community participation. Secondary impairments in body structures and function, such as ROM limitations, disuse atrophy, and impaired aerobic capacity, may further limit functional motor skills and ability for activities and participation. Multiple episodes of physical therapy management are frequently warranted as the child attempts more complex functional skills and as the risk for secondary impairments increases. The goal of physical therapy intervention for children and young adults with CP is to maximize the individual's ability to participate in age-appropriate activities within the home, school, and community settings.

Children with CP present with a variety of functional abilities, reflecting the location and severity of their original neurological insult. Distribution of motor involvement varies and may include hemiplegia, diplegia, or quadriplegia. The degree to which the neurological insult impacts motor ability and function also varies. The Gross Motor Function Classification System (GMFCS) provides a mechanism to classify these children, based on their gross motor abilities and limitations (Palisano, Rosenbaum, Bartlett, & Livingston, 2008; Palisano et al., 1997). Based on Kayla's ability to ambulate with an assistive device and need to use power mobility for community mobility, she would be classified as functioning at the GMFCS level III through elementary and high school.

Based on the American Physical Therapy Association (APTA)'s *Guide to Physical Therapist Practice* (2001), Kayla's physical therapy needs may best be addressed by Preferred Practice Pattern 5C: Impaired Motor Function and Sensory Integrity Associated with Nonprogressive Disorders of the Central Nervous System—Congenital Origin or Acquired in Infancy or Childhood. This pattern was chosen because the pathology leading to the presenting impairments occurred in the prenatal, neonatal, or infancy period, and therefore involves the immature motor cortex. The resulting impaired motor function will potentially have a negative effect on the developing muscular, skeletal, cardiovascular, and pulmonary systems. The practice pattern chosen should most comprehensively address the developmental issues brought about by abnormal motor control from infancy and throughout childhood and adolescence. Kayla's physical therapy at ages 6 and 13 years is summarized, as well as a discussion of her potential lifelong physical therapy needs. Physical therapy is being provided by therapists working in educational settings and in accordance with the federal Individuals with Disabilities Education Act Amendments of 1997 (IDEA 97) in both episodes of care reported. In the first episode of care, Kayla is also receiving home health physical therapy services because she has recently had orthopedic surgery, and additional physical therapy services are indicated to address her postsurgical needs.

Examination: Age 6 Years

History

Kayla is the youngest of four children. She was born prematurely, at 34 weeks' gestation, and, as reported by her mother, had a fairly uneventful neonatal course. She was hospitalized for 2 weeks after birth because she had difficulty sucking and experienced periods of bradycardia. She did not have respiratory problems and was not noted to have had an intraventricular hemorrhage at that time. Her family became concerned when at 10 months of age she could not sit or crawl. When held in standing position, she was very stiff and could not balance. She was diagnosed at that time with spastic, diplegic CP.

Kayla was enrolled at a center-based early intervention program at 1 year of age. She was seen by a physical therapist, an occupational therapist, a speech-language pathologist, and an early childhood educator. Her primary areas of difficulty were gross motor function, fine motor function, and visual perception. At 3 years of age, Kayla began attending an early childhood program in her local school district and has continued in this setting until the present. She is now transitioning into a full-day, first-grade setting. Kayla has also received occupational and physical therapy services outside the school setting, after neurosurgical and orthopedic surgical procedures. Kayla's family has been very active in her intervention program and has strongly advocated for Kayla to be an active participant in community activities for children her age. She has participated in a local preschool at ages 3 and 4 years and in library programs and a park district day camp, and she is now beginning in Brownies.

Medically, Kayla's history includes ocular surgery at 18 months of age to correct a muscular imbalance, a selective dorsal rhizotomy at 4 years of age to decrease spasticity, bilateral derotational femoral osteotomies and medial hamstring release to improve lower extremity alignment at $5\frac{1}{2}$ years of age, and a right tibial plateau fracture at age 5 years after a fall from her swing set. At age $4\frac{1}{2}$ years, she was diagnosed with a mild temporal lobe seizure disorder, which is controlled with medication (Tegretol).

Systems Review

Cardiovascular and Pulmonary

No problems are noted in cardiovascular or pulmonary function. Kayla is very active physically and has good endurance. She does not have problems with respiratory infections. Kayla's blood pressure (100/70 mm Hg) and her heart rate (100 beats per minute) are within normal limits (WNL) for her age (Cech & Martin, 2012).

Integumentary

Kayla wears bilateral hinged ankle-foot orthoses (AFOs), and her parents report that she occasionally has areas of redness and irritation related to them. At this time, however, no problems with skin condition are noted.

Musculoskeletal

Kayla demonstrates muscle atrophy and weakness of her lower extremities, especially distally. Trunk weakness is also noted. The family reports that the weakness is especially noticeable since her recent orthopedic surgery, but has been noted ever since her dorsal rhizotomy. Bilateral hip flexion and knee flexion muscle contractures were reported before the recent orthopedic surgery, but at this time, functional ROM appears to be WNL. Further examination of muscle strength and ROM is warranted.

Neuromuscular

Hypertonicity and increased muscle stiffness are noted in the lower extremities. Some tremor is noted in the upper extremities during reaching and fine manipulative activities. Kayla cannot balance in standing position, does not walk without an assistive device, and has difficulty with coordination. Further examination of gait, motor function, and self-care is needed.

Cognition, Language, and Communication

Kayla's language development and communication skills are good. She may demonstrate a mild cognitive delay, but this might be related to visual perceptual difficulties. These areas will be further evaluated by the educational team and current classroom staff.

Tests and Measures

In completing a physical therapy examination with Kayla at 6 years of age, baseline function was determined in several areas. In the following discussion, areas of function that were found to be normal or identified an impairment that did not strongly affect function are briefly described. Tests and measures for areas that were thought to be affecting motor function are discussed in more detail.

Aerobic Capacity and Endurance

Kayla is able to keep up with her friends on the playground, even though she is using a walker. She does not get short of breath and does not appear to have problems with aerobic capacity or endurance.

Assistive and Adaptive Devices

Kayla uses a variety of assistive devices to aid mobility. She uses a motorized cart for community locomotion, a walker when walking for long distances or in more active environments (i.e., recess), and bilateral quad canes for short distances within her home. All devices currently fit appropriately and are in good repair. Kayla can use the cart and walker very safely in all environments. She can use the quad canes only for short distances (10 to 15 feet) and with close supervision.

Gait, Locomotion, and Balance

Kayla safely uses a wheeled rear-walker in all terrains and environments (school, home, and community). She has begun to use quad canes, but she fatigues quickly and has difficulty picking her feet up high enough, causing her to trip when using the canes. For community mobility, Kayla uses a motorized cart and safely navigates curb cuts and school hallways. She drives it approximately two blocks to or from school. Before her recent orthopedic surgery, Kayla had a full computerized gait assessment with and without her orthotics. This examination was performed at a gait laboratory affiliated with the hospital where she sees her orthopedic surgeon and had her surgery.

Kayla has difficulty with sitting and standing balance. She cannot stand without support. She can sit on the floor independently, but she does not reach too far outside of her base of support or reach over her head. When sitting on a bench, she cannot reach out of her base of support to the right or the left. She also demonstrates a loss of balance when she reaches above shoulder level. In most sitting positions, Kayla's posture is kyphotic, with rounded shoulders and a forward head position. Her most stable and favored sitting position is W-sitting.

Examination Update: If Kayla's balance were being evaluated today, sitting balance ability could be quantified using the pediatric modification of the functional reach test (Bartlett & Birmingham, 2003), which would measure her ability to reach laterally and forward from the sitting position. The Timed Up & Go (TUG) test has also been found to be reliable and responsive to change in children with cerebral palsy (Williams, Carroll, Reddihough, Phillips, & Galea, 2005). Kayla would use her assistive device during the TUG test. To monitor improvements in standing balance when using her canes, Kayla could perform this test with the walker, and the results could be compared to results with the canes. Over time, progress would be shown if scores with the canes improved. The Berg Balance test (Berg, Wood-Dauphinée, Williams, & Gayton, 1989) and Pediatric Balance Scale (Franjoine, Gunter, & Taylor, 2003) have also been recommended as valid measures of balance for children with CP, functioning at the GMFCS level III (Gan, Tung, Tang, & Wang, 2008; Kembhavi, Darrah, Magill-Evans, & Loomi, 2002).

Motor Function

Kayla creeps easily, using a reciprocal lower extremity pattern, and can knee-walk for 3 to 5 feet. She has difficulty grading movements, often initiating the movement quickly. In fine motor activity, she demonstrates fine tremors with both hands when reaching for a target and grasping. She frequently overshoots the target. She uses a pincer grasp to pick up many types of small objects but stabilizes her wrist on the surface for very small objects, such as beads.

In standing, Kayla keeps her weight shifted forward onto the balls of her feet, with an increased lumbar lordosis, and her shoulders back. If her weight is shifted onto her full foot, her lordosis is reduced, but her lower extremities buckle into flexion and she falls to the floor. When falling forward or to the side from sitting, kneeling, or standing, her protective reactions are good. No protective reactions are seen when she falls backward.

Examination Update: Use of either the original 88-item Gross Motor Function Measure (GMFM-88) or the GMFM-66 (Russell, Rosenbaum, Avery, & Lane, 2002) would provide a quantified measure of Kayla's abilities in motor skills such as sitting, crawling, standing, and walking. The computerized scoring format of the GMFM-66 would also provide the therapist with specific information to use in the intervention planning process.

Muscle Performance

Kayla's upper extremity muscular strength is very good. When she stabilizes by stiffly extending or adducting her lower extremities, she can maintain an upright trunk position. Isolated strength of the trunk extensor and flexor muscles is approximately 3/5. Lower extremity hip flexion and quadriceps strength are good (4/5), reflecting that Kayla can move the lower limb through the full range of motion with some resistance. Hip extension, hip abduction, and knee flexion strength are 2-3/5, whereas distally at the foot, strength in dorsiflexion and

plantarflexion are 1-2/5. Functionally, Kayla is able to perform concentric muscle contractions easily, but she has more difficulty with eccentric muscle control. For example, she cannot lower herself slowly from standing back down to sitting.

Examination Update: Handheld dynamometry would be a better method of measuring muscle performance, as it provides a quantifiable score and is reliable and valid with children as young as 2 years of age (Gajdosik, 2005). Handheld dynamometry has been found to be a reliable test of hip flexor, hip extensor, knee flexor and extensor, and ankle dorsiflexor muscles in children with CP (Crompton, Galea, & Phillips, 2007).

Neuromotor Development and Sensory Integration

Kayla demonstrates delays in fine motor development, with skills reflective of the 4- to 5-year age level based on the Peabody Developmental Motor Scale (PDMS), Fine Motor subsection (Folio & Fewell, 1983). She has difficulty using scissors with precision, manipulating and controlling a pencil, and manipulating small objects (e.g., coins, small pellets). In the area of gross motor development, Kayla is functioning significantly below her age level because she cannot balance in standing, walk, run, and so on. She has difficulty using her lower extremities reciprocally when she is walking. Based on the PDMS, Gross Motor subsection (Folio & Fewell, 1983), she is functioning at less than the second percentile compared with age-matched peers.

Examination Update: The PDMS was significantly revised and the Peabody Developmental Motor Scale, second edition (PDMS-2), was published in 2000 (Folio & Fewell, 2000). The newer edition of this standardized test has been normed on a sample reflective of the U.S. population and stratified to age. Improved scoring criteria better differentiate between possible scores on items; item revision and administration revisions have been made. The PDMS-2 is appropriate for children between birth and 6 years.

Orthotic Devices

Kayla's recent AFOs are hinged with a plantarflexion stop. Before receiving these orthotics, Kayla used a solid ankle AFO. She appears to be able to control the hinged ankle during gait. No knee hyperextension is seen during the stance phase. The orthotics fit well, and Kayla and her family are very good at monitoring skin condition after using the orthotics.

Range of Motion

Hamstring tightness is noted, with a popliteal angle of 15° on the left and 20° on the right. Even though muscle tightness is noted in the hip adductors, hip internal rotators, and plantarflexor muscles, passive ROM is WNL, with the following exceptions: dorsiflexion is limited to neutral on the right and hip flexion is 5° to 110° bilaterally. Hypermobility is noted in lumbar extension, hip internal rotation, and knee extension.

Reflex Integrity

Muscle tone is increased in the lower extremities, the right greater than the left. The left lower extremity hip adductor, hip internal rotator, quadriceps, and plantarflexor muscle groups were scored at a grade of 2 on the Modified Ashworth Scale (Bohannon & Smith, 1987), indicating motion possible, but resistance noted. The same muscle groups of the right lower extremity were scored at a grade of 1 on the Modified Ashworth Scale, indicating a "catch" of resistance at the initiation of the movement. The Modified Ashworth Scale has been found to be reliable in documenting resistance to passive motion in adults with a variety of neurological conditions (Gregson et al., 2000; Allison, Abraham, & Petersen, 1996).

Examination Update: The Modified Ashworth Scale has been reported to correlate with other muscle tone measures in children, but poor test-retest and interrater reliability of this test with children has been demonstrated (Clopton et al., 2005; Fosang, Galea, McCoy, Reddihough, & Story, 2003). The Modified Tardieu Scale (Boyd & Graham, 1999) may provide a more reliable measure of spasticity in children, but has a fairly large margin of error. (Fosang et al., 2003; Scholtes, Becher, Beelen, & Lankhorst, 2006).

Self-Care and Home Management (Including Activities of Daily Living and Instrumental Activities of Daily Living)

Kayla is fairly independent in basic activities of daily living (ADLs) and instrumental activities of daily living (IADLs). She is independent in bathing, toileting, and eating. She needs some assistance with putting on her socks and shoes but otherwise is independent in dressing. Kayla uses a walker for independent ambulation at school. She is also beginning to use bilateral quad canes for walking short distances in her home. She uses a motorized cart for community mobility. She often "walks" to school with her older brother and safely drives the cart two blocks to and from school. At home, Kayla helps with age-appropriate household chores, such as folding laundry and making her bed. At school, she is able to participate in classroom activities, but her handwriting is slow and requires a lot of concentration. With modified lesson plans and assistance from a classroom aide, Kayla is able to work with her classmates.

When evaluated with the Pediatric Evaluation of Disability Index (PEDI) (Haley, Coster, Ludlow, Haltiwanger, & Andrellos, 1992), Kayla demonstrates age-appropriate skills in social function and independence in all areas of function. Mild difficulty is seen in self-care skills, especially related to precise fine motor control (e.g., buttering bread, parting hair). Significant functional limitations are noted in activities, such as transitioning into or out of sitting without arm support, walking without support, stair climbing, and dynamic balance activities in standing. As a result, her performance in the mobility functional skill domain is well below that in other areas.

Examination Update: If Kayla's physical therapy examination were being completed today, it would be appropriate to include a measure of her participation in activities at home, school, and in the community. Some appropriate assessments include the Canadian Occupational Performance Measure (COPM), the School Function Assessment (SFA), the Pediatric Quality of Life Inventory (PedsQL) or PedsQL-CP (a specific version of the PedsQL for children with CP), the Pediatric Outcomes Data Collection Instrument (PODCI), or the Children's Assessment of Participation and Enjoyment (CAPE). These instruments are described in Chapter 3.

Evaluation, Diagnosis, and Prognosis
Including Plan of Care

In a review of the data collected from the examination, Kayla was found to be an active first grader in her local school program. She successfully uses adaptive equipment to participate in home, school, and community activities. She does present with impaired muscle function (muscle strength, muscle endurance, and muscle tone); motor function (motor control and motor learning); gait, locomotion, and balance; coordination; and functional ROM. These impairments contribute to functional limitations in activities, such as ambulation, sitting and standing, posture/control, fine motor manipulations, and restrictions in community participation such as playing on the playground and walking to school. Based on her ability to walk with assistive devices and her ability to sit independently, Kayla would be rated at Level III on the GMFCS (Palisano et al., 1997).

Kayla recently underwent bilateral lower extremity orthopedic surgery and subsequent casting for 6 weeks, resulting in increased lower extremity weakness, increased muscle tightness, and decreased endurance. Because of the chronicity of Kayla's condition, she has been followed for physical therapy on a regular basis since she was 1 year old. Services have been provided in school, home, and outpatient settings. She has continued to make functional gains despite her motor limitations. Growth, development, and medical interventions (i.e., selective dorsal rhizotomy, bilateral femoral osteotomies) have affected her ability to function motorically. With periods of growth in height, muscle tightness has increased, affecting her balance and mobility skills. Orthotic needs have become apparent, and orthotic modifications have been necessary to accommodate growth. Throughout the course of normal development, she has been encouraged to explore her environment and participate in her community, even though she had gross and fine motor activity restrictions. After surgery, she has participated in intensive physical therapy (at home and at school), both to regain presurgical functional status and to learn to move within the context of altered muscle performance and bony alignment.

Prognosis

It is anticipated that with therapy Kayla will return to presurgical levels of function at home, at school, and in her community. The focus of Kayla's therapy program will be on helping her function as independently as possible in her local school program and at home. As Kayla learns to use less restrictive assistive devices in a more energy-efficient manner, she should be better able to access her school environment. Assistance will still be needed to adapt curriculum and assist with fine manipulative activities. In addition, it is anticipated that Kayla will be able to participate in age-appropriate leisure activities (tricycle/bicycle riding).

Goals

The following goals will be achieved within the current school year (within 8 months), with physical therapy provided twice weekly (30 minutes per session) at school, and 60 minutes per week at home:

- Kayla will use bilateral quad canes to independently walk 20 feet, within her home and classroom environment, in 2/3 trials.
- Kayla will ascend/descend three stairs, using a railing and standby assistance, in 2/3 trials.
- Kayla will independently pedal a tricycle or a bicycle with training wheels for one block in 2/3 trials.
- Kayla will independently put on her socks in 2/3 trials.

Intervention

Coordination, Communication, and Documentation

Frequent communication among Kayla, her family, her teachers, her physicians, and her therapists is very important. Progress should be communicated to her orthopedic surgeon as she continues to recover from her bilateral femoral osteotomies. In Kayla's case, therapists at both home and school should communicate to coordinate care. The school therapist also needs to communicate with teachers, classroom aides, and other school personnel.

In addition to written physical therapy evaluations and progress notes, therapists will contribute to Kayla's individualized education plan (IEP) and daily education plans (e.g., position suggestions) and develop a home program. Collaboration with Kayla and her parents is important to adequately meet their needs with the therapy plan and home program.

Expected outcomes of this comprehensive coordination and communication will include coordination of care among Kayla and her family, school personnel, and physical therapists; collaboration and coordination among school, home, and home-health therapist; and enhanced decision making and case management.

Patient/Client-Related Instruction

Within Kayla's physical therapy management, Kayla and her parents, teachers, classroom aides, and siblings will all benefit from patient/client-related instruction. Instruction strategies must be designed appropriately for each person, focusing on the person's learning style and the activities in which he or she will be assisting Kayla. Instruction strategies for Kayla and her siblings, parents, and classroom staff members may be very different from one another, but all should include an opportunity for the learner to demonstrate to the therapist what he or she has learned.

For caregivers, instructions regarding specific activities, such as putting on AFOs or climbing stairs with a railing, should be presented verbally and reinforced in writing and/or pictures. The therapist should also demonstrate activities and watch the caregiver perform the activity. Feedback can be given to reinforce or revise the caregivers' participation in the activity.

Expected outcomes of this patient/client-related instruction include improved mobility, increased functional independence, and improved safety in home, school, and community settings.

Procedural Interventions

Therapeutic Exercise

The prime focus of Kayla's therapeutic exercise program is on balance and coordination training, lower extremity- and trunk-strengthening activities, and gait training. Balance and coordination activities are done in kneel-standing, sitting on a bench, and standing. Use of these and other functional activities also result in lower extremity and trunk strengthening. As multiple repetitions of activities are completed, muscle endurance is increased. Kayla's family has been encouraged to take her to indoor playgrounds for climbing, pulling, and ambulation activities (Fig. 19.1).

When sitting on a bench, Kayla can reach forward but cannot easily reach to the side outside of her base of support. Therapy activities, including having Kayla reach for objects, catch and throw a ball, and throw beanbags at targets in various locations, make therapy sessions fun. When performing these activities, Kayla is challenged to shift her weight and reach just outside her base of support, requiring active trunk control, while the upper extremities are involved in another activity.

Kneel-standing balance activities are included, as well as lower extremity-strengthening exercises, such as lowering to side-sitting and then back up. This activity also improves active control of trunk rotation and ROM (hip internal and external rotation) of the lower extremities. Other functional activities, such as slowly moving from standing to sitting, are included to improve eccentric muscle control and strengthening.

In the area of gait training, Kayla is learning a 4-point gait with bilateral quad canes. Use of the canes will ultimately allow her greater access at school, at home, and in the community, as she learns to use them on the stairs (which is not possible with the walker). The canes are also less bulky than the walker and will make locomotion around the crowded classroom more effective. The 4-point gait pattern should reinforce more active trunk control during walking and reciprocal upper and lower extremity function.

Functional Training in Self-Care

The areas of focus for Kayla in ADLs and IADLs are lower extremity dressing activities, gait and locomotion training in school and community environments, and age-appropriate play activities (pumping a swing, pedaling a bike). Safety is emphasized as a wide variety of school and community environments are explored.

Taking off shoes, orthotics, and socks is practiced in sitting, both on a bench and on the floor. In bench sitting, Kayla must shift her weight, use both hands in the activity, and actively balance her trunk. This is a challenging activity because of the amount of balance required, and standby assistance is needed. For more independent doffing of shoes and socks, Kayla ring-sits on the floor, which requires a lesser amount of trunk control and balance. She is practicing putting on socks in floor sitting and also in supine. These positions require less balance and allow her to practice precision in bimanual activities (placing sock correctly on her foot) while increasing functional ROM in hip flexion and external rotation.

Both pumping a swing and pedaling a tricycle or bicycle are difficult for Kayla because she must activate lower extremity muscles in a different way from the one she usually uses. In tricycle or bicycle riding, her feet

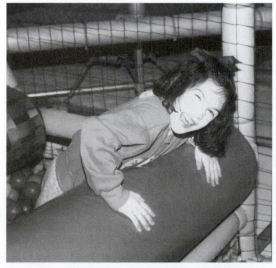

Figure 19.1 Strengthening and coordination emphasized during activities at indoor playground.

frequently push into plantarflexion and off the pedal. When her feet are secured onto the pedals, she actively uses lower extremity muscles to pedal herself. Kayla has been using a tricycle, but it is becoming too small for her. She is now trying a bicycle with wide-base training wheels. It is hoped that these wheels will provide a more stable base as she turns corners (Fig. 19.2).

Manual Therapy/Range of Motion

Therapy sessions are initiated with activities designed to increase soft tissue mobility and ROM of the lower extremities. Not only does this provide increased circulation to the tissues that will be used in functional activities, but also it is hoped that increased mobility will improve Kayla's motor control and function. Active ROM activities are included, emphasizing slow, prolonged stretch. Avoiding quick stretch activities will minimize activating the stretch reflex and eliciting spasticity.

Electrotherapy

Even though Kayla is only 6 years old, biofeedback is being used to help her isolate muscle activation in the lower extremities and volitionally relax muscles. Both auditory and visual feedback from the biofeedback unit let Kayla experience actively contracting or relaxing a muscle. Surface electrodes are placed on muscles that

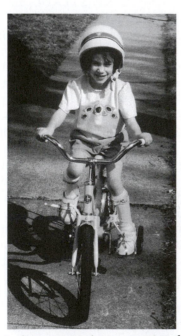

Figure 19.2 Age-appropriate recreational activity (bike riding) contributes to lower-extremity strengthening and balance training.

initiate knee flexion, knee extension, plantarflexion, and dorsiflexion, and Kayla is asked to focus on which muscles she should make work to complete a motion, as well as which muscles must be quiet during the motion.

Summary of Procedural Interventions

Expected outcomes of procedural interventions include decreased risk of secondary impairments, increased safety, development and improvement of functional motor skills, and independence in these activities. Impaired strength, ROM, and balance should also be improved. Kayla will be able to assume her self-care, home, school, and community roles.

Termination of Episode of Care

This episode of care will be terminated when Kayla has achieved the stated goals. Within her school-based setting, it is anticipated that the goals would be achieved during the current school year. If the goals are achieved sooner, the episode of care will be terminated and a new episode of care initiated if new goals are identified.

For children with CP, it is anticipated that they may "require multiple episodes of care over the life span to ensure safety and effective adaptation following changes in physical status, caregivers, environment, or task demands" (APTA, 2001, p. 345). For Kayla, it is anticipated that additional episodes of physical therapy care will be indicated as musculoskeletal growth occurs, classroom tasks change throughout her elementary school career, teachers and caregivers change, additional medical or surgical issues arise, or level of impairment, functional limitation, or activity restrictions change.

Episodes of physical therapy maintenance (APTA, 2001), which include a series of occasional clinical, educational, or administrative services necessary to maintain the child's level of function, may be required to monitor fit, repair, and determine the appropriateness of adaptive equipment and orthotics.

Episodes of physical therapy prevention (APTA, 2001) may also be useful to focus on primary and secondary prevention and health promotion. Secondary impairments of ROM, muscle strength/endurance, integumentary integrity, and aerobic conditioning often occur as skeletal growth continues. Not only does increased bone length frequently cause increased muscle tightness, but also increases in extremity and trunk length may biomechanically challenge the child. Larger amounts of weight must be moved or balanced over longer lever arms.

Examination: Age 13 Years

History

Kayla is now 13 years old and continues to live at home with her parents and three siblings (aged 14 to 18 years). She has been enrolled at her local elementary school in inclusive classroom settings from first through sixth grade. Kayla actively participated in Girl Scouts until she was in the fifth grade and has participated in various clubs at school. This is her first year at the junior high school, where she is a seventh grader. Some adaptations have been made to the curriculum every year to accommodate Kayla's needs, and she has participated in an adaptive physical education class.

Kayla has been relatively healthy over the past 6 years. She has developed some allergies to dust and mold, which have resulted in seasonal sinus infections. At age 10 years, she had increased respiratory difficulty with her allergies and was diagnosed with asthma. In addition to regular allergy medication, Kayla will use breathing treatments when her asthma is triggered. Last year she also underwent a right tibial derotational osteotomy. Respiratory issues and growth have resulted in Kayla adopting a less physically active lifestyle. As she has gotten more homework, she also has less time to actively ride her bike or exercise after school, contributing to a more sedentary lifestyle. She has continued to receive physical and occupational therapy as part of her school program. She has also participated in adapted swimming, aerobic exercise, and karate programs offered in her community. This year she is enrolled to participate in a peer group at a local outpatient center for individuals with disabilities, where she will have a chance to socialize and talk with other teenage girls with physical disabilities.

Kayla's goals are to transition successfully to junior high school, where she will have to change classrooms every period and carry her books. She is also hoping that she will be able to walk without her AFOs and transition to a less noticeable orthotic. Kayla's parents are concerned about her level of fitness and increased weight gain over the past year. They have noticed that it is harder for her to walk long distances at the shopping mall.

Systems Review

Cardiovascular and Pulmonary

Kayla's heart rate and blood pressure are WNL for her age. Her resting respiratory rate is 25 breaths per minute, but this increases to 32 breaths per minute with moderate amounts of activity (e.g., walking between rooms at school) and Kayla reports that she gets "short of breath" easily. Further examination of aerobic conditioning is indicated, especially with her history of asthma.

Integumentary

Kayla does not demonstrate any areas of redness or skin breakdown under her AFOs.

Musculoskeletal

Kayla's height is within the 30th percentile and her weight is in the 60th percentile for her age. Hip flexion and knee flexion contractures are noted. Kayla also presents with a thoracic kyphosis and increased lumbar lordosis. Muscle strength and endurance of the lower extremities are decreased. More detailed examination of ROM and muscle strength is indicated.

Neuromuscular

Kayla continues to demonstrate impaired motor control with hypertonicity and increased muscle stiffness of the lower extremities. She can balance in standing position for short periods of time (2 to 3 minutes), which is helpful during ADLs, and can walk independently with bilateral forearm crutches. Further examination of motor function and motor control is indicated.

Communication, Affect, Cognition, Language, and Learning Style

Kayla's communication skills are good. She has mild cognitive delays and continues to demonstrate some problems with visual perception. She learns best by demonstration and feedback during task performance.

Tests and Measures

Aerobic Capacity and Endurance

Kayla becomes fatigued and short of breath after walking short distances. Lower extremity muscle weakness appears to contribute to this problem. After walking for 2 minutes, her heart rate increases to 168 beats per minute, returning to a resting heart rate of 110 beats per minute within 1 minute of rest.

Assistive and Adaptive Devices

Kayla uses forearm crutches when walking in her home and classroom settings (Fig. 19.3). She will also use a walker for long distances to increase her speed and decrease her fatigue. For community locomotion, Kayla uses a motorized cart (Fig. 19.4). At this time, all adaptive equipment fits well and is in good repair.

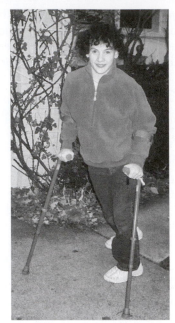

Figure 19.3 Walking with bilateral forearm crutches is functional for short distances.

Gait, Locomotion, and Balance

Kayla walks with bilateral forearm crutches, using a 4-point gait pattern, within her home and classroom settings. As she becomes fatigued, she begins dragging her right toe and occasionally trips. She safely uses a walker for longer distances but tends to use a swing-to

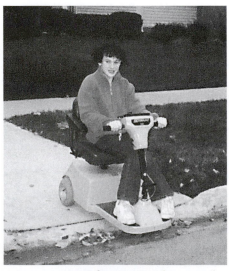

Figure 19.4 Motorized cart provides a mode of age-appropriate community mobility.

gait pattern and support herself primarily on her upper extremities if she is in a hurry. Kayla safely drives her motorized cart within her community, using curb cuts. Occasionally she will drive off the sidewalk. She usually quickly corrects herself and can get the cart back on the sidewalk, but occasionally her wheel gets stuck in the grass or dirt and she needs assistance.

Kayla can balance in static standing position for 2 to 3 minutes. When participating in dynamic standing activities, she often places her hand on a surface for support or leans against a stable object. This is sufficient for her to participate in ADLs, such as combing her hair and securing fasteners after toileting. She can also independently transition from sitting to standing and back to sitting, using her hands for support. The Berg Balance Test (Berg et al., 1989), although originally designed as a measure of balance in elderly individuals, has been suggested as a measure of functional balance in children with CP (Kembhavi et al., 2002). Kayla's score on the Berg Balance Test was 29 of a possible 56 points.

Examination Update: As discussed earlier, the TUG, Pediatric Balance Test, and Functional Reach Test could also be used to assess Kayla's balance at this age.

Motor Function (Motor Control and Motor Learning)

In addition to walking with assistive devices as described above, Kayla moves efficiently through her home by either creeping or cruising holding onto furniture or walls. She can ascend and descend stairs using a railing.

Mild intention tremor persists during activities such as buttoning or putting toothpaste on her toothbrush.

Examination Update: The GMFM would be appropriate to include in Kayla's examination and would quantify her motor function.

Muscle Performance

Pelvic and lower extremity weakness persists, especially distally (Table 19.1). Manual muscle testing has been chosen as an examination method because no special equipment is needed and it is a well-recognized method of muscle strength examination used by a variety of health-care providers. Recent literature has suggested that myometry, using a handheld dynamometer, is more reliable and valid for quantifying the muscle strength of children with a variety of conditions (Sloan, 2002; Stuberg & Metcalf, 1988). Because Kayla's body

Table 19.1 Lower Extremity Muscle Strength as Measured by Manual Muscle Test

Muscle Group	Right	Left
Hip abduction	2/5	2/5
Hip extension	2/5	3/5
Knee extension	3/5	3/5
Knee flexion	3/5	4/5
Dorsiflexion	1/5	2/5

mass and height have increased, it is more difficult for her to fully extend her lower extremities against gravity and support her body weight. Muscle endurance also is decreased.

Orthotic Devices

Kayla uses bilateral, hinged AFOs with a dorsiflexion stop at 5° and a plantarflexion stop at neutral. The orthotics fit well and appear to be appropriate for her current needs.

Range of Motion

Kayla presents with hip and knee flexion contractures bilaterally; external rotation is also limited. Goniometric measurements are listed in Table 19.2. The reliability of goniometric measurements in children with CP has been questioned because of wide variations in both intrasession and intersession measurements, even by experienced therapists (Kilgour, McNair, & Stott, 2003; Stuberg, Fuchs, & Miedaner, 1988). It has been suggested that goniometry is most reliable when completed by the same tester in subsequent tests. In this case, because measurements even on repeated tests can vary by several degrees, it is suggested that use of the average score from two consecutive measurements improves reliability (Stuberg, Fuchs, & Miedaner, 1988; Watkins, Darrah, & Pain, 1995).

Table 19.2 Lower Extremity Range of Motion

Motion	Right	Left
Hip flexion	15°–120°	0°–120°
Hip external rotation	0°–15°	0°–30°
Knee flexion	5°–120°	5°–120°
Dorsiflexion	0°	0°–3°

Reflex Integrity

In standing position and when stabilizing herself during sitting, Kayla demonstrates increased hip adduction and internal rotation. Muscle tone is increased in the bilateral lower extremities, the right greater than the left. During passive abduction and external rotation motion, the left leg has a score of 1 on the Ashworth Scale and the right leg a score of 2. These scores are very similar to the scores recorded when Kayla was 6 years old.

Self-Care and Home Management

Kayla is independent in dressing, bathing, toileting, transferring, and locomotion (using assistive devices). She has difficulty walking and carrying objects, which will be a difficulty in junior high school. She also has difficulty pouring beverages from a container while sitting.

Although she is older than recommended for the PEDI, her level of functional independence was measured using the scaled score for this test. Her skill level still falls within the parameters of the test, and use of the tool allows comparison with earlier performance. Scaled scores in functional skills, self-care, and social function domains have improved from Kayla's performance at 6 years of age. Kayla has achieved all items on the PEDI in these areas. In the area of the functional skills mobility domain, her scaled score has improved from 68.7 at 6 years of age to 75.2 at this time, continuing to reflect difficulty in walking or transferring without hand support, as well as ascending or descending stairs.

Work, Community, and Leisure Integration

Kayla functions well in school and community settings. She is able to participate in karate classes, school clubs, swimming, and so on. She also continues to ride an adult-size three-wheel bike, which provides more stability than her two-wheel bike. This is important because her height and weight have increased, and leisure time physical activity should be a regular part of her day.

Examination Update: If Kayla were being examined today, a measure of participation would be included. Some age-appropriate instruments include the COPM, PODCI, CAPE, and PedsQL (or PedsQL-CP).

Evaluation, Diagnosis, and Prognosis
Including Plan of Care

Although Kayla functions independently in her home, school, and community settings, she presents with activity and participation restrictions. These restrictions are related to functional limitations in standing balance, walking, and fine motor function. She is able to walk only by holding onto furniture and walls or with an assistive device (bilateral forearm crutches or wheeled walker). The energy cost of balance and ambulation is high. Movement patterns are inefficient, and she requires more time than is typical to complete activities. Her most efficient means of community mobility is with a motorized cart, but she cannot use this in all weather conditions (e.g., snow and ice) or in nonaccessible environments.

Kayla presents with impaired aerobic capacity, muscle performance (strength and endurance), motor function (motor control), and ROM, which interfere with her ability to efficiently complete ADLs.

Prognosis

Kayla is expected to function in the junior high school setting as independently as possible. Improved muscle strength, ROM, and endurance will assist in accomplishing tasks more efficiently, and Kayla will actively participate in her educational experience.

Goals

The following goals will be achieved within the current school year (within 8 months), with physical therapy services provided once weekly (30 minutes per session) at school:

- Kayla will independently open her locker and store or retrieve items from a standing position in 90% of trials.
- Kayla will move between classrooms within the 5-minute changing period, 6 periods per school day.

Intervention

Coordination, Communication, and Documentation

Services among home, school, and community settings should be coordinated. Regular communication must occur with Kayla, school personnel, Kayla's parents, and her physician. As Kayla enters the junior high school setting, coordination and communication with previous elementary school therapy and classroom staff should take place. Personnel at the high school should also be aware of Kayla's programming needs in anticipation of her enrollment 2 years from now.

In addition to written physical therapy evaluation and progress notes, therapists will also contribute to Kayla's IEP and daily education plan and develop a home program with Kayla. Kayla's parents remain an important part of the team; however, at this time Kayla will begin playing a more prominent role and should be encouraged to assume some of the responsibility for her therapy program.

Expected outcomes of this comprehensive coordination and communication will include increased effectiveness of case conferences, coordination of services, development of Kayla's IEP, and effective transition between the elementary and junior high schools.

Patient/Client-Related Instruction

With Kayla's transfer to a new school setting, personnel at the junior high school who will be interacting with Kayla should be instructed in how to assist Kayla in functional mobility within the school setting, positioning requirements (e.g., type and size of classroom chair), and any other elements of her program in which they may be involved.

Kayla and her parents should be well informed with regard to functional expectations and safety in the junior high school setting and any expected developmental changes as Kayla progresses through puberty (impact of growth spurts, importance of continued weight-bearing activities to promote bone growth). Kayla should take a more active role in developing her goals, objectives, and functional mobility program. Increased emphasis on fitness and maintaining an active lifestyle should be included.

Expected outcomes of patient/client-related instruction will include reduced risk of secondary impairments; increased functional independence in home, school, and community settings; and improved safety for Kayla and her caregivers.

Procedural Interventions

Therapeutic Exercise

The prime focus of Kayla's therapeutic exercise program at this time is on improving muscle performance, aerobic capacity/endurance, and ROM. As increasing height and body weight have negatively affected Kayla's ability to efficiently perform ADLs and ambulation, it is important for her to maximize her muscle strength and endurance. Although muscle weakness does limit her activities at this time, her more sedentary lifestyle may also negatively affect aerobic capacity.

Muscle-strengthening activities include weight training with light weights and multiple repetitions. Resistive exercise has been demonstrated to be beneficial and appropriate for children with CP, especially when maximal resistance or overloading of the muscle is avoided (Damiano, Dodd, & Taylor, 2002; Dodd, Taylor, & Damiano, 2002; Mockford & Caulton; 2008, Williams & Pountney, 2007). At Kayla's age, she is motivated by tracking her progress as she performs more repetitions and uses more weight. The main muscle groups targeted in the weight-training program are hip extensors, hip abductors, hip flexors, knee extensors, and knee flexors. Active ROM is used to strengthen musculature at the ankle. Kayla is encouraged to perform both concentric and eccentric muscle contraction. Strengthening programs have been found to contribute to positive outcomes for children with CP. Some of the functional changes seen have been increased gait speed, improved walking/running/jumping skills, and improved endurance (Damiano & Abel, 1998).

Kayla's adaptive physical education program is focused on encouraging development of lifelong physical activity. Presently Kayla is participating in a walking program, with her crutches or walker. With the crutches, she works harder at actively using lower extremity musculature and this reinforces the weight-training program. With the walker, Kayla is able to walk longer distances at a faster pace, fostering aerobic conditioning.

Active ROM activities are included at the beginning of each therapy and exercise session to improve alignment during functional mobility and "warm up" the muscle before beginning to exercise it.

Biofeedback

Biofeedback is used to help Kayla actively contract ankle plantarflexor and dorsiflexor muscle groups. Both auditory and visual feedback reinforce correct muscle group contraction.

Functional Training in Work, Community, and Leisure Integration

Kayla will be encouraged to continue in leisure activities, such as swimming, riding her bike, and walking. These activities can be carried on throughout the life span and will encourage a physically active lifestyle.

Summary of Procedural Interventions

Expected outcomes of these procedural interventions are improved muscle strength and endurance; improved ROM; improved balance; increased functional independence in self-care, home, school, and community activities; increased safety during activity; and

prevention of secondary impairments. More specifically, improved muscle performance and motor control will help Kayla meet her goals to access her locker and change classes with her peers. Kayla's aerobic capacity should also be improved, and she will assume a role in maintaining a physically active lifestyle.

Termination of Episode of Care

The present episode of care will be terminated when Kayla meets the goals/objectives listed previously. If her status changes (e.g., health issues, task demands), the episode of care may be modified. A new episode of care may be initiated as new goals/objectives are written. It is anticipated that additional episodes of physical therapy care will be required until skeletal maturity is reached, when she must transition into the high school setting, and in preparation for work. It is also anticipated that secondary impairments (muscle weakness, ROM limitations, and decreased aerobic capacity) may negatively affect her ability to function optimally and independently in her community.

Kayla will benefit from therapy until she can function efficiently and independently in home, school, and community settings. She is entitled to physical therapy services within her educational program until she is 21 years of age, as long as she has difficulty meeting her educational objectives because of a movement dysfunction. After the age of 21 years, future episodes of physical therapy care, physical therapy maintenance, and physical therapy prevention are likely to be required. Individuals with CP may need multiple episodes of care over their lifetime to ensure safe and optimal functioning as they assume new roles and responsibilities, as caregiver changes occur, and as they function in new environments. Frequently an episode of physical therapy maintenance, consisting of occasional visits to maintain function, is appropriate. Episodes of physical therapy prevention also contribute to improved fitness, wellness, and function. These occasional services may include education regarding prevention of secondary impairments, revision of a fitness program, and monitoring condition and appropriateness of assistive devices and orthotics.

Kayla: 20 Years of Age

Kayla is now a college sophomore, majoring in social work. She selected a college campus several hundred miles from her family's home. The college is in the southern United States, where snow and ice do not interfere with Kayla's mobility and participation in college activities. Two of her siblings had relocated to a nearby city prior to Kayla's college selection. Even though she is far away from her parents, Kayla can call upon her brothers if necessary.

Kayla independently lives in the dormitory and is able to walk throughout her campus. She often chooses to walk using her forearm crutches, although for long distances she will use her motorized cart. When selecting her dormitory, Kayla chose not to limit her room selection by indicating her disability. Subsequently, she lived on a higher floor of the dorm and was even able to safely evacuate the building (using the stairs, with a railing) when necessary (fire drills, hurricane warnings).

Kayla does not report significant limitations in her ability to participate in college or community activities. She does occasionally report foot or back pain following a lot of activity. She currently has supramalleolar orthotics (SMO) for both feet, which she wears when she will be doing a lot of walking.

Interventions

Physical therapy intervention plans for children with CP may include a wide variety of activities, based on any one of several theoretical approaches. It is difficult to determine the effectiveness of physical therapy intervention for the child with CP based on available evidence. Research evidence is difficult to interpret because of methodological issues, variety of outcome measures, and wide diversity of subjects (age, severity, and type of involvement). Recent research evidence related to physical therapy interventions for children with CP is summarized in Table 19.3. When designing intervention plans for an individual child, it is important to consider how similar that child is to subjects in the research studies.

Table 19.3 Evidence-Based Interventions for Cerebral Palsy

Intervention	Author (date)	Study Design	No. of Subjects/ Articles	Question	Findings
General Interventions	Antilla, Autti-Ramo, Suoranta, Makela, & Malmivaara, 2008	Systematic review (SR) of only randomized controlled trials (RCT)	$n = 22$ articles	Assess the effectiveness of physical therapy (PT) interventions on function in children with cerebral palsy (CP)	Limited evidence for effectiveness of PT interventions studied by RCT (Adeli suite, functional therapy, neurodevelopmental treatment , sensorimotor training) Moderate evidence for effectiveness of upper extremity training with therapy or constraint induced therapy
Therapeutic Exercise: Aerobic Capacity/ Endurance Training	Vershuren et al., 2007	RCT,	$n = 65$ children with CP gross motor function classification system (GMFCS) level I or II, 7–18 years of age	Can an exercise program increase aerobic and anaerobic capacity of children with CP?	Training program of aerobic and anaerobic activities leads to increased aerobic capacity, increased anaerobic capacity, increased gross motor function measures (GMFM-88 Dimension D scores; increased participation (CAPE scores)
	Butler, Scianni, & Ada 2010	SR	$n= 3$ studies	Does training increase aerobic capacity and carryover to function?	Training may improve aerobic capacity, but minimal carryover is seen into function

Table 19.3 Evidence-Based Interventions for Cerebral Palsy—cont'd

Intervention	Author (date)	Study Design	No. of Subjects/ Articles	Question	Findings
Therapeutic Exercise: Gait and Locomotion Training	Dodd & Foley, 2007	Nonrandom-ized controlled trial	$n = 14$, 6-12 years of age, GMFCS level III or IV	Can in-school partial body-weight–supported treadmill train-ing (PBWSTT) improve gait speed and en-durance for chil-dren with CP?	PBWSTT leads to increase in gait speed (large effect size, $d = 1.84$); 10-minute walk distance
Therapeutic Exercise: Strength, Power, and Endurance Training for Muscles	Mattern-Baxter, 2009	SR	$n = 10$ articles; 1 controlled trial, 6 small cohort studies, 3 case reports	Examine the effects of PBW-STT on balance, gait, and en-durance in chil-dren with CP	Limited conclusions on PBW-STT for infants/toddlers possi-bly due to small number and size of studies For preschool and school-age children, PBWSTT increases gait speed and endurance
	Mockford & Caulton, 2008	SR, experimen-tal and quasi-experimental studies	$n = 13$ articles	Can progres-sive strength training im-prove function and gait in chil-dren with CP?	Strength training produces mod-erate to strong improvement in mm strength and function for children with CP (4–20 years); improves function; mild to mod-erate improvement in gait
	Dodd et al., 2002	SR	$n = 23$ articles	Is strength training benefi-cial in individu-als with CP?	Strength training increased muscle strength and may im-prove motor activity without adverse effects
	Williams & Pountney, 2007	Nonrandom-ized A-B-A design	$n = 11$ children (GMFCS level IV or V, 11-15 years of age)	Can a static bicycling pro-gram improve function in chil-dren who are nonambulant?	Graded-resistance strength training on stationary bike im-proved function: GMFM-66, GMFM-88 Dimensions D (standing) and E (walking, running, and jumping)
Manual therapy techniques: Passive range of motion (PROM)	Pin, Dyke, & Chan, 2006	SR related to passive stretching	$n = 7$ articles	Investigate the effectiveness of passive stretching in spastic CP	Weak support for effective-ness of passive stretching found. Sustained stretching appears to be more effective than manual stretching
	Wiart, Darrah, & Kembhavi, 2008	SR of passive and active stretching	$n = 7$ articles (3 single sub-ject design, 3 small ($n = $ 15-21) RCT, 1 quasi-experimental design)	Review the ef-fectiveness of stretching in children with CP	Only 3 studies had significant finding (30 minutes on tilt table to stretch triceps surae), show-ing decreased EMG response to stretch up to 35 minutes after stretch, improved activa-tion of tibialis anterior

Continued

■ **Table 19.3** Evidence-Based Interventions for Cerebral Palsy—cont'd

Intervention	Author (date)	Study Design	No. of Subjects/ Articles	Question	Findings
Electrotherapeutic modalities: Biofeedback/ electrical stimulation	Seifart, Ungri, & Burger, 2009	SR	$n = 5$ articles of all level of articles available (3 case reports, 1 single subject design, 1 crossover study)	Assess the effectiveness of lower extremity functional electrical stimulation (FES) in children and adolescents with CP	Wide variety of protocols used, small subject size, lack of experimental design, very weak evidence. Seems to indicate stimulation of triceps surae with or without tibialis anterior leads to improved gait parameters
Physical agents and mechanical modalities: Gravity-assisted compression devices (standing frame)	Kecskemethy et al., 2008	Descriptive study of weight bearing in different standers	$n = 14$	Assess actual amount of weight borne in a stander, comparing 2 different standers	Weight bearing can vary by as much as 29% based on type of stander Personal characteristics impact amount of weight bearing in a stander
	Pin, 2007	SR	$n = 10$ studies	Examine the effectiveness of static upper and lower extremity weight bearing in children with CP	Evidence exists that static standing leads to increased bone mineral density in lumbar spine and femur Static weight bearing on lower extremities may decrease spasticity for short periods of time (30 minutes), small effect size

DISCUSSION QUESTIONS

1. Hypothesize Kayla's current and future level of participation restriction. Discuss how her childhood development, family, and community resources have shaped her current level of participation.

2. Identify potential secondary impairments of body function and structure that Kayla may develop at 6 years and 12 years of age. What possible prevention strategies should be integrated into her therapy program to minimize development of these impairments?

3. Hypothesize potential limitations in activities and participation and secondary impairment of body

function and structure at 25 years of age and 40 years of age.
   a. What aspects of prevention could have been emphasized throughout childhood to minimize these impairments and restrictions in adulthood?
   b. What aspects of prevention should be emphasized now that Kayla is a college student?

4. What impairments in body functions and structures contribute to Kayla's difficulty with sitting and standing balance at 6 years of age and 13 years of age?

5. Identify intervention strategies for each impairment that would contribute to improved sitting and standing balance at 6 years of age and 13 years of age.

Recommended Readings

Carlon, S., Shields, N., Yong, K., Gilmore, R., Sakzewski, L., & Boyd, R. (2010). A systematic review of the psychometric properties of Quality of Life measures for school aged children with cerebral palsy. *BMC Pediatrics, 10*, 81.

Kerr, C., McDowell, B.C., Parkes, J.H., Stevenson, M., Cosgrove, A.P. (2011). Age-related changes in energy efficiency of gait, activity, and participation in children with cerebral palsy. *Developmental Medicine and Child Neurology, 53*, 61-67.

Palisano, R.J., Chiarello, L.A., Orlin, M., Oeffinger, D., Polansky, M., Maggs, J., Bagley, A., Gorton, G. (2011). Determinants of intensity of participation in leisure and recreational activities by children with cerebral palsy. *Developmental Medicine and Child Neurology, 53*,142-149.

Smits, D., Ketelaar, M., Gorter, J.W., van Schie, P., Dallmeijer, A., Jongmans, M., & Lindeman, E. (2011). Development of daily activities in school-age children with cerebral palsy. *Research in Developmental Disabilities, 32*, 222-234.

References

Allison, S.C., Abraham, L.D., & Petersen, C.L. (1996). Reliability of the Modified Ashworth Scale in the assessment of plantar flexor muscle spasticity in patients with traumatic brain injury. *International Journal of Rehabilitation Research, 19*(1), 67–78.

American Physical Therapy Association (APTA) (2001). Guide to physical therapist practice (2nd ed.). *Physical Therapy, 81*, 9–744.

Antilla, H., Autti-Ramo, I., Suoranta, J., Makela, M., & Malmivaara, A. (2008). Effectiveness of physical therapy interventions for children with cerebral palsy: A systematic review. *BMC Pediatrics, 8*, 14.

Bartlett D., & Birmingham, T. (2003). Validity and reliability of the pediatric reach test. *Pediatric Physical Therapy, 15*, 84–02.

Berg, K., Wood-Dauphinée, S.L., Williams, J., & Gayton, D. (1989). Measuring balance in the elderly: Preliminary development of an instrument. *Physiotherapy Canada, 41*, 304–311.

Bohannon, R., & Smith, M. (1987). Interrater reliability of a Modified Ashworth Scale of muscle spasticity. *Physical Therapy, 67*, 206–207.

Boyd, R., & Graham, H. (1999). Objective measurement of clinical findings in the use of botulinum toxin type A in the management of spasticity in children with cerebral palsy. *European Journal of Neurology, 6*, 523–536.

Butler, J.M., Sianni, A., & Ada, L. (2010). Effect of cardiorespiratory training on aerobic fitness and carryover to activity in children with cerebral palsy: A systematic review. *International Journal of Rehabilitation Research, 33*(2), 97–103.

Cech, D., & Martin, S. (2012). *Functional movement development across the life span* (3rd ed.). Philadelphia: W.B. Saunders.

Clopton, N., Dutton, J., Featherston, T., Grigsby, A., Mobley, J., & Melvin, J. (2005). Interrater and intrarater reliability of the Modified Ashworth Scale in children with hypertonia. *Pediatric Physical Therapy, 17*, 268–274.

Crompton, J., Galea, M.P., & Phillips, M.P. (2007). Hand-held dynamometry for muscle strength measurement in children with cerebral palsy. *Developmental Medicine & Child Neurology, 49*, 106–111.

Damiano, D.L., & Abel, M.F. (1998). Functional outcomes of strength training in spastic cerebral palsy. *Archives of Physical Medicine and Rehabilitation, 79*, 119–125.

Damiano, D.L., Dodd, K., & Taylor, N.F. (2002). Should we be testing and training muscle strength in cerebral palsy? *Developmental Medicine and Child Neurology, 44*, 68–72.

Dodd, K.J., & Foley, S. (2007). Partial body-weight supported treadmill training can improve walking in children with cerebral palsy: A clinical controlled trial. *Developmental Medicine and Child Neurology, 49*, 101–105.

Dodd, K., Taylor, N., & Damiano, D. (2002). A systematic review of the effectiveness of strength-training programmes for people with cerebral palsy. *Archives of Physical Medicine and Rehabilitation, 83*, 1157–1164.

Engel-Yeger, B., Jarus, T., Anaby, D., & Law, M. (2009). Differences in patterns of participation between youths with cerebral palsy and typically developing peers. *American Journal of Occupational Therapy, 63*(1), 96–104.

Folio, M.R., & Fewell, R.R. (1983). *Peabody Developmental Motor Scales*. Austin, TX: DLM Teaching Resources.

Folio, M.R., & Fewell, R.R. (2000). *Peabody Developmental Motor Scales* (2nd ed.). Austin, TX: Pro-Ed.

Fosang, A., Galea, M.P., McCoy, A.T., Reddihough, D.S., & Story, I. (2003). Measures of muscle and joint performance in the lower limb of children with cerebral palsy. *Developmental Medicine and Child Neurology, 45*, 664–670.

Franjoine, M.R., Gunter, J.S., & Taylor, M.J. (2003). Pediatric balance scale: A modified version of the Berg Balance Scale for the school-age child with mild to moderate motor impairment. *Pediatric Physical Therapy, 15*, 114–128.

Gajdosik, C.G. (2005). Ability of very young children to produce reliable isometric force measurements. *Pediatric Physical Therapy, 17*, 251–257.

Gan, S., Tung, L., Tang, Y., & Wang, C. (2008). Psychometric Properties of functional Balance Assessment in children with Cerebral Palsy. *Neurorehabilitation Neural Repair, 22*, 745–753.

Gregson, J.M., Leathley, M.J., Moore, A.P., Smith, T.L., Sharma, A.K., & Watkins, C.L. (2000). Reliability of measurements of muscle tone and muscle power in stroke patients. *Age and Ageing, 29*(3), 223–228.

Haley, S.M., Coster, J., Ludlow, L.H., Haltiwanger, J.T., & Andrellos, P.J. (1992). *Pediatric Evaluation of Disability Inventory (PEDI)*. Boston: New England Medical Center Hospitals, Inc.

Kecskemethy, H.H., Herman, D., May, R., Paul, K., Bachrach, S.J., & Henderson, R.C. (2008). Quantifying weight bearing while in passive standers and a comparison of standers. *Developmental Medicine and Child Neurology, 50*, 520–523.

Kembhavi, G., Darrah, J., Magill-Evans, J., & Loomi, J. (2002). Using the Berg Balance Scale to distinguish balance abilities in children with cerebral palsy. *Pediatric Physical Therapy, 14*, 92–99.

Kilgour, G., McNair, P., & Stott, N.S. (2003). Intrarater reliability of lower limb sagittal range-of-motion measures in children with spastic diplegia. *Developmental Medicine and Child Neurology, 45,* 391–399.

Maher, C.A., Williams, M.T., Olds, T., & Lane, A.E. (2007). Physical and sedentary activity in adolescents with cerebral palsy. *Developmental Medicine and Child Neurology, 49,* 450–457.

Mattern-Baxter, K. (2009). Effects of partial body weight supported treadmill training on children with cerebral palsy. *Pediatric Physical Therapy, 21,* 12–22.

Mockford, M., Caulton, J.M. (2008). Systematic review of progressive strength training in children and adolescents with cerebral palsy who are ambulatory. *Pediatric Physical Therapy, 20,* 318–333.

Palisano, R.J., Rosenbaum, P., Bartlett, D., & Livingston, M.H. (2008). Content validity of the expanded and revised Gross Motor Function Classification System. *Developmental Medicine and Child Neurology, 50,* 744–450.

Palisano, R., Rosenbaum, P., Walter, S., Russell, D., Wood, E., & Galuppi, B. (1997). Development and reliability of a system to classify gross motor function in children with cerebral palsy. *Developmental Medicine and Child Neurology, 39,* 214–223.

Pin, T.W. (2007). Effectiveness of static weight-bearing exercises in children with cerebral palsy. *Pediatric Physical Therapy, 19,* 62–73.

Pin, T., Dyke, P., & Chan, M. (2006). The effectiveness of passive stretching in children with cerebral palsy. *Developmental Medicine and Child Neurology, 48,* 855.

Russell, D.J., Rosenbaum, P.L., Avery, L.M., & Lane, M. (2002). Gross Motor Function Measure (GMFM-66 & GMFM-88) Users Manual. *Clinics in Developmental Medicine No. 159.* London: Mac Keith Press.

Scholtes, V.A.B., Becher, J.G., Beelen, A., & Lankhorst, G.J. (2006). Clinical assessment of spasticity in children with cerebral palsy: A critical review of available instruments. *Developmental Medicine and Child Neurology, 48,* 64–73.

Seifart, A., Ungri, M., & Burger, M. (2009). The effect of lower limb functional electrical stimulation on gait of children with cerebral palsy. *Pediatric Physical Therapy, 21,* 23–30.

Shikako-Thomas, K., Majnemer, A., Law, M., & Lach, L. (2008). Determinants of participation in leisure activities in children and youth with cerebral palsy: Systematic review. *Physical and Occupational Therapy in Pediatrics, 28*(2), 155–169.

Sloan, C. (2002). Review of the reliability and validity of myometry with children. *Physical and Occupational Therapy in Pediatrics, 22*(2), 79–93.

Stuberg, W.A., Fuchs, R.H., & Miedaner, J.A. (1988). Reliability of goniometric measurements of children with cerebral palsy. *Developmental Medicine and Child Neurology, 30,* 657–666.

Stuberg, W.A., & Metcalf, W.K. (1988). Reliability of quantitative muscle testing in healthy children using a hand-held dynamometer. *Physical Therapy, 68*(6), 977–982.

Vershuren, O., Ketelaar, M., Gorter, J.W., Helders, P.J.M., Uiterwaal, C.S.P.M., & Takken, T. (2007). Exercise training program in children and adolescents with cerebral palsy: A randomized controlled trial. *Archives of Pediatric and Adolescent Medicine, 161*(11), 1075–1081.

Watkins, B., Darrah, J., & Pain, K. (1995). Reliability of passive ankle dorsiflexion measurements in children: Comparison of universal and biplane goniometers. *Pediatric Physical Therapy, 7,* 3–8.

Wiart, L., Darrah, J., & Kembhavi, G. (2008). Stretching with children with cerebral palsy: What do we know and where are we going? *Pediatric Physical Therapy, 20,* 173–178.

Williams, E.N., Carroll, S.G., Reddihough, D.S., Phillips, B.A., & Galea, M.P. (2005). Investigation of the timed "Up & Go" test in children. *Developmental Medicine and Child Neurology, 47,* 518–524.

Williams, H., & Pountney, T. (2007). Effects of a static bicycling programme on the functional ability of young people with cerebral palsy who are non-ambulant. *Developmental Medicine and Child Neurology, 49,* 522–527.

CHAPTER **20**

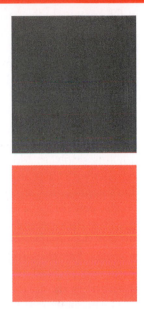

Case Study

Cystic Fibrosis

—Carole A. Tucker, PT, PhD, PCS, RCEP

Cystic fibrosis (CF) is an autosomal recessive condition affecting approximately 30,000 Americans and 60,000 people worldwide. According to the Centers for Disease Control and Prevention (CDC), approximately 1,000 new cases are diagnosed yearly in the United States, with a known incidence of 1 per 3,900 live births. The disease prevalence varies greatly by ethnicity, with the highest prevalence occurring in Western European descendants and within the Ashkenazi Jewish population.

The cystic fibrosis gene, located on chromosome 7, was first identified in 1989. The disease process is caused by a mutation to the gene that encodes for the cystic fibrosis transmembrane conductance regulator (CFTR) protein. This mutation alters the production, structure, and function of cAMP (cyclic adenosine monophosphate), a dependent transmembrane chloride channel carrier protein found in the exocrine

mucus glands throughout the body. The mutated carrier protein is unable to transport chloride across the cell membrane, resulting in an electrolyte and charge imbalance. Diffusion of water across the cell membrane is thus impaired, resulting in the development of a viscous layer of mucus. The thick mucus obstructs the cell membranes, traps nearby bacteria, and incites a local inflammatory response. Subsequent bacterial colonization occurs at an early age and ultimately this repetitive infectious process leads to progressive inflammatory damage to the organs involved in individuals with CF.

CF involves the exocrine mucous glands and typically affects the lungs, liver, pancreas, gastrointestinal tract, sweat glands, and genitourinary tracts. The severity of the disease and the organs affected depends largely on the specific type of genetic mutation involved. To date there are more than 1,200 known mutations of the CFTR gene, not all of which cause CF.

655

The specific type of mutation dictates the organ systems involved, the pathology observed, and the disease severity. The most prevalent mutation to the CFTR gene is the Delta-F508 mutation, accounting for 66% of CF patients worldwide. The Delta-F508 mutation is a deletion of only three nucleotide base pairs in the CFTR gene, resulting in the absence of the amino acid phenylalanine in the protein. Patients with the Delta-F508 mutation have predominant impairments in body structure and function of both the respiratory and gastrointestinal tracts. The respiratory system impairments in CF may include airway obstruction with recurrent and progressive lung infections (such as recurrent pneumonia), chronic bronchitis, asthma, chronic cough, and nasal polyps. Gastrointestinal system impairments may include pancreatic enzyme insufficiency, fat and protein malabsorption, type 1 or 2 diabetes mellitus, failure to thrive, abdominal pain, increased flatulence, intestinal obstruction, cirrhosis, pancreatic inflammation, and bulky, greasy, foul-smelling stools. In addition, the genitourinary systems in males with CF is impaired, with a 97% infertility rate due to congenital absence of the vas deferens, with a smaller percentage of men having obstructive azoospermia. The incidence of infertility of females with CF is not well documented but appears to be much less then in males. Female infertility in CF is primarily due to thickened cervical mucus, ovulation disruption, or amenorrhea secondary to the effects of malnutrition.

The median predicted life expectancy for individuals with CF has increased from 32 years in the year 2000 to 37.42 years in the year 2008, according to data from the Cystic Fibrosis Patient Registry. The primary factors that contribute to the improvements in the predicted survival age of individuals having CF include improved early detection methods and the evolution of more effective treatment protocols—in particular, the development of pharmacological interventions directed at ameliorating the impaired cellular functions caused by the genetic defect, as well as medications to reduce lung infection and inflammation.

In 2003, the CDC conducted a panel review of all the literature regarding newborn screening programs worldwide. Based on the evidence, the CDC recommended implementing newborn screening throughout the United States. They found that children diagnosed at birth by newborn screening had less morbidity, improved growth, less chronic malnutrition, improved cognitive development, and fewer hospitalizations in childhood than those children with a delayed diagnosis. Mandatory newborn screening for CF is now required in every state in the United States. Newborn screening is accomplished by examination of the newborn's blood for a pancreatic product called immunoreactive trypsinogen (IRT). IRT levels are elevated in infants with CF but are nonspecific (i.e., infants with other disease processes may have elevated IRT levels), so if levels of IRT are high, genetic testing is performed. Since it is not feasible to test for all 1,200 suspected CFTR genetic mutations, each state tests for the most likely mutations. Finally, to differentiate CF gene carriers from those afflicted with CF, a sweat test, known as pilocarpine iontophoresis, is performed. The test quantifies the concentration of chloride in the sweat, and a chloride sweat test value of 60 mmol/L or greater is positive for CF.

Based on the American Physical Therapy Association (APTA)'s *Guide to Physical Therapist Practice* (APTA, 2001), the impairments presented by individuals with CF may be best addressed by the physical therapy management described in the Preferred Practice Patterns 6C: Impaired Ventilation, Respiration/Gas Exchange, and Aerobic Capacity/Endurance Associated with Airway Clearance Dysfunction; 6E: Impaired Ventilation and Respiration/Gas Exchange Associated with Ventilatory Pump Dysfunction or Failure; and 6F: Impaired Ventilation and Respiration/Gas Exchange Associated with Respiratory Failure. The practice pattern 6C best represents the changes in body structure and function with mild disease severity, often encountered throughout infancy and early childhood. The practice patterns 6E and 6F best address limitations associated with greater disease severity.

This case study focuses on the physical therapy management of a boy named Jerry, who was diagnosed with CF at 2 months of age. As with most children diagnosed with CF, Jerry required repeated episodes of physical therapy services throughout his childhood and adolescence. Jerry was followed monthly at an outpatient cystic fibrosis clinic at a comprehensive care center and received physical therapy at every inpatient admission. This case study describes Jerry's episodes of inpatient care at an acute-care facility at 2 months (initial diagnosis), 8 years of age, and 16 years of age, with a focus on the physical therapy examination and interventions. These descriptions highlight the evolution in patient education to support his growing independence in self-care.

Examination: Age 2 Months

History

Jerry was referred to the hospital at 2 months of age for work-up related to poor weight gain and severe gastroesophageal reflux (GER). Initially diagnosed with failure to thrive, a positive sweat test ultimately confirmed the diagnosis of CF. Jerry and his family were referred to physical therapy for family instruction in airway clearance techniques.

General Demographics

Jerry is a 2-month-old white male infant of Northern European descent who lives with his mother, father, and 8-year-old half-sister. Both parents smoke in the home. English is the primary language spoken by his family. Further pedigree analysis reveals no family history of CF.

Growth and Development

Jerry was born at full term, with a normal spontaneous vaginal delivery, weighing 8 pounds 3/4 ounce at birth (50th percentile). Maternal iron deficiency anemia complicated the pregnancy. He went home on day 2 of life, at which time he experienced nonprojectile emesis after every feed. No weight gain was noted despite trials on various infant formulas including Enfamil (cow's milk based), Isomil (soy based), and Nutramigen (elemental formula). Despite a voracious appetite, at 3 weeks of age, Jerry weighed 7 pounds 14 ounces, and at 8 weeks of age, he weighed 9 pounds, below the 5th percentile for weight. The parents reported he had frequent yellow, greasy stools. A sweat test revealed a sodium level of +150 mg, thus confirming his diagnosis of CF.

Medications and Diet

Jerry's medications include Coenzyme-S, a pancreatic enzyme replacement; Poly-Vi-Sol, a liquid multivitamin; and the fat-soluble vitamins E and K. He is currently fed Similac with iron, a cow's milk–based formula.

Other Tests and Measures

Jerry's chest radiograph displays hyperinflation with mild lower airway disease. Pulmonary markings are slightly prominent. Bowel gas pattern appears normal. His laboratory values are provided in Table 20.1.

Systems Review

A systems review of Jerry's integumentary, neuromotor, and sensory (vision and hearing) systems were normal. His gross motor development is age appropriate.

Cardiovascular and Pulmonary

Jerry's cardiovascular and pulmonary systems appear to be functioning within normal limits (WNL) (see Chapter 9, Fig. 9.8) at this time. Jerry's heart rate is

Table 20.1 Laboratory Values at 2 Months of Age*

Laboratory Value	Jerry's Values	Normal Values for Age
Hemoglobin	**8.5 g/dL**	10–13 g/dL
Hematocrit	**25%**	30–40%
White blood cell count	9,500 cells/µL	3,000–10,000 cells/µL
Sodium	139 mEq/L	135–144 mEq/L
Potassium	5.1 mEq/L	3.6–5.2 mEq/L
Chloride	105 mEq/L	97–106 mEq/L
Bicarbonate	**17 mEq/L**	24–34 mEq/L
Blood urea nitrogen	15 mg/dL	5–18 mg/dL
Creatinine	**0.6 mg/dL**	<0.5 mg/dL
Glucose	**101 mg/dL**	60–100 mg/dL
Prothrombin time	12.1 seconds	11–13 seconds
Partial prothrombin time	25.3 seconds	20–30 seconds

Source: Normal values obtained from Children's Liver Association for Support Services, http://www.classkids.org/library/ref/liverlabs.htm.
*Bold indicates abnormal value.

138 beats per minute (bpm), blood pressure (BP) is 88/63 mm Hg, and oxygen saturation (Sao_2) is 95% on room air at rest. His respiratory rate (RR) is 30 breaths per minute with no increased work of breathing. Heart rate (HR) and rhythm are regular and without murmur.

Musculoskeletal

Jerry presents with asymmetrical length, weight, and head circumference parameters. Jerry's body length is 57.5 cm (50th percentile of age), weight is 3.99 kg (10th percentile for age), and head circumference is 37.5 cm (20th percentile for age).

Tests and Measures
Aerobic Capacity and Endurance

A normal diaphragmatic breathing pattern is observed at rest and feeding. At times his bottle feeds take longer than expected as he pauses to breathe during feedings. A small increase in HR and mild nasal flaring are seen during sucking, but there is no drop in Sao_2. The feeding team found his bottle feed ability to be WNL. He possesses a robust cry.

Muscle Performance

At this age, muscle performance is evaluated through observation of the infant's movements in supine and prone to assess neck, trunk, and extremity strength and underlying tone. Jerry initiates movement symmetrically against gravity in all positions, but he appears to be less vigorous than would be expected for a baby his age. This seems to imply age-appropriate muscle strength, but perhaps endurance limits his performance.

Neuromotor Development

In prone, Jerry is able to lift and turn his head and briefly fix visually on a toy. He holds his head in midline when held at the shoulder in supported sit and will briefly hold a small rattle placed in his hand in supine. These skills reflect age-appropriate performance on the Peabody Developmental Motor Scales (Folio & Fewell, 2000).

Range of Motion

Jerry's active range of motion (AROM) and passive range of motion (PROM) are WNL for his age.

Ventilation and Respiration/Gas Exchange

Auscultation reveals equal and clear breath sounds, with no rhonchi, rales, or wheezes. No chest wall retractions or nasal flaring are noted. Jerry is pale, but no skin mottling or cyanosis is observed. No head bobbing is seen on inspiration at rest or during bottle feeds, reflecting the absence of accessory respiratory muscle use.

Examination Update: If Jerry were being evaluated today, many of the same outcome measures would be appropriate. In some major CF centers, the use of pulmonary function tests to assess lung volumes and airflow in infants may be included as part of routine evaluation. In the near future, more discriminative genetic testing that may direct emerging focused gene–based therapies may be included in the medical evaluations of young infants with CF.

Evaluation, Diagnosis, and Prognosis
Including Plan of Care

Jerry presents with malabsorption and poor weight gain. Because of his diagnosis of CF, impaired airway clearance and inefficient gas exchange are anticipated to emerge in the future. During this episode of care, his family will become proficient with techniques to maximize airway clearance and gas exchange, thereby enhancing his ability to function within his environment. Jerry will demonstrate optimal ventilation to support developmental skill acquisition and weight gain.

Goals

The following family-centered goals will be achieved during this hospitalization:

1. Jerry's parents will verbalize understanding of the CF disease process.
2. Jerry's parents will verbalize the necessity for daily use of regular airway clearance techniques for prevention of secondary pulmonary complications.
3. Jerry's parents will independently and appropriately perform non-Trendelenburg postural drainage, percussion, and vibration on all lobes of Jerry's lungs for 1.5 minutes per segment.
4. Jerry's parents will verbally commit to eliminating his exposure to secondhand smoke and identify a location outside of the home for their smoking.

Intervention

Coordination, Communication, and Documentation

Coordination, communication, and documentation of physical therapy management will be directed toward the family and CF clinic personnel. With appropriate communication, coordination of care will be enhanced, risk reduction will be improved, and the family will understand the goals and objectives of the physical therapy management protocol. The family verbalizes knowledge about the hospital's outpatient CF clinic and the medical team members to contact for future needs related to CF.

Patient/Client-Related Instruction

At this time, it is of the utmost importance that the caregivers demonstrate independence with postural drainage, percussion, and vibration (PDPV). The family is given materials with both written descriptions and illustrations delineating the appropriate postural drainage positions and areas for percussion (see Chapter 9). PDPV is to be performed at home two times daily, either before or an hour and a half after bottle feeds. PDPV will be increased to three times daily if Jerry experiences a pulmonary exacerbation. The Trendelenburg position is avoided during PDPV in infancy to reduce GER. The importance of encouraging play activities after an airway clearance session, to promote further expectoration of mucus in the larger airways, is also discussed. The parents demonstrate independence with the airway clearance techniques and demonstrate a clear understanding of the disease progression and preventive strategies to minimize future complications. The parents verbalize the importance of preventing their son's exposure to secondhand smoke and verbally commit to smoke outside the home only.

Procedural Interventions

As anticipated since Jerry has negligible lung pathology at this time, postural abnormalities are not observed, and Jerry has appropriate gross motor developmental skills for his age. Therefore no specific intervention is necessary, and a referral to community-based early intervention service is not indicated at this time.

Airway Clearance Techniques

PDPV is performed two times daily, incorporating five alternative positions for each session, without implementation of the Trendelenburg position secondary to reflux. The anticipated outcomes of this intervention are improved airway clearance, prevention of accumulation of mucus, and maximized ventilation/respiration.

Examination Update: The importance of a physically active lifestyle, optimal body composition, and weight maintenance being instilled in childhood has emerged as a critical component of health management, and perhaps even slowing of disease progression, in individuals with CF. In addition to the focus on airway clearance techniques as part of the outpatient physical therapy program, a focus on the promotion of active lifestyle choices that include both strengthening and aerobic activities would be emphasized. Though Jerry is currently an infant, parent education concerning healthy lifestyle choices and promotion of physical activity starting in early childhood not only help ensure Jerry's later compliance but may influence his activity preferences.

Termination of Episode of Care

The family achieved all goals during Jerry's first hospitalization. He was discharged from physical therapy with a daily home program. The parents demonstrated knowledge of the outpatient cystic fibrosis clinic and the medical team members to contact for future needs related to CF. A physical therapist will follow Jerry through the outpatient clinic to provide continual family support and screen Jerry's motor development. When Jerry reaches 12 months of age, the physical therapist will progress PDPV instruction to include all 12 positions secondary to his increased chest wall surface area. Factors that would indicate a need for a new episode of physical therapy care include pulmonary exacerbation, delayed acquisition of developmental milestones, and the need to oversee education of additional family members for PDPV.

Examination: Age 8 Years

Jerry is now followed quarterly in the cystic fibrosis clinic. He has had no hospitalizations from the time of his initial diagnosis at 2 months of age until 8 years of age. At this time he presents to the clinic with a 1-week history of persistent cough, increased work of breathing, and weight loss. He is admitted for his first acute pulmonary exacerbation. Inpatient physical therapy is consulted secondary to Jerry's impaired endurance.

History

General Demographics

Jerry is 8 years old and currently in second grade. He lives with his mother, father, and 16-year-old half-sister. Both parents continue to smoke in the home.

Medical/Surgical History

Jerry was diagnosed with asthma at 7 years of age in the outpatient cystic fibrosis clinic.

History of Current Condition

Two weeks prior to this admission, Jerry contracted varicella (chickenpox). Since this exposure, he has had a worsening cough, associated posttussive emesis, increased volume and thickness of secretions, as well as decreased exercise tolerance. In addition, over the past year, his pulmonary function tests have gradually declined. On admission, he is found to test positive for colonized mucoid and nonmucoid *Pseudomonas aeruginosa* and coagulase-positive *Staphylococcus* bacteria.

Functional Status and Activity Level

Jerry reports independence in his functional activities. He participates without restrictions in gym class, in after-school play with friends, and in league ice hockey throughout the year. Jerry reports daily physical exercise, which is corroborated by his parents. He reports the ability to keep up with his friends' activity level without compromise, until two weeks ago.

Medications

Jerry takes several medications on a regular basis to improve his nutritional status and improve ventilation, such as Pancrease, Mucomyst, Albuterol, and Intal. Pancrease is a pancreatic enzyme replacement supplement necessary for the proper digestion and absorption of fats, proteins, and carbohydrates. Mucomyst is a mucolytic that helps to thin pulmonary secretions to facilitate airway clearance. Albuterol (Ventolin) is a bronchodilator that decreases airway resistance. Intal is an antiasthmatic medication that can help prevent bronchospasm. Jerry also regularly takes vitamin E and multivitamin supplements.

During Jerry's hospital admission the antibiotics tobramycin, oxacillin, and ticarcillin in intravenous form were prescribed.

Other Tests and Measures

Pulmonary function test results (Table 20.2) reflected small airway involvement with a mildly reduced forced expiratory volume in 1 second (FEV_1), $FEV_{25-75\%}$, and FEV_1/forced vital capacity (FVC). A chest radiograph, taken on admission, displays moderate hyperinflation, increased anterior posterior thoracic diameter, and moderate peribronchial thickening in the central portions of the lungs. No focal atelectasis, infiltrate, or effusion is noted. The soft tissue shadow of the liver is not enlarged. Five days later, a chest radiograph displays mildly hyperinflated lungs with peribronchial thickening. No focal parenchymal infiltrate, pleural effusion, or pneumothorax is noted. No other cystic changes are observed. The radiographs in Figure 20.1 display common findings in children with CF.

Systems Review

Systems review of the integumentary and neuromuscular systems are WNL.

Cardiovascular and Pulmonary

Cardiovascular and pulmonary system functions are an area of concern because Jerry has elevated resting vital signs of HR, 92 bpm; BP, 130/80 mm Hg; and RR, 24 breaths per minute. See Chapter 9, Table 9.8, for a review of normally expected vital sign values in children. HR and rhythm are regular and without murmur. Minimal lateral intercostal and suprasternal retractions are observed at rest. Mild clubbing of the digits is observed, but no cyanosis is noted. Pulses are brisk throughout all extremities.

Musculoskeletal

Jerry's height is 49 inches (124 cm), and his weight is 50 pounds (23 kg), both falling within the 25th percentile for his age.

Tests and Measures

Aerobic Capacity and Endurance

Jerry is able to ambulate on the treadmill at 2.2 mph for 18 minutes but is limited by shortness of breath. Vital signs during exercise are SaO_2 of 94% to 96%; HR, 110 to 126 bpm; and RR, 32 to 44 breaths per minute. All values return to values equal to or below baseline levels within 9 minutes postexercise (SaO_2 of 98%; HR, 85 bpm; and RR, 15 breaths per minute). Jerry reports a rate of perceived exertion (RPE) of 6/10 on the modified Borg scale (Borg, 1982) (see Chapter 9, Fig. 9.11) during exercise with a maximum HR of 126 bpm. The RPE is reported to be a reliable measure of exertion with individuals of any age or gender (American College of Sports Medicine, 1991; Yankaskas & Knowles, 1999).

Muscle Performance

Muscle strength appears to be WNL, with strength throughout all extremities graded with a score of 5/5.

Table 20.2 Pulmonary Function Tests*

Age	FEV_1	$FEF_{25-75\%}$	FVC	FEV_1/FVC	PO_2
Admission: 8 years	71	68	110	67	96%
Discharge: 8 years	86	72	117	70	100%
Admission: 16 years	83	49	71	86	95%
Discharge: 16 years	92	54	97	89	98%

*Values are reported as a percentage of expected value. Expected values are greater than or equal to 80 for FEV_1, $FEF_{25-75\%}$, FVC, and FEV_1/FVC.

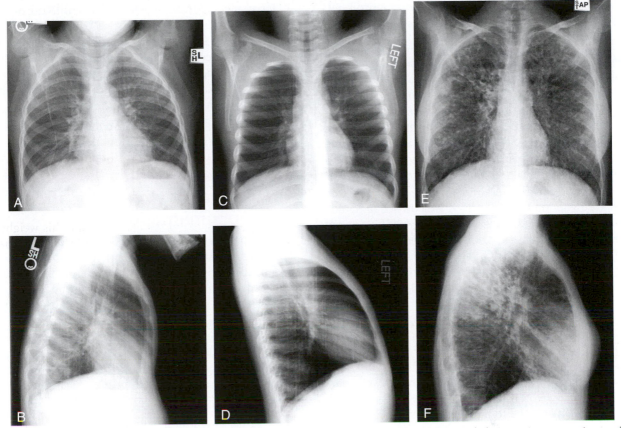

Figure 20.1 Radiographs of lungs of children having cystic fibrosis at different ages: (*A*) Anterior posterior and (*B*) medial lateral radiograph of 3-year-old with cystic fibrosis showing mild interstitial changes. (*C*) Anterior posterior radiograph of 9-year-old with cystic fibrosis with bronchiectatic changes visible. (*D*) Medial lateral radiograph of 9-year-old with cystic fibrosis with infiltrate visible in the upper lobe. (*E*) Anterior posterior and (*F*) medial lateral radiograph of 16-year-old with cystic fibrosis with diffuse infiltrates visible.

Neuromotor Development and Sensory Integration

All neuromotor development areas appear to be WNL.

Posture

No postural deformities are observed.

Range of Motion

Jerry demonstrates full AROM throughout all extremities.

Self-Care and Home Management

Jerry reports a mild increase of his work of breathing related to activities at school and home during the 2 weeks before this admission. He has not participated in ice hockey in the 2 weeks before this admission because of a persistent nonproductive cough and increased work of breathing.

Ventilation and Respiration/Gas Exchange

Minimal suprasternal and intercostal retractions with some accessory muscle use are noted at rest. On auscultation, good air movement is noted bilaterally, with minimal adventitious sounds including soft rales on the right only. The adventitious sounds clear with a cough. Pulmonary function testing completed at the hospital admission (see Table 20.2) indicates that Jerry has mild small airway disease. Jerry does present with a chronic cough. At this time there is increased congestion and the cough is productive of light yellow sputum.

Work, Community, and Leisure Integration

Jerry has no chronic limitations or restrictions in his activities or participation related to his disease. Prior to contracting varicella 2 weeks ago, he reports full participation in all school activities including competitive extracurricular endeavors with his peers.

Examination Update: If Jerry were evaluated today, standardized assessments of his physical function capability, activity, and participation would most likely be included in his examination. A 6-minute walk test or standardized submaximal exercise treadmill test could be performed. Objective ambulatory monitoring of his physical activity level using actigraphy or step monitors, or a self-report of physical activity would be useful tools to better quantify the amount and pattern of physical activity. Patient-reported outcomes that include dyspnea and fatigue as well as social participation (peer relationships), subjective well-being, and performance of physical activity are emerging as potential clinical tools. Quality of life assessment through self-reported measures would also be appropriate for a child 8 years of age or older.

Evaluation, Diagnosis, and Prognosis
Including Plan of Care

Since the age of 2 months, Jerry has been followed quarterly in the cystic fibrosis clinic and has not had significant problems related to his chronic disease. This is his first acute pulmonary exacerbation requiring an inpatient admission. Pulmonary function tests have declined slightly over time, indicating the gradual emergence of mild small airway disease. For this admission, Jerry presents with impaired pulmonary endurance primarily related to his acute exacerbation. By termination of this episode of care, it is anticipated that he will demonstrate optimal ventilation, optimal respiration/gas exchange, and optimal aerobic capacity, enabling him to fully participate in school, home, community, and leisure activities. It is also anticipated that he will assume more responsibility for his airway clearance management.

Goals

The following goals will be achieved during his hospitalization:

1. Jerry will perform all bathing, grooming, and dressing independently and without increased work of breathing.
2. Jerry will demonstrate adequate aeration of bilateral lung fields, without adventitious sounds.
3. Jerry's parents will demonstrate independence in postural drainage, percussion, and vibration for all segments for 1.5 minutes each segment.

4. Jerry will demonstrate independence with use of a positive expiratory pressure (PEP) device. He will perform the following with a proper sitting posture: breathe in deeply and slowly and hold breath for 2 to 3 seconds, then exhale slowly through the device. After repeating the above for 8 to 10 breaths he will cough with huffing 2 to 3 times to expectorate the mucus. The above set will be repeated 4 to 6 times.

Intervention

Coordination, Communication, and Documentation

The two paramount issues discussed during the care conference include the need for Jerry to possess the skills for independence with an airway clearance technique and the need to reinforce with the parents the importance of elimination of secondhand smoke within their home. The physical therapist educated the school nurse on the protocol for use of the PEP device. The nurse was aware that Jerry would use the device in the nurse's office as needed. The case manager is directed to procure a mechanical percussor and PEP device for the home.

Patient/Client-Related Instruction

Jerry is instructed in alternative airway clearance techniques. A handheld mechanical percussor and sonic percussor are introduced. He elects to use the mechanical percussor and independently manages clearance of his anterior and lateral segments. The family continues to perform manual percussion with vibration of his posterior segments.

Jerry is also instructed to supplement the primary airway clearance technique of manual or mechanical percussion with the use of the PEP or the Flutter device (see Chapter 9, Figs. 9.17 and 9.18). The PEP and Flutter devices are easily transportable and enable him to clear his airway immediately before or during a sport or gym activity. In addition, the PEP or Flutter gives him the opportunity to increase the number of daily independent airway clearance sessions, as needed. Jerry chose to use the PEP device.

Previously, in the cystic fibrosis clinic, the family was instructed to implement vibration immediately after percussion to each lung segment while Jerry performed a pursed-lipped, slow, and protracted exhalation. During this admission, the family is instructed in proper use of the mechanical percussor and PEP device. The family prefers manual percussions to mechanical percussion on Jerry's posterior segments to be able to palpate fremitus. All of the techniques are reviewed and the family demonstrates the ability to perform these activities appropriately. Child and family instruction related to the prevention of complications and the impact of smoking on Jerry's pulmonary status are reiterated.

Procedural Interventions

Therapeutic Exercise

Aerobic Capacity/Endurance Training

In light of his failure-to-thrive comorbidity, closed-chain activities, such as ice hockey, are encouraged to promote increased bone density. Physical activity will also assist in attaining peak oxygen consumption and aerobic capacity. During any physical activity, ventilation will increase and assist in secretion clearance.

Airway Clearance Techniques

Jerry is instructed on how to differentiate diaphragmatic breathing from accessory muscle breathing. Diaphragmatic breathing exercises are performed twice daily when he is at rest and during the vibration portion of his airway clearance protocol.

Jerry is instructed on the proper use of the mechanical percussor as a primary airway clearance technique on his anterior and lateral segments, in the respective postural drainage positions. The duration of percussion per segment remains at 1.5 minutes, twice daily. The family elects to continue manual percussion and vibration to Jerry's posterior segments. Jerry and the family are instructed how to properly use the PEP device as a supplement to the primary airway clearance technique. The PEP is to be used at school, as well as whenever else Jerry deems it necessary.

Examination Update: The importance of participation in regular physical activity has emerged as a potential adjunctive method for airway clearance method as well as more directly impacting disease progression in CF at the cellular level. Strengthening and weight-bearing activities build body and bone mass, which have been correlated with less severe disease progression. Jerry enjoys playing ice hockey, and should be encouraged to continue as this activity is meaningful to him. Jerry should add strengthening and more consistent aerobic conditioning components to his program of physical activity. Ice hockey is typically performed in cold, dry environments (ice hockey rinks), which may exacerbate Jerry's asthma. While ice hockey is a closed-chain activity, the necessary forces for bone growth stimulus may be inadequate given the minimal vertical forces that occur. Higher-impact activities (e.g., jumping rope, hopping, running) should be encouraged as they provide more adequate bone accretion than lower-impact activities.

Examination: Age 16 Years

Jerry has had numerous hospitalizations from the age of 8 until the age of 16 years old because of pulmonary exacerbations and failure to thrive. Over the past year, his pulmonary function tests have shown a progressive decline (see Table 20.2).

History

General Demographics

Jerry is 16 years old and continues to live with his father and 24-year-old half-sister. His parents are now amicably separated. The father works nights. Both the sister and father smoke in the home. He is in the 10th grade and regularly plays organized ice hockey in an after-school league.

Medical/Surgical History

Jerry has had multiple admissions to the hospital for pulmonary exacerbations within the past 8 years. His most recent admission was 3 months before this admission, during which he had a gastrostomy tube placed for overnight feeding secondary to failure to thrive. Before the gastrostomy tube placement, he received night feeding through a nasogastric tube. At that time a high-frequency chest wall oscillator (HFCWO) was also ordered for him as he needed complete independence with his airway clearance.

History of Current Condition

One month before this admission, Jerry reported symptoms of increased coughing, fever, weight loss, and posttussive emesis. He was treated with tobramycin, ciprofloxacin, and prednisone over a 4-week period while at home. His pulmonary function tests showed no improvement at home, so he is now admitted to the hospital for more aggressive therapy.

Growth and Development

Jerry is below the fifth percentile for height and weight. His height is 60.12 in (152.7 cm) and his weight is 90.7 lbs (37.8 kg).

Living Environment

Discharge to the home is anticipated.

Medications

Jerry continues to take Albuterol, Intal, Flonase, and Mucomyst to assist in control of bronchospasm and improve airway clearance. He also regularly takes sinus and allergy medications such as Sudafed, Flovent, and Claritin. He is prescribed Cisapride to control reflux and Fosamax and calcium carbonate to minimize bone loss. To reduce the frequency of respiratory infections and improve pulmonary function he is taking Pulmozyme, a medicine designed to thin and loosen mucus. Lastly he is prescribed Ultrase, a pancreatic enzyme supplement, and the fat-soluble vitamins A, D, E, and K.

During his hospital stay, Jerry is also taking to-bramycin, an antibiotic used specifically to treat *Pseudomonas* infection. Prolonged use of tobramycin may result in irreversible ototoxicity (dizziness and tinnitus) and neurotoxicity (headache, dizziness, and tremors). Although he does not report any of these symptoms at this time, these concerns should be considered during the physical therapy reexamination. Other medications taken during the admission include prednisone to reduce inflammation and Ceftazidime to minimize stomach upset and diarrhea.

Jerry's diet now includes Scandishake (3 times a week) and Nutren (ingested via gastrostomy tube). His total caloric intake per day is 3,408 kcal.

Other Tests and Measures

The chest radiograph demonstrated bilateral bronchiectasis, mucus plugging, peribronchial thickening, increased interstitial markings, and flattening of bilateral diaphragms. Pulmonary function tests (see Table 20.2) revealed FEV_1 of 83% and FVC of 71%. Sputum cultures revealed mucoid and nonmucoid *P. aeruginosa* bacteria. Laboratory studies included a DEXA scan, which revealed no change from a scan performed 3 months earlier. Jerry's scores on the scan showed bone mass to be –3.67 SDs below the mean, indicating a 60% predicted bone mass. The DEXA scan revealed a bone age of 13, which is considered a significant delay.

Systems Review
Cardiovascular and Pulmonary

Function of the cardiovascular and pulmonary systems is of concern during this admission attributable to the chest radiographic changes, which display worsening cystic changes and poor pulmonary function tests (see Table 20.2).

Integumentary

The gastrostomy tube site with button is clean and dry.

Musculoskeletal

Musculoskeletal development is an area of concern because of Jerry's significantly poor bone density, as well as his failure to display appropriate weight and height gain. Jerry is 60.12 in tall (152.7 cm) and weighs 90.7 lbs (37.8 kg). Both measurements are below the 5th percentile for his age.

Tests and Measures
Aerobic Capacity and Endurance

Jerry's vital signs at rest are HR of 104 bpm; RR, 22 breaths per minute; and BP, 107/76 mm Hg. Based upon expected values for his age, HR and RR are slightly increased (see Chapter 9, Table 9.8). His Sao_2 is 94% on room air, which is lower than the expected Sao_2 of 97% to 98%. HR is regular, and the rhythm is without murmurs. Jerry is able to ambulate on a treadmill at 2.5 mph with 5% incline for 12 minutes maximally. His exercise vital signs are HR of 120 bpm; RR of 38 breaths per minute, and Sao_2 of 97%.

Muscle Performance

Bilateral lower and upper extremity strength is grossly 5–/5 throughout. Decreased trunk strength is also noted.

Range of Motion

Jerry presents with AROM that is within functional limits. Passively, he has decreased hamstring flexibility evidenced with popliteal angles of 55° bilaterally. There is no limitation of functional upper extremity ROM.

Posture

Postural deviations include an increased thoracic kyphosis, forward head, rounded shoulders, winging scapula on the left greater than the right, posterior pelvic tilt, and elevated shoulder girdles with the left greater than the right. Hypertrophied accessory breathing musculature is also evident, with poor thoracic cage mobility and a barrel-shaped chest.

Ventilation and Respiration/Gas Exchange

Jerry uses his accessory muscles for quiet breathing. On auscultation, he has bilateral rales, which clear with a cough. The right middle lobe has predominant rales and the right lower lobe has decreased breath sounds.

Moderate clubbing of all the digits is noted bilaterally. His pulses are normal throughout.

Work, Community, and Leisure Integration

Jerry continues to fully participate in all school activities and to compete in extracurricular endeavors. He has no limitations or restrictions related to CF. He is independent with all of his activities of daily living; however, he reports that when a pulmonary exacerbation occurs he requires a longer time to finish daily living tasks around the house and school. For instance, he will take the elevator at school if he is feeling too fatigued to take the stairs. Jerry reports that he modifies his activities as needed such as taking longer recovery times during his hockey games.

Examination Update: As noted at 8 years the use of standardized health outcomes that include patient-reported measures of activity and participation, and quality of life would most likely be included. Given the increase in lifespan, work-related capacity evaluations and preferences would be appropriate to support Jerry's transition into young adulthood.

Evaluation, Diagnosis, and Prognosis
Including Plan of Care

Jerry's primary areas of concern include impairments in ventilatory capacity, decreased muscular endurance, decreased bone mineralization, and postural deviations with concomitant decreased muscular flexibility. In addition, Jerry knows no alternative airway clearance technique to the HFCWO and PDPV. The physical therapy diagnosis is as follows: decreased cardiorespiratory endurance, decreased muscular endurance and strength, decreased muscular flexibility, decreased independence with alternative airway clearance techniques, and postural deviations related to increased work of breathing.

Goals

The following goals will be achieved during six 1-hour-long physical therapy sessions per week for the duration of 2 weeks or until medical discharge:

1. Jerry will demonstrate independence with the PEP device as an alternative airway clearance technique.
2. Jerry will demonstrate independence with monitoring vital signs of HR and RR before, during, and after exercise.
3. Jerry will demonstrate independence with a home exercise program that will include:
   a. A weight-bearing endurance activity 3 to 4 times per week to achieve 60% HR maximum for 20 minutes.
   b. A strengthening protocol throughout all extremities that include spinal extension.
4. Jerry will demonstrate increased muscular endurance and ventilatory capacity in tolerance of treadmill for 25 minutes with 4-minute warm-up and cool-down, maintaining SaO_2 of greater than 94%, achieving 60% HR maximum.

Intervention
Patient/Client-Related Instruction

Jerry demonstrates independence with the HFCWO, his primary airway clearance technique. He continues to be quite active in school sports and extracurricular activities such as ice hockey. He did, however, complain recently of the inability to participate in a full period of ice hockey because of his poor ventilatory capacity. He will, therefore, greatly benefit from the implementation of an additional airway clearance technique, such as the PEP, to use independently before and during his sport engagement. His family continues to recognize the benefit of not smoking in the home in order for Jerry to avoid secondhand smoke, but they have failed to comply. This issue continues to be a focus of the team.

Procedural Interventions
Therapeutic Exercise
Aerobic Capacity/Endurance Training

Jerry is instructed to participate daily in an aerobic activity that is weight bearing in nature for a minimum of 30 minutes, as weight-bearing exercise will improve bone mineral density. He will continue to work on diaphragmatic breathing exercises to minimize accessory muscle use.

Flexibility Exercises

Jerry is given instruction on stretching exercises, including hamstring and thoracic cage stretches. An emphasis is placed on stretching his neck, shoulder girdle, and trunk muscles, which all contribute to current postural deviations seen.

Strength, Power, and Endurance Training

Of concern is his recent diagnosis of moderate osteopenia, evidenced on DEXA scans. Jerry's exercise program was modified to implement weight training to improve muscle strength while continuing to emphasize the preference of closed-chain to open-chain activities to foster ossification. Breathing exercises for respiratory muscle strengthening is also included in his program.

Examination Update: Given the concern over Jerry's bone density and his decreased exercise tolerance, higher-impact activities of shorter duration may be preferred over longer-duration, moderate-impact aerobic activities. Such activities include drop-jumping off an 8-inch step 10 to 20 times daily, or jumping rope in an interval (anaerobic) mode as tolerated. The importance of and balance between passive airway clearance techniques and active techniques, including aerobic physical activity, may be seen in a different perspective given the positive changes at the cellular and tissue levels induced by exercise adaptation in individuals with CF. In addition, strength training to not only promote muscle strength gains but also improve body mass would be emphasized as these have been shown to be correlated with slower disease progression. Jerry's pharmacological regime would most likely now include more gene therapy–based medications. Finally, Jerry may also be considered a candidate for a partial or full lung or heart-lung transplant.

Discussion

The most important goal when treating a child with CF is to achieve early independent airway clearance strategies. The specific intervention strategies that the therapist and child elect to use are dependent on the age of the child, the caregivers' training, and the manifestation of the disease process. Jerry originally presented at 2 months of age with emesis, voracious appetite, pancreatic dysfunction, and failure to thrive. Deficits that emerged later in his life included osteopenia, asthma, a decline in his ventilatory capacity, and the persistence of failure to thrive, which required the placement of a gastrostomy tube for night feedings.

Because the lungs of an infant with CF are normal at birth, lung pathology will not present until later. Jerry was, in fact, diagnosed with CF secondary to failure to thrive. His therapist performed a developmental evaluation to ensure that he was achieving his developmental milestones despite poor nutritional metabolism and episodes of emesis with feedings. If, at that point, a developmental delay were identified, then an early intervention referral would have been made. The primary goals at 2 months of age are ensuring the family's

independence with PDPV and the monitoring of the child's ability to meet developmental milestones.

After Jerry's initial diagnosis, he was followed in the cystic fibrosis clinic regularly through adolescence. The airway clearance techniques were progressed to include percussion of additional lung fields and vibration. By the age of 8 years, he was instructed in an alternative airway clearance technique to PDPV. He should have performed at least one of the three required daily airway clearance sessions independently. This could have been with the handheld mechanical percussor or an HFCWO. In addition, by 8 years of age Jerry should be able to demonstrate the ability to supplement the primary airway clearance technique of PDPV, with the use of the PEP or Flutter device. The PEP and Flutter devices are easily transportable and would enable him to clear his airway immediately before or during his sport activity or gym class. In addition, the PEP or Flutter would give him the opportunity to increase the number of airway clearance sessions he could have in a day independently, if the necessity arose.

At 16 years of age, Jerry's DEXA scan reveals a significant decrease in bone mineralization. He would greatly benefit from the promotion of both a rigorous strength-training program as well as closed-chain exercises to enhance bone density. A 16-year-old should also be able to monitor his cardiovascular status during exercise, through the use of the Borg perceived exertion scale (Borg, 1982), and to measure his vital signs in order to achieve and maintain an optimal aerobic workout.

The intervention strategies used upon entering young adulthood do not vary significantly from those mandated in adolescence. It will be important to ensure that he adheres to his chosen airway clearance techniques and that he is continually exposed to other airway clearance strategies as his lifestyle and needs change.

Examination Update: The scientific evidence continues to build with regards to airway clearance techniques, pharmacological interventions, and exercise testing and interventions in individuals with CF. Recent evidence has improved our understanding that impairments in activity tolerance and muscle strength may have a basis in specific muscle metabolic defects in addition to the more commonly appreciated pulmonary system impairments. In particular, we have learned that the CFTR genetic mutation can impact the regulation of adenosine triphosphatases in the sarcoplasmic reticulum that are essential to excitation-contraction coupling.

In reference to Jerry's physical therapy management, the recent literature supports earlier inclusion of more structured aerobic and strengthening activity in his physical therapy management—perhaps warranting as much emphasis as do more standard airway clearance techniques and pulmonary hygiene. In particular, strength training, high-intensity interval training, and the inclusion of short-duration high-impact activities to promote improved body composition would be of great value. The capability to provide improved ambulatory monitoring and pharmacological interventions in the home setting has become more common and may improve preventative care and health maintenance in individuals with CF. Recent evidence is highlighted in the recommended readings.

Acknowledgments

The author wishes to express appreciation to the authors of the first edition of this chapter: Heather Lever Brossman, MS, DPT, CCS, and Coleen Schrepfer, PT, MD.

DISCUSSION QUESTIONS

1. What do Jerry's vital signs during his exercise test tell you about his aerobic capacity?

2. What does a muscle strength grade of 3/5 tell you about a 2-month-old?

3. How would you work on the strength of a 2-month-old?

4. What are the purposes of the various medications taken by a child with CF?

5. For what purpose is an HFCWO prescribed? When would you order one?

6. How would you convince this family to provide a smoke-free environment for Jerry?

7. In a chronic disease such as CF, what are potential barriers to the child participating in his or her own care?

8. What is the role of exercise, aerobic and strengthening, in the health management of a child with CF? How can physical therapy influence activity preferences?

9. What patient-reported health outcomes are available and appropriate to use in an 8-year-old, 16-year-old, or young adult with CF? How would the information from such standardized assessments influence physical therapy management?

10. The pharmacological management of CF has evolved to more routinely include drugs based on genetic therapeutic principles. How does this influence Jerry's medical care?

Recommended Readings

Brannon, F.J., Foley, M.W., Starr, J.A., & Saul, L.M. (1998). *Cardiopulmonary rehabilitation: Basic theory and application* (3rd ed.). Philadelphia: F.A. Davis.

Cystic Fibrosis Foundation, available at http://www.cff.org

de Jong, W., van Aalderen, W.M., Kraan, J., Koeter, G.H., & van der Schans, C.P. (2001). Inspiratory muscle training in patients with cystic fibrosis. *Respiratory Medicine, 95*(1), 31–66.

Dwyer, T.J., Alison, J.A., McKeough, Z.J., Daviskas, E., & Bye, P.T. (2011). Effects of exercise on respiratory flow and sputum properties in cystic fibrosis. *Chest, 139*(4), 870–877.

Gondor, M., Nixon, P., Mutich, R., Rebovich, P., & Orenstein, D. (1999). Comparison of flutter device and chest physical therapy in the treatment of cystic fibrosis during pulmonary exacerbation. *Pediatric Pulmonology, 28*, 255–260.

Flume, P.A., Robinson, K.A., O'Sullivan, B.P., Finder, J.D., Vender, R.L., Willey-Courand, D.B., White, T.B., & Marshall, B.C. (2009). Clinical Practice Guidelines for Pulmonary Therapies Committee. Cystic fibrosis pulmonary guidelines: Airway clearance therapies. *Respiratory Care, 54*(4), 522–537.

Hommerding, P.X., Donadio, M.V., Paim, T.F., & Marostica, P.J. (2010). The Borg scale is accurate in children and adolescents older than 9 years with cystic fibrosis. *Respiratory Care, 55*(6), 729–733.

Hulzebos, H.J., Snieder, H., van der Et, J., Helders, P.J., & Takken, T. (2011). High-intensity interval training in an adolescent with cystic fibrosis: A physiological perspective. *Physiotherapy Theory and Practice, 27*(3), 231–237.

Lamhonwah, A.M., Bear, C.E., Huan, L.J., Kim Chiaw, P., Ackerley, C.A., & Tein, I. (2010). Cystic fibrosis transmembrane conductance regulator in human muscle: Dysfunction causes abnormal metabolic recovery in exercise. *Annals of Neurology, 67*(6), 802–808.

Nixon, P. (2003). Cystic fibrosis. In J.L. Durstine & G.E. Moore (Eds.), *ACSM's exercise management for persons with chronic diseases and disabilities* (pp. 111–116). Champaign, IL: Human Kinetics.

Radtke, T., Stevens, D., Benden, C., & Williams, CA. (2009). Clinical exercise testing in children and adolescents with cystic fibrosis. *Pediatric Physical Therapy, 21*(3), 275–281.

van Doorn, N. (2010). Exercise programs for children with cystic fibrosis: A systematic review of randomized controlled trials. *Disability and Rehabilitation, 32*(1), 41–49.

Wilkes, D.L., Schneiderman, J.E., Nguyen, T., Heale, L., Moola, F., Ratjen, F., Coates, A.L., &Wells, G.D. (2009). Exercise and physical activity in children with cystic fibrosis. *Paediatric Respiratory Review, 10*(3), 105–109.

Williams, C.A., Benden, C., Stevens, D., & Radtke, T. (2010). Exercise training in children and adolescents with cystic fibrosis: Theory into practice. *International Journal of Pediatrics*, pii: 670640.

Ziegler, B., Rovedder, P.M., Oliveira, C.L., de Abreu e Silva, F., & de Tarso Roth Dalcin, P. (2010). Repeatability of the 6-minute walk test in adolescents and adults with cystic fibrosis. *Respiratory Care, 55*(8),1020–1025.

References

American College of Sports Medicine (1991). *Guidelines for exercise testing and prescription* (4th ed.). Philadelphia: Lea & Febiger.

American Physical Therapy Association (APTA). (2001). Guide to physical therapist practice (2nd ed.). *Physical Therapy, 81*, 6–746.

Borg, G.V. (1982). Psychophysical basis of perceived exertion. *Medicine and Science in Sports and Exercise, 14*, 377.

Children's Liver Association for Support Services (2011). Pediatric Lab Values. Retrieved from http://www.classkids.org/library/ref/liverlabs.htm

Folio, M.R., & Fewell, R.R. (2000). *Peabody Developmental Motor Scales* (2nd ed.). Austin, TX: Pro-Ed.

Yankaskas, J.R., & Knowles, M.R. (1999). *Cystic fibrosis in adults*. Philadelphia: Lippincott-Raven.

CHAPTER 21

Case Study

Down Syndrome

—Alyssa LaForme Fiss, PT, PhD, PCS

—Susan K. Effgen, PT, PhD, FAPTA

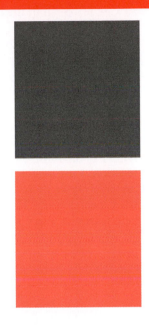

This case study focuses on the ongoing physical therapy management of Carrie, a child with Down syndrome. Carrie has received physical therapy services from the age of 4 weeks to the present. For individuals with Down syndrome, episodes of physical therapy services may be necessary across the life span to address changing issues as growth occurs and as the child gains increasing independence in various environments. Functional demands change as the individual moves from infancy, through the school years, and into adulthood.

Individuals with Down syndrome commonly present with impairments in strength (Stemmons-Mercer & Lewis, 2001), range of motion (ROM) (Zausmer & Shea, 1984), tone (Shea, 1991), balance and coordination (Connolly & Michael, 1986; Lauteslanger, Vermeer, & Helders, 1998), and sensory processing (Uyanik, Bumin, & Kayihan, 2003) leading to delays in acquisition of motor skills and to functional limitations. Associated impairments, such as mental retardation (Hayes & Batshaw, 1993; Henderson, Morris, & Ray, 1981), cardiovascular pathology (Freeman et al., 1998), and frequent middle ear infections, may also have a negative impact on motor skill acquisition and activities.

The impairments of body structure and function and limitations in activities and participation presented by Carrie led the health-care team to consider the physical therapy management options described in Preferred Practice Patterns 5B: Impaired Neuromotor Development and 4C: Impaired Muscle Performance as outlined in the American Physical Therapy Association (APTA)'s *Guide to physical therapist practice* (APTA, 2001). Ultimately, Pattern 5B: Impaired Neuromotor Development was selected because of Carrie's delayed motor skill development, impaired cognition, and sensory integration impairments. This case study will focus on episodes of care at 3 years and 16 years of age, with a brief review of Carrie's transition into adulthood. Physical therapy services at ages 3 and 16 were provided by therapists working in educational settings in accordance with the federal legislation Individuals with Disabilities Education Act (IDEA) (2004).

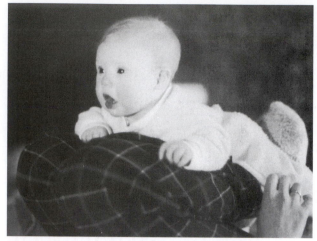

Figure 21.2 Prone position on mother's legs.

Examination: Age 3 Years

History

At Carrie's birth in the late 1970s, doctors were suspicious of a potential diagnosis of Down syndrome. She presented with soft signs, including slanted eyes, poor sucking reflex, and hypotonia (Fig. 21.1). When Carrie was 2 days old, she was transferred from her local rural hospital to a major urban hospital for genetic testing. At this time, a diagnosis of Down syndrome was confirmed. Her parents, Tim and Peggy, were both 35 years old and had three other children: Wendy, 12 years; Jamie, 9 years; and Thea, 4 years. Tim and Peggy's initial reactions were love for Carrie, fear of the unknown, and uncertainty of their capabilities as parents of a child with special needs. However, they were determined to help Carrie in every way they could.

When Carrie was 4 weeks old, her family began the process of early intervention (EI) to help them foster Carrie's development. The EI services team included an educator, a speech therapist, and a physical therapist. Carrie received weekly home visits from a physical therapist to assist the family with facilitating her gross motor development. During this period of Carrie's development, the physical therapist gave the family different activities to work on with Carrie, including spending time in the prone position, maintaining her sitting balance while playing with toys, transitioning through various positions, and propelling a ride-on toy (Figs. 21.2 through 21.4).

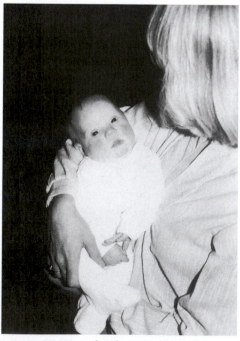

Figure 21.1 Carrie at birth.

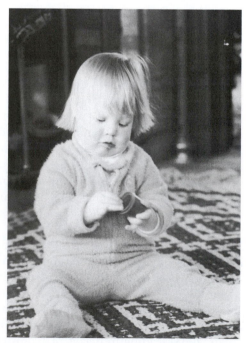

Figure 21.3 Maintaining sitting position during play.

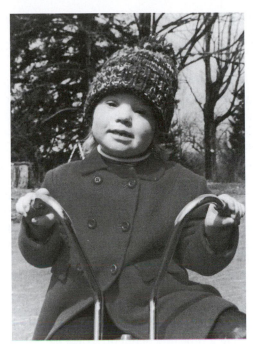

Figure 21.4 Propelling a ride-on toy.

Table 21.1 Age at Which Carrie Achieved Gross Motor Milestones

Gross Motor Milestones	Age Achieved (mo.)
Lift head to 90° in prone prop	4.5
Roll from stomach to back	5
Roll from back to stomach	6
Pivot in prone	9
Sit with arms propped for support	9
Sit unsupported	10
Belly crawling	11
Transition from prone to quadruped	12
Pull to stand from sitting	13
Creep on hands and knees	14
Transition from prone to sitting	15
Transition from supine to sitting	15
Cruise	15
Stand independently for 10 seconds	17
Walk 10 feet with two-hand support	17
Walk 20 feet with a push toy	18
Walk five steps without support	20
Creep up stairs independently	22
Independent household ambulation	24
Crawl down stairs independently	25
Walk up stairs with two-hand support	28
Walk down stairs with two-hand support	29

At 2 years of age, Carrie had open-heart surgery to repair a persistent patent ductus arteriosus that never closed on its own when she was an infant. Before the surgery, Carrie was continuously sick. She had frequent ear infections, scarlet fever (twice), and pneumonia. These illnesses hindered her progress in the areas of speech, cognition, fine motor, and gross motor development. After the surgery, Peggy and Tim noticed a significant improvement in Carrie's health. She recovered well from her heart surgery. The ages at which Carrie achieved her gross motor milestones from birth to 29 months are listed in Table 21.1. These milestones are consistent with the typical gross motor skill acquisition milestones for children with Down syndrome as outlined by the motor growth curves created by Palisano and colleagues (2001). According to these growth curves, children with Down syndrome are typically able to roll by 6 months, sit by 12 months, crawl by 18 months, and walk by 24 months (Palisano et al., 2001). Because of the recurrent ear infections, Carrie had tympanostomy tubes put in her ears when she was 30 months old. No known hearing loss is evident at this time.

Carrie is presently attending her mother's preschool 1 day per week. She also attends Sunday school at church, where she is with typically developing peers. After Carrie chooses her own toy, she occasionally plays near the other children at preschool and with her siblings at home. She engages in pretend play at home and at school.

Carrie will turn 3 years old in a few weeks, and she will transfer out of her EI program and into her local school district program. Peggy and Tim want to make sure that they maintain a high level of participation in Carrie's therapy sessions and in the design of her Individualized Educational Plan (IEP). They are concerned about Carrie's continued development in all areas. Although she has recovered well from her surgery a year ago, they are still concerned about her health and how it affects her development. Peggy and Tim would like to see Carrie integrated into all areas of their local community, as their other children have been, to the level that Carrie can effectively sustain participation. Their major gross motor concern is related to Carrie's limited ability to participate independently in the community, specifically with endurance, ambulation on uneven surfaces, playground independence, and stair negotiation.

Systems Review

Cardiovascular and Pulmonary

Carrie's cardiovascular and pulmonary systems appear to be functioning within normal limits with a pulse of 76 beats per minute (bpm), blood pressure (BP) of 90/60 mm Hg, and respiratory rate (RR) of 19 breaths per minute. (All measurements were taken at rest.)

Integumentary

A well-healed scar from the open-heart surgery is noted between ribs 6 and 7, beginning at the anterior portion of the left upper chest and following along the ribs to the posterior portion of the left upper chest. It measures 7 inches long and 0.25 inch wide.

Musculoskeletal

Height and weight are within the 40th percentile for her age. Joint hypermobility and generalized weakness with hypotonia are noted.

Neuromuscular

Impaired balance and coordination are noted, and development of functional motor skills is delayed.

Cognition

Carrie is typically alert and aware of her surroundings. She manipulates toys to explore their novel features and demonstrates an attention span of at least 15 minutes when playing with one of her favorite toys, especially with anything musical. Carrie demonstrates keen observation skills that allow her to deduce the location of a hidden object and to anticipate the path of a rolling ball.

Carrie's family and therapists have noticed that Carrie is a visual learner. They use pictures to label objects to assist Carrie in learning new words and skills (e.g., brushing teeth, eating, and putting on socks).

Carrie's receptive language appears age appropriate, but she has a delay with expressive language and has articulation problems. She uses sign language along with verbal expression to communicate her wants and needs with two-word sentences.

Tests and Measures

Aerobic Capacity and Endurance

Carrie demonstrates enough endurance to walk for at least 300 feet at a time and to "run" stiffly for 50 feet. This is a significant improvement occurring after her recovery from open-heart surgery. Before surgery she was limited to walking 50 feet because of fatigue, shortness of breath, and generalized muscle weakness.

Gait, Locomotion, and Balance

In standing position, Carrie exhibits a wide base of support, hip external rotation, and flat feet. She ambulates with a heel strike followed by a foot slap because of poor eccentric control of her dorsiflexors. She has a wide base of support and holds her arms at her sides. She attempts to "run" stiffly when playing with her siblings and peers. She negotiates up and down stairs with two hands on the railing and placing both feet on each step. Carrie demonstrates delayed equilibrium reactions in sitting and in standing. She demonstrates protective reactions forward and to the sides in sitting and standing. This skill is emerging to the rear. Carrie leads with one foot and needs both hands for support when attempting to jump in place. She balances on one foot for 3 seconds with both hands held. Carrie propels a ride-on toy up to 5 feet at a time independently, on a flat surface.

Motor Function (Motor Control and Motor Learning)

Carrie's resting sitting posture is ring sitting with external hip rotation, flexed spine, and a forward head (Fig. 21.5). She can ambulate and climb stairs, as noted

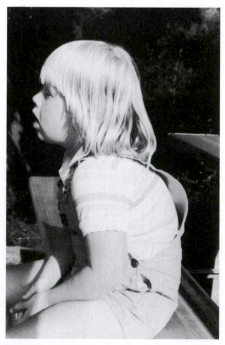

Figure 21.5 Resting posture in sitting.

previously. She has mastered simple fine motor activities, including using a pincer grasp for small objects, manipulating push/pull levers, and completing a four-piece shape puzzle.

Carrie has difficulty developing motor plans for novel, multistep tasks. She needs to have the tasks broken down into steps. After a demonstration of each of the steps, she can put them together once she has mastered the individual steps. Carrie still has difficulty grading the amount of force she needs when performing fine motor and gross motor tasks.

Muscle Performance

Carrie has low muscle tone throughout her body. This low tone is more prevalent proximally compared with distally. Although she demonstrates enough strength to move her upper and lower extremities through full ROM against gravity, she has poor midrange control. She has difficulty extending her neck and back musculature against gravity for long periods of time (e.g., sitting during circle time). She is unable to sit straight up from a supine position, indicating weak abdominal muscles. This functional, general assessment of muscle strength was chosen for Carrie's evaluation because other more standardized methods are difficult to use reliably with children as young as 3 years of age and with children who have cognitive impairments (Westcott, Lowes, & Richardson, 1997).

Carrie's decreased muscle strength and limited midrange motor control limit her abilities to keep up with her peers during gross motor play, including running, climbing on playground equipment, negotiating stairs independently, and propelling a riding toy. In addition to the decreased muscle strength and motor control issues, Carrie's muscle endurance is limited. Her mother reports that Carrie will often sit down after about 15 minutes of gross motor play and remain seated for up to 10 minutes at a time until she returns to activities with her peers.

Neuromotor Development and Sensory Integration

Carrie's equilibrium is good when she is able to anticipate her environment (e.g., negotiating up a grassy knoll that she is practicing on). However, when surrounded by peers, which alters her ability to predict her environment (e.g., traversing the same grassy knoll with her friends and getting bumped), she will lose her balance 50% of the time.

Carrie seeks out light touch by lightly rubbing her fingers on her palms and forearms, suggesting that this

sense is diminished. She demonstrates limitations in activities and participation by getting distracted by her need to provide this sensory feedback for herself. Her mother notes that Carrie's occupational therapist gave them light-touch activities to do before Carrie needs to concentrate on activities.

Carrie has difficulty articulating her sounds when attempting to produce words. It is hard for her to produce the consonant sounds /k/, /t/, /g/, /l/, /tr/, /d/, and /s/. She uses one- to two-word sentences to convey her wants and needs. When she is unable to articulate, she uses Signed English to help others understand her. She knows approximately 90 Signed English words.

Range of Motion

Carrie presents with joint hypermobility, especially proximally, throughout all of her joints. Specific goniometric measurements for these joints are listed in Table 21.2. Because of the concern of atlantoaxial instability in individuals with Down syndrome (see Chapter 6, Fig. 6.20, for a discussion relative to this topic), Carrie had radiographs taken of her atlantoaxial joint, and the results were negative for hypermobility.

Self-Care and Home Management (Including Activities of Daily Living and Instrumental Activities of Daily Living)

Carrie drinks from a cup without assistance and takes a few sips through a straw. She uses a spoon independently with some spilling. She demonstrates a pincer grasp to pick up small objects (e.g., raisins) and uses a palmar grasp with a spoon. She uses the same palmar grasp with crayons to make vertical and circular scribbles on either a flat surface or an easel.

Examination Update: A standardized assessment of function was not completed during Carrie's

Table 21.2 Goniometry Measurements

Joint motion	Right	Left
Hip flexion	0–136°	0–138°
Hip extension	0–10°	0–8°
Hip external rotation	0–80°	0–86°
Shoulder flexion	0–200°	0–202°
Shoulder extension	0–66°	0–64°
Shoulder external rotation	0–114°	0–110°

examination at age 3 years. Today, measurement instruments are readily available to test the functional mobility and self-help skills of children:

- Carolina Curriculum for Infants and Toddlers with Special Needs (2nd ed.) (Johnson-Martin, Jens, Attermeier, & Hacker, 1991)
- Functional Independence Measure for Children (WeeFIM) (Granger et al., 1991)
- Gross Motor Function Measure (GMFM) (Russell, Rosenbaum, Avery, & Lane, 2002)
- Pediatric Evaluation of Disability Inventory (PEDI) (Haley, Coster, Ludlow, Haltiwanger, & Andrellos, 1992)

See Chapter 3 for a more complete listing of measurement tools.

Work, Community, and Leisure Integration

Carrie enjoys playing with other children at school, on the playground, and at home. She does her best at keeping up but struggles to do so. At school she needs assistance negotiating the stairs to get in and out of her school, climbing onto various gross motor climbing structures in the gym, and propelling ride-on toys. When on the playground, Carrie falls 50% of the time while transitioning from one surface to another (e.g., pavement, sand, and grass). Because her home environment is more familiar to her, she falls there only 30% of the time. This trend suggests that Carrie needs repetition to help her generalize gross motor skills to new environments.

Examination Update: Although unavailable at the time of Carrie's 3-year examination, participation level assessments are now available to help define a child's abilities in this area:

- Miller Function and Participation Scale (M-FUN) (Miller, 2006)
- Pediatric Quality of Life Inventory (PedsQL) (Varni, Seid, & Rode, 1999)
- Children's Assessment of Participation and Enjoyment (CAPE) (King et al., 2005)
- Preferences for Activities of Children (PAC) (King et al., 2005)

Evaluation, Diagnosis, and Prognosis
Including Plan of Care

At age 3, Carrie presents with overall developmental delays in the following areas: gross motor, fine motor, cognition, self-help, social/emotional, and language.

Her gross motor and fine motor functional limitations lead to participation restrictions in her life role as a family member by limiting her independence.

Diagnosis

Carrie has demonstrated impairments of motor function, balance, motor planning, sensory integration, cognition, and expressive language, decreasing her functional independence and restricting her activities and participation. Specific impairments in muscle strength, low muscle tone, and increased ROM negatively affect mid-range control of the lower extremities during ambulation and limit her ability to use stairs.

Activity Limitations

Carrie's decreased muscle strength and balance are major contributing factors to her gross motor developmental delay, including delays in independent stair negotiation, ambulation on uneven surfaces, climbing onto and off of various surface levels, independent jumping skills, independent propulsion of ride-on toys, and ball skills.

Participation Limitations

Carrie's gross motor delays limit her ability to keep up with her peers during activities such as playing with peers on playground equipment, participating in gross motor gym and classroom activities, and participating with neighborhood peers in outdoor gross motor play.

Prognosis

Over the course of 12 months, Carrie will demonstrate an increased level of independent motor function at home, school, and in her community. She will also demonstrate ongoing neuromotor development of gross motor skills typical of preschoolers.

Goals/Objectives

Suggested gross motor goals (Table 21.3) are developed as a result of this evaluation. They are expected to be achieved within 1 year, with the assistance of weekly physical therapy visits. These suggested gross motor goals will be shared at Carrie's upcoming IEP team meeting for further discussion and modification by all team members (Peggy, Tim, the physical therapist, speech therapist, occupational therapist, psychologist, educator, and others). The focus and location of service delivery will change as Carrie moves from receiving EI services to school-based services.

Table 21.3 Suggested Gross Motor Goals for Carrie's IEP at Age 3 Years

Functional Independence Goals

1. Carrie will negotiate up stairs with alternating feet without support with close supervision 80% of the time.

2. Carrie will negotiate down stairs with alternating feet with one hand on the railing 80% of the time.

3. Carrie will ambulate on uneven surfaces independently without falling 80% of the time, including but not limited to:
   (a) grass
   (b) sand
   (c) gravel
   (d) sidewalk
   (e) soft surface (i.e., mattress or foam)

4. Carrie will independently climb onto and off of a variety of surface level heights without falling to increase her independence 80% of the time, including but not limited to:
   (a) chair at the kitchen table
   (b) step stool at the bathroom sink
   (c) family room furniture
   (d) toddler playground equipment

Advanced Motor Skill Goals

1. Carrie will jump off the floor with both feet together with one hand for support to play hopscotch 80% of the time.

2. Carrie will propel a riding toy 50 feet using a reciprocal pattern with her feet on the floor with close supervision 80% of the time.

3. Carrie will negotiate a playground-type ladder up and down with contact guarding 100% of the time.

Ball Skill Goals

1. Carrie will kick a playground-sized ball at least 5 feet with accuracy 80% of the time.

2. Carrie will throw a playground-sized ball at least 5 feet with accuracy 80% of the time.

Intervention

Coordination, Communication, and Documentation

Carrie will be served by an interdisciplinary team that will have monthly case conferences for all of the therapists and educators involved. In addition, Carrie's family will be able to schedule meetings when they deem it necessary.

Carrie's weekly physical therapy visits will alternate between home and preschool. The physical therapist will have direct communication with Carrie's mother, Peggy, and other caregivers present at the two settings. Written material is given to Peggy to share with caregivers not present at home visits to ensure maximum carryover. A copy of this material is placed in Carrie's file for other team members to review. An annual report will be sent to Carrie's developmental pediatrician to keep him informed of Carrie's progress and current goals.

Carrie's family is given information about the National Down Syndrome Congress (NDSC) and a local parent support group for further resources about issues related to Carrie's specific needs.

Expected outcomes of this comprehensive coordination and communication include collaboration between those at home and at school and the therapists and educators working with Carrie; supplementary information specific to children with Down syndrome (available through NDSC and the local parent support group) provided to family, therapists, and teachers; and referrals to appropriate professionals when necessary.

Patient/Client-Related Instruction

During the examination, the physical therapist found it useful to use a variety of instructional methods, including visual cues, verbal cues, and hands-on facilitation, when teaching Carrie new skills. All three methods in combination will be necessary to help Carrie gain new skills (Table 21.4).

In addition, the team will provide Carrie's family with information about the differences between EI and school-based services. (See Chapters 11 and 12 for further details regarding the federal regulations governing these services.)

Table 21.4 Example of Instructional Cues for a New Skill

New skill	Jumping off floor with two feet together
Visual cue	Demonstrate the skill
Verbal cue	"Bend your knees and jump."
Hands-on facilitation	Two-hand support at her hips to facilitate the movement

Procedural Interventions

Therapeutic Exercise

Therapeutic exercise focuses on improving aerobic capacity and endurance; balance, coordination, and agility training; neuromotor development training; and muscle strengthening. Use of task-specific activities within the intervention plan will allow for increased practice of desired skills. Table 21.5 includes therapeutic exercises for Carrie to perform in a variety of settings (shown in Fig. 21.6 and Fig. 21.7).

Expected outcomes of these therapeutic exercises include increased aerobic capacity and endurance, increased balance and coordination, increased neuromotor development, and increased strength.

Functional Training in Self-Care

A proper seating position for Carrie is determined for use during mealtimes. Fine motor activities are aimed at providing the proper support needed to allow the highest level of independent functioning. Appropriate-sized step stools will be placed in front of the bathroom sinks to allow for independence with hand washing and tooth brushing.

To help Carrie become more independent with dressing, the physical therapist instructs her family and primary caregivers on teaching her to balance on one leg. This intervention will ultimately help Carrie put on her pants and shoes and take them off while standing.

Another activity to work on with Carrie is the negotiation of stairs and curbs, both up and down, as well as getting on and off various playground equipment and toys. She currently requires assistance, making her dependent on others.

Expected outcomes of this functional training in self-care include increased independence in daily tasks and activities, increased balance and coordination, increased neuromotor development, and increased strength.

Table 21.5 Therapeutic Exercise

Aerobic Capacity/Endurance Conditioning	
Running	Run in the yard with her siblings to catch bubbles.
Swimming	Motor boat—Carrie kicks her legs while she is supported by her arms.
Building with blocks to build a fort	Move building blocks of various sizes and shapes from one corner of her classroom to the other.
Balance Coordination and Agility Training	
Ball activity	Kick ball at a target.
Sitting	Sit on a small ball (kickball-size) during circle time.
Obstacle course	Negotiate over, under, up, down, and around through various play structures (see Fig. 21.6).
Bean bag toss	Throw bean bags at designated target; have Carrie stand on a piece of foam as her aim improves to increase the challenge.
Water game	Balance while sitting on a small raft in the water.
Neuromotor Development Training	
Jumping	Jump on a small trampoline then on the floor.
Stairs	Learn an alternating feet pattern to negotiate stairs.
Climbing	Use alternating pattern between feet and hands when climbing on various structures.
Strength and Endurance Training	
Abdominal exercises	Do sit-ups (see Fig. 21.7).
Stairs	Negotiate up and down stairs with the least amount of support.
Ride-on toy	Propel ride-on toy between classrooms at school.
Walking	Walk home from school and in the grocery store instead of riding in the stroller or shopping cart.

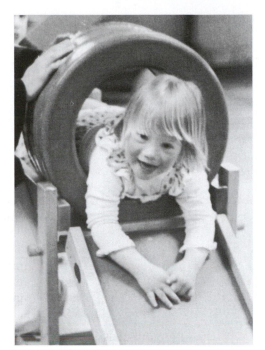

Figure 21.6 Obstacle course.

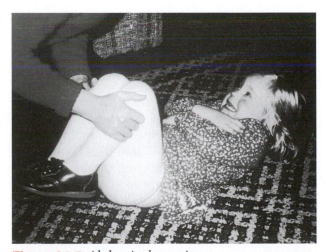

Figure 21.7 Abdominal exercises.

Termination of Episode of Care

This episode of care will be terminated when Carrie has achieved the stated goals and outcomes. Within the early childhood practice settings, goals are anticipated to be achieved in approximately 1 year. If the goals are achieved sooner, the episode of care would be terminated and a new episode of care initiated if new goals are identified by the IEP team.

It is anticipated that individuals with Down syndrome may "require multiple episodes of care over the lifetime to ensure safety and effective adaptation after changes in physical status, caregivers, environment, or task demands" (APTA, 2001, p. 334). Additional episodes of physical therapy care for Carrie will be indicated as musculoskeletal growth occurs, classroom task requirements change, teachers and caregivers change, medical or surgical issues arise, or level of impairment or physical function changes. As Carrie continues to have educationally relevant needs, as determined under IDEA, related services, including physical therapy, will be provided in the school setting. As Carrie becomes older, her physical therapy may need to be transitioned to an outpatient setting if the goals are no longer educationally based.

Examination: Age 16 Years

History

Carrie is now 16 years old. She has been relatively healthy medically over the past 13 years. She still struggles with her balance, endurance, strength, and weight control. Carrie has attended her local public elementary, junior high, and high school programs in inclusive settings each year. She is now a ninth grader in high school. At 12 years of age, Carrie's IQ was 68 and her educational classification of multiply handicapped (educable mentally retarded and speech impairment) was established. She has received speech therapy and physical therapy services as part of her educational program. Carrie is a member of the high school choir, and in the past, she participated in the elementary and junior high choirs. Carrie will participate in the annual high school musical production this year as a member of the chorus. Her family is very musical, and all of her siblings participated in these activities when they were in high school. Carrie is proud to participate in the same activities as her siblings. Her parents allow her to participate in school activities that are appropriate for her because it helps her interact socially with her peer group.

To help facilitate friendships for Carrie, last year her parents enrolled her in a weekly program for teenagers with disabilities, the Resource Center for Independent Living. This program helps Carrie develop self-esteem, self-advocacy, friendships with others with all types of mental and physical disabilities, and awareness of other disabilities. Interviewing skills, job shadowing, and technology training are also provided through the program. Carrie and her family are also active members of both the NDSC and their local parent-support group. Both organizations have provided information to Carrie's parents and siblings and have served as a support network for the family, especially for Carrie.

Carrie had several ear infections throughout her early childhood. She had tubes placed in both ears when she was 6 years old; however, they were not effective. Because of her numerous ear infections, her right ossicle was corroded and her right eardrum was perforated, yielding a 60% hearing loss in her right ear. There is no hearing loss in her left ear. Carrie is near-sighted and has astigmatism. She wears glasses to correct these problems.

At the age of 14 years, Carrie developed hand and then full body tremors. She also had a "seizurelike" episode with unconsciousness. She was diagnosed with Graves' disease (hyperthyroidism), which caused these symptoms. Because children with Down syndrome often have hypothyroidism (Pueschel & Bier, 1992), Carrie's condition is unusual. She initially took medication to decrease her thyroid hormone levels, but then required radioactive iodine treatments to regulate the thyroid hormone levels. She is monitored monthly by an endocrinologist.

Carrie has maintained a physically active lifestyle. She participated in community soccer programs from ages 8 to 10 years and gymnastics from the ages of 9 to 12 years. Her endurance became limited with extreme heat and humidity. In these weather conditions, she had multiple fainting episodes when she pushed herself to continue participating.

Carrie now monitors her heart rate before, during, and after any type of exercise. She has a blue belt in karate and attends karate classes twice weekly. She wants to continue with her karate classes to ultimately achieve her black belt (Fig. 21.8). She realizes that she needs to exercise and eat well-balanced meals to continue to develop her endurance, balance skills, and strength and to maintain a healthy weight. She has just started taking cardio-kickboxing, which focuses more specifically on her aerobic endurance.

Functionally, Carrie is able to care for herself independently in the areas of dressing and hygiene. She still needs assistance in making healthy choices for meals. She is also learning a variety of home management skills, such as cooking, housecleaning, and doing laundry. For the past 2 years, Carrie has participated in a county-funded program that provides a one-on-one assistant for adolescents with disabilities to learn life skills. Carrie's assistant comes to her house for 20 hours per week to help Carrie increase her independence with

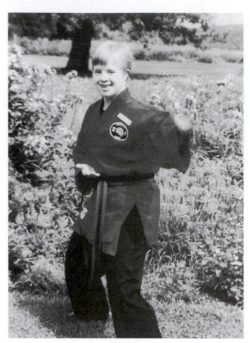

Figure 21.8 Carrie in karate uniform.

household chores. They focus on cleaning, cooking simple meals, doing laundry, keeping her checkbook updated and balanced, and using socialization skills when out in the community. Carrie's mother is especially grateful for this program because she believed that her relationship with Carrie was being strained. Peggy felt that she was always nagging Carrie to do things instead of being a source of encouragement for her.

Carrie's goal is to become a special education teacher's assistant when she graduates from high school. This goal was included in her IEP, and the school set up a special program for Carrie to participate in this school year. She tutors in the elementary school self-contained classroom 3 days per week for 45 minutes. Her responsibilities include tutoring the children in reading and math. This program helps Carrie increase her self-esteem, and it gives her great joy and confidence to help others.

Systems Review

Cardiovascular and Pulmonary

Carrie's cardiovascular and pulmonary systems appear to be functioning within normal limits, with a pulse of 64 bpm, BP of 115/65 mm Hg; and RR of 16 breaths per minute. All measurements were taken at rest. When Carrie has fainting episodes in the heat and humidity, her pulse and blood pressure usually increase.

Integumentary

Carrie's scar from her surgery is well healed and does not present any problems.

Musculoskeletal

Carrie's height and weight are within the 50th percentile for age. Joint hypermobility with hypotonia are still noted.

Neuromuscular

With high-level vestibular activities, such as riding a bicycle, Carrie is unable to balance herself. She feels dizzy, does not know where her body is in space relative to the bicycle, and then gets very anxious about the activity. Even with training wheels attached, she is still afraid of attempting to pedal because of her lack of body-in-space awareness when on the bicycle. Her family and therapists have encouraged her to try again every spring, with no improvement. To support Carrie's desire to ride a bike, her family purchased an adult-sized tricycle for her last year. The increased base of support of the tricycle (28 inches versus 12 inches with training wheels) provides enough stability for Carrie to be able to negotiate on the pavement (Fig. 21.9). She is now learning traffic safety rules for riding on the streets.

Cognition

Carrie requires repetition for learning and does so at a slower pace relative to her peers. She is included in English and science classes with her peers but needs a self-contained classroom setting for math.

Carrie stopped using Sign Language completely at 5 years of age. She now has difficulties with dysfluency and articulation. However, most people understand her as long as she concentrates on what she is saying and takes her time.

Tests and Measures

Aerobic Capacity and Endurance

Carrie's involvement in sports over the years has given her a fun and social way to work on increasing her endurance. As mentioned, she is working toward her black belt in karate. Carrie currently completes a 1-mile walk-run in 14 minutes, which is slightly higher than the average for her age of 10:30 minutes (Ross, Dotson, Gilbert, & Katz, 1985). One of the criteria for achieving her black belt is to complete a 9-minute mile.

Arousal, Attention, and Cognition

Carrie's reported IQ is 68. She is motivated to do her best in school and in her athletic endeavors. Following multistep auditory directions is difficult for Carrie. She can complete the first step but often needs to ask for the latter steps to be repeated.

Circulation

Carrie monitors her pulse during exercise. She understands the need to vary the intensity of her workout to maintain her target heart rate between 65% and 80% (33 and 41 beats per 15 seconds, respectively).

She was also trained to use the Original Borg Scale (Borg, 1982) to track her perceived exertion during her exercise routines. The following are average scores for Carrie over the past year:

- Karate class: Sparring = 15
- Karate class: Kata Demonstrations = 9
- Cardio-kickboxing = 14
- Running = 16
- Weight training = 12

Gait, Locomotion, and Balance

Carrie's equilibrium is good for most basic activities requiring balance. She is able to maintain her balance during walking, running, and karate; however, intricate balancing activities are difficult for Carrie. Her current gait is characterized with excessive foot pronation during the stance phase when walking without shoes. When Carrie ambulates with inframalleolar orthotics in her shoes, the pronation is significantly reduced. A forward head, rounded shoulders, and a pronounced kyphotic spinal column characterize Carrie's upper body positioning during ambulation and other activities.

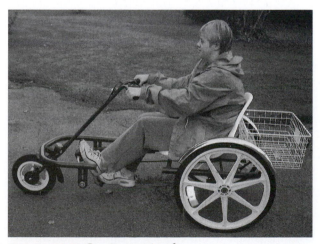

Figure 21.9 Carrie on tricycle.

Motor Function (Motor Control and Motor Learning)

Carrie is able to demonstrate muscle control throughout her body through extensive strength and coordination training in her karate classes. Carrie continues to be a visual learner. She masters skills with some type of visual representation coupled with repetition.

Muscle Performance

Carrie's overall muscle strength has improved. She can move against gravity with her whole body. Muscle strength examination with a handheld dynamometer is valid and reliable for use in individuals with Down syndrome (Stemmons-Mercer & Lewis, 2001). Muscle strength for large muscle groups was evaluated with a handheld dynamometer and was as follows:

- Hip extension = 30 lb (133.4 N)
- Hip flexion = 28 lb (124.6 N)
- Hip abduction = 43 lb (191.3 N)
- Hip adduction = 28 lb (124.6 N)
- Knee extension = 56 lb (249.1 N)
- Knee flexion = 45 lb (200.2 N)
- Ankle dorsiflexion = 17 lb (75.6 N)
- Ankle plantarflexion = 23 lb (102.3 N)
- Shoulder flexion = 32 lb (142.3 N)
- Shoulder extension = 25 lb (111.2 N)
- Elbow flexion = 27 lb (120.1 N)
- Elbow extension = 24 lb (106.8 N)
- Wrist flexion = 16 lb (71.2 N)
- Wrist extension = 12 lb (53.4 N)

Carrie's muscle endurance has also improved. She is able to participate in karate class for 1 hour without breaks. Three years ago, she needed to sit and rest 30 minutes into the class. Her 14-minute mile is also an improvement from her 17-minute mile 3 years ago. She walks 3 miles home from school with ease.

Range of Motion

Carrie still presents with hypermobility in her shoulders, but it does not affect her functionally.

Self-Care and Home Management

Carrie is independent with dressing and hygiene. She can cook independently in the microwave but needs supervision when using the stove.

Examination Update: Few assessment tools were available to measure self-care when Carrie was 16. Measurement instruments available today to test self-help skills include the Canadian Occupational Performance Measure (COPM) (Law et al., 1998) and Functional Independence Measure (FIM) (Smith, Hamilton & Granger, 1990).

Work, Community, and Leisure Integration

Carrie would like to achieve independent community mobility, including driving. She had difficulty learning to ride a two-wheel bike because of decreased balance and anxiousness about the task. She has an adult-sized tricycle that she rides in the driveway and is learning to ride in the street.

Carrie is aware of basic dangers to the children she tutors. She knows to keep sharp objects away from the children, to use proper body mechanics when assisting with transfers, and never to leave the children unattended.

Examination Update: Tools to assess participation and quality of life during a client's adolescent years that weren't available during Carrie's examination at age 16 include the Children's Assessment of Participation and Enjoyment (CAPE) (King, et al., 2005), Preferences for Activities of Children (PAC) (King, et al., 2005), and the Youth Quality of Life Instrument—Research Version (YQOL-R) (Patrick, Edwards, & Topolski, 2002).

Evaluation, Diagnosis, and Prognosis
Including Plan of Care

Carrie remains partially dependent on her family, friends, and one-on-one assistant to participate in the community. She still has difficulties in the areas of gross motor, speech, cognition, and self-help. She will continue to receive physical therapy in school because she has educationally relevant needs; however, she will also be seen in an outpatient setting to address goals that are not related to her educational needs.

Diagnosis

Carrie demonstrates impairments of motor planning attributable to her need for repetitious verbal and visual cues for multistep tasks. Muscle weakness, decreased balance, and decreased endurance make it difficult for her to complete the 9-minute mile required for karate or to ride a bike.

Prognosis

Over the course of this episode of care, it is anticipated that Carrie will demonstrate improved motor planning, balance, strength, and endurance, allowing her to achieve increased levels of independence in work, community, and leisure activities. At Carrie's present age, it is important to strive for maximal independence as she begins to transition from school to work environments.

Goals/Objectives

Carrie will receive outpatient physical therapy consultation once per month in a variety of settings (i.e., home, school, recreation/gym facilities) to assist in achieving Goals 1 to 3 listed in Table 21.6. She will also receive monthly physical therapy consultation at school to focus on Goal 4.

Intervention

Coordination, Communication, and Documentation

Services are coordinated among home, school, and community recreation settings. Consultation services are provided in all settings to ensure that appropriate supervision can be given and that Carrie safely participates in activities. Direct communication with Carrie, her respective trainers, and school personnel is given at each site. Written material is given to Carrie to share with her parents at each monthly visit.

Expected outcomes of this comprehensive coordination and communication include collaboration between Carrie, home, school, and the physical therapist, and referrals to appropriate professionals when necessary.

Patient/Client-Related Instruction

Carrie and her family are already discussing her transition from high school, which is anticipated in 4 years. She would like to get a certificate at the local community college to be a teacher's assistant for preschoolers with special needs. She needs to remain healthy and physically fit in order to interact easily with preschoolers.

With Carrie's learning style, visual aids should be used when teaching her new tasks and reviewing learned skills. Expected outcomes of this patient/client-related instruction include a plan to help Carrie meet her transitioning goals and increased ability to learn new skills and tasks.

Procedural Interventions

Therapeutic Exercise

Carrie attends karate class two to three times per week. She works on increasing balance, endurance, strength, and coordination during her Kata routines, a series of choreographed movements that work on these areas. Sparring (staged offensive and defensive maneuvers) also helps Carrie to develop these skills. Six months ago, Carrie inquired about adding cardio-kickboxing to her regimen to get more endurance training.

Carrie also completes a strength-training circuit on machines that use concentric, eccentric, and isometric muscle contractions for her arms, legs, abdominals, and back muscles. She focuses on her weaker muscle groups: triceps, rhomboids, trapezius, latissimus dorsi, deltoid, pectoralis major, rectus abdominis, gluteus maximus, hip adductors, and tibialis anterior. Carrie's trainer at the gym immediately relays any changes in weight, repetitions, or sets of this routine to the physical therapist.

Expected outcomes of these therapeutic exercises are increased balance and coordination, increased neuromotor development, increased strength, increased endurance, and maintenance of health and physical condition.

Functional Training in Work, Community, and Leisure Integration

Transfer techniques are reviewed with Carrie monthly so that she can assist with transfers in the preschool classroom. Body mechanics, specific scenarios, and emergency procedures are demonstrated to Carrie. She is then required to repeat the specific steps from memory.

Carrie loves water sports. It is recommended that she alternate between cardio-kickboxing and water aerobics for variety.

Expected outcomes of functional training in work, community, and leisure integration are that Carrie will maintain safety standards during transfers at a preschool work setting and vary endurance and strength-training activities to keep interest level high.

Table 21.6 Physical Therapy Goals for Carrie at Age 16 Years

Functional Independence Goals

1. Carrie will increase her aerobic endurance in order to run a 9-minute mile, a requirement for her karate classes.

2. Carrie will increase her balance to ride a bicycle independently on the road, following traffic rules.

3. Carrie will maintain high-level balance skills by completing the appropriate Kata (choreographed routine) for each karate level.

4. Carrie will maintain safety standards during student transfers in the classroom.

Termination of Episode of Care

Carrie will be discharged from outpatient physical therapy when she functions within her home, school, and community in an independent and safe manner, meeting all of her goals. Other situations that may change Carrie's physical therapy episode of care are a change in the status of her Graves' disease, medical complications, a decision by Carrie or her caregiver to terminate services, or Carrie no longer benefitting from the services.

Carrie and her family, along with her medical professionals, will review annually the need for outpatient physical therapy. As Carrie becomes older, her weight and physical endurance will continue to be struggles for her. The physical therapist's role is to help Carrie with prevention activities and continue her exercise programs in a safe manner to address these areas of need.

Carrie has an established diagnosis of Down syndrome and has the right to receive educationally based services from her local school district until the age of 21 years, as long as she has difficulty functioning independently within the education setting.

Adulthood and Associated Transition Considerations

As a young adult, Carrie has worked hard to create an independent and productive lifestyle. She has become an advocate for individuals with Down syndrome and speaks at many national meetings, area schools, and colleges about living with Down syndrome. Carrie earned a certificate as a teacher's assistant from a community college and previously worked as a volunteer aide in a daycare classroom. Recently, her volunteering position has changed to a paid substitute teacher's aide position. Carrie loves her teaching position and was nominated by the family of one of her students for the 2008 Accent on Excellence Award. She was one of the recipients of the award among fellow recipients that are at various executive levels of companies in the area. Carrie has also continued her active lifestyle and has completed her black belt in karate.

Carrie has married a young man with Down syndrome whom she met through the NDSC. They live together independently in an apartment with support from family and community resources. They also have Support Staff five days a week to assist them with life skills (i.e., grocery shopping, cleaning, laundry, etc.) as part of their state Individualized Initiatives Program (Self-Determination). Carrie hopes that sharing her story with others will encourage individuals with

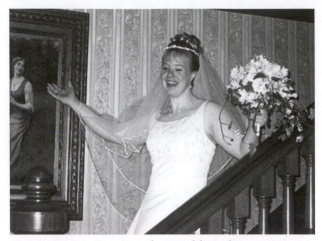

Figure 21.10 Carrie on her wedding day.

Down syndrome to advocate for their needs and dreams for the future.

Although resources for employment and supported living have greatly increased over the past few decades, making independence more attainable for individuals with Down syndrome, the transition to adulthood poses new challenges.

Age-Related Changes

Maintaining a healthy, active lifestyle is important for young adults with Down syndrome who are at an increased risk for numerous age-related changes. For example, adults with Down syndrome have an increased risk of developing hyperthyroidism and hypothyroidism, with up to 40% of all people with Down syndrome developing hypothyroidism by adulthood (Finesilver, 2002; Smith, 2001). Symptoms of hypothyroidism may include low energy level, weight gain, constipation, bradycardia, and dry skin (Finesilver, 2002).

Possible cardiovascular changes for adults with Down syndrome include mitral valve prolapse (Smith, 2001) and low cardiovascular capacity (Pitetti et al., 1992). These changes can lead to increased risk of heart failure, heart disease, and cerebrovascular accident (Finesilver, 2002).

Studies have also found increased rates of obesity in adults with Down syndrome, with 79% of males and 69% of females noted as overweight or obese in one study (Prasher, 1995). Prasher hypothesized potential reasons for this higher obesity rate, including poor dietary habits (Jackson & Thorbecke, 1982), depressed metabolic rate (Chad, Jobling, & Frail, 1990), reduced exercise (Sharav & Bowman, 1992), hypotonia, and hypothyroidism (Finesilver, 2002). Higher rates of obesity may also contribute to an increased risk of diabetes in adults with Down syndrome (Anwar, Walker, Frier, 1998).

Musculoskeletal changes may be noted at an earlier age for individuals with Down syndrome as compared with the general population (Finesilver, 2002). These changes may include arthritis (Barnhardt & Connolly, 2007; Finesilver, 2002), hip dysplasia (Finesilver, 2002), and osteoporosis (Center, Beange, & McElduff, 1998), and place individuals with Down syndrome at a higher risk for bone fractures than the general population.

High rates of Alzheimer's disease and dementia are also noted in adults with Down syndrome, with rates of these diseases increasing with age. As many as 75% of adults with Down syndrome between 60 and 65 years of age have Alzheimer's disease (Shamas-Ud-Din, 2002). Symptoms of dementia and Alzheimer's disease observed in adults with Down syndrome may include memory loss, weight loss, decreased adaptive skills, personality changes, and loss of conversation skills (Barnhardt & Connolly, 2007).

Other age-related changes may include sensory impairments such as conductive hearing loss and vision impairments (Barnhardt & Connolly, 2007; Finesilver, 2002). These sensory impairments have been reported at rates of 70% in adults with Down syndrome (Finesilver, 2002; Kapell et al., 1998).

Rates of depression are higher in individuals with Down syndrome than in the general population (McGuire & Chicoine, 1996). Carrie reports that she still feels lonely and isolated from her peers who do not have disabilities. Carrie attempts to stay involved with her family and community to combat feelings of loneliness and isolation.

Intervention

Exercise is advocated for individuals with Down syndrome to improve physical fitness and to decrease the impact of many of the age-related changes affecting this population (Barnhardt & Connolly, 2007), but additional research is needed in this area. Participation in exercise programs for individuals with Down syndrome was found to be related to caregivers' perceptions of exercise outcomes and access barriers to exercise (Heller, Hsieh, Rimmer, 2002). Carrie, however, continues to be active, as evidenced by her black belt in karate.

One role of the physical therapist working with individuals with Down syndrome in the transition to adulthood is to improve access to and provide education about exercise programs available in the community. Other physical therapy interventions for individuals with Down syndrome may vary widely depending on the age and specific needs of the individual. Additional research on various interventions for children and adults with Down syndrome has become available since Carrie was a child. Table 21.7 details current evidence-based interventions for individuals with Down syndrome.

Table 21.7 Evidence-Based Interventions for Down Syndrome (DS)

Intervention	Author (date)	Study Design	No. of Subjects/ Articles (SR)	Question	Findings
General Interventions	Connolly, Morgan, Russell, & Fulliton (1993)	Longitudinal controlled trial	*n* = 20	What is the long-term impact of participation in an early intervention program on motor, cognitive, and adaptive functioning of children with DS?	Adolescents with DS who participated in early intervention had significantly higher scores on measures of intellectual and adaptive functioning as compared to adolescents with DS who had not participated in early intervention.

Continued

Table 21.7 Evidence-Based Interventions for Down Syndrome (DS)—cont'd

Intervention	Author (date)	Study Design	No. of Subjects/ Articles (SR)	Question	Findings
	LaForme Fiss (2007)	Nonrandomized controlled trail	*n* = 11	Do young children with DS who participate in 10 weekly sensori-motor group sessions in addition to individual physical therapy intervention display greater improvements in gross motor skill acquisition than young children with DS who received individual intervention only?	Young children with DS who participated in the sensorimotor group sessions in addition to individual physical therapy demonstrated significant improvement as compared to the control group on selected domains of the GMFM, PEDI, and Goal Attainment Scaling. Parent satisfaction with group sessions was high.
Therapeutic Exercise: Aerobic Capacity/ Endurance Training	Angulo-Barroso, Burghardt, Lloyd, & Ulrich (2008)	Randomized controlled trial (RCT)	*n* = 30	Does a higher-intensity, individualized treadmill training protocol elicit immediate and short-term higher physical activity levels in infants with DS than a lower-intensity, generalized treadmill training program?	Infants with DS receiving higher-intensity treadmill training demonstrated higher activity levels than infants with DS receiving lower-intensity treadmill training.
	Rimmer, Heller, Wang, & Valerio (2004)	RCT	*n* = 52	What is the effect of a cardiovascular and strength-training program on endurance, muscle strength, and body weight for adults with DS?	Adults with DS who participated in a cardiovascular and strength-training program demonstrated significant improvements in cardiovascular fitness, muscle strength and endurance, and body weight as compared to a control group.
Therapeutic Exercise: Gait and Locomotion Training	Looper & Ulirch (2010)	RCT	*n* = 17	What is the difference in developmental outcomes for early orthotic	Children with DS who received treadmill training alone demonstrated higher GMFM

Table 21.7 Evidence-Based Interventions for Down Syndrome (DS)—cont'd

Intervention	Author (date)	Study Design	No. of Subjects/ Articles (SR)	Question	Findings
				use in combination with treadmill training as compared to treadmill training alone for infants with DS?	scores than children who received early orthotic use and treadmill training in combination.
	Looper & Ulrich (2006)	RCT	$n = 9$	Does the use of prefabricated foot orthoses improve the quality of gait in new walkers with DS?	No significant differences were found in step length, step width, and relative double support time in infants with DS who wore orthotics as compared to wearing shoes only.
	Martin (2004)	Repeated measures design	$n = 17$	What are the effects of flexible supramalleolar orthoses (SMOs) on postural stability in children with DS?	Young children with DS showed immediate and longer-term (7 week) improvement in postural stability with the use of flexible SMOs.
	Selby-Silverstein, Hillstrom, & Palisano (2001)	Nonrandomized controlled trial	$n = 26$	Do foot orthoses (FOs) immediately affect gait of children with DS and excessively pronated feet?	FOs improved gait parameters during gait for children with DS and excessively pronated feet.
	Ulrich, Ulrich, Angulo-Kinzler, & Yun (2001)	RCT	$n = 30$	Does practice stepping on a motorized treadmill help reduce the delay in walking onset normally experienced by infants with DS?	Infants with DS who participated in treadmill training 5 days per week for 8 minutes per day learned to walk with help and to walk independently significantly earlier (73.8 days and 101 days respectively) than the control group.
	Ulrich, Lloyd, Tiernan, Looper, & Angulo-Barroso (2008)	RCT	$n = 30$	Does a higher-intensity, individualized treadmill training program lead to increased	Infants with DS in the higher-intensity, individualized training group increased their stepping more

Continued

Table 21.7 Evidence-Based Interventions for Down Syndrome (DS)—cont'd

Intervention	Author (date)	Study Design	No. of Subjects/ Articles (SR)	Question	Findings
				stepping frequency and earlier independent walking for infants with DS as compared to a lower-intensity, generalized treadmill training program?	dramatically and attained motor skills at an earlier age than infants with DS who participated in a lower-intensity, generalized treadmill training program.
	Wu, Looper, Ulrich, Ulrich, & Angulo-Barroso (2007)	RCT	$n = 45$	What are the effects of three intervention protocols (high-intensity treadmill training, low-intensity treadmill training, and no treadmill training) on the development of walking for infants with DS?	Infants with DS who participated in high-intensity treadmill training walked independently earlier than infants with DS who participated in low-intensity treadmill training or no treadmill training (19.2 months, 21.4 months, and 23.9 months, respectively). Infants receiving high-intensity treadmill training also demonstrated significantly increased stride length when compared to the control group.
Therapeutic Exercise: Strength, Power, and Endurance Training for Muscles	Shields, Taylor, & Dodd (2008)	RCT	$n = 20$	Does progressive resistance training improve muscle strength, muscle endurance, and physical function in adults with DS?	Adults with DS participating in progressive resistance training demonstrated significant improvement in upper extremity limb endurance compared to the control group. No difference was found for muscle strength, lower-limb muscle performance, or physical function measures.

Acknowledgments

The authors wish to express their appreciation to the authors of the first edition of this chapter, Katie Bergeron, PT, MS, and the late Carol Gildenberg Dichter, PT, PhD, PCS.

DISCUSSION QUESTIONS

1. What are some common characteristics of the gait pattern of a child with Down syndrome?

2. At what ages might a child with Down syndrome benefit the most from physical therapy intervention?

3. What might be the role of the physical therapist during transition periods (early intervention to preschool, preschool to school, and high school to work) in the life of a child with Down syndrome?

4. Discuss appropriate recreational activities for children with Down syndrome at different ages.

5. What are some common secondary impairments in body structure and function for children with Down syndrome that may be addressed by the physical therapist at different ages?

Recommended Readings

Barnhardt, R.C., & Connolly, B. (2007). Aging and Down syndrome: Implications for physical therapy. *Physical Therapy, 87*(10), 1399-1406.

Palisano R.J., Walter, S., Russell, D.J., Rosenbaum, P., Gemus, M., Galuppi, B., et al. (2001). Gross motor function of children with Down syndrome: Creation of motor growth curves. *Archives of Physical Medicine and Rehabilitation, 82,* 494–500.

Ulrich, D., Lloyd, M.C., Tiernan, C.W., Looper, J.E., & Angulo-Barroso, R.M. (2008). Effects of intensity of treadmill training on developmental outcomes and stepping in infants with Down syndrome: A randomized trial. *Physical Therapy, 88,* 114–122.

References

American Physical Therapy Association (APTA). (2001). Guide to physical therapist practice (2nd ed.). *Physical Therapy, 81*(1), 6–746.

Angulo-Barroso, R., Burghardt, A.R., Lloyd, M., & Ulrich, D.A. (2008). Physical activity in infants with Down syndrome receiving a treadmill intervention. *Infant Behavior and Development, 31*(2), 255–269.

Anwar, A.J, Walker, J.D., & Frier, B.M. (1998). Type 1 diabetes mellitus and Down's syndrome: Prevalence, management and diabetic complications. *Diabetes Medicine, 15,* 160–163.

Barnhardt, R.C., & Connolly, B. (2007). Aging and Down syndrome: Implications for physical therapy. *Physical Therapy, 87*(10), 1399-1406.

Borg, G.V. (1982). Psychological basis of perceived exertion. *Medicine and Science in Sports and Exercise, 14,* 377–381.

Center, J., Beange, H., & McElduff, A. (1998). People with mental retardation have an increased prevalence of osteoporosis: A population study. *American Journal of Mental Retardation, 103,* 19–28.

Chad, K., Jobling, A., & Frail, H. (1990). Metabolic rate: A factor in developing obesity in children with Down syndrome? *American Journal of Mental Retardation, 95,* 228–235.

Connolly, B.H., & Michael, B.T. (1986). Performance of retarded children, with and without Down syndrome, on the Bruininks-Oseretsky Test of Motor Proficiency. *Physical Therapy, 66*(3), 344–348.

Connolly, B.H., Morgan, S.B., Russell, F.F., & Fulliton, W.L. (1993). A longitudinal study of children with Down syndrome who experienced early intervention programming. *Physical Therapy, 73*(3), 179–181.

Finesilver, C. (2002). A new age for childhood diseases: Down syndrome. *RN, 65,* 43–48.

Freeman, S.B., Taft, L.F., Dooley, K.J., Allran, K., Sherman, S.L., Hassold, T.J., Khoury, M.J., & Saker, D.M. (1998). Population-based study of congenital heart defects in Down syndrome. *American Journal of Medical Genetics, 80,* 213–217.

Granger, C., Braun, S., Griswood, K., Heyer, N., McCabe, M., Msau, M., et al. (1991). *Functional independence measure for children.* Buffalo, NY: Medical Rehabilitation, State University of New York, Research Foundation.

Haley, S.M., Coster, W.J., Ludlow, I.H., Haltiwanger, J.T., & Andrellos, P. (1992). *Pediatric Evaluation of Disability Inventory.* Boston: Department of Rehabilitation Medicine, New England Medical Center Hospital.

Hayes, A., & Batshaw, M.L. (1993). Down syndrome. *Pediatric Clinics of North America, 40,* 523–535.

Heller, T., Hsieh, K., & Rimmer, J. (2002). Barriers and supports for exercise participation among adults with Down syndrome. *Journal of Gerontological Social Work, 38*(1–2), 161–178.

Henderson, S.E., Morris, J., & Ray, S. (1981). Performance of Down syndrome and other retarded children on the Cratty Gross Motor Test. *American Journal of Mental Deficiency, 85,* 416–424.

Individuals with Disabilities Education Improvement Act (IDEA) of 2004, Pub. L. No. 108-466, 20 U.S.C. §§ 1400 (2004).

Jackson, H.J., & Thorbecke, P.J. (1982). Treating obesity of mentally retarded adolescents and adults: An exploratory program. *American Journal of Mental Deficiency, 87,* 302–308.

Johnson-Martin, N.M., Jens, K.A., Attermeier, S.N., & Hacker, B.J. (1991). *Carolina curriculum for infants and toddlers with special needs* (2nd ed.). Baltimore: Paul H. Brookes.

Kapell, D., Nightingale, B., Rodriguez, A., Lee, J.H., Zigman, W.B., & Schupf, N. (1998). Prevalence of chronic medical conditions in adults with mental retardation: comparison with the general population. *Mental Retardation, 36,* 269–279.

King, G., Law, M., King, S., Hurley, P., Hanna, S., Kertoy, M., Rosenbaum, P., & Young, N. (2005). *Children's Assessment of Participation and Enjoyment (CAPE) and Preferences for Activities of Children (PAC)*. San Antonio, TX: Harcourt Assessment, Inc.

LaForme Fiss, A.C. (2007). Effect of increased task practice using sensorimotor groups on gross motor skill acquisition for young children with Down syndrome. Unpublished doctoral dissertation, University of Kentucky.

Lauteslager, P.E.M., Vermeer, A., & Helders, P.J.M. (1998). Disturbances in the motor behavior of children with Down syndrome: The need for a theoretical framework. *Physiotherapy, 84,* 5–13.

Law, M., Baptiste, S., Carswell, A., McColl, M.A., Polatajko, H., & Pollock, N. (1998). *Canadian Occupational Performance Measure* (2nd ed. Rev.) Ottawa, ON: CAOT Publications ACE.

Looper, J.E., & Ulrich, D.A. (2006). The effects of foot orthoses on gait in new walkers with Down syndrome. *Pediatric Physical Therapy, 18*(1), 96–97.

Looper, J., Ulrich, D. A. (2010) Effect of treadmill training and supramalleolar orthosis use on motor skill development in infants with Down syndrome: a randomized clinical trial. *Physical Therapy, 90*(3), 382–390.

Martin, K. (2004). Effects of supramalleolar orthoses on postural stability in children with Down syndrome. *Developmental Medicine and Child Neurology, 46*(6), 406–411.

McGuire, D.E., & Chicoine, B. (1996). Depressive disorders in adults with Down syndrome. *Habilitative Mental Healthcare Newsletter, 15*(1), 26–27.

Miller, L.J. (2006). *The Miller Function and Participation Scale.* San Antonio, TX: The Psychological Corporation.

Palisano R.J., Walter, S., Russell, D.J., Rosenbaum, P., Gemus, M., Galuppi, B., et al. (2001). Gross motor function of children with Down syndrome: Creation of motor growth curves. *Archives of Physical Medicine and Rehabilitation, 82,* 494–500.

Patrick, D.L., Edwards, T.C., & Topolski, T.D. (2002). Adolescent quality of life, part II: Initial validation of a new instrument. *Journal of Adolescence, 25,* 287–300.

Pitetti, K.H., Climstein, M., Campbell, K.D., et al. (1992). The cardiovascular capabilities of adults with Down syndrome: A comparative study. *Medicine & Science in Sports Exercise,* 24, 13–19.

Prasher, V.P. (1995). Prevalence of psychiatric disorders in adults with Down syndrome. *European Journal of Psychiatry, 9,* 77–82.

Pueschel, S.M., & Bier, J.A. (1992). Endocrinologic aspects. In S.M. Pueschel & J.K. Pueschel (Eds.), *Biomedical concerns in patients with Down syndrome* (pp. 259–272). Baltimore: Paul H. Brookes.

Rimmer, J.H., Heller, T., Wang, E., & Valerio, I. (2004). Improvements in physical fitness in adults with Down syndrome. *American Journal of Mental Retardation, 109*(2), 165–174.

Ross, J.G., Dotson, C.O., Gilbert, C.G., & Katz, S.J. (1985). The National Youth and Fitness Study. 1: New standards for fitness measurement. *Journal of Physical Education, Recreation and Dance, 56,* 62–66.

Russell, D., Rosenbaum, P., Avery, L., & Lane, M. (2002). The Gross Motor Function Measure (GMFM-66 & GMFM-88) User's Manual. *Clinics in Developmental Medicine No.159 ed.* United Kingdom: Mac Keith Press.

Selby-Silverstein, L., Hillstrom, H.J., & Palisano, R.J. (2001). The effect of foot orthoses on standing foot pressure and gait of young children with Down syndrome. *NeuroRehabilitation, 16*(3), 183–193.

Shamas-Ud-Din, S. (2002). Genetics of Down's syndrome and Alzheimer's disease. *British Journal of Psychiatry, 181,* 167–168.

Sharav, T., & Bowman, T. (1992). Dietary practices, physical activity, and body-mass in a selected population of Down's syndrome children and their siblings. *Clinical Pediatrics,* 31, 341–344.

Shea, A.M. (1991). Motor attainments in Down syndrome. In M.J. Lister (Ed.), *Contemporary management of motor control problems: Proceeding of the II step conference* (pp. 225–236). Alexandria, VA: Foundation for Physical Therapy.

Shields, N., Taylor, N.F., & Dodd, K.J. (2008). Effects of a community-based progressive resistance training program on muscle performance and physical function in adults with Down syndrome: A randomized controlled trial. *Archives of Physical Medicine and Rehabilitation, 89*(7), 1215–1220.

Smith, D.S. (2001). Health care management of adults with Down syndrome. *American Family Physician, 64,* 1031–1038.

Smith P., Hamilton, B.B., Granger, C.V. (1990). Functional in-dependence measure decision tree. The FONE FIM. Research Foundation of the State University of New York, Buffalo, New York.

Stemmons-Mercer, V., & Lewis, C.L. (2001). Hip abductor and knee extensor muscle strength of children with and without Down syndrome. *Pediatric Physical Therapy, 13*(1), 18–26.

Ulrich, D., Lloyd, M.C., Tiernan, C.W., Looper, J.E, & Angulo-Barroso, R.M. (2008). Effects of intensity of treadmill training on developmental outcomes and stepping in infants with Down syndrome: A randomized trial. *Physical Therapy, 88,* 114–122.

Ulrich, D., Ulrich, B., Angulo-Kinzler, R., & Yun, J. (2001). Treadmill training of infants with Down syndrome: evidence-based developmental outcomes. *Pediatrics, 108,* e84–90.

Uyanik, M., Bumin, G., & Kayihan, H. (2003). Comparison of different therapy approaches in children with Down syndrome. *Pediatrics International, 45,* 68–73.

Varni, J.W., Seid, M., & Rode, C.A. (1999). The PedsQL: Meas-urement model for the Pediatric Quality of Life Inventory. *Medical Care, 37*(2), 126–139.

Westcott, S.L., Lowes, L.P., & Richardson, P.K. (1997), Evalua-tion of postural stability in children: Current theories and assessment tools. *Physical Therapy, 77*(6), 629–645.

Wu, J., Looper, J., Ulrich, B.D., Ulrich, D.A., & Angulo-Barroso, R.M. (2007). Exploring effects of different treadmill inter-ventions on walking onset and gait patterns in infants with Down syndrome. *Developmental Medicine and Child Neurology, 49*(11), 839–945.

Zausmer, E., & Shea, A. (1984). Motor development. In S.M. Pueschel (Ed.), *The young child with Down syndrome* (pp. 143–206). New York: Human Sciences Press.

CHAPTER 22

Case Study
Pediatric Leukemia

—Victoria Gocha Marchese, PT, PhD

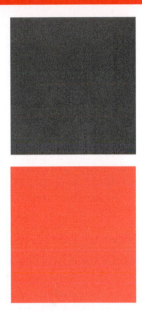

In 2007, in the United States, approximately 10,400 children younger than 15 years of age were diagnosed with cancer, and leukemia accounted for approximately one-third of these childhood cancer cases (American Cancer Society 2007; Ries et al., 2008). The diagnostic groups and specific diagnoses of pediatric leukemia are outlined in Table 22.1. These percentages are determined from data collected from the Surveillance, Epidemiology, and End Results 2001–2005 Program of the National Cancer Institute (Ries et al., 2008).

Medical intervention for children with leukemia varies according to the type of leukemia and the protocol. Each medical institution uses specific protocols to guide the drugs and dosages that children will receive. All children with leukemia receive chemotherapy and in some cases radiation. If a child with acute lymphoblastic leukemia (ALL) has a relapse, meaning that the cancer has returned, a stem cell transplant (SCT) or bone marrow transplant (BMT) is typically administered. Children with acute myeloid leukemia (AML) often receive chemotherapy for a few months and then receive a BMT or SCT. SCT includes only the most immature type of cell, given before the cell has differentiated to a specific type. BMT involves administering marrow, including all types of cells. The protocols for children with leukemia commonly include some or all of the following phases:

1. *Induction,* which lasts approximately 4 to 6 weeks. High doses of a combination of chemotherapy agents are given to eliminate the leukemia cells, with the goal of achieving remission.
2. The *consolidation* and *intensification phases,* which last 1 to 2 months. High doses of chemotherapy are given to eliminate any remaining cancerous cells.

■ **Table 22.1** Common Types of Pediatric Leukemia

Lymphocytic Leukemia	Myeloid and Nonlyphocytic Leukemia
• Accounts for 79% of all childhood leukemia cases	• Accounts for 18% of all childhood leukemia cases
• Acute lymphoblastic leukemia accounts for 99% of the lymphocytic leukemias	• Acute myeloid leukemia accounts for 76% of the nonlymphocytic leukemias
• Chronic lymphocytic leukemia accounts for <1% of the lymphocytic leukemias	• Acute monocytic leukemia accounts for 11% of the nonlymphocytic leukemias
• Nearly 80% survival rate for children with acute lymphoblastic leukemia older than 1 year and younger than 10 years of age. Infant and adolescent survival rates are not as favorable.	• Chronic myeloid leukemia accounts for 10% of the nonlymphocytic leukemias
	• Approximately 40% survival rate for acute myeloid leukemia

Source: Ries, L.A.G., Melbert, D., Krapcho, M., et al. (2008). *SEER Cancer Statistics Review, 1975–2005*. Bethesda, MD: National Cancer Institute. http://seer.cancer.gov/csr/1975_2005/, based on November 2007 SEER data submission, posted to the SEER website, 2008.

3. *Maintenance therapy,* which for children with ALL lasts approximately 2 calendar years for girls and 3 calendar years for boys. Low doses of chemotherapy are given with the goal of preventing relapse. In the future boys may begin to participate in protocols where the length of time is only 2 years.

4. *BMT* or *SCT,* which is performed after a child has received chemotherapy. Children are admitted to the hospital approximately 1 week before receiving the transplant for what is called *conditioning.* This is the time when children receive chemotherapy agents, such as thiotepa or Cytoxan, and total body irradiation with the goal of depressing their bone marrow. The child's age will determine whether the child will receive the total body irradiation or just chemotherapy due to the risk of irradiation to the developing nervous system. During this period, the children are at risk for infection, bruising, and fatigue.

Certain chemotherapy agents cause secondary complications such as myelosuppression, peripheral neuropathy, myopathy, and osteonecrosis. Myelosuppression is a process in which bone marrow activity is inhibited, resulting in decreased production of platelets, red blood cells (RBCs), and white blood cells (WBCs), thus increasing the risk for bleeding, anemia, and infection. Vincristine is a chemotherapy agent known to cause peripheral neuropathy, affecting primarily ankle dorsiflexion and the intrinsic musculature of the feet and hands (Vanionpaa, 1993). Studies have identified that children who receive vincristine are susceptible to decreased ankle dorsiflexion active range of motion (AROM) and strength (Marchese, Chiarello, & Lange,

2003, 2004; Wright, Halton, & Barr, 1999; San Juan et al., 2007). Dexamethasone and prednisone may cause proximal muscle weakness and osteonecrosis (DeAngelis, Gnecco, Taylor, & Warrell, 1991; Mattano, Sather, Trigg, & Nachman, 2000). Osteonecrosis occurs in 15% to 38% of children with ALL and is more common in children aged 10 years or older (Ribeiro et al., 2001; Mattano et al., 2000; Karimova et al., 2006). Marchese et al. (2008) suggest that children, adolescents, and young adults with ALL may have hip or knee osteonecrosis without clinical symptoms. Methotrexate is another chemotherapy agent that interferes with skeletal growth and causes osteoporosis and fractures, primarily in the lower extremities (Schwartz & Leonidas, 1984; Mandel, Atkinson, Barr, & Pencharz, 2004).

Physical therapists receive consultations for children with cancer for many reasons. A child may have decreased active and passive ankle dorsiflexion range of motion (ROM), reduction in muscle strength, pain, delayed gross motor development, limited functional mobility requiring an assistive device such as crutches, and decreased participation in school, social activities, or sports functions because of fatigue. Considering that children with cancer are at risk for blood levels that are below normal, the physical therapist must be cognizant of these numbers and modify the examination and interventions accordingly. See Tables 22.2 and 22.3 for examples of exercise guidelines.

This case study focuses on the physical therapy management of a 6-year-old girl, Emily, who has ALL. The medical management of her disease may result in the secondary complications discussed earlier, which may negatively affect her motor function.

■ **Table 22.2** Exercise Guidelines Used by the
■ Physical Therapists at the Children's Hospital
of Philadelphia for Children Before and After
Bone Marrow Transplantation

Platelet Counts	Recommended Activity Level
>50,000/mm^3	Resistive exercises (e.g., weights and exercise bands)
10,000–50,000/mm^3	Active exercise (e.g., riding a stationary bike, walking, and performing squats while playing)
<10,000/mm^3	Active and passive range of motion, gentle stretching, and light exercise (e.g., shooting hoops)

Based on the side effects of chemotherapy, deconditioning secondary to several months of chemotherapy, and Emily's inability to keep up with her peers at school, the American Physical Therapy Association's *Guide to physical therapist practice* (2001) Preferred Practice Pattern 6B: Impaired Aerobic Capacity/Endurance Associated with Deconditioning was chosen.

Examination: Age 6 Years

History

Emily was a healthy 6-year-old girl when diagnosed 10 months earlier with ALL. A lumbar puncture identified central nervous system (CNS) disease in the cerebrospinal fluid. Emily is receiving medical treatment according to the Children's Oncology Group (COG) protocol. She is in the maintenance phase of her medical intervention, with 3 months of chemotherapy remaining. Emily has a central line, called a Broviac.

The indwelling catheter is under the skin just below the clavicle and enters into a major vein of the heart. Central lines, such as a Port-a-Cath, Hickman, or Broviac, are used for the administration of chemotherapy agents and for withdrawing blood. These catheters are used because they decrease frequent needle sticks and allow large doses of toxic medication to be delivered. However, there are risks of infection and the formation of clots in the line.

Emily's medical treatment has included a possible combination of the following agents: vincristine sulfate, crisantaspase, leucovorin calcium, cytarabine, pegaspargase, thioguanine, filgrastim, prednisone, mercaptopurine, dexamethasone, daunorubicin, doxorubicin, cyclophosphamide, and methotrexate.

Emily has no significant medical history and has achieved age-appropriate motor milestones. She lives with her mother, father, and 8-year-old brother in a two-story home. Emily is in the second grade and enjoys roller skating, bike riding, coloring, cheerleading, and playing with her friends in the neighborhood.

Emily was referred to outpatient physical therapy because she was tripping at the end of the day and twisted her ankle twice while roller skating. Her mother noticed her daughter not running as smoothly and not keeping up with the other children. Emily's goals were to keep up with her friends and to regain her roller skating skills and advance her cheerleading techniques. Her mother's goals were for Emily to avoid a serious fall and to return to her previous level of function. She also expressed concern with her daughter's ability to focus on tasks for a long period of time.

Systems Review
Cardiovascular and Pulmonary

Heart rate, respiratory rate, blood pressure, and temperature are all within normal limits (WNL).

■ **Table 22.3** American Physical Therapy Association Acute-Care Clinical Practice Section
■ Exercise Guidelines

Parameter	No Exercise	Light Exercise	Resistive Exercise
White blood cells (/mm^3)	<5,000 with fever	>5,000	>5,000 (as tolerated)
Platelets (mm^3)	<20,000	20,000–50,000	>50,000
Hemoglobin (g/100 mm)	<8	8–10	>10
Hct	<25%	25%–30%	>30%

Source: Garritan, S., Jones, P., Kornberg, T., & Parkin, C. (1995). Laboratory values in the intensive care unit. *Acute Care Perspectives, The Newsletter of the Acute Care/Hospital Clinical Practice Section of the American Physical Therapy Association,* p.10. Adapted with permission.

Integumentary

The skin around Emily's central line is clean and dry. No other skin problems are noted.

Musculoskeletal

Emily presents with decreased active and passive ROM in her ankles and decreased strength in her lower extremities.

Neuromuscular

Deep tendon reflexes are decreased at the patellar and Achilles tendons. Vision, auditory, and other sensations are WNL.

Communication, Affect, Cognition, Language, and Learning Style

Emily's communication skills are WNL. Cognitive, language, and learning skills were recommended for examination by a psychologist.

Tests and Measures

Before beginning further specific tests and measures in the examination process, it is important to review Emily's blood count levels. The day of the physical therapy examination, Emily's blood counts were WNL (WBCs, 6,000 [normal range, 5,000 to 13,000]; RBCs, 4.2 [normal range, 4.1 to 5.70]; hemoglobin, 13 [normal range, 11.0 to 16.0]; and platelets, 200,000 [normal range, 140,000 to 450,000]).

Aerobic Capacity and Endurance

Emily performed the 9-minute walk-run test, a measure of maximal functional capacity and endurance of the cardiorespiratory system, completing 650 yards. This score places her below the 5th percentile for her age and gender (American Alliance for Health, Physical Education, Recreation, and Dance, 1980). Emily's heart rate was 88 beats per minute (bpm) at rest and ranged from 145 to 160 bpm during the 9-minute walk-run test. Emily did not demonstrate any nasal flaring or increased work of breathing.

Gait, Locomotion, and Balance

Emily walks and runs independently in a variety of environmental settings. Gait was characterized by a mild steppage pattern and flat foot at initial contact caused by her limitations in ankle dorsiflexion AROM and strength. While Emily was running, the therapist noted increased upper body rotation and decreased flight phase (time when both feet were off the floor). Within the first 5 minutes of performing the 9-minute walk-run test, Emily caught her left toe on the ground twice. She was able to catch herself independently, thus avoiding a fall to the ground. However, during the final minute of the 9-minute walk-run test, Emily was running and again caught her left toe on the ground and fell without injury.

She can start and stop ambulation on cue without extra steps and perform a dual task, such as walking on grass for 50 feet while answering math problems. She turned 180° without loss of balance. Emily performed single-limb stance on the left foot for 8 seconds and the right foot for 11 seconds. She was unable to tandem walk on a 3-inch balance beam without loss of balance.

Motor Function

Emily independently transitioned from ring sitting to standing position and from standing to sitting on the floor, requiring the use of her upper extremities. She independently ascended and descended 12 steps with the use of a rail within 10 seconds, placing one foot on a step at a time.

Muscle Performance

Emily presented with upper extremity strength grossly WNL (5/5) and bilateral lower extremity strength 5/5, except for bilateral hip flexion (4/5), knee flexion and extension (4/5), and bilateral ankle dorsiflexion (3+/5), within Emily's available AROM. Considering that Emily is 6 years old and follows directions very well, manual muscle testing and handheld dynamometry measurements were performed. Dynamometry testing in children 6 years of age is a reliable and valid outcome measure (Backman, Odenrick, Henriksson, & Ledin, 1989; Marchese et al., 2003; Stuberg & Metcalf, 1988). Handheld dynamometer measurements identified that Emily's left ankle dorsiflexion strength was 1.7 kg (16.6 N), and on the right ankle it was 2.2 kg (21.5 N). According to Backman and colleagues (1989), ankle dorsiflexion strength for a girl 5.5 to 7 years of age should be 12.6 kg (124 N).

Emily performed 4 sit-ups in 60 seconds, placing her below the 5th percentile for her age (American Alliance for Health, Physical Education, Recreation and Dance, 1980). She performed bilateral heel rises 5 times in standing position, using her upper extremities to assist with balance.

Pain

The Faces Pain Scale (FPS) was used to document Emily's pain level (Wong & Baker, 1988). This scale has

6 pictures of faces, ranging from 0 with a very happy face to 6 with a crying face. The FPS is typically used for children 3 to 7 years of age. Emily reported a dull ache in her ankles and rated the pain as 4 on the FPS. This pain occurred after Emily walked long distances or played in the yard. She also reported pain of 3 in the proximal muscles in her legs.

Range of Motion

Emily presented with full active ROM in all extremities, except ankle dorsiflexion active and passive ROM. She achieved actively 2° of left ankle dorsiflexion with her knee extended, and 3° on the right. Passive ankle dorsiflexion with her knee extended on the left was 6°, and 8° on the right. With the knee flexed, Emily achieved active dorsiflexion on the left 6° and right 7°; passively, left 7° and right 9°.

Self-Care and Home Management (Including Activities of Daily Living)

Emily is independent with activities of daily living such as brushing her teeth and dressing herself. Emily's mother carries her daughter upstairs (11 stairs) to bed at least 3 nights a week because Emily reports her legs hurt too badly, and she is too tired.

Work, Community, and Leisure

Emily rides the bus to school. She holds the bus driver's hand and a rail while ascending the bus steps. All of Emily's classes are on the first floor except music and art, which are on the second floor. The school's principal has expressed concern about Emily's ability to climb the school steps. On two occasions, Emily tripped while ascending the steps and bruised her knee. The school nurse reported seeing Emily three times this year for falling on the playground. During gym class, the teacher reported that Emily was not included in play activities and cried numerous times because of not keeping up with her friends while running. She also frequently misses school because of physician appointments and not feeling well.

Evaluation, Diagnosis, and Prognosis
Including Plan of Care

Evaluation

Emily is a cooperative, sociable, and active little girl with great family support. She presents with pain in her proximal and distal lower extremities, decreased active and passive ankle dorsiflexion ROM, decreased lower extremity muscle strength, decreased endurance, decreased high-level gross motor skills, and limitations in participation in school recess, gym class, and neighborhood activities.

Diagnosis

Emily's diagnosis consists of pain, impaired ankle ROM, impaired lower extremity strength, and impaired endurance. These body function impairments contribute to activity limitations in her gait pattern and in her ability to participate in school and neighborhood activities.

Prognosis

Emily has a good prognosis from a medical standpoint (>80% 5-year survival rate). Through stretching, strengthening, aerobic conditioning, and family consultation, she has a good prognosis to demonstrate improvements in motor functional activity and participate fully in school and community activities.

The recommended frequency of physical therapy is 3 times per week for the first week, 2 times per week for the second week, and 1 time during the third week, followed by 3 months of monthly physical therapy sessions to advance Emily's home program.

Goals

1. Increase right and left active ankle dorsiflexion ROM to WNL to prevent tripping while ambulating.
2. Increase lower extremity strength so that Emily can ascend and descend the school bus stairs independently without holding the bus driver's hand.
3. Increase endurance so that Emily is able to keep up with her peers in school and her neighborhood and does not demonstrate signs of fatigue such as sitting down or becoming short of breath. Endurance was also improved as demonstrated by Emily placing greater than 25th percentile on the 9-minute run-walk.

Intervention

Coordination, Communication, and Documentation

Communication and coordination of activities with Emily and her parents, nurses, physician, schoolteacher, and gym coach are important. Communication with Emily's physician confirmed that she did not have osteonecrosis in the sites where she complained of pain.

Frequency and duration of physical therapy services were also discussed with her insurance company. Recommendations were made for referral to a psychologist for further evaluation of Emily's limited attention span.

Clear documentation of Emily's physical therapy management and outcomes is important to measure progress and to assist in modifying the intervention program. A notebook was used to send suggestions to school personnel.

The expected outcomes of effective coordination, communication, and documentation of services are improved collaboration with all individuals working with Emily; coordination of care with Emily, her family, and other health-care professionals; and assurance that appropriate referrals are made to other care providers as necessary.

Patient/Client-Related Instruction

Emily, her parents, and school personnel were informed regarding Emily's present status, including strength and ROM limitations. Common side effects of medications influencing motor performance were discussed, and a plan of care was developed to address impaired strength and ROM. Health, wellness, and fitness programs were also discussed, with emphasis on aerobic activity for someone with Emily's health problems. The plan of care is summarized in Table 22.4.

The expected outcomes of the patient/client-related instruction are improved physical function and health status; improved safety in home, school, and community settings; and decreased risk of secondary impairments (Fig. 22.1 and Fig. 22.2).

Procedural Interventions
Therapeutic Exercise

Aerobic capacity/endurance conditioning activities focused on bike riding and roller skating, which were Emily's activity selections. While Emily was in the physical therapy clinic, the therapist assisted her in determining her level of exercise intensity when performing her aerobic activities at home. Recommended exercise heart rate was 70% of maximum heart rate and was calculated with the equation $(220 - age) \times 70\%$ (American College of Sports Medicine, 2006). Perceived exertion was rated on a 1 to 10 scale, with 1 = very, very easy and 10 = so hard I'm going to stop (Williams, Eston, & Furlong, 1994; Marinov, Mandadjieva, & Kostianev, 2007). Both heart rate and perceived exertion were monitored during bike riding and roller skating while working at 70% of her maximum heart rate. Emily roller skated with kneepads, elbow pads, and a helmet in the physical therapy clinic and while at home with her mother present. The skates laced up tightly over Emily's ankles, providing stability and deep pressure. She skated continuously for 20 minutes with her heart rate between 65% and 70% of her maximum heart rate and her perceived exertion of 2 without complaints of ankle pain.

Table 22.4 Summary of Plan of Care

Area of Focus	Activity	Frequency	Comments
Stretching	• Ankle dorsiflexion stretch with a towel	• 1 repetition holding for 30 seconds, 5 times per week	• This exercise can be performed in standing lunge position with shoes on to support the arch. • Emphasis on form and proper body alignment while stretching to prevent secondary complications.
Strengthening	• Squatting to pick up a large ball and toss overhead/mid-chest/underhand • Ankle pumps in the bathtub • Jumping (like a frog)	• 20 repetitions, 3 sets, 3 times per week • 20 repetitions, 3 sets, 3 times per week • 20 feet, 3 sets, 3 times per week	• Other activities the child enjoys may be performed to accomplish strengthening of the trunk, and upper and lower extremities.
Aerobic exercise	• Bike riding • Roller skating	• 30 minutes daily	• Perform the aerobic activity continuously even if it requires slowing down.

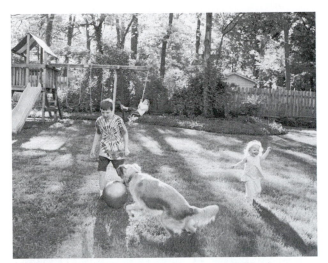

Figure 22.1 After 3 years of long and difficult treatments for acute lymphoblastic leukemia, 10-year-old Devin, who had the same diagnosis and course of treatment as Emily, enjoys a healthy life and playing outside with his sister.

Strengthening exercises were performed on the lower extremities. These exercises included Emily tapping her feet to music, heel walking, and ankle dorsiflexion with resistance (offered by water or the therapist's hand). Outcomes of the flexibility and strengthening program were monitored with goniometric measurements and dynamometry of lower extremity strength.

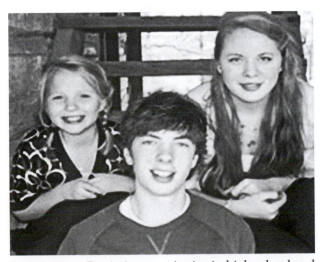

Figure 22.2 Devin is now a junior in high school and enjoying his sisters and planning to attend college.

Manual Therapy

Passive ROM yielded improved ankle joint mobility. This intervention contributed to improved balance and coordination when Emily was walking in the home, school, and community settings.

Gentle massage of Emily's proximal and distal lower extremities was performed to assist with pain relief. Emily did require bilateral solid ankle-foot orthoses during ambulation and play for 3 months. It was also recommended that Emily wear sneakers versus sandals to help with foot alignment and support, with the expectation of increasing safety during gait and decreasing pain.

Termination of Episode of Care

Emily was discharged after 4 months of physical therapy. Her active ankle dorsiflexion ROM on the left had increased from 2° to 10°, and on the right from 3° to 14°. Her bilateral lower extremity strength was grossly 5/5, except for bilateral ankle dorsiflexion, which was 4/5. She increased the distance traveled on the 9-minute walk-run by 100 yards from 650 to 750 yards, placing her performance in the 5th percentile. Emily also increased her number of sit-ups performed in 60 seconds from 4 to 6, placing her in the 5th percentile. Emily did not require her mother's assistance to go up the steps in her home. Her teacher reported no incidences of tripping at school. Most important, Emily reported to her mother and teachers that she felt bigger and stronger and that she could keep up with her friends. With her increased ankle ROM and lower-extremity strength, Emily decreased her chances of falling, thus preventing a possible fracture. Progression of further ROM limitations was prevented, which could have required surgical intervention. Emily's overall physical wellness and her family's awareness of their daughter's general physical abilities increased.

Emily and her family were also made aware of what issues might trigger a need for additional physical therapy services. Long-term side effects from Emily's medical treatment may include the following: a lower-extremity fracture from the radiation and chemotherapy agents, especially methotrexate; osteonecrosis from the steroids; musculoskeletal pain, especially in the ankles from the peripheral neuropathy caused by the chemotherapy agent vincristine; and obesity caused by irradiation. It would not be unusual for Emily to develop a secondary cancer as a progression of her original disease.

Emily is now a healthy second grader who enjoys cheerleading and jumping rope. She continues to return to yearly follow-up appointments with her oncologist while receiving favorable news each time that her cancer has not returned and that she does not demonstrate any secondary complications at this time (Fig. 22.3).

Examination Update: The literature continues to support the benefits of physical therapy intervention

for children with ALL (see Table 22.5). The role of the physical therapist in caring for children with ALL is broadening greatly from interventions that focused on impairments and activity limitations that had already developed to now seeing the children earlier in the treatment phase with the goal of prevention.

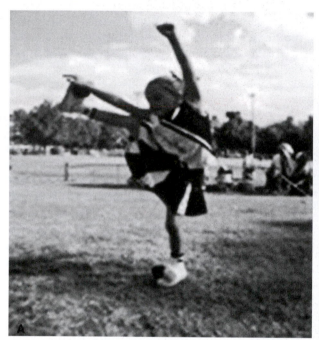
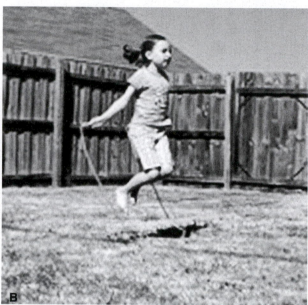

Figure 22.3 Emily is a second grader enjoying cheerleading and jumping rope. She is the little girl that the case study was modeled after from initial diagnoses to the present.

Table 22.5 Evidence-Based Interventions for Pediatric Leukemia

Intervention	Author (Date)	Study Design	No. of Subjects	Question	Findings
Therapeutic Exercise: Aerobic Capacity/ Endurance Training; Balance, Coordination, Flexibility, Strength, Power	San Juan et al., 2007	Time-series; quasi experimental	7	To determine whether a 16-week intrahospital supervised conditioning program including both resistance and aerobic-type training would improve functional capacity, dynamic muscular strength of the upper and lower extremities, muscle functional mobility, ankle range of motion, and quality of	Children with ALL in the maintenance phase of treatment who participated in 3 sessions per week for 16 weeks of resistance and aerobic training followed by 20 weeks where no structured exercise program was performed, after training, significantly increased VO_{2peak}, ventilator threshold, upper-and lower-body muscular strength, and all

Table 22.5 Evidence-Based Interventions for Pediatric Leukemia—cont'd

Intervention	Author (Date)	Study Design	No. of Subjects	Question	Findings
				life in children receiving treatment for acute lymphoblastic leukemia (ALL).	measures of functional mobility (p<0.05). This study supports that it is safe for children with ALL to participate in an aerobic and resistance training program during medical treatment.
	Aznar et al., 2006	Nonexperimental (observational)	7	To measure physical activity levels in children undergoing treatment for ALL.	Children with ALL as compared to healthy controls presented with significantly lower levels of total weekly time of moderate to vigorous physical activity (p<0.05). The authors conclude that children with ALL must be encouraged to participate in sports, games, and physical activities, in both the family and school environments.
	Wright, Galea, & Barr, 2005	Nonexperimental (observational)	99	To compare the balance skills of children and youth who have had ALL with those of comparable subjects and explore the associations with demographics, therapy, physical activity, and health-related quality of life.	Children and youth who had ALL had poorer balance than the comparison subjects as demonstrated on the Bruininks-Oseretsky Test of Motor Proficiency, and lower Children's Self-Perceptions of Adequacy and Predilection for Physical Activity Scale, and Health Utilities Index. Factors such as exposure to cranial irradiation and being overweight may contribute to the balance deficits.
Musculoskeletal: Bone	Marchese et al., 2008	Nonexperimental (observational)	33	To explore the relationships among severity of osteonecrosis, pain, range of motion, and functional mobility in children, adolescents, and young adults with ALL	Correlations were observed between Association Research Circulation Osseous (hip osteonecrosis staging scale) and hip pain (r = –0.34) and between knee pain and time on the Timed Up and Down Stairs test (r = –0.34). Physical therapists should consider that people with ALL may have hip and knee osteonecrosis without clinical symptoms.

Continued

Table 22.5 Evidence-Based Interventions for Pediatric Leukemia—cont'd

Intervention	Author (Date)	Study Design	No. of Subjects	Question	Findings
Education	Gurney et al., 2007	Nonexperimental (observational)	70	To evaluate the degree to which adult survivors of childhood ALL differed in symptom knowledge from that of a population-based, frequency-matched comparison group who completed the same module of the Centers for Disease Control and Prevention's Behavioral Risk Factor Surveillance Study.	Survivors of ALL scored worse on symptom knowledge than did their population comparison group. The results of this study indicate an important gap in knowledge and underscore the need for health education among survivors of childhood leukemia that includes information about symptoms of myocardial infarction and stroke.

DISCUSSION QUESTIONS

1. Explain why Emily is a good candidate for ankle-foot orthoses.

2. Describe the types of difficulties Emily is at risk for in the future.

3. List three of Emily's physical, family, and environmental characteristics that will guide her into a healthy and happy young-adult life.

4. What are a few questions a physical therapist must consider before providing physical therapy services to a child with cancer?

Recommended Readings

Gohar, S.F., Marchese, V., & Comito, M. (2010). Physician referral frequency for physical therapy in children with acute lymphoblastic leukemia. *Pediatric Hematology and Oncology, 27*(3), 179-187.

Huang, T.-T., & Ness, K. K. (2011). Exercise interventions in children with cancer: A review. *International Journal of Pediatrics, 2011*, 461512-461512. Available at: http://www.hindawi.com/journals/ijped/2011/461512/

McGrath, P., & Rawson-Huff, N. (2010). Corticosteroids during continuation therapy for acute lymphoblastic leukemia: the psycho-social impact. *Issues in Comprehensive Pediatric Nursing, 33*(1), 5-19.

Ness, K.K., Baker, K.S., Dengel, D.R., Youngren, N., Sibley, S., Mertens, A.C., & Gurney, J.G. (2007).

Body composition, muscle strength deficits and mobility limitations in adult survivors of childhood acute lymphoblastic leukemia. *Pediatric Blood and Cancer, 49*(7), 975-981.

References

American Alliance for Health, Physical Education, Recreation, and Dance (1980). *Health related physical fitness test manual.* Reston, VA: American Alliance for Health, Physical Education, Recreation, and Dance.

American Cancer Society (2007). *Cancer facts and figures.* Atlanta: Author.

American College of Sports Medicine (2006). *Guidelines for exercise testing and prescription* (7th ed.). Philadelphia: Lippincott Williams & Wilkins.

American Physical Therapy Association (2001). *Guide to physical therapist practice* (2nd ed.). *Physical Therapy, 81*, 6–746.

Aznar, S., Webster, A.L., San Juan, A.F., Mate-Munoz, J.L., Moral, S., Perez, M., Lucia, A. et al. (2006). Physical activity during treatment in children with leukemia: a pilot study. *Applied Physiology Nutrition and Metabolism, 31*, 407–413.

Backman, E., Odenrick, P., Henriksson, K.G., & Ledin, T. (1989). Isometric muscle force and anthropometric values in normal children aged between 3.5 and 15 years. *Scandinavian Journal of Rehabilitation Medicine, 21*, 105–114.

DeAngelis, L.M., Gnecco, C., Taylor, L., & Warrell, R.P. (1991). Evolution of neuropathy and myopathy during intensive vincristine/corticosteroid chemotherapy for non-Hodgkin's lymphoma. *Cancer, 67*, 2241–2246.

Garritan, S., Jones, P., Kornberg, T., & Parkin, C. (1995). Laboratory values in the intensive care unit. *Acute Care Perspectives: The Newsletter of the Acute Care/Hospital Clinical Practice Section of the American Physical Therapy Association.*

Gurney, J.G., Donohue, J.E., Ness, K.K., Leary, M., Glasser, S.P., & Baker, K.S. (2007). Health knowledge about symptoms of heart attack and stroke in adult survivors of childhood acute lymphoblastic leukemia. *Annuals of Epidemiology, 17*, 778–781.

Karimova, E.J., Rai, S.N., Ingle, D., Ralph, A.,C., Deng, X., Neel., M.D., Kaste, S.C., et al. (2006). MRI of knee osteonecrosis in children with leukemia and lymphoma, part 2: Clinical and imaging patterns. *American Journal of Roentgenology, 186*, 477-482.

Mandel, K., Atkinson, S., Barr, R., & Pencharz, P. (2004). Skeletal morbidity in childhood acute lymphoblastic leukemia. *Journal of Clinical Oncology, 22*(7), 1215–1221.

Marchese, V.G., Chiarello, L.A., & Lange, B.J. (2003). Strength and functional mobility in children with acute lymphoblastic leukemia. *Medical and Pediatric Oncology, 40*(4), 230–232.

Marchese, V.G., Chiarello, L.A., & Lange, B.J. (2004). Effects of physical therapy intervention for children with acute lymphoblastic leukemia. *Pediatric Blood and Cancer, 42*(2), 127–133.

Marchese, V.G., Connolly, B., Able, C., Booten, A.R., Bowen, P., Porter, B.M., Rai, S.N., Hancock, M.L., Pui, C.H., Howard, S., Neel, M.D., & Kaste, S.C. (2008). Relationships among severity of osteonecrosis, pain, range of motion, and functional mobility in children, adolescents, and young adults with acute lymphoblastic leukemia. *Physical Therapy, 88*, 341–350.

Marinov, B., Mandadjieva, S., & Kostianev, S. (2007). Pictoral and verbal category-ratio scales for effort estimation in children. *Child: Care, health and development, 34*, 35–43.

Mattano, L.A., Sather, H.N., Trigg, M.E., & Nachman, J.B. (2000). Osteonecrosis as a complication of treating acute lymphoblastic leukemia in children: A report from the children's cancer group. *Journal of Clinical Oncology, 18*(18), 3262–3272.

Ribeiro, R.C., Fletcher, B.D., Kennedy, W., Harrison, P.L.,Neel, M.D., Kaste, S.C., Pui C.H., et al. (2001). Magnetic resonance imaging detection of avascular necrosis of the bone in children receiving intensive prednisone therapy for acute lymphoblastic leukemia or non-Hodgkin lymphoma. *Leukemia, 15*, 891–897.

Ries, L.A.G., Melbert, D., Krapcho, M., Stinchcomb, D.G., Howlanders, N., Mariotto, A., Edwards, B.K., et al. (2008). *SEER Cancer Statistics Review, 1975–2005*. Bethesda, MD: National Cancer Institute. http://seer.cancer.gov/csr/1975_2005/, based on November 2007 SEER data submission, posted to the SEER website, 2008.

San Juan, A.F., Fleck, S.J., Chamorro-Vina, C., Mate-Munoz, J.L., Moral, S., Perez, M., Lucia, A., et al. (2007). Effects of an intrahospital exercise program intervention for children with leukemia. *Medical & Science in Sports & Exercise, 39*(1), 13–21.

Schwartz, A.M., & Leonidas, J.C. (1984). Methotrexate osteopathy. *Radiology, 11*, 13–16.

Stuberg, W.A., & Metcalf, W.K. (1988). Reliability of quantitative muscle testing in healthy children and in children with Duchenne muscular dystrophy using a hand-held dynamometer. *Physical Therapy, 68*(6), 977–982.

Vanionpaa, L. (1993). Clinical neurological findings of children with acute lymphoblastic leukemia at diagnosis and during treatment. *European Journal of Pediatrics, 152*, 115–119.

Williams, J.G., Eston, R., & Furlong, B. (1994). CERT: A perceived exertion scale for young children. *Perceptual & Motor Skills, 79*, 1451–1458.

Wong, B.L., & Baker, C.M. (1988). Pain in children: Comparison of assessment scales. *Pediatric Nursing, 14*(1), 9–17.

Wright, M.J., Galea, V., & Barr, R.D. (2005). Proficiency of balance in children and youth who have had acute lymphoblastic leukemia. *Physical Therapy, 85*(8), 782–790.

Wright, M.J., Halton, J.M., & Barr, R.D. (1999). Limitations of ankle range of motion in survivors of acute lymphoblastic leukemia: A cross-sectional study. *Medical and Pediatric Oncology, 32*, 279–282.

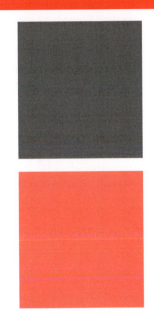

Case Study
Duchenne Muscular Dystrophy

CHAPTER 23

—Shree Devi Pandya, PT, DPT, MS

—Marcia K. Kaminker, PT, DPT, MS, PCS

Pediatric physical therapists can make important contributions to the care of children with inherited neuromuscular disorders. These conditions may include Duchenne muscular dystrophy (DMD), a muscle disorder; spinal muscular atrophy, an anterior horn cell disorder; Charcot-Marie-Tooth disease, a neuropathic disorder; and many other congenital and/or pediatric forms of muscular dystrophies and neuropathies. Common elements are their (1) genetic/inherited etiology, (2) progressive nature, (3) primary impairment of muscle weakness, (4) resulting activity limitations and participation restrictions, and (5) secondary complications leading to increased morbidity and mortality. However, they differ in their (1) associated impairments of body structures and functions, (2) secondary complications, (3) natural history, (4) prognosis, and (5) medical management.

In addressing the needs of these children and their families, the role of the physical therapist varies by setting. As a team member in a multidisciplinary specialty clinic, the therapist may perform evaluations and make recommendations over extended periods of time. The school-based physical therapist may serve as consultant, educator, and coordinator, facilitating the provision of services to meet the student's educational needs and prepare for the transition to adulthood. The outpatient therapist may intervene for brief episodes of care after surgical interventions or to assist in the acquisition of and training regarding orthoses, wheelchairs, and other adaptive equipment. Home care may involve procedural interventions, patient/client-related instruction with the family, and recommendations for adaptive equipment and home modifications.

This case study of a boy with DMD will describe the process for developing appropriate plans for evidence-based intervention and management that reflect parent and child preferences and are based on available evidence or, in the absence of evidence, expert consensus. These decisions should also be consistent with the American Physical Therapy Association (APTA)'s *Guide to Physical Therapist Practice* ("*Guide*") (2001).

To meet the varying needs of these children, practice patterns for examination, evaluation, and intervention can be found in the *Guide* (APTA, 2001) under all four systems. Some common examples include 4C: Impaired Muscle Performance; 5G: Impaired Motor Function and Sensory Integrity Associated with Acute or Chronic Polyneuropathies; 6B: Impaired Aerobic Capacity/ Endurance Associated with Deconditioning; and 6E: Impaired Ventilation and Respiration/Gas Exchange Associated with Ventilatory Pump Dysfunction or Failure.

DMD is the most common inherited muscle disease of childhood. It is an **X-linked inherited disorder** with an incidence of 1:3,500 to 1:6,000 male births (Emery, 1991). A recent survey of four states in the United States documented a prevalence of 1.3 to 1.8 per 10,000 males aged 5 to 24 years (Centers for Disease Control and Prevention, 2009). A third of the cases arise from new mutations and therefore may not have a family history of the disorder.

The condition was first described in the late 1800s (Duchenne, 1868; Gowers, 1879), the gene lesion was discovered in 1985 (Kunkel, Monaco, Middlesworth, Ochs, & Latt, 1985), and the protein product was described in 1987 (Hoffman, Brown, & Kunkel, 1987). The mutation is located on the short arm of the X chromosome in the Xp-21 region, affecting the gene that codes for dystrophin. Boys with DMD have an absence of **dystrophin**, a protein normally present in skeletal muscle, smooth muscle, and the brain. In skeletal muscle, dystrophin is located in the sarcolemmal membrane and is believed to play a role in maintaining the integrity of the muscle fibers as part of the dystrophin-sarcoglycan complex. The absence of dystrophin and associated structural proteins leads to a breakdown of muscle fibers, resulting in progressive weakness and loss of function (Bushby et al., 2010a).

Although DMD is inherited, and the gene defect is present from birth, most boys are not identified until 3 to 7 years of age unless there is a family history of the disorder (Ciafaloni et al., 2009). Early motor milestones, such as rolling, sitting, and walking, are usually achieved at expected ages, though some children show delays in ambulation and speech. Some children exhibit marked hypertrophy of the calf muscles; this is often referred to

as *pseudohypertrophy* because it is composed of enlarged muscle fibers as well as fat and connective tissue. The symptoms that lead parents to seek medical attention include difficulty with running, jumping, hopping, climbing stairs, and keeping up with peers in daycare, school, and community settings. The *primary impairment* causing activity limitations in DMD is muscle weakness. All muscles are not affected equally, but there is a predictable proximal-to-distal pattern of involvement (Bushby et al., 2010a). The natural progression of weakness in DMD has been well documented by the Clinical Investigation of Duchenne Dystrophy (CIDD) Group (Brooke et al., 1981, 1983). More than 100 boys aged 5 to 15 years were followed for a year in this multicenter study. Pertinent findings from this study are described below.

Weakness is present early in the neck flexors and abdominal muscles, and the child has difficulty attempting a sit-up. Next to be affected are the pelvic girdle muscles (hip extensors and abductors) and the knee extensors, resulting in the need to use **Gowers' maneuver/sign** to rise from the floor, in which the boy pushes with his hands on the floor and onto his legs to assume a standing position (Fig. 23.1, Fig. 6.15). Progressive weakness of the lower limb muscles eventually leads to the loss of independent ambulation by about 12 years of age. Weakness of the shoulder girdle muscles results in difficulty with overhead activities by the early teens. Eventually, the distal muscles of the

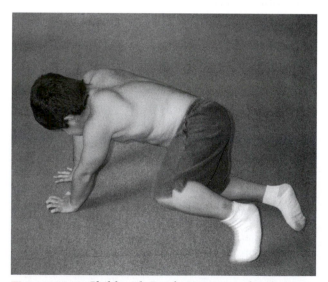

Figure 23.1 Child with Duchenne muscular dystrophy attempting to rise from the floor. He will use a Gowers' maneuver/sign where he will use his hands and arms to "walk" up his legs to come to standing (see Fig. 6.15).

upper extremities become involved as well, causing problems with feeding, grooming, and writing. The muscles that are notably spared are the gastrocnemius/soleus muscles, facial and eye muscles, muscles involved in speech and swallowing, and sphincters (Brooke et al., 1981, 1983).

The early pattern of unequal muscle involvement (extensors weaker than flexors) leads to the *secondary problem* of progressive muscle tightness and joint contractures. In the CIDD study, contractures were present by 6 years of age at the ankles and hips, attributable to tightness in the gastrocnemius/soleus, iliotibial band/tensor fasciae latae (ITB/TFL), and hip flexors.

By 9 years of age, contractures develop at the knee, caused by tightness of the hamstrings, and at the elbows and wrists, caused by elbow flexor and wrist flexor tightness. Contractures at the hips, knees, elbows, and wrists worsen as a consequence of prolonged sitting in a wheelchair. The weakness and contractures lead to restrictions in activities and participation. Between the ages of 8 and 10 years, more than 50% of the boys in the CIDD study had lost the ability to rise from the floor or climb stairs (Brooke et al., 1981, 1983). Several worldwide studies have documented the loss of independent ambulation between the ages of 8 and 12 years (Emery, 2003).

As the boys start to spend increasing amounts of time in a wheelchair, the development of scoliosis becomes a major concern. More than 80% develop significant scoliosis by their late teens. Several factors are hypothesized to contribute to the development of scoliosis, including asymmetric trunk muscle involvement, handedness, and the loss of normal lumbar lordosis with prolonged sitting. The progression of scoliosis can adversely affect pulmonary function, comfort in sitting, and use of the upper extremities for functional activities. Loss of standing leads to a greater risk of osteopenia and resultant fractures, especially in the lower extremities; this is a particular concern for boys who are on corticosteroid therapy (King et al., 2007).

Respiratory and cardiac muscles are also involved in DMD. Involvement of respiratory muscles results in lower than normal respiratory function during the first decade and a gradual decline in the second decade (Rideau, Jankowski, & Grellet, 1981). With decreased respiratory reserves, even a simple cold can lead to severe respiratory problems. More than 70% of boys with DMD die as a result of pulmonary complications (Emery, 2003). Cardiac manifestations include arrhythmia and/or cardiomyopathy (Chénard, Bécane, Tertrain, de Kermadec, & Weiss, 1993; de Kermadec, Bécane, Chénard, Tertrain, & Weiss, 1994). Although a majority

of boys will develop cardiac involvement, the severity of the problem varies greatly; fewer than 30% of boys die as a result of cardiac complications (Emery, 2003). The smooth muscle in the gastrointestinal (GI) tract is also involved, causing GI motility problems, especially in the later stages of the disease, leading to problems with constipation and impaction (Barohn, Levine, Olson, & Mendell, 1988). The exact role of dystrophin in the brain is not well understood, but about 30% of boys with DMD have learning problems and require special education and related services (Anderson, Head, Rae, & Morley, 2002; Dubowitz, 1995; Hinton, De Vivo, Nereo, Goldstein, & Stern, 2000).

Over the past two decades, not only have advances occurred in our understanding of the genetics, molecular mechanisms, and natural history of DMD, but also there have been major advances in the medical, surgical, and rehabilitation interventions available. Ambulation can be prolonged for up to 3 years, and standing thereafter for up to another 2 years, through an aggressive program that includes daily stretching, functional activities, swimming, bracing with knee-ankle-foot orthoses (KAFOs), and contracture-release surgery (Brooke et al., 1989; Harris & Cherry, 1974; Heckmatt, Dubowitz, & Hyde, 1985; Vignos, Wagner, Karlinchak, & Katirji, 1996). Prolonged walking and standing delay the development of contractures and scoliosis. Surgical correction of scoliosis and spinal stabilization with the Luque procedure (Luque, 1982) delay the decline in pulmonary function (Galasko, Delaney, & Morris, 1992, Eagle et al., 2007), improve sitting comfort, and allow continued use of the upper extremities for functional activities (Miller, Moseley, & Koreska, 1992). The advantage of the Luque procedure is that it does not require external stabilization with an orthosis, allowing the patient who is medically stable to be sitting upright within 24 hours, thus reducing problems from disuse atrophy. Aggressive use of noninvasive mechanical ventilation improves life expectancy. The mean age of death in the 1960s was 14.4 years; whereas, since the 1990s, it has been about 25.3 years for those who choose ventilation (Eagle et al., 2002).

The use of corticosteroids—prednisone and deflazacort—is also changing the natural history and prognosis of DMD. The effects of each of these medications have been well documented in several short-term randomized controlled trials (Angelini et al., 1994; Backman & Henriksson, 1995; Griggs et al., 1991, 1993; Mendell el al., 1989; Mesa, Dubrovsky, Corderi, Maarco, & Flores, 1991). Corticosteroids improve muscle mass, strength, and function within the first 6 months of treatment. With continued treatment, the improvement is maintained for up to 18 months (Griggs et al., 1993), and the subsequent decline is slower than predicted, as documented in patients followed for up to 3 years (Fenichel et al., 1991). Several open follow-up cohort studies of long-term corticosteroid use have reported delays in the loss of independent ambulation, development of scoliosis, decline in pulmonary function, and development of cardiomyopathy (Biggar, Gingras, Feblings, Harris, & Steele, 2001; Biggar, Harris, Eliasoph, & Alman, 2006; DeSilva, Drachman, Mellits, & Kunel, 1987; Houde et al., 2008: King et al., 2007: Markham, Spicer, & Khoury et al., 2005: Markham et al., 2008; Moxley, Pandya, Ciafaloni, Fox, & Campbell, 2010; Schara, Mortier, & Mortier, 2001). Therefore, corticosteroids are now recommended in the management of children with DMD (Bushby et al., 2010a; Manzur, Kuntzer, Pike, & Swan, 2004, 2008; Moxley et al., 2005). Clinics across the country have been prescribing these medications more readily, though wide variations continue to exist. While about 20% of patients were on corticosteroid regimens in 1991, that percentage increased to 44% in 2005. Despite the documented benefits, some families choose not to initiate this intervention or it is discontinued because of remaining concerns about side effects of long-term use, including weight gain, Cushingoid facies, behavioral issues, short stature due to decreased growth, cataracts, and vertebral fractures (Matthews et al., 2010).

Although this disorder remains "incurable," the available supportive and symptomatic interventions have substantially improved the life span and quality of life of affected patients (Manzur, Kinali, & Muntoni, 2008). These advances are changing the description of this disorder from "fatal" to "chronic" and are creating both optimism and new challenges (Rahbek et al., 2005; Arias, Andrews, Pandya, et al., 2011; Moxley et al., 2010; Vinna et al., 2007; Wagner, Lechtzin, & Judge, 2007).

This case study of a boy with DMD illustrates (1) the long-term approach to the management of children with inherited neuromuscular disorders, (2) the role of the physical therapist as a member of a multidisciplinary team of care providers, (3) the role of the school-based physical therapist, and (4) an evidence-based approach that integrates high-quality research with clinical expertise and child/family preferences. To demonstrate the issues encountered in the ongoing care of these children, the case covers a follow-up period of almost 15 years. For the sake of brevity, not all encounters are presented, and within the visits described, not all elements from the *Guide* (APTA, 2001) are covered. Only highlights of specific elements pertinent to that encounter are provided.

Sam is a 20-year-old young man with DMD. Since he was 5 years old, he has been followed by a clinic for children with progressive neuromuscular disorders, funded by the Muscular Dystrophy Association (MDA). The core team includes a pediatric neurologist, a nurse, and a physical therapist. Access to other specialists is available as necessary, including genetic counselors, dieticians, occupational therapists, orthopedists, orthotists, pulmonologists, respiratory therapists, and cardiologists. The role of the physical therapist includes coordination of care among all of the clinic providers and with the team at school. Sam has been seen at the clinic at least twice per year. This schedule of visits is based on the nature of the condition and the changing needs of the child. Recent care recommendations developed by a panel of experts convened by the Centers for Disease Control and Prevention (CDC) offer detailed information regarding the evaluation and management of children with DMD. The intent of these guidelines is to minimize the nationwide variation in services for patients and their families and to provide teams with the best available evidence for decision making (Bushby et al., 2010a, 2010b). The synopses of specific visits, described below, emphasize essential elements of Sam's physical therapy examinations, interventions, and plans of care.

Examination: Age 5 Years

History

Sam was brought to medical attention because his daycare providers reported to his parents that he was unable to keep up with his peers on the playground. He had difficulty running, jumping, and climbing the jungle gym and the steps to the slide. No problems had been noted during pregnancy or childbirth or in the development of early milestones, such as rolling, sitting, ambulation, or speech. The pediatrician observed Sam's enlarged calf muscles and his difficulty in rising from the floor, requiring him to use Gowers' maneuver. There was no family history of muscular dystrophy or, more specifically, DMD. The pediatrician ordered a screening blood test, which revealed a level of creatine kinase (CK/CPK) that was more than 1,000 times normal. This led to a referral to a pediatric neurologist, who performed a blood test for the chromosomal abnormality specific to DMD. The genetic test reported a deletion of exon 51, confirming the diagnosis. Sam's mother is awaiting the results of her genetic tests to see if she is a carrier. Sam has an older sister, and his mother is worried that her daughter might be a carrier.

She is also concerned about her two sisters, who are of child-bearing age and are planning families.

Parent Interview

Sam is independent in age-appropriate self-care activities at home. He enjoys books, knows the alphabet, numbers, and colors, and looks forward to starting school. Currently, Sam is in daycare full-time. Except for the problems noted on the playground and the fact that he needs to push with his hands to rise from the floor, he plays well with his peers.

Systems Review

Growth and Development

Height and weight are within normal limits (WNL).

Cardiovascular and Pulmonary

Sam's vital signs are WNL, showing no obvious dysfunction of the cardiovascular or pulmonary systems. However, pulmonary involvement is common in DMD; therefore, Sam will undergo a forced vital capacity (FVC) measurement today. Because of the possibility of cardiac involvement, Sam is also scheduled for a baseline electrocardiogram (ECG).

Integumentary

The integumentary system is WNL.

Musculoskeletal

On musculoskeletal examination, Sam exhibits a lordotic posture with slight winging of the scapulae. He also has enlargement of the calf muscles (pseudohypertrophy) similar to that in the child in Fig. 23.2. Given the medical diagnosis, a detailed examination of ROM and muscle strength will be performed.

Neuromuscular

Neuromuscular examination is WNL in terms of motor control, sensory integrity, and tone. Specific functional activities known to be affected will be examined in detail.

Cognition and Communication

Sam is a friendly 5-year-old who has been cooperative through all the tests he has undergone today with the various providers. He communicates at an age-appropriate level and follows instructions well.

Mobility

Sam ambulates safely indoors and outdoors and negotiates curbs independently. He keeps up with his peers when walking around the neighborhood and when riding his tricycle, though he has difficulty in running.

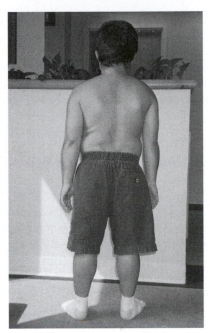

Figure 23.2 Posterior view of a child with Duchenne muscular dystrophy displaying "winging" of the scapula and enlargement of the calf muscles (pseudohypertrophy).

Gait is characterized by brisk knee extension, rapid progression from heel strike to foot-flat, and mildly increased arm swing. Sam holds a railing when walking up and down stairs.

Tests and Measures

Considering Sam's age and diagnosis, the elements for detailed examination were chosen based on the findings from studies of the natural history of DMD. The items included muscle force measurements by manual muscle tests (MMTs) and range of motion (ROM) measurements by goniometric tests, timed function tests, and measurements of FVC. Studies have shown that these items can be reliably documented in children with DMD aged 5 years and older (Florence et al., 1984), and that they are sensitive to disease progression (Brooke et al., 1983) and therapeutic interventions.

Muscle Performance

Muscle force measurements with MMTs were performed on selected muscles that are known to show early involvement: neck flexors, hip extensors, hip abductors, hip flexors, and knee extensors. The MMT procedures used are those described by Daniels and Worthingham (Hislop & Montgomery, 2002), and the scoring system is a modification of the Medical Research Council

(MRC) scale (normal strength 5, 5-, 4+, 4, 4-, 3+, 3, 3-, 2, 1, 0 no movement) (MRC, 1976), as reported in the CIDD studies (Florence et al., 1984). The intrarater and interrater reliabilities of the procedures, the scoring system, and the sensitivity are high and have been well documented in this population (Florence et al., 1984, 1992; Griggs et al., 1993; Mendell et al., 1989).

Range of Motion

ROM measurements were performed for ankle dorsiflexion and knee extension, the Thomas test for hip flexor tightness, and the Ober test for ITB/TFL tightness. Goniometric tests followed the procedures described in the CIDD study, which have shown high levels of reliability (Pandya et al., 1985).

Motor Function

Three timed function tests were conducted: (1) time to rise from a supine position on the floor, (2) time to go 30 feet (walk, jog, run), and (3) time to climb four steps. Sam was instructed to perform all of these tests "as quickly as you can." The timed function tests are the simplest objective measure of progress and they are meaningful to the child and his parents. These tests have also been found to be highly reliable and sensitive in this patient population (Brooke et al., 1983; Florence et al., 1984).

Ventilation and Respiration

FVC has been recommended as a simple measure to document respiratory function in the muscular dystrophies (Rideau et al., 1981). It has been shown to be highly reliable and sensitive in children aged 5 years and older (Brooke et al., 1983; Florence et al., 1984).

Results of Sam's MMT, ROM, timed function tests, and FVC are presented in Table 23.1. The findings from these tests allow us to establish a baseline against which progression can be documented in the future.

Table 23.1 Results of Longitudinal Follow-up Examinations

	July 1990	July 1991*	July 1995	July 2000	July 2003
Age (yr)	5	6	10	15	18
Height (cm)	113	115	120	133	157
Weight (kg)	18.6	20.2	33.4	50.9	69.1
Vital signs	WNL	WNL	WNL	WNL	WNL
Timed Tests (seconds)					
Stand from supine	3	2*	3	7	Unable
Run 30 feet	5	3	3	5 (walk)	7 (walk)
Climb 4 stairs	3	2*	3	4	Unable
Neuromuscular (Muscle Performance)					
Neck flexors	2	3*	3	3	3
Hip extensors	4–	4+*	4	4–	3–
Hip abductors	4–	4+*	4	4–	3–
Hip flexors	4	4+*	4+	4	4–
Knee extensors	4	4+*	4	4–	3–
Musculoskeletal (Range of Motion)					
Ankle/dorsiflexion	+10	+10	0	–10	–15
Hip/extension	+20	+20	+10	0	–10
Knee/extension	WNL	WNL	WNL	WNL	–10
ITB/TFL	WNL	WNL	WNL	–10	–20
Pulmonary					
FVC (mL)	600	1,000	1,600	1,900	2,600†

*Improvements secondary to initiation of prednisone 6 months ago.
†FVC (forced vital capacity) continues to improve and does not show a plateau yet.

Examination Update: Practice today would include other recommended tests of function, participation, and quality of life such as the 6-minute walk test (6MWT) and the Pediatric Quality of Life (PedsQL) test. The reliability, sensitivity, predictive validity, and relevance of these tests in the DMD population remain to be documented.

Evaluation, Diagnosis, and Prognosis
Including Plan of Care

Evaluation

Sam's height, weight, and vital signs are all WNL. Strength is decreased in the neck flexors, hip flexors, hip extensors, hip abductors, and quadriceps. His ROM is WNL, except at the ankle, where he is beginning to show tightness in the gastrocnemius/soleus group. Sam rises from the floor using Gowers' maneuver because of his pelvic girdle weakness. He walks normally, but when attempting a run assumes a wide base and a Trendelenburg "waddle" attributable to the weakness of his hip abductors. Sam prefers to use the railing when climbing stairs and is unable to go step-over-step as would be expected for his age. His FVC is 1.2 liters, which is 80% of normal for his age. All of these findings are consistent with his medical diagnosis of DMD.

Diagnosis

Physical therapy diagnoses at this stage include impaired posture, ROM, muscle performance, respiratory function, and locomotion, associated with activity limitations and participation restrictions within the daycare and community environments.

Prognosis

Based on Sam's medical diagnosis, his long-term prognosis for improvement is poor. Progressive ROM restrictions can be delayed with a daily program of stretching, positioning, and splinting (Scott, Hyde, Goddard, & Dubowitz, 1981; Vignos, 1983; Vignos et al., 1996). Insufficient evidence is available to determine whether these interventions can ultimately prevent or delay the need for contracture-release surgery or can prolong ambulation. The expert consensus, reported in the 2010 multidisciplinary care recommendations, is that stretching, splinting, and positioning should be performed at least 4 to 6 times per week (Bushby et al., 2010b). In the short term, muscle performance can be improved with submaximal strengthening exercises (deLateur & Giaconi, 1979). Unfortunately, longitudinal studies of the effects of strengthening have not been conducted in patients with DMD or in other muscular dystrophy populations. To avoid disuse atrophy, the expert consensus recommendations encourage submaximal strengthening exercises, functional movement, and recreational activities such as swimming (Bushby et al., 2010b). Respiratory function, although below age-expected levels, will continue to increase during the first decade of life and is not expected to plateau or decline until the teens (Rideau et al., 1981).

Goals

Given an understanding of the etiology of this condition, the knowledge about its natural history, and the effectiveness of various interventions, the following goals were developed collaboratively with Sam and his parents.

Long-term goals: Maximize Sam's functional abilities and participation in the home, school, and community settings within the limitations imposed by his progressive disorder. Delay and/or prevent the loss of strength and ROM.

Short-term goals (by the next clinic visit in 6 months):

1. Sam will maintain his ankle ROM through passive stretching exercises performed at least once daily, assisted by his parents.
2. Sam will maintain his passive hip extension by lying prone for at least one 30-minute session each day.
3. Sam will maintain present strength and functional status by exercising in a community pool program.

Examination Update: While having goals related to limitations in body structures and functions is important in a clinical setting, it is equally important to have functional goals related to activities and participation, consistent with the ICF model. Based on current practice, the following short-term goals are projected to be achieved by the next clinic visit in 6 months:

1. Sam will maintain his present levels of ROM and strength to be able to perform functional activities.
2. Sam will maintain the ability to walk independently without restrictions in his home, school, and community, on level surfaces and uneven outdoor terrain.
3. Sam will continue to be able to walk up and down stairs independently.
4. Sam will maintain the ability to negotiate the outdoor playground equipment at his school, to participate with his peers during recess.
5. Sam will continue to be able to ride his tricycle, to participate with his neighborhood friends.

Intervention

Coordination, Communication, and Documentation

The clinic physical therapist and Sam's parents agreed that as soon as he enters kindergarten and the personnel working with him are identified, his parents will help to establish communication between the physical therapists in school and clinic. The school therapist will convey pertinent information to the other members of the educational team, including the classroom teacher, physical education teacher, and school nurse.

Patient/Client-Related Instruction

Sam's parents have been diligent in seeking information about DMD from the health-care professionals whom they have encountered. They have talked with the MDA services coordinator about the agency's services and the child support groups available in their area. They also receive information and support through the online community of Parent Project Muscular Dystrophy, a nonprofit organization devoted to providing information, resources, and advocacy for patients and their families who are affected by DMD. The clinic team discussed Sam's short-term prognosis, in addition to explaining the roles of the various team members and coordination among the clinic team, the pediatrician, and the school. Sam will continue to be followed by the pediatrician for his regular medical needs, such as annual checkups, immunizations, and booster shots. Unless specific concerns require more frequent visits, Sam will be followed every 6 months in the MDA clinic.

The clinic physical therapist advised Sam's parents to encourage him to engage in functional physical activities and low-intensity exercise. He should avoid overexertion, especially eccentric or high-resistance exercise, because of the potential for contraction-induced muscle damage (Eagle, 2002). Muscle pain within the 24-hour period after exercise and myoglobulinuria are considered symptoms of overuse that would signal the need to reduce the level of future exercise (Eagle, 2002). Sam's parents were asked to explore opportunities for a swimming program, which can be an enjoyable method of generalized muscle strengthening. These recommendations are based on empirical consensus; limited evidence exists to support specific exercise protocols in humans with DMD, though animal research has been performed, principally on dystrophin-deficient *mdx* mice. The literature suggests that submaximal exercise may be beneficial early in the disease process, but probably not in the later stages when contractile muscle has been replaced by adipose and connective tissue (Bushby et al., 2010b; Eagle, 2002; Grange & Call, 2007; Vignos, 1983).

Procedural Interventions

The physical therapist demonstrated for Sam and his parents the passive stretching exercises to maintain ROM at the ankle, as well as prone positioning for when he is watching television, to prevent tightness from developing at the hip.

Termination of Episode of Care

Sam was seen for a regularly scheduled episode of physical therapy prevention (APTA, 2001, p. 679) as part of the MDA clinic in his local community. The purpose of these visits was to support maintenance of optimal function, health, wellness, and fitness. His parents were advised to contact the clinic if they have any questions or concerns before the next regularly scheduled visit. Sam will also be followed by a physical therapist at school, who will develop a specific plan of care for the school setting. While the clinic physical therapist sees Sam in an isolated setting, the school therapist interacts with him in his natural educational environment, observing his daily function, activity limitations, and participation restrictions. This enables the school-based therapist to appropriately assist Sam and his school team in addressing his unique needs.

Examination: Age 6 Years

History

Sam has been healthy over the past year. He completed kindergarten, performing well both academically and in his regular physical education class. Sam did not require any type of assistance or services in the classroom; therefore, he was not eligible for special education and related services under the Individuals with Disabilities Education Act (IDEA). However, he was entitled to school-based physical therapy services under Section 504 of the Rehabilitation Act of 1973. The school physical therapist periodically conferred with the physical education teacher about Sam's physical education program, developing modifications necessary to accommodate his limitations in activity and participation secondary to his muscle weakness. They have also incorporated Sam's stretching needs into the physical education program. The family has joined the local YMCA, and Sam goes swimming at least twice a week, once during a weeknight and once over the weekend. They continue to perform the stretching exercises and positioning as instructed at least 5 times a week.

Six months ago Sam began taking prednisone, 0.75 mg/kg/day, as recommended by the pediatric neurologist and based on the findings from several randomized controlled trials (Griggs et al., 1991, 1993; Mendell et al., 1989). His parents have noticed an improvement in Sam's functional abilities since he started on prednisone. He no longer needs the railing to climb stairs and uses a reciprocal (step-over-step) pattern. He rises from the floor more easily and seems to be able to run faster. Sam has learned to ride a bicycle without training wheels and is able to keep up with the neighborhood children. He is hungrier (a known side effect of prednisone), but his parents have been successful in following the clinic dietician's recommendations to restrict sugar, salt, and unnecessary calories.

Systems Review

Growth and Development

Height and weight remain WNL. It is extremely important to monitor height and weight, because decreased growth and weight gain are among the side effects associated with steroid therapy (Fenichel et al., 1991).

Cardiovascular and Pulmonary

Vital signs are WNL. Sam's baseline ECG performed last year showed abnormal Q waves and prominent R waves, suggesting ventricular hypertrophy. This abnormality on ECG, in the absence of clinical signs of cardiomyopathy, is not uncommon and requires monitoring. Pulmonary function will be evaluated through FVC testing, as recorded in Table 23.1.

Integumentary

The integumentary system is WNL. Sam does not show striae (stretch marks), a side-effect of prednisone that has been reported for some boys, especially on the abdomen (Fenichel et al., 1991, 1993).

Musculoskeletal

Sam's posture is unchanged from last year. Muscle performance and ROM will be examined in detail.

Neuromuscular

Neuromuscular examination is WNL in terms of motor control, sensory integrity, and muscle tone. Specific functional activities documented previously will be examined in detail.

Cognition and Communication

Sam continues to communicate at an age-appropriate level and follows instructions well.

Tests and Measures

Items include the same tests that were performed last year: muscle performance, ROM, timed motor function tests, and FVC (see Table 23.1). Sam has improved his performance on all of the timed tests and is even able to run for short distances without assuming a wider base and Trendelenburg gait. He is keeping up with his friends on the playground at school and in the community.

Evaluation, Diagnosis, and Prognosis
Including Plan of Care

Evaluation

As expected, Sam shows improvement since his examination 1 year ago. The randomized controlled trials of corticosteroid management have shown that during the first 6 months, patients show an increase in muscle strength and an improvement in timed function tests and functional abilities (Mendell et al., 1989). These improvements last 18 months or more and, although the disease progresses thereafter, the progression is slower than would be expected without steroid therapy (Fenichel et al., 1991). With the tests and measures described above, physical therapists can assist the medical team in monitoring the effects of medications on muscle performance and functional abilities.

Diagnosis

Sam's physical therapy diagnoses continue to be impaired posture, ROM, and muscle performance, with minimal activity limitations and participation restrictions in the areas of physical education and community sports.

Prognosis

In general, Sam's condition is associated with a progressively poor prognosis. However, it is difficult to make specific short-term prognostic statements regarding muscle performance and functional skills because of the unpredictable response to long-term prednisone therapy.

Goals

Long-term goals include maintaining ROM, strength, and maximizing functional abilities and participation.

Examination Update: To promote Sam's assuming responsibility for his personal health-care needs, short-term goals for this visit include teaching Sam techniques for self-stretching and incorporating these into his daily routine. Short-term goals for the next 6 months based on current practice would include the following:

1. Sam will correctly perform self-stretching of the gastrocnemius/soleus muscles.
2. Sam will assume a prone position to stretch his hip flexors for 30 minutes once daily.
3. Sam will maintain his ability to walk independently on level indoor surfaces and uneven outdoor terrain. He will monitor the distances he is able to walk without getting overly tired.
4. Sam will continue to be able to walk up and down stairs independently with one hand on a railing, using a reciprocal pattern (step-over-step) to ascend and a nonreciprocal pattern (step-to-step) to descend.
5. Sam will ride his bicycle around the neighborhood for up to 30 minutes daily during his summer vacation.

Intervention

Coordination, Communication, and Documentation

During the past year, the school physical therapist continued to monitor Sam and to work with the classroom teacher and the physical education teacher to modify his activities based on his recent improvements in mobility. In the fall, the clinic physical therapist will communicate with the school therapist, either in writing or by telephone, to coordinate care for the new school year.

Patient/Client-Related Instruction

The clinic physical therapist encouraged Sam's parents to continue the program of stretching, positioning, and swimming to maximize the gains achieved through steroid therapy. Sam was instructed in self-stretching exercises for the gastrocnemius/soleus and the proper position for prone stretching of the hip flexors, which he can do while watching television or reading. The therapist reminded his parents not to restrict Sam's activities unless he complained of being tired after a good night's sleep or of cramps in specific muscles. They were also encouraged to increase the frequency of swimming over the summer to replace some of the exercise he typically engages in at school. High-intensity aerobic activities are not recommended

because of musculoskeletal constraints (Bushby et al., 2010b).

Episode of Physical Therapy Prevention

Sam will continue to be followed in the MDA clinic at 6-month intervals, where physical therapy services will include examination, instruction, and education. He and his parents reported regular adherence to his home exercise program and seemed to appreciate its benefits. The family was advised to contact the clinic if they had any questions or concerns before the next visit.

Examination: Age 10 Years

History

Sam has been healthy since his last clinic visit 6 months ago. He continues the prednisone therapy and has developed Cushingoid facies, a typical side effect of corticosteroid use (Griggs et al., 1991). Sam has maintained most of the functional gains he had made when he started on medication, showing only a minimal decline. Both Sam and his parents are extremely pleased with the maintenance of his physical capabilities, as they are aware of the natural history of DMD. Sam attended the 1-week summer camp sponsored by the MDA last month and is already looking forward to attending next year.

Systems Review
Growth and Development

Sam is short in stature and has gained weight over the past year; when compared to typical boys his age, he is in the 20th percentile for height and the 90th percentile for weight. This is of some concern to him and his parents, as he prepares to enter middle school this fall. Sam and his parents know that both growth retardation and weight gain are side effects of prednisone, as documented in long-term studies of corticosteroid use (Biggar et al., 2006).

Cardiovascular and Pulmonary

Sam's ECG at this clinic visit showed signs of cardiomyopathy, such as abnormal Q waves, prominent R waves, and elevation of the ST segment. These findings do not require any new activity restrictions, but he will be referred to a cardiologist for long-term management of the cardiomyopathy. Pulmonary function tests will be conducted to monitor his FVC. Sam's respiratory rate is WNL, but his heart rate is at the upper limit of normal at 100 beats per minute. Resting tachycardia is a common finding in boys with DMD (Bushby et al., 2010b).

Integumentary

The integumentary system is WNL.

Musculoskeletal

Sam's standing posture exhibits increased lumbar lordosis, with a slightly wider base of support as compared to 6 months ago. ROM and muscle performance will be examined in detail.

Neuromuscular

Neuromuscular examination is WNL in terms of motor control, sensory integrity, and muscle tone. Specific functional activities documented previously will be examined in detail.

Communication and Cognition

Sam continues to communicate at an age-appropriate level. He remains outgoing, and he reports an interest in history and geography. Unlike about 30% of boys with DMD, Sam performs well academically and does not exhibit any problems with learning (Anderson et al., 2002; Dubowitz, 1995; Hinton et al., 2000).

Tests and Measures

Results of the examination of ROM, muscle performance, timed functional activities, and FVC are presented in Table 23.1. Sam is slower on all timed function tests and is no longer able to run. His gait is wide-based; weakness of the quadriceps causes inconsistent terminal extension on heel strike and requires him to negotiate stairs using a nonreciprocal pattern. Sam cannot keep pace with his peers in the school and community environments because of difficulty on uneven surfaces and fear of falling.

Evaluation, Diagnosis, and Prognosis

Evaluation

Results of Sam's examination support the observations made by him and his parents. Although there are some declines compared with previous examinations, he continues to perform well above expectations as reported in the natural history studies. Sam has resumed using Gowers' maneuver when rising from the floor. He tends to toe-walk more than he did at his last clinic visit. Although he is able to climb stairs without holding

a railing, he reports feeling safer when using it. Sam's participation in his physical education class is becoming quite limited, and the school physical therapist has discussed the option of adaptive physical education for next year when he starts middle school. Architectural barriers will be of concern, too, as the middle school is a two-story building that is much larger than his elementary school. The school therapist will address the implications for Sam's mobility within the school building, including emergency evacuation procedures. Sam's FVC continues to show an increase and is nearly normal. Natural history studies of pulmonary function in boys with DMD indicate that FVC continues to increase until about 10 to 12 years of age, plateaus for a couple of years, and then begins to decline (Rideau et al., 1981).

Prognosis

Sam has done extremely well, given the natural history of DMD. Reports of the effects of corticosteroids beyond a decade are currently unavailable, making it difficult to predict the long-term future. Sam and his parents are aware of this and appreciate that we are learning from his follow-up visits. In the short term, decreasing muscle performance, ROM, and functional abilities continue to be the main concern.

Goals

Long-term goals continue to be the maximizing of Sam's functional abilities and participation within the limitations of his progressive disorder.

Short-term goals for the next 6 months include maintaining ROM and strength through daily stretching exercises and participation in an adaptive physical education program and/or a community pool program.

Goal Update: Short-term goals for Sam based on current practice would include the following:

1. Sam will correctly perform self-stretching of the gastrocnemius/soleus muscles.
2. Sam will assume a prone position to stretch his hip flexors for 30 minutes once daily.
3. Sam will maintain his ability to walk independently on level indoor surfaces.
4. Sam will continue to be able to walk up and down stairs independently with one hand on a railing.
5. Sam will ride his bicycle around the neighborhood for up to 30 minutes daily during his summer vacation.
6. Sam will swim at least twice per week, at the YMCA or community pool.

Intervention

Coordination, Communication, and Documentation

The middle school that Sam will attend has planned to accommodate him by ensuring that all his classes will be on the entry level, avoiding the need to climb stairs. A school-owned manual wheelchair will be available if necessary for long-distance mobility and field trips, though Sam is reluctant to use it. An assistance plan is already in place for emergency evacuation, and he will practice those procedures during fire drills. Sam and his parents are concerned that he may not be able to participate fully in physical education. A program of regular and adaptive physical education will be developed by the school physical therapist and the physical education teacher. Sam has expressed a desire to participate in team sports in some capacity, perhaps as scorekeeper or timekeeper; although he would prefer to play, he will enjoy the socialization. He will explore the possibility of being transported to the community's indoor pool to swim while the high school swim team practices there. The physical therapist has also discussed the importance of standing and weight bearing. Sam's classroom teacher has agreed to allow him to stand while doing class work over several short sessions throughout the school day.

Patient/Client-Related Instruction

Sam and his father described his exercise routine. Sam does self-stretching for the heel cords and ITB/TFL as part of his physical education routine at school, and he follows the positioning instructions when he comes home and watches television or reads a book. His father performs the stretches for the heelcord and ITB/TFL at bedtime. Sam also understands the importance of standing and weight bearing and spends 3 to 4 hours a day on his feet between the school and home settings (Bushby et al., 2010b; Vignos, 1983).

Synopsis of Visit at Age 15 Years

History

Sam has been healthy over the past year. He continues on prednisone, although at a reduced dose of 0.5 mg/kg/day because of his weight gain. Sam has developed punctate cataracts in both eyes, a long-term side effect of steroid use (Fenichel et al., 1991; Moxley et al., 2005; Biggar et al., 2006). Although they do not affect his vision or require surgery at this time, he will be followed annually by an ophthalmologist. The orthopedist obtained a baseline spine radiograph today to start monitoring him for development of scoliosis. Sam is having greater difficulty walking long distances, and he chose to use a wheelchair during the family's recent trip to Disney World. His parents are planning to obtain a manual wheelchair from MDA's "loan closet" for occasional family trips this summer. Sam has trouble climbing stairs, and the family is exploring the option of either adding or converting space on the first floor of their house into a bedroom and an accessible bathroom for Sam. They also plan to add a ramp to the side entrance from the garage. Sam's mobility limitations have decreased his participation with his peers in the neighborhood and in the community. He continues to enjoy school and to do well academically. He is interested in history and computer sciences, and he is already beginning to explore options for college.

Systems Review

Growth and Development

Sam's growth rate has slowed since he started on prednisone. He has been struggling to manage his weight, but he hopes to be more successful with the reduction in his prednisone dose and more vigilant attention to his diet. Anecdotal data from our clinic suggests that some boys on prednisone have shown delayed secondary sex characteristics, and these findings have been shared with Sam and his parents.

Cardiovascular and Pulmonary

Vital signs are WNL. Sam has no cardiac or pulmonary symptoms. Annually, he continues to be monitored by the cardiologist and to have formal pulmonary function evaluations. Results of the FVC are noted in Table 23.1. His FVC is still continuing to improve; therefore, any further tests or preventive measures are not necessary at this stage.

Integumentary

The integumentary system is WNL.

Musculoskeletal

Increased tightness is noted at all joints in the lower extremities, especially the ankles.

Neuromuscular

Sam's muscle weakness has increased, and he had more difficulty with the timed function tests at this clinic visit. When asked to run, he increased his pace to a fast walk without demonstrating the period of double float that defines running. When climbing stairs, Sam relies heavily on the railing for support. At home, he goes downstairs in the morning and does not go upstairs to his room until the evening. He is no longer able to rise from the floor without pulling himself up on the furniture and rarely performs this transfer at home.

Tests and Measures

Results of the ROM, muscle performance tests, timed function tests, and FVC are detailed in Table 23.1.

Mobility

Sam's gait is now characterized by more consistent toe walking, a markedly lordotic posture, and a wide base of support, as he seeks to maintain stability. He is aware that his weakness compromises his balance, and he needs to be careful, especially in the crowded school hallways. KAFOs are helpful in maintaining mobility during the first decade, but by the second decade they are not as appropriate for maintaining walking and are usually used only for therapeutic standing. Standing tables/standers may be another option to prolong standing while providing appropriate support (Bushby et al., 2010b; Eagle, 2002). Sam does not need a stander at this time, because he is still able to stand and to ambulate for short distances.

Intervention

Coordination, Communication, and Documentation

The high school has accommodated Sam by clustering his classes and locker in one wing of the building. A manual wheelchair is available for him for emergency evacuations and to travel long distances, such as to the cafeteria or library; the school physical therapist advised him to ask a friend to push him for long distances, as excessive self-propelling may cause too much muscular exertion. Sam has chosen to continue to walk even though it takes him longer than it did in previous years. He is released a few minutes early from each class to allow him unobstructed passing time between classes. Safety is a concern because his muscle weakness could cause him to fall easily.

Patient/Client-Related Instruction

Sam works out in the training room with his peers. The school physical therapist and the physical education teacher developed an exercise routine for the upper extremities using mild resistance. Sam also performs pulmonary exercises daily with an incentive spirometer. Although there is a paucity of evidence for long-term benefits of respiratory exercises, short-term studies support respiratory muscle training (Finder et al., 2004). The clinic physical therapist instructed Sam and his parents in assisted coughing techniques to be used when he has an upper respiratory infection.

Sam is having difficulty continuing his self-stretching of the ankles. The clinic physical therapist met with him and his father to review his stretching exercises for the heel cords, ITB/TFL, and hamstrings. Sam reported that he continues to spend 45 to 60 minutes prone daily when watching television or reading. The therapist discussed the option of using night splints to maintain his ankle ROM. The clinic does not routinely provide them because most boys do not tolerate them all night. Also, they do not extend above the knee, stretching only the soleus and the distal portion of the gastrocnemius muscles. With an understanding of their benefits, Sam agreed to try the splints.

The physical therapist explained the options of power mobility, either a scooter or a motorized wheelchair, comparing their costs and ease of transportation. Sam and his parents decided that they would discuss the issue and speak with the school personnel, other families who had made these decisions, and the MDA services coordinator. They will investigate how much of the costs would be covered by their medical insurance and what out-of-pocket expenses they would incur. The clinic social worker will assist them in seeking alternative sources of funding.

Synopsis of Visit at Age 18 Years
History

Sam graduated from high school in May. He will attend a college that is located about a 4-hour drive from home. The college is well known for its services and environmental adaptations to meet the special needs of students with disabilities. Sam is excited about living on campus, where a personal care assistant (PCA) will help him with his activities of daily living and his stretching program an hour in the morning and at bedtime. Sam also plans to work out in the wheelchair-accessible pool on campus, 2 to 3 times per week. His PCA will help him in the changing room at the pool and will assist him in getting in and out of the pool. In preparation for his move to college, Sam obtained a motorized wheelchair this spring. The family purchased a van and equipped it with a lift so that they can transport Sam and his chair back and forth from college. At some point during the next 2 years, Sam hopes to have the van adapted to his needs and to pursue driver training so that he can drive the van himself.

Examination

Sam is unable to get up from the floor or climb stairs. He continues to be able to walk around the house, though he often uses the furniture and walls for support. He needs assistance with some self-care activities but otherwise is fairly independent, with adaptations in the bathroom (a shower seat, raised toilet seat, grab bars) and bedroom (railings on the side of his bed). Sam has difficulty with overhead activities such as shampooing his hair and pulling a shirt over his head. He is still able to feed himself, use his computer keyboard, and write. The shoulder girdle muscles are in the 3– range. The elbow flexors and extensors are 4–, and the distal hand muscles are in the 4 range. His grip is fair. Results of ROM and FVC tests and measures are detailed in Table 23.1.

Coordination, Communication, and Documentation and Patient/Client-Related Instruction

Sam and his family are very knowledgeable about his condition and the various intervention and management options. They have attended seminars and support groups offered by the MDA and Parent Project

Muscular Dystrophy. Sam has attended MDA camp every summer for the past 7 years, where he has met other children and adolescents with inherited neuromuscular disorders. Therefore, he is well aware of the progression that occurs in these disorders; he knows that without corticosteroid therapy, he would have lost the ability to ambulate 6 to 10 years ago. The whole family has been involved in Sam's care and management: (1) helping him adhere to his home program of stretching, positioning, and swimming, (2) obtaining equipment as needed, (3) planning home modifications, and (4) supporting his desire to live a productive life. Because Sam is going away to college, the clinic team again reviewed the (1) plan for continuing visits with the multidisciplinary team at least once a year, (2) importance of a pulmonary workout to maintain respiratory function, (3) need to seek immediate care in case of even minor respiratory problems, and (4) emergency plan in case of a fall when Sam is alone. They discussed future equipment needs, including mechanical transfer devices for use in the bedroom and bathroom, a mobile arm support to assist with feeding and writing, and a mechanical ventilatory apparatus to assist inspiration, expiration, and coughing (Table 23.2).

Synopsis at Age 21 Years

Since Sam started college, his medical management has been coordinated by a clinic serving adults with neuromuscular disorders that is located near the college. Even

Table 23.2 Adaptive Equipment Recommended Based on Vignos Functional Rating Scale for Duchenne Muscular Dystrophy

Vignos Level	Adaptive Equipment Required
1. Walks and climbs stairs without assistance.	• None
2. Walks and climbs stairs with aid of railing.	• Railings for stair climbing
3. Walks and climbs stairs slowly with aid of railing (over 25 seconds for 8 standard steps).	• Railings for stair climbing • Ankle foot orthoses (AFO) for night splints
4. Walks unassisted and rises from chair but cannot climb stairs	• AFOs for night splints
5. Walks unassisted but cannot rise from chair or climb stairs.	• Manual wheelchair for long distances • AFOs or knee-ankle-foot orthoses (KAFOs) for night splints • May need resting hand splints for tight finger flexors
6. Walks only with assistance or walks independently with KAFOs.	• Manual wheelchair for long distances with assistance for propelling • AFOs or KAFOs for night splints • May need resting hand splints for tight finger flexors

Table 23.2 Adaptive Equipment Recommended Based on Vignos Functional Rating Scale for Duchenne Muscular Dystrophy—cont'd

Vignos Level	Adaptive Equipment Required
7. Walks with KAFOs but requires assistance for balance.	• Manual wheelchair with assistance for propelling, motorized scooter, or power wheelchair for long distances • AFOs or KAFOs for night splints • May need resting hand splints for tight finger flexors
8. Stands with KAFOs but cannot walk even with assistance.	• Power wheelchair (may include power standing) • Mechanical transfer device for use in bedroom and bathroom • Devices to assist with feeding and writing • May need mechanical nocturnal ventilatory support and mechanical cough assistance • AFOs and KAFOs for night splints • May need resting hand splints for tight finger flexors
9. Is in wheelchair full-time. Strength of elbow flexors is >3/5.	• Power wheelchair (may include power standing) • Mechanical transfer device for use in bedroom and bathroom • Devices to assist with feeding and writing • Mechanical ventilatory apparatus to assist inspiration, expiration, and cough • AFOs and KAFOs for night splints • May wear AFOs while seated in wheelchair • May need resting hand splints for tight finger flexors
10. Is in wheelchair or bed. Strength of elbow flexors is <3/5.	• Power wheelchair (may include power standing) • Mechanical transfer devices for use in bedroom and bathroom • Mobile arm support to assist with feeding and writing • Mechanical ventilatory apparatus to assist inspiration, expiration, and cough • AFOs and KAFOs for night splints • May wear AFOs while seated in wheelchair • May need resting hand splints for tight finger flexors

Source: Adapted from Vignos, P.J., Spencer, G.E., & Archibald, K.C. (1963). Management of progressive muscular dystrophy of childhood. *Journal of American Medical Association, 184* (2), 89–110.

if he had continued to live at home, eventually his care would have needed to be transferred from the pediatric MDA clinic to providers serving adult patients. This transition in care can be stressful for patients and families who have developed close and long-standing relationships with their providers since the diagnosis was confirmed. Sam's parents have continued to encourage him to take more responsibility for his health and well-being and to manage the coordination of his health-care needs. They have supported him in completing the necessary directive documents, such as health-care proxies and a living will.

Sam is pursuing a degree in communication and hopes to become a sportswriter. He is still able to feed himself and to use his computer keyboard. His college provides accommodations during exams and assistance in completing papers.

Discussion

This case report of a boy with DMD highlights the responsibilities of the physical therapist in the care of children with inherited neuromuscular disorders. When preparing to conduct an examination and provide intervention for a child with a medical diagnosis that is uncommon or unfamiliar, it is important to review the following information about the condition: (1) etiology, (2) pathophysiology, (3) natural history or prognosis, (4) resulting impairments in body structures and functions, (5) common activity limitations and participation restrictions, and (6) current medical, surgical, and rehabilitative management. A comprehensive review of the literature regarding physical therapy interventions that have been shown to be effective, combined with expert consensus, can lead to the development of evidence-based plans of care.

Physical therapy for children with progressive disorders is different from intervention for those with a condition that is expected to show some improvement (e.g., cerebral palsy) or complete recovery (e.g., fracture). Although all of these children may have "impaired muscle function" as one of their physical therapy diagnoses, the medical prognosis and natural history will determine the appropriate goals and interventions. In the case of a child with a progressive neuromuscular disorder, the goals may not be to normalize strength and activities of daily living but to prevent and/or delay activity limitations and participation restrictions, to maximize function and quality of life within the imposed constraints.

School-Based Physical Therapy

Although the multidisciplinary clinic is generally the primary service provider for boys with DMD, the school-based physical therapist plays a complementary role and, therefore, should be knowledgeable about all aspects of the continuum of care. An essential responsibility is to teach other members of the school team and the student's peers about the nature of the disability, to promote understanding, develop realistic goals, and support the psychosocial needs of the student. The school therapist works collaboratively with the physical education teacher, classroom teacher, school nurse, occupational therapist, and teaching assistants regarding mobility issues, access and participation in the educational program, and assistive technology.

During the ambulatory stage, the school therapist may reinforce the regimen of stretching, positioning, and splinting to maintain range of motion of the gastrocnemius/soleus group, ITB/TFL, hamstrings, and hip flexors. Exercise is promoted in the form of functional activities in school and community recreation, including swimming (Bushby et al., 2010b).

As ambulation deteriorates, the school-based physical therapist should encourage the family to obtain a manual wheelchair for family outings and emergency evacuation at school. The school and clinic therapists may work together to prescribe a power wheelchair, which will become the student's primary means of mobility around the school, retaining the manual wheelchair as backup. Features of the power wheelchair should include "headrest, solid seat and back, lateral trunk supports, power tilt and recline, power-adjustable seat height, and power-elevating leg rests (with swing-away or flip-up footrests to facilitate transfers) . . . along with pressure-relieving cushion, hip guides, and flip-down knee adductors" (Bushby et al., 2010b, p. 179). For some boys, power standing chairs may be appropriate. A mechanical lift for toileting may be needed for use in school. The student may also require a computer for academic work, as it may be less fatiguing than handwriting.

Students who are not treated with corticosteroids may develop respiratory insufficiency during their late teenage years, in contrast to the mid-20s for those who are treated. For adolescents who are untreated, parents and school staff should be aware of signs of declining respiratory function, such as morning headaches, daytime sleepiness, and excessive fatigue. These symptoms are not likely to arise until the FVC falls below 1 liter; nighttime oximetry is recommended when the FVC is below 1.25 liters.

Transition Planning

The school physical therapist should serve as a key member of the transition team, to assist the student and his family in preparing for life after high school. Early in the process, a student seeking postsecondary education should meet with the college's Office of Disability Services to discuss services that are available and those that should be implemented. He will need to consider whether he will live at home or on campus. In either case, a PCA may be required to help manage transportation, books and supplies, toileting, and mobility around the campus (e.g., navigating among buildings, opening doors). A student who lives on campus will also need a PCA for other activities of daily living.

Preparation for employment, too, is the role of the transition team, to assist with choosing an appropriate job, training the student to perform required tasks, assessing architectural barriers, and anticipating future needs for equipment and personnel. The physical therapist can offer a valuable perspective in this process.

Summary

Sam's case history illustrates the improved prognosis for boys with DMD, attributable to advances in medical, surgical, and rehabilitative management. As a result, many of these young men are graduating from high school and college, and they are looking forward to living independently, being employed, and becoming productive members of society (Bushby et al., 2010a, 2010b). The role of the physical therapist should expand to meet the changing needs of this older population of patients with DMD and their families, serving as consultants, coordinators, and educators, as well as direct-service providers. The patient needs to learn to advocate for himself and to teach his caregivers how to assist him, in order to navigate the adult world of health care, employment, residential life, transportation, and recreation (Campbell, 1997).

Interventions Update: Physical therapy for children with Duchene muscular dystrophy is well described in consensus documents previously described in this chapter (Bushby, 2010b). Only a few recent research studies of physical therapy interventions have been conducted with this population and most of the sample sizes have been small. Recent evidence related to physical therapy interventions for children with muscular dystrophy is summarized in Table 23.3.

Table 23.3 Evidence-Based Interventions for Muscular Dystrophics

Intervention	Author (Date)	Study Design	No. of Subjects	Question	Findings
Therapeutic Exercise: Aerobic Capacity/ Endurance Training	Sveen et al., 2008	Pre-post outcome	18 (11 with Becker muscular dystrophy, 7 matched controls)	Will participation in 30-minute exercise program at 65% max oxygen uptake for 12 weeks improve VO_{2max}?	Boys with muscular dystrophy had 47% increase in VO_{2max} with no evidence of increased muscle damage.
Therapeutic Exercise: Strength, Power, and Endurance Training for Muscles	Topin et al, 2002	Randomized control trial, double blinded	16 (Duchenne Muscular Dystrophy)	Will home inspiratory muscle training increase respiratory muscle endurance?	Training group increased respiratory muscle endurance.
	Yeldan, 2008	Prospective outcome study	23 (17 with limb girdle dystrophy, 6 with Becker muscular dystrophy)	Will inspiratory muscle training and breathing exercises improve respiratory function in a 12-week home program?	Inspiratory muscle training increased inspiratory muscle strength more than breathing exercises. Breathing exercises increased both inspiratory and expiratory muscle strength.

DISCUSSION QUESTIONS

1. Discuss the difficulty in developing and writing appropriate objectives for a child whose ability to function is expected to deteriorate over time.

2. What are some aids for activities of daily living that might commonly be used to help a child with DMD?

3. What are some obstacles you would look for when evaluating a high school for a student with DMD who uses a power wheelchair?

4. What are some of the transitional issues faced by young men with DMD in the educational, health-care, and independent-living settings? What is the role of the physical therapist in preparing them for this transition?

Recommended Readings

Glanzman, A.M., & Flickinger, J.M. (2008). Neuromuscular disorders in childhood: Physical therapy intervention. In J.S. Tecklin (Ed.), *Pediatric physical therapy* (4th ed., pp. 335–363). Philadelphia: Lippincott Williams & Wilkins.

Harris, S.E., & Cherry, D.B. (1974). Childhood progressive muscular dystrophy and the role of physical therapy. *Physical Therapy, 54* (1), 4–12. (Even though published 30 years ago, this article is still pertinent today in terms of physical therapy examination, intervention, and management. It is a classic!)

Stuberg, W.A. (2012). Muscular dystrophy and spinal muscular atrophy. In S.K. Campbell, R.J. Palisano, & M. N. Orlin (Eds.), *Physical therapy for children* (4th ed., pp. 353-384). St. Louis: Elsevier Saunders.

Web Resources

The following websites are recommended for information regarding the latest research findings, clinical management, support groups, and advocacy initiatives.

National Institute of Neurological Disorders and Stroke
   http://www.ninds.nih.gov

National Institute of Child Health and Human Development
   http://www.nichd.nih.gov

Muscular Dystrophy Association
   http://www.mdausa.org

Parent Project Muscular Dystrophy
   http://www.parentprojectmd.org

References

American Physical Therapy Association (APTA). (2001). Guide to physical therapist practice (2nd ed.). *Physical Therapy, 81*, 6–746.

Anderson, J.L., Head, S.I., Rae, C., & Morley, J.W. (2002). Brain function in Duchenne muscular dystrophy. *Brain, 125*, 4–13.

Angelini, C., Pergoraro, E., Turella, E., Intino, M.T., Pini, A., & Costa, C. (1994). Deflazacort in Duchenne dystrophy: Study of long-term effect. *Muscle and Nerve, 17*, 386–391.

Arias R., Andrews J., Pandya S. et al. (2011). Palliative care services in families of males with Duchenne muscular dystrophy. *Muscle and Nerve 44*(1): 93-101.

Backman, E., & Henriksson, K.G. (1995). Low-dose prednisolone treatment in Duchenne and Becker muscular dystrophy. *Neuromuscular Disorders, 5*, 233–241.

Barohn, R.J., Levine E.J., Olson J.O., & Mendell, J.R., (1988). Gastric hypomobility in Duchenne's muscular dystrophy. *New England Journal of Medicine, 319* (1), 15–18.

Biggar, W.D., Gingras, M., Feblings, D.L., Harris, V.A., & Steele, C.A. (2001). Deflazacort treatment of Duchenne muscular dystrophy. *Journal of Pediatrics, 138*, 45–50.

Biggar, W.D., Harris, V.A., Eliasoph, L., & Alman, B. (2006). Long-term benefits of deflazacort treatment for boys with Duchenne muscular dystrophy in their second decade. *Neuromuscular Disorders, 16*, 249–255.

Brooke, M.H., Fenichel, G., Griggs, R., Mendell, J.R., Moxley, R., Miller, J.P., et al. (1983). Clinical investigations in Duchenne dystrophy. Part 2. Determination of the "power" of therapeutic trials based on the natural history. *Muscle and Nerve, 6*, 91–103.

Brooke, M.H., Fenichel, G., Griggs, R., Mendell, J.R., Moxley, R., Miller, J.P., et al. (1989). Duchenne muscular dystrophy: Patterns of clinical progression and effects of supportive therapy. *Neurology, 39*, 475–481.

Brooke, M.H., Griggs, R.C., Mendell, J.R., Fenichel, G.M., Shumate, J.B., et al. (1981). Clinical trial in Duchenne dystrophy: Design of the protocol. *Muscle and Nerve, 4*, 186–197.

Bushby, K., Finkel, R., Birnkrant, D.J., Case, L.E., Clemens, P.R., Cripe, L., et al. (2010a). Diagnosis and management of Duchenne muscular dystrophy, part 1: Implementation of multidisciplinary care. *Lancet Neurology, 9*, p. 77–93.

Bushby, K., Finkel, R., Birnkrant, D.J., Case, L.E., Clemens, P.R., Cripe, L., et al. (2010b). Diagnosis and management of Duchenne muscular dystrophy, part 2: Implementation of multidisciplinary care. *Lancet Neurology, 9*, p. 177–189.

Campbell, S.K. (1997). Therapy programs for children that last a lifetime. *Physical and Occupational Therapy in Pediatrics, 1*, 1–15.

Centers for Disease Control and Prevention. (2009). Prevalence of Duchenne/Becker muscular dystrophy among males aged 5–24 years—four states, 2007. *Morbidity and Mortality Weekly Report, 58*(40), 1119–1122.

Chénard, A.A., Bécane, H.M., Tertrain, F., de Kermadec, J.M., & Weiss, Y.A. (1993). Ventricular arrhythmia in Duchenne muscular dystrophy: Prevalence, significance and prognosis. *Neuromuscular Disorders, 3*(3), 201–206.

Ciafaloni, E., Fox, D.J., Pandya, S., Westfield, C.P., Puzhankara, S., Romitti, P.A., et al. (2009). Delayed diagnosis in Duchenne muscular dystrophy: Data from the Muscular

Dystrophy Surveillance, Tracking, and Research Network (MD STARnet). *Journal of Pediatrics, 155*(3), 380–385.

de Kermadec, J.M., Bécane, H.M., Chénard, A., Tertrain, F., & Weiss, Y.A. (1994). Prevalence of left ventricular systolic dysfunction in Duchenne muscular dystrophy: An echocardiographic study. *American Heart Journal, 127*(3), 618–623.

deLateur, B.J., & Giaconi, R.M. (1979). Effect on maximal strength of submaximal exercise in Duchenne muscular dystrophy. *American Journal of Physical Medicine, 58*, 26–36.

DeSilva, S., Drachman, D.B., Mellits, D., & Kunel, R.W. (1987). Prednisone treatment in Duchenne muscular dystrophy: Long-term benefit. *Archives of Neurology, 44*, 818–822.

Dubowitz, V. (1995). *Muscle disorders in childhood* (2nd ed.). London: W.B. Saunders.

Duchenne, G.B. (1868). Recherches sur la paralysie musculaire pseudohypertrophique ou paralysie myosclérosique. *Archives Générales de Médecine (11)*5, 179, 305.

Eagle, M. (2002). Report of the Muscular Dystrophy Campaign Workshop: Exercise in neuromuscular diseases. *Neuromuscular Disorders 12*(10), 975–988.

Eagle, M., Baudouin, S.V., Chandler, C., Giddings, D.R., Bullock, R., & Bushby, K. (2002). Survival in Duchenne muscular dystrophy: Improvements in life expectancy since 1967 and the impact of home nocturnal ventilation. *Neuromuscular Disorders, 12*(10), 926–930.

Eagle, M., Bourke, J., Bullock, R., Gibson, M., Mehta, J, Giddings, D., et al. (2007). Managing Duchenne muscular dystrophy: The additive effect of spinal surgery and home nocturnal ventilation in improving survival. *Neuromuscular Disorders, 17*(6), 470–475.

Emery, A.E.H. (1991). Population frequencies of inherited neuromuscular diseases: A world survey. *Neuromuscular Disorders 1*, 19–29.

Emery, A.E.H. (2003). *Duchenne muscular dystrophy* (2nd ed.). Oxford: Oxford University Press.

Fenichel, G.M., Florence, J.M., Pestronk, A., Mendell, R.T., Griggs, R.C., Miller, J.P., et al. (1991). Long-term benefit from prednisone in Duchenne muscular dystrophy. *Neurology, 41*, 1874–1877.

Finder, J.D., Birnkrant, D., Carl, J., Farber, H.J., Gozal, D., Iannacone, S.T., et al., (2004). Respiratory care of the patient with Duchenne muscular dystrophy: ATS consensus statement. *American Journal of Respiratory Critical Care Medicine, 170*(4), 456–465.

Florence, J.M., Pandya, S., King, W.M., Robinson, J.D., Baty, J., Miller, J.P., Signore, L.C., et al. (1992). Intrarater reliability of manual muscle test (Medical Research Council Scale) grades in Duchenne's muscular dystrophy. *Physical Therapy, 72*(2), 115–122.

Florence, J.M., Pandya, S., King, W.M., Robinson, J.D., Signore, L.C., Wentzell, M., et al. The CIDD Group. (1984). Clinical trials in Duchenne muscular dystrophy: Standardization and reliability of evaluation procedures. *Physical Therapy, 64*(1), 41–45.

Galasko, C.S., Delaney, C., & Morris, P. (1992). Spinal stabilisation in Duchenne muscular dystrophy. *The Journal of Bone and Joint Surgery (British), 74B*, 210–215.

Gowers, W.R. (1879). Clinical lecture on pseudohypertrophic muscular paralysis. *Lancet, 2*, 73–75.

Grange, R.W., & Call, J.A. (2007). Recommendations to define exercise prescription for Duchenne muscular dystrophy. *Exercise & Sport Sciences Reviews, 35*(1), 12–17.

Griggs, R.C., Moxley, R.T., Mendell, J.R., Fenichel, G.M., Brooke, M.H., Pestronk, A., et al. (1991). Prednisone in Duchenne dystrophy. A randomized controlled trial defining the time course and dose response. *Archives of Neurology, 48*, 383–388.

Griggs, R.C., Moxley, R.T., Mendell, J.R., Fenichel, G.M., Brooke, M.H., Pestronk, A., et al. (1993). Duchenne dystrophy: Randomized controlled trial of prednisone (18 months) and azathioprine (12 months). *Neurology, 43*, 520–527.

Harris, S.E., & Cherry, D.B. (1974). Childhood progressive muscular dystrophy and the role of physical therapy. *Physical Therapy, 54*(1), 4–12.

Heckmatt, J.Z., Dubowitz, V., & Hyde, S.A. (1985). Prolongation of walking in Duchenne muscular dystrophy with lightweight orthoses: Review of 57 cases. *Developmental Medicine and Child Neurology, 27*, 149–154.

Hinton, V.J., De Vivo, D.C., Nereo, N.E., Goldstein, E., & Stern, Y. (2000). Poor verbal working memory across intellectual level in boys with Duchenne dystrophy. *Neurology, 54*(11), 2127–2132.

Hislop, H.J., & Montgomery, J. (2002). Techniques of manual examination. In *Daniels and Worthingham's Muscle Testing* (7th ed.). Philadelphia: W.B. Saunders.

Hoffman, E.P., Brown, R.H., & Kunkel, L.M. (1987). Dystrophin: The protein product of the Duchenne muscular dystrophy locus. *Cell, 51*, 919–928.

Houde, S., Filiatrault, M., Fournier, A., Dube, J., D'Arcy, S., Berube, D., et al. (2008). Deflazacort use in Duchenne muscular dystrophy: An 8-year follow-up. *Pediatric Neurology, 38*(3), 200–206.

King, W.M., Ruttencutter, R., Nagaraja, H.N., Matkovic, V., Landoll, J., Hoyle C., et al. (2007). Orthopedic outcomes of long-term daily corticosteroid treatment in Duchenne muscular dystrophy. *Neurology, 68*(19), 1607–1613.

Kunkel, L.M., Monaco, A.P., Middlesworth, W., Ochs, S.D., & Latt, S.A. (1985). Specific cloning of DNA fragments absent from the DNA of a male patient with an X chromosome deletion. *Proceedings of the National Academy of Science USA, 82*, 4778–4782.

Luque, E.R. (1982). Segmental spinal stabilization for the correction of scoliosis. *Clinical Orthopedics, 163*, 192–198.

Manzur, A.Y., Kinali M., & Muntoni F. (2008). Update on the management of Duchenne muscular dystrophy. *Archives of Disease in Childhood* published online 30 July 2008.

Manzur, A.Y., Kuntzer, T., Pike, M., & Swan, A. (2004). Glucocorticoid corticosteroids for Duchenne muscular dystrophy (Review). In *The Cochrane Library*, Issue 3. Chichester, UK: John Wiley & Sons.

Manzur, A.Y., Kuntzer, T., Pike, M., & Swan, A. (2008). Glucocorticoid corticosteroids for Duchenne muscular dystrophy. *Cochrane Database of Systematic Reviews. Issue 1*.

Markham, L.W., Kinnett, K., Wong, B.L., Woodrow Benson, D., & Cripe, L.H. (2008). Corticosteroid treatment retards development of ventricular dysfunction in Duchenne muscular dystrophy. *Neuromuscular Disorders, 18*(5), 365–370.

Markham, L.W., Spicer, R.L., Khoury, P.R., Wong, B.L., Mathews, K.D., & Cripe, L.H. (2005). Steroid therapy and cardiac function in Duchenne muscular dystrophy. *Pediatric Cardiology, 26* (6), 768–771.

Matthews, D.J., James, K.A., Miller, L.A., Pandya, S., Campbell, K.A., Ciafaloni, E., et al. (2010). Use of corticosteroids in a population based cohort of boys with Duchenne and Becker muscular dystrophy. *Journal of Child Neurology,* e-pub 5 March 2010.

Medical Research Council, Memorandum # 45. (1976) *Aids to the examination of the peripheral nervous system.* Her Majesty's Stationery Office, Government Bookshops, London

Mendell, J.R., Moxley, R.T., Griggs, R.C., Brooke, M.H., Fenichel, G.M., Miller, J.P., et al. (1989). Randomized double-blind six-month trial of prednisone in Duchenne's muscular dystrophy. *New England Journal of Medicine, 320,* 1592–1597.

Mesa, L.E., Dubrovsky, A.L., Corderi, J., Maarco, P., & Flores, D. (1991). Steroids in Duchenne muscular dystrophy: Deflazacort trial. *Neuromuscular Disorders, 1,* 261–266.

Miller, F., Moseley, C.F., & Koreska, J. (1992). Spinal fusion in Duchenne muscular dystrophy. *Developmental Medicine and Child Neurology, 34,* 775–786.

Moxley, R.T., III, Ashwal, S., Pandya, S., Connolly, A., Florence, J., Mathews, K., et al. (2005). Practice parameter: Corticosteroid treatment of Duchenne dystrophy. Report of the quality standards subcommittee of the American Academy of Neurology and the Practice Committee of the Child Neurology Society. *Neurology, 64,* 13–20.

Moxley, R.T.,III, Pandya,S.,Ciafaloni, E., Fox, D. J., Campbell, K. J., (2010). Change in natural history of Duchenne muscular dystrophy with long-term corticosteroid treatment: Implications for management. *Journal of Child Neurology, 25*(9):1116-29

Pandya, S., Florence, J.M., King, W.M., Robinson, V.D., Wentzell, M., Province, M.A., & The CIDD Group. (1985). Reliability of goniometric measurements in patients with Duchenne muscular dystrophy. *Physical Therapy, 65,* 1339–1342.

Rahbek, J., Werge, B., Madsen, A., Marquardt, J., Steffensen, B.F., & Jeppesen, J. (2005). Adult life with Duchenne muscular dystrophy: Observations among an emerging and unforeseen patient population. *Pediatric Rehabilitation 8*(1), 17–28.

Rideau, Y., Jankowski, L.W., & Grellet, J. (1981). Respiratory function in the muscular dystrophies. *Muscle and Nerve, 4,* 155–164.

Schara, U., Mortier, J., & Mortier, W. (2001). Long-term steroid therapy in Duchenne muscular dystrophy: Positive results versus side effects. *Journal of Clinical Neuromuscular Disease, 2,* 179–183.

Scott, O.M., Hyde, S.A., Goddard, C., & Dubowitz, V. (1981). Prevention of deformity in Duchenne muscular dystrophy: A prospective study of passive stretching and splintage. *Physiotherapy, 67,* 177–180.

Sveen, M.L., Jeppesen, T.D., Haverdev, S., Kober, L., Krag, T.D., & Vissing, J. (2008). Endurance training improves fitness and strength in patients with Becker muscular dystrophy. *Brain, 131,* 2824–2831.

Topin, N., Matecki, S., LeBris, S., Rivier, F., Echenne, B., Prefaut, C., & Ramonatxo, M. (2002). Dose-dependent effect of individualized respiratory muscle training in children with Duchenne muscular dystrophy. *Neuromuscular Disorders, 12*(6), 576–583.

Vignos, P.J., Jr. (1983). Physical models of rehabilitation in neuromuscular disease. *Muscle and Nerve, 6,* 323–338.

Vignos, P.J., Jr., Spencer, G.E., Jr., & Archibald, K.C. (1963). Management of progressive muscular dystrophy of childhood. *Journal of American Medical Association, 184* (2), 89–110.

Vignos, P.J., Jr., Wagner, M.B., Karlinchak, B., & Katirji, B. (1996). Evaluation of a program for long-term treatment of Duchenne muscular dystrophy: Experience at the University Hospitals of Cleveland. *The Journal of Bone and Joint Surgery (British), 78,* 1844–1852.

Vinna, R., La Donna, K., Koopman, W., Campbell, C., Schulz, V., Venance, S., (2007). Pilot study to determine the transition needs of adolescents and adults with Duchenne muscular dystrophy. (Abstract) *Neuromuscular Disorders 17,* 864.

Wagner, K.R., Lechtzin, N., & Judge, D.P. (2007). Current treatment of adult Duchenne muscular dystrophy. *Biochimica et Biophysica Acta, 1772*(2), 229–237.

Yeldan, I. (2008). Comparison study of chest physiotherapy home training programmes on respiratory functions in patients with muscular dystrophy. *Clinical Rehabilitation, 22,* 741–748.

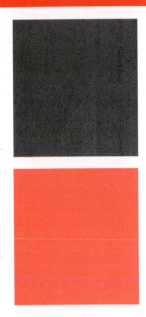

CHAPTER 24

Case Study

Developmental Coordination Disorder

—DEBORAH ANDERSON, PT, MS, PCS

Children who have developmental coordination disorder (DCD) have previously been given a wide variety of diagnoses, including but not limited to developmental apraxia, motor impaired, clumsy child syndrome, perceptual motor difficulties, and sensory integrative dysfunction (Baxter, 2012; Blank, Smits-Engelsman, Polatajko, & Wilson, 2012; Sugden & Chambers, 2005; Barnhart, Davenport, Epps, & Nordquist, 2003;). Over the past several years, physicians, therapists, and school personnel have identified common characteristics that apply to most of these children. Common characteristics include but are not limited to low muscle tone, balance deficits, awkward running pattern, difficulty following two- to three-step motor commands, learning difficulties, poor interactive play skills, perceptual deficits, slower response time, and decreased fitness levels (Blank et al., 2012; Cairney Hay, Veldhuizen, & Faught, 2011; Sugden & Chambers, 2005). In 1994, the American Psychiatric Association (APA) identified a *Diagnostic and Statistical Manual of Mental Disorders* (*DSM-IV*) diagnostic category for DCD for children who meet the following three qualifying conditions: (1) marked impairment in development of motor coordination, (2) impairment that interferes with academic achievement or activities of daily living (ADL), and (3) coordination difficulties that are not due to a general medical condition or pervasive developmental disorder (APA, 1994). In 2000, the *DSM-IV* was updated to include "If mental retardation is present, the motor difficulties are in excess of those usually associated with it," (APA, 2000).

The prevalence of DCD is estimated to be 5% to 6% of all school-age children (Blank et al., 2012; Pieters et al., 2012). Because of this high prevalence, physical therapists are called upon frequently to provide assessments and interventions for children with DCD.

Children with DCD often exhibit multiple comorbidities (Pieters et al., 2012). Because of the complexity of DCD, physical therapists address not only impairments in strength, balance, and coordination, but also impairments in respiration and endurance (Cairney et al., 2011). Boys with DCD have been found to spend less time participating in activities that require moderate to vigorous physical activity and more time in low-intensity physical activities (Poulsen, Barker, & Ziviani, 2011; Poulsen, Ziviani, & Cuskelly, 2008). Parents of children with DCD have identified additional concerns as their children have matured. For example, early concerns in the areas of motor ability and play evolved into concerns with self-care, academic performance, and the inability to successfully participate in organized sports and social activities (Jarus, Lourie-Gelberg, Engel-Yeger, & Bart, 2011; Missiuna, Moll, King, King, & Law, 2007).

This case study focuses on the physical therapy management of Mark, a 6-year-old boy who has DCD, over the course of a yearlong episode of care. It was determined that Mark's impairments of body structure and function and limitations in activities and participation would be best addressed by the Preferred Practice Pattern 5B: Impaired Neuromotor Development from the American Physical Therapy Association's *Guide to Physical Therapist Practice* (2001). Pattern 5B was selected because of Mark's delayed gross motor skills, impaired sensory integration, and clumsiness during play.

Examination: Age 5 Years

History

Mark was born after a full-term pregnancy. He weighed 7 lb. 11 oz. at birth. Congenital nystagmus was noted soon after birth, and Mark was examined by a pediatric ophthalmologist while in the hospital. Developmental motor milestones of sitting, creeping, standing, and walking were all achieved within expected ranges. An occupational therapy report from when Mark was 2 years old indicated that Mark was slow to learn utensil use as a result of a severe head turn resulting from the nystagmus. Mark underwent eye surgery at 2 years of age to reposition his eye muscles. Following the surgery, Mark's vision was reported to be 20/50 and his head turn improved significantly.

When Mark was 2 years old, he began receiving outpatient occupational therapy services. At the age of 3 years, Mark was evaluated by his local school system. Mark was recommended to enroll in an Early Childhood Program at that time to help foster his kindergarten readiness skills. School-based physical and occupational therapy were provided as part of the educational program to address concerns with Mark's coloring and writing skills as well as concerns with gross motor performance. Mark has also received outpatient speech/language services to address speech production and articulation difficulties.

At the age of 5 years, Mark was referred for outpatient physical therapy due to concerns of muscle weakness, atypical posture, poor endurance, poor respiratory control, and uncoordinated movement patterns. The primary parental concerns reported at the evaluation were Mark's asymmetrical head posture, his uncoordinated movements, and his inability to participate in peer motor activities due to fatigue. Mark's mother reports that school-based occupational therapy services are provided once per week and focus on fine motor performance with cutting and handwriting. Mark also participates in structured motor activities in the classroom and on the playground, which are supervised by the physical therapist.

Mark is currently enrolled in an Early Childhood Program through his local school district. He has an Individualized Educational Plan (IEP) with goals to improve in the areas of peer socialization, academic readiness, fine motor skills, and gross motor skills. Mark's mother reports that at school Mark has a difficult time making eye contact and does not recognize the members of his class after several months into the school year. Mark has a younger sister with whom he appears to enjoy cooperative play.

Systems Review

Cardiovascular and Pulmonary

Mark's vital signs are within normal limits with a heart rate of 96 beats per minute and a resting respiratory rate of 29 breaths per minute taken in a supine position. Because of concerns of poor endurance and poor respiratory control, further evaluation of fitness and respiration will be made.

Integumentary

Mark does not have any apparent skin breakdown, contusions, bruises, or other skin problems.

Musculoskeletal

Mark exhibits increased range of motion (ROM) in his upper and lower extremities. His posture exhibits a slight left head tilt with right rotation, an increased lumbar lordosis, and slight winging of the scapula. Because of these postural deviations, further assessment of posture and strength will be made.

Neuromuscular

Mark presents with hypotonia throughout his trunk and extremities. Decreased muscle tone impacts Mark's movement and function. Mark exhibits nystagmus of both eyes, which appears to increase with attempts to focus in the midline. Mark is getting glasses to help with his midline vision.

Communication, Affect, Cognition, Language, and Learning Style

Mark has good communication skills, but he appears to "run out of breath" when talking. "Low normal" cognitive skills were reported by the school psychologist at the time of Mark's initial school evaluation at 3 years of age. Mark is a very active child and has difficulty remaining focused on structured physical therapy tasks. He follows multistep directions and relies heavily on auditory cues. Mark has difficulty with midline visual activities because of his nystagmus. Mark has difficulty sustaining eye contact and does not routinely visually scan the environment when he enters a room.

Tests and Measures

The components for a detailed examination were chosen based on Mark's age and the areas of concern identified by his parents.

Aerobic Capacity and Endurance

Upon respiratory examination, Mark presents with a breathing pattern that lacks rhythm and consistency. He exhibits a weak cough. Mark reportedly has good sleeping and eating habits; however, talking has been limited to short phrases due to lack of breath support. Quick, shallow breaths, shoulder elevation, and an audible breathing pattern are observed during low-level gross motor activity. When asked to perform a full inhalation followed by a full exhalation, Mark has difficulty performing a smooth inhalation and instead takes several short inhalations. He is able to maintain a controlled exhalation for 9.13 seconds as measured with a standard stopwatch. Ribcage mobility appears to be appropriate in all planes.

The Timed Up and Down Stairs (TUDS) test (de Campos, da Costa, & Rocha, 2011; Zaino, Marchese, & Wescott, 2004) was used as a reference measure of endurance and speed. Eighteen steps located in the clinic were used for this assessment. Mark utilized a reciprocal lower extremity pattern to ascend and descend 18 steps in 24.9 seconds. Currently, there is minimal normative outcome data for the use of the TUDS with children.

Gait, Locomotion, and Balance

Mark walks independently on level surfaces and stairs. He moves quickly throughout the environment with his arms abducted, externally rotated and swinging randomly. A footprint analysis (Shores, 1980) of Mark's gait pattern demonstrates a wide base of support and Mark's inability to progress his legs in a straight line. Running is characterized by a forward trunk posture, arms extended behind trunk, and plantarflexion of both ankles. Mark appears to have difficulty stopping his forward progression when running 25 feet and takes up to five additional steps after receiving the verbal command to stop. Mark's balance is examined using the balance items of the Bruininks-Oseretsky Test of Motor Proficiency, second edition (BOT2) (Bruininks & Bruininks, 2005). Mark scores within the average range for males in his age group on items involving standing on one foot and walking on a line.

Motor Function (Motor Control and Motor Learning)

Mark's motor skills were evaluated using the BOT2 (Bruininks & Bruininks, 2005). The BOT2 has been identified in the literature as a discriminative and descriptive measure of motor performance in children with DCD (Cairney et al., 2011; Rivilis et al., 2012; Slater, Hillier, & Civetta, 2010; Watter, Marinac, Woodyatt, Ziviani, & Ozanne, 2008). Mark's scores were compared using same-sex norms and a 95% confidence interval. Mark completed the test over one 90-minute session. Mark utilized his preferred right hand, right arm, and right leg to complete the items. Mark's scores on the BOT2 at the age of 5 years can be found in Table 24.1.

Mark sits on the floor independently with widely abducted and flexed lower extremities and excessive trunk flexion (forward bending). He assumes standing through half-kneeling and stands independently, but he has difficulty maintaining quiet independent standing for more than a few minutes. Mark walks independently on level surfaces and stairs, moving quickly throughout the environment. Mark long jumps and jumps off of elevated surfaces. He walks backward without difficulty. Mark can throw a tennis ball 8 feet with his right arm and a 10-inch ball 6 feet using two hands over his head. Mark is unable to catch a ball thrown to him or bounce a ball on the floor and catch it regardless of ball size. Mark rides a tricycle independently the length of his neighborhood block.

Muscle Performance

Mark presents with decreased muscle tone throughout his trunk and proximal extremities, as exhibited

Table 24.1 Mark's Scores on the BOT2 at Age 5 Years

Motor Composites	Standard Score	Percentile Rank	Age Equivalents	Descriptive Category
Fine Motor Control	44	27		Average
Fine motor precision			4:8–4:9	Average
Fine motor integration			5:2–5:3	Average
Manual Coordination	25	1		Well below average
Manual dexterity			<4	Well below average
Upper-limb coordination			<4	Well below average
Body Coordination	38	12		Below average
Bilateral coordination			<4	Below average
Balance			5:0–5:1	Average
Strength and Agility	40	16		Below average
Running speed and agility			4:0–4:1	Below average
Strength			4:6–4:7	Average
Total Motor Composite	35	7		Below average

by a rounded sitting posture; increased flexibility at his shoulder, elbow, hip, and knee joints; and an increased lumbar lordosis. Muscle weakness is evident throughout Mark's shoulder girdle musculature as his scapulae are positioned in abduction, with winging of the scapula noted during throwing activities and reaching above 90 degrees. Abdominal muscle weakness and spinal extensor muscle weakness is apparent in Mark's excessive trunk flexion and wide base of support in sitting, anterior pelvic tilt in standing, and scapular adduction during running. Lower extremity muscle weakness results in knee hyperextension in standing.

Neuromotor Development and Sensory Integration

Mark exhibits impairments in neuromotor development as documented by his below-average total motor composite score on the BOT2. Mark has particular difficulty in the areas of manual dexterity and upper limb and bilateral coordination. Mark's visual deficit and his decreased muscle tone impact his ability to interact with and gain feedback from his environment. Mark assumes postures and demonstrates motor behaviors that provide him with increased sensory feedback, such as extending his arms for stability during running, walking on the stairs with "heavy feet," and spinning behavior. Mark appears to respond positively to sensory feedback that provides input to his system in a consistent and organized fashion. For example, following repetitive jumping on a trampoline or walking with

roller skates, Mark exhibits increased attention to task and decreased compensatory postures such as arm extension with running.

Range of Motion/Posture

Mark exhibits bilateral elbow and knee hyperextension during passive ROM of his extremities. Elbow hyperextension is also noted during upper extremity weight bearing in sitting. Knee hyperextension is present during static standing. All other joint motions are within normal limits. There is no evidence of scoliosis. Mark's posture in sitting is characterized by increased thoracic rounding and sacral sitting. In standing, Mark exhibits an increased lumbar lordosis. Mark is able to correct his posture with verbal and manual cues.

Self-Care and Home Management

Mark's self-care skills are examined using the Pediatric Evaluation of Disability Inventory (PEDI)—Self-Care Domain (Haley, Coster, Ludlow, Haltiwanger, & Andrellos, 1992). Mark exhibits a self-care domain raw score of 55, which correlates to a normative standard score of 32.3 + 1.9 based on a mean of 50. Mark's standard score falls below the mean but is within +2 SD; therefore, his score is within the average range for his age group. Mark participates in dressing by removing his shirt, pants, socks, and shoes. He has difficulty donning his shirt because he frequently gets tangled up in the sleeves. Mark requires assistance to don his shoes and socks. Mark is independent with eating except for cutting meats. Mark requires minimal assistance for bathing and toileting primarily because of difficulty with fine motor control and manipulation of fasteners.

Work, Community, and Leisure Integration

Mark enjoys playing outside. He is frustrated with his inability to ride a two-wheeled bike without training wheels. Mark participated in a park district soccer class but, per parent report, he had difficulty maintaining focus on the game and was frequently distracted by the activity around him. Mark also fatigued quickly during soccer and was not able to participate in a complete game. Mark has requested that his mom not sign him up for any park district activities next year.

Evaluation, Diagnosis, and Prognosis
Including Plan of Care

Diagnosis

Mark is an active 5-year-old child who is unable to participate in motor activities at the level of his peers within his family, his school, or the community because of impairments in muscle strength, endurance, coordination, and vision.

Activity Limitations

Mark exhibits unsafe and inefficient mobility throughout his environment and does not always visually attend to objects on the floor or in his path. Mark has had difficulty maneuvering within the classroom setting, which has resulted in his bumping into objects and classmates as well as tripping over objects on the floor. Mark continues to have difficulty coordinating both sides of his body, manipulating small balls or toys while standing, and visually attending to motor tasks that require repetitive eye-hand or eye-foot coordination. Decreased fine motor control limits Mark's independence in ADLs. Mark's decreased endurance has also resulted in limited play on the playground and the need for use of a stroller during family outings to the zoo.

Participation

Mark has difficulty participating in age-appropriate recreational activities such as soccer. He is currently unable to keep up with the physical demands of his peers and may be excluded from play activities. Due to Mark's difficulty with speech production, he is not always able to carry out a conversation with his peers and may become frustrated.

Prognosis

Mark is a happy, active child who is interested in his environment and cooperative with adult interactions. Mark's prognosis for improvement with physical therapy is good because of Mark's enjoyment of motor activities, motivation to learn new skills, and ability to follow directions. Over the course of this episode of care, it is expected that Mark will demonstrate improved strength, coordination, and endurance, allowing him to achieve increased independence in his home and school environments as well as with recreational activities.

Goals/Objectives

The following goals will be achieved during weekly physical therapy sessions over the next 6 months:

1. Mark will independently don and doff shoes with Velcro closures 100% of the time during three consecutive physical therapy sessions.
2. Mark will catch a ball when thrown to him from a distance of 7 feet 75% of the time.
3. Mark will ride a two-wheeled bike without training wheels a distance of 100 feet three out of four trials.
4. Mark will walk from his house to the neighborhood park (four blocks away) without stopping for a break three times over a 2-week period.

Intervention

Mark receives outpatient physical therapy once per week for 6 months. Physical therapy is provided utilizing a top-down approach, which focuses on motor skill training through cognitive and task-oriented strategies (Bernie & Rodger, 2004; Blank et al., 2012; Niemeijer, Smits-Engelsman, & Schoemaker, 2007; Polatajko, Missiuna, Miller, & Sugden, 2007; Polatajko, Mandich, Miller, & Macnab, 2001) as well as traditional physical therapy interventions (Hillier, 2007; Pless & Carlsson, 2000). Motor tasks considered priorities for therapy are identified by Mark's mom, Mark, and the evaluation process. This approach begins with an analysis of Mark's current competency in performing each motor skill, practice of the skill with variations to specific conditions, and use of visualizations such as a "soldier" and "Christmas tree" during the teaching of jumping jacks.

After 6 months, Mark's physical therapy is decreased to rechecks, and suggestions for home and community fitness activities are provided to the family. Mark's physical therapy is decreased because of improvements in strength, endurance, and coordination, which have allowed Mark to achieve his physical therapy goals as well as participate successfully in a karate class offered by the park district.

Coordination, Communication, and Documentation

To ensure that Mark's therapeutic needs are being addressed in multiple settings, the outpatient therapists and the school therapist must develop an ongoing method of communication. Several avenues of communication are used, including telephone calls, e-mail, and a notebook provided by Mark's mother. Mark's mom also shares IEP documentation, therapy progress reports, and periodic updates from the pediatrician and the ophthalmologist with all members of Mark's team.

Patient/Client-Related Instruction

Mark's mom is given ongoing information concerning Mark's condition as well as specific instructions for home programming. Pictures are taken and provided to Mark's family to enhance his accuracy and success with home program activities (Fig. 24.1 and Fig. 24.2). Mark's mom is given examples of verbal prompts to assist Mark's ability to self-assess his achievement of a motor skill (Niemeijer

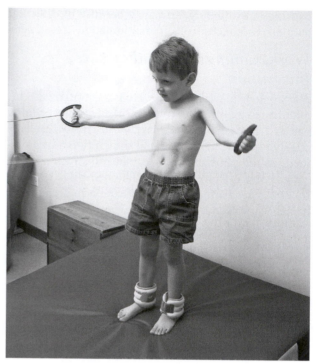

Figure 24.2 Bilateral arm activity.

et al., 2003, 2006, 2007). Mark's mom practiced these verbal prompts with Mark during a physical therapy session.

Procedural Interventions

Recent studies have identified problems with muscle weakness, decreased energy expenditure, and decreased cardiorespiratory fitness in children with DCD as contributing factors to poor body awareness, decreased motor skill development, and diminished participation in leisure time physical activities (Cairney, et al., 2011; Poulsen et al., 2008; Raynor, 2001).

Mark participates in weekly therapeutic exercise, which includes endurance, coordination, posture, strength, respiratory, and task-specific activities (Blank et al., 2012; Hillier, 2007; Kaufman & Schilling, 2007; Missiuna, Mandich, Polatajko, & Malloy-Miller, 2001; Pless & Carlsson, 2000).

Body Mechanics and Postural Stabilization

Mark participates in posture exercises at home and in the clinic. These exercises focus on midline head and body orientation. Mark uses a mirror for feedback on correct alignment and engages toys that require bilateral upper or lower extremity activation (Fig. 24.2). Mark also attends a weekly karate class where he learns

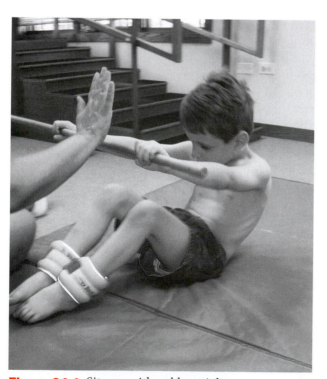

Figure 24.1 Sit-ups with ankle weights.

controlled kicking and practices repetitive arm and leg multijoint movements.

Neuromotor Development Training

Repetition and variability are used as part of the neuromotor task training (NTT) approach to increase Mark's ability to throw, catch, and kick a ball. As age-appropriate motor tasks are attempted, Mark is prompted to discuss his performance. He is also provided with immediate feedback from the therapist. Mark's family explores additional means for teaching Mark how to ride a bike without training wheels. They discover an approach in which the bike's pedals are removed until the child develops the ability to maintain his balance and glide on the two wheels (Nix, 2007). Mark's parents work with Mark without pedals on his bike for 1 week. At the end of the week, Mark learns how to successfully negotiate a two-wheeled bike safely.

Strength, Power, and Endurance Training

Body weight and low-load strengthening activities have been found to be safe and effective for young children (Council on Sports Medicine and Fitness, 2008; Faigenbaum, 2000). Mark participates in strengthening activities, including sit-ups, wheelbarrow walking, sitting on a small therapy ball, negotiating inclined surfaces with 1-pound weights on his ankles, and pushing heavy objects.

Cardiorespiratory fitness (CRF) has been found to be decreased in older children with DCD (Cairney et al., 2011); however, interventions to increased CRF have not yet been studied in this population. Mark's CRF is addressed through activities intended to increase the efficiency and effectiveness of Mark's breathing pattern, strengthen his ventilatory muscles, and promote participation in endurance activities.

Mark's breathing pattern is addressed during each therapy session. Coordination of breathing is cued through verbal instruction and manual input to the rib cage. Inhaling through a straw to pick up a tissue is one technique used to increase coordination and effectiveness of Mark's inhalations. An inspirometer is introduced as a progression of the inhalation activities when Mark is able to sustain an inspiration of enough strength and endurance to raise the stopper. Various breathing toys are utilized to promote and lengthen expiration. A standard recorder is introduced as a home exercise program to further promote coordinated inspirations and expirations. Practice of forced

exhalation is combined with motor activities such a kicking a ball to further strengthen the diaphragm and abdominal musculature. A variety of speech patterns are utilized during motor play to expand Mark's breathing repertoire and ultimately increase breath support for the production of uninterrupted longer sentences. Mark also participates in a home exercise program, which includes aerobic exercise at least three times per week in such forms as family walks, swimming, or bike riding.

Termination of Episode of Care

After 6 months of interventions, Mark achieves the ability to ride a two-wheeled bike without training wheels and begins taking bike rides with his father several times per week. He no longer requires a rest break when walking to the park in his neighborhood and has no further playground concerns at school. Mark is now able to catch a ball thrown to him from 7 feet away. Mark participates in a weekly karate class and seems to enjoy this activity. Fatigue no longer limits Mark's participation in any activity. Increased vocalizations are observed during motor activities. Mark's successful achievement of 75% of physical therapy goals and his participation in weekly endurance and agility activities results in outpatient physical therapy being decreased to rechecks as needed. Mark continues to work on independent dressing skills at home, including donning and doffing his shoes.

Examination: Age 6 Years

At age 6, Mark returns to physical therapy to have his fine and gross motor function reevaluated.

History

Mark will enter a first-grade educational program next year. His school therapists are recommending discharge from educational physical and occupational therapy services at that time.

Systems Review

Vision

Mark's vision has improved. His mom reports a change in his prescription to 20/30. Mark has difficulty maintaining eye contact with the therapist but is able to focus on the fine motor tasks presented. Frequent prompting is required to improve Mark's ability to visually attend during the gross motor activity part of the evaluation.

Cardiovascular and Pulmonary

Mark now appears to have adequate respiration for conversational speech and gross motor play. Mark's resting heart rate is 88 beats per minute and his resting respiratory rate is 20 breaths per minute.

Integumentary

Mark does not have any apparent skin breakdown, contusions, bruises, or other problems.

Musculoskeletal

Mark exhibits increased range of motion in his upper and lower extremities. Mark exhibits slight neck rotation to the left during fine and gross motor activities. This posture may be related to Mark's vision. Mark presents with greater definition of muscle throughout his trunk; however, proximal weakness continues to be present as indicated by Mark's inability to perform sit-ups at peer levels.

Neuromuscular

Mark presents with hypotonia throughout his trunk and extremities. Mark is exhibiting improvement in overall motor control and sensory processing; however, decreased quality of movement and decreased coordination continue to impact his function.

Communication, Affect, Cognition, Language, and Learning Style

Mark shows improvement with communication between his family, the therapists, and his peers. He now makes spontaneous eye contact approximately 50% of the time. Mark is engaged in motor tasks and now attends for longer periods. Per parent report, Mark is completing kindergarten tasks at the level of his peers. Mark has an extended vocabulary and continues to use speech as a distraction from motor performance when tasks become difficult.

Tests and Measures

Aerobic Capacity and Endurance

Upon respiratory examination, Mark presents with a coordinated breathing pattern without shoulder elevation. His cough is strong. His mom reports no respiratory illnesses over the past 6 months. Mark is able to maintain a controlled exhalation for 11.24 seconds and completes a 10-syllable sentence without requiring a breath. Mark did not require a rest between motor activities during the 75-minute evaluation session. The TUDS test is repeated for comparison with previous measures. Mark utilizes a reciprocal lower extremity pattern to ascend and descend 18 steps in 20.20 seconds (Table 24.2).

Gait, Locomotion, and Balance

Mark negotiates his environment safely with adequate balance, speed, and coordination. Mark has developed a reciprocal arm swing during running activities. Mark has improved his ability to stop his forward progression when running 25 feet by taking only two additional steps after receiving the verbal command to stop. Despite Mark's apparent progress in the area of dynamic balance, his score on the balance items of the BOT2 has not significantly changed over the past year.

Motor Function (Motor Control and Motor Learning)

Mark's motor skills are reevaluated using the BOT2 (Table 24.3). His performance of skills in the fine motor and manual coordination composites items on the BOT2 have improved since he was age 5. These composites include items related to coloring, drawing, cutting, and copying as well as timed items such as transferring pennies and sorting cards. Although Mark's performance in the body coordination and strength and agility composites have not significantly changed, he does exhibit improvement in several items in the bilateral coordination subtest as well as in the running speed and agility subtest.

Table 24.2 Initial and Follow-Up Examination Measures

	At 5 Years	After 6 Months of Intervention	At 6 Years
Respiratory rate (breaths per minute)	29	21	20
Heart rate (beats per minute)	96	84	88
Timed Up and Down Stairs Test	24.90 seconds	21.66 seconds	20.20 seconds
Exhalation	9.13 seconds	10.54 seconds	11.24 seconds

Table 24.3 Mark's Scores on the BOT2 at Age 6 Years

Motor Composites	Standard Score	Percentile Rank	Age Equivalents	Descriptive Category
Fine Motor Control	59	82		Average
Fine motor precision			7:0–7:2	Average
Fine motor integration			8:3–8:5	Above average
Manual Coordination	35	7		Below average
Manual dexterity			4:0–4:1	Below average
Upper-limb coordination			4:10–4:11	Below average
Body Coordination	40	16		Below Average
Bilateral coordination			4:10–4:11	Average
Balance			4:4–4:5	Below Average
Strength and Agility	39	14		Below average
Running speed and agility			4:8–4:9	Below average
Strength			4:4–4:5	Below Average
Total Motor Composite	41	18		Average

Muscle Performance

Mark presents with decreased muscle tone throughout his trunk and proximal extremities, as exhibited by increased flexibility at the shoulder, elbow, hip, and knee joints. Mark's scapulae no longer exhibit winging but instead are maintained in a stable position on his thorax during upper extremity reaching and weight-bearing activities. Mark no longer exhibits a lumbar lordosis or knee hyperextension in standing. Mark's muscle strength is additionally assessed as a component of the BOT2. Mark exhibits the ability to perform a 35-inch long jump. He performs 1 push-up and 8 sit-ups with ankles supported in 30 seconds. Mark sustains prone extension against gravity for 9 seconds, but he is unable to sustain the wall-sit posture. Mark has made functional improvements in muscle strength over the past year as indicated by his improved posture and overall motor function. These improvements in strength occurred over a period in which Mark grew 3 inches in height and gained 7 pounds. Despite Mark's functional improvement in muscle strength, he continues to exhibit muscle weakness as compared with his peers of the same age.

Neuromotor Development and Sensory Integration

Mark exhibits improved midline orientation of his head and trunk. Left neck rotation is observed during challenging gross motor tasks, but Mark is able to spontaneously resume a midline head position following the activity. Mark's movements are quick and his extremities are held close to his body. The therapist notes that Mark appeared to be distracted by the surrounding environment (for example, the noise from cars passing by on the street outside of the clinic) during his reevaluation.

Mark appears to have difficulty with test items that include visual motor skills and coordination of his body around a central axis, such as standing on one leg while looking at a circle on the wall. Although Mark's visual acuity has improved, his visual motor skills are still impacted by nystagmus and his tendency to use his right eye for better focus.

Mark's total motor composite score of 41 on the BOT2 falls within 1 SD below the mean of 50 and is considered within the average range of motor performance when compared to his same age peers.

Range of Motion

Mark exhibits increased mobility in his upper and lower extremities. Mark no longer exhibits lumbar lordosis and he maintains an erect spine without kyphosis in all antigravity positions.

Self-Care and Home Management

Mark's self-care skills are examined utilizing the PEDI–Self-Care Domain. Mark exhibits a self-care domain raw score of 69, which correlates to a normative standard score of 39.7 ± 3. Mark's PEDI score increased by 14 points over the past year. Mark's standard score is within the average range for his age group. Mark now fully dresses and undresses himself, including donning and doffing shoes with Velcro closures, but he is not yet able to tie his shoes. Mark requires assistance for thorough teeth brushing and combing his hair.

Work, Community, and Leisure Integration

Mark has attended weekly karate classes to work on strength, balance, and coordination. Mark appears to enjoy his karate classes and his mother has observed consistent improvement in his karate skills since the beginning of the program. Mark continues to take long-distance bike rides with his father during good weather. Over the winter months, Mark participated in a sports skills class with his sister through the local park district. Mark was able to fully participate in this 60-minute class without requiring a rest.

Evaluation, Diagnosis, and Prognosis
Including Plan of Care

Mark is currently enrolled in a kindergarten program through his school district. As part of his kindergarten program, Mark receives educationally based physical and occupational therapy. Mark is having a successful kindergarten year in academic and motor pursuits. Mark has not received additional outpatient physical or occupational therapy since the beginning of the school year because no concerns were identified by the family or the school district.

Diagnosis

Mark is a 6-year-old child who exhibits muscle weakness, decreased coordination, and delays in motor development.

Activity Limitations

Mark continues to have difficulty coordinating both sides of his body, manipulating small balls or toys, and visually attending to motor tasks that require repetitive eye-hand or eye-foot coordination.

Participation

Mark's overall participation with motor tasks at home, school, and in the community has improved. As Mark advances to first grade and beyond, he will encounter greater demands on fine motor and gross motor performance. Mark's participation in physical education as well as recreational activities needs to be closely monitored.

Prognosis

Mark enjoys movement and gross motor play. He has a very supportive family environment and parents who enjoy sharing activities such as bike riding with Mark.

For this reason, Mark has a good prognosis for continued improvement of his motor skills as well as continued success with overall fitness.

Goals/Objectives

The current goal is to promote recreational activities to foster strength, coordination, and overall fitness.

Intervention

Direct physical therapy is not warranted at this time. Mark is now capable of and interested in participating in peer-appropriate motor activities. The physical therapist and Mark's mother discuss options for summer activities when Mark is not in school, including swimming, bike riding, soccer, and an art class. Mark will again enroll in a karate class in the fall.

The role of the physical therapist has now become that of a consultant and evaluator. The physical therapist will continue to consult with Mark's family, physician, and school personnel about Mark's participation in the classroom and physical education class. Physical therapy re-assessments will be performed twice per year to monitor Mark's progress with his gross motor performance and to provide suggestions and recommendations to enhance Mark's gross motor success with a growing musculoskeletal system, especially in the areas of fitness, strength, and coordination.

Termination of Episode of Care

Mark's diagnosis of DCD may require Mark to receive multiple episodes of physical therapy intervention throughout his life span. Termination of each episode of care will be based on the successful resolution of the individualized goals and objectives that have been established by Mark and his family.

Longitudinal research on children and young adults with DCD has documented ongoing impairments in the areas of motor control and coordination as well as participation issues resulting from decreased strength and poor endurance (Hill, Brown, & Sophia Sorgardt, 2011; Jarus et al., 2011; Kirby, Edwards, & Sugden, 2011). Mark will need to make choices about vocation, recreation, and leisure activities across his life span to prevent the development of secondary impairments and maximize positive functional outcomes.

Summary

This case study summarizes the examination, intervention, and outcomes for a child with DCD. Information on DCD has multiplied in the literature over the past 10 years as more and more children are being diagnosed with this condition. Physical therapists, as experts in the field of movement dysfunction, play a crucial role in early diagnosis of these children. Physical therapists have a primary role in diagnosis, intervention, and advocacy in the educational system as well as in clinical settings. Special consideration to the social and emotional development of children with DCD is necessary. Such consideration must focus on evaluation of self-perception and quality of life measures as well as advocacy for ongoing leisure time and participation in fitness activities (Hill et al., 2011; Poulsen et al.,

2008). As evidence-based practitioners, physical therapists should explore the literature for the wide variety of interventions being successfully utilized with children who have DCD. Table 24.4 provides a synopsis of the available literature. What appears to be evident in this table is a focus on the top-down approach to intervention for children with DCD. The literature on cognitive and task-oriented strategies continues to grow and gives new insight on physical therapy instruction of new motor tasks. Future research should focus on how therapeutic outcomes affect quality of life and self-perception as these children grow into adulthood and assume their roles in society.

Table 24.4 Evidence-Based Interventions for Developmental Coordination Disorder (DCD)

Intervention	Author (Date)	Study Design	No. of Subjects/ Articles	Question	Findings
General Interventions	Hillier (2007)	Systematic review (SR)	28 studies	Is there evidence of the effectiveness of interventions to improve movement capability of children with developmental coordination disorder (DCD)?	There is strong evidence to support perceptual motor training and sensory integrative therapy, physiotherapy, and incorporation of mastery concepts. Moderate evidence supports the use of kinesthetic training.
	Pless & Carlsson (2000)	SR and meta-analysis	21 studies reviewed, 13 studies analyzed	Does evidence exist in published research from 1970 to 1996 to support motor skill intervention for children with DCD?	Motor skill intervention is most effective when applied to children with DCD who are older than age 5 utilizing the specific skill theoretical approach in a group setting or home exercise program, three to five times per week.
	Mandich, Polatajko, Macnab, & Miller (2001)	SR	32 studies reviewed	What are the results of various treatment approaches to DCD?	Bottom-up approaches: **1.** Sensory integration (SI) is as effective as other interventions in improving motor skills; however, impact of SI on functional performance is unknown.

Continued

Table 24.4 Evidence-Based Interventions for Developmental Coordination Disorder (DCD)—cont'd

Intervention	Author (Date)	Study Design	No. of Subjects/ Articles	Question	Findings
General Interventions *(continued)*					**2.** Evidence regarding process-oriented treatment is inconclusive. Some studies have indicated that process-oriented treatment is as effective as other interventions to improve motor skills; in contrast, other studies have indicated that it is not any better than no treatment at all. **3.** Perceptual motor training—the preferred method for many clinicians to treat children with DCD—has been found to be ineffective in improving motor skills in children with learning disabilities, found to have equal effect on DCD as all other approaches. **4.** Limited evidence exists to support combined approaches. *Top-down approaches:* **1.** Task-specific intervention results in gains of task worked on without transfer to other skills. **2.** Cognitive approaches are shown to be effective with DCD, but evidence is just beginning to accumulate.

Table 24.4 Evidence-Based Interventions for Developmental Coordination Disorder (DCD)—cont'd

Intervention	Author (Date)	Study Design	No. of Subjects/ Articles	Question	Findings
Therapeutic Exercise: Aerobic capacity/endurance training, balance, coordination, agility training; body mechanics/ postural stabilization; gait and locomotion training; neuromotor development training; strength, power, and endurance training	Peters & Wright (1999)	Time series quasi-experimental study (one group with pretest and posttest)	*n* = 14 subjects	What is the effectiveness of a group exercise program for DCD on the Movement Assessment Battery for Children (M-ABC), and Forced Vital Capacity increased (FVC)?	Study showed that 12 out of 14 subjects improved on the M-ABC and FVC. No change in competence scores occurred.
	Kaufman & Schilling (2007)	Case report	*n* = 1 subject	What is the impact of strength training with DCD?	Strength training improved muscle strength, gross motor function, and proprioception in an individual with DCD.
	Pless, Carlsson, Sundelin, & Persson (2000)	Randomized controlled trial (RCT)	*n* = 37 subjects	Does group physical therapy once per week for 10 weeks lead to improved motor skill performance?	Group motor skill intervention does not show significant improvement.
Top-down approaches: Task-oriented and cognitive strategies	Wilson, Thomas, & Maruff (2002)	RCT	*n* = 54 subjects	What are the effects of motor imagery versus traditional perceptual motor training versus no intervention?	Improvement occurred in M-ABC for both intervention groups but not the control group.
	Miller, Polatajko, Missiuna, Mandich, & Macnab (2001)	Time series quasi-experimental design (one group with pretest and posttest)	*n* = 20 subjects	This study compared a new treatment approach, the Cognitive Orientation to Daily Occupational Performance (CO-OP) to the Contemporary Treatment Approach (CTA) to treat children with DCD.	Children were randomly assigned to CO-OP or CTA group. All children received intervention through 10 individualized sessions lasting approximately 50 minutes. Results indicated that both groups had improved scores on the Canadian Occupational Performance Measure (COPM), the Performance Quality Rating Scale (PQRS), and the Vineland Adaptive Behavior Scales

Continued

Table 24.4 Evidence-Based Interventions for Developmental Coordination Disorder (DCD)—cont'd

Intervention	Author (Date)	Study Design	No. of Subjects/ Articles	Question	Findings
Top-down approaches: Task-oriented and cognitive strategies *(continued)*					(VABS), but gains were greater in the CO-OP group on all of the above tests. Significant treatment differences were not recorded on the Bruininks-Oseretsky Test of Motor Proficiency (BOTMP) or the Developmental Test of Visual-Motor Integration-Revised. Both groups improved.
	Niemeijer et al. (2006)	Time series quasi-experimental design (one group with pretest and posttest)	$n = 19$ children, 11 therapists	Are teaching principles of neuromotor task training (NTT) associated with improved motor performance?	NTT may be associated with improved movement performance.
	Schoemaker, Niemeijer, Reynders, & Smits-Engelsman (2003)	Nonrando-mized controlled group trial, quasi-experimental design	$n = 15$ subjects	What is the effectiveness of NTT for DCD?	NTT improved performance on the M-ABC.
	Niemeijer et al. (2007)	Nonrando-mized controlled group trial, quasi-experimental design	$n = 26$ subjects	What is the effectiveness of NTT for DCD?	NTT improved performance on the M-ABC.
	Polatajko, Mandich, Miller, & Macnab (2001)	Review of five studies	Data from five studies: Study 1: single case experiments, $n = 10$ subjects Study 2: systematic replication of the single case	Use of CO-OP for treatment of DCD was studied. Could results from study 1 be replicated by a different therapist? How does CO-OP compare with current treatment for DCD? What is the clinical replicability of CO-OP?	Children with DCD could learn to use problem-solving strategies to acquire skills. Another therapist had similar results to study 1. CO-OP is an effective treatment for DCD as measured by the COPM, PQRS, VABS, Evaluation Tool of Children's Hand-writing (ETCH), and

Table 24.4 Evidence-Based Interventions for Developmental Coordination Disorder (DCD)—cont'd

Intervention	Author (Date)	Study Design	No. of Subjects/ Articles	Question	Findings
			experiment, $n = 4$ subjects Study 3: informal follow-up and videotape analysis Study 4: RCT pilot, $n = 20$ subjects Study 5: retrospective chart audit, $n = 25$ subjects		BOTMP. CO-OP positively affects direct skill acquisition.
	Mandich, Polatajko, Missiuna, & Miller (2001)		$n = 80$ videotaped interventions	What are the cognitive strategies used during verbal self-guided (VSG) intervention sessions?	Confirm the use of the global, executive strategy, Goal-Plan-Do-Check (GPDC) and components of the Good Strategy User (GSU) model as cognitive learning strategies used to treat children with DCD. GPDC is a problem-solving strategy that consists of the child identifying a motor task that they are having difficulty with (goal) and want to change, establishing a plan to work on that goal with help from the physical therapist, carrying out the plan with guided revision from the physical therapist, and assessing the results.

Continued

■ **Table 24.4** Evidence-Based Interventions for Developmental Coordination Disorder (DCD)—cont'd

Intervention	Author (Date)	Study Design	No. of Subjects/ Articles	Question	Findings
					The GSU model combines the GPDC with supplementation of task knowledge and the addition of domain-specific strategies: 1. task specification 2. motor mnemonic 3. body position 4. feeling the movement 5. attention to doing 6. verbal guidance 7. verbal self-guidance 8. verbal rote script

DISCUSSION QUESTIONS

1. What impairments in body structure and function contribute to Mark's difficulty with bilateral coordination?

2. Identify intervention strategies for each of Mark's impairments that would contribute to improved bilateral coordination.

3. What are some secondary impairments that Mark might develop as he goes through significant periods of growth in high school?

4. Identify potential barriers to participation that Mark may encounter as he progresses through school.

Recommended Readings

Blank, R., Smits-Engelsman, B., Polatajko, H., & Wilson, P. (2012). European Academy for Childhood Disability (EACD): Recommendations on the definition, diagnosis and intervention of developmental coordination disorder (long version). *Developmental Medicine and Child Neurology, 54*(1), 54-93.

Hillier, S. (2007). Intervention for children with developmental coordination disorder: A systematic review. *Internet Journal of Allied Health Sciences and Practice, 5*(3), 1–11.

Slater, L. M., Hillier, S. L., & Civetta, L. R. (2010). The clinimetric properties of performance-based gross motor tests used for children with developmental coordination disorder: A systematic review. *Pediatric Physical Therapy, 22*(2), 170-179.

Sugden, D., & Chambers, M. E. (2005). *Children with developmental coordination disorder*. London, England: Whurr Publishers.

References

American Physical Therapy Association (APTA). (2001). Guide to physical therapist practice (2nd ed.). *Physical Therapy, 81*, 6–746.

American Psychiatric Association (APA). (1994). *Diagnostic and statistical manual of mental disorders* (4th ed.). Washington, DC: Author.

American Psychiatric Association (APA). (2000). *Diagnostic and statistical manual of mental disorders* (4th ed., text revision.). Washington, DC: Author.

Barnhart, R.C., Davenport, M.J., Epps, S.B., & Nordquist V.M. (2003). Developmental coordination disorder. *Physical Therapy, 83*, 722–731.

Baxter, P. (2012). Developmental coordination disorder and motor dyspraxia. *Developmental Medicine and Child Neurology, 54*(1), 3-3.

Bernie, C., & Rodger, S. (2004). Cognitive strategy use in school-aged children with developmental coordination disorder. *Physical and Occupational Therapy in Pediatrics, 24*(4), 23–45.

Blank, R., Smits-Engelsman, B., Polatajko, H., & Wilson, P. (2012). European Academy for Childhood Disability

(EACD): Recommendations on the definition, diagnosis and intervention of developmental coordination disorder (long version). *Developmental Medicine and Child Neurology, 54*(1), 54-93.

Bruininks, R.H., & Bruininks, B.D. (2005). *Bruininks-Oseretsky Test of Motor Proficiency* (2nd ed.). Circle Pines, MN: American Guidance Service.

Cairney, J., Hay, J., Veldhuizen, S., & Faught, B.E. (2011). Trajectories of cardiorespiratory fitness in children with and without developmental coordination disorder: A longitudinal analysis. *British Journal of Sports Medicine, 45,* 1196-1201.

Cairney, J., Hay, J.A., Faught, B.E., Flouis, A., & Klentou, P. (2007). Developmental coordination disorder and cardiorespiratory fitness in children. *Pediatric Exercise Science, 19,* 20–28.

Council on Sports Medicine and Fitness. (2008). Strength training by children and adolescents. *Pediatrics, 121,* 835–840.

de Campos, A., da Costa, C.N., & Rocha, N.F. (2011). Measuring changes in functional mobility in children with mild cerebral palsy. *Developmental Neurorehabilitation, 14*(3), 140-144.

Faigenbaum, A.D. (2000). Strength training for children and adolescents. *Clinics in Sports Medicine, 19*(4), 1–20.

Haley, S.M., Coster, W.J., Ludlow, L.H., Haltiwanger, J., & Andrellos, P. (1992). *Pediatric Evaluation of Disability Inventory (PEDI): Development, standardization and administration manual.* Boston: PEDI Research Group, New England Medical Center Hospitals.

Hill, E., Brown, D., & Sophia Sorgardt, K. (2011). A preliminary investigation of quality of life satisfaction reports in emerging adults with and without developmental coordination disorder. *Journal of Adult Development, 18,* 130-134.

Hillier, S. (2007). Intervention for children with developmental coordination disorder: A systematic review. *Internet Journal of Allied Health Sciences and Practice, 5*(3), 1–11.

Jarus, T., Lourie-Gelberg, Y., Engel-Yeger, B., & Bart, O. (2011). Participation patterns of school-aged children with and without DCD. *Research in Developmental Disabilities, 32,* 1323-1331.

Kaufman, L.B., & Schilling, D.L. (2007). Implementation of a strength training program for a 5-year-old child with poor body awareness and developmental coordination disorder. *Physical Therapy, 87*(4), 455–467.

Kirby, A., Edwards, L., & Sugden, D. (2011). Emerging adulthood in developmental co-ordination disorder: Parent and young adult perspectives. *Research in Developmental Disabilities, 32*(4), 1351-1360.

Mandich, A.D., Polatajko, H.J., Macnab, J.J., & Miller, L.T. (2001). Treatment of children with developmental coordination disorder: What is the evidence? *Physical and Occupational Therapy in Pediatrics, 20*(2/3), 51-68.

Mandich, A.D., Polatajko, H.J., Missiuna, C., & Miller, L.T. (2001). Cognitive strategies and motor performance in children with developmental coordination disorder. *Physical and Occupational Therapy in Pediatrics, 20*(2/3), 125-143.

Miller, L.T., Polatajko, H.J., Missiuna, C., Mandich, A.D., & Macnab, J.J. (2001). A pilot trial of a cognitive treatment for children with developmental coordination disorder. *Human Movement Science, 20,* 183–210.

Missiuna, C., Mandich, A.D., Polatajko, H.J., & Malloy-Miller, T. (2001). Cognitive orientation to daily occupational performance (co-op): Part I—theoretical foundations. *Physical and Occupational Therapy in Pediatrics, 20*(2/3), 69–81.

Missiuna, C., Moll, S., King, S., King, G., & Law, M. (2007). A trajectory of troubles: Parents' impressions of the impact of developmental coordination disorder. *Physical and Occupational Therapy in Pediatrics, 27*(1), 81–101.

Niemeijer, A.S., Schoemaker, M.M., & Smits-Engelsman, B.C.M. (2003). Verbal actions of physiotherapists to enhance motor learning in children with DCD. *Human Movement Science, 22*(4–5), 567–581.

Niemeijer, A.S., Schoemaker, M.M., & Smits-Engelsman, B.C.M. (2006). Are teaching principles associated with improved motor performance in children with developmental coordination disorder: A pilot study. *Physical Therapy, 86*(9), 1221–1230.

Niemeijer, A.S., Smits-Engelsman, B.C.M., & Schoemaker, M.M. (2007). Neuromotor task training for children with developmental coordination disorder: A controlled trial. *Developmental Medicine and Child Neurology, 49,* 406–411.

Nix, H.A. (2007). *Learning to ride with "the bits."* Indianapolis: Reading Matter.

Peters, J.M., & Wright, A.M. (1999). Development and evaluation of a group physical activity programme for children with developmental co-ordination disorder: An interdisciplinary approach. *Physiotherapy Theory and Practice, 15,* 203–216.

Pieters, S., De Block, K., Scheiris, J., Eyssen, M., Desoete, A., Deboutte, D., Van Waelvelde, H., & Roeyers, H. (2012). How common are motor problems in children with a developmental disorder: Rule or exception? *Child: Care, Health and Development, 38*(1), 139-145.

Pless, M., & Carlsson, M. (2000). Effects of motor skill intervention on developmental coordination disorder: A meta-analysis. *Adapted Physical Activity Quarterly, 17,* 381–401.

Pless, M., Carlsson, M., Sundelin, C., & Persson, K. (2000). Effects of group motor skill intervention on five- to six-year old children with developmental coordination disorder. *Pediatric Physical Therapy, 12,* 183–189.

Polatajko, H.J., Mandich, A.D., Miller, L.T., & Macnab, J.J. (2001). Cognitive orientation to daily occupational performance (co-op): Part II—the evidence. *Physical and Occupational Therapy in Pediatrics, 20*(2/3), 83–106.

Polatajko, H.J., Missiuna, C., Miller, L.T., & Sugden, D. (2007). Current approaches to intervention in children with developmental coordination disorder. *Developmental Medicine and Child Neurology, 49,* 467–471.

Poulsen, A.A., Barker, F.M., & Ziviani, J. (2011). Personal projects of boys with developmental coordination disorder. *Occupational Therapy Journal of Research: Occupation, Participation & Health, 31*(3), 108-117.

Poulsen, A.A., Ziviani, J.M., & Cuskelly, M. (2008). Leisure time physical activity energy expenditure in boys with developmental coordination disorder: The role of peer relations self-concept perceptions. *Occupational Therapy Journal of Research: Occupation, Participation and Health, 28*(1), 30–39.

Raynor, A.J. (2001). Strength, power, and coactivation in children with developmental coordination disorder. *Developmental Medicine and Child Neurology, 43,* 676–684.

Rivilis, I., Liu, J., Cairney, J., Hay, J. A., Klentrou, P., & Faught, B.E. (2012). A prospective cohort study comparing workload in children with and without developmental coordination disorder. *Research in Developmental Disabilities, 33,* 442-448.

Schoemaker, M.M., Niemeijer, A.S., Reynders, A.S., & Smits-Engelsman, B.C.M. (2003). Effectiveness of neuromotor task training for children with developmental coordination disorder: A pilot study. *Neural Plasticity, 10*(1–2), 155–163.

Shores, M. (1980). Footprint analysis in gait documentation. *Physical Therapy, 60*(9), 1163–1167.

Slater, L.M., Hillier, S.L., Civetta, L.R. (2010). The clinimetric properties of performance-based gross motor tests used for children with developmental coordination disorder: A systematic review. *Pediatric Physical Therapy, 22*(2), 170-179.

Sugden, D., & Chambers, M.E. (2005). *Children with developmental coordination disorder.* London, England: Whurr Publishers.

Watter P.R.S., Marinac, J., Woodyatt, G., Ziviani, J., & Ozanne, A. (2008). Multidisciplinary assessment of children with developmental coordination disorder: Using the ICF framework to inform assessment. *Physical & Occupational Therapy in Pediatrics, 28*(4), 331-352.

Wilson, P.H., Maruff, P., Butson, M., Williams, J., Lum, J., & Thomas, P.R. (2004). Internal representation of movement in children with development coordination disorder: A mental rotation task. *Developmental Medicine and Child Neurology, 46,* 754–759.

Wilson, P.H., Thomas, P.R., & Maruff, P. (2002). Motor imagery training ameliorates motor clumsiness in children. *Journal of Child Neurology, 17*(7), 491–498.

Zaino, C.A., Marchese, V.G., & Wescott, S.L. (2004). Timed up and down stairs test: Preliminary reliability and validity of a new measure of functional mobility. *Pediatric Physical Therapy, 16,* 90–98.

CHAPTER 25

Case Study

Myelodysplasia

—MARY JO PARIS, PT, DPT

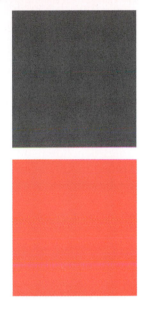

This case study will focus on the school-based physical therapy provided for Salomon, a 7-year-old boy with myelodysplasia at the thoracolumbar level. He is currently attending a public school, receiving services by a special education teacher in a pullout model for part of his day, and he attends regular first-grade classes for the rest of his day. Salomon's physical therapy will be discussed from age 15 months through 7 years of age, with consideration of possible physical therapy needs in adolescence and transition to adulthood.

Children with myelodysplasia present many challenges for the pediatric physical therapist working in the school setting. The role of the physical therapist includes evaluating and implementing appropriate environmental adaptations and assistive technology for the child in collaboration with the school personnel. The physical therapist will provide direct intervention

services to maximize function and promote optimal positioning to prevent skin breakdown and deformity. School personnel may not be familiar with the particular problems these students have. The physical therapist must provide information concerning not only the medical and physical issues that the student with myelodysplasia presents with, but also how these issues can impact the student's success in the school environment.

Salomon's physical therapy evaluation/diagnosis was addressed based on the American Physical Therapy Association's *Guide to Physical Therapist Practice* (2001) by Preferred Practice Pattern 5C: Impaired Motor Function and Sensory Integrity Associated with Nonprogressive Disorders of the Central Nervous System—Congenital Origin or Acquired in Infancy or Childhood. This pattern was selected because the impairments occurred in the prenatal period and the resulting manifestations affect the muscular, sensory, neurological, and skeletal systems. Practice Pattern 7A: Primary Prevention/Risk Reduction for Integumentary Disorders will also be included due to the presence of neuromuscular dysfunction, obesity, vascular disease, and spinal cord involvement.

Working with students in their natural environment can provide the therapist with an opportunity not only to be creative in intervention planning but also to be innovative in finding solutions to problems. Ideally, the physical therapist uses a collaborative model in this natural setting and provides the necessary ecological modifications and assistive technology to promote the maximal independence for the student (Palisano, 2006). Along with considerations in the school setting, the impact of the home setting also needs to be considered.

The model of collaboration within the natural setting can be challenging. There can be funding issues involved with implementing ecological changes. Assistive technology within the school environment is sometimes dependent on outside resources to make the needed modifications. Despite these obstacles, there can be simple solutions to immediate problems that require creativity, innovation, and staff collaboration to accomplish the stated goals. School staff and teacher attitudes concerning independence need to be considered, especially with preschool-aged children, as there can be tendencies to foster dependence in areas of daily living. The physical therapist relies on the classroom staff to follow through with mobility and transfer activities on a daily basis, and it is important for all members of the team to work toward common goals. A key component of the physical therapy interventions in this case study was to not only provide instruction to the student but, more importantly, to collaborate with the teachers and paraprofessionals during daily routines.

Examination: Age 3 Years

History

Salomon was delivered via caesarean section at 33 weeks' gestation and weighed 10 pounds. He was diagnosed with myelodysplasia at the thoracolumbar level and underwent a ventriculoperitoneal shunt placement and myelomeningocele closure following his birth. Hydrocephalus is one of the complications that can occur in children with myelodysplasia, and it often presents as a complication after the surgical closure of the hydrocele (Hinderer, Hinderer, & Shurtleff, 2006). A ventriculoperitoneal shunt is frequently inserted to assist in draining the excess fluid from the brain to the peritoneal space. Children with shunts need to be monitored for possible signs of infection or blockage of the shunt. There are early warning signs and symptoms of shunt dysfunction (see Table 7.10), and it is essential to share this information with the classroom teacher and school personnel who will be working with the student. The child will need medical attention if he or she displays any of these adverse symptoms.

Salomon was evaluated by a pediatric orthopedist at the age of 3 months. The orthopedist's impression was that there was good closure of the myeloid defect with no spinal deformity, even with the level of lesion at the thoracolumbar level. The orthopedist noted that there was a tendency for the hips to be laterally rotated but that the feet were flexible and easily placed in plantigrade. He recommended the initiation of physical therapy, as well as a referral to the neurosurgeon for follow-up.

Salomon gained weight rapidly in the next few months and weighed 25 pounds at 5 months of age. He had frequent episodes of bronchitis over the next year and was seen by his pediatrician for treatment. He was given the diagnosis of obesity at age 9 months when he weighed 32 pounds.

At age 15 months a prescription was written for Salomon to receive physical therapy through an early intervention program. The emphasis of his early therapy was independence in rolling, transitions to sitting, and commando crawling. At 2 years of age he attempted hands and knees positioning with support. The physical therapist indicated that Salomon's movement was limited due to the thoracolumbar level of his lesion; however, he was independent in moving his wheelchair on flat surfaces. He is able to play a game incorporating wheelchair push-ups to strengthen his arms and to encourage pressure relief. He is working on transfers from his wheelchair to the sofa. He is able to get off the sofa independently, using his upper body strength. Salomon is pulling himself up onto low surfaces.

In the adaptive area, he can feed himself and drink from a sippy cup. The family is working with a nutritionist who helps monitor his weight, and recommendations for a healthy diet have been provided. He enjoys bath time and assists with dressing by holding out his arms and removing his socks. He is able to complete a simple puzzle, stack 4 blocks, and assemble toys. Salomon enjoys playing with his cousins, shares toys easily, and helps with simple household tasks. By the age of 2 years, he used 30 to 40 words in Spanish to communicate with family members, including some two-word phrases.

Salomon had two shunt replacements by the time he was 2 years old. He continues to be followed as needed by his pediatrician for colds, bronchitis, pneumonia, and a urinary tract infection. He has problems associated with nonpitting edema of his lower extremities, and he is described as having poor circulation in his legs with purplish discoloration. Salomon was referred to a vascular surgeon and was diagnosed with vasculopathy when he was 3 years old. He had previously been prescribed a wheelchair with dependent footrests but needs to have his legs and feet elevated for periods during the day to promote improved lower extremity circulation.

System Review

Cardiovascular and Pulmonary

Salomon had frequent colds, bronchitis, and pneumonia from the age of 4 months to 3 years of age. He had a respiratory rate (RR) of 36 breaths per minute and his blood pressure was 95/63 mm Hg.

Integumentary

There is nonpitting edema, purplish coloration of the skin of both lower extremities. He has a scar in the thoracolumbar area where the myeloid defect was closed. He has erythema and skin breakdown in the skin folds of his knees, inguinal area, and axilla due to his obesity, which is being addressed at home and by the school nurse. Latex allergy precautions were recommended.

Musculoskeletal

Active range of motion (AROM) was within normal limits in the upper extremities as well as the upper and lower trunk. The lower extremities tend to be externally rotated at the hips and there are limitations in internal rotation of the hips. His feet are fixed in approximately 30 degrees of plantar flexion. He exhibits full passive range of motion (PROM) of knee flexion and extension. There is good strength in the upper extremities but marked weakness in the lower extremities. He has the ability to hike his hips bilaterally and there is trace hip flexion. At the time of the exam, he weighed 70 pounds and was 37 inches tall.

Neuromuscular

Normal muscle tone was noted in the upper extremities and trunk to the T12 level. Some pelvic control and hip hiking were noted, as well as trace hip flexion bilaterally. There was flaccid paralysis of the lower extremities.

Cognition, Language, and Communication

Salomon is learning English as a second language. He is able to talk in short sentences and can understand simple commands and requests, though he sometimes requires physical demonstration. A speech language pathologist sees him for a speech and language impairment. He is learning letters, numbers, colors, and the names of objects.

Because Salomon has a Hispanic background, there are communication challenges for him as well as his family. There is a need for interpreters for all aspects of communication, and written communication is translated by interpreters or by utilizing free online translation programs.

An Individualized Education Program (IEP) was developed with the diagnostics staff, the service coordinator from the early intervention program, and Salomon's mother. The speech language diagnostician is Spanish speaking and performed the diagnostic testing. She also helped to translate all of the proceedings of the IEP meeting into Spanish for the parent. Future IEP meetings were all conducted with the assistance of a translator. All written communication and telephone calls utilized the translation line or were done with the assistance of Spanish-speaking staff at school.

Salomon was initially evaluated by the school system's diagnostic department for screening and placement recommendations. The initial screening and tests included American Guidance Service (AGS) Early Screening Profiles, the Batelle Developmental Inventory (BDI-2), Vineland, and a speech language assessment. The Preschool Language Scale (PLS-4) was administered in Spanish by a Spanish-speaking speech-language pathologist. The AGS Early Screening Profiles, BDI-2, Vineland, and speech language assessment are all standardized on a mean of 100 and a standard deviation of 15.

The screening information was summarized, and Salomon was given the eligibility of significant developmental delay (SDD). To be given the eligibility of SDD in this school district, a child must score at least 2 standard deviations below the mean in one or more of the five skill areas (cognition, communication, physical development—gross and fine motor, adaptive domain, and social/emotional development). Salomon had scores of at least 2 standard deviations below the mean in cognition and communication. The diagnostics team recommended that he receive special education services at an early childhood public school 2 days per week for a total of 7 hours per week in a self-contained classroom. It was recommended that he be transported to school in his wheelchair on a lift bus.

Tests and Measures

Aerobic Capacity and Endurance

Salomon is able to move his manual wheelchair in the school environment as well as on the playground, keeping pace with his classmates. Distances from the classroom to the cafeteria are more than 500 feet. He does not appear to have any difficulties with aerobic capacity or endurance.

Assistive and Adaptive Devices

Salomon required immediate accommodations to allow him independence in his transfers at school. He quickly learned to move from the wheelchair to the table, using the sliding board with adult assistance. He also needed accommodations in the cafeteria, as the tables were too low. Salomon is able use a desk at an appropriate height for eating. Additionally, a large wedge was utilized for transfers from his wheelchair to the floor during motor activities or in the classroom for rest time. He utilizes the wedge to move from the floor back into his wheelchair, although he requires physical assistance with this activity.

Gait, Locomotion and Balance

Salomon is nonambulatory, and standing has not been attempted because of his past problems with cellulitis, poor circulation, and lack of past weight-bearing activity. He does not wear shoes due to difficulties with trying to fit his feet. Salomon is learning to move his wheelchair with good speed and accuracy and exhibits safety with his wheelchair mobility in the classroom and hallways, as well as on the playground and a variety of terrains.

Motor Function

Salomon is able to scoot forward on his arms in prone. He can also push up into a 4-point position with moderate assist given to support his legs in midline. He demonstrates the ability to sit independently on the mat or floor, but when reaching forward or to the side, he displays postural instability and a loss of balance.

Muscle Performance

Salomon has a thoracolumbar lesion and in sitting is able to move forward or to the side by hip hiking and using his upper extremities to lift his body. He has trace ability to flex at the hip, as he can initiate slight hip flexion when gravity is eliminated. Standardized manual muscle tests are difficult to use reliably on 3-year-olds, especially with Salomon who has difficulties understanding specific requests due to his limited English proficiency and extreme shyness. A functional assessment of Salomon's strength was done. Salomon demonstrates the ability to lift his body, pushing up on his arms to assist with sliding board transfers. He can also push his manual wheelchair without difficulty and at an appropriate walking speed. He is able to lift his arms above his head to catch and throw a ball and demonstrates the ability to perform modified push-ups using his arms for 5 repetitions. He displays weakness in his trunk, as he is able to sit only briefly without upper extremity support.

Neuromotor Development and Sensory Integration

Salomon has good manipulation skills as he is able to stack at least 6 cubes, make linear marks, and use a neat pincer grasp. Sensory testing was not initiated due to difficulties with accurate assessment at this age. It was assumed that there could be a lack of sensation below the level of T12 and safety precautions were implemented. Salomon has a neurogenic bowel and bladder.

Orthotic Devices

Salomon did not have any orthotics at this time.

Range of Motion

Salomon exhibits full PROM of his upper extremities. His feet are fixed in approximately 30 degrees of plantar flexion.

Self-Care and Home Management (Including Activities of Daily Living and Instrumental Activities of Daily Living)

Salomon is able to feed himself with a spoon, eating a variety of foods. He drinks from an open cup without spillage. He assists with dressing. He can transfer from his wheelchair to another chair or low mat table with assist. He is learning how to use a transfer board for transitions. At home, he is dependent in his transfers to the bathtub and needs bathing equipment to assist with independence in this area. He has a neurogenic bowel and bladder and is not involved in an intermittent catheterization program. He is being diapered frequently during the school day.

Examination Update: If being seen today, it would be appropriate to evaluate Salomon using the Pediatric Evaluation of Disability Inventory (Haley, Coster, Ludlow, Haltiwanger, & Andrellos, 1992).

Evaluation, Diagnosis, and Prognosis
Including Plan of Care

Salomon is not only shy and fearful in his new environment but also unwilling to communicate with new adults or other children. He has quickly learned sliding board transfers from his wheelchair to the low mat table for diaper changes. He has motor impairments (muscle strength, muscle endurance), sensory loss (T12 and below with neurogenic bowel and bladder), obesity, and integumentary disorder (skin breakdown around the knees, inguinal area, and axilla; history of cellulitis). These impairments pose challenges for optimal wheelchair positioning, with the potential to impact his level of activity and his ability to play with his peers.

Prognosis

Salomon will be independent in his wheelchair mobility in the school environment with appropriate environmental modifications. His wheelchair positioning will be an ongoing need as he continues to grow. His weight management will be critical to his health and mobility. There will also need to be a coordinated effort between the school nurse, child, and family along with possible intermittent catheterization procedures implemented at school and at home. This will help to prevent skin breakdown as a result of ammonia burns. Salomon will need to maintain the motor skills to assist with transfers, and wheelchair accommodations may be necessary to promote this process. Adaptations will be necessary to allow participation in physical education (PE) and playground activities (see Table 25.1).

Goals

Salomon will work on the goals and objectives listed in Table 25.2 and Table 25.3 for the current school year, with physical therapy provided once weekly for 30-minute sessions at school. Initially, there will be more physical therapy involvement to instruct the teachers and to coordinate with the nurse and PE teacher for needed adaptations. The family, school personnel, and the wheelchair vendor will meet to coordinate recommendations for wheelchair positioning and adaptations. A task analysis will be followed for teaching sliding board transfers to the school personnel, Salomon, and his family.

Intervention

Coordination, Communication, and Documentation

Initially, there was a need for frequent communication with the school personnel, teachers, and nurses for ongoing positioning needs and adaptations for Salomon. The physical therapist also communicated with the parents and wheelchair vendors to provide optimal seating

Table 25.1 Adaptations of Preschool Environment

Location	Environmental Adaptations/Assistive Technology
Bus	Lift bus necessary for wheelchair transport. Assist student initially to move into school and roll wheelchair to classroom. Work on moving on and off lift independently.
Classroom	Open areas to allow for ease of wheelchair mobility. Assess alternative positioning and transfers to a mat via wedge.
Bathroom	Changing table/sliding board/lifting and transfer training are of immediate concern for the student and staff. Grab bar necessary to assist with rolling activity. Evaluate for use of a sliding board and begin to instruct staff and student in technique. Rolling stool needed to promote good body mechanics for staff due to low changing table.
Cafeteria	Check height of table to allow sufficient wheelchair clearance for eating lunch and provide desk or tray as needed.
Playground	Areas for wheelchair mobility, ability to access playground equipment, including paved track around playground, cushioned-synthetic rubber surface to play structure, ramp to one level of equipment.

Table 25.2 IEP Goal at Age 3 Years

IEP Goal—The student will improve in the gross motor area

Short-Term Objective	Strategy
Salomon will assist with transfers from the chair to the floor with physical and verbal prompts, 3 out of 5 trials.	Use large wedge to move from chair to floor. Needs assist when going back up wedge as he tends to slide back down; needs support at feet.
Salomon will perform sliding board transfers with verbal cues and physical assistance (adult places sliding board and provides support for lower extremities), 3 out of 5 trials.	Task analysis as described below. Practice done with teacher/staff/student daily at first, then monitor/return demonstration weekly.
Salomon will propel his wheelchair on even surfaces, up and down ramps, and over thresholds with appropriate speed, keeping pace with his peers with distant supervision, 80% of the school day.	Practice in natural setting—moving with class to all school locations (including playground). Monitor speed. Move in line with other classmates, avoiding obstacles/people with accurate stop/starts.

Table 25.3 Task Analysis for Sliding Board Transfer

Goal	Task Analysis
Independent sliding board transfer	Salomon moves wheelchair to table. Salomon sets brakes. Salomon unfastens seat belt. Classroom teacher places sliding board under front of chair (with new chair, he can use the seat as a sliding board). Salomon pushes up and scoots forward, hiking his hips and using the grab bar to help pull onto the changing table. (Minimal assist is provided by the teacher to help position his legs.) Salomon uses the grab bar to assist in rolling over to help with diapering.

for Salomon. After Salomon was evaluated by the physical therapist, an IEP meeting was held to discuss the results of the evaluation with the parents and team members. Physical therapy began and daily program planning was implemented. Positioning and transfers were addressed with all staff members who worked with Salomon. Salomon's mother observed him transferring at school and also provided input on his performance at home.

Patient/Client-Related Instruction

It was initially necessary to schedule direct individual physical therapy sessions to correspond with the transfers needed for diaper changes and to reinforce the activity in the natural environment. This provided instruction to Salomon as well as the teachers and the support staff. Salomon's teacher was not familiar with sliding board transfers, and initial instruction required repeated trials of this activity to instruct both the teacher and the assistants in proper technique. Salomon learned the technique with a few repetitions, but the staff needed to learn to allow him to be as independent as possible in his attempts. There was a tendency for the staff to lift him rather than promote the sliding board transfer. The physical therapist worked closely with the staff to promote Salomon's independence in transfers. With repeated trials, he was able to perform this activity with minimal assistance.

Procedural Interventions

Initial Environmental Modifications

The process to secure the initial environmental modifications for Salomon in the school was initiated by the physical therapist. These modifications included sliding board, wedge, grab bar, changing table, and a large wedge for classroom transfers to the floor. A request was made for a specific length and placement of the grab bar in the bathroom. The school provided a transfer sliding board and a wedge to help with the height difference between the chair and low mat table that would be used for diaper changes. An electric changing table was also requested, and a year after Salomon arrived at school, additional funding became available to order it. The electric changing table was used for transfers and could be elevated to encourage better body mechanics for the staff changing his diaper. Physical therapy intervention was provided in the classroom and natural environment (hallways, cafeteria, playground, bathroom, and gym) as much as possible.

Therapeutic Exercise

Exercise and conditioning have been incorporated into Salomon's daily routine. He is working on his sitting balance during transfer activities. His motor skills of rolling over and sitting up from supine are being addressed during his twice-daily diaper changes. His endurance in wheelchair ambulation has increased with continued practice. During motor or PE class, modifications are being made to incorporate pressure relief exercises along with strengthening exercises using activities such as reaching to retrieve a ball at the side of his wheelchair. He is able to push his wheelchair around the outside track, follow his friends on their tricycles, and maintain good speed and direction, which improves his endurance.

Assistive/Adaptive Equipment

Wheelchair Modifications

It is important to consider the following goals for optimal wheelchair seating for students with myelodysplasia: protect the skin integrity, promote optimal mobility, and assure good alignment, especially of the spine (Hastings, 2000). Another important consideration for children who will be lifelong wheelchair ambulators is the reduction of forces needed to propel the wheelchair. Recent studies suggest that lightweight and ultralight wheelchairs are preferred by children and their families (Meiser & McEwen, 2007). A lightweight wheelchair was selected, but the extended seat, which incorporated a sliding board, added additional weight. The physical therapist and seating specialist, incorporating parental input, made recommendations for wheelchair modifications as outlined in Table 25.4.

Salomon's wheelchair does not have armrests. An adjustable easel is used in the classroom for schoolwork. A desk is used in the cafeteria, as the chair does not fit under the cafeteria table.

Summary of Procedural Interventions

Salomon improved in his independence during transfers. With adaptations made to the wheelchair, his lower extremities were supported, further skin

Table 25.4 Wheelchair Modifications

Wheelchair Description	Positioning Problem With Old Wheelchair	Recommendations Made and Equipment Provided With New Wheelchair
Custom seating system— manual wheelchair	Seat-to-back angle was reclined. He needed 90-90 angle.	New wheelchair base accommodates upright 90-90 seat-to-back angle. Seat: 15 inches wide, 22 inches long Back (from original chair): 12 inches × 12 inches
New manual wheelchair	Footrest: one-piece footrest, which is difficult to remove and swing out of the way; feet need to be elevated.	Custom wood/foam seat was fabricated to provide leg support and allow for sliding transfers to changing table. Base also provided protection for legs and feet (especially a concern due to lack of sensation). Base will help prevent swelling of legs.

Continued

Table 25.4 Wheelchair Modifications—cont'd

Wheelchair Description	Positioning Problem With Old Wheelchair	Recommendations Made and Equipment Provided With New Wheelchair
	Hip pads: small and difficult to remove, difficult to set brakes	Custom hip pads were made that are longer and larger with optimal placement (not impacting setting brakes); this will protect legs from rubbing on wheels and promote midline positioning of legs.
	Poor wheel placement for propulsion	New frame allows wheel placement for better propulsion.
	Chair needs to be larger to accommodate weight gain	New wheelchair has larger frame.

breakdown was prevented, and there was improved lower extremity circulation. The school nurse monitored his skin for breakdown and coordinated his medical care with the family and primary physician. She also assisted with his appointments at the spina bifida clinic at the local children's hospital. Intermittent catheterization procedures were discussed with the family.

While Salomon achieved his objective of transferring from his wheelchair to the changing table, due to changes in school personnel and the need for continuity of care, this skill will need to be maintained. It will also need to be monitored, due to possible changes in his medical condition. The positioning needs will be ongoing as he grows. Salomon will also need to have modifications made for participation in PE and continue to have access to participate in appropriate exercises to encourage activity. He will need to continue to participate in exercises to provide pressure relief throughout his school day to prevent skin breakdown.

Examination: Age 5 years

History

Salomon is in kindergarten in the same school where he attended preschool. He continues to be monitored daily for skin breakdown by the school nurse. He is utilizing intermittent catheterization for bladder management twice daily in the nurse's clinic as well as at home. He was seen in the spina bifida clinic this past year, and his mother was instructed in catheterization procedures and given nutrition counseling for Salomon. During a hospitalization for cellulitis, it was noted that his shunt was cracked and a shunt revision was done. A physical therapy consult in the hospital was done, and it was

recommended that Salomon receive a bath transfer chair and a sliding board. He was diagnosed with asthma and has inhalation treatments as needed. He has been closely monitored during exercise as this sometimes exacerbates his asthma.

System Review

Cardiovascular and Pulmonary

Salomon was diagnosed with asthma, which appeared to be exacerbated with exercise. This needs to be monitored closely at school, especially when he is playing outside. His heart rate and blood pressure were within normal limits (WNL) for his age.

Integumentary

Salomon continues to be monitored closely for skin erythema in the skin folds of his knees, inguinal area, and axilla. His skin irritation has lessened with the introduction of intermittent catheterization. He has some incontinence between catheterizations, and a trial of Ditropam was initiated to possibly help with this problem. He has been on a diet and has successfully lost weight, which will potentially help with his skin condition.

Musculoskeletal

Since the age of 9 months, Salomon has had a diagnosis of obesity. The usual method used to assess body mass index (BMI) is height-weight ratios, but for individuals with myelodysplasia, arm span–weight ratios are considered more appropriate (Shurtleff, 1986). The arm-span measurement is considered to be a more accurate measure due to the short stature of individuals with myelodysplasia, which is a result of the decreased growth of the paretic limbs (Shurtleff, 1986). Due to the level of his lesion (thoracic and high lumbar), there is a 0.9 correction factor "to avoid underestimating body fat content" (Del Gado & Del Gaizo, 1999).

Salomon was 43 inches tall and weighed 103 pounds at age 5. He had an arm span of 50 inches, and when this was calculated with the 0.9 correction factor, it was determined that he had a BMI of 36 (in the range of obesity). He has been on a diet and, according to his mother, is aware of what he can and cannot eat. He has been able to lose weight and his doctor was pleased with his progress. Salomon continues to improve in his trunk strength and balance. He is able to reach to either side of his wheelchair to retrieve a ball from the floor, and then sit back up in his wheelchair.

Neuromuscular

Sensory testing was done, which indicated sensation was intact through T12 but absent below this level.

Communication, Affect, Cognition, Language, and Learning Style

Salomon is a friendly boy, and he initiated greetings and responded to greetings from friends and familiar staff. He continues to be shy with new teachers and students. He is always eager to please and has a smile on his face. He is working on letter recognition and recognizes 13 of 26 letters. He recognizes numerals 1 to 5 and is able to name the letters in his name. He has improved in his ability to comprehend and respond correctly to questions during a story. He has made gains with understanding and verbally expressing new vocabulary words. The school speech language pathologist describes him as shy and not a risk taker with language. When he is unsure of an answer, he will not attempt a response. He is working on verbalizations to indicate that he needs help or does not know.

Tests and Measures

Aerobic Capacity and Endurance

Salomon experiences shortness of breath during periods of increased effort when moving his wheelchair at a fast speed while on the playground. He is being monitored for exercise-induced asthma when he is engaged in aerobic activities.

Assistive and Adaptive Devices

Salomon has a new wheelchair with an extended seat to assist with sliding transfers to the electric changing table. The new wheelchair has armrests that can be used for his lap tray or can be lifted up to provide better access to his wheels for improved mobility. The lap tray is used in the classroom for writing assignments and in the cafeteria for meals.

Gait, Locomotion, and Balance

Salomon continues to propel his wheelchair independently throughout the school and can now move his chair up the ramp on the playground and across the grassy areas as well. He enjoys moving around the track with his classmates chasing him. He is able to move his wheelchair on and off the bus lift. Salomon continues to exhibit good upper extremity strength, and his trunk strength has improved with daily practice and exercise. (Fig. 25.1). He is able to sit comfortably on the changing table without upper extremity support.

Motor Function

Salomon has improved in his ability to move his trunk forward and from side to side without a loss of balance. He is able to assist with rolling to either side while on the changing table as well as pull up to sit independently using the grab bars. He is able to move from

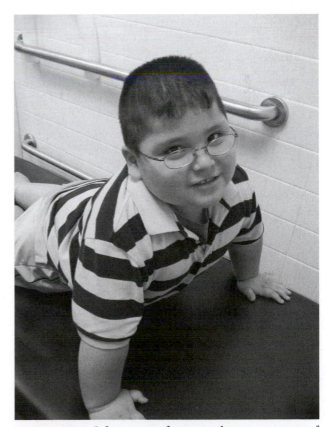

Figure 25.1 Salomon performs push-ups as a part of his daily exercise routine.

sitting to backlying, roll from side to side, and move back up to sitting. He can now sit without losing his balance. He lifted a 3-pound bar weight to perform a daily exercise routine while on the changing table.

Muscle Performance

Salomon continues to exhibit good upper extremity strength. He exhibits good trunk strength, which has improved with daily practice and exercise. He exhibits some pelvic control in sitting, which might indicate abdominal or paraspinal muscle innervation. He can perform hip hiking, which possibly indicates activity in the quadratus lumborum muscle. He exhibits slight hip flexion with gravity eliminated, which might indicate iliospoas activity. This would support the level of the lesion at the thoracolumbar motor level, possibly T12, L1.

Orthotic Devices

Salomon was evaluated by an orthotist and has bilateral custom ankle-foot orthosis (AFOs). The AFOs provide protection and positioning for his legs, particularly his feet.

Range of Motion

Through observation it was noted that Salomon has a possible hip dislocation. He has adduction of the right hip with the femur moving in and out of the acetabulum. This is addressed by keeping his legs in an abducted position. He was discouraged from falling forward over his legs into a prone position, as this tends to loosen the hip joint by overstretching the capsule. The information concerning the possibility of a dislocating hip was given to Salomon's parents. Surgery is probably not indicated since there is no indication of pain and no deformity (Asher & Olson, 1983). The right hip dislocation will need to be monitored and addressed with his wheelchair positioning. PROM remains WNL in the upper extremities and trunk. No other ROM limitations were noted in the lower extremities.

Self-Care and Home Management (Including Activities of Daily Living and Instrumental Activities of Daily Living)

Salomon is independent in all transfers at home. He is able to move easily from his wheelchair to the bed. He can also transfer independently to the bath chair in the tub. He is able to assist with lower extremity dressing and puts on a shirt and jacket independently. Salomon continues to assist with simple chores at home, such as setting the table and picking up his toys.

When evaluated with the School Function Assessment (SFA) (Coster, Deeney, Haltiwanger, & Haley, 1998), Salomon has difficulties in cognitive tasks, as well as written work and functional communication. His strengths are noted in the areas of following directions, behavior regulation, and safety. In the classroom he is working on writing his letters and numbers. He can copy sentences with lined paper.

Salomon is being catheterized at school and at home and is beginning to participate in this procedure.

He is able to move safely and efficiently in his wheelchair to all areas of the school and is transferring independently at home and at school (Fig. 25.2).

Evaluation, Diagnosis, and Prognosis
Including Plan of Care

Salomon is making friends and is eager to learn new things. He continues to follow a diet for weight reduction and has lost 3 pounds this past year. He enjoys

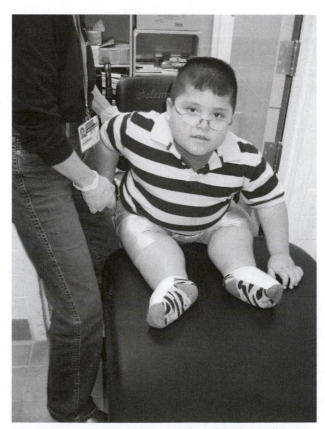

Figure 25.2 Transfers are made safely from the wheelchair to the hi-low table.

playing ball and moves around the outside track, chasing his friends. He continues to need monitoring for skin erythema and breakdown. He participates in weight-shift exercises and wheelchair push-ups to prevent pressure areas. He participates in PE with typical peers with modifications for some of the activities.

Prognosis

Salomon will continue to need monitoring for his wheelchair positioning. He will also need to continue to participate in his exercise program to prevent skin breakdown and to encourage activity. He would benefit from a community program to participate in wheelchair sports activities, such as basketball or soccer. His weight will continue to be a major concern. It will possibly impact his ability to maintain transfer skills and will affect endurance and cardiovascular health, as well as his skin integrity. He will need family and school support to assist him in following an exercise program and with eating a healthy diet.

Goals

Salomon will be transitioning to a new school for first grade. The environmental modifications, in particular the electric changing table, will need to be available to him at his new school. See Table 25.5.

Intervention

Coordination, Communication, and Documentation

There continues to be regular communication between teachers, nurses, physical therapists, and Salomon's physician and family. Progress notes and annual evaluations are done by the physical therapist and treatment is provided during PE or, as needed, in the classroom or the playground. Salomon continues to receive direct physical therapy; however, he is seen for less time and requires only occasional monitoring for progress on his goals. The physical therapist continues to be involved in IEP meetings. Salomon will be transitioning to another school and recommendations will be made for a smooth transition.

Patient/Client-Related Instruction

Personnel at his new school will be instructed in transfers and a new changing table may need to be ordered to accommodate his needs. Salomon will need to become familiar with the layout of the school and access will be monitored. Wheelchair positioning will continue to be monitored and exercises for weight shift and mobility will continue in his new setting. Nursing services will be necessary to provide continued instruction in self-catheterization. A picture program of exercises was provided for Salomon and his family to encourage continuation of his exercise routine at home.

Procedural Interventions

Therapeutic Exercise

Salomon is working on improving his upper extremity strength. He is lifting light weights and performing push-ups, as well as moving frequently during the day for transfers. He continues to work on improving his trunk strength during his transitions from his wheelchair to the changing table. He is continuing to participate in a modified PE program. He enjoys pushing his wheelchair around the track and can play basketball on a lower hoop

---

Table 25.5 IEP Goals and Strategies at 5 Years of Age

Goal	Strategy
Salomon will propel his wheelchair on even surfaces, up and down ramps, and on and off the bus with appropriate speed, 90% of the school day.	• Continue to monitor and encourage pushing wheelchair laps around playground. • Monitor access on/off bus lift.
Salomon will lean to either side of his wheelchair to pick up an 8-inch playground ball from the floor, 3 out of 5 attempts.	• Instruct and collaborate with PE coach to encourage during motor class. • Hold onto armrest for support. • Lift ball alongside of chair.
Health-related objective: Salomon will perform wheelchair push-ups or lean forward for pressure relief, with verbal prompts as needed.	• Teacher will remind student to do push-ups or to lean forward with changes in activity or schedule.

with his classmates (Fig. 25.3 and Fig. 25.4). He also enjoys hitting a baseball off a baseball T.

Functional Training in Work, Community, and Leisure Integration

Salomon has been encouraged to participate in an adapted sports program in his county. This program will offer him the opportunity to participate in group sports including wheelchair handball, basketball, and football to provide physical activity and to promote social interactions and team skills.

Summary of Procedural Interventions

Salomon has shown improved endurance and muscle strength in his trunk and upper extremities. He is now independent in his transfers at home and at school, with the appropriate modifications. He can now transfer to and from his bed and bathtub at home and to the changing table with standby assist.

Salomon will continue to be monitored as he transitions from preschool to elementary school for first

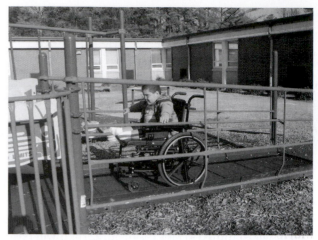

Figure 25.4 Negotiating the ramp to the playground structure is easier using the rail.

through fifth grades. His new school will need to be evaluated for access to all areas of the school. There may be a need to order an electric changing table to continue independent wheelchair transfers. His exercise program and pressure relief exercises will need to be continued and monitored. Nursing will continue to be involved with his catheterization.

Examination: Age 7 Years

History

Salomon has transitioned to an elementary school and is attending first grade. He had another hospitalization for cellulitis this year. He continues to be catheterized by the nurse as well as monitored for skin breakdown.

System Review

Cardiovascular and Pulmonary

Salomon has a blood pressure of 124/70 mm Hg, and his heart rate is 104 beats per minute. Salomon requires infrequent inhalation treatments for his asthma while at school. He is able to participate in PE without any problems with endurance.

Integumentary

Salomon was hospitalized this year for cellulitis. The school nurse reported that his skin has been improving, and he is doing well with the intermittent catheterization program. She continues to encourage Salomon to drink water throughout the day. He continues to exhibit nonpitting edema and purplish color in both feet when his feet are dependent.

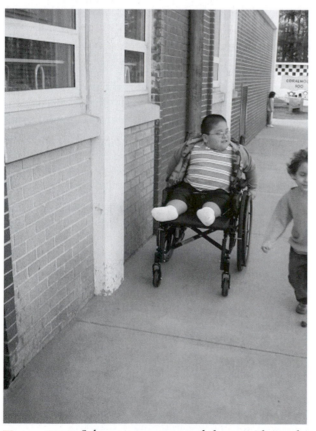

Figure 25.3 Salomon races around the outside track with a friend.

Musculoskeletal

Salomon weighs 120 pounds, with an arm span of 54 inches. He has a BMI of 35.2, which is in the range of obesity. He continues to exhibit good trunk and upper extremity strength. There is continued emphasis on functional movement during catheterization when Salomon transfers to the changing table and moves from sitting to backlying and back to sitting. He also participates in PE twice per week. With the increasing demands for academics, there is less opportunity for playtime outside, and this elementary school does not have a paved outdoor track for wheelchair mobility. Salomon does participate in walks around the campus with his class, which provides outdoor science activities.

Neuromuscular

There have been no changes in this area. He continues to display sensory and motor loss below the T12 level.

Communication, Affect, Cognition, and Learning Style

Salomon has made gains in his knowledge of letters, sounds, numbers, and counting. He has received intensive support from the special education teacher in a pull-out model of co-teaching. Although Salomon made significant academic progress, his skills are at the kindergarten level. It was recommended by the IEP team that he repeat first grade. He will continue to benefit from this coteaching model when he repeats first grade next year. His teacher stated that he has improved in his verbal expression as well as his comprehension.

Tests and Measures

Aerobic Capacity and Endurance

He is able to propel his wheelchair with adequate speed for distances of 500 feet without difficulty.

Examination Update: It would be appropriate to evaluate wheelchair propulsion using either the rate of perceived exertion (pediatric version) or energy expenditure index.

Assistive and Adaptive Devices

The new school received an electric changing table this year, which allows Salomon to continue his independent transfers. He has a wheelchair desk that he uses in his first-grade classroom and one in the special education classroom. He is able to pull up under the table in the cafeteria (Fig. 25.5).

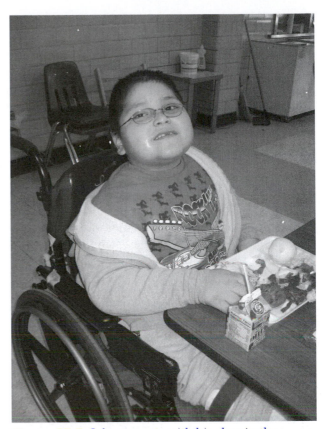

Figure 25.5 Salomon eats with his class in the cafeteria.

He has a manual wheelchair with custom hip pads, and a custom wood/foam seat for leg support that allows for sliding transfers to the changing table. He continues to be monitored for growth and fit of his wheelchair. The wheel placement was adjusted to promote optimal ability to push the chair and to prevent strain to his shoulders and arms.

Gait, Locomotion, and Balance

Salomon continues to be independent in his wheelchair mobility in all areas of his new school.

Motor Function

Salomon continues to perform push-ups and pressure relief exercises throughout the day. He continues to perform independent transfers to the changing table, and he is able to roll from side to side during catheterization procedures. He continues to work on his trunk exercises when he moves from supine to sitting.

Neuromotor Development and Sensory Integration

There have been no changes in this area.

Orthotic Devices

He continues to wear solid ankle AFOs and is monitored for fit and skin breakdown.

Range of Motion

Salomon has hip flexion contractures, which were measured in the prone position. The prone extension test (Staheli, 1977) has been shown to have better reliability as compared to the Thomas test (Bartlett, Wolf, Shurtleff, & Staheli, 1985). He has lack of full knee flexion as well as limitations in internal rotation of the hips. Both hips can be passively positioned in neutral (0 degrees) rotation with passive movement. He has external rotation of both hips with the left to 30 degrees and the right to 25 degrees. He does not have any internal rotation of the hips. There is full knee extension on the right and 30 degrees lacking in full extension on the left. Both the right and left knees flex to 65 degrees. Goniometric measurements are listed in Table 25.6.

Self-Care and Home Management (Including Activities of Daily Living and Instrumental Activities of Daily Living)

Salomon has maintained all of his previous skills. He continues to exhibit independent transfers to the changing table (Fig. 25.6). Salomon is able to put on his jacket independently. He continues to work on pulling up his shorts during the catheterization procedure. He is able to independently don and doff his AFOs. He continues to work on pushing his wheelchair from the lower level of the parking lot to the upper level.

Examination Update: It would be appropriate to update the SFA to provide information about his function in the new school setting. Other appropriate

Table 25.6 Lower Extremity Range of Motion

Joint motion	Right	Left
Hip flexion	20–120 degrees	20–120 degrees
Hip external rotation	0–25 degrees	0–30 degrees
Knee flexion	0–65 degrees	30–65 degrees

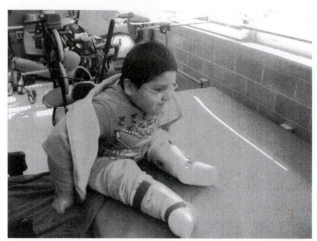

Figure 25.6 Salomon transfers independently to the mat table.

assessments that would address Salomon's level of participation in activities in the home, school, and community would include the Canadian Occupational Performance Measure or the Children's Assessment of Participation and Enjoyment.

Evaluation, Diagnosis, and Prognosis
Including Plan of Care

Salomon transitioned to a new school and is independent in his mobility and transfers. He had gained weight and his diet will continue to be monitored. He needs to be reminded to perform weight-shift exercises and wheelchair push-ups to prevent pressure areas.

Prognosis

In spite of his weight gain, Salomon continues to move easily to the changing table. An adapted sports program would promote fitness, but he has not participated in this program. There were possible support system issues that precluded Salomon's participation in this program. It would be beneficial to explore this with his family and school personnel to determine whether this could be implemented.

Goals

Salomon is independent in his mobility and transfers. He continues to require reminders to perform wheelchair push-ups and pressure relief exercises. There are no goals or short-term objectives identified during this episode of care that require physical therapy support. There will continue to be consultative services to address positioning and modifications that might be needed.

Intervention

Coordination, Communication, and Documentation

The physical therapist will continue to monitor Salomon for his positioning and equipment needs. The physical therapist continues to provide input as needed during PE and in the classroom or cafeteria.

Patient/Client-Related Instruction

Salomon continues to need reminders to perform weight-shift exercises. He should begin to be involved in skin inspection for breakdown, especially his feet and legs.

Procedural Interventions

Therapeutic Exercise

Salomon was receiving consultative physical therapy services at this time. The physical therapist provided consultation during PE and also during his school day. Recommendations were made to the classroom teachers for encouraging pressure relief exercises with every subject change or hourly during the school day. The physical therapist encouraged participation in the regular PE program with modifications made for the activities as needed. Upper extremity strengthening was emphasized during the warm-up exercises at the beginning of the PE classes. For example, when the students are performing push-ups, Salomon can perform wheelchair armrest push-ups. Flexibility warm-up exercises were performed, incorporating toe touches and side bends while sitting in his wheelchair. Salomon engages in aerobic conditioning during relay races, as well as when the students run daily laps around the gym. Peer helpers assist Salomon during PE if help is needed to participate in the games. There continue to be challenges for Salomon to work on improving his endurance and aerobic capacity during the school day.

Examination Update: One method for encouraging and monitoring Salomon's aerobic capacity and endurance would be participation in a laps program around the school. Using a pulse oximeter, his pulse and O_2 saturation could be monitored following completion of the required laps. A stopwatch could be used to determine the time required for lap completion. This could be monitored on a monthly basis and the laps program could be completed on a daily basis. In addition to promoting increased fitness, Salomon could chart his progress as part of a math lesson.

Functional Training in Work, Community, and Leisure Integration

Physical therapy was provided in a consultative model. There continues to be training in wheelchair mobility with emphasis on moving from the lower parking lot to the upper parking lot.

Summary of Procedural Interventions

Salomon demonstrates maintenance of his ability to transfer and moves his wheelchair easily to all locations at his new school.

Termination of Episode of Care

There will continue to be a need to monitor Salomon in the area of positioning and follow-up to ensure his compliance with the pressure relief exercises. His classroom teacher will need to assist in monitoring this program. Physical therapy was recommended for consultative services to address any positioning concerns, to monitor his transfers, and to provide modifications as needed during PE.

Adolescence and Associated Transitions/Considerations

It will continue to be imperative to monitor Salomon's wheelchair positioning and transfers in the school and home environment as he transitions from elementary school into middle and high school. Travel in typical middle and high schools involves increased distances, and he may encounter more environmental obstacles. Access will be needed to public transportation and also training and adaptations for driving a car. Power wheelchair mobility may be an option at that time.

With increased growth during adolescence, it will be particularly important to monitor Salomon for scoliosis and contractures of the hips and knees. He will need to continue to inspect his feet and lower extremities for any sign of skin lesions. The physical therapist will also continue to monitor Salomon for any decreases in trunk or upper extremity strength, as this might be related to a progression in neurologic deficit.

Salomon should continue to be monitored for overuse syndromes, as this may occur with manual wheelchair mobility and transfers.

Salomon will need to monitor his weight and will need encouragement to maintain healthy eating habits. He will need opportunities for ongoing fitness activities to continue to be functional in the activities of daily living (Fragala-Pinkham, Haley, & Goodgold, 2006).

Intervention Update: Physical therapy intervention for individuals with myelodysplasia may vary widely depending on the age and specific needs of the individual. Children with thoracic, lumbar, or sacral level lesions have very different functional abilities and participation restrictions. In the years since Salomon was a young child, additional research on various interventions for children and adults with myelodysplasia has become available. Table 25.7 details current evidence-based interventions for individuals with myelodysplasia.

Table 25.7 Evidence-Based Interventions for Myelomeningocele (MMC)

Intervention	Author (Date)	Study Design	No. of Subjects	Question	Findings
Therapeutic Exercise: Aerobic capacity/ endurance training	Buffart, Roebroeck, Rol, Stam, & Berg-Emons (2008)	Cross-sectional	51	What is the relationship between physical activity, aerobic fitness, and body fat in adolescents & young adults with myelomeningocele (MMC)?	39% inactive, 37% extremely inactive, 35% obese, 42% lower than normal values for aerobic fitness, ambulatory status related to physical activity.
	Bartonek, Eriksson, & Saraste (2002)	Cohort study	8	What is the heart rate and walking velocity of children with low- and mid-lumbar MMC using 2 types of orthoses?	All children showed higher heart rate than nondisabled peers. No difference between 2 orthoses. Pause when heart rate reaches strenuous activity level.
	De Groot et al. (2009)	Cross-sectional	20	Determine whether VO_2 peak can be measured during incremental treadmill test. What is the maximum O_2 uptake (VO_{2max}) in ambulatory children with spina bifida?	VO_2 peak measured: Incremental treadmill test seems to reflect true VO_{2max} in ambulatory children with spina bifida, validating use of treadmill test.
Therapeutic Exercise: Gait and locomotion training	Franks, Palisano, & Darbee (1991)	Alternating condition; single subject	2	What are the effects of walking with an assistive device or wheelchair on school performance in students with MMC?	All subjects had significantly lower visuomotor accuracy scores during assistive-device ambulation phase than wheelchair phase, manual dexterity variable results, reading fluency not affected.

Table 25.7 Evidence-Based Interventions for Myelomeningocele (MMC)—cont'd

Intervention	Author (Date)	Study Design	No. of Subjects	Question	Findings
Therapeutic Exercise: Neuromotor development training	Mazur, Shurtleff, Menelaus, & Colliver (1989)	Cohort study	72	Is it worthwhile to encourage high-level individuals with MMC to walk at an early age? Compared two groups: one nonambulatory and one early ambulators.	Early walkers had fewer fractures, were more independent, and had better transfer skills. Wheelchair users had fewer hospitalizations. No difference in activities of daily living, hand function, obesity.
Therapeutic Exercise: Strength, power, and endurance training for muscles	Fragala-Pinkham, Haley, & Goodgold, (2006)	Quasi-experimental clinical study, pre/post test design	28	What is the feasibility of community-based group fitness program for children with disabilities?	Improvements in all clinical outcomes. Most clinically meaningful was improved functional mobility.
	Liusuwan, Widman, Abresch, Johnson, & McDonald (2007)	Case report/case series	20	What are the effects of nutrition/exercise intervention on health and fitness of adolescents with mobility impairment due to spinal cord dysfunction/myelomeningocele and spinal cord injury?	16-week intervention of BENEfit program increased strength, and improved aerobic capacity and endurance of overweight, obese children with mobility impairments and helped them adopt a healthy diet. No significant changes in weight and BMI. There were improvements in body composition, but no change in blood lipids.
Assistive, adaptive, orthotic, protective, supportive, or prosthetic equipment	Meiser & McEwen (2007)	Single subject A-B-A design	2	How do two wheelchair types compare in propulsion and preference?	Supports use of ultralightweight, rigid-frame wheelchair by young children.

DISCUSSION QUESTIONS

1. Identify environmental accommodations needed for Salomon at each transition: elementary school to middle school, middle school to high school, high school to postsecondary environments.

2. Discuss how to address the medical issues that children with myelodysplasia have with teachers and school personnel, such as latex allergy, shunt precautions, need for pressure relief, catheterization procedures, and obesity. How can this information be presented to assist the classroom teacher in monitoring and implementing medical interventions during the school day?

3. What is the role of the physical therapist in designing and implementing exercise programs for children with myelodysplasia and obesity? What type of exercise program can be implemented for wheelchair-dependent children in the school or community setting?

4. How can the physical therapist assist with simple modifications when no funding is available? What resources can be implemented?

5. What factors should be considered in making recommendations for lower extremity orthotics for children with myelodysplasia?

6. How can the physical therapist assist in coordinating and communicating with families where English is not the primary language? What resources are available, and how reliable are these in assisting with communication with families?

Acknowledgment

This case was originally submitted as a requirement for completion of the Doctor of Physical Therapy program at Shenandoah University under the mentorship of Patricia Chippendale, PT, DPT.

Recommended Readings

Bartonek, A. (2010). Motor development toward ambulation in preschool children with myelomeningocele-a prospective study. *Pediatric Physical Therapy, 22,* 52-60.

Hinderer, K.A., Hinderer, S.R., & Shurtleff, D.B. (2012). Myelodysplasia. In S.K. Campbell, R.J. Palisano, & M.N. Orlin, (Eds.) *Physical therapy for children* (4th ed., pp. 703-755). St. Louis: Elsevier Saunders.

Pantall, A., Teulier, C.. Smith, B., Moerchen, V.. & Ulrich, B. (2011). Impact of enhanced sensory input on treadmill step frequency: Infants born with myelomeningocele. *Pediatric Physical Therapy, 23,* 42-52.

References

American Physical Therapy Association (APTA). (2001). Guide to physical therapist practice (2nd ed.). *Physical Therapy, 81,* 9–744.

Asher, M., & Olson, J. (1983). Factors affecting the ambulatory status of patients with spina bifida cystica. *The Journal of Bone & Joint Surgery, 65,* 350-356.

Bartlett, M.D., Wolf, L.S., Shurtless, D.B. & Staheli, L.T. (1985). Hip flexion contractures: A comparison of measurement methods. *Archives of Physical Medicine and Rehabilitation, 66,* 620-625.

Bartonek, A., Eriksson, M., & Saraste, H. (2002). Heart rate and walking velocity during independent walking in children with low and midlumbar myelomeningocele. *Pediatric Physical Therapy, 14,* 185–190.

Buffart, L., Roebroeck, M., Rol, M., Stam, H., & Berg-Emons, R., (2008). Triad of Physical activity, aerobic fitness and obesity in adolescents and young adults with myelomeningocele. *Journal of Rehabilitation Medicine, 40,* 70–75.

Coster, W., Deeney, T., Haltiwanger, J. & Haley, S. (1998). *School Function Assessment.* San Antonio, TX: The Psychological Corporation.

De Groot, J., Takken, T., de Graaff, S., Gooskens, H., Helders, P., & Vanhees, L. (2009). Treadmill testing of children who have spina bifida and are ambulatory: Does peak oxygen uptake reflect maximum oxygen uptake? *Physical Therapy, 89,* 679–687.

Del Gado, R., & Del Gaizo, D., (1999). Obesity and overweight in a group of patients with myelomeningocele. In S. Matsumoto & H. Sato, *Spina Bifida* (pp. 474–475). New York: Springer Verlag.

Fragala-Pinkham, M.A., Haley, S.M., & Goodgold, S. (2006). Evaluation of a community-based group fitness program for children with disabilities. *Pediatric Physical Therapy, 18,* 159–167.

Franks, C., Palisano, R., & Darbee, J. (1991). The effect of walking with an assistive device and using a wheelchair on school performance in students with myelomeningocele. *Physical Therapy, 8,* 570–577.

Haley, S.M., Coster, W.J., Ludlow, L.H., Haltiwanger, J.T., & Andrellos, P.J. (1992). *Pediatric Evaluation of Disability Inventory (PEDI).* Boston: New England Medical Center Hospitals.

Hastings, J., (2000). Seating assessment and planning. *Physical Medicine and Rehabilitation Clinics of North America, 11,* 185.

Hinderer, K.A., Hinderer, S.R., & Shurtleff, D.B. (2006). Myelodysplasia. In S. Campbell, D. Vander Linden, & R. Palisano, R. (Eds.). *Physical therapy for children* (3rd ed., pp. 736–740). St. Louis: Saunders Elsevier.

Liusuwan, R., Widman, L., Abresch, R., Johnson, A., & McDonald, C. (2007). Behavioral intervention, exercise, and nutrition education to improve health and fitness (BENEfit) in adolescents with mobility impairment due to spinal cord dysfunction. *Journal of Spinal Cord Medicine, 30*(S1), S119–S126.

Mazur, J.M., Shurtleff, D., Menelaus, M., & Colliver, J., (1989). Orthopaedic management of high-level spina bifida. Early walking compared with early use of a wheelchair. *The Journal of Bone & Joint Surgery, 71,* 56–61.

Meiser, M.J., & McEwen, I. (2007). Lightweight and ultralightweight wheelchairs: Propulsion and preferences of two young children with spina bifida. *Pediatric Physical Therapy, 19,* 245–253.

Palisano, R. (2006). A collaborative model of service delivery for children with movement disorders: A framework for evidence-based decision making. *Physical Therapy, 86,* 1301.

Shurtleff, D.B. (1986). Dietary management. In D.B. Shurtleff (Ed). *Myelodysplasias and exstrophies:Significance, prevention and treatment* (pp. 258–298). Orlando, FL: Grune & Stratton.

Stahelli, L.T. (1977). The prone hip extension test: A method of measuring hip flexion deformity. *Clinical Orthopaedics and Related Research, 12,* 12-15.

Index

Note: Page numbers followed by f indicate figures and page numbers followed by t indicate tables.